Mental Health in Nursing

Theory and practice for clinical settings

6th edition

Mental Health in Nursing
Theory and practice for clinical settings
6th edition

Kim Foster, RN, DipAppSc, BN, MA, PhD, FACMHN
Professor and Eileen O'Connor Chair of Mental Health Research
Australian Catholic University, Melbourne, Victoria
Australia

Peta Marks, RN, BN, MPH, MCFT, CMHN, FACMHN
National Programs Manager
InsideOut Institute, The University of Sydney and Sydney Local Health District,
Sydney, NSW

Chief Operating Officer, Australian Eating Disorders Research and
Translation Centre, Sydney, InsideOut Institute, Sydney, NSW
Mental Health Consultant, Australian Health Consulting, Byron Bay, NSW
Australia

Anthony J O'Brien, RN, BA, MPhil(Hons), PhD, FNZCMHN, ONZM
Associate Professor, Te Huarahi Waiora School of Health
University of Waikato, Hamilton
New Zealand

John Hurley, MSc(Nurs), PhD, FACMHN
Professor of Mental Health
Faculty of Health,
Southern Cross University, Coffs Harbour, NSW
Australia

ELSEVIER

ELSEVIER

Elsevier Australia. ACN 001 002 357
(a division of Reed International Books Australia Pty Ltd)
Tower 1, 475 Victoria Avenue, Chatswood, NSW 2067

ISBN: 978-0-7295-4468-9

National Library of Australia Cataloguing-in-Publication Data

A catalogue record for this book is available from the National Library of Australia

Senior Content Strategist: Natalie Hunt
Content Project Manager: Shivani Pal
Editor: Margaret Trudgeon
Proofreader: Tim Learner
Cover and internal designer: Gopalakrishnan Venkatraman
Index by SPI
Typeset by GW Tech
Printed in Singapore by Markono Print Media Pte Ltd

Last digit is the print number: 9 8 7 6 5 4 3 2 1

CONTENTS

FOREWORD

Mental Health Nursing: Theory and practice for clinical settings, 6th edition, is a text with welcome differences because it draws upon the narratives of people with lived experience of mental health issues who have been under the care and treatment of nurses. It also, bravely, brings into the open lived experience narratives of nurses who themselves have experienced trauma and mental health issues. Because of this, and because of the focus placed on recovery and the humane treatment of people who have experienced trauma and psychological distress, it is an honour to write the foreword for this text. In doing so, I hope to enthuse students and nurses to consider the important role they play in the lives of each person they treat, care for, support and work with. Whether the care is offered in primary, community, in-patient or other clinical settings, the impact of nurses with lived experience on people can have lasting positive (or detrimental) effects on their lives, their sense of self, recovery and subsequent outcomes.

This edition focuses on nursing practices embedded in the Code of ethics for nurses, the healing power of dedicated nurses and the recognition that every person has a unique and innate value. The authors and editors recognise that great nurses contribute to a person's healing and recovery, and to living socially and emotionally satisfying lives, contributing to the person's family, workplace and community.

My career in mental health has had wide dimensions. I have been a lived experience volunteer, peer worker, manager of peer workers and a director of a large public mental health service. I founded Vision in Mind, a national systemic advocacy, consultancy and training body. I was the inaugural Deputy Commissioner with the NSW Mental Health Commission and an executive member of a large specialist community-managed organisation. For years I have written policies, issues papers, strategic plans, guidelines and protocols, and have always undertaken these utilising co-design practices. I am also a person with lived experience of trauma and subsequent mental health issues. Through all these experiences I have had the personal and professional honour of working with great mental health nurses who work from a strong human rights base and use strengths-based language, and who practise empathy and holistic care with each person. Nurses working in this way regard people with mental health issues as individuals, not as a diagnosis or as a constellation of problematic behaviours. They do not pathologise the human experience. High-quality mental health services and nurses work in respectful, multidisciplinary teams, including all clinical staff and peer workers. The individual needs of each person in their care are central to everything good nurses do and they respect the lived experience mantra of "Nothing about me, without me". The power dynamic is recognised and smoothed out, providing a respectful, holistic and therapeutic alliance with the people they care for and, where appropriate, with their family.

I have also had the unfortunate and traumatising experience of working with nurses who do not practise holistic, therapeutic and empathic care. They use the nurse's station as just one tool in the unequal power dynamic they enjoy, and use seclusion and restraint far more often than is needed; they see this as a win, rather than a failure of care. When I was working in the public system I could look at the roster and know if there were going to be instances of seclusion and restraint by the particular staff who were rostered on. I implore student nurses and practising nurses to work together to ensure these attitudes and outcomes do not prevail in their services. Please work within the spirit of this text and create holistic healing instead of further trauma for all people and staff involved.

I have had the great honour of speaking at conferences and workshops for the ANZ Nurses and Midwives Association over a number of years. The focus over the past 12 months has been on the mental health and wellbeing of nursing staff. One strategy I encourage nurses to embrace is to change the victimhood narratives they may have fallen into – where nurses feel like they are victims of underfunding, unrealistic expectations, understaffing, bullying and intimidation from colleagues (including other nurses, registrar, doctors and executive decision-makers), as well as experiencing trauma during "take downs" and incidents of seclusion and restraint.

As a person who has experienced a great deal of trauma and powerful feelings of victimhood, I know the value of changing your worldview and personal narrative away from being a victim, and into claiming your agency and leadership. Not focusing on what has happened and what you can't do, but rather focusing on your strengths and capabilities and what you can do; what you can impact; what you can change. I ask you to imagine yourself as a leader, each nurse engaging with the feeling of being a leader rather than a victim; to cultivate narratives that leaders use in self-talk, to own these narratives for yourself and to approach problem-solving from the perspective and demeanour of a leader to create the changes you know are needed for all stakeholders, especially the people you care for and colleagues. Don't leave this important work up to a handful of people; Everyone needs to claim their leadership and go forward in hope and strength and create the light at the end of the tunnel.

Indigenous healing circles and the Open Dialogue model of care are practices that work in holistic ways utilising the community, family, kin, whānau and multidisciplinary teams working together to provide healing supports for individuals, families and communities. I would encourage all services to engage with these practices. I would also encourage nurses to become familiar with the different cultural beliefs around mental health issues and connection to country and community, spirituality and body language. Recognising all aspects of a person's needs and making allowances for these demonstrates respect and care, and builds a stronger therapeutic alliance between patients/consumers/people with lived experience, their families and communities.

Until recently, the interconnection between mental and physical health was generally ignored. Doctors and nurses could often be dismissive of consumers' concerns about their physical health and attribute symptoms to "paranoia", "being all in their mind", "hypochondria" or "just attention seeking". Discrimination has led to the physical health needs of people with mental health conditions being seen as less important than their mental health, than other people's physical health, and the community's discomfort about "the behaviour" of the person. Also, the negative impact of mental distress and pharmaceutical treatment on a person's health was underestimated and downplayed. Clinicians often point to a person's life choices, such as diet, lack of exercise, drugs, cigarettes and alcohol use, as being the causes of their physical health issues. However, ethical clinical treatment is transparent about the unwanted effects of prescribed psychiatric medications on people's short- and long-term health. Ethical clinical treatment is also transparent about the risks that electroconvulsive therapy (ECT) may have on people's memory and physical health. To achieve holistic care, preserving memory and the physical health of people with mental health issues must also be seen as a priority in all services, including acute, stepped, community and primary healthcare settings. Ethical practices ensure that people know what their treatment involves and the possible unwanted side effects of medication, which often includes obesity, metabolic syndrome and a major gap in life expectancy. Physical illness that is untreated, or inadequately treated, increases the burden of disease on the community and on individuals, and diminishes the speed and likelihood of recovery, and increases the gap in life expectancy. The relationship between personal and family trauma, social dynamics and environmental impacts on mental and physical health are being increasingly understood.

This text outlines a social and ecological approach that integrates the various influences on mental health from biological through to environmental and social. Valuable nurses recognise that the causes of mental health issues include external factors and rarely lie solely within the individual. Childhood and adult abuse, harsh environments, the impact of global warming (fire, floods, drought, earthquakes and destruction of nature), neglect and intergenerational trauma, including the destruction of family and communities through war, stolen lands, stolen children, sexual abuse and poverty, all contrive to undermine people's lives and wellbeing.

Epidemiological studies show that mental health and addiction issues affect up to 50% of people in their lifetime. It would seem obvious by this figure that mental health issues can no longer be seen as "crazy", disordered or abnormal, but rather on the spectrum of normal responses to trauma, abuse, neglect and harsh living conditions.

As this text points out, the World Health Organization recommends that mental health care be based in primary care. While this trend is increasing in Australia and New Zealand, a large percentage of clinical and acute treatment takes place in psychiatric wards. Throughout my career I have worked in and attended mental health settings across Australia, New Zealand and internationally, amid diverse cultures with varying degrees of wealth and poverty. Some services have been exciting, empathic environments exuding hope and healing, even when resources have been scarce and the facilities poor. Sadly, my excitement has often been overwhelmed by shame, anger and painful questioning as to why all clinical and community mental health services are not holistic, therapeutic, trauma-informed and person-centred/person-led environments.

I have consulted multiple stakeholders about the reasons for the variations in service quality and outcomes. While mental health certainly needs more funding and resources, contrary to popular narratives, I believe the variants do not relate to resources and finances; rather, they are based in individual nurse and clinician attitudes and the collective culture of the services. This can be evidenced by comparisons between services within the same states of Australia. State public services are working under the same funding models and the same policies and protocols, yet vary dramatically in culture and outcomes. Interactions between nurses, clinical staff and the people they care for are either empathic, hopeful and respectful cultures engaged in respectful multidisciplinary teams producing outcomes desired by the people accessing the service and staff, or that of a culture with inequitable power dynamics, in which nurses and clinicians primarily pathologise the human experience and see people as the diagnosis, disorder or "problem behaviour". The latter culture produces detrimental outcomes, including higher instances of seclusion, restraint and suicide, with people feeling further marginalised and traumatised by the so-called "trauma-informed treatment and care" they receive. Such detrimental cultures are also often characterised by workplace bullying, increased staff trauma and burnout.

This text speaks to the importance of respect, care and wellbeing for all stakeholders. As previously mentioned, *Mental Health Nursing: Theory and practice for clinical settings* takes the brave and wonderful step of including not only the voices of people accessing services with lived experience, but also nurses' stories of their own lived experience.

This deserves to be applauded. While the practices of nursing and mental health peer work are very different, nurses with lived experience have a positive impact on service culture and outcomes. Nurses and clinical staff with lived experience are valued and celebrated in this text, as they should be in all workplaces. The stigma and discrimination shown against people with mental health issues has, in the past, driven nurses to hide their lived experience. This, coupled with workplace bullying and incidents of seclusion, restraint and enforced treatment, leads to trauma for both people being "treated" and staff, and burnout among good nurses. Cultures such as these intimidate good staff and breed fear in people who need to access mental health services. People often turn to alcohol and drugs to self-medicate and to self-harm or suicide rather than return to a service where they feel unsafe, traumatised and humiliated.

Australia and New Zealand are signatories to the United Nations' declarations and conventions on human and disability rights. Nurses who focus on human rights and the innate value and needs of each person build healing, trusting relationships and workplaces for all stakeholders. Coercion, bullying, seclusion and restraint are non-existent or rare in services that are focused on respectful interactions. Nurses working in this culture see incidents of seclusion and restraint as failures of the service, rather than the fault of the person in distress. While this text points out that current laws allow for seclusion and restraint in New Zealand and Australia, it also speaks to the need for these practices to be used as a last resort. However, lived experience advocates declare restrictive practices as abuses against human rights. I hope you will permit me to challenge all nurses to work as if seclusion and restraint were illegal and to consider alternative protocols to meet individual needs, such as the support of peer workers. Peer workers use mutual experiences to connect with people and provide a calming and hope-filled influence that can lead to a positive shift in the power dynamic between the multidisciplinary team and the people they care for.

The editors of this edition of *Mental Health Nursing: Theory and practice for clinical settings* have engaged chapter authors who focus on the particular aspects of ethical nursing practice. They have used vignettes written from different perspectives and consulted people with lived experience, peer workers, family/carers, clinicians and academics. The use of "Critical thinking challenges" engages nurses in reflective thinking, learning and practice. This text draws on lived experience, professional experience and tools to produce a learning experience based in ethical practices and the therapeutic alliances built between caring, respectful nurses and the people they treat and care for, their families and communities.

I commend this text to students and practising nurses at all stages of their careers. I thank the editors and authors for valuing lived experience and producing such a strong human rights-based, recovery-focused mental health guide to good nursing. Working in the ethical way this text demonstrates will, I hope, lead to improved outcomes, increased rates of recovery and healing, decreased rates of suicide and enforced treatment, and the cessation of seclusion and restraint.

May nurses' careers be filled with a sense of pride, coupled with respect and humility as they witness how their practices and interactions with people contribute to the positive reframing of lived experience, enriched sense of self, healing and recovery and the ability to lead contributing, meaningful, respected lives.

Fay Jackson, DipEd, BCVA, LEA, EBE
Founder of Vision In Mind
Lived Experience Advocate
Inaugural Deputy Commissioner, NSW Mental Health Commission
NSW, Australia

ABOUT THE AUTHORS

Kim Foster is a registered nurse with specialist mental health nursing qualifications. She is currently Professor of Mental Health Nursing and leads the Mental Health Nursing Research Unit at the Royal Melbourne Hospital, a joint research partnership between Australian Catholic University and NorthWestern Mental Health. Kim has extensive experience as a mental health nurse academic and educator, having developed and taught mental health curricula at the undergraduate and postgraduate levels across several Australian universities and in Fiji. She has consulted to AusAID and the World Health Organization, and has an international reputation as a mental health researcher, with more than 120 publications. Her key research interests include: the resilience and wellbeing of the health workforce; the resilience of individuals and families with challenging health conditions; and the experiences and needs of families where a person has mental illness.

Peta Marks is a credentialled mental health nurse and family therapist working in private practice, who specialises in working with people who have eating disorders and their families. Peta has extensive experience undertaking mental health project management at the national level and as a mental health writer and subject matter expert for online learning platforms. She is currently working as the National Programs Manager for InsideOut Institute and is the Chief Operating Officer for the Australian Eating Disorders Research and Translation Centre.

Anthony J O'Brien graduated as a registered nurse in Dunedin in 1977 and as a psychiatric nurse in Auckland in 1982. Anthony is currently employed at the University of Waikato as an Associate Professor in nursing and has clinical expertise in liaison psychiatry with the Auckland District Health Board. Anthony's PhD research investigated variation in the use of mental health legislation, including the roles of social deprivation, ethnicity, clinical decision-making and service provision. Anthony's research interests are in social issues related to mental health, police and mental health, and advance directives. In 2020 Anthony was made an Officer of the New Zealand Order of Merit in recognition of services to mental health nursing.

John Hurley is a credentialled mental health nurse, counsellor, gestalt psychotherapist, educator and researcher. Currently a professor of mental health at Southern Cross University, his research interests focus on the preparation and worth of the mental health nursing discipline, emotional intelligence and youth mental health. John has worked in the United Kingdom and Australia, and continues to clinically practise mental health nursing through a regular headspace clinic.

Scott Brunero, DipApSc, BAHsc, MA(Nurs Prac), PhD
Academic, Nursing, Western Sydney University, Campbelltown, NSW, Australia
Clinical Nurse Consultant, Mental Health Liaison, Prince of Wales Hospital, Randwick, NSW, Australia

Michelle Cameron, BN(Hons)
Senior Lecturer, Nursing, University of Waikato, Hamilton, New Zealand

Katrina Campbell, BNSci, MN(MentHlth)
Lecturer, School of Health and Human Sciences, Southern Cross University, Bilinga, Qld, Australia

Andrew Cashin, DipAppSci, BHSC, GCertPTT, GCert HPol, MN, PhD
Professor of Autism and Intellectual Disability, Faculty of Health and Human Sciences, Southern Cross University, Lismore, NSW, Australia
Honorary Professor, School of Nursing, The University of Sydney, Sydney, NSW, Australia

Justin Chia, BSci(Psych), BN, MN(MentHlth)
Nurse Practitioner, Community Mental Health, Sydney Local Health District, Camperdown, NSW, Australia

Greg Clark, BHSc(MHN), MN(Adv Prac), MN(NP), PhD
Academic Program Adviser, Post Graduate Mental Health, School of Nursing and Midwifery, Western Sydney University, Rydalmere, NSW, Australia

Elizabeth Currie, RPN, BPN, BAppScNurs, MMHN
Mental Health Nurse, North Western Mental Health Program, University of Melbourne, Parkville, Vic, Australia

Catherine Daniel, RPN, BPsychNurs, PGDipN(MentHlth) MN, PhD, CMHN
Department of Nursing, The University of Melbourne, Melbourne, Victoria, Australia
Consultation Liaison Psychiatry, The Royal Melbourne Hospital, Melbourne, Victoria, Australia

Cynthia Delgado, MNurs(MentHlthNursPrac), GradCertResMethDesign
Nurse Manager, Research and Education, Sydney Local Health District Mental Health Services, Camperdown, NSW, Australia

Andrea E. Donaldson, MSc, PhD, CATE, RCN
School of Nursing, Massey University, Palmerston North, Manawatu, New Zealand

Anna Louise Elders, PGCertChildAdolMentHlth, PGDipCogTher, MN
Clinical Lead, Just a Thought Wise Group, Hamilton, New Zealand
Nurse Practitioner/CBT Therapist, Tamaki Health, Auckland, New Zealand

Honorary Teaching Fellow, School of Nursing, University of Auckland, Auckland, New Zealand

Julie Ferguson, GradDipHSM, MN(AdvPracMentHlth), MN(NursePrac)
School of Nursing, Midwifery and Indigenous Health, Charles Sturt University, Bathurst, NSW, Australia

Jane Ferreira, RN, DipNsg, PGDipHC
Nurse Advisor, Aged Care, Bupa NZ, Wellington, New Zealand

Kim Narelle Foster, RN, DipAppSc, MA, PhD, FACMHN
Professor and Eileen O'Connor Chair of Mental Health Research
School of Nursing, Midwifery and Paramedicine, Australian Catholic University, Melbourne, Victoria, Australia

Patrick Gould, BN(Hon), MCN
Project Officer Psychiatry, Mindgardens Neuroscience Network, Randwick, NSW, Australia
Clinical Nurse Educator, Mental Health, South Eastern Sydney Local Health District, Randwick, NSW, Australia
Project Officer, Department of Psychiatry and Mental Health, University of NSW, Kensington, NSW, Australia

Nicole Denise Graham, RN, BN, MAdvPrac, CMHN
Lecturer, Faculty of Health, Southern Cross University, Bilinga, Qld, Australia

Monica D. Guha, MN(MntlHlth), BScMentHlthNurs, BScBiomedSci, CMHM
The Thriving Spirit Project, Orange, NSW, Australia

Elizabeth Jane Halcomb, RN, BN(Hons), GradCertICNurs, GradCertHE, PhD, FACN
Professor of Primary Health Care Nursing, School of Nursing, University of Wollongong, Wollongong, NSW, Australia

Graham Holman, MN
Senior Lecturer, Te Huataki Waiora School of Health, University of Waikato, Hamilton, New Zealand

John Hurley, MSc(Nurs), PhD, FACMHN
Professor of Mental Health, Faculty of Health, Southern Cross University, Coffs Harbour, NSW, Australia

Sophie Isobel, BN, PhD, CFHN, CAMH
Associate Professor of Mental Health Nursing, Faculty of Medicine and Health, University of Sydney, Camperdown, NSW, Australia

Elissa-Kate Jay, BN(Hons), GradCertMentHlthNurs
School of Nursing, Faculty of Science Medicine and Health, University of Wollongong, Wollongong, NSW, Australia
Illawarra Health and Medical Research, University of Wollongong, Wollongong, NSW, Australia

Chantel Jurcevic, BAComm(WritCultSt)
Family and Carer Peer Worker, Mental Health, Sydney Local
    Health District, Sydney, NSW, Australia

Richard Lakeman, BN, BA(Hons), GradDipMentHlth,
MMH(Psych)
Associate Professor, Faculty of Health, Southern Cross
    University, Bilinga, Qld, Australia
Adjunct Associate Professor, School of Nursing & Midwifery,
    Edith Cowan University, Perth, WA, Australia

Scott Lamont, RMN, RN, MN(Hons), PhD
Clinical Nurse Consultant, Mental Health Liaison Nursing,
    Prince of Wales Hospital, Sydney, NSW, Australia
Associate Professor, Faculty of Health, Southern Cross
    University, NSW, Australia

Tessa Maguire, RN, GradDipFBS, GradDipFMHN,
MMentHlthSc, PhD
Senior Lecturer, Forensic Mental Health Nursing, Centre for
    Forensic Behavioural Science, Swinburne University of
    Technology, Melbourne, Victoria, Australia
Forensicare, Melbourne, Victoria, Australia

Peta Marks, RN, BN, MPH, MCFT, CMHN, FACMHN
National Programs Manager, InsideOut Institute, The
    University of Sydney and Sydney Local Health District,
    Sydney, NSW, Australia
Chief Operating Officer, Australian Eating Disorders Research
    and Translation Centre, Sydney, InsideOut Institute, Sydney,
    NSW, Australia
Mental Health Consultant, Australian Health Consulting,
    Byron Bay, NSW, Australia

Megan McKechnie, PGDipAddictMentHlth,
PGDipMentHlthNurs, MAdvNursPrac(NP), MAddictStud(Sci)
Addiction Psychiatry Nurse Practitioner, Consultation and
    Liaison Psychiatry and Addiction Services, Alfred Health,
    Melbourne, Victoria, Australia
Addiction Psychiatry Nurse Practitioner, Medically Supervised
    Injecting Rooms
North Richmond Community Health, Richmond, Victoria,
    Australia

Brian McKenna, RN, BA, MHSc(Hons), PhD
Professor, Forensic Mental Health, School of Clinical Sciences,
    Auckland University of Technology, Auckland, New Zealand
Adjunct Professor, Centre of Forensic Behavioural Sciences,
    Swinburne University of Technology, Melbourne, Victoria,
    Australia
Associate Clinical Director for Improvement, Auckland Regional
    Forensic Psychiatry Services, Auckland, New Zealand

Luke Molloy, PhD
Senior Lecturer Nursing, University of Wollongong,
    Wollongong, NSW, Australia

Bridget Anne Mulvey, DipHlthSci(Nurs),
MMentHlth(ChildAdol)
Clinical Nurse Consultant, Child and Adolescent Mental
    Health, Sydney Children's Hospital Network, Randwick,
    NSW, Australia

Irene Ngune, PhD, RN, CMHN, FHEA
Senior Lecturer, School of Nursing and Midwifery, Edith
    Cowan University, WA, Australia

Anthony J. O'Brien, RN, BA, MPhil(Hons), PhD, FNZCMHN,
ONZM
Associate Professor, Te Huarahi Waiora School of Health,
    University of Waikato, Hamilton, New Zealand

Lucie Ramjan, RN, BN(Hons), PhD
Associate Professor, School of Nursing and Midwifery, Western
    Sydney University, Penrith, NSW, Australia

Sharon Elizabeth Rydon, BEd, MPhil(Nurs)
Clinical Professional Development Lead, Clinical Services
    Improvement Team, Bupa New Zealand, Auckland, New Zealand

Bryce Samuel, BN
School of Nursing, University of Waikato, Kirikiriroa, Waikato,
    New Zealand

Matthew Scott, BN, GradCertAddictStud
Aboriginal Mental Health Drug and Alcohol Services, Western
    NSW Local Health District, Bloomfield Hospital, Orange
    (Wiradjuri Country), NSW, Australia

Julie Sharrock, RN, CertCritCare, CertPsychNurs, BEd,
AdvDip(GestaltTher), MHSc(PsychNurs), FACMHN, MACN,
MACSA
Mental Health Nurse Consultant, Private Practice, Ocean
    Grove, Victoria, Australia

Sophie Temmhoff, AdvDipVA
Art mentor, Disability Support Worker and Advocate, Western
    Sydney, NSW, Australia

Scott Trueman, BCom(Acc), LLB, GDLP, MMHN, GMHN, PhD
Senior Lecturer, School of Nursing & Midwifery, Flinders
    University, Adelaide, SA, Australia

Marika Kris Van Ooyen, MAEPESC, BN(IndigAustHlth),
GradCertSpecNurs(MentHlth),
Nurse Educator, Centre for Education and Workforce
    Development, Sydney Local Health District, Sydney, NSW,
    Australia

Stephen Van Vorst, BAppSc(Nurs), MN(Res)
Faculty of Health, Nursing, Southern Cross University, Bilinga,
    Qld, Australia

Andrew Watkins, BN, GradCert(ChildAdolMH), Grad
Dip(MentHlthNurs), MNurs(NP), PhD
Nurse Practitioner, Mindgardens Neuroscience Network,
    University of NSW, Randwick, NSW, Australia

Jim Xu, MN
Community Mental Health Services for Older People, Health
    New Zealand Auckland, Auckland, New Zealand

Taylor Yousiph, BRes(Hons), BNursAdvMentHlth
School of Nursing, University of Wollongong, Wollongong,
    NSW, Australia

REVIEWERS

Karen-Ann Clarke, RN, GradDipPsych, MMHlthNurs, PhD
Lecturer in Nursing (Mental Health)
Program Coordinator, Nursing
School of Nursing, Midwifery and Paramedicine
University of the Sunshine Coast, QLD

Russell James, PhD
Lecturer, School of Nursing
University of Tasmania
Mental Health Nurse, Royal Hobart Hospital, TAS

Diana Jeffries, BA, PhD
Academic Program Advisor – Postgraduate, Nursing
School of Nursing and Midwifery
Western Sydney University, NSW

Tracey MacGregor, PGCertHealthSci, PGCertPHCSN
Nursing Lecturer
School of Nursing
Te Kura Kaupapa Tapuhi
Eastern Institute of Technology,
New Zealand

Elijah Marangu, GradCertHE, PhD
Lecturer
School of Nursing and Midwifery
Deakin University, VIC

Shirley McGough, RN, MNurs, PhD, RMHN, SFHEA
Director of Work Integrated Learning
Curtin School of Nursing, Faculty of Health Sciences, Perth,
    Australia

Loma-Linda Tasi, RN, PGCertNursSci, MProfPract
Senior Nurse Lecturer
Bachelor of Nursing Pacific (Samoan)
Pacific Strategy Team
Wellington Institute of Technology & Whitireia Polytechnic
New Zealand

INTRODUCTION

Welcome to the sixth edition of this popular text on mental health in nursing. This edition continues the direction followed by its predecessor, reflected in the title – *Mental Health in Nursing: Theory and practice for clinical settings*. Mental health is increasingly recognised as part of the holistic care provided by nurses in every clinical setting, as well as a diverse area of specialist practice. Nurses respond to mental health needs of consumers across the lifespan and across different practice settings, including emergency departments, aged care, acute medical and surgical services and primary care. Specialist settings include acute in-patient care, eating disorders, forensic mental health and addiction services. The text is intended to appeal to undergraduate nursing students and to nurses in their early years of clinical practice. It is also intended as a resource for nursing teachers charged with introducing students to mental health concepts.

For this edition, John Hurley of Southern Cross University has joined the editorial team of Kim Foster, Peta Marks and Anthony O'Brien. John is a Professor of Mental Health at Southern Cross University and is a credentialled mental health nurse with 30 years' experience. He maintains his clinical practice at headspace and is a Fellow of the Australian College of Mental Health Nurses. John is a widely published academic whose expertise covers education, clinical practice and professional issues. John has contributed to several chapters in this edition and has brought an extensive professional background to the editing role. We acknowledge the contribution of former editor Toby Raeburn to the fifth edition of the text. Toby maintains a presence in the sixth edition through the historical anecdotes that appear in Parts 1 and 2.

The editorial team is once again thankful to Jarrad Hickmott, who contributed to the text as a lived experience consultant. With an established reputation as a mental health advocate, Jarrad is a peer support worker at Prince of Wales Hospital in Sydney, and has served as a youth adviser to the national board of headspace, Australia's national youth mental health foundation. As with the fifth edition, Jarrad has reviewed numerous chapters and authored several lived experience commentaries throughout. Jarrad's story of recovery journey is available in both written and video materials associated with this publication. The text also contains contributions from many others with lived experience who have been involved as co-authors. Their contributions remind us that lived experience is central to mental health care and to the practice of nursing.

The fifth edition introduced the socio-ecological approach to mental health nursing practice, which remains in this current edition. The socio-ecological approach provides a model for integrating the many influences on mental health at the levels of individual, society and environment, expressed in the relationship between nurse and service user and in the skills of the practising nurse. The socio-ecological approach is used to frame all chapters of the text, reflecting our belief that this approach can assist nurses to understand mental health within a broad framework, and that it can support nurses in developing skills of holistic practice.

The change of direction introduced in the fifth edition, where we extended the range of clinical contexts to include many generalist settings, has remained for this sixth edition. This change was in recognition of the centrality of mental health to the health encounter, and to the practice of nursing. Part 3 provides seven chapters on nursing in a range of generalist and specialist health settings, with a focus on the mental health needs of health consumers in settings such as primary care, older adult care and emergency care. These chapters have been contributed by clinical experts in each area. We trust that the clinical scenarios in Part 3 provide students and nurses who work in generalist contexts with knowledge and confidence by providing information focused on the practical application of mental health nursing skills.

A new inclusion in the sixth edition are the two chapters on Indigenous mental health. The chapters on Aboriginal and Torres Strait Islander mental health and Māori mental health speak to the experience of the Indigenous populations of Australia and Aotearoa New Zealand, and the impacts of colonisation and dispossession on the mental health of Indigenous peoples. The chapters have been contributed by Indigenous nurses and reflect the dual clinical and cultural skills of the authors. In these chapters, readers will find a historical background to Indigenous mental health and advice for culturally safe nursing practice.

Another inclusion for this edition is the chapter on preparation for mental health clinical placement. *Mental Health in Nursing* is widely used in preparing undergraduate students for placement in mental health specialist settings and this chapter is intended to help students ready themselves for their clinical experience in mental health. We hope the chapter will provide the student with strategies for engaging with their mental health placement and developing the mental health skills that are fundamental to nursing.

The current concepts of mental health have deep roots, requiring nurses to have historical knowledge in order to be informed members of the profession and to formulate views and opinions grounded in understanding past practices and beliefs. The historical anecdotes of the fifth edition are once again included throughout Parts 1 and 2. Through these glimpses into our past we aim to promote awareness of how current practices and beliefs have parallels and precedents with previous historical periods. Historical understanding provides an important lens of critique and promotes different readings and interpretations of what is accepted as contemporary knowledge.

The language of mental health is a contested domain, and the different terminology used to describe the experience of mental distress and illness, and the people nurses care for, is reflected across the text. As students and as nurses, you will hear a wide range of terms used, reflecting the preferences and experience of consumers and professionals. We have not taken a position on what the "correct" language is, and we encourage students and nurses to follow this approach in their own professional practice. Nurses need to develop flexibility of thinking, rather than adopt a fixed approach to language. Many different terms can be used to describe a person with lived experience of mental illness, including consumer, patient, client, service user and person with (or experiencing) a mental illness. You will hear all these terms (and more) in clinical practice, depending on the setting and people's preferences, and you will read them all in this text too. The language we use needs to reflect the preferences of the people we care for, and at times, the requirements of services, health policies and legal frameworks. One practice we do promote is that health consumers are referred to in person-centred language rather than as diagnostic labels such as "schizophrenic" or "a psychotic". For example, we might describe someone as "a person with a lived experience of psychosis", reminding us that this is a person experiencing an illness or set of symptoms, rather than as "a schizophrenic", which is an objectifying label implying that the individual's identity is defined by the disorder. Person-centred language also reflects the view that although someone may experience mental distress or illness, they might not identify as a consumer of mental health services. In every clinical context, mental health is part of nursing, but may not be the primary reason the person seeks health care.

Mental Health in Nursing is organised into three sections. Specialist mental health nursing knowledge and skills are a key focus, particularly in Parts 1 and 2, with Part 3 outlining mental health skills for practice in generalist settings.

Part 1 *Positioning Practice* introduces the context for nursing in mental health, describes the importance of mental health, introduces the social-ecological approach to mental health in nursing that frames the text, and explores the mental health nursing knowledge, skills and attitudes needed to provide effective mental health care for individuals and their family or carers. Part 1 also addresses the need for nurses to engage in professional self-care, as this is an essential but often neglected aspect of the nursing role.

Part 2 *Knowledge for Practice* is a core feature of the text, examining specific mental health conditions that people experience, and providing a comprehensive description of major mental health problems, their assessment, nursing management and relevant treatment approaches. This section specifically addresses the specialist practice of mental health nursing. It will be of particular interest to nursing students on mental health clinical placements as part of their undergraduate education, and to nurses in their first years of specialist clinical practice in mental health.

Part 3 *Contexts of Practice* is a new section of the text, with chapters demonstrating how mental health nursing knowledge and skills can be integrated into the nursing role and applied across a range of clinical settings – both generalist and mental health settings. This does not mean that mental health knowledge and skills are *only* applicable in these settings – we have included these settings because they are common clinical settings and areas where nurses frequently practice.

Familiar features of the text have been retained, including lists of useful websites, nurses' and consumers' stories, key points, key terms and learning outcomes, critical thinking exercises and exercises for class engagement. Part 2 chapters, as in previous editions, include the language of diagnosis but not sets of diagnostic criteria, which are easily available elsewhere. Although diagnosis is a major concern of clinical services, it is also imprecise, contested, and can be unreliable. In addition, diagnosis does not capture individuals' subjective experiences. The focus of nurses is on people's experiences and their responses to adversity, stress and distress, rather than on diagnosis and symptoms. Our aim is to emphasise the nursing role in responding to the experience of individuals, rather than to a diagnostic label.

The new chapters of this text have been externally reviewed, and all previously included chapters have been revised to include references to contemporary research and scholarship while retaining core references that situate the text within the scholarly history of mental health and nursing.

We warmly thank all the chapter authors, authors with lived experience, family/carers, clinicians and academics who contributed to this edition, as well as the reviewers who have provided helpful and constructive feedback. We hope the text continues to be widely used because of its contemporary focus and integration of theory and practice.

Kim Foster
John Hurley
Peta Marks, and
Anthony J O'Brien

Positioning Practice

Why Mental Health Matters

Anthony J. O'Brien, Peta Marks, Kim Foster and John Hurley

KEY POINTS

- There is no health without mental health.
- Mental distress and mental illness are relatively common in Australia and Aotearoa New Zealand, and rates vary between different population groups.
- Nurses care for people who have mental health needs in every practice setting.
- Nurses do not need to be a specialist mental health nurse to respond to fundamental mental health needs.

KEY TERMS

Cultural safety

Mental distress

Mental health

Mental health care

Mental health legislation

Mental illness

Physical health

Prevalence of mental illness

Scope of practice

Self-harm

Suicide

LEARNING OUTCOMES

The material in this chapter will assist you to:
- understand the importance of mental health in every clinical practice setting
- understand the prevalence of mental distress and illness
- identify how physical health problems can affect mental health
- discuss how mental health is seen in Aotearoa New Zealand and Australia's Indigenous cultures
- describe the provision of mental health care.

INTRODUCTION

Mental health matters. When individuals can live socially and emotionally satisfying lives, families, communities and whole nations benefit. The term "mental health" refers to a range of experiences that affect the health and functioning of individuals, families, communities, societies and nations. These experiences include everything from happiness and wellbeing through to mild distress, anxiety and mental illness. The term "mental health" is often used as a synonym for "mental illness", but the term properly refers to a state of wellbeing, not illness. It is important to keep this distinction in mind as you read this chapter. Effects of mental ill health can extend to economic impacts through healthcare costs and loss of economic productivity. These impacts are not just from mental illness, although mental illness does have a considerable impact on employment, productivity and quality of life, but also from distress and impaired function. In Chapter 2 we will outline a social ecological approach to mental health nursing that integrates the various influences on mental health, from biological through to social. Health planners are increasingly recognising that mental health problems can also lead to physical illness, slow or incomplete recovery from physical illness and impaired social functioning. Successive epidemiological studies have shown that mental health problems are relatively common, with high proportions of the population experiencing a mental health problem at some point in their lives.

Nurses care for people who may be experiencing mental distress or ill health in every clinical setting and in the work of many social agencies, such as schools, police services, social welfare services and correctional services. For this reason, mental health and wellbeing are increasingly regarded as issues for all health professionals and social agencies. For nurses, therefore, mental health skills form an essential part of their clinical skill set.

This chapter begins with an overview of the prevalence of mental distress and illness internationally and in Australia and Aotearoa New Zealand. The chapter then outlines some of the central mental health issues, including the range of nursing responses available for people with mental health problems and the place of mental health in the nursing scope of practice. Reading this chapter should help you understand why mental health matters in nursing.

EPIDEMIOLOGY OF MENTAL DISTRESS AND ILLNESS

To understand the impact of mental health problems it is important to consider their epidemiology, or distribution in the population. Distribution is measured by prevalence and incidence. Prevalence is a measure of the rate of mental illness over a given time period – for example, at a single point in time (point prevalence) or over a year (12-month prevalence). Incidence is the measure of new cases of a disorder – for example, the number of new cases in a year. Both the

Australian and Aotearoa New Zealand governments have conducted extensive research into the prevalence of mental health problems. The following sections review reports on the prevalence of mental distress and illness internationally and in Australia and Aotearoa New Zealand.

Prevalence of Mental Distress

Mental distress is an unpleasant mental or emotional state that can impact on enjoyment of life and on personal and social functioning. The experience of distress is a common part of life, although if severe or prolonged it can impact on health and is a risk factor for mental distress and mental illness. Mental distress can be measured using standardised scales, the most common of which is the Kessler Psychological Distress Scale (K10). Using the K10, the 2020–21 New Zealand Household Survey found that 11.2% of adults and 23.6% of young people (15–24) experienced high levels of distress, with younger people, Māori and Pacific people and women reporting higher levels (Ministry of Health 2022). In a similar national survey, also using the K10, Australians reported higher levels of distress, with 15.6% of the Australians aged 16–85 reporting very high levels (Australian Bureau of Statistics 2020–21). Rates were twice as high (20%) in those aged 16–34 compared to Australians aged 65–85 (9.6%).

Rates of mental distress have been reported to be high in countries as diverse as Norway (Sterud & Hanvold 2021), the United States (Blanchflower & Oswald 2020) and Germany (Müller et al 2021), and even higher in developing countries such as Bangladesh (Islam 2019) and in conflict zones (Brown et al 2020; Summers et al 2019). Distress is also common in people with physical illness – for example, people with diabetes (McCarthy et al 2019), cancer (Kirk et al 2021), cardiac disease (McPhillips et al 2019) or renal disease (Damery et al 2019) – and for people experiencing adverse events, such as trauma (Skinner et al 2019), victimisation (Boyle et al 2022), fire (Maybery et al 2019) or natural disaster (West et al 2020). Nurses can also experience high rates of distress as "second victims" following their involvement in patients' adverse events (Huang et al 2022).

Increased rates of distress have been reported in the context of the global COVID-19 pandemic (Leung et al 2022), although rates reduced as the pandemic abated (McGinty et al 2022) and the anticipated increase in rates of suicide did not occur (Sinyor et al 2022). An Australian study showed no difference in rates of distress over two time points during the pandemic (Wright et al 2022). Despite being a common experience, however, attempts to reduce levels of mental distress in the community are not always successful. Western countries, including Australia and Aotearoa New Zealand, have made substantial increases in mental health care provision in recent decades, but there has been little change in population rates of distress (Tomitaka et al 2019).

Costs of Mental Illness

According to the World Health Organization (WHO), "mental, neurological and substance use disorders make up 10% of the global burden of disease and 30% of non-fatal disease burden" (WHO 2019), with one in five children and adolescents experiencing a mental disorder. WHO also reports that depression alone affects 280 million people worldwide and is one of the leading causes of disability (WHO 2023). Depression is also associated with higher rates of unemployment, incarceration and homelessness (Grech & Raeburn 2019).

In developed nations, total government spending on mental health is substantial. In Australia, the quantifiable costs of mental ill health and suicide in 2018–19 were estimated to be from $43 billion to $51 billion and include healthcare, education, housing and justice, with healthcare alone estimated at $18 billion (Productivity Commission 2019). The main societal costs related to mental illness are lost productivity, caused by high unemployment and under-employment of people with mental illness, along with impacts on quality of life and other non-quantifiable costs, such as the cost of stigma. In addition, there are social participation impacts, as well as the pain and suffering of family and friends who have lost a loved one to suicide.

Australia's 2019 Productivity Commission Inquiry into Mental Health identifies that the cost of lost productivity due to lower employment, absenteeism and presenteeism (working while unwell) ranges from $10 billion to $18 billion. Informal care costs to family and friends has been valued at $15 billion per annum. There is a cost of approximately $130 billion associated with diminished health and reduced life expectancy for people with mental ill health. On an individual level, for example, the annual costs for a person who experiences psychosis in Australia have been evaluated as comprising $40,941 in lost productivity, $21,714 in health sector costs and $14,642 in other costs.

In Aotearoa New Zealand there are similar costs associated with mental illness. A recent inquiry into mental health and addiction (Ministry of Health 2018) received submissions on the personal, social and economic impacts of mental illness. The Ministry of Health (2017) estimates that the annual cost of the burden of serious mental illness, including addiction, in Aotearoa New Zealand is $12 billion or 5% of gross domestic product. In addition to this economic impact, there is an estimated $1.5 billion annual cost across government agencies associated with the nearly 60,000 health and disability benefit recipients whose primary barrier to work is mental illness. Poor mental health has other indirect costs – for example, the cost of housing for those who cannot work because of mental health problems. This cost is estimated at $1.2 billion over the lifetime of Aotearoa New Zealand's 6700 social housing tenants receiving benefits whose primary barrier to work is mental health (Ministry of Health 2018). Health system, social and financial costs of mental illness were demonstrated in an Aotearoa New Zealand study of people with schizophrenia (Gibb et al 2021). People with schizophrenia were found to be significantly more likely to have a general hospital admission, a mental health in-patient admission or to attend the emergency department (ED). They were also more likely to be receiving a social welfare benefit, to be living in social housing or to be involved with the criminal justice system. In addition, individuals with schizophrenia were significantly less likely to be employed. Their average annual income was less than half that of those without schizophrenia, and they were significantly more likely to live in areas of high socioeconomic deprivation (Gibb et al 2021).

✳ HISTORICAL ANECDOTE 1.1
Early Descriptions

Experiences of mental ill health have been described since the beginning of human history in ancient documents such as Egyptian papyri, the Indian Ramayana and the Old Testament of the Bible. The longest lasting historical theory regarding mental ill health was developed by ancient Greek philosophers Pythagoras (570–495 BCE) and Hippocrates (460–377 BCE), who proposed that the human body contains four "humors": blood, phlegm, yellow bile and black bile. Black bile and phlegm were thought to cause mental ill health, which was believed to be more common in spring and beginning of winter when the humors were "active". Humoral theory dominated medical treatment for more than 2000 years, informing the administration of several painful remedies such as blisters to the head, castor oil, a solution of lilac emetic and bloodletting. Each of these "treatments" was designed to purge the body of the "black bile and phlegm" thought to be causing mental ill health. Today, we still see the relic of humoral theory in our modern terms "choleric" and "sanguine" used to describe different personality types.

Read More About It
Davison, K. 2006, Historical aspects of mood disorders. Psychiatry 5(4), 115–118.

Australian National Survey of Mental Health

The Australian Bureau of Statistics (ABS) conducted a national survey of mental health and wellbeing in 2020–2022, which collected information on lifetime and 12-month prevalence of selected mental health problems among people aged 18–65 years. The following information was obtained from the survey report (ABS 2023).

Almost half of all Australians aged 18–65 reported a mental health problem at some point in their life, and one in five (21%) experienced a mental health problem within the preceding 12 months. Analysis of survey results showed that anxiety disorders (16.8%) were the most commonly experienced type of mental health problem in Australia, with the most frequently reported anxiety disorder being social phobia (7%) followed by post-traumatic stress disorder (PTSD) (5.7%). Affective disorders were reported by 7.5% of respondents, with the most common affective disorder being depression (4.6%). Substance use disorders affected 3.3% of respondents, the most common being harmful or dependent use of alcohol, reported by 2.5% of respondents.

While the most recent survey has not reported comorbid or co-associated mental and physical illness, the 2008 ABS survey highlighted significant connections between mental and physical conditions; 11.7% of respondents had both a mental and a physical health problem, and 8.5% reported two or more mental disorders. In line with prevalence of discreet mental health problems, the most common comorbidity was anxiety disorder and a physical condition (6%). Comorbidity compounds the impact of individual disorders, resulting in higher rates of relapse, greater impairment, higher use of health services and higher risk of suicidal behaviour.

The 2020–22 survey showed the gendered distribution of mental disorder in Australia. Women (24.6%) were more likely to experience mental disorders than men (18%). Compared with men, women reported higher rates of anxiety disorder than men (21% vs 12.4%) and higher rates of affective disorders (78.5% vs 6.2%). Compared to 2008, rates of substance use reduced for both men and women, but, as in 2008, men had more than twice the rate of substance use disorders (4.4%) compared with women (2.3%). Rates of mental disorder varied across age groups, with younger people more likely to have a mental illness than older people. Almost 40% of people aged 16–24 reported a mental disorder in the past year compared with 12% of those aged 65–85. Substance use disorders were more common among younger people (16–34) than in other age groups, with a reported rate of 13.5%, while anxiety disorders (31.5%) were more common in people aged 16–24. Social factors associated with mental illness have not been reported in the 2020 survey; however, in 2008 family and housing status were associated with rates of mental disorder. One-third (34%) of people living in one-parent families reported a mental health problem compared with 19% of those living in couple families. More than half of those who had ever been homeless had a mental health problem, almost three times the rate of those who had never been homeless. Mental health problems were more common among unemployed people (29%) and in people who had ever been incarcerated (41%). Recent Australian research has shown relationships between mental illness and homelessness (Moschion & van Ours 2021) and between social adversities and mental illness (Hashmi 2020).

Rates of psychotic disorder were examined in the 2010 Survey of High Impact Psychosis, Australia's second national psychosis survey (Morgan et al 2012). That survey reported a 12-month prevalence of psychotic disorder of 4.5 in 1000. Of those diagnosed with a psychotic disorder, the most common diagnosis was schizophrenia spectrum disorder (63%). While the overall rate might seem relatively low, especially compared with the rates of depression and anxiety, the impacts of psychotic disorder can be profound. Morgan and colleagues reported that 49.5% of those with a psychotic disorder had attempted suicide over their lifetime, 63.2% experienced significant social impairment and 78.5% were unemployed. The relationship between mental and physical illness is marked, with 54.8% of this sample having metabolic syndrome and therefore at significant risk of developing type 2 diabetes and cardiovascular disease.

Te Rau Hinengaro: the New Zealand Mental Health Survey

Te Rau Hinengaro ("the many minds"), the New Zealand Mental Health Survey (Oakley Browne et al 2006), aimed to describe the mental health state of the entire Aotearoa New Zealand population. The survey data is now two decades old, but remains the basis for much of the planning of mental health services (Lockett et al 2022). Like its Australian counterpart, Te Rau Hinengaro did not collect data on psychotic disorders. Specific objectives of Te Rau Hinengaro were to describe:

- the one-month, 12-month and lifetime prevalence rates of major mental disorders among those aged 16 or older living in private households, overall and by sociodemographic correlates
- patterns of and barriers to health service use for people with a mental disorder
- the level of disability associated with a mental disorder.

The survey reported a 44.6% lifetime prevalence of mental disorder, with a 12-month prevalence of 20.7%. The latter figure is very close to the 20% 12-month prevalence reported in Australia. In addition to overall prevalence, the survey presented specific findings on age, gender, ethnicity and socioeconomic status.

Mental disorders are more common in young people in Aotearoa New Zealand, with younger people reporting a higher prevalence of disorder in the past 12 months and more likely to report having ever had a disorder. In terms of gender, females reported a higher prevalence of anxiety disorder, major depression and eating disorders than males, whereas males reported substantially higher prevalence for substance use disorders than females. Social disadvantage is also associated with mental disorders, with higher rates for people who are disadvantaged in terms of educational qualification, household income or social deprivation. Comorbidity of mental disorders is common, with 37.0% of those experiencing 12-month mental disorders having two or more disorders. Mood disorders and anxiety disorders are most likely to co-occur. The survey also noted that rates of mental and physical comorbidity are high and cause compounding disability, but these rates of comorbidity are not reported in Te Rau Hinengaro.

The prevalence of disorder in any period is higher for Māori and Pacific people than for the "Other" composite ethnic group. For disorder, in the past 12 months the prevalence rates are 29.5% for Māori, 24.4% for Pacific people and 19.3% for "Other", which indicates that Māori and Pacific people have a greater burden due to mental health problems. Much of this burden appears to be due to the youthfulness of the Māori and Pacific populations and their relative socioeconomic disadvantage.

Suicidality was also reported in Te Rau Hinengaro. Of the Aotearoa New Zealand population, 15.7% reported ever having thought seriously about suicide. In total, 5.5% had ever made a suicide plan and 4.5% had ever made an attempt. These rates are comparable with those of several other developed countries. In the 12 months preceding the survey, 3.2% experienced suicidal ideation, 1.0% made a suicide plan and 0.4% made a suicide attempt. Higher rates of suicidality were reported for women, younger people and for people experiencing social deprivation. Individuals with a mental disorder had elevated risks of suicidal behaviour, with 11.8% of people with any mental disorder reporting suicidal ideation, 4.1% making a suicide plan and 1.6% making a suicide attempt. It is important to remember, however, that many of the individuals reporting suicidal thoughts, plans and even attempts will not have sought professional support. Others will have attended a primary care service for a physical health problem, but will not have reported their suicidal thoughts.

 CRITICAL THINKING EXERCISE 1.1

Epidemiological studies show that mental illness and addiction problems are relatively common in our communities, with up to 50% of people experiencing a mental illness (including addiction) in their lifetime. Yet the belief persists that mental illness is uncommon and experienced by only a small minority of people. Why does the belief persist that only a small minority of people experience mental illness? What effect does this belief have on nurses and other primary care clinicians who regularly see many patients with mental health and addiction problems?

Physical and Mental Health

In 1954 Dr Brock Chisholm, the first Director-General of WHO, stated that "without mental health there can be no true physical health" (Kolappa et al 2013). Conversely, it has been argued that "there is no true mental health without (physical) health" (Kolappa et al 2013).

Health is defined in the WHO constitution as:

A state of complete physical, mental and social wellbeing and not merely the absence of disease or infirmity.

(WHO 2014, p. 1)

As can be seen from the above quote, people are holistic beings with both physical and mental health needs. However, generalist and mental health services are often separated, which has led to an artificial divide between physical and mental health care. This means that the mental health needs of patients in generalist health settings can be overlooked. Similarly, the physical health of people with mental illness in mental health settings may not be prioritised.

People with mental illness have higher rates of physical illness than the general population (Richmond-Rakerd et al 2021) and do not always receive adequate screening, assessment and treatment for their physical health (Roberts et al 2018). In addition, people with mental illness have high rates of chronic physical illness, which contributes to higher morbidity and mortality rates. It is therefore important in every practice setting that nurses respond to both the physical health and the mental health needs of people with mental illness. Both Australia and Aotearoa New Zealand have strategies to address the health disparities experienced by people with mental illness. The *Equally Well* consensus statements (Mental Health Commission of NSW 2016; Te Pou o Te Whakaaro Nui 2014) express the commitment of multiple organisations to improving the physical health of people with mental illness. These statements reflect the view that mental health is "everybody's business", including the whole health sector, as well as social agencies, employers, housing providers and police. The physical health of people with mental illness is discussed in detail in Chapter 20.

Nowhere is the relationship between mind and body more evident than in the area of chronic conditions. People with mental illness experience chronic disease at greater rates than the general community in areas including but not limited to respiratory disease, cardiovascular disease, diabetes, chronic pain and cancer. Mental illness is also associated with a reduction in life expectancy of up to 25 years (Firth et al 2019). People with the more enduring forms of psychotic illness struggle to have even their most basic physical health needs met and experience very poor access to regular physical review by a general

practitioner (GP) and health promotion services (e.g. smoking cessation programs and cancer screening) (Bos et al 2022; Solmi et al 2020). This lack of appropriate health care contributes significantly to increased risk of chronic disease and premature death.

The relationship between physical and mental health is also important in understanding causes and treatment of physical illness. For example, depression can precede a physical disease. It has been linked to diseases such as cardiovascular disease, stroke, colorectal cancer, epilepsy, chronic obstructive pulmonary disease and type 2 diabetes (Sartorius 2018). In addition, people with any chronic physical disease tend to feel more mental distress than do healthy people (Gold et al 2020). Poor physical health brings an increased risk of depression (Thom et al 2019), as do the social and relationship problems that are common among chronically ill patients (Gürhan et al 2019). Understanding the relationship between physical and mental health is crucial for nurses in order to develop strategies to reduce the incidence of co-existing conditions and support those already living with mental illnesses and chronic physical conditions. Modifiable behaviours with the potential to positively or negatively affect physical and mental health include sleep, diet, alcohol/drug use and physical exercise (Wickham et al 2020).

Assisting patients to manage their physical health and mental health is a role for all nurses. Simple ways we can observe a person's physical health status include taking note of their body shape, skin, central adiposity, weight, height, body mass index, blood pressure, heart rate, cholesterol, blood sugar levels, abdominal circumference and fitness level. See Chapter 20 for further nursing strategies.

 CRITICAL THINKING EXERCISE 1.2

Metabolic syndrome is a cluster of risk factors that predicts development of type 2 diabetes and cardiovascular disease. Rates of metabolic syndrome are high in people taking antipsychotic medication, yet nurses in mental health and primary care settings do not always provide routine screening for metabolic syndrome. Consider your own area of practice or your current clinical placement. Are mental health consumers in that area screened for metabolic syndrome? Do nurses consider this to be part of their practice? If consumers are screened, what interventions are used to reduce the risk of metabolic syndrome?

Self-Harm and Suicide

As identified earlier, in addition to mental disorders, self-harm and suicidality are behaviours that nurses commonly encounter in settings such as primary care and ED , as well as mental health services. Suicide is a prevalent mental health problem in both Australia (Yousiph 2022) and Aotearoa New Zealand (Ministry of Health 2019), and for every person who completes suicide there are many more who self-harm (Mars et al 2019). Self-harm can vary from cutting to relieve distress, to overdoses of prescribed or over-the-counter medication and potentially lethal attempts at suicide. Depression is a common mental disorder and is associated with self-harm and suicidal thoughts.

In general hospital settings, patients may sometimes express a sense of hopelessness when faced with ill health, pain, lost function or an adverse prognosis. Such patients may then have passive suicidal thoughts – ideas that they would be better off dead or a wish that they would die from their illness. Passive suicidal thoughts are relatively common and may respond to the listening skills and validation of an empathic nurse (Sisler et al 2020). If passive suicidal thoughts worsen and develop into active suicide plans, the nurse may need to consider referral to a mental health specialist.

Although suicide is statistically rare, it leaves an emotional impact on the lives of hundreds of thousands of friends and relatives of people who complete suicide each year. Research suggests many people who complete suicide had recent contact with a health professional (Chiang et al 2021), indicating that those considering suicide are not always receiving the psychological support they seek. Certain population groups are at higher risk of suicide. These groups currently include men and young people. In fact, suicide is a leading cause of death in adolescents and young adults in Australia (Australian Institute of Health and Welfare 2019) and Aotearoa New Zealand (Te Rōpū Arotake Auau Mate o te Hunga Tamariki, Taiohi 2021); men over the age of 85 have the highest suicide rate of all age groups (ABS 2021). Other groups that have been identified as being at higher risk of suicide include people from rural and remote communities and Aboriginal and Torres Strait Islander people (Cutler et al 2021).

MENTAL HEALTH CARE

Australian mental health service delivery is guided by a national mental health strategy that comprises a national policy and plan (the *Fifth National Mental Health and Suicide Prevention Plan* was published in 2017). Each of the states and territories develops and reforms services in accordance with this national strategy. In Aotearoa New Zealand, the Ministry of Health provides national direction for mental health services. In both countries the aim is to provide mental health care in a stepped care arrangement (see below), with the majority of care provided in primary care settings, and to the least restrictive standard. In keeping with this, mental health care is provided in a wide range of clinical settings from generalist health settings and primary care through to specialist mental health services, with the preferred setting for service delivery being in the community wherever possible.

WHO recommends that mental health care should be based in primary care. This is because general practice is usually the first point of contact for people seeking assistance for all health problems – including mental health problems – and a significant number of people with severe mental illness and high care needs receive their mental health care from a GP working in a primary care setting and/or a psychiatrist working in private practice. In addition, the high prevalence of comorbid illnesses and the side effects of psychotropic medications make the need for strong and well-established links with general practice important. A systematic review by Perkins and colleagues (2017) identified that generalist healthcare providers in Australia, including nurses, undertake recognition and identification of illness, assessment and care planning, patient education, pharmacotherapy, psychological therapies (and other therapies), ongoing management, physical care and referral for people with mental health problems.

The "stepped care" model of mental health care is an evidence-based, staged system that includes a hierarchy of interventions that are matched to a person's needs – ranging from least to most intensive (Australian Government Department of Health 2019; Cornish 2020). Box 1.1 provides some descriptors around the intervention hierarchy in the stepped care model.

In a stepped care arrangement, it's not necessary to start at level 1. The care that people need depends on the severity of their problems, the impact of their experiences on their functioning and how any problems identified may have responded to initial (first-line) interventions. For example, for some people interventions such as relaxation training, sleep hygiene and moderating the use of alcohol may be effective in reducing mild anxiety, while others might need

---

BOX 1.1 Stepped Care Model of Mental Health Care in Primary Health

Level 1: Self-management – for people with no or mild mental illness, designed to prevent the development of illness (or prevent illness from progressing) and focused on helping individuals to manage symptoms themselves. This might include pamphlets about mental health and well-being, workbooks about a specific problem or online self-help programs.

Level 2: Low-intensity services – for people with mild to moderate mental illness and might include guided self-help or brief psychological interventions designed to last for a few short sessions.

Level 3: Moderate-intensity services are for people with mild to moderate mental illness but provide more structured, frequent and intensive interventions.

Level 4: High-intensity services are for people with more severe mental illness that is persistent or episodic, but that doesn't carry a high level of risk, complexity or disability. This includes high-intensity services and intensive interventions that might include multidisciplinary support.

Level 5: Acute and specialist community mental health services are for people with severe and persistent needs and those with complex multi-agency needs or conditions that include high levels of risk, disability or complexity. These services include intensive team-based specialist assessment and intervention provided by mental health professionals across disciplines.

---

specialist assessment, psychological therapy or pharmacological treatment. In addition to improving access to mental health care, as well as detection, early intervention and outcome for consumers, stepped care aims to improve the efficiency and effectiveness of mental health service delivery.

Within mental health services, there are many settings in which a nurse may practise. The most common of these include in-patient services in general hospitals, crisis teams, community mental health teams and recovery-focused services. Specialist mental health services are delivered in mental health settings by health professionals with specialist mental health qualifications and training, including mental health nurses, psychiatrists, psychologists and mental health-trained social workers and occupational therapists.

Increasingly, people with a lived experience of mental illness are undertaking peer worker roles across primary care, community and in-patient settings (Shin 2020) (see Perspectives in Practice: Nurse's Story 1.1). The essence of these roles is to provide support based on mutual respect, shared responsibility and mutual agreement about what support is needed (Cleary et al 2018). Similarly, community-managed organisations (also known as non-government organisations or NGOs) are increasingly playing a key role in providing support to people with a lived experience of mental illness – through direct service delivery (Balagopal & Kapanee 2019). They complement existing mental health services and strengthen community supports and partnerships. The main types of support provided include: accommodation support and outreach; employment and education; leisure and recreation; family and carer support; self-help and peer-support; helpline and counselling services; and promotion, information and advocacy. While it is critical for nurses to work in an integrated way with community-managed organisations, it is important to remember that NGOs do not provide whole-of-life services, but rather are stepping stones for those people who choose to use them. The aim is for people to develop naturally occurring supports within the community or to use other created supports that are accessed by all members of the community.

PERSPECTIVES IN PRACTICE

Nurse's Story 1.1

When I started nursing, I didn't really have any idea what area of specialisation I wanted to go into. There's so much choice in nursing and I really enjoyed my first clinical placement, which was in a paediatric ward. At the start of my second year, I had a really hard break-up with my partner of three years. It was very traumatic for me, mostly because it was so sudden. My partner was particularly nasty and made some very unkind comments about my appearance. I became quite depressed. I come from a rural area, so I was living on campus in college accommodation at the time. You would think living with so many other people that everyone would have noticed me getting more and more unhappy, but shared living with hundreds of other students provided quite a lot of anonymity and I hadn't really made all that many friends during the first year. I went to my classes, did a fair bit of work online and stayed in my room most of the time. I wasn't someone who partied, and I didn't confide in my parents about how upset I was. My mother had suffered from depression for many years and I didn't want to burden her or my dad. I also didn't want to be like her, so I pretended nothing was wrong.

Eventually I did talk to one of my friends from home and he encouraged me to go and see a GP at the university, which I did. The GP was really helpful and referred me to one of the counsellors there. Being able to talk about the break-up and how I was feeling made a big difference, although it was hard and sometimes emotional. It took me quite a while to fully recover.

I never thought I wanted to work in mental health. To be honest, I was a bit scared of the idea, but when I did my mental health placement in third year, I loved it. It was nothing like I expected it to be and I do think my personal journey really helped to create a curiosity and understanding of the experience people with mental health problems face. When it was time to do my graduate year, people said I shouldn't do mental health, that I should consolidate my general skills somewhere first, but mental health was for me and I'm so pleased to have made the decision to just do it. I have never looked back.

? CRITICAL THINKING EXERCISE 1.3

Nurses meet people with mental health and addiction problems in every clinical setting. For some people, their mental health needs can be met within a general health setting, such as primary care or in a medical ward of a general hospital. Others need referral to a specialist mental health service. How would you assess the mental health needs of a patient in a general health setting? When would you consider referral for a specialist mental health assessment?

Cultural Considerations

Australia and Aotearoa New Zealand are culturally diverse countries originally peopled by Indigenous populations. Following colonisation and migrant settlement over two centuries, both countries now embrace multiple cultures, although the dominant culture in both countries reflects a Western worldview and values. This dominant worldview has been found to be inadequate in the face of the cultural diversity of both countries.

The Indigenous peoples of Australia and Aotearoa New Zealand experience high rates of mental disorder that reflects the history and modern legacy of colonisation (Rhodes 2019). "Mental illness" is a Western construct, however, and so for many Indigenous people represents Western ideas of the individual and the relationship between the individual and society. These ideas may be profoundly different from people from non-Western cultures. Aboriginal and Torres Strait Islanders and Aotearoa New Zealand Māori have views of health and illness that are informed by their wider cultural beliefs and that

support practices unique to those cultures. The way people express mental distress and illness will reflect their cultural beliefs. In Aotearoa New Zealand, for example, the phenomenon of *whakamaa* (shame, self-abasement, shyness, excessive modesty and withdrawal describe some aspects of this concept) is unique to the Māori culture (Mooney et al 2020). For Australian Aboriginal and Torres Strait Islander peoples, individuals who spend long periods of time away from their country (place of birth/Dreaming) can be vulnerable to episodes of unwellness due to their weakened spiritual link with country and community (Westerman 2021). Symptoms of a cultural syndrome known as "longing for country" commonly include feelings of weakness, nausea and general "sickness" and somatic complaints, identity confusion and disorientation, which if cultural background is not considered may be misinterpreted by clinicians reliant on Western interpretations as forms of clinical depression or anxiety. Not being able to go home and settle these feelings can lead Aboriginal and Torres Strait Islanders to further health deterioration. The importance of country might partially explain the profound effect that prison has on many First Nations people and the high rate of deaths in custody among Aboriginal and Torres Strait Islanders compared with non-Indigenous Australians (Westerman 2021). Connection with land, culture and community is central to many Indigenous people and is often related to issues of mental health.

The increasing ethnic and cultural diversity of Western societies means that diverse individuals attend Western health services with presentations influenced by cultural beliefs and practices different from those of clinicians trained in Western models. Nurses respond to this diversity by developing an understanding of the diversity of cultures in their own societies and by developing cross-cultural communication skills (Minton et al 2022). Services also attempt to provide clinicians from the cultural group of the service user and, in some cases, develop specialty services based on a culturally specific model of treatment. Collaborations between traditional and Western practitioners in mental health care have been further described by NiaNia and colleagues (2017).

? CRITICAL THINKING EXERCISE 1.4

Consider the cultural influences on your own identity. What insights does your cultural experience give you into the experience of people from cultures other than your own? In what ways does your cultural background limit your understanding of the cultures of others? What skills and strategies can you use to ensure barriers to cross-cultural communication are effectively addressed?

CULTURAL SAFETY AND MENTAL HEALTH CARE

Nursing is about people of all cultures. Consumers and nurses have diverse cultural backgrounds, and while this diversity makes for rich and rewarding experiences it also brings the possibility of misinterpretations and misunderstandings. Experiences of distress and emotional conflict are embedded in cultural beliefs and traditions, so it is important that every nursing encounter is regarded as one that occurs with the cultural contexts of the nurse and consumer. The populations of Australia and Aotearoa New Zealand are characterised by increasing cultural diversity, and it is important that this diversity is acknowledged by nurses. Australian professional standards for mental health nurses recognise the need for nurses to work with consumers from all cultures (Australian College of Mental Health Nurses 2010), and Aotearoa New Zealand standards require nurses to provide care that is culturally safe (Te Ao Maramatanga 2012). The term "cultural safety" (kawa whakaruruhau) was developed by Aotearoa New Zealand nurse

Irihapeti Ramsden and can be considered the effective nursing of a person/family from another culture by a nurse who has undertaken a process of reflection on their own cultural identity and recognises the impact of their own cultural identity on their nursing practice (adapted from definition provided by Nursing Council of New Zealand 2011).

The concept of cultural safety has been widely adopted across many countries and health settings (Tremblay et al 2020), and has been promoted as a model for nursing in Australia (McGough et al 2022). More recently there has been increasing recognition that individuals carry multiple cultural and other identities (De Sousa et al 2022), making cultural safety a more complex construct, but also one that is more sensitive to the realities of nurses' and consumers' multiple cultural beliefs, values and practices. For this reason, the Nursing Council of New Zealand's definition of "culture" extends to "age or generation; gender; sexual orientation; occupation and socioeconomic status; ethnic origin or migrant experience; religious or spiritual belief; and disability" (Nursing Council of New Zealand 2011, p. 5). As can be seen from that definition, culture is regarded as a construct that applies to many possible identities. A key to cultural safety is the nurse's own self-awareness and sensitivity to the impact of their cultural identity on the care they provide to others. (See Case study 1.1.)

As we have discussed above, the mental health experience of First Nations Australians and New Zealanders is shaped by the historical and contemporary experience of colonisation. Awareness of this history and how it continues within contemporary society is a critical aspect of cultural safety if nurses are to avoid reinforcing the colonial relationship within their nursing practice. This historicising approach provides a foundation for culturally safe practice with all the diverse cultures of Australia and Aotearoa New Zealand. Cultural safety does not require that nurses "understand" the cultures of all consumers and communities. Such an approach is naive and risks the nurse assuming cultural expertise they do not have. See Chapters 6 and 7 for further information on Indigenous and Māori mental health and culture.

CASE STUDY 1.1: Zahra

Zahra is a 30-year-old Somalian woman who police found wandering on a busy road. They were unable to engage her in conversation and were also unclear as to whether she was under the influence of alcohol or drugs. They took her to a mental health facility where mental health clinicians were asked to assess her.

The mental health team approached Zahra and introduced themselves. At that moment Zahra became more aware of her surroundings and became agitated. She kept repeating that she was not a prisoner and not to hurt her. Her English was limited, but her meaning was clear to all. The mental health team attempted to calm her and requested that the police remain in the area but be unseen. This had a short-term calming effect.

Using an interpreter, the mental health team undertook their assessment and mental state examination. It became evident that Zahra was using multiple substances, including cannabis and alcohol. She stated that she was using these substances more and more because they helped her forget the past.

Zahra had experienced terrible hardship, including rape, separation from her family and living in a detention centre for 3 years. As a result, she had developed PTSD.

Many refugees have experienced and witnessed appalling conditions, often perpetrated by people in authority. In Zahra's case, staff could not have predicted her response. However, when working with refugees and asylum seekers, nurses need to be mindful of the possibility of traumatic stress and the associated sequelae, including substance use.

✴ HISTORICAL ANECDOTE 1.2
Ancient Treatments

Communities as early as 5000 BCE associated mental ill health with mythological and spiritual beliefs, such as demonic possession, sorcery and curses. Archaeologists have found the remains of prehistoric human skulls that had holes chipped into them using stone instruments (a treatment known as trephining) in the belief that by opening the skull an evil spirit, thought to be inhabiting a person's head and causing mental ill health, might be released and the individual would be cured. Some who underwent such procedures appear to have survived and lived for many years afterwards as trephined skulls of early humans show signs of healing. Pressure on the brain may have also been incidentally relieved.

Read More About It
Prioreschi, P. 1991. Possible reasons for neolithic skull trephining. Anecdotes in Biology and Medicine, 34(2), 296–303.

MENTAL HEALTH LEGISLATION

Mental health is unique within the healthcare environment in providing legislation that can compel people to accept treatment and, in some cases, to remain in hospital. Treatment without consent under mental health legislation is known as "compulsory treatment" or "civil commitment". Informed consent is normally considered fundamental to providing care in every clinical setting, and treatment without consent is considered unethical. The usual rationale for providing compulsory treatment under mental health legislation is given in terms of risk to the person with mental illness or to another person. It is not enough for risk to be present; the risk must be due to mental illness. Examples include impaired judgement due to mania that might lead people to take actions that are very unsafe, suicidal thoughts together with intentions to act due to depression, or thoughts of harming others in response to voices telling the person to act in a harmful way. In these circumstances, people may temporarily lose their capacity to make decisions. These high-risk situations are exceptional and require clinicians to act within the definitions of mental disorder contained in legislation. The purpose of compulsory treatment is to protect the person or others from potential harm. In addition to compulsory treatment in hospital, mental health legislation can also compel patients to accept treatment in community settings under a community treatment order. Although mental health legislation limits some rights of consumers, it also provides protections through the right to consult a lawyer and to appeal to a court for a review of legal status. Several Australian states have amended their mental health legislation in recent years to give greater effect to human rights through processes such as supported decision-making and advance directives. Mental health legislation is further explored in Chapter 10.

MENTAL HEALTH AND THE SCOPE OF NURSING PRACTICE

In Australia and Aotearoa New Zealand nursing is regulated by statutory bodies that determine the responsibilities and obligations of nurses. One of the main mechanisms of statutory bodies is through statements of the scope of nursing practice (Cross et al 2021). Another mechanism is through statements of competencies, which are descriptions of the skills every nurse is expected to demonstrate. Nurses are legally and professionally responsible for working within their nursing scope of practice and for meeting all competencies of their regulatory bodies. There is no regulated scope of practice for mental health nursing in either Australia or Aotearoa New Zealand. Instead the scope is stated in broad terms and applies in every clinical setting.

The Nursing and Midwifery Board of Australia (2023) advises that the nursing scope of practice:

includes the health needs of people, the level of competence and confidence of the nurse [...] and the policy requirements of the service provider. As the nurse [...] gains new skills and knowledge, their individual scope of practice changes.

The Nursing Council of New Zealand (2023) also identifies a broad scope of practice for nurses:

Registered nurses use nursing knowledge and complex nursing judgment to assess health needs and provide care, and to advise and support people to manage their health [...]. This occurs in a range of settings in partnership with individuals, families, whānau and communities.

Statements of the scope of nursing practice make it clear that mental health care is every nurse's business. Together with the competencies for practice, they encompass the whole range of health care, meaning that nurses are expected to respond appropriately to the full range of patient needs. When we understand how common mental health issues are in the community, and how commonly people experience both mental and physical health problems, it is clear that there is a professional obligation for nurses to respond to the whole person, including their physical and mental health needs. The nursing scope of practice reflects that obligation.

NURSING AND MENTAL HEALTH

As a nurse you will meet people with mental health issues in every area of clinical practice, from primary care through to specialist settings such as intensive care and surgery, and in prisons, schools, workplaces and aged care services. Mental health is both a specialised field of nursing practice and a fundamental part of every nurse's scope of practice. Yet you do not need to be a mental health specialist to respond to people's mental health needs. Fundamental mental health knowledge and skills can (and should) be used by all nurses, regardless of setting (O'Brien 2014).

Caring for people's mental health is a vital part of nursing. Patients in every clinical setting have mental health needs that may or may not contribute to their reasons for accessing health services. For many people nurses work with, mental health care is about helping a person maintain a sense of social and emotional wellbeing and seeking to optimise their mental health, which they normally experience as being positive. For others, mental health care may involve some short-term assistance to overcome mild experiences of mental health challenges such as anxiety or low mood. Nurses also commonly care for people who have long-term experience of mental illness such as schizophrenia

or bipolar disorder that requires support of varying levels of intensity over many years. It is important for nurses to consider the whole of each person's health needs. Just as a patient with a long-term mental illness might present to their GP with asthma or high blood pressure, a patient with a chronic physical illness such as diabetes might experience episodes of low mood or anxiety.

Responding to a person's mental health needs requires a variety of nursing skills, including listening, exploring emotional issues and troubling thoughts, showing empathy, offering encouragement and building on strengths. See Chapter 2 for a discussion of holistic mental health nursing practice and therapeutic mental health nursing skills. Such actions can be incorporated into regular nursing care; they do not have to wait until other needs have been attended to. A nurse who practises holistically will be aware of the needs of each person at the time, will be open to discussing emotional and physical health issues and will be comfortable in responding in an informed and helpful way. This may involve seeking guidance from other professionals or making a referral to a specialist service. Such referral or advice seeking is an integral part of the nurse's practice and an acknowledgement of the scope of nursing practice. Mental health is part of the core business of every nurse, whether by the direct care the nurse provides or by referral to a specialist service. See Personal perspectives: Consumer's Story 1.1: Maria.

PERSONAL PERSPECTIVES
Consumer's Story 1.1: Maria

I had a difficult childhood and found myself on the streets at the age of 13 doing what I had to do to survive. I married young to a violent man and had four children. I didn't start using drugs until I was in my mid-40s when I was told that speed (methamphetamine) wasn't addictive! Before too long I was injecting and had a $300 a day habit. I even injected it into my neck when I couldn't find a vein in my arm. I was always chasing the dragon (trying to get that incredible feeling of elation experienced at the first taste). I was a junkie, and nothing mattered more than getting my next hit. Not even my kids. Eventually I realised I had a problem, so I walked down to my local GP and asked for some help. I was told they didn't work with people like me. I was stunned, but I walked further along the street to another GP and was standing at the reception desk asking if someone would see me when one of the doctors, who just happened to be standing near the desk, invited me into his office right there and then. He referred me to the mental health nurse working at the practice and I saw both of them for the next several years. She (the mental health nurse) would see me at home even when I didn't want to see her! There were times when I wouldn't see her because I'd started using again and I was too ashamed to look her in the eye. But she kept coming back. After 10 years of addiction I've now been clean for more than 2 years. I now have a "normal" life. I work two jobs, but, more importantly, I have a pretty good relationship with my kids and a fantastic relationship with my three gorgeous grandkids. And now I've been cigarette-free for almost 11 months.

CHAPTER SUMMARY

Mental health matters because mental health problems are prevalent in our society, have significant personal, social and economic impacts, present in every clinical setting, and form part of the nursing scope of practice. Mental health is part of health. Mental health problems impact on the course and severity of physical health problems and are associated with worse health outcomes. Mental health consumers experience high rates of physical health disorders, are less likely to have physical health issues attended to and die younger than those in the general population. People with physical illnesses experience worse mental health than those

without illness, and mental health problems adversely affect treatment, recovery and quality of life. Nurses have opportunities to use mental health skills to improve consumers' mental and physical health.

Responding to the mental health needs of patients is a professional obligation of nurses. Nurses do not need to be specialists to respond to patients' mental health needs. Fundamental mental health nursing skills, such as listening, validating and responding empathically, can help to meet some of the mental health needs of patients in all clinical settings. Nurses can also learn and develop skills in specific therapeutic modalities. In some cases, nurses will feel they need to ask for further advice about a patient's needs or to refer them to a mental health specialist. Every nurse is not a *specialist* mental health nurse, just as every nurse is not a specialist in diabetes care, coronary care or primary care. But just as mental health is part of health, mental health is part of every nurse's scope of practice.

REVIEW QUESTIONS

After reading this chapter discuss the following scenarios in small groups.

Scenario 1
Mental health is part of the scope of practice of every nurse. However, the mental health needs of consumers in general health settings (such as medical and surgical wards and primary care) are frequently overlooked. Discuss the possible barriers to nurses in general settings responding to consumers' mental health needs. Make a list of the six most important barriers. Consider individual, system and policy-level barriers.

Scenario 2
Taking the list made in discussing Scenario 1 above, identify strategies that would help nurses in addressing the identified barriers. The strategies may need support from others to implement.

Scenario 3
Many individual, social and political factors can influence mental health. Conversely, mental distress and illness can impact on employment, social organisation and the economy.
1. Identify five social factors that can influence a person's mental health.
2. For each factor, discuss how that factor can be addressed.
3. Identify five social impacts of mental distress or illness.
4. For each factor, discuss how the impact of mental distress or illness could be reduced.

Scenario 4
Rebecca is a 32-year-old woman who has been feeling increasingly tired and "strung out" after the birth of her first child 5 months ago. When she visits her GP to ask for medication to help her sleep the GP asks a primary care nurse to interview Rebecca and assess her mood, safety and sleep. Rebecca is surprised to learn that the nurse considers she may be depressed.
1. What initial support and intervention could be considered for Rebecca?
2. What areas of assessment would you consider in interviewing Rebecca?
3. What would you consider before recommending to the GP that Rebecca is prescribed medication for her mood?
4. At what point would you consider referring Rebecca to a specialist mental health clinician for further assessment and treatment? (See stepped care model in Box 1.1.)

USEFUL WEBSITES

Australian Government, Department of Health and Aged Care. Primary Health Networks (PHN) collection of primary mental health care resources: www.health.gov.au/resources/collections/primary-health-networks-phn-collection-of-primary-mental-health-care-resources?utm_source=health.gov.au&utm_medium=callout-auto-custom&utm_campaign=digital_transformation

Black Dog Institute, Australia: www.blackdoginstitute.org.au/

Healthify He puna Waiora New Zealand. Mental health conditions: https://healthify.nz/health-a-z/m/mental-health-conditions/

Mental Health Australia: https://mhaustralia.org

Mental Health Coordinating Council: mhcc.org.au

Mental health data and statistics (Aotearoa New Zealand): www.health.govt.nz/nz-health-statistics/health-statistics-and-data-sets/mental-health-data-and-stats

Mental Health Foundation of New Zealand: www.mentalhealth.org.nz

National Mental Health Commission, Australia: www.mentalhealthcommission.gov.au/

Wellplace New Zealand: ignite.org.nz/learn?searchFilters=Mental%20health

REFERENCES

Australian Bureau of Statistics (ABS), 2023. National Study of Mental Health and Wellbeing 2020–2022. Online. Available at: www.abs.gov.au/statistics/health/mental-health/national-study-mental-health-and-wellbeing/latest-release

Australian Bureau of Statistics (ABS), 2021. Causes of Death, Australia. ABS. Online. Available at: www.abs.gov.au/statistics/health/causes-death/causes-death-australia/latest-release

Australian Bureau of Statistics (ABS), 2008. National Survey of Mental Health and Wellbeing: Summary of results. Cat. No. 4326.0. Commonwealth of Australia, Canberra.

Australian College of Mental Health Nurses, 2010. Standards of Practice for Mental Health Nursing in Australia. Australian College of Mental Health Nursing, Canberra.

Australian Government Department of Health, 2019. PHN Mental Health Flexible Funding Pool Programme Guidance: Stepped Care. Australian Government Department of Health, Canberra.

Australian Institute of Health and Welfare, 2019. Deaths in Australia. Cat. no. PHE 229. AIHW, Canberra. Online. Available at: www.aihw.gov.au/reports/life-expectancy-deaths/deaths-in-australia/contents/about

Balagopal, G., Kapanee, A.R.M. 2019. Lessons learnt from NGO approaches to mental healthcare provision in the community. In: Balagopal, G., Kapanee, A.R.M. Mental Health Care Services in Community Settings. Springer, Singapore.

Blanchflower, D.G., & Oswald, A.J. 2020. Trends in extreme distress in the United States, 1993–2019. Am J Pub Health, 110(10), 1538–1544.

Bos, D., Gray, R., Meepring, S., White, J., Foland, K., et al., 2022. The Health Improvement Profile for people with severe mental illness: Feasibility of a secondary analysis to make international comparisons. J Psychiatric Ment Health Nurs, 29(1), 86–98.

Boyle, M., & Murphy-Tighe, S. 2022. An integrative review of community nurse-led interventions to identify and respond to domestic abuse in the postnatal period. J Adv Nurs, 78(6), 1601–1617.

Brown, F.L., Aoun, M., Taha, K., Steen, F., Hansen, P., et al., 2020. The cultural and contextual adaptation process of an intervention to reduce psychological distress in young adolescents living in Lebanon. Front Psychiatry, 11, 212.

Chiang, A., Paynter, J., Edlin, R. & Exeter, D.J. 2021. Suicide preceded by health services contact – A whole-of-population study in New Zealand 2013–2015. PLOS ONE, doi.org/10.1371/journal.pone.0261163

Cleary, M., Raeburn, T., West, S., et al., 2018. Two approaches, one goal: How mental health registered nurses perceive their role and the role of peer support workers in facilitating consumer decision-making. Int J Ment Health Nurs, 27(4), 1212–1218.

Cornish, P. 2020. Stepped Care 2.0: A Paradigm Shift in Mental Health. Springer Nature.

Cross, J., De Carlo, P., Lennon, K., Peregrina, M. & Viney, J. 2021. Creating a proactive and dynamic nursing profession In: Crisp, J., Douglas, C., Rebeiro, G., & Waters, D. Potter and Perry's Fundamentals of Nursing, 6th ed. Elsevier, Sydney.

Cutler, T., Pirkis, J., Eades, S., Gibberd, A., & Gubhaju, L. 2021. 1457 Aboriginal and/or Torres Strait Islander deaths by suicide in Australia. Int J Epidemiol, 50(Supp 1), 168–148.

Damery, S., Brown, C., Sein, K., et al., 2019. The prevalence of mild-to-moderate distress in patients with end-stage renal disease: Results from a patient survey using the emotion thermometers in four hospital trusts in the West Midlands, UK. BMJ Open, 9(5), e027982.

Davison, K., 2006. Historical aspects of mood disorders. Psychiatry 5(4), 115–118.

De Sousa, I., & Varcoe, C. 2022. Centering black feminist thought in nursing praxis. Nurs Inq, 29(1), e12473.

Firth, J., Siddiqi, N., Koyanagi, A., et al., 2019. The Lancet Psychiatry Commission: A blueprint for protecting physical health in people with mental illness. Lancet Psychiatry, 6(8), 675–712.

Gibb, S., Brewer, N., & Bowden, N. 2021. Social impacts and costs of schizophrenia: A national cohort study using New Zealand linked administrative data. NZMJ (Online), 134(1537), 66–83.

Gold, S.M., Köhler-Forsberg, O., Moss-Morris, R., Mehnert, A., Miranda, J.J., et al., 2020. Comorbid depression in medical diseases. Nature Rev Dis Primers, 6(1), 69.

Grech, E., Raeburn, T. 2019. Experiences of hospitalised homeless adults and their health care providers in OECD nations: A literature review. Collegian, 26(1), 204–211.

Gürhan, N., Beşer, N.G., Polat, Ü., et al., 2019. Suicide risk and depression in individuals with chronic illness. Comm Ment Health J, 55(5), 840–848.

Hashmi, R., Alam, K., & Gow, J. 2020. Socioeconomic inequalities in mental health in Australia: Explaining life shock exposure. Health Policy, 124(1), 97–105.

Huang, R., Sun, H., Chen, G., Li, Y. & Wang, J. 2022. Second-victim experience and support among nurses in mainland China. J Nurs Manage, 30(1), 260–267.

Islam, F.M.A. 2019. Psychological distress and its association with socio-demographic factors in a rural district in Bangladesh: A cross-sectional study. PLoS ONE, 14(3), e0212765.

Kirk, D., Kabdebo, I., & Whitehead, L. 2021. Prevalence of distress, its associated factors and referral to support services in people with cancer. J Clin Nurs, 30(19–20), 2873–2885.

Kolappa, K., Henderson, D.C. & Kishore, S.P. 2013. No physical health without mental health: Lessons unlearned? Bull WHO, 91, 3–3A.

Kopua, D.M., Kopua, M.A. & Bracken, P.J. 2020. Mahi a Atua: A Māori approach to mental health. Transcult Psychiatry, 57(2), 375–383.

Leung, C.M., Ho, M.K., Bharwani, A.A., Cogo-Moreira, H., Wang, Y., et al., 2022. Mental disorders following COVID-19 and other epidemics: A systematic review and meta-analysis. Translat Psychiatry, 12(1), 205.

Lockett, H., Lacey, C., Jury, A., Postelnik, T., Luckman, A., et al., 2022. Whakairo: Carving a values-led approach to understand and respond to the mental health and substance use of the New Zealand population. NZMJ (Online), 135(1567), 8–12.

Mars, B., Heron, J., Klonsky, E.D., Moran, P., O'Connor, R.C., et al., 2019. Predictors of future suicide attempt among adolescents with suicidal thoughts or non-suicidal self-harm: A population-based birth cohort study. Lancet Psychiatry, 6(4), 327–337.

Maybery, D., Jones, R., Dipnall, J.F., et al., 2019. A mixed-methods study of psychological distress following an environmental catastrophe: The case of the Hazelwood open-cut coalmine fire in Australia. Anxiety Stress Coping, 33(2), 216–230.

McCarthy, M.M., Whittemore, R., Gholson, G., et al., 2019. Diabetes distress, depressive symptoms, and cardiovascular health in adults with type 1 diabetes. Nurs Res, 68(6), 445–452.

McGinty, E.E., Presskreischer, R., Han, H., & Barry, C.L. 2022. Trends in psychological distress among US adults during different phases of the COVID-19 pandemic. JAMA Network Open, 5(1), e2144776.

McGough, S., Wynaden, D., Gower, S., Duggan, R., & Wilson, R. 2022. There is no health without cultural safety: Why cultural safety matters. Contemp Nurse, 58(1), 33–42.

McPhillips, R., Salmon, P., Wells, A., et al., 2019. Cardiac rehabilitation patients' accounts of their emotional distress and psychological needs: A qualitative study. J Am Heart Assoc, 8(11), e011117.

Mental Health Commission of NSW, 2016. Physical health and mental wellbeing: Evidence guide. Mental Health Commission of NSW, Sydney.

Ministry of Health (NZ), 2022. Annual Update of Key Results 2020/21: New Zealand Health Survey. Ministry of Health, Wellington.

Ministry of Health (NZ), 2019. Every life matters – He Tapu te Oranga o ia tangata: suicide prevention strategy 2019–2029 and suicide prevention action plan 2019–2024 for Aotearoa New Zealand. Ministry of Health, Wellington.

Ministry of Health (NZ), 2018. He Ara Oranga. Report of the Government Inquiry into Mental Health and Addiction, Ministry of Health, Wellington.

Ministry of Health (NZ), 2017. Briefing to the Incoming Minister of Health 2017: The New Zealand Health and Disability System. Ministry of Health, Wellington.

Minton, C., Burrow, M., Manning, C., & van der Krogt, S. 2022. Cultural safety and patient trust: The hui process to initiate the nurse–patient relationship. Contemp Nurse, 58(2–3), 228–236.

Mooney, H., Watson, A., Ruwhiu, P., & Hollis-English, A. 2020. Māori social work and Māori mental health in Aotearoa New Zealand. Ment Health Soc Work, 259–279.

Morgan, V.A., Waterreus, A., Jablensky, A., et al., 2012. People living with psychotic illness in 2010: the second Australian national survey of psychosis. A N Z J Psychiatry, 46(8), 735–752.

Moschion, J., & van Ours, J.C. 2021. Do transitions in and out of homelessness relate to mental health episodes? A longitudinal analysis in an extremely disadvantaged population. Soc Sci Med, 279, 113667.

Müller, G., Bombana, M., Heinzel-Gutenbrenner, M., Kleindienst, N., Bohus, M., et al., 2021. Socio-economic consequences of mental distress: quantifying the impact of self-reported mental distress on the days of incapacity to work and medical costs in a two-year period: A longitudinal study in Germany. BMC Public Health, 21(1), 1–14.

NiaNia, W., Bush, A., Epston, D., 2017. Collaborative and Indigenous Mental Health Therapy. Tataihono – Stories of Māori Healing and Psychiatry. Routledge, New York.

Nursing and Midwifery Board of Australia (NMBA), 2023. Fact sheet: Scope of practice and capabilities of nurses. Online. Available at: www.nursing-midwiferyboard.gov.au/Codes-Guidelines-Statements/FAQ/Fact-sheet-scope-of-practice-and-capabilities-of-nurses.aspx

Nursing Council of New Zealand, 2023. Tapuhi Kua Rēhitatia Registered Nurse: Scope of Practice. Online. Available at: www.nursingcouncil.org.nz/Public/Nursing/Scopes_of_practice/Registered_Nurse/NCNZ/nursing-section/Registered_nurse.aspx

Nursing Council of New Zealand, 2011. Guidelines for Cultural Safety, the Treaty of Waitangi and Māori Health in Nursing Education and Practice. Wellington. Nursing Council of New Zealand.

O'Brien, A., 2014. Every nurse is a mental health nurse. Nurs NZ, 20(8), 2.

Oakley Browne, M.A., Wells, J.E., Scott, K.M., et al., 2006. Lifetime prevalence and projected lifetime risk of DSM–IV disorders in Te Rau Hinengaro: the New Zealand Mental Health Survey. ANZ J Psychiatry, 40(10), 865–874.

Perkins, D., Williams, A., McDonald, J., et al., 2017. What is the place of generalism in mental health care in Australia?: A systematic review of the literature. Australian Primary Health Care Research Institute. Online. Available at: https://openresearch-repository.anu.edu.au/handle/1885/119238.

Prioreschi, P. 1991. Possible reasons for neolithic skull trephining. Perspect Biol Med, 34(2), 296–303.

Productivity Commission, 2019. Mental Health, Draft Report, Australian Government, Canberra.

Rhodes, L. 2019. The colonising effect of western mental health discourses. Soc Work Policy Stud: Soc Justice, Pract Theory, 2(2), https://openjournals.library.sydney.edu.au/index.php/SWPS/article/view/14182.

Richmond-Rakerd, L.S., D'Souza, S., Milne, B.J., Caspi, A., & Moffitt, T.E. 2021. Longitudinal associations of mental disorders with physical diseases and mortality among 2.3 million New Zealand citizens. JAMA Network Open, 4(1), e2033448.

Roberts, R., Lockett, H., Bagnall, C., Maylea, C. & Hopwood, M. 2018. Improving the physical health of people living with mental illness in Australia and New Zealand. Aust J Rural Health, 26(5), 354–362.

Sartorius N. 2018. Depression and diabetes. Dialogues Clin Neurosci, 20(1), 47–52.

Shin, S., & Choi, H. 2020. A systematic review on peer support services related to the mental health services utilization for people with severe mental illness. J Korean Acad Psychiatric Ment Health Nurs, 29(1), 51–63.

Sinyor, M., Knipe, D., Borges, G., Ueda, M., Pirkis, J., et al. & International COVID-19 Suicide Prevention Research Collaboration, 2022. Suicide risk and prevention during the COVID-19 pandemic: One year on. Arch Suicide Res, 26(4), 1944–1949.

Sisler, S.M., Schapiro, N.A., Nakaishi, M. & Steinbuchel, P. 2020. Suicide assessment and treatment in pediatric primary care settings. J Child Adolesc Psychiatric Nurs, 33(4), 187–200.

Skinner, H.K., Rahtz, E., & Korszun, A. 2019. Interviews following physical trauma: A thematic analysis. Intern Emerg Nurs, 42, 19–24.

Solmi, M., Firth, J., Miola A., Fornaro, M., Frison, E., et al., 2020. Disparities in cancer screening in people with mental illness across the world versus the general population: Prevalence and comparative meta-analysis including 4 717 839 people. Lancet Psychiatry, 7(1), 52–63.

Sterud, T., & Hanvold, T.N. 2021. Effects of adverse social behaviour at the workplace on subsequent mental distress: A 3-year prospective study of the general working population in Norway. Int Arch Occ Env Health, 94, 325–334.

Summers, A., Leidman, E., Periquito, I.M.P.F., et al., 2019. Serious psychological distress and disability among older persons living in conflict-affected areas in eastern Ukraine: A cluster-randomized cross-sectional household survey. Confl Health 13(1), 10.

Te Ao Maramatanga (New Zealand College of Mental Health Nurses), 2012. Standard of Practice for Mental Health Nursing in New Zealand. Auckland: Te Ao Maramatanga.

Te Pou o Te Whakaaro Nui, 2014. Take action to improve physical health outcomes for New Zealanders who experience mental illness and/or addiction. A consensus position paper. Te Pou o Te Whakaaro Nui, Auckland.

Te Rōpū Arotake Auau Mate o te Hunga Tamariki, Taiohi | Child and Youth Mortality Review Committee. 2021. 15th data report: 2015–19. Health Quality & Safety Commission, Wellington.

Thom, R., Silbersweig, D.A. & Boland, R.J. 2019. Major depressive disorder in medical illness: A review of assessment, prevalence, and treatment options. Psychosomat Med, 81(3), 246–255.

Tomitaka, S., Kawasaki, Y., Ide, K., et al., 2019. Distribution of psychological distress is stable in recent decades and follows an exponential pattern in the US population. Sci Rep, 9(1), 1–10.

Tremblay, M.-C., Graham, J., Porgo, T.V., Dogba, M.J., Paquette, J.-S., et al., 2020. Improving cultural safety of diabetes care in Indigenous populations of Canada, Australia, New Zealand and the United States: A systematic rapid review. Can J Diabetes, 44(7), 670–678.

Westerman, T. 2021. Culture-bound syndromes in Aboriginal Australian populations. Clin Psychologist, 25(1), 19–35.

Wickham, S.R., Amarasekara, N.A., Bartonicek, A., & Conner, T.S. 2020. The big three health behaviors and mental health and well-being among young adults: A cross-sectional investigation of sleep, exercise, and diet. Front Psychol, 11, 579205.

World Health Organization (WHO), 2023. Depressive disorder (depression). Online. Available at: www.who.int/news-room/fact-sheets/detail/depression

World Health Organization (WHO), 2019. Mental health. Online. Available at: who.int/news-room/facts-in-pictures/detail/mental-health.

World Health Organization (WHO), 2014. Constitution of the World Health Organization. WHO, Geneva.

Wright, A., De Livera, A., Lee, K.H., Higgs, C., Nicholson, M., et al., 2022. A repeated cross-sectional and longitudinal study of mental health and wellbeing during COVID-19 lockdowns in Victoria, Australia. BMC Public Health, 22(1), 1–14.

Yousiph, T. 2022. Let's talk about suicide. Aust Nurs Midwif J, 27(8), 43.

2

Nursing and Mental Health in Context

Kim Foster, Peta Marks, Anthony J. O'Brien and John Hurley

KEY POINTS

- Developing therapeutic relationships is the key to effective nursing practice in mental health.
- Together, nurses and mental health consumers develop therapeutic alliances as a basis for consumers' growth and recovery.
- A social ecological approach to mental health nursing practice provides a framework for holistic practice.
- Self-awareness, insight and reflexivity are fundamental skills for nursing practice in mental health.
- Nursing practice occurs in the broader context of mental health, including the social determinants of mental health.

KEY TERMS

Compassion
Empathy
Emotional intelligence
Healing
Hope

Professional boundaries
Recovery
Reflection
Self
Self-awareness

Self-disclosure
Social determinants
Social ecological
Spirituality
Therapeutic alliance

LEARNING OUTCOMES

The material in this chapter will assist you to:
- describe the social ecological approach to effective mental health nursing practice
- identify the social determinants of mental health
- describe therapeutic relationships and how they are developed in the context of a person's mental health
- describe the three components of empathy
- define self-awareness and describe a strategy for developing self-awareness.

INTRODUCTION

Mental health nursing is one of the most interesting and challenging areas of nursing practice. It requires a fusion of personal characteristics, professional knowledge and experience, and clinical and interpersonal skills. The challenge of mental health nursing is working with people who are experiencing mental and emotional distress and may doubt themselves, the environment and the people around them. The reward of this work is often the satisfaction of using knowledge and skills to provide a context of safety and care where trust in self and others can be re-established.

People with mental illnesses may have complex and long-term needs, engage in frequent and regular encounters with the healthcare system or have a one-off experience that brings them briefly into contact with mental health services or providers. The long-term and cyclic nature of some more complex mental illnesses means that the therapeutic relationship between mental health nurses and consumers can last for long periods. This relationship will also vary in intensity as consumers move along a continuum between periods of high dependence at one end (in acute phases when they are experiencing acute distress or illness) and independence at the other (when their

symptoms are less troublesome or they are mentally healthy). This health–illness continuum is explored in depth in Chapter 3.

This chapter outlines the social ecological framework for mental health nursing practice that frames the text. This is a holistic framework for practice and the various elements of the framework are described: therapeutic relationships and consumer–nurse partnership; personal and contextual factors influencing practice; identities, including gender and culture (nurse and consumer); and the context of practice (including social determinants of health and major approaches to mental health care – recovery-oriented care and trauma-informed care). The remainder of the chapter explores the interpersonal relationship as the essential foundation of effective mental health nursing practice and the knowledge, attitudes and skills needed to work with people in mental distress. Key concepts and issues that are fundamental to effective and safe mental health nursing practice are also introduced.

Holistic and skillful mental health nursing requires a sound knowledge of human physiology, health and illness, as well as a biopsychosocial understanding of mental illnesses and their treatments, including pharmacology. In addition, to practise effectively, nurses working in mental health need to be open-minded and reflective and to have developed an understanding of concepts such as compassion, empathy, spirituality and hope. Personal qualities, such as responsiveness, self-awareness and insight, are essential for effective therapeutic relationships. Nurses in all settings care for the mental health and wellbeing of consumers, and mental health skills are required of all nurses and can be applied in all clinical settings.

SOCIAL ECOLOGICAL APPROACH TO MENTAL HEALTH NURSING PRACTICE

In this text we take a social ecological approach to mental health nursing practice. A social ecological perspective refers to the dynamic interactions between a person and their environment that influence their health and wellbeing. This person–environment interaction involves a number of factors and processes. Mental health can be understood as involving a person's physical, mental, emotional and spiritual characteristics, and the interactive processes that occur between them and their environment or ecology (including their social and family context). This includes being able to access available resources that help sustain their mental health (Ungar & Theron 2020) and support their recovery. These resources can be human, such as relationships and supports in the form of family and friends, and/or healthcare resources, including nursing and mental healthcare (hospital or community-based), and/or practical resources such as financial support and housing. A social ecological or holistic perspective is relevant to understanding mental health and mental health nursing practice because mental health problems can challenge people across every aspect of their life, including relationships, healthcare and finances. Equally, mental health problems can be worsened or mitigated by these factors. Similarly, nursing practice is shaped by our personal characteristics and skills, and the health service context we work in. This dynamic person–environment interaction involves personal and contextual factors that influence nurses' practice and their relationships with consumers.

Therefore, from an ecological perspective, nursing practice includes:
- nurses' personal characteristics (e.g. their personality, interpersonal style, cultural and gender identity, emotional intelligence and nursing knowledge, attitudes and skills)
- therapeutic relationships and interpersonal interactions between nurses and consumers
- cultural and practice context within which a nurse and consumer are based
- available people and resources that can be accessed to support consumers' recovery.

Fig. 2.1 provides a diagrammatic representation of all these elements and their interactions. The following section outlines each of the elements.

Social Determinants of Health

In relation to the context or environment of mental health, the social determinants of health are the social and economic circumstances within which we are "born, grow, work, live and age" (World Health Organization (WHO) 2022). These determinants are shaped by social norms, policies and systems relating to the distribution of power and resources in society and can lead to health inequities because they have a direct influence on the prevalence and severity of mental health conditions, which can extend across the life course (WHO 2022).

In respect to mental health, key social determinants that directly influence health and quality of life include:
- early childhood development
- mental health stigma
- poverty (employment, education)

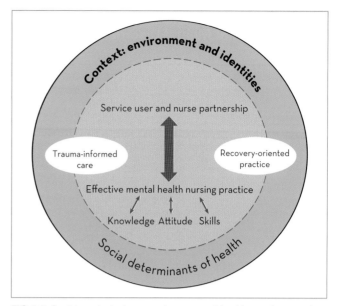

FIG 2.1 Social ecological approach to mental health nursing practice.

- violence
- forced migration
- insecure living conditions, including homelessness (WHO 2022).

Because mental ill health is strongly influenced by these factors, mental health problems are not able to be improved by mental health treatments alone. The social factors that have contributed to these problems also need to be addressed and, wherever possible, eliminated. Social determinants can be either proximal or distal. Proximal factors are those that act directly to influence health (e.g. ongoing trauma), whereas distal factors act more indirectly (e.g. social deprivation). There is a need for targeted reduction of social determinants. To reduce the burden of mental ill health, Lund and colleagues (2018), using an ecological framework, identified the proximal and distal social determinants that are risk and/or protective factors for mental ill health according to five domains (see also Table 2.1):
- demographic
- economic
- neighbourhood
- environmental
- social and cultural.

An ecological approach to nursing therefore requires that nurses understand and respond to the social contexts within which people live. Nurses working clinically do not necessarily have the capacity to influence, prevent or intervene with all these factors, but it is vitally important when working with mental health consumers, and as relevant for the person, that these factors are considered and identified during history-taking and assessment. Indeed, the nurse needs to position and understand the consumer as a person within these social contexts, rather than being simply a person with symptoms. Then, as part of the work of the multidisciplinary team, wherever possible and relevant, various factors can be directly addressed to help decrease risk and increase protection against further ill health. This may be negotiating adequate housing for consumers (and ensuring people are not discharged if they have nowhere to go), helping to build social support for consumers who are isolated and/or providing psychological support for the psychological impacts of trauma and associated distress, such as a trauma-informed approach to care. An ecological approach to nursing also requires that nurses understand the environments within which they practise.

TABLE 2.1 Social and Cultural Determinants of Mental Disorders

Domain	Proximal	Distal
Demographic	Age Gender Ethnicity	Community diversity Population density Longevity Survival
Economic	Income Debt Assets Financial strain Relative deprivation Unemployment Food security	Economic recessions Economic inequality Macroeconomic
Neighbourhood	Safety and security Housing structure Overcrowding Recreation	Infrastructure Neighbourhood deprivation Built environment Setting Safety and security
Environmental	Natural disasters Industrial disasters War or conflict Climate change Forced migration	Trauma Distress
Social and cultural	Community social capital Social stability Cultural	Individual social capital Social participation Social support Education

Adapted from Lund et al 2018.

Contexts of Mental Health: Environment and Identities

It is important to understand that the models of care and the health service approach within which nurses work directly influence our practice. Equally, nursing practice can influence and shape the environments within which we work. Working with people who experience mental illness can pose unique ethical challenges to nurses; for example, where a person experiences episodes of mental ill health that necessitate compulsory admission under mental health legislation, removing part or all of their autonomy due to considerations of risk and safety. Involuntary admission often makes it difficult for nurses to apply recovery-oriented approaches that seek to provide people with choice and opportunity to develop strengths. Working in such challenging environments means that nurses need not only have an up-to-date working knowledge of health conditions and interventions, but also need to be able to empathise with the difficulties consumers face as they navigate their recovery from experiences of mental ill health within what are often disconnected and under-resourced healthcare systems (State of Victoria 2019).

Cultural, Sexual and Spiritual Identities

The concept of identity. Identity can be thought of as an individual's enduring sense of themselves as a person. It is the answer people give to the question: "Who am I?" Psychologists have traditionally defined identity in individualistic terms, with an emphasis on developing stable personality traits. However, identity is deeply influenced by belonging to, or difference from, significant social groups – for example, cultural groups, religious faiths and peer groups. By identifying with the values and beliefs of a social group we come to define our own

unique sense of who we are. Others have argued that identity is inherently unstable, constantly in transition and made up of multiple components or identities. Some examples of identity are outlined below, but it is important to remember that individuals will have multiple identities and that these may change over the course of their lives. Nurses should not presume to know what a consumer's identities are and should not expect individuals to conform to stereotyped ideas about what a particular identity means.

Cultural identity. Cultural identity refers to a person's sense of belonging to one or more cultural groups. For Aboriginal and Torres Strait Islanders and Māori, Indigenous culture may be the most important source of identity, but they may also identify, through ancestry or association, with non-Indigenous cultures. Most healthcare providers support consumers to declare their own cultural identity, and clinicians should respect this statement. Cultural identity is an important source of beliefs, values and practices that impact on mental health and assist individuals to develop their own frameworks for recovery. As nurses, it is important that we reflect on our own cultural identities and how these may influence our interactions with consumers (cultural awareness). We cannot be knowledgeable or skilled in all the cultures of a health service's consumers, but it is important that we ask about and respectfully acknowledge consumers' culture, seek to listen, learn and respond to their cultural preferences (cultural sensitivity), and work in a culturally safe way (Best 2021). See Chapters 6 and 7 for a discussion of Aboriginal and Torres Strait Islander and Māori mental health.

Spiritual identity. Mental health theorists have a long tradition of scepticism towards spirituality and religion. Individualistic models of mental health (e.g. rational emotive therapy) have valued rationalism over faith and belief, and have seen spirituality as a source of pathology, rather than a resource for mental health. The increasing diversity of our communities challenges this view and for some people leads to spirituality and religious faith being regarded as central to identity and to psychosocial functioning. While clinical support can help people manage distress and develop coping strategies, spirituality can provide a sense of hope and acceptance in the face of seemingly insurmountable life problems. Although spirituality is often associated with religious faith, many people have a non-religious worldview while still maintaining spiritual beliefs and values. Others have both religious and non-religious worldviews. As nurses we will not always share the spiritual beliefs of consumers. However, as with cultural identity, it is important that consumers feel their spiritual beliefs and values are recognised as an important part of their identity and that they are supported in maintaining their spirituality as part of their recovery.

Gender identity. Gender is another source of identity where previous mental health practice has treated difference as pathology and sought to impose compulsory treatment on individuals whose gender identity and sexual preferences did not fit dominant social norms. From being perceived as a fixed function of biology (individuals assigned either male or female gender at birth with no anticipation of change), gender is now understood as a fluid, socially constructed concept, and gender identity as reflective of the person's own internal sense of being a man, woman or someone outside that gender binary. A range of terms reflects the changing perspectives on gender in contemporary society, seen in the term LGBTIQA+, which incorporates a range of sexual orientations and gender identities. Specific terms related to gender include transgender, non-binary, gender diverse and cis-gender. Gender should not be confused with sexual preference, which refers to an individual's gender preferences in intimate relationships in the acronym above – lesbian, gay, bisexual. Preferences are not necessarily fixed and can change over the course of psychosocial development.

As a nurse you will meet people with gender identities and sexual preferences that are different from your own. It is important that you become comfortable with relating to gender diverse consumers, including using appropriate pronouns and terminology, as the stigma and prejudice commonly experienced in response to a person's gender and/or sexuality may be a source of distress.

Identity, stress and mental illness. While a strongly developed sense of who we are as a person is important to our mental health, identity can also be a source of stress for those whose identities are disvalued and subject to stigmatising views and prejudice. The term "minority stress" (Spittlehouse et al 2019) refers to the experience of stigma and discrimination encountered by people in relation to their identity. This can relate to social and cultural dimensions of gender, race, ethnicity, religious affiliation, sexuality and other aspects of identity (e.g. ability, age, socio-economic status) (Victorian Transcultural Mental Health [VTMH] 2021). Micro-aggressions, overt rejection and discrimination can create a hostile environment in which minority stress leads to cognitive and affective changes that increase susceptibility to symptoms of mental illness, including depression, anxiety, suicidal ideation and harmful substance use (Bailey 2019). People who are subject to one form of marginalisation are more likely to also experience other forms of marginalisation, a concept referred to as "intersectionality" (Grzanka & Brian 2019; VTMH 2021).

Nurses encounter many consumers who experience one or more forms or marginalisation and need to be aware of how these experiences shape the person's health experience and the responses of clinicians. Supporting consumers to negotiate what may be viewed as "contested" identities enhances their mental health and helps build resilience for living in an environment in which stigma and discrimination are regrettably common. From a service level, an intersectional response ensures that a multiplicity of identities and experiences are considered when designing services, gathering information or analysing data.

✳ HISTORICAL ANECDOTE 2.1

Stigma and Mental Illness

In his 1963 book, *Stigma: Notes on the Management of Spoiled Identity*, sociologist Erving Goffman identified three types of stigma, each of which led to disvalued identity. Goffman argued that people with mental illness experience character stigma as they are perceived as weak, unreliable and possibly dangerous, and social stigma through which disvalued aspects of being labelled "mentally ill" lead to the person being seen as associated with a disvalued group. Goffman's work led to a focus on the negative effects of stigma on people with mental illness, including the internalisation of stigma by which individuals come to believe the negative stereotypes of the dominant social group. Goffman also argued that people who work in mental health, such as nurses, are subject to "courtesy stigma" because their identity is influenced by their association with a socially disvalued group.

Read More About It
Goffman, E. 1963. Stigma: Notes on the Management of Spoiled Identity. Prentice-Hall, Englewood Cliffs.

Mental health nurse identity. Finally, mental health nursing also has a distinct identity. The identity of the mental health nurse can be understood as possessing both technical skills, such as delivering psychological interventions and undertaking complex assessments, and interpersonal or non-technical skills, such as those supporting interpersonal relationship building, communication and emotional intelligence. Mental health nursing identity includes a considerable component of interpersonal therapeutic work and the use of a personal and professional self, all directed at enhancing the wellbeing of consumers. This identity is at odds with how the discipline is sometimes understood by those outside of it, who can construe that the identity of mental health nursing is limited to simply dispensing medications (Hurley et al 2022). However, the social ecological approach and consumer identity factors previously outlined should alert you that mental health nursing work has significant complexities necessitating a wider identity role than pharmacology alone.

Concepts of Recovery
Clinical Recovery

A significant amount of research has explored outcomes experienced by people with mental illness over the past 100 years. Most of these studies have used an approach to understanding recovery developed by mental health professionals, referred to as "clinical recovery" (Slade et al 2012). This concept considers mental illness as a health condition that is in need of clinical treatment. As such, in common with recovery from most physical illnesses, working from this perspective involves the expectation that recovery from mental illness should include a substantial reduction of symptoms and restoration of function in work and relationships. The conceptualisation of clinical recovery is objective (rather than subjective), it is rated by the clinician (who is considered the "expert") and it enables researchers to measure recovery in terms of "hard" data, such as numbers of people who cease to need medication, avoid (re-)hospitalisation or regain paid employment. Studies that have used the paradigm of clinical recovery suggest that little improvement has been made in rates of recovery over the past 100 years. For example, a meta-analysis that reviewed the results of 50 studies published between 1921 and 2010 suggested that only 13% of people diagnosed with schizophrenia experience clinical recovery (Jääskeläinen et al 2012). Despite the poor outcomes identified in this research, people with a lived experience of mental illness (consumers) often have more hopeful stories to tell about their recovery journey.

As people with lived experience of mental illness gained political influence over the past few decades, they challenged the concept of clinical recovery and models of care that focus on medical treatment alone (Cleary et al 2018). This led to a review of how recovery from mental illness is understood, including the concept of personal recovery. Recent research suggests that clinical and personal recovery are overlapping constructs and that recovery from one perspective is associated with recovery from the other (Dubreucq et al 2022). While there are distinct differences between conceptualisations of clinical and personal recovery, they can be considered complementary (van Weeghel et al 2019). For many people, symptom change is important, but it's not the only indicator of recovery, or the most important one.

Personal Recovery

The concept of "personal recovery" emerged from the consumer movement that developed in the second half of the 20th century to advocate for the rights of people living with mental illness. People with lived experience have emphasised that recovery is a transformational, deeply personal journey of reclaiming the right to a meaningful life, even if symptoms of mental illness persist. It is a subjective, multidimensional, continuous process that is defined by the person (who is considered the "expert"). It is unique and means different things to different people (Slade & Wallace 2017).

There is no single definition of mental health recovery; however, one of the most commonly used explanations was written by Bill Anthony in 1993 (p. 15), who described it as:

A deeply personal, unique process of changing one's attitudes, values, feelings, goals, skills and/or roles. It is a way of living a satisfying, hopeful, and contributing life even with limitations caused by the illness. Recovery involves the development of new meaning and purpose in one's life as a person grows beyond the catastrophic effects of mental illness.

Beginning with personal accounts of recovery journeys published by people with a history of mental illness, such as Deegan (1988) and Leete (1989), a large body of literature has developed describing the lived experience of mental health recovery. Personal narratives are essential to recovery-informed perspectives and for determining what is important for any individual in their journey of recovery. Case Study 2.1, about the recovery of Mary O'Hagan, a prominent international consumer "survivor", educator and consultant, illustrates the tension between what people say is important to them and what professionals and the system focus on. This tension is underscored by the fact that although many people find meaning in their "madness", the people they turn to for support often view it primarily as pathological and something to be managed and medicated. Table 2.2 draws a distinction between recovery-informed practice and traditional practice.

CASE STUDY 2.1: Mary O'Hagan

In common with so many people who experience mental distress, Mary describes her madness as the loss of self, the solid core of her being. While this core is not evident during times of madness, it returns stronger, renewed and ready to go again. Madness is a crisis of being that is a part of the full range of human experience. Mary explains:

My self is the solid core of my being. It is like an immutable dark sun that sits at the centre of things while all my fickle feelings, thoughts and sensations orbit around it. But my self goes into hiding during madness. Sometimes it slides into the great nothingness like a setting sun. Sometimes it gets trampled in the dust by all the whizzing in my body and mind ... Sometimes my madness strips me bare but it is also the beginning of renewal; every time I emerge from it I feel fresh and ready to start again.

Mary had to make friends with rather than fight her madness, to get to know, understand and respect it – a complex process.

My madness was like a boarder coming to live in my house, who turned out to be a citizen from an enemy country. Knowing I might not get rid of him meant I had to make peace with him and learn to understand his language. Once I got to know the boarder, he was no longer the stereotypical enemy, but a complex character that deserved some respect.

Mental health professionals did not find any value in helping Mary to understand the meaning in her madness. Nor did they allow her to tap into her own power, her own resourcefulness. Mary's experience of care within mental health services was one of being "skilled in lowered expectations" – for example, repeatedly being told that things such as studying or working would be too stressful and she would not be able to do them. The way mental health care was provided to Mary encouraged passivity rather than autonomy. She found the capacity to tap into her own resourcefulness only by coming across the consumer/survivor literature that inspired her. She was then able to find and use her own power to get out of the cycle of madness. Mary went on to be appointed as a mental health commissioner in New Zealand and has been an international consultant on mental health since that time.

What was most difficult for Mary was not the symptoms but how people regarded her. In retrospect, her madness was a place of beauty and difficulty, madness filled with soul. Mary talks about the terrible suffering and the desperate struggle of her madness, but she also talks about the richness in her experience that she could interpret as filled with purpose and meaning. She wanted acceptance of her reality. For Mary, the best thing people could have done was to be kind and accept her reality – a basic human response.

We encourage you to visit Mary's website at www.maryohagan.com to learn more about her story.

❓ CRITICAL THINKING EXERCISE 2.1

Is Mary O'Hagan's experience an isolated one? Is it an "old" story that would not happen today?

In 2012, Glover presented the stories of two women and their personal experiences of mental distress managed in Australia by involuntary inpatient admissions. The women's perceptions of their care included that they were not helped to make sense of their experiences, felt stripped of their power and were not responded to as people but as "diagnostic categories". Their experiences were described using the language and meaning of the professional knowledge base; their own meaning and language for their experiences were not encouraged or valued. What makes Glover's work so powerful is that while both women had very similar experiences, one story took place in 1985 and the other in 2010. The latter occurred at a time when services were promoting their model of care as "recovery-informed", leading Glover to ask, what has actually changed in the previous 25 years?

The next section of this chapter overviews recovery-oriented and trauma-informed care approaches that have been developed to support people with mental illness in their personal recovery. These approaches are increasingly used in mental health care and can be used by nurses in all settings to better support people who are experiencing mental distress or illness.

Recovery-Oriented Care

In 2011 Leamy and colleagues undertook a systematic literature review to identify experiences commonly associated with personal recovery. After screening more than 5000 papers, the authors identified five processes that are common in personal recovery, known by the acronym CHIME: Connectedness; Hope and optimism; Identity; Meaning in life; and Empowerment (Leamy et al 2011). Not only have experiences associated with personal recovery been well explored, but the concept is increasingly incorporated into government mental health policies, including Australia's national mental health service policy and framework for recovery approaches to service provision (Commonwealth of Australia 2013) and the *Fifth National Mental Health and Suicide Prevention Plan* (Department of Health 2017; see also Progress Report 4 – Australian Government National Mental Health Commission 2021). Concepts of recovery have also influenced mental health policy in New Zealand (Ministry of Health 2021).

TABLE 2.2 Key Differences Between Recovery-Informed and Traditional Practice

Recovery-Informed Practice	Traditional Practice
Person is central	Illness and symptoms are central
Driven by a human rights agenda	Driven by the medical model
Connecting with and maintaining meaningful roles, relationships and community is key; many things contribute to recovery	Propensity for person's life to revolve around and be taken over by illness
Looks for possibilities and promotes hope	Looks for constraints and sets limits and lower expectations
Collaborative risk management with the person	Focuses on risk control by others
Learns from people's narratives of recovery	Personal narratives not a focus of care
The person has expertise gained from their experience of mental health challenges	The professional is the expert on the person's experience
Medication is a small part of management; types and doses are titrated for the individual	Treatment of symptoms, usually with medications, is the main form of intervention
The person is the change agent	The program is the change agent
Takes a stance of "unknowing" and curiosity to help uncover the meaning people make of their experience	Takes a stance of "knowing" and looks for confirmation of symptoms to make a diagnosis
Empowering for the person to be acknowledged for their expertise	Symptoms are more important than personal meaning
Promotes self-directed care requiring the active involvement of the person	Promotes passivity and compliance
Explores what is important to the person; recognises unique experience and takes spirituality into account	Recovery primarily involves the active involvement of others
Connects with the person's strengths and draws on them to overcome challenges	Informs people about illness and what is important to them to manage it; spirituality not taken into account
Choice and ability to connect with a broad range of services in community	Focuses on deficits to treat and manage
Peer support or peer-run services are essential	Choice of services can be limited
Trauma-informed care asks: "What has happened to you?"	Peer support limited or non-existent
	Not trauma-informed – the background issues ("What is wrong with you?") are more important
Recovery is moving beyond premorbid functioning towards thriving and developing a new sense of self	Recovery is, at best, returning to a premorbid level of functioning
Non-linear process	Linear process of interventions
Timeframes meaningless – ongoing process	Recovery is the end point of the process
Crisis is a time of learning how to thrive; an active recovery space	Crisis is viewed as a relapse and failure

In respect to mental health recovery, there are five key domains that health professionals and mental health services are expected to practise within:

- promoting a culture and language of hope and optimism
- putting the person first and at the centre of practice and viewing their life holistically
- supporting personal recovery and placing it at the heart of practice
- organisational commitment and workforce development for skilled practitioners and an environment that is conducive to recovery
- action on social inclusion and social determinants of health, mental health and wellbeing (Commonwealth of Australia 2013).

To better understand the sort of practices promoted in government guidelines, Le Boutillier and colleagues (2011) undertook a qualitative analysis of 30 recovery policy documents from governments in England, Scotland, Ireland, Denmark, New Zealand and the United States. They found that the policies promoted four common practice domains, including organisational commitment, supporting personally defined recovery, working relationship and promoting citizenship. Despite these findings, the authors concluded that a key challenge for mental health services is the continued lack of clarity about what constitutes service-level recovery-oriented practice (Raeburn et al 2017). This lack of clarity has remained an ongoing knowledge gap, with researchers observing that while government policy may promote the concept of personal recovery, most mental health interventions still aim to reduce symptoms and improve a person's functioning rather than promote personal recovery (Leendertse et al 2021); and that evidence is lacking regarding how recovery practices are implemented and whether (and how) this is achieved in practice within individual services (Slade et al 2015).

Greater collaboration and co-design of services, service planning, policy and research by people with a lived experience of mental illness is required for better recovery-oriented care (Gordon & O'Brien 2018). This requires a purposeful shift away from paternalistic and authoritative ways of treating people towards more mutually respectful person-centred care (Reid et al 2018). Consumers and carers understand the inadequacies and opportunities that exist within the health and mental health system (Banfield et al 2018) – after all, they are the ones who are attempting to navigate it! Transforming the health and mental health system to be fully recovery-oriented requires genuine integration of lived experience perspectives, addressing discrimination and factors that inhibit consumer participation at all points in the healthcare continuum. Transformation of the mental health system means focusing more on enhancing hope, empowerment and life meaning in mental health interventions, to support personal recovery (Leendertse et al 2021).

Trauma-Informed Care

An essential component of a recovery-oriented approach is to practise within a framework that recognises many people experiencing mental health challenges have a background that includes trauma experience(s). A trauma or traumatic event can be described as a distressing event – for example, a severe physical injury or a specific experience that triggers mental and emotional distress. Trauma is often linked with loss and grief, which are a universal part of life. Loss can be described as an event where something that belongs to you, is either precious or has meaning for you, has been taken away or destroyed. This encompasses a range of losses, from a "minor" loss, such as losing your wallet, to a "devastating loss", such as losing your home and all your belongings in a bushfire. Bereavement generally refers to being deprived of an object or a person – usually used in the context of losing someone you love through death. Grief has been defined as "the response to the loss in all of its totality – including its physical, emotional, cognitive, behavioural and spiritual manifestations – and as a natural and normal reaction to loss" (Hall 2014, p. 182).

Research demonstrates clear links between trauma and the onset of a range of mental health problems (Green et al 2018). This makes it imperative for nurses to be sensitive to the vulnerabilities and potential triggers that may give rise to re-traumatisation and to be aware that this could impede recovery. While a single-incident traumatic event, such as a severe car accident, an unexpected death of a close family member or natural disaster, may result in an acute crisis, where the person's ability to cope is overwhelmed for a time, it does not necessarily result in mental illness. Research indicates that most people exposed to a traumatic event recover after an initial period of destabilisation, followed by adjustment and recovery. In fact, some people describe positive changes, such as a renewed appreciation for life and loved ones, personal growth and enhanced coping strategies (van Weeghel et al 2019). See Chapter 3 for more information about the mental health and illness continuum.

In respect to trauma, the US Adverse Childhood Experiences (ACE) study began in the late 1990s and explored the relationship between adverse effects in childhood and health problems experienced in adulthood (Felitti et al 1998). Participants were asked to report on adverse events experienced during childhood. Adverse childhood events included: experiencing psychological, physical or sexual abuse as a child; living with a mother who was in a domestic violence situation; or living in a household where there were people who abused substances, had mental illness, were suicidal and/or had ever been in prison. Researchers found that the greater the number of these adverse events a child experienced, the greater the burden of physical illnesses such as chronic obstructive pulmonary disease and heart disease, and mental illnesses such as depression. The researchers have continued to collect data documenting the health status from these initial participants (see the Useful websites list at the end of this chapter for more details). The initial findings have been confirmed in subsequent research, demonstrating that early adversity has lasting impacts – increasing the risk of both physical and mental illness over the course of the person's life (Javier et al 2019). Children exposed to trauma are less likely to develop resilience and have a more than 50% increased risk of depression (Jones et al 2018).

Despite the negative effects of trauma and mental ill health, the human brain has a remarkable ability to adapt. Research (some of which dates back more than 100 years) has demonstrated how individuals with significant brain damage arising from physiological disorders, such as stroke (cerebral vascular accident) and traumatic brain injury, can recover and regain function that seemed to have been lost as a result of the damage (Turolla et al 2018). The mechanism for this process is the brain's capacity to generate new brain cells (neurogenesis) and to establish alternative neural pathways. The term "neuroplasticity" was introduced in the 1960s as a way of understanding this reorganisation of neuronal anatomy affecting the structure and function of the brain in response to many external and internal events (Voss et al 2017).

You will recall from your nursing education that the brain consists of three parts that develop from the bottom up. These parts "talk" to one another via trillions of neural pathways. The "reptilian brain" (brain stem) is responsible for the automatic functions, such as breathing, heart rate and survival. The "mammalian brain" (limbic system) is responsible for emotions and memory; it is about survival and safety. The "primate brain" (cerebral cortex) is responsible for higher order tasks, such as thinking, learning, decision-making, reasoning, organising, planning, meaning-making, gaining control over emotions and language. When people experience trauma and/or severe emotional stress, it can be much harder to engage the cerebral cortex. Instead, they "loop" in the limbic cortex and this builds stronger neural pathways, making it more likely they will experience distressing emotions in the future when challenges arise.

Consider how this information might be relevant when someone comes into a mental health inpatient unit. Personal safety is an important basis for effective nursing care; the key here is the absolute necessity for people to feel safe so they can effectively engage with others in their ongoing care. Often, people will be frightened of the inpatient environment, including acute mental health units, particularly if it is their first experience of admission to a mental healthcare setting. It is important to take time to find out how the person feels and what they need to feel safe and secure. This may be listening to them or helping them consider strategies they could use to increase feelings of safety – for example, calling for help if someone enters their room. Do not assume that the person experiencing mental distress will feel safe in the healthcare setting just because you feel comfortable in the environment as a nurse.

The essentials of trauma-informed care include recognising the following (Sweeney et al 2018):

- Trauma and its effects have been historically unrecognised in the design of mental health systems. To counteract this, it is necessary to take a universal precaution approach that assumes all people who seek mental health care may have experienced trauma.
- Services need to ensure early assessment of trauma history and supervision for staff in responding sensitively and appropriately to disclosures of trauma.
- Reiterating the necessity for the person to feel safe, so that nurses can help the person to respond more effectively to the distressing emotions; for example, sitting, listening or walking with the person; using basic mindfulness or relaxation techniques; and ensuring a calm environment can all help. When this occurs, people are more likely to be able to engage their thinking brain and find ways that work for them to feel safe.
- Impacts of trauma can affect how people react to potentially helpful relationships. Building trust is essential so you can work with the person. Remember, trauma often occurs when a person's trust in people or situations has been severely violated. Nurses need to understand how trauma and abuse may have shaped difficulties in relationships and affect therapeutic relationships.
- Coercive interventions may re-traumatise people. Be mindful that nurses are often seen as figures of authority. Using the power that comes with this to exercise control over the person to do what you think they "should" do will be counterproductive and coercive, and may even re-traumatise the person. Recognise the person's strengths and support them by collaboratively developing a care plan that validates their experience and affirms their preferences for care and how they can manage their distress.
- Avoid interventions that may be perceived as shaming and humiliating. Nurses are responsible for maintaining the dignity and individual rights of the person at all times and providing services in ways that are flexible, individualised, culturally competent, respectful and based on best practice.
- There is a strong need to focus on *what happened* to the person rather *what is wrong* with the person, which pathologises the person in response to their presenting symptoms (where the focus is on). Nurses need to develop an understanding of presenting behaviour and symptoms in the context of past experiences.

In summary, trauma-informed services are informed by key principles to guide practice (Wilson et al 2021):

- People need to feel connected, valued, informed and hopeful about their recovery from mental illness.

- Staff understand the connection between childhood trauma and adult mental health issues.
- Staff practise in empowering ways with consumers and their family and friends and other services to promote consumers' autonomy.

While these principles focus on the needs of consumers and their family and friends, a trauma-informed approach to care can also provide support for managing workplace stress (Isobel & Edwards 2017). Trauma-informed practice does not replace recovery-oriented practice, but is complementary and provides another perspective from which people (staff and consumers) may view recovery and therapeutic engagement. See Perspectives in practice: Nurse's story 2.1.

PERSPECTIVES IN PRACTICE

Nurse's Story 2.1: Katrina

Why I Chose Mental Health Nursing

I did not start my nursing education with a plan to work in mental health nursing. Like many of my fellow students I thought about paediatric nursing, or maybe cardiac nursing. I enjoyed all my clinical placements and my greatest pleasure was talking to consumers in whatever setting they were in. I found the most interesting theoretical study was of understanding people from a psychological, sociological and cultural perspective: how people came to be like they were; how they responded to health and illness and stress. My understanding about mental illness had been coloured by common community attitudes, by media depictions of psychiatric hospitals, and by the experience of an aunt being forcibly admitted for treatment. It was not really talked about in the family and I am not sure if anyone visited her while she was in hospital.

There have been two "lightbulb moments" that led me to choose to work in mental health following graduation. The first was a visiting lecturer who was a "mental health consumer", someone who had experienced mental illness and its treatment. I left that tutorial with a mixture of feelings: sadness for the experience of stigmatisation; admiration for the bravery to speak up and for the resilience to re-establish a life that was satisfying; an awful awareness of the way my family had silenced my aunt by acting like her experience had not happened; and a new compassion for people with mental illness.

When it came to my mental health clinical placement I was rather anxious. I really did not know what to expect. My mental health clinical placement was a second "lightbulb moment". I found the consumers had interesting stories to tell and that they wanted to tell me about their lives. I watched the staff as they interacted with consumers. I admired their capacity to remain calm and to intervene early when someone became upset. The staff taught me a lot about how mental illness is manifested and experienced, and what treatments were used. I enjoyed the interdisciplinary discussions and felt that nurses' observations about consumers were taken seriously.

I have now been working in an acute mental health inpatient unit for a year and I have found this time to be a steep learning curve. The biggest challenge has been developing an understanding of me and how I respond to various people and situations. At times I found myself getting upset or angry with consumers if things did not go according to my plan and I really needed to make sure I did not get into negative talk with other staff who were also frustrated. I attend group clinical supervision sessions every 2 weeks and this is helpful in keeping us focused on the person and their needs. The group has provided a safety net that we can use between sessions. I had a preceptor assigned when I first started and that helped with day-to-day skill development. I have an informal arrangement with a mentor who is an experienced nurse that I identified as someone I want to emulate in my practice. She has been very supportive in helping me identify knowledge that I need to gain, what further education would be helpful, where my career path might lead and what kind of clinical experience would be beneficial to me. I would like to work on one of the community mental health teams in the future.

HISTORICAL ANECDOTE 2.2

We Were Convicts

The first nurses involved in mental health care in Australia were convict nurses assigned to care for patients sent to Castle Hill and Liverpool "lunatic asylums" in colonial New South Wales. In spite of their pioneering role, contemporary nurse historians often skip over them without any acknowledgement. Such a generalised approach to nursing history may be tied to a desire to eradicate the memory of a so-called "convict stain" from modern nurses' professional identity. It perpetuates a tradition started in early healthcare journals promoting the myth that nursing in Australia was "rescued" by Lucy Osbourne and her Nightingale nurses in 1863. Nurses prior to Osbourne were characterised as "gamps", which was a reference to the fictional character of the coarse, fat, drunken nurse "Sarah Gamp" in Charles Dickens' novel, *Martin Chuzzlewit*. By contrast, early convict nurses, such as Martha Entwistle at Castle Hill Lunatic Asylum and Mary Coughlen at Liverpool Lunatic Asylum, were resilient women who overcame traumatic experiences in their own lives while caring for others in harsh colonial environments, short of adequate resources, during an era of fast-paced industrial and technological change. We should be more proud of our convict nursing roots.

Read More About It
Raeburn, T., Liston, C., Hickmott, J., Cleary, M. 2018. Life of Martha Entwistle: Australia's first convict mental health nurse. Int J Ment Health Nurs 27(1), 455–463.

EFFECTIVE MENTAL HEALTH NURSING PRACTICE

A central element of the social ecological framework for practice is effective mental health nursing practice. To practise effectively in their roles, mental health nurses need sound theoretical knowledge of mental health and illness and associated treatments, positive attitudes towards mental illness and people living with mental illness, and effective mental health nursing skills. In their practice, mental health nurses consider the person's physical, psychological, social, cultural and spiritual healthcare needs; that is, they take a holistic or comprehensive approach.

A holistic approach to mental health nursing includes knowledge and skills in:

- preventive and early intervention strategies for mental health and mental illness
- biological processes that may underpin mental illness
- the impacts of social determinants of health on the development and course of mental illness
- the importance of social connections and relationships for mental health and illness
- psychological processes associated with mental health and illness
- cultural practices and beliefs and their relationship to mental health
- spiritual beliefs and faith and their relationship to mental health
- communication and interpersonal relationship knowledge and skills
- the physical health care of people with mental illness
- psychotherapeutic approaches and strategies for mitigating mental distress and mental illness
- the physiological effects and side effects of psychotropic medications and physical treatments for mental illness.

Therapeutic Relationship – Consumer and Nurse Partnership

As nurses, we bring our knowledge and attitudes to mental health/illness, our identities (e.g. cultural and gender) and our values, knowledge, experience and skills in nursing. This shapes how we develop a therapeutic relationship with consumers. The therapeutic relationship is the foundation of effective mental health nursing practice (Peplau 1997). We consider this relationship to be one of equal partnership. Partnership involves working with the person and their family/carers to provide support in a way that makes sense to them, including sharing information and working in a positive way to help them reach their goals (Commonwealth of Australia 2010). The therapeutic relationship is underpinned by the nurse's use of self. Key knowledge and skills for an effective therapeutic relationship include developing a therapeutic alliance, self-awareness and empathy.

LIVED EXPERIENCE COMMENT BY JARRAD HICKMOTT
The framing of nursing around the therapeutic use of self and therapeutic alliance is very important. A lot of times it can be difficult to maintain these aspects in an environment where a heavily medicalised model is dominant. Discussing the very human side of nursing and the different domains of life that interplay with the mental ill health of consumers is very enriching and of great benefit.

Therapeutic Use of Self

As mentioned, therapeutic relationships are the central activity of mental health nursing. The therapeutic relationship provides a healing connection between the nurse and the consumer through a caring, emotional connection and narrative, and with this process, potentially having a powerful neurobiological impact on the mental health of the person (Wheeler 2011). Therapeutic relationships are the foundation upon which all other activities are based. Mental health nursing is therefore primarily an interpersonal process that uses self as the means of developing and sustaining nurse–consumer relationships. Therapeutic use of self involves using aspects of the nurse's personality, background, life skills and knowledge to develop a connection with a person who has a mental health problem or illness. Nurses intentionally and consciously draw on ways of establishing human connectedness in their encounters with service users. The process is based on a genuine interest in understanding who the consumer is and how they have come to be in their current situation – separating the person from the illness (Wyder et al 2017). Lees and colleagues (2014, p. 310) describe therapeutic engagement as the "establishment of rapport, active listening, empathy, boundaries, relating as equals, genuineness, compassion, unconditional positive regard, trust, time and responsiveness", and suggest that most of these elements need to be present for engagement to occur.

The purpose of using self therapeutically is to establish a therapeutic alliance with the service user – who may not only be experiencing frightening symptoms or perhaps overwhelming mood changes or overwhelming thoughts and feelings, but may also be experiencing alienation and isolation. They may be fearful of talking to others about their symptoms or difficulties because they fear being rejected and seen as "crazy", or they may have had experiences of rejection because the mental illness makes it difficult for them to form relationships. Studies of consumers' experiences of mental health services provide evidence that being understood and listened to in a thoughtful, sensitive manner confirms their humanity and provides hope for their future (Gunasekara et al 2014). In the process of using self therapeutically, the nurse develops a dialogue with the person to understand their predicament. Consumers need to feel safe enough to disclose personal, difficult and distressing information. It is in the way in which the nurse conveys genuine interest, concern and desire to understand that a therapeutic alliance can be established. How the nurse relates to, and what prior understandings they bring to, the encounter will affect this relationship (Wyder et al 2015).

Studies of the experiences of both mental health nurses and service users of mental health services overwhelmingly attest to the importance of therapeutic relationships. Consumers have identified the need to feel compassionately cared for, to have meaningful contact with nurses, to be listened to, and for nurses to know them as people and understand their predicament (Hurley et al 2023; Lakeman et al 2022). Similarly, studies of nurses' experiences identify that they see therapeutic engagement as the hallmark of good practice in mental health settings (Hurley et al 2022; Lakeman & Hurley 2021).

Empathy and Therapeutic Use of Self

Empathy is underpinned by caring and compassion and is positively linked with the ability to develop therapeutic relationships and the desire to alleviate suffering. As indicated earlier, the ability to engage empathically with consumers is highly valued. Empathy is not merely a feeling of understanding and compassion. Empathy, as used in the therapeutic relationship, is underpinned by intentional actions that are aimed at reducing the person's distress. Empathic interactions have a number of components:

- First, empathy involves an attempt to understand the person's predicament and the meanings they attribute to their situation. This means the nurse makes a conscious attempt to discuss with the person their current and past experiences and the feelings and meanings associated with these experiences.
- Second, the nurse verbalises the understanding that they have developed back to the person. The understanding that the nurse has of the service user's situation will be at best tentative; we can never really know what life is like for another. However, the process of seeking to understand, and of conveying the desire to understand, creates the opportunity for further exploration in a safe relationship. In addition, maintaining a stance of curiosity rather than making assumptions averts the tendency to make judgements about the person and their behaviour.
- Third, empathy involves the person's validation of the nurse's understanding. One of the most important aspects of developing the therapeutic relationship through empathic understanding is that the nurse can convey to the person a desire to understand. This level of empathic attunement enables the person to participate in identifying those aspects of their illness and healthcare experience that are problematic.

The Therapeutic Alliance

The value of a therapeutic alliance, developed through therapeutic use of self, has been clearly identified from the perspective of nurses and service users in international studies (Zugai et al 2015). A therapeutic alliance is characterised by the development of mutual partnerships between consumers and nurses, and has been linked with greater consumer satisfaction with care (Zugai et al 2015). Several studies have indicated that a therapeutic alliance can have a significant impact on consumer outcomes and that it is possibly one of the most important factors contributing to the effectiveness of a mental health service (Stewart et al 2015). People who have a positive relationship with the clinician have better outcomes (Pilgrim et al 2009). However, a therapeutic relationship alone may not be sufficient to sustain health improvements, and so a combination of both a therapeutic relationship and the technical skill of specific therapeutic approaches may provide the best outcomes (e.g. see Hurley et al 2022).

HISTORICAL ANECDOTE 2.3

Mental Health Nurse of the Century!

Hildegard Peplau (1909–1999) has been cited as the most influential mental health nurse of the 20th century. She was trained and began her career in the United States, where she was heavily influenced by psychologist Harry Stack Sullivan's work on interpersonal therapy. During World War II she moved to England where she served in an army hospital involved in the mental health rehabilitation of soldiers. After returning to North America after the war she contributed to developing the 1946 *National Mental Health Act*, which involved a major reconfiguration of mental health services away from asylums towards community-based care. In 1952 Peplau published an influential book titled *Interpersonal Relations in Nursing*. In it she described the essential skills, functions and roles of mental health nurses of her era. The book is viewed as being the first systematic, theoretical framework for the practice of modern mental health nursing. Later in her career Peplau was appointed to various influential roles with the World Health Organization, the American Nurses Association and various universities in the United States and around the world.

Read More About It
Peplau, H. 1997. Peplau's theory of interpersonal relations. Nurs Sci Quarterly, 10(4), 162–167.

Self-Awareness

The process of working together and understanding others begins with understanding oneself. "Self" is a concept that describes the core of our personality. We use the concept of self when we want to convey our uniqueness as a human being. The self has consistent attributes that pervade the way we live in and experience the world. It is awareness of these attributes of self that can enhance the way we relate to others. A strong sense of self allows us to develop resilience in dealing with the difficulties and complexities of human communication and experience. Self-awareness is about knowing how you might respond in specific situations, about your values, attitudes and biases towards people and situations, and about knowing how your human needs might manifest in your work. The purpose of being self-aware is to identify those things in our background and in our way of relating that might affect how we relate to others. The way we view people is always subjective. The lens through which we look at the world is always our own. Although there can be no true objectivity, knowledge of the experiences that influence our subjective view of the world allows us to identify how they influence our thinking. Nurses need to be aware of the belief systems and values that arise from their cultural, social and family backgrounds. Everyone develops biases that affect the way they view other people's behaviour. Behaviour that is understandable to one nurse might not be understandable to another. However, the self is not static, but constantly evolving and sensitive to experience. We bring values, biases and beliefs to nursing and to our relationships with consumers, and in turn those relationships offer the opportunity for self-development. It is through the process of self-reflection and the examination of particular experiences that nurses can learn and flourish (Fowler 2019).

Working in the mental health field requires the ability to listen to, respond to and empathise with people from a range of backgrounds and with multiple identities. Unexamined belief systems can become obstacles to developing a therapeutic alliance. Lack of self-awareness can cause nurses to respond to a person's distress and behaviour in ways that may not be helpful. For example, it might cause nurses to use power coercively in the belief that what they are doing is best for the service user. Lack of self-awareness can also lead to nurses being overly concerned, refusing to allow consumers choice or overwhelming them with advice, in an attempt to protect them. Alternatively, nurses may avoid contact with particular service users or fail to respond to distress. This growing self-awareness needs to take place against a background of self-compassion, and to develop the ability to empathise with others requires "the ability to be sensitive, non-judgemental and respectful to oneself" (Gustin & Wagner 2013, p. 182). See Personal perspectives: Consumer's Story 2.1.

PERSONAL PERSPECTIVES

Consumer's Story 2.1: Therese

You are a new nurse working in an emergency department and have been assigned Therese. You are aware of the other staff's negative feelings about this consumer. Some of the staff know her from previous presentations and see her problems as self-inflicted. However, as you take the necessary observations, you ask Therese about what has happened to her.

Therese then tells her own story:

I am 28 years old and have had lots of presentations to emergency departments. I used to cut myself often or take overdoses. However, in the past 3 years I have hardly had any presentations and no admissions to hospital. I have two children aged 4 and 2 and I am trying to get my act together for them. I do not want to lose my children. My childhood was chaotic with lots of foster care. I spent time in refuges and took drugs for a while. I do not take drugs or drink alcohol now. I have had a community mental health nurse who has been seeing me regularly for more than 3 years. Tonight I took an overdose of antidepressants that I had been prescribed. I feel ashamed because it was impulsive and stupid. I can see the staff talking about me and saying all the old things. They do not think I deserve care because I inflicted this on myself and everyone else here is physically ill or has had an accident. I just got to the end of my tether. I had a boyfriend who moved in and I didn't like how he treated the kids, so he has gone now. My community nurse is on leave. I couldn't contact anyone; I just felt so alone, empty and lost. I thought the kids would be better off without me.

If my community nurse was here, she would ask me what happened, how I was feeling. She would treat me with respect without condoning what I did. She would help me identify how I can get out of this mess I have made. We would talk about the crisis plan that is on my fridge and how I can get through the next few days keeping myself and my children safe.

? CRITICAL THINKING EXERCISE 2.2

Consider Consumer's Story 2.1: Therese.
What are your thoughts and feelings on reading about Therese's self-harm? How do you think this might impact your relationship and nursing practice with her?

Emotional Intelligence

Skills such as self-awareness, communicating empathy and therapeutically engaging with others can be collectively understood as enacting emotional intelligence. Although there are several different models of emotional intelligence, they all share core features. *Emotional intelligence* is the ability to be aware of and correctly identify our emotions, and then integrate those emotions with our cognitive knowledge to best meet our needs, or desired outcomes (Dugué et al 2021). Other core skills of emotional intelligence include identifying and regulating the emotions of self and others, displaying authentic behaviours, such as honest emotional communication, and positively influencing others through support, effective helping and problem-solving. The applications of emotional intelligence to mental health nursing, and nursing more broadly, are quickly evident. The capacity for self-awareness is intrinsic to emotional intelligence and supports an understanding of complex emotional and physiological responses to challenging work environments, trauma and distress. This skill of coping with our own emotions, as well as those of others, enables clinicians to manage stress more effectively, which subsequently supports their own health, as well as the individuals for whom they are providing care (Soto-Rubio et al 2020). This is especially relevant in relation to the high level of emotional work or burden of caring for consumers with high levels of suffering, pain, trauma and emotional distress. The concept of emotional intelligence also includes the ability to recognise the emotional states of others (Dugué et al 2021).

Emotional intelligence is integral to nursing, in the context of addressing risks to mental health, as well as the genesis of core nursing skills, including effective communication, sensitivity and creativity, self-discipline, assertiveness and awareness of self (Soto-Rubio et al 2020). Effective therapeutic relationships are founded on emotional intelligence, as the ability to understand the emotions of others, as well as knowledge and regulation of our own emotional response is the foundation of acknowledging the experience of others, thus supporting empathy (Hofmeyer et al 2020). Significantly, emotional intelligence is something that you can increase with practice, unlike your IQ. Being more self-reflective, seeking feedback about yourself from trusted others and developing your understanding of the emotions of others, are a few simple ways towards achieving this end.

Hope and Spirituality

In respect to health, there is still much that we do not know about recovery, healing and how people manage long-term problems. Why do some people pull through an illness, while others do not? How is it that some people seem to cope well with even the most invasive treatments, while others suffer terribly? How do some people with life-long mental illnesses function well in the community, while others are in and out of hospital? We know that factors such as personality, resilience, social support, general health and access to acceptable (to the service user) health services all play crucial roles in service user outcomes. But the importance and value of concepts such as hope, and the role that hope plays in the lives of service users and their families, is an area of increasing interest. "Hope" is a taken-for-granted term and, although it is used widely in the literature, it is seldom clearly defined. Hope is considered essential in dealing with illness and can be described as an act by which the temptation to despair is actively overcome. We know hope is a complex and multidimensional variable that has optimistic and anticipatory dimensions and involves looking ahead to the future. Hope has been linked to emotional healing and better adaptation to life stress (Carretta et al 2014) and is a central component in personal recovery from mental illness (Slade et al 2015).

In a study of qualitative literature related to hope in older people with chronic illnesses, Carretta and colleagues (2014, p. 1211) identified characteristics of hope as including "transcending possibilities" and "positive reappraisal". Transcending possibilities involves finding meaning through searching and connecting with others. The positive role of health professionals in maintaining hope is described as supporting hope and the search for meaning. Positive reappraisal depends on the ability to seek and find meaning in the illness experience, and health professionals also have a role in supporting service users in this

search. Hope has particular relevance to mental health nursing practice, and there is growing recognition of the concept of hope and its relationship to health, wellbeing and recovery from illness or traumatic life events. Closely linked with hope, Hemingway and colleagues (2014) describe therapeutic optimism in mental health nurses as a belief that they can make a difference and that the people they work with can recover.

The need for further research to generate knowledge and enhance understanding about suffering, hope and spirituality in relation to mental health nursing is acknowledged in the literature (Cutcliffe et al 2015). However, the emphasis on the biomedical understanding of mental illness is a barrier to such research. The biomedical model values things that can be seen, measured and quantified. Although hope and spirituality can be felt, they cannot be seen, touched or smelt, and cannot always be clearly articulated, and so occupy what Crawford and colleagues (1998, p. 214) termed "an embarrassed silence". However, if we recognise that spirituality underpins the meanings that people make of illness and other life events, and that hope is a variable that has some form of healing potential, then we cannot ignore the importance of spirituality and the search for meaning in practice. Indeed, Cutcliffe and colleagues (2015) reinforce the importance of recognising and responding to the spiritual care needs of service users and calls for nurses to develop skills in supporting consumers to understand and search for meaning in their experience. The ability to maintain hope and to make meaning of the experience of illness is central to recovery, and it is important for mental health nurses to maintain hope for consumers' recovery and to support them in maintaining hope and finding meaning in their experiences. This leads to the question: What skills do nurses need if we are to care for the spiritual needs of consumers? The short answer is that we need to develop effective interpersonal skills. Being open to the belief systems of other people, intuitiveness, active listening, being alert to the cues that tell us the things that matter to a person, self-awareness, spiritual awareness and reflective skills, are crucial in providing spiritual care (Ramezani et al 2014).

Compassion and Caring

Compassion is a concept closely associated with and underpinning caring. Compassion is linked with sensitivity to suffering and a desire to alleviate distress (Sawbridge & Hewison 2015). Gustin and Wagner (2013) suggest that compassion inspires "the act of the conscious intention of being present in moments of another's despair" (p. 175). Compassion underpins concepts of acceptance, a non-judgemental attitude, awareness, being present and listening. To be able to provide compassionate nursing care, we need to be able to imagine what it would be like to be in the person's situation, what it would be like to experience the world as they are experiencing it and to imagine what might help.

Caring is considered to be central to nursing theory and practice (Schofield et al 2013). Although the word "caring" is simple, its use in complex healthcare situations has rendered it problematic. Following a meta-synthesis of research, Finfgeld-Connett (2008) conceptualised caring as a "context-specific interpersonal process that is characterised by expert nursing practice, interpersonal sensitivity and intimate relationships" (p. 196). Finfgeld-Connett further elaborated on the concept to make explicit factors related to the roles of the consumer and the nurse, and to the working environment, discussing the "recipient's need for and openness to caring, and the nurse's professional maturity and moral foundations … [as well as] a working environment that is conducive to caring" (p. 196). However, providing nursing care in mental health settings can be even more complex as people with mental illnesses may not acknowledge the need for care, or be open to caring interventions, especially in acute phases of illness. Nurse scholars have invested much time and energy in trying to explain what it is that makes nurse caring special or different from informal caring, and from the caring provided by medical practitioners. There have also been many attempts to find a "fit" between caring as a construct and the biomedically dominated and economically driven healthcare sectors within which nursing is situated. From a mental health perspective, there are even more issues to consider in relation to caring. For example, there are special issues associated with caring for consumers who are compelled to accept professional care under mental health legislation.

Historically, mental health nursing was associated with custodial care and control. Godin (2000) captured the dilemma of mental health nurses when he raised questions about the *dis*-ease between the caring and coercive roles that mental health nurses assume. Godin positioned caring as "clean" and constructed the coercive control elements of mental health nursing (a term he used for forced treatment, community orders and so on) as "dirty" (Godin 2000, p. 1396). While Godin's argument focused on service users and nurses in the community, many of the issues he raised (related to forced administration of medication, seclusion and detention) are still relevant to nurses in inpatient and community settings. From the perspective of people who have been involuntarily detained for treatment, Wyder and colleagues (2015) found that having staff willing to listen empathically was important and that the person's involuntary legal status should not be an impediment to nurses providing compassionate care and forming therapeutic relationships. The absolute vulnerability of service users who can be detained against their will and subjected to various treatments that they may vigorously and robustly resist means that elements of the caring role, such as consumer advocacy, are critical to skillful and compassionate mental health nursing practice.

Professional Boundaries

In nursing, professional boundaries are invisible yet powerful lines that mark the territory of the nurse. They define a role and allow the nurse to say: "This is what I do. This is the purpose of my presence here." Professional boundaries are important in all areas of healthcare, but in mental health nursing they have an increased importance due to the highly personal nature of the work of mental health nurses and the vulnerability of consumers. Clear boundaries provide consumers and nurses with a safe interpersonal context in which therapeutic work can take place. Over time, there has been a decrease in formal divisions between staff and service users in mental health settings, with the encouragement of friendliness and collaborative partnerships. However,

a power imbalance is always present in clinician–consumer encounters, and there are a number of ways that boundary violations can occur. Boundary violations can involve exerting power through coercion, use of force, over-treatment or under-treatment, or inappropriate intimate relationships. Maintaining professional boundaries while being involved in therapeutic relationships is a skill that cannot be underestimated in importance.

Mental health nurses have to be able to maintain professional boundaries while simultaneously developing close therapeutic relationships with service users based on empathy and positive connectedness. While many of the interactions and interventions of mental health nurses may appear social in nature (e.g. playing table tennis, cards or volleyball with a service user, or going for a walk or having a coffee with a service user), it is the therapeutic intent and the conscious awareness of the purpose of the relationship that puts them within the professional role. It is when interventions and interactions lose their therapeutic intent and are instead primarily for the benefit of the nurse that professional boundaries are breached. Any breach of professional boundaries has the potential to cause serious harm to service users and is a violation of professional ethics.

Professional boundaries are maintained by nurses having a clear understanding of their therapeutic role, being able to reflect on therapeutic interactions and being able to document and narrate their interventions. Maintaining professional boundaries is always the responsibility of the nurse.

Self-Disclosure

Mental health nurses use self-disclosure as a way of developing therapeutic relationships with service users. Many of the relationships that nurses have with service users are long term, either by repeated admissions to hospital or by continued contact in community or primary care/ private practice settings, so nurses and service users may come to know each other well. In a study of nurses in mental health, nurses often used self-disclosure. The most common reason they shared personal information was to impact the nurse–consumer relationship, and try to make it more open and honest, reciprocal and equal (Unhjem et al 2018).

However, self-disclosure should be used consciously and carefully. The boundary issue is not about whether disclosure of information occurs or does not occur. The issue is the nature of the disclosure and whether the nurse burdens the service user with their own personal problems. The decision about what to disclose to service users about your life needs to be made in advance. Self-disclosure does not include unburdening your personal problems. The focus always needs to be on the needs of the consumer and building the relationship with them.

CHAPTER SUMMARY

This chapter has introduced the social ecological approach to practice used throughout this text and some of the core concepts and ideas that shape and inform mental health nursing practice. Therapeutic relationships lie at the heart of mental health nursing and include the use of emotional intelligence skills. A clear understanding of professional boundaries is crucial to developing and sustaining such relationships. To be effective and therapeutic in caring for others, nurses must understand concepts such as compassion, caring, hope and spirituality.

Mental health nursing is an exciting and challenging area of nursing practice. Effective mental health nursing requires the culmination of all your skills, as well as your professional and life experiences, and in return it offers a stimulating and rewarding career path. As we strive to meet the complex needs of diverse communities and to provide care within increasingly restrictive economic environments, there are many challenges before us. Developing positive personal qualities, such as self-awareness, and fostering productive and supportive collegial relationships will help us to meet the challenges that lie ahead.

ACKNOWLEDGEMENT

This chapter was adapted and extended from a chapter written by Louise O'Brien in the 4th edition of this text.

REVIEW QUESTIONS

Consider the social ecological approach to mental health nursing described in this chapter.

1. What personal characteristics (including strengths) do you bring to your nursing practice?
2. How can these be used to develop an effective partnership with consumers and their family/carers?

3. In respect to social determinants of health, which determinants do you think nurses can have an influence on? How might they do this?

USEFUL WEBSITES

Emotional Intelligence
Genos International: www.genosinternational.com/emotional-intelligence/

Professional Boundaries
Australian Nurses and Midwives Council: www.nursingmidwiferyboard.gov.au/Codes-Guidelines-Statements/Codes-Guidelines.aspx

Te Kaunihera Tapuhi o Aotearoa, Nursing Council of New Zealand – Guidelines: professional boundaries: www.nursingcouncil.org.nz/Public/Nursing/Standards_and_guidelines/NCNZ/nursing-section/Standards_and_guidelines_for_nurses.aspx?hkey=9fc06ae7-a853-4d10-b5fe-992cd-44ba3de

Recovery
A National Framework for Recovery-Oriented Mental Health Services – Guide for Practitioners And Providers: www.health.gov.au/sites/default/files/documents/2021/04/a-national-framework-for-recovery-oriented-mental-health-services-guide-for-practitioners-and-providers.pdf

National Standards for Mental Health Services – Principles of recovery oriented mental health practice: apmha.com.au/wp-content/uploads/practice-priniciples.pdf

Trauma
Adult Survivors of Child Abuse: www.ascasupport.org/

Adverse Childhood Experiences (ACE) study: acestudy.org/

Australian Government National Indigenous Australians Agency: Closing the Gap implementation plan: www.niaa.gov.au/2023-commonwealth-closing-gap-implementation-plan#:~:text=The%20Minister%20for%20Indigenous%20Australians,next%2012%20to%2018%20months

Domestic Violence Services New Zealand. Help for family violence: www.police.govt.nz/advice/family-violence/help

Mental Health Coordinating Council (MHCC) – Trauma-informed care and practice (including Trauma-informed Care and Practice Organisational Toolkit, Trauma-Informed Leadership for Organisational Change Framework and Trauma-informed Events Checklist and Policy and Protocol) search: www.mhcc.org.au/our-work/resources/

NSW Service for the Treatment and Rehabilitation of Torture and Trauma Survivors (STARTTS): www.startts.org.au/

Phoenix Australia, Centre for Posttraumatic Health: www.phoenixaustralia.org/

Transcultural Mental Health Centre: www.dhi.health.nsw.gov.au/transcultural-mental-health-centre

REFERENCES

Anthony, W.A. 1993. Recovery from mental illness: The guiding vision of the mental health service system in the 1990s. Psychiatr Rehabil J, 16(4), 11–23.

Australian Government, National Mental Health Commission 2021. The Fifth National Mental Health and Suicide Prevention Plan – Progress Report 4. Commonwealth of Australia. Online. Available at: www.mentalhealthcommission.gov.au/getmedia/d3688adf-4cf7-4f0a-93e1-a3fa79743956/NMHC_Fifth_Plan_2021_Progress_Report_Accessible.PDF

Bailey, M. 2020. The minority stress model deserves reconsideration, not just extension. Arch Sexual Behav, 49(7), 2265–2268.

Banfield, M.A., Morse, A.R., Gulliver, A. et al., 2018. Mental health research priorities in Australia: A consumer and carer agenda. Health Res Policy Syst, 16, 119.

Best, O. 2021 The cultural safety journey: An Aboriginal Australian nursing and midwifery context. In: Best, O. & Fredricks, B. (eds). Yatdjuligin. Aboriginal And Torres Strait Islander Nursing and Midwifery Care. 3rd edition. Cambridge University Press, Port Melbourne.

Carretta, C.M., Ridner, S.H., Dietrich, M.S. 2014. Hope, hopelessness, and anxiety: A pilot instrument comparison study. Arch Psychiatr Nurs, 28, 230–234.

Cleary, M., Raeburn, T., West, S., et al., 2018. "Walking the tightrope": The role of peer support workers in facilitating consumers' participation in decision-making. Int J Ment Health Nurs, 27(4), 1266–1272.

Commonwealth of Australia 2013. A National Framework for Recovery-Oriented Mental Health Services: Guide for Practitioners and Providers. Online. Available at: www.health.gov.au/sites/default/files/documents/2021/04/a-national-framework-for-recovery-oriented-mental-health-services-guide-for-practitioners-and-providers.pdf

Commonwealth of Australia 2010. National Standards for Mental Health Services. Online. Available at: www.health.gov.au/sites/default/files/documents/2021/04/national-standards-for-mental-health-services-2010-and-implementation-guidelines-national-standards-for-mental-health-services-2010.pdf

Crawford, P., Nolan, P., Brown, B., 1998. Ministering to madness: the narratives of people who have left religious orders to work in the caring professions. J Adv Nurs, 28(1), 212–220.

Cutcliffe, J.R., Hummelvoll, J.K., Granerud, A., et al., 2015. Mental health nurses responding to suffering in the 21st century occidental world: Accompanying people in their search for meaning. Arch Psychiatr Nurs, 29, 19–25.

Deegan, P.E., 1988. Recovery: The lived experience of rehabilitation. Psychiatr Rehabil J, 11(4), 11–19.

Department of Health 2017. The Fifth National Mental Health and Suicide Prevention Plan. Commonwealth of Australia. Online. Available at: www.mentalhealthcommission.gov.au/getmedia/0209d27b-1873-4245-b6e5-49e770084b81/Fifth-National-Mental-Health-and-Suicide-Prevention-Plan.pdf

Dubreucq J, Gabayet F, Godin O, Andre M, Aouizerate B, et al., 2022. Overlap and mutual distinctions between clinical recovery and personal recovery in people with schizophrenia in a one-year study. Schizophren Bull, 48(2), 382–394.

Dugué, M., Sirost, O., & Dosseville, F. 2021. A literature review of emotional intelligence and nursing education. Nurse Educ Pract, 54, 103124.

Felitti, V.J., Anda, R.F., Nordenberd, D., et al., 1998. Relationship of childhood abuse and household dysfunction to many of the leading causes of death in adults. The Adverse Childhood Experiences (ACE) Study. Am J Prev Med, 14(4), 245–258.

Finfgeld-Connett, D. 2008. Meta-synthesis of caring in nursing. J Clin Nurs, 17(2), 196–204.

Fowler, J. 2019. Reflection and mental health nursing. Part one: Is reflection important? BJMHN, 8(2), 68–69.

Glover, H. 2012. Recovery, Life-long learning, social inclusion and empowerment: Is a new paradigm emerging? In: Ryan, P., Ramon, S., Greacen, T. (eds), Empowerment, Lifelong Learning and Recovery in Mental Health: Towards a New Paradigm. Palgrave Macmillian, London.

Godin, P. 2000. A dirty business: Caring for people who are a nuisance or a danger. J Adv Nurs, 32(6), 1396–1402.

Goffman, E., 1963. Stigma: Notes on the Management of Spoiled Identity. Prentice-Hall, Englewood Cliffs.

Gordon, S., O'Brien, A.J. 2018. Co-production. Power problems and possibilities. Int J Ment Health Nurs, 27(4), 1201–1203.

Green, M., Linscott, R.J., Laurens, K.R., et al., 2018. Latent profiles of developmental schizotypy in the general population: Associations with childhood trauma and familial mental illness. Schizophr Bull, 44(Suppl. 1), S229.

Grzanka, P.R., Brian, J.D. 2019. Clinical encounters: The social Justice question in intersectional medicine. Am J Bioeth, 19(2), 22–24.

Gunasekara, I., Pentland, T., Rodgers, T., et al., 2014. What makes an excellent mental health nurse? A pragmatic inquiry initiated and conducted by people with lived experience of service use. Int J Ment Health Nurs, 23, 101–109.

Gustin, L.W., Wagner, L. 2013. The butterfly effect of caring – clinical nurse teachers' understanding of self-compassion as a source of compassionate care. Scand J Caring Sci, 27, 175–183.

Hall, C. 2014. Bereavement theory: Recent developments in our understanding of grief and bereavement. Bereave Care, 33(1), 7–12.

Hemingway, S., Rogers, M., Elsom, S. 2014. Measuring the influence of a mental health training module on the therapeutic optimism of advanced nurse practitioner students in the United Kingdom. J Am Assoc Nurse Pract, 26, 155–162.

Hofmeyer, A., Taylor, R. & Kennedy, K. 2020. Knowledge for nurses to better care for themselves so they can better care for others during the Covid-19 pandemic and beyond. Nurse Educ Today, 94, 104503.

Hurley, J., Foster, K., Campbell, K., Eden, V. Hazelton, M. 2023. Mental health nursing capability development: Perspectives of consumers and supporters. Int J Ment Health Nurs, 32(1), 172–185.

Hurley, J., Lakeman, R., Linsley, P., McKenna- Lawson, S., & Ramsay, M. 2022. Utilizing the mental health nursing workforce: A scoping review of mental health nursing clinical roles and identities. Int J Ment Health Nurs, 31(4), 796–822.

Isobel, S., Edwards, C. 2017. Using trauma informed care as a nursing model of care in an acute inpatient mental health unit: A practice development process. Int J Ment Health Nurs, 26(1), 88–94.

Jääskeläinen, E., Juola, P., Hirvonen, N., et al., 2012. A systematic review and meta-analysis of recovery in schizophrenia. Schizophr Bull, 39(6), 1296–1306.

Javier, J.R., Hoffman, L.R., Shah, S.I., Pediatric Policy Council 2019. Making the case for ACEs: Adverse childhood experiences, obesity, and long-term health. Pediatr Res, 86(4), 420–422.

Jones, T., Nurius, P., Song, C., et al., 2018. Modeling life course pathways from adverse childhood experiences to adult mental health. Child Abuse Negl, 80, 32–40.

Lakeman, R. & Hurley, J. 2021. What mental health nurses have to say about themselves: A discourse analysis. Int J Ment Health Nurs, 30(1), 126–135.

Lakeman, R., Foster, K, Campbell, K. & Hurley, J. 2022. Helpful encounters with mental health nurses in Australia: A survey of service users and their supporters. J Psychiatr Ment Health Nurs, 30(3), 515–525.

Le Boutillier, C., Leamy, M., Bird, V.J. 2011. What does recovery mean in practice? A qualitative analysis of international recovery-oriented practice guidance. Psychiatr Serv, 62(12), 1470–1476.

Leamy, M., Bird, V., Le Boutillier, C., et al., 2011. Conceptual framework for personal recovery in mental health: Systematic review and narrative synthesis. Br J Psychiatry, 199(6), 445–452.

Lees, D., Procter, N., Fassett, D. 2014. Therapeutic engagement between consumers in suicidal crisis and mental health nurses. Int J Ment Health Nurs, 23(4), 306–315.

Leete, E., 1989. How I perceive and manage my illness. Schizophr Bull, 15(2), 197.

Leendertse, J.C.P., Wierdsma, A.I., van den Berg, D., Ruissen, A.M., Slade, M., et al., 2021. Personal recovery in people with a psychotic disorder: A systematic review and meta-analysis of associated factors. Front Psychiatry, 23(12), 622628.

Lund, C., Brooke-Sumner, C., Baingana, F., et al., 2018. Social determinants of mental disorders and the Sustainable Development Goals: A Frontiers Psychiatry systematic review of reviews. Lancet Psychiatry 5(4), 357–369.

Ministry of Health. 2021. Kia Manawanui Aotearoa: Long-term pathway to mental wellbeing. Ministry of Health, Wellington.

Peplau, H., 1997. Peplau's theory of interpersonal relations. Nurs Sci Q, 10(4), 162–167.

Pilgrim, D., Rogers, A., Bentall, R. 2009. The centrality of personal relationships in the creation and amelioration of mental health problems: The current interdisciplinary case. Health (London), 13, 235–254.

Raeburn, T., Liston, C., Hickmott, J., et al., 2018. Life of Martha Entwistle: Australia's first convict mental health nurse. Int J Ment Health Nurs, 27(1), 455–463.

Raeburn, T., Schmied, V., Hungerford, C., et al., 2017. Autonomy support and recovery practice at a psychosocial clubhouse. Perspect Psychiatr Care, 53(3), 175–182.

Ramezani, M., Ahmadi, F., Mohammadi, E., et al., 2014. Spiritual care in nursing: A concept analysis. Int Nurs Rev, 61, 211–219.

Reid, R., Escott, P., Isobel, S. 2018. Collaboration as a process and an outcome: Consumer experiences of collaborating with nurses in care planning in an acute inpatient mental health unit. Int J Ment Health Nurs, 27(4), 1204–1211.

Sawbridge, Y., Hewison, A. 2015. Compassion costs nothing – the elephant in the room? Pract Nurs, 26(4), 194–197.

Schofield, R., Allan, M., Jewiss, T., et al. 2013. Knowing self and caring through service learning. Int J Nurs Educ Scholarsh, 10(1), 267–274.

Slade, M., & Wallace, G. 2017. Recovery and mental health. In: Slade, M., Oades, L., & Jarden, A. (eds), Wellbeing, Recovery and Mental Health. Cambridge University Press.

Slade, M., Bird, V., Clarke, E., et al., 2015. Supporting recovery in patients with psychosis through care by community-based adult mental health teams (REFOCUS): A multisite, cluster, randomised, controlled trial. Lancet Psychiatry, 2(6), 503–514.

Slade, M., Leamy, M., Bacon, F., et al., 2012. International differences in understanding recovery: Systematic review. Epidemiol Psychiatr Sci, 21(4), 353–364.

Soto-Rubio, A., Giménez-Espert, M.D.C. & Prado-Gascó, V. 2020. Effect of emotional intelligence and psychosocial risks on burnout, job satisfaction, and nurses' health during the COVID-19 pandemic. Int J Environ Res Public Health, 17(21), 7998.

Spittlehouse, J.K., Boden, J.M., Horwood, L.J. 2019. Sexual orientation and mental health over the life course in a birth cohort. Psychol Med, 1–8.

State of Victoria. 2019. Royal Commission into Victoria's Mental Health System, Interim Report, Parl Paper No. 87 (2018–19). finalreport.rcvmhs.vic.gov.au

Stewart, D., Burrow, H., Duckworth, A., et al., 2015. Thematic analysis of psychiatric patients' perceptions of nursing staff. Int J Ment Health Nurs, 24(1), 82–90.

Sweeney, A., Filson, B., Kennedy, A., et al., 2018. A paradigm shift: Relationships in trauma-informed mental health services. BJ Psych Adv, 24(5), 319–333.

Turolla, A., Venneri, A., Farina, D., et al., 2018. Rehabilitation induced neural plasticity after acquired brain injury. Neural Plast, 2018, 6565418.

Ungar, M., and Theron, L. 2020. Resilience and mental health: How multisystemic processes contribute to positive outcomes. Lancet Psych, 7(5), 441–448.

Unhjem, J.V., Vatne, S. & Hem, M.H. 2018. Transforming nurse–patient relationships. A qualitative study of nurse self-disclosure in mental health care. J Clin Nurs, 27(5–6), e798–e807.

van Weeghel, J., van Zelst, C., Boertien, D., et al., 2019. Conceptualizations, assessments, and implications of personal recovery in mental illness: A scoping review of systematic reviews and meta-analyses. Psychiatr Rehabil J, 42(2), 169–181.

Victorian Transcultural Mental Health (VTMH) 2021. An Integrated Approach to Diversity Equity and Inclusion in Mental Health Service Provision in Victoria: A Position Paper. Victorian Transcultural Mental Health. Online. Available at: vtmh.org.au/reports-and-publications/

Voss, P., Thomas, M.E., Cisneros-Franco, J.M., de Villers-Sidani, E. 2017. Dynamic brains and the changing rules of neuroplasticity: Implications for learning and recovery. Front Psychology, 8, 1657.

Wheeler, K. 2011. A relationship-based model for psychiatric nursing. Perspect Psychiatr Care, 47(3), 151–159.

Wilson, A., Hurley, J., Hutchinson, M., & Lakeman, R. 2021. Can mental health nurses working in mental health inpatient units really be trauma-informed? An integrative review of the literature? J Psychiatr Ment Health Nurs, 28(5), 900–923.

World Health Organisation (WHO), 2022. Social determinants of health. Online. Available at: www.who.int/health-topics/social-determinants-of-health#tab=tab_1

Wyder, M., Bland, R., Blythe, A., et al., 2015. Therapeutic relationships and involuntary treatment orders: service users' interactions with health-care professionals on the ward. Int J Ment Health Nurs, 24(2), 181–189.

Wyder, M., Ehrlich, C., Crompton, D., et al., 2017. Nurses experiences of delivering care in acute inpatient mental health settings: a narrative synthesis of the literature. Int J Ment Health Nurs, 26(6), 527–540.

Zugai, J.S., Stein-Parbury, J., Roche, M. 2015. Therapeutic alliance in mental health nursing: An evolutionary concept analysis. Issues Ment Health Nurs, 36(4), 249–257.

3

The Mental Health and Illness Continuum

John Hurley, Peta Marks, Kim Foster and Anthony J. O'Brien

KEY POINTS

- All nursing work will bring you into encounters with people experiencing mental health challenges.
- Consequently, all nurses need foundational mental health nursing skills to be helpful towards the mental and emotional wellbeing of the people they work with. These foundational skills begin with developing therapeutic relationships that enable wellbeing.

- Understanding that every individual's mental wellbeing fluctuates across a continuum of mental health and illness, from everyday stress to acute mental disorders, informs the nurse's responses to the person's needs.
- Most people who experience episodes of mental ill health will also move towards and experience recovery.

KEY TERMS

Crisis

Healing relationships

Lived experience

Mental illness recovery and trauma informed care

Stress and coping

LEARNING OUTCOMES

The material in this chapter will assist you to:

- understand the continuum of mental health and illness that people may experience during their lives
- understand stress and coping and the impact they have on wellbeing

- identify the various types of crisis
- form an understanding of the therapeutic value of working in partnership with patients
- describe how to take a strengths focus in practice.

LIVED EXPERIENCE COMMENT BY JARRAD HICKMOTT
This chapter expertly covers the important areas of the strengths model, recovery model and trauma-informed care. These models are the cornerstones of the lived experience and consumer movements. I very much appreciate the acknowledgement of mental distress as being a "human experience", in that we all experience it to varying degrees and for different reasons.

INTRODUCTION

Mental health is crucial to everybody's quality of life and influences the social and economic fabric of whole communities, states and nations (Department of Health and Ageing 2022). It is that important.

Importantly, mental health and illness are neither static nor absolute states. Mental health, which can also be termed mental wellbeing, and mental illness, are not turned on and off like a light switch. Rather, all people will move along a continuum of mental health and illness in response to biological, psychological, environmental and social influences. People can move along the continuum of mental health and illness (see Fig. 3.1) and remain in various states for shorter or longer periods (Chen et al 2020). As discussed in Chapter 2, in this book we promote a 'social ecological' understanding of mental health nursing practice that views mental health as existing within these influences. In the same way that any physically healthy person may become unwell or a physically unwell person may become well, there is always the opportunity for a person who is mentally healthy to develop mental

ill-health or for a person who is experiencing mental illness to recover and regain mental health. Understanding the continuum of mental health and illness is therefore crucial if nurses are to assist the people to whom they deliver care effectively.

Mental health cannot be separated from the concept of overall health, which is defined by the World Health Organization (WHO) (2022) as:

Mental health is a state of mental well-being that enables people to cope with the stresses of life, realize their abilities, learn well and work well, and contribute to their community. It is an integral component of health and well-being that underpins our individual and collective abilities to make decisions, build relationships and shape the world we live in. Mental health is a basic human right.

Conversely at the other end of the continuum is mental illness, defined as:

A mental illness is a health problem that affects people's thoughts, mood, behaviour or the way they perceive the world around them. A mental illness causes distress and may affect the person's ability to function at work, in relationships or in everyday tasks.

(Health Direct 2021)

When the focus is more on assessing people for mental illness rather than assisting them towards recovery, mental *health* can be overlooked. This one-dimensional search for illness situates the "patient" as being "sick" and ignores the strengths they will most certainly have. The illness approach inevitably ends up in an ongoing cycle of assessment, diagnosis, treatment and discharge, resulting in poor outcomes for consumers and families, with high rates of relapse (Rosenberg & Hickie 2019). Identifying where a person may be situated on the continuum of mental health and illness enables more effective targeting of nursing interventions, and supports the formation of the therapeutic relationship.

It is important to acknowledge that there are a wide variety of words and concepts used to explain various stages of the continuum of mental health and illness. The following sections synthesise several major concepts in mental health and illness.

MENTALLY HEALTHY

The earlier definition from the WHO (2022) communicates that mental health is an essential and significant component of wellbeing and that being mentally healthy enables us to function effectively in relationships and other social roles. There is no clear point at which mental health ends and physical health begins; they are intertwined, each impacting the other. As evident in the model in Figure 3.1, being mentally healthy also includes the capacity to respond effectively to everyday challenges.

Descriptions of mental health have differed throughout history and continue to vary in the modern era due to factors such as language, culture and the influence of particular interest groups. A more recent phenomenon in mental health is the concept of "thriving" (Sorgente et al 2021). Here, an individual is functioning at their absolute maximum potential across physical, social and mental domains. While there are some variations as to what helps people thrive, common factors include:
- having positive relationships and community connection
- being able to fully immerse yourself into experiences
- attaining skills and achieving realistic goals
- having life purpose, to give service to something bigger than ourselves
- adopting optimistic perspectives.

It is important to recognise that being mentally healthy or thriving is not a permanent state, nor is it an all-perfect, all-positive life. As evident in the list of common factors that influence thriving, being mentally healthy does not happen in isolation from others or our social roles. Fig. 3.2 shows how our environment, who we are (our identity) and social factors (such as employment or housing) have a direct relationship on our mental health, problems with mental health and in triggering mental illness. As environmental and social factors shift and change over days, weeks and months, people's capacity to cope (or not cope) in response to those changes impacts their mental health. Consequently, most human beings living a mentally healthy life will display a wide range of personal and social characteristics. Personal characteristics exhibited by people who are mentally healthy may mean that they appear to be accepting or angry, hopeful or hateful, active or anxious, humble or humourless, brave or bullying, successful or sad, compassionate or conniving, wise or naive. Similarly, the social circumstances of people who are mentally healthy vary tremendously. People who are employed or unemployed, introverted or extroverted, or who are with or without family and friends can live mentally healthy lives. Mental health helps a person to live a life that is satisfying to them and the community they live in; how this is achieved or what the person's life looks like is of no consequence at all.

Importantly, Figure 3.2 also communicates where nurses can assist individuals and communities across the continuum, from mental health through to mental illness, to improve the modifiable environmental, relational, psychological and physical determinants that can affect mental health. At the public health level, nurses may work to influence the development of service models and advocate for fairer distribution of resources that impact on mental health, such as affordable housing, access to education, income equality and employment. Clinically, nurses work to enhance people's mental health using practices such as mental health assessment, psychotherapy, promotion of physical health care, social advocacy and promotion of ethical medication management (Hurley et al 2022).

Mental Health Continuum Model			
Healthy	**Reacting**	**Injured**	**ILL**
Normal fluctuations in mood Takes things in stride Good sense of humour Consistent performance Physically and socially active Confident in self and others Drinking in moderation	Nervousness, irritability Sadness, overwhelmed Displaced sarcasm Procrastination Forgetfulness Trouble sleeping Low energy Muscle tension, headaches Missing an occasional class or deadline Decreased social activity Drinking regularly or in binges to manage stress	Anxiety, anger Pervasive sadness, tearfulness, hopelessness, worthlessness Negative attitude Difficulty concentrating Trouble making decisions Decreased performance, regularly missing classes/deadlines, or over-work Restless, disturbed sleep Avoidance, social withdrawal Increase used of alcohol – hard to control	Excessive anxiety Panic attacks Easily enraged, aggressive Depressed mood, numb Cannot concentrate Inability to make decisions Cannot fall asleep/stay asleep Constant fatigue, illness Absent from social events/classes Suicidal thoughts/intent Unusual sensory experiences (hearing or seeing things) Alcohol or other addiction
Nurture support systems.	Recognise limits, take breaks, identify problems early, seek support.	Tune into own signs of distress. Talk to someone, ask for help. Make self-care a priority. Don't withdraw.	Seek professional care. Follow recommendations.

FIG. 3.1 Mental Health Continuum Model. Chen et al 2020 (adapted from Canadian Armed Forces).

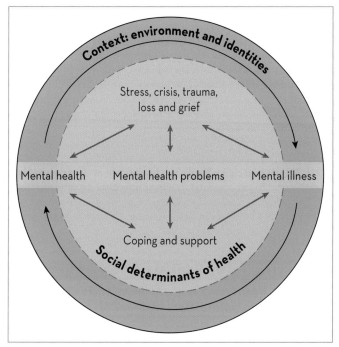

FIG. 3.2 Socio-Ecological Factors Influencing the Mental Health Continuum.

In describing aspects of the continuum of mental health, parts of a mental health journey are used for illustrative purposes. In describing aspects of the continuum of mental health, we share parts of the mental health journey of Mary and Jarrad (below) to illustrate the various personal perspectives that individuals bring.

PERSONAL PERSPECTIVES

Consumer's Story 3.1 Part 1: Mary

Mental Health
Growing up in regional Australia was pretty easy going for me really. I never thought about whether I was "mentally healthy" or not; the idea never crossed my mind to dismiss it. I had my friends and other family living nearby. I don't recall much about primary school, except it was not something I dreaded. Home was OK, Mum and I were close and still are. My dad left when I was really young and never came back into our lives again until I was much older. I never knew any different, so that was not a problem for me. Mum had a new partner, who was kind enough and left me pretty much alone. I had friends, went to Nippers and was pretty good at dance and gymnastics. All in all, I was happy most of the time.

PERSONAL PERSPECTIVES

Consumer's Story 3.2 Part 1: Jarrad

Mental Health
It seems that when things are going well and we are experiencing what is referred to as "mental health" we tend to kind of take it for granted and don't really think much about it. Blessed with a happy childhood in a safe and loving family home, I performed well at primary school. In my final year of primary I was school captain, debating team captain, school sports representative, involved in and achieving all that I could.

Stress and Coping

Stress

A key common factor that influences where an individual sits within the mental health continuum is stress. Stress can trigger dramatic movement towards illness, while for others it can equally be something that triggers significant personal growth. Indeed, stress is an utterly normal part of being human. The term "Eu-stress" is widely used in positive psychology to describe an essential and helpful type of stress that improves wellbeing and performance (Bienertova et al 2020). Common examples of Eu-stress include having a first child or moving into new accommodation. In contrast, the term "Dis-stress" is used to describe unpleasant experiences of stress that can manifest in anxiety and irritability, and potentially culminate in a mental health crisis. Common examples include bereavement and living with chronic pain.

Every individual responds to stressors differently, depending on factors including their appraisal of the stressor and their existing coping strategies. This appraisal will be of their actual and perceived ability to cope measured against the actual and perceived demands of the stressor. Where coping strategies are equal to or stronger than the stressor demands, Eu-stress is a likely response. However, when the stressor demands are perceived by the individual as exceeding their coping capacity, dis-stress will likely result.

The significance of distress is seen when we consider that although distress is experienced psychologically, it has profound effects on brain functioning, in some cases establishing neural pathways that predispose individuals to responses that become automatic and can be resistant to change (Everly & Lating 2019). These stress responses, while they are adaptive ways of meeting the immediate challenges of the external environment, can be persistent over time, prevent new learning and become maladaptive. Chronic stress can lead to hypersensitivity of the limbic system of the brain, with the result that any experience resembling those that caused the initial stress can trigger an acute stress reaction, including the associated patterns of thinking and behavioural responses. In such cases, the stress response becomes encoded in our memories and is activated automatically (Goldfarb et al 2019). Chronic stress is mediated by the sympathetic nervous system and higher neural functions in the pituitary and hypothalamus, resulting in high levels of cortisol, which maintain a heightened sense of arousal. If you consider the case of a child raised in an environment of physical and emotional abuse, the constant exposure to high levels of psychological distress will cause a sustained stress response that becomes the child's way of living with their adverse experiences. In time they become less able to return to a non-aroused emotional baseline, and even minor stimuli such as words associated with a traumatic experience can trigger an acute stress response. Adverse events of childhood are further discussed below.

For the most part, a person presenting in mental distress needs empathy, understanding and emotional support, rather than a diagnosis, treatment and medication (Craig et al 2020). In order for nurses to effectively respond to distress with empathy and support, it is essential they suspend their own negative judgements. This non-judgemental nursing approach is enabled by understanding some basic reasons as to why some people are more vulnerable to stress than others. Referring to Figure 3.2, it is evident that individuals are impacted by a range of environmental and social factors. Factors such as insecure accommodation or financial burdens will both add to a person's stress burden and simultaneously reduce their capability to cope effectively with any additional demands. A less obvious but equally important factor that makes some more vulnerable to stress is their childhood exposure to adverse events, widely known as Adverse Childhood Events (ACEs).

Compelling research powerfully indicates that when children experience neglect or parental divorce or witness domestic abuse, they may experience psychological trauma as a result. This psychological trauma can manifest itself throughout their lives and has been shown to directly and negatively impact on physical health, social outcomes and mental health (Loxton et al 2021). It is important for all nurses to acknowledge that the adults they are supporting are quite likely to have long standing emotional trauma. In mental health settings nearly two thirds of those receiving in-patient mental health care in Australia have been exposed to trauma. Consequently, mental health nurses need to communicate and relate with non-judgmental empathy in order to best respond to the person's needs (Wilson et al 2023).

Coping

Human beings are remarkably resilient, and generally people are able to cope adaptively with the life stressors they experience and move back along the continuum towards mental health relatively quickly (Sax Institute 2020). Coping refers to people's capacity to adjust effectively to life stressors without experiencing significant ongoing mental and emotional disturbances. The risk and protective factors that influence stress and coping vary, and depend upon factors such as age and ethnicity. Sedentary lifestyle inhibits coping in children, while for young adults, being in a sexual minority is a factor. For older adults, being a carer has a more significant negative impact on coping, while separation from country and culture is significant for Indigenous peoples (Sax Institute 2020). Despite these variances, common protective factors include those that also promote thriving, such as regular physical exercise, a close relationship with a partner or parental figure; risk factors might include a lack of safe housing and biological stressors. Table 3.1 provides some illustrative examples of factors that are

TABLE 3.1 Protective and Risk Factors

	Protective Factors	Risk Factors
Social environment	Safe housing Access to education Employment Economic stability Access to social welfare support if needed	War Poverty and crime LGBTIQA+, Insecurity Homelessness Discrimination Lack of support services
Relationships	Positive childhood attachment Supportive family and friends Communication skills Sense of personal autonomy Community participation	Abuse (physical, psychological, sexual, financial, spiritual) or exposure to abuse (e.g. domestic violence) Neglect Separation and loss Peer rejection Social isolation
Psychological factors	Positive sense of self Good coping skills Attachment to family Social skills Good physical health	Low self-esteem Low self-efficacy Poor coping skills Insecure attachment in childhood Physical and intellectual disability
Physical health	Access to clean air and water Adequate nutrition Regular physical exercise Access to quality physical health care	Low-quality nutrition High consumption of alcohol/drugs Cigarette smoking Low access to healthcare services

protective and those that are often risks across social environments, relationships, and psychological and physical health. Importantly, in the same way that distress can create hypersensitivity of the limbic system and higher levels of cortisol, effective coping responses can trigger adaptive changes in brain function. Resilience in adolescents who have experienced adversity is associated with changes in prefrontal structures (Gee 2021) showing that the brain changes in response to both negative and positive life experiences. The concept of neuroplasticity refers to the capacity of the brain to change in response to new experiences and to develop new neural pathways that replace those that have become maladaptive or unhelpful (Smith & Merwin 2021). Yet the process of change can be difficult, as the brain tends to revert to established responses, however unhelpful or unwanted these are. Psychological interventions and even physical interventions, can lead to sustained changes in brain function and can help the person over time (Bishop et al 2021).

✴ HISTORICAL ANECDOTE 3.1

Humane Responses Towards Mental Health Problems: Philippe Pinel (1745–1826)

> Across cultures and over time people who displayed unusual behaviours have been shunned from society and treated cruelly. Much of this was driven by fear and superstition. In European cultures those in mental distress were considered to be possessed by the devil or implicated in witchcraft. Indeed, up to the 1700s thousands of distressed people were executed or died in response to the 'treatments' offered such as trephining.
>
> Philippe Pinel (1745–1826) was a French physician who instigated humane and compassionate approaches to those in mental distress as a method of treatment. He is most well-known for unchaining asylum inmates (Kendler 2020), but it is less well-known that Pinel was also a biological scientist and trained philosopher. Pinel's humane approaches were based upon his growing understanding of different types and classifications of distress achieved by scientific (for the era) observations and repeated assessments. Philosophically, he challenged the common beliefs of the causes of mental distress and made the first links between emotions and decision-making. He attributed mental illnesses to distressed people being exposed to social and psychological stressors.

Mental Health Injuries

Whether at home, at school, at work or in any other situation, if a person experiences an inability to cope and adapt to life stressors, they are at risk of experiencing challenges to their mental wellbeing. The distress experienced can be understood as a social and/or emotional wound(s) that negatively affects a person's life, but not to the extent that their relationships or normal daily activities are seriously disrupted. As indicated in Figure 3.1, the individual can be "injured", without necessarily deteriorating further and moving along the continuum into mental illness. The list of "symptoms" within the orange "Injured" segment of the model can be viewed as lived experiences of people in distress, including ongoing sadness and intense emotional upset that persists for extended periods of time, and poor sleep, which has the consequence of tiredness, concentration difficulties and a drop in performance of social roles. For example, by underperforming as a student, parent or partner, the person may feel less worthwhile and lose a sense of their own self-worth. If ignored, these experiences will add even more distress, risking movement along the continuum towards illness (Chen et al 2020).

The role of the nurse is to work collaboratively with the person to create a sense of safety and hope that they can and will move back towards better mental health. The nurse can support them to find the correct help and identify self-care strategies. Communicating empathy, compassion and non-judgemental attitudes will by themselves help the injured person to make a move towards better health. It is essential that nurses seek to assist people experiencing mental health problems on an individual basis. Keep in mind that some groups – such as infants, children and those who struggle to communicate due to disability, serious physical illness, frailty or extreme age – are vulnerable and need a high degree of care and support. Likewise, people arriving as refugees or seeking asylum after exposure to war and other traumatic events, such as physical or sexual violence and assault, being kidnapped, tortured and seeing family members killed, are extremely vulnerable and also in need of extensive care and support.

PERSONAL PERSPECTIVES
Consumer's Story 3.1 Part 2: Mary

Mental Health Injury

At the start of high school, we moved town for my stepfather's work, which triggered my first real experience of struggling. I was around 14 at the time. I found it hard to fit in and experienced a lot of bullying at school. Most of it was just being excluded by the other girls, but there were a couple of occasions where it was physical. I hung out with the boys or mostly just kept to myself at break times. I wasn't a great student either, so would sit in the back of classes not to get noticed. School became a lonely place for me and I began thinking that there was something unlikeable about me as a person. I was sad most of the time and was anxious whenever I left to go to school. I began making scratches on my arm at night with a pair of scissors, just to do something with all the emotions I was holding onto. It all came to a head when Mum saw the marks. Everyone sort of rallied around and I ended up getting some counselling at Headspace. The thing that struck me at the time was that my family, Headspace and the school were all just trying to help and weren't judging me.

PERSONAL PERSPECTIVES
Consumer's Story 3.2 Part 2: Jarrad

Mental Health Injury

I don't remember much about what went on, but my parents had marriage trouble towards the end of primary school and by the time high school rolled around I didn't want to attend. It remains inexplicable to me, but on my first day at high school aged 12 my mother drove me to school and I panicked about her leaving me there. A teacher had to restrain me because I was crying, kicking and screaming while my mother left. From that day on, high school was a difficult experience for me. I often managed to avoid school from Year 7 (age 12) to Year 10 (age 16) and the school rarely seemed to notice. When I did attend, I coasted without much attention to education. I found that being of a younger age I was able to avoid social engagements with little to no fallout or effort. When asked to attend a friend's party or event I would make excuses that I was playing sport or that I was helping a grandmother move or whatever else I could fabricate in order to avoid invitations. Not only was I trying to avoid the invitations out, but also the awkwardness of a group of friends talking about something they all did on the weekend at an event I hadn't attended. People would often talk about their plans for after they graduated from high school and what universities they were planning to attend, where my only concern was just surviving the high school experience. Counselling support at our school was provided by an old Irish priest. His kind approach was that if I didn't want to go to class, I could just sit in his room in the office instead. That often involved random casual chats, which a lot of the time I found helpful to avoid the social anxiety I experienced when sitting in class.

Crisis

The social and environmental stressors that people experience can gradually overwhelm their coping, or can also impact them more acutely. This more acute onset is felt as a *crisis*. Nurses regularly support people who are experiencing crisis, trauma, loss and grief across all clinical settings. To be effective at supporting people in crisis, nurses require some beginning understandings of how crises may occur and their common characteristics. It is also important to remember that for some people, crisis can be transformational and lead to increased capacity for coping and resilience.

Most current theories and responses to crisis are based upon the earlier work of Gerald Caplan from the United States (Caplan 1964). While there are many different theories and models, the common features of a crisis situation include the following:
- The person is presented with a sudden precipitating event that is actually, or is perceived to be, beyond their usual levels of coping.
- This event is actually, or is perceived to be, a threat or a danger.
- High levels of emotional disturbance are evident.
- The person will seek to find new or novel ways of coping as their habitual approaches are overwhelmed.

In contrast to a stressful event, such as a job interview or an exam, a specific experience that the person perceives to be threatening, such as loss of employment, the death of a loved one, assault (physical, emotional or sexual) or divorce, may trigger a state of acute crisis. In this state, usual coping strategies can be seriously challenged and a person's ability to manage the demands of everyday life can be disrupted, resulting in disorganisation and disequilibrium. Without relief, severe emotional, cognitive and behavioural disfunction can occur, which in turn can precipitate the person to break from reality or be a risk to themselves or others

A simple breakdown of common crisis situations that you as a nurse may encounter are shown in Table 3.2 (Kanel 2019).

Considering the type of crisis can help to deepen understanding of what may have triggered the crisis and what course of action may assist the person. The initial role of the nurse in crisis situations is to ensure the physical and emotional safety of the person in crisis. This role is undertaken with the same approach as taken to those in distress, with clearly communicated empathy, professional calmness and compassion. Offering emotional reassurance, and seeking and clarifying what the person's needs are in the current moment are also useful strategies. People in crisis will often be unable to access coping strategies they have used successfully in the past or will have unused external coping resources, such as friends or family. Encouraging the person to identify and utilise these strategies and coping resources increases the possibility that the crisis will be an opportunity for personal growth and greater future resilience.

TABLE 3.2	Common Types of Crisis
Type of Crisis	**Key Features**
Developmental crisis	These have precipitating events that emerge from normal life changes and are typified by transitional moments in a person's development. For example, moving into puberty, moving into living away from home, or retirement.
Situational crisis	These have precipitating events that are uncommon, unpredictable and mostly not preventable. Within nursing contexts these may be the onset of sudden serious illness or an unexpected cancer diagnosis. In wider social and ecological contexts precipitants can include disasters, unexpected death of a loved one or relationship breakdown.

Consumer's Story 3.3: Nathan

Nathan in Crisis

Twenty-five-year-old Nathan presented to an emergency department (ED) distraught and overwhelmed. Several recent losses had caused him considerable grief and eroded his usual resilience and pragmatic coping style. He felt helpless to instigate any previously used problem-solving strategies. Nathan was distressed and tearful as he recounted the sequence of events that had led him to think ending his life was his best course of action. The nurse's initial assessment concluded that Nathan was displaying depressive symptoms with suicidal thoughts. Nathan had no specific plan to harm himself, but he did admit that his suicidal thoughts had scared him because he had never previously experienced such thoughts. Given his risk of self-harm, the nurse felt concerned about his ability to keep himself safe, and her first inclination was to admit him to hospital, if necessary, against his will.

Slowly, Nathan calmed himself a little, but still felt helpless and hopeless and unable to see any way through his distress. The nurse reassured Nathan that he was safe, and he agreed to continue with the assessment. As the nurse talked with Nathan, she raised her concerns and discussed how they might work together to keep him safe through this challenging time. Admission to hospital was a possible option. Although Nathan did not refuse hospitalisation, he was clearly not keen about the suggestion. Together they considered other options as the nurse attempted to tap into Nathan's strengths and help him utilise his now disrupted coping strategies. The nurse asked Nathan what he thought he needed to overcome his distress. "I don't know", he replied. This response is typical of a person whose thinking is affected by the emotional upset of an acute crisis. The nurse reframed the question, asking Nathan what his life and circumstances would look like if none of these events had happened. He described in some detail how life would be without such overwhelming grief and loss. Nathan rapidly became discouraged again when he could not think of how to live without feeling overwhelmed by grief and loss.

A shift in focus was needed again. Calming her own anxiety, the nurse expressed her curiosity about his efforts and past successes in overcoming adversities in his life. Nathan recalled several difficult events and described how he had overcome these difficulties. The nurse reflected aloud on the strength and resilience he had demonstrated in overcoming these challenges. As Nathan acknowledged his own capacity to overcome adversity, the change in him was almost tangible. The nurse witnessed an "aha" moment. When he realised he was already working hard to recover, Nathan's level of distress dissipated markedly and he began to think of other strategies he could employ to continue his recovery.

Nathan was very thankful for the nurse's help. While the nurse accepted his thanks, at the same time she was humbled as she really hadn't worked miracles, nor did she have easy answers for Nathan. Rather, it had been a process of listening (really listening and asking the right questions), while allowing Nathan the time required to reconnect with his own strength and resilience. Instead of letting anxiety overwhelm her, the nurse had been able to avoid reinforcing Nathan's sense of helplessness and circumvented an admission to hospital. Nathan was able to leave with renewed strength and hope for his future. Before leaving, Nathan was happy to make an appointment for follow-up and note down phone numbers that he could call if he needed to talk before they met again.

MENTAL ILLNESS

A key feature of the mental health continuum (Fig. 3.1) is that it is dynamic. By this we mean that a person does not remain static in one segment of the continuum, but will move across it, often influenced by social and psychological factors, which are identified in Figure 3.2.

Many people who experience mental health injuries never access a mental health professional for assistance and so never interpret their problems as mental ill health.

In the same way that descriptions of mental health have varied throughout history, so too have ideas about mental illness. The number of categories of mental illness are steadily growing. When the first diagnostic manual was published in the 1950s there were just over 100 categories of mental illness. This grew to 265 categories in 1980 and in the most modern diagnostic manuals there are now just over 300 (Leggatt 2022). While the number of disorders has risen, there have also been significant changes to what is and what is not considered to be a mental illness. These descriptions of mental illness can vary according to culture and over time. For example, homosexuality was only delisted as a mental illness in 1974.

Historical Views of Mental Illness

In the 18th and 19th centuries, the so-called "mental institutions" in New Zealand and in Australia strongly reflected the cultural norms of England. Such norms considered that any behaviour of women that was not aligned with society's expectations of the men was in fact mental illness. Women were considered by nature to be dependent, of gentle disposition and highly prone to illness. Women who were assertive, sought to be independent or who disagreed with their husband, could be admitted to an asylum simply on the word of their spouse or family. Morality, or rather, failure to conform to expected norms of female behaviour in women, was also considered to be mental illness. Female biology was considered to be connected to mental illness in this era and as a result a hysterectomy was performed to correct the "mental illness" in the woman and ready her to return to society.

Read More About It

Milne-Smith, A. 2022. Gender and madness in nineteenth-century Britain. History Compass, e12754.

Modern definitions of mental illness vary considerably depending on the culture, language and interests of particular groups. Earlier in this chapter we cited a recent definition of mental illness from the Australian Government website (Health Direct 2021). Importantly, this definition highlighted that mental illness has impacts on thoughts, emotions and behaviour, as well as the person's ability to socially function in day-to-day life. When examining the illness segment of the mental health continuum (Fig. 3.1), it is evident that those experiencing illness are in marked distress that impacts a significant proportion of their lives. Intense emotional states and impaired capability to undertake sustained logical thinking are evident, along with experiencing sensory perceptions without the normal associated stimuli. Social dislocation is also evident, which when considered alongside the discomfort caused by the other symptoms, can lead to suicidal thinking, potentially as a way of escaping distress. Accurately counting those with a mental illness is difficult, as there is no clear boundary between what is an "illness" and what is considered to be "mentally unwell". However, we can get some sense of the prevalence of those experiencing illness by looking at the available data. According to the *National Study of Mental Health and Wellbeing*, one in five (21%) people who had experienced a mental disorder in their lifetime had symptoms in the 12 months before the survey interview; and 16–24-year-olds (40%) were most likely to have experienced symptoms of a mental disorder in the previous 12 months, while those aged 75–85 years were the least likely (4%) (Australian Institute of Health and Welfare 2022). See Chapter 1 for further information.

While reporting of data for New Zealand varies from that in Australia, the picture is similar, with some 28% of the population reporting poor wellbeing. Youth followed by those in the LGBTIQA+ community and those from socially deprived settings, were the most likely to have experienced symptoms in the previous year (Stats New Zealand 2022). What we can conclude from the available data is that those who are significantly impacted by mental illness are among the most vulnerable people in our communities.

It is important to acknowledge that the mental health continuum described in this chapter is an attempt to simplify exceptionally complex human phenomena. Providing simple models of understanding can be both useful and detrimental, depending on how they are applied. The reality is that people's emotional and psychological experiences are in a constant state of change as they react to life experiences, thereby affecting their social functioning. In line with this understanding, the statement is often made that "no one has absolute health" or is "completely normal". Contrary to this, however, when a person is described as experiencing mental illness, they tend to be described as either mentally ill or not; that is, the person is identified as having a specific set of symptoms and is therefore labelled as having a specific clinical condition. It is helpful to consider that although population surveys identify the proportion of the population experiencing mental illness in the course of a year, the individuals making up that proportion change from year to year, with people moving out of or into the group identified as experiencing mental illness. A binary distinction between mental health and illness, however, is overly simplistic because it fails to address the range of human experiences of everyday life. In the end, mental health and illness are complex social constructs that vary in each society and cultural group as we attempt to describe differences we perceive in life experiences.

PERSONAL PERSPECTIVES
Consumer's Story 3.1 Part 3: Mary

Mental Illness

I can't point to one particular reason, but by my early 20s I was really struggling. I had moved away to try out for a career in fashion and the arts, but unluckily experienced some medium-term physical health problems. As a consequence, I had to move back home where work was scarce other than casual and low paid hospitality jobs. Living at home was stressful and there were lots of arguments. We all loved each other, but just couldn't live in the same house together. I really needed to live independently, so moved out as soon as I could, but that just created a new set of problems. I was in perpetual financial stress having inconsistent work but consistent bills for rent, car and phone etc. I could feel my levels of anxiety really begin to rise, so that I felt uneasy most days and was arguing with housemates. Around the same time, I kept bumping into people I had gone to school with and came to realise I had buried a lot of trauma, especially over the physical assaults I had experienced at school. There seemed to be no happiness in my life. I remember thinking that just 18 months earlier I was living in the city, dreaming of a career and feeling positive about myself. I withdrew and the smaller my world became, the more depressed I became until I was not even getting out of bed for days on end. Suicide seemed like a realistic solution to a pretty empty life that I could not see an end to. It took all my energy simply not to kill myself.

PERSONAL PERSPECTIVES
Consumer's Story 3.2 Part 3: Jarrad

Mental Illness

By age 17 my anxieties about social interactions became very pronounced. From age 16 to 18 there was a lot of added pressure to go out socially, which would make me anxious and fearful of experiencing further panic. I cared very little for academic or social pursuits; every day presented a difficulty just to get through without having a full-blown panic attack.

I had been missing school, missing assessments and avoiding going to the doctor's … Eventually something had to give, and that time came halfway through Year 11. I attended a mental health service where I was diagnosed with social phobia and, on reflection, I suppose it was at that point that society labelled me with a mental illness.

Eventually the school decided that I had missed too many days and would be unable to complete the academic year and progress to Year 12. It was not a great shock to me or my family, but we didn't really have any plan for what to do for the next 6 months and how to use the time productively. My family was under the impression that it just meant I would return the next year and do the year over again.

I spent the next 6 months in my bedroom at home with little to no engagement with the world, including my family. The only times I would leave my room would be to go to the bathroom or to eat. Rather than attend the dinner table for meals like the rest of my siblings, I would instead leave my room to collect a plate of food then return to my room to eat. It was no way to live.

Looking back, I view my life in those days as akin to a mouse scurrying from the safety of its dark crevice to fill its stomach, depending on the guise of night or its own agility and low profile, so as not to be disturbed by unwanted guests. The mouse is concerned not to cross paths with the family pet or a conveniently placed piece of food in the jaws of a trap. For me, I was trying to avoid crossing paths with members of my family and the anxieties that such interactions could cause. I had to avoid what often felt like a trap (the dinner table), which, to me, seemed like an attempt to be lured into social interaction by food.

Working with People who Experience Mental Health Distress

As discussed in Chapter 2, nursing care for people who experience mental ill health needs to be both recovery-oriented and trauma-informed. There are national and multiple state and territory recovery guiding policies and frameworks, as well as a range of non-government organisations, both in Australia and internationally (Gyamfi et al 2022). In essence, these policies and frameworks articulate that in order to be helpful to people with mental health difficulties, nurses and other health professionals need to:
- use language that communicates hope and optimism
- see *the person* you are working with – not "a patient" or diagnostic label
- work in partnership with the person to reach their identified goals
- help mitigate the sociological impacts on mental health and wellbeing.

Although not as well established as recovery approaches, trauma-informed care helps define and shape best practice in contemporary mental health nursing care, as well as the future delivery of mental health services. As for "recovery", a number of trauma-informed care frameworks and guidelines exist. Some of these inform how entire services should be structured, while others direct nurses on how to best interact with consumers within therapeutic relationships. Importantly, trauma-informed care and recovery approaches are not two different or competing guides to best nursing practice in mental health contexts. Rather, together they collectively guide the nurse on how to work effectively alongside people experiencing mental health challenges (Agency for Clinical Innovation 2022). While not exhaustive, key features of a trauma-informed approach for nurses include:

- working from a strength-based rather than an illness approach to care
- knowing that the person you are working with has trauma history and helping to build a sense of safety when working with them
- co-constructing care plans with the person and their loved ones
- communicating that you value and respect the person (Isobel et al 2021).

What should be becoming apparent is that working in mental health is an evidence-based and highly inter-personal endeavour. Rather than using nursing instruments, such as thermometers and blood pressure monitors, or focusing on assessing levels of consciousness and pain, mental health nursing work is deeply relational. Where nurses work in partnership and alongside individuals drawing from recovery and trauma-informed principles, they will be actively helping the person move closer to wellbeing.

Work in Partnership-Based Relationships

We know relationships are fundamentally important, from our earliest attachment experiences, for our emotional, social and physical wellbeing. Research on the outcomes of psychotherapy has consistently found that the "non-specifics of psychotherapy" (genuineness, empathy, warmth, positive regard, flexibility and the therapeutic alliance) are the most important factors in determining outcome (Cuijpers et al 2019).

When the therapeutic relationship and client factors are considered, the importance of working in partnership and considering the person's perspective of what is helpful appears to be more important than what the nurse believes might work. Research shows that partnership-based relationships are key to the transformation needed in recovery, and that patients and their supporters want nurses to have the capabilities to build and maintain therapeutic relationships. In a recent Australian study, consumers reported wanting nurses to be self-aware, calm and compassionate, as well to be able to listen effectively, communicate empathy and build relationships (Hurley et al 2022). This relational focus of effective mental health nursing directs the nurse to identify that consumers have strengths, talents and confidence, as well as opportunity for personal growth (Pullman et al 2023), rather than be focused on the illness, to the exclusion of the person experiencing the illness.

Although still in need of full implementation, contemporary and evidence-based mental health practice is increasingly informed by the expertise of those who have experienced mental health challenges. Where nurses draw from this expertise to guide their practice as clinicians and in informing therapeutic relationships, the outcomes are better for all (Happell et al 2022). The evidence emerging from lived experience expertise reflects recovery and trauma-informed care principles, and puts high value on nurses forming respectful therapeutic relationships with consumers. People with lived experience of mental ill health can be key supports for each other in terms of recovery, self-help and responsibility. This includes nurses who have lived experience of mental illness (Oates et al 2018). Sharing experiences and stories of overcoming with others who have had similar experiences can be powerful, because people learn they are not alone in their experience, that there is hope and that there are many different options and opportunities for recovery that may be helpful. Within Australia and New Zealand, consumer organisations provide advice, advocacy, support and service delivery; and many other organisations that provide broader supports operate at the local community level. There are also a growing number of peer workers and peer-run services emerging. Several alternative groups have been established to support those consumers who hold firmly to their experiences, such as voice-hearing groups and groups to support people to explore unusual beliefs without having to label their experiences in professional jargon.

PERSONAL PERSPECTIVES

Consumer's Story 3.1 Part 4: Mary

Experiencing Recovery

I still have weeks where I am incredibly depressed and life's challenges simply overwhelm me, but I know I have things to live for. I consider myself as being on a recovery journey. I have bad weeks, yeah, but suicide is not an option. I know I have depression and have also been diagnosed with attention deficient hyperactive disorder and low-level autism, but I also know what I am good at. I am focused and creative and have been developing social programs to help people with disability. I am super proud, I just started my first-ever permanent job. It's been a long journey.

PERSONAL PERSPECTIVES

Consumer's Story 3.2 Part 4: Jarrad

Therapeutic Relationships for Recovery

Things really started to change for me when I was referred to a local Headspace youth centre. Rather than a psychologist, I was given an appointment with a mental health nurse practitioner.

Unlike other clinicians I had seen, the nurse didn't ask me what was wrong and how he could help straightaway; he seemed to realise that that approach was never going to work with me. I had sat through many appointments with psychologists where I just stared at the ground incommunicado. I was crying and I remember the nurse reaching out without delving into anything too personal. I was wearing a black New Zealand rugby jersey and at that first appointment after receiving some brief information from my mother and asking her to leave the two of us in the room alone, the nurse began with some friendly banter about the Australian and New Zealand rugby team, which proved an easy way to get me to interact. Rather than the relationship with the mental health nurse practitioner forming as "expert and patient", it was almost like "teacher and student". He taught me that my experiences were not uncommon and that they could be explained with reference to my body, brain, and various biological and social interactions I had been having. A kind of partnership developed between us where I had real input into my own care. There were times when I would suggest a way to move forwards because I had that insight into his mindset as well as my own. At times I would disagree with his perspective and recommendations because I knew they wouldn't work for me. And there were times where he would suggest an approach that I would disagree with because it made me uncomfortable, but, based on my mindset, he knew that it was the right direction. The chance to negotiate in a kind of team as I sought to recover led to far better outcomes than previous services, which had felt very prescriptive. This relationship was a catalyst for significant progress on the social side of things and also in terms of my longer term goals. I ended up entering Sydney University through a mature entry scheme where I completed a short course for a year in preparation for entering a bachelor's degree.

PERSPECTIVES IN PRACTICE

Nurse's Story 3.1: Pamela

Sarah, a 22-year-old university student, was brought in for involuntary admission after having walked in front of traffic, unable to explain what had happened or to communicate what she was thinking or feeling. Sarah had been sexually assaulted the previous year and more recently had witnessed a woman falling in front of a train. She had also recently experienced sleeplessness and poor appetite, could not study and had great fears about herself and her family members dying. She had a very close and loving relationship with her parents and her twin brother.

Using principles of recovery-informed care, the nurse took considerable time to assist Sarah in establishing a sense of safety and control in the inpatient environment. This was achieved by allowing her family members to stay with her until she went to sleep. This involved the nurse negotiating for the hospital's visiting policy to be interpreted more flexibly, as well as arranging with other staff to spend as long with Sarah as she required to establish a sense of safety.

Sarah had difficulty talking directly with the nurse, but talking with family members in Sarah's presence about their lives, their strengths as a family and how they had supported each other through difficult times was an approach that seemed to permit Sarah to calm herself. Eventually she was able to communicate what her family could do to help her feel in control. She was able to make arrangements for the next day with her family and asked for her belongings to be brought into the hospital and for friends to be contacted. Family members were able to tell stories of times they had overcome problems and the strengths they all brought to support each other. Sarah's admission was very brief, and she reported feeling that the nurse and her family were encouraging, reminding her of the resources she had in her family and friends, and how they were there to support her. She appreciated the time the nurse took to patiently wait for her to be able to communicate.

CRITICAL THINKING EXERCISE 3.1

- Develop a concept map that answers the question: How do people who are mentally well/healthy become mentally ill?
- Now develop a concept map that answers the question: How do people who experience mental illness become mentally well/healthy?

- Are there similarities between the two maps? What are the differences?
- What do these concept maps suggest about mental health and illness?
- What do these concept maps suggest about the maintenance of mental wellbeing?

CHAPTER SUMMARY

This chapter has provided a platform on which you can continue to build your understanding of the continuum of mental health and illness. You now have a beginning understanding of the long-lasting impact of trauma on a person's development and the ways in which this may influence their response to difficulties over their lifetime. Mental distress is a part of the human experience: it may vary in severity, but it will happen to all of us at times. The journey of healing and recovery is salient for everyone. There is a need to talk about recovery in more humane terms because it is not something that happens to "the other" – we are all vulnerable to mental distress under certain circumstances. Nurses need to be with people in this humane context rather than in a context of pathology, difference and a reductionist focus on symptoms and diagnosis (Lakeman et al 2020).

We encourage you to reflect on how the principles of mental health practice are fundamental to all nursing practice, regardless of setting. We hope we have encouraged you to think about how you can participate more fully in your practice by developing your awareness of the complexities and realities of the context in which practice occurs. More specifically, we hope you appreciate how your attitudes, values and beliefs play a crucial role in your everyday practice.

Mental health nursing practice is influenced by an ever-evolving knowledge base; hence, the principles informed by this knowledge base continue to change and to evolve. Practice is time- and context-specific, making the ability to tolerate and incorporate change vital. Consequently, the way you think about your practice will be continually influenced by your developing self-awareness, your incorporation of new ideas into practice as your professional and personal experiences increase. The primary focus of mental health nursing practice is people with lived experience of mental health challenges. Nurses can help facilitate recovery by working in trauma-informed partnership with consumers to help them realise their potential and tap into a wide range of community resources and supports, of which mental health services are just one. Just as importantly, we hope you find the experience of mental health nursing as rewarding as we have.

REVIEW QUESTIONS

Clinical nursing work of all types is an interpersonal undertaking that utilises the self in relationship with the person in order to improve their health; we bring our knowledge and our emotions into all those endeavours. We often forget the role our emotions play in achieving better clinical outcomes, better team work between nurses and better health for the nurse. Ask students to reflect and write down as many emotions as they can recall over the last 24-hour period. When they are done, get them to share the list and everyone can add emotions they had not originally thought of. Finally, have them classify the feelings as either unhelpful or helpful for their own wellbeing or the wellbeing of others. The record for most emotions listed by a nurse in this exercise is 21!

USEFUL WEBSITES

Adverse Childhood Events
https://acestoohigh.com/aces-101/

General Mental Health Sites
Mental Health Australia: mhaustralia.org/about-us
Multicultural Mental Health: embracementalhealth.org.au
National Mental Health Commission: www.mentalhealthcommission.gov.au/
World Health Organization. Mental Health: www.who.int/news-room/facts-in-pictures/detail/mental-health

Lived Experience Experts
Lived experience: www.betterhealth.vic.gov.au/amy-corcoran-lived-experience-worker-melbourne
NSW Mental Health Commission: Lived experience (contains consumer stories): nswmentalhealthcommission.com.au/lived-experience

Mental Health Nursing
Australian College of Mental Health Nurses. Standards of Practice: www.acmhn.org/common/Uploaded%20files/PDFs/Best%20practice/standards_2010_web.pdf
New Zealand College of Mental Health Nurses: https://nzcmhn.org.nz

Wellbeing
www.mentalhealth.org.uk/our-work/research/our-top-tips-connecting-nature-improve-your-mental-health

REFERENCES

Agency for Clinical Innovation, 2022. Trauma-informed care in mental health services across NSW: A framework for change. Online. Available at: https://aci.health.nsw.gov.au/networks/mental-health/trauma-informed-care

Australian Institute of Health and Welfare (AIHW), 2022. Mental health: prevalence and impact of mental illness. Online. Available at: www.aihw.gov.au/reports/mental-health-services/mental-health#Common

Bienertova-Vasku, J., Lenart, P., & Scheringer, M. 2020. Eustress and distress: neither good nor bad, but rather the same? BioEssays, 42(7). Online. Available at: https://doi.org/10.1002/bies.201900238

Bishop, J., Shpaner, M., Kubicki, A., & Naylor, M. 2021. Structural Neuroplasticity Following Cognitive Behavioral Therapy for the Treatment of Chronic Musculoskeletal Pain: A Randomized Controlled Trial with Secondary MRI Outcomes. medRxiv. Online. Available at: www.medrxiv.org/content/10.1101/2021.07.13.21260466v1.full.pdf

Caplan, G. 1964. Principles of preventive psychiatry. Basic Books, New York.

Chen, S.P., Chang, W.P., & Stuart, H. 2020. Self-reflection and screening mental health on Canadian campuses: validation of the mental health continuum model. BMC Psychol, 8(1), 1–8.

Craig, C., Hiskey, S., & Spector, A. 2020. Compassion focused therapy: A systematic review of its effectiveness and acceptability in clinical populations. Expert Rev Neurotherapeutics, 20(4), 385–400.

Cuijpers, P., Reijnders, M., & Huibers, M.J. 2019. The role of common factors in psychotherapy outcomes. Ann Rev Clin Psychol, 15(1), 207–231.

Department of Health and Ageing. 2022. About mental health. Online. Available at: www.health.gov.au/health-topics/mental-health-and-suicide-prevention/about-mental-health

Everly, G. S., & Lating, J. M. 2019. The anatomy and physiology of the human stress response. In: Everly, G.S., & Lating, J.M. (eds). A Clinical Guide to the Treatment of the Human Stress Response. Springer, New York, NY.

Gee, D.G. 2021. Early-life trauma and resilience: Insights from developmental neuroscience for policy. Biolog Psychiatry: Cogn Neurosci Neuroimag, 6(2), 141–143.

Goldfarb, E.V., Tompary, A., Davachi, L., et al., 2019. Acute stress throughout the memory cycle: Diverging effects on associative and item memory. J Exp Psychol Gen, 148(1), 13.

Gyamfi, N., Bhullar, N., Islam, M.S., & Usher, K. 2022. Models and frameworks of mental health recovery: A scoping review of the available literature. J Ment Health, 1–13.

Happell, B., Warner, T., Waks, S., O'Donovan, A., Manning, F. et al., 2022. Something special, something unique: Perspectives of experts by experience in mental health nursing education on their contribution. J Psychiat Ment Health Nurs, 29(2), 346–358.

Health Direct 2021. Mental illness. Online. Available at: www.healthdirect.gov.au/mental-illness

Hurley, J., Foster, K, Campbell, K., Edin, V. Hazelton, M. et al., 2023. Mental health nursing capability development: Perspectives of consumers and supporters. Int J Ment Health Nurs, 32, 172–175.

Hurley, J., Lakeman, R., Linsley, P., McKenna-Lawson, S., & Ramsay, M. 2022. Utilizing the mental health nursing workforce: A scoping review of mental health nursing clinical roles and identities. Int J Ment Health Nurs, Online. doi.org/10.1111/inm.12983

Isobel, S., Wilson, A., Gill, K., & Howe, D. 2021. What would a trauma-informed mental health service look like? Perspectives of people who access services. Int J Ment Health Nurs, 30(2), 495–505.

Kanel, K. 2019. A Guide to Crisis Intervention, 6th ed. Brookes/Cole, CA.

Kendler, K.S. 2020. Philippe Pinel and the foundations of modern psychiatric nosology. Psychol Med, 50(16), 2667–2672.

Lakeman, R., Cashin, A., Hurley, J., & Ryan, T. 2020. The psychotherapeutic practice and potential of mental health nurses: An Australian survey. Aust Health Rev, 44(6), 916–923.

Leggatt, M. 2022. DSM: A history of psychiatry's bible by Allan V. Horwitz. Health Hist, 24(1), 144–148.

Loxton, D., Forder, P.M., Cavenagh, D., Townsend, N., Holliday, E., et al., 2021. The impact of adverse childhood experiences on the health and health behaviors of young Australian women. Child Abuse Neglect, 111, 104771.

Milne-Smith, A. 2022. Gender and madness in nineteenth-century Britain. History Compass, e12754.

Oates, J. 2018. Interwoven histories: Mental health nurses with experience of mental illness, qualitative findings from a mixed methods study. Int J Ment Health Nurs, 27(5), 1383–1391.

Pullman, J., Santangelo, P., Molloy, L., & Campbell, S. 2023. Impact of strengths model training and supervision on the therapeutic practice of Australian mental health clinicians. Int J Ment Health Nurs, 32(1), 236–244.

Rosenberg, S., Hickie, I. 2019. No gold medals: assessing Australia's international mental health performance. Australas Psychiat, 27(1), 36–40.

Sax Institute. 2020. Evidence check: Mental wellbeing risk and protective factors. Online. Available at: www.vichealth.vic.gov.au/sites/default/files/VicHealth-Attachment-1—-Evidence-review-of-risk—protective-factors.pdf

Smith, P.J., & Merwin, R.M. 2021. The role of exercise in management of mental health disorders: An integrative review. Ann Rev Med, 72, 45.

Sorgente, A., Zambelli, M., Tagliabue, S., & Lanz, M. 2021. The comprehensive inventory of thriving: A systematic review of published validation studies and a replication study. Current Psychology, 42, 7920–7932.

Stats New Zealand. 2022. New Zealanders' mental wellbeing declines. Online. Available at: www.stats.govt.nz/news/new-zealanders-mental-wellbeing-declines

Wilson, A., Hurley, J., Hutchinson M. & Lakeman, R. 2023. Trauma-informed care in acute mental health units through the lifeworld of mental health nurses: A phenomenological study. Int J Ment Health Nurs, 32 (3), 829–838.

World Health Organization (WHO), 2022. Mental health: Strengthening our response. Online. Available at: www.who.int/news-room/fact-sheets/detail/mental-health-strengthening-our-response

4

Safety in Care, Safety at Work

Scott Brunero and Scott Lamont

KEY POINTS

- Creating safety in care and a safe work environment is essential in the context of mental health.
- Challenges to safe care and work can occur in the context of staff knowledge, skills and attitudes, and in consumer distress, anxiety and past experiences of mental health care.
- Behaviours associated with a safe caring and work environment include empathy, compassion, reflective practice, high-level

- de-escalation skills, violence prevention, behavioural risk assessment and management.
- Nurses need to practise reflectively and be mindful of their own behaviour.

KEY TERMS

Difficult behaviour
Empathy
Legal issues
Limit setting

Manipulation
Person-centred care
Reflection
Risk analysis

Safe care
Safe work
Self-harm
Trauma

LEARNING OUTCOMES

The material in this chapter will assist you to:
- develop and maintain therapeutic relationships with consumers
- understand nursing staff, consumer and environmental factors contributing to safety in care and safety at work
- understand risk in the context of safe care and work

- understand general principles of creating a safe care and work environment
- identify specific approaches to managing behaviour that challenges a safe care and work environment.

INTRODUCTION

The nurse–consumer relationship is central to nursing care. Nurses, in general, are in continuous and direct contact with consumers, and, as such, spend extended periods of time with them. Continuous contact places nurses in a unique position to develop therapeutic relationships with consumers through processes of collaboration, inclusiveness, mutuality and respect. However, there may be times when the relationship nurses have with consumers is tested, placing nurses in a difficult position and facing behaviours that challenge safe care and work (Gerace et al 2020; Stein-Parbury 2021).

Behaviours that challenge safe care and work include aggression, manipulation, self-harm, suicide and psychosis-related behaviour. These types of behaviour occur in inpatient units, community settings, emergency departments (EDs), general hospitals and primary care settings. Within the social ecological model that underpins this book, the nurse and consumer are engaged in a partnership which is informed by the nurse's knowledge skills and attitudes, and is situated within a context of social determinants of health.

This chapter will help you to engage in healthy relationships with consumers and to understand the most common types of behaviour that challenge safe care and work encountered by nurses. It will make you more aware of the antecedents of challenging behaviour, help you to recognise when they are present and guide you in developing responses and strategies. Finally, it will help you understand what people mean when they engage in these behaviours and become self-aware regarding your own emotions and care needs.

Types of Behaviour that Challenge Safety in Care and Safety at Work

A key skill of mental health nurses is to interpret and understand consumers with high levels of distress, to assist them in their navigation of healthcare systems, to monitor and manage their own distress and to manage conflict in interpersonal relationships (Stein-Parbury 2021). Knowing whether behaviour is a challenge or not can be subjective and individual; it may depend on the skill of the nurse or the social setting the nurse is in. Commonly encountered behaviours that challenge safe care and work reported in the literature include:
- aggression (verbal and physical threats, shouting, conflict, non-adherence, absconding)
- manipulation ("splitting" or demanding attention or that special conditions are met)
- self-harm and suicidal behaviour (cutting, ingesting poisons, overdose).

✳ HISTORICAL ANECDOTE 4.1
Gone Battie?

William Battie (1703–1776) was a pioneer in the care of mental health patients. As a physician of high repute with a scientific background and distinguished social position, he helped to turn mental health care into a respectable medical specialty. While observing patients, Battie noted that some would recover without treatment or only after treatment had been stopped. This observation led him to consider the powerful therapeutic effects of a caring environment. He was one of England's first public figures to recognise that carers in "mental asylums" needed to be specially selected and trained. Considering all the good he did for people with mental health problems, it is ironic that the modern derogatory term "gone batty" was derived from his name!

Read More About It
Bynum, W.F. 1974. Rationales for therapy in British psychiatry: 1780–1835. Medical History, 18(4), 317–334.

These behaviours are not mutually exclusive – they may occur in combination, or all at once, frequently or infrequently, and can be seen across the diagnostic groups in mental health settings. Nurses working within the mental health setting will experience some or a range of these behaviours in the course of their clinical practice. Responding requires a wide range of nursing skills. It is therefore essential to understand the social context and circumstances of behaviours that nurses find challenging (Cutler et al 2021).

UNDERSTANDING THE CONTEXT OF SAFETY IN CARE AND SAFETY AT WORK

An understanding of the social context within which safe care and work occurs is essential in identifying the numerous factors that precede and influence safety. For example, staff and consumers often have different perceptions of why a safe work environment is challenged; while staff may cite consumer factors, consumers may cite staff factors. The reality is that a range of socially determined factors, including staff, consumer, environmental, cross-cultural and social factors, act as precipitants that can challenge a safe care and work environment (Cutler et al 2020; SICSAW 2019).

Staff Factors

A safe care and work environment often occurs as a result of what we as nurses do, or, in some circumstances, don't do. We may not always be conscious of how we are perceived by consumers, or how our behaviour influences the behaviour of consumers. Our knowledge, skills and attitudes and subsequent behaviours become important aspects of preventing, mitigating and managing how we deliver care.

Developing therapeutic relationships with consumers is essential in maintaining safety at work. This requires commitment from you as a nurse to engage purposefully with consumers in a person-centred manner: developing intimate knowledge of the consumer as a person; showing respect and being courteous; actively listening to concerns, fears and frustrations; responding in an empathic way; looking for meaning behind the behaviour (anger is directed at me, but seems to be coming from being locked up in hospital!); and communicating a genuine desire to help. Nurses who are unable or unwilling to facilitate effective therapeutic relationships are likely to encounter difficulties in delivering care (Stein-Parbury 2021).

Developing therapeutic relationships can be easier said than done and may be compromised by a range of personal factors. For example, nurses may have personal issues that compromise their ability to engage therapeutically. This includes the nurse's own mental health and personality style, current stressors in the nurse's life, previous experience (or inexperience), tiredness and illness. Any of these factors can contribute to an interaction style that leads to a perception that nurses are not interested or are simply ignoring the needs of consumers. Furthermore, nurses who are impatient, controlling, authoritarian or coercive in their interactions with consumers are less likely to build positive relationships and to achieve desirable outcomes in care (Kwame & Petrucka 2020).

Consumer Factors

Mental illness and disorders can influence a consumer's ability to engage purposefully in the healthcare that nurses provide. Such conditions include: psychotic disorders; adjustment disorders; mood, anxiety and personality disorders; organic disorders; drug and alcohol intoxication or withdrawal; intellectual disability; and brain injury. Other issues which can make engagement difficult include discrimination, being stigmatised or marginalised; and experiences of trauma or trauma-related mental health care.

A range of experiences associated with psychotic disorders may increase the likelihood of difficulties with consumers engaging in safe care delivery. These experiences can include thought disorder, hallucinations and delusions – in particular, where consumers may be paranoid, suspicious, fearful or frightened. Consumers who are cognitively compromised may present with anxiety, confusion and disorientation. Behaviours that challenge accepting care have been linked to the increased energy, disinhibition and irritability associated with mood disorders (mania), making care delivery challenging. This may lead to frustration, helplessness or catastrophic thinking and to difficulties engaging with consumers. Consumers with a low mood typically seen in depressive disorder may have difficulty engaging in their own self-care and other daily activities, which may require constant prompting from the nurse. Consumers at risk of self-harm behaviours may need close monitoring and observations of behaviour, with constant efforts to engage in dialogue. Consumers with personality vulnerabilities may have a heightened perception of rejection or humiliation, particularly when healthcare concerns or requests are ignored or dismissed. Some consumers may have poor impulse control as a feature of their personality, while consumers with narcissistic personality styles may present with excessive demands or entitlement of nurses' time. Factors such as fatigue, pain and physical comorbidities influence consumers' quality of life and subsequently their psychological and emotional wellbeing.

If consumers are not involved in planning and discussions about their care, they will be unaware of what is expected of them. Mental health problems often adversely influence a person's control over aspects of their life; therefore, processes of partnership, inclusion and engagement can help mitigate some of the consumer factors mentioned in this section.

Environmental Factors

Health staff in general are often unaware of the effect of the environment on the wellbeing of consumers. Environmental factors become part of our contextual understanding of a safe workplace. However, the physical environment should not be viewed in isolation from system or operational aspects, such as the infrastructure, policies and procedures that govern its operation. Coercive or restrictive processes that limit inclusion and choice for consumers, suboptimal communication with unclear care plans, and staff caught in a reactive bind because of busy workloads and competing systemic demands, are likely to experience increased frustration.

Many aspects of the environments in which nurses work are beyond our control: we may practise in ageing facilities that are no longer commensurate with modern care, and capital works funding may be scarce in relation to maintenance, improvement and renovation. Frustration, high expressed emotion and anger are more likely to be present in poorly structured environments that are aesthetically unappealing, noisy and crowded, too hot/too cold, devoid of natural light and lacking in private space (dormitories versus single rooms) (Cutler et al 2021). There is a need to balance the design of inpatient wards so as not to overstimulate aroused or agitated consumers while not understimulating withdrawn or depressed consumers. Person-centred design, using the aforementioned attributes, can lead to better cognitive, motivational and emotive processes in both consumers and staff. Sensory modulation or using specific equipment and modifying the physical and social environment have been shown to assist consumers in reducing their high expressed emotions (Wright et al 2020).

Cultural Factors

Diverse cultures have behavioural and communication nuances that may be interpreted variously by nurses from different cultural backgrounds. Behaviours that appear challenging within one culture may be acceptable within another. Therefore, the need to be culturally aware has significant implications for nurses in the context of safe care and work (Kaihlanen et al 2019). In some Asian societies, it is not culturally appropriate to show overt emotional reactions in public, and in some Arab cultures, women may not be allowed in the same room as a man unless accompanied by a relative. Both situations, if poorly managed by nurses, may be precursors to a conflicted work environment. Indigenous Australians' experience of mental health services, and in particular their experience of seclusion, suggests that there is a need for social and cultural factors to be considered when engaging in these practices (Barr et al 2022). Indigenous Australians may have had historical traumatic experiences of governmental control and coercion and their perception of care may be influenced by this. Nurses need to be aware of their own cultural biases and potential misconceptions and tendencies to subscribe to myths about particular cultural groups. Providing culturally congruent care may give the nurse an opportunity to understand why someone is behaving the way they are, to prevent the behaviour from escalating, and to gain the knowledge to approach the behaviour with confidence. Factors related to cultural and gender identity are further explored in Chapter 2. Specific factors related to Australian and New Zealand Indigenous peoples are discussed in chapters 6 and 7.

Social Factors

Mental illness in our society is impacted by the media and public perceptions, and this has resulted in consumers with mental illness being labelled as at risk, dangerous, difficult, absconders and/or frequent flyers. The power of these negative labels can influence how we as professionals engage with people. When labels are attributed to people, they can consequently be adopted by them, and individuals may therefore engage in behaviours that perpetuate these labels (Foster et al 2019; Volkow et al 2021). As nurses, we must be mindful of the language we use when relating to consumers and how we engage with them, by not proliferating negative labels relating to mental illness that exist more broadly in society.

MODELS OF CARE

Care cultures that are risk-focused, coercive or restrictive in nature are likely to lead to negative interpersonal relationships and dynamics. An awareness of your own identity and practice within such cultures is essential to achieving optimum care outcomes (Cutler et al 2020; Cutler et al 2021). Consumer-focused frameworks adopt strengths-based approaches to care. Models underpinned by such a framework seek to actively involve consumers as partners in all aspects of care provision and not as passive recipients of care. Thus, shared decision-making and consumer-led decision-making enhance goal planning, care options and subsequent outcomes (Horgan et al 2021).

Consumer-focused models of care operate on the premise that only consumers can understand the real experience and journey of being a consumer. Therefore, consumers are the key stakeholders in planning and discussions about care and so need to be active, valued and empowered throughout. Studies exploring strengths-based approaches have identified that these approaches are associated with improvements in quality-of-life indicators, confidence, self-esteem, self-advocacy and self-care. Strengths-based approaches unsurprisingly focus on strengths, abilities and empowerment – a shift from traditional problem-based care approaches, which largely ignore strengths and positive abilities that help fulfil wellbeing. Strengths-based approaches result in more purposeful engagement with consumers, help maintain a sense of control over their decision-making and lead to more positive experiences of care.

There are various specific consumer-focused models:

- The **recovery model** (or recovery approach) adopts an approach whereby the consumer's potential for recovery is paramount and supported by a network of personal and professional relationships. Recovery has less of an emphasis on clinical outcomes and instead focuses on the consumer's personal journey, instilling and maintaining hope, a positive sense of self and meaning, a secure base and social inclusion within a paradigm of empowerment and flourishing (Gyamfi et al 2020).
- The **tidal model** focuses on the ebb and flow of personal human experience and aims to empower consumers in their own recovery, with an emphasis on the power of their own self and wisdom, as opposed to health professionals directing this (Barker 2001; Turgut et al 2020).
- **Solution-focused (brief) therapy** is a goal-directed psychotherapeutic partnership that focuses on what consumers want to achieve in the here and now and in the future. While the relevance of past experience is not ignored, it is not an emphasis or focal point of care (Smith & Macduff 2017).
- **Trauma-informed care** adopts the principle that only a consumer who has experienced trauma can truly understand the journey of healing. The unique skills, attributes and resilience that have enabled trauma survivors to survive are emphasised within a strengths-based framework and supported by health professionals (Palfrey et al 2019).

These consumer-focused frameworks can be adopted as collaborative models of care or as individual philosophical frameworks for interpersonal relationships with consumers. Nurses must be mindful that to engage purposefully with consumers, they must engage in activities that promote their own self-care.

Case study 4.1, by Irene Gallagher, reflects the importance of looking beyond the external behaviour. Note the interactions between the people in Irene's story, how the nurse moved beyond the initial "labels" given to the consumer, and how the nurse was able to use objects in the environment to develop a social bond or therapeutic rapport. Adaptive and flexible frameworks of care will enhance relationships with individual consumers.

CASE STUDY 4.1: Irene Gallagher
The Importance of Therapeutic Engagement

As a peer worker, I place great value on supporting a person with lived experience of mental distress with their own personal recovery journey, which may include fostering hope, self-determination, choice, and intrinsically supporting them to connect with others in developing trusting relationships. Some may proclaim this to be the essence of the peer-to-peer relationship as mutuality and reciprocity. Having said this, I don't see that fostering relationships which support an individual's personal recovery journey as belonging solely to peer workers; in fact, I have both personal experience as well as having been witness to seeing the wonderful connections that begin and unravel in the therapeutic relationship.

One such therapeutic engagement which comes to mind is a client who had been labelled by the system as challenging and hard to engage with – lost in their own world of what the medical profession would label as "delusional". This individual was in fact difficult to engage with, loud and verbally abusive to everyone around them. No one wanted to engage with this person, staff or clients, for fear of verbal backlash or perhaps a fear of not knowing what approach to use with someone in this situation.

However, one nurse chose to find a way of working with and connecting with this person on some different level. Curiously, I asked the nurse how she had established these connections, how was it that she was able to communicate and work with this person? Interestingly, the nurse responded by noting that she had worked out that the client liked to have their hair brushed, and when the nurse brushed the client's hair, the client would come into "our" reality. From there, the two were able to communicate in a way that they were previously unable to. Similarly, the nurse discovered that a gentle touch on the client's forearm had a similar effect and they were able to have meaningful discussions, such as talking about the client's hopes and dreams for their future and what treatments worked and did not work for them during their hospitalisation.

Those around perhaps put this positive alliance down to luck; however, the reality was that this nurse had taken the time to connect with the client, to spend quality time getting to know the individual, using the therapeutic relationship to actively engage and involve the client in their own care. Time was taken to listen intently, to explore the client's values and what made meaning for them, while supporting the individual to participate in their recovery journey.

Engaging in reflective practice with the nurse supported how much the nurse had gained from working in this way and prioritising the development of the therapeutic relationship for all it holds: working from an empathic approach, developing rapport and trust, and approaching the collaborative work ahead as a team with mutual understanding and respect. Everyone has that connection waiting to be found – and in this scenario, one nurse found it.

SELF-PREPAREDNESS FOR CREATING SAFETY IN CARE AND SAFETY AT WORK

Professional Boundaries

Nurses are bound by professional practice guidelines through their nurse registration bodies. Professional boundaries can be thought of as the space between the professional's power and the consumer's vulnerability. This space needs to be observed and maintained to ensure a beneficial outcome for the consumer. Table 4.1 outlines some of the differences between social and professional relationships.

So, what occurs within professional relationships that makes a safe and effective practitioner? An expectation of the nurse is that they have a professional body of knowledge, skills and attitudes that can be used to improve the consumer's health status. The following elements could describe a poor professional relationship: cynicism, judgemental attitudes, personal intimacy, being patronising, developing dependency, showing favouritism, playing one person off against another ("splitting"), showing minimal care, neglect or punitiveness (Stein-Parbury 2021). Nurses need to emphasise creating safe, therapeutic relationships with consumers based on openness, collaboration, respect and trust.

Nurses' Self-Care

It may come as no surprise that for nurses to engage therapeutically in relationships with consumers, they must be aware of and take care of their own emotional and psychological wellbeing. The stressful nature of nursing in general is well recognised and may be more prominent when attempting to create a safe work environment (López-López et al 2019).

Being self-aware and being able to evaluate your own actions and behaviours will help you to engage therapeutically with consumers. This may be easier said than done, however, as we are often unaware of the emotional labour and stress that the competing demands involved in contemporary mental health care place upon us. Some individuals naturally engage in reflective thinking to enhance self-awareness, while others require some formal structure to engage in this practice. It may be that as mental health nursing is your chosen specialty, you have a natural tendency for critical thinking, challenge and reflection.

The following workload practices can help in maintaining psychological and emotional wellbeing: working collaboratively where the workload is shared and delegated appropriately; being honest and transparent about your limitations (we all have bad days), but also maintaining professional conduct; and engaging in more formal, structured processes of reflective practice and clinical supervision. Clinical supervision within mental health is a practice endorsed across all professional groups, particularly nursing. The process has a focus on personal and professional development in the context of safe and effective consumer care. Although there is a dearth of research within this area, attention to its effects and benefits is growing and is proposed as a key feature in reducing the emotional labour associated with nursing practice. Central to clinical supervision is the opportunity for protected "time out" from clinical activity spent with an experienced nurse, who supports and guides processes of reflection and structured discussion. Reflection involves processes of enlightenment as to what nurses do and how we behave. During these processes, the nurse may reflect on what they did, why they did it and implications for consumers, colleagues

TABLE 4.1 Differences Between Social and Professional Relationships

Social Relationships	Professional Relationships
Open-ended time period	Restricted to period of care
Personal choice	Restricted choice
Both parties' needs considered	Consumer's need predominant
Multipurpose	Primary purpose is care
Sympathy	Empathy
Confiding	Confidential
Tolerant to personal limit	Professional tolerance
Inconsistent	Consistent
Judgemental	Non-judgemental
Unstructured	Structured
Personal responsibility	Professional responsibility
Personal boundaries	Professional boundaries

and wider professional and ethical practice (Delgado et al 2020). There is a role for nurses to engage with each other about the emotions evoked in them: the more transparent we are about these emotions, the more adaptive and self-aware we become.

How Nurses Behave

As nurses, we need to be aware of our own expectations of consumers' behaviour. Having high levels of expectation that a consumer will change their behaviour completely and quickly, and/or express gratitude for your help may be unhelpful to you. How you respond can have a significant impact on the outcome of the strategies employed to help consumers change these behaviours. Unhelpful nursing responses include avoiding consumers and minimising issues. Such responses may be seen with consumers who are demanding of care, constantly approaching the nurse's office space or persistently phoning a nurse in a community setting. Taking the avoidance approach often leads the consumer to escalate their behaviour as they feel that their needs are not being met. While nurses may not want to encourage some behaviours, there is still a need to engage with the consumer. If you respond to anger from a consumer by being angry yourself or respond to manipulative behaviour by being punitive in return, these responses are unhelpful. Therefore, being aware of your own emotional responses to consumers is an integral part of creating a safe work environment (Delgado et al 2020).

How to Manage Your Own Emotions

In any relationship you will need to be able to make sense of and manage your own emotions and behaviour. The natural response we have, known as the "fight or flight response", is often evoked when people are threatening, angry and/or manipulative, resulting in an immediate natural response to defend yourself. Nurses should be aware that the fight or flight response is normal, and you should expect it to occur. Some of the physical signs that you may experience include:

- increased pulse rate and blood pressure
- shallow, rapid respirations
- muscular tension
- dry mouth
- excessive perspiration.

There is also a range of psychological symptoms that you may experience following a fight or flight response:

- irritability and impatience
- frequent ruminating, worry and anxiety
- moodiness
- feeling sad or upset
- poor concentration, memory lapses
- ambivalence and feeling overwhelmed, or unable to face even minor problems.

To assist you in managing your fight/flight response, a self-management plan can be helpful. For example, concentrating on your breathing or counting to five before you engage with someone may help you to respond in a calm and measured way. Inner dialogues are also suggested as a strategy for successfully approaching challenging situations. For example, if you approach a situation with a negative attitude that things are not going to go well, this will probably influence your behaviour and resulting outcome. Be aware of what you are telling yourself or thinking to yourself. Thinking the worst, or catastrophic thinking, can lead you to behave in a negative way (e.g. "This patient will never change" or "I can't nurse this patient anymore"). You can also take time out for a few minutes to reflect on your own behaviour: "Am I being too angry here?" or "Do I need to calm myself down before interacting with this consumer again?". In addition, conveying how you feel and reflecting on your behaviour with a colleague can be helpful (Simpson & Sawatzky 2020).

ORGANISATIONAL PREPAREDNESS FOR CREATING SAFETY IN CARE AND SAFETY AT WORK

Infrastructure and Governance

Organisational capacity building, which includes infrastructure, governance and training, is an integral component to organisations that are safe for all. Dedicated workplace violence positions and personnel (including consumers, work health and safety, clinicians and security services) will ensure a visible and coordinated approach to safety for all. Policy and guidance that incorporate zero tolerance approaches and emergency response procedures underpin effective practices relating to safety, as do quality and review processes at both local department and organisational levels. Assessing the climate of violence in a clinical specialty can enable the monitoring of violence prevalence and culture, while measuring the effectiveness of workplace violence prevention strategies (Brunero et al 2021b). See Table 4.2 for components of organisational readiness and effectiveness in maintaining safety for all. The checklist highlights key elements that can be used across different organisations (Lamont & Brunero 2018).

Education and Training

Violence prevention and management training content should seek to increase confidence, attitude and knowledge of nurses. Training components of workplace violence programs traditionally involve theoretical aspects of identifying and managing risk factors associated with violence, verbal de-escalation techniques, legal issues, breakaway techniques and restraint training. These training programs are often delivered face to face as they require the teaching of verbal and physical skills and often occur over several days (Lamont & Brunero 2018). Tabletop exercises have also been used to educate staff on violence prevention and management. Tabletop exercises are short (45 minute) "tabletop discussions" of a scenario typically seen in the workplace and focus on nurses talking through their response to a violent scenario in the context of their local workplace policies and processes (Brunero et al 2021b).

PRINCIPLES FOR ENGAGING CONSUMERS IN SAFE CARE

It is important to understand some general principles in creating safety in care and work (Beattie et al 2019; McAllister et al 2019).

Verbal Interactions

How we say things can often be more important than what we say. Using an appropriate tone of voice, the rate at which you talk, and the volume and pressure in your speech, can influence how you engage consumers. You need to make adjustments to the "how" of speaking. Ask yourself "Am I speaking loud enough?", "Am I too loud, and do I sound threatening?" You will need to fine-tune your tone of voice as the interaction with the consumer occurs, testing and retesting your approach. Linking your words with actions can give the consumer a sense that you are interested in engagement and can help maintain therapeutic rapport. Alternatively, if you show incongruence between your words and actions, the consumer and others may interpret this as you being untrustworthy and lacking authenticity.

Non-Verbal Interactions

Your non-verbal communication, how you hold yourself or behave, is an important aspect of engaging consumers. Through body language we constantly (and sometimes unconsciously) send and receive non-verbal signals. Awareness of the non-verbal signals you are sending may be particularly useful. Your words might convey one message, but the movements and gestures you make might convey another, potentially

TABLE 4.2   Workplace Violence Organisational Checklist

Workplace Violence Organisational Checklist	Yes	No
Governance		
1. Identify key stakeholders; hospital executive, nursing, medicine, allied health, occupational health/work health and safety, quality assurance, security services, police liaison, employee assistance program.		
2. Convene organisational workplace violence committee involving key stakeholders.		
3. Develop workplace violence guidance and emergency response protocol, which aligns with relevant national, state and local policy. This should include identifying a dedicated emergency response team for violent incidents.		
4. Locate workplace violence prevention and management within new staff orientation programs.		
5. Develop memorandum of understanding with external services (e.g. police) relating to response and liaison.		
Training		
1. Develop training capacity via attendance at workplace violence "Train the Trainer" programs.		
2. Implement training program of workplace violence workshops for relevant staff.		
3. Facilitate table top simulations (e.g. bi-monthly or quarterly) which reflect like–like violence scenarios. These help facilitate incident preparedness and effective response to escalating incidents.		
4. Implement "refresher" programs which incorporate key aspects of workplace violence workshops.		
Quality and Review		
1. Develop and implement a consistent, uniform approach to the assessment and management of violence risk across the organisation.		
2. Undertake violence prevention climate assessments prior to, during, and following interventions and programs of work.		
3. Implement audit systems which identify violent incident trends.		
4. Implement multidisciplinary review of workplace violent incidents.		
5. Incorporate violence risk into existing safety huddles.		
6. Undertake rigorous evaluation of workplace violence training and initiatives, via the use of validated instruments and qualitative inquiry.		

creating confusion, misunderstanding and an array of negative feelings. The following are some ways of non-verbally responding:

- While you are talking, try to be aware of how you are sitting or standing, the expression on your face and what your hands and legs are doing.
- Allow the consumer to determine the distance between yourself and them. This may help the consumer to feel some sense of control. Personal space or distance can vary according to cultural or personal nuances.
- Keeping a relaxed open posture with your hands visible at either waist height or below can make you appear less threatening.
- The way you make eye contact can help. It is helpful to make intermittent eye contact and to avoid prolonged staring.
- Using appropriate facial expressions for the situation can be important – seek a balance between smiling and looking concerned. Expressions of warmth and acceptance can help. Be mindful that your position, movements and gestures may need to vary depending on the clinical situation.

Being Flexible

Nursing requires the ability to be flexible and engage in different approaches. Nurses are often tempted to take control, when a more helpful approach is to consider how you can help the consumer to maintain or regain internal self-control – care versus control is a good mantra to keep in mind. You may be required to restructure requests and allow time for information to be processed. This requires qualities, such as being patient and empathic, as well as skills in redirecting and negotiating.

Active Listening

Mental health nurses use active listening skills in most of their daily work with consumers. Active listening shows that we are attending to someone's needs. The act of active listening starts a process of being empathic and may give you more time to formulate your response. Reflecting what the consumer is saying while taking a position of not offering advice but expressing acceptance without agreeing, may offer the consumer a more comfortable position to reflect on their behaviour. Active listening demonstrates the presence of empathy and helps consumers to acknowledge their emotions, while enabling consumers to talk about them as opposed to negatively acting upon them (Stein-Parbury 2021).

Empathy

A sense of openness can be developed by disclosing your concerns and issues with the consumer openly and honestly. Being empathic or entering into the feelings of the consumer and trying to appreciate their point of view gives the consumer a sense that you are acknowledging their concerns and trying to connect with them (Gerace 2020). Respecting different points of view does not mean you agree with them; for example, "I understand that you would like to visit your family tonight, and I can see that you are angry about not being able to do that". This position demonstrates that you can accept someone's experience, without the need to agree with what they may be asking for (Gerace 2020).

Assertiveness

Being assertive is a skill that requires careful consideration so as not to appear punitive or indeed aggressive. Being assertive may involve reflecting your own experience while simultaneously setting expectations about behaviour from others. This approach involves displaying high levels of empathy while setting clear limits or boundaries. The following are examples of assertiveness statements that demonstrate showing empathy and setting limits in a way that is non-judgemental and therefore humanistic:

- "You are speaking very loudly, and I am finding it hard to understand how I can help you."
- "You seem distressed and angry. Can we talk more when you are ready?"

Combining these assertiveness statements with statements such as "I realise you don't want to do this" and "I appreciate you are trying" can also be helpful. It is important to avoid argument, conflicting advice and long-winded explanations. Some situations may also require a firm and concise request about what needs to happen; for example:

- "I appreciate you want your visitors to stay after hours, but unfortunately it is hospital policy that they leave by 7.30."
- "I need you to spend some time in this area because some people are finding your behaviour upsetting."

Initially, a consumer may continue with the same behaviour, but as you repeat your expectations your message is reinforced. Provided that your demeanour is not aggressive, and your response is consistent, this offers the best opportunity to change the problematic behaviour. Be mindful to acknowledge any satisfactory outcome – saying "thank you" and showing humility are extremely powerful tools in any nurse–consumer relationship.

CRITICAL THINKING EXERCISE 4.1

Think about a situation of conflict that you were involved in or observed that was approached safely or you believe could have been treated differently. Write down some notes to the following questions:

1. What was the context preceding the situation?
2. What were the safety issues? Who was involved and what was each person's role? What was the outcome?
3. Could the situation have been approached differently from a safety point of view? If so, how?
4. What are the safety implications for the consumer or other consumers?
5. What safety issues have you learnt from this situation? Have you identified any learning needs?
6. How can you incorporate your new learning into future practice?

SAFETY IN CARE DURING AGGRESSION

Nurses often use the word "agitated" to describe some of the behaviours they see. Agitation is a signal that something has happened for the consumer. It can be a consumer's reaction to an abnormal situation, distress or trauma (Beattie et al 2019). Aggression or aggressive behaviour is frequently perceived to be hostile, injurious or destructive and is often caused by frustration. Sometimes, despite our best attempts at being empathic and actively listening, consumers become frustrated and agitated. While the anger may be directed at you as the nurse, it is not directed at you as a person. Although this difference appears subtle, the implications can be significant. By not personalising the behaviour, but rather seeing it through the eyes of your professional role, this will help you to remain objective. When someone is angry, they are often unaware of their own emotional state (Beattie et al 2019). An integral part of mental health nursing is the observation of consumers' demeanour and interactions with others. Some physiological observations that may require early intervention include:

- flushed or red face
- gritted teeth, tense facial features
- increased muscle tone, such as clenched fists
- increased motor activity, such as pacing or shuffling
- prolonged eye contact or staring.

Consumers who are frustrated or agitated may refuse to communicate or even withdraw from you. It is on these occasions that you may be required to intervene to prevent these physiological observations from escalating.

CRITICAL THINKING EXERCISE 4.2

What might be your emotional response when someone is aggressively shouting, intimidating and demanding your attention? Can you describe in words how you would feel? What physical reaction would you have? What thoughts would go through your mind? How could you approach the situation in a safe manner?

Safety in Care and De-escalation Techniques

De-escalation aims to bring about resolution through effective communication techniques (not force) and its success is underpinned by an empathic, respectful and collaborative approach by the nurse (Haefner et al 2021). This approach involves understanding common signs of escalating behaviours and an ability to use communication skills to purposefully engage anxious, emotionally aroused or agitated individuals. Several elements of de-escalation have been identified in the literature and these may be helpful in preparing you to de-escalate situations. These primary elements of de-escalation are outlined in Table 4.3.

Variously known as "talking down", de-fusion or diffusion, de-escalation is widely considered a first-line intervention for escalating behaviour. General principles involve non-provocatively engaging someone using short-term psychosocial interventions that minimise restriction and enable a mutually satisfactory outcome for both parties (Hallett & Dickens 2017).

Themes, Principles and Attributes of De-escalation

A multitude of techniques, domains, themes and validated scale items have been identified within the international literature suggesting the principal components of de-escalation. However, a recent concept analysis of de-escalation in healthcare settings, which included 79 studies, has attempted to resolve concerns over clarity by proposing the following theoretical definition:

> … a collective term for a range of interwoven staff-delivered components comprising communication, self-regulation, assessment, actions, and safety maintenance which aims to extinguish or reduce patient aggression/agitation irrespective of its cause, and improve staff–patient relationships while eliminating or minimising coercion or restriction.
>
> **(Hallett & Dickens 2017, p. 16)**

This definition arguably provides the most comprehensive understanding of de-escalation as a concept and provides an opportunity to explore theory–practice translational aspects of de-escalation. Successful de-escalation, therefore, comprises a complex set and interaction of skills and behaviours, which can be helpful in addressing challenging behaviour and workplace violence exposure, and may prevent the need for more restrictive practices, such as restraint and sedation.

Restraint and Seclusion

There may be occasions when your attempts to de-escalate are unsuccessful and consequently a decision is made to physically intervene. It should be emphasised that physical restraint of consumers is an intervention of last resort and should be carried out only by health professionals trained in safely facilitating this. Programs such as "Safewards" (see Useful websites) have been developed to minimise the use of restraint and seclusion in mental health units (Bowers 2014; Mullen et al 2022). You should always consider whether any alternative strategies are available and, if so, have these been exhausted? Also, what would happen if you did nothing? These questions may be asked in the context of alleged assault when considering whether reasonable force was applied, either in a consumer's best interests or as a basis for self-defence. Restraint carries with it significant risks of injury to consumers and staff and, in some cases, even death (Kennedy et al 2019). Seclusion also carries with it significant trauma and distress for consumers and staff alike. Some guiding principles for use of safe restraint and seclusion are summarised in Box 4.1 (Al-Maraira & Hayajneh 2018; SICSAW 2019).

Perspectives in practice: Nurse's story 4.1, by Natalie Cutler, on p. 48, illustrates the complexities and emotional and psychological issues associated with using consumer restraint and seclusion. Narrated by an experienced mental health nurse, who reflected upon her

TABLE 4.3   De-escalation, Themes, Principles, Attributes and Interventions

Themes and Principles	How You Could Do This	What You Could Say
Communication		
Establish contact early in escalation	One person should engage in a calm and measured way because it can be confusing and counterproductive when more than one person is speaking. Use the person's name and yours, and use tactful language and humour sensitively (only if you feel it safe to do so).	*"Hello, John. My name is Jane. That looks painful. Can I take a look at it?"*
Non-provocative engagement	Display a calm demeanour and appropriate tone of voice and engage assertively (not emotively or confrontationally). Eye contact should be intermittent to avoid staring. Awareness of one's own body language and adoption of an open, non-threatening posture with arms visible (not folded or behind back). Humour can help but only when appropriate.	Avoid saying: *"You need to calm down", "Don't speak to me like that"* or *"You're upsetting other people"*. Try: *"Let's sit down and talk so I can understand what's happening."*
Identify wants and feelings	Violent behaviour is a primitive form of communicating that something is wrong or a need is not being met. Look beyond the external manifestation of this and ask how you can help.	*"I understand you're frustrated. Let's sit down and discuss that"* or *"We're here to help you. How best can we do that?"*
Active listening	Convey through body language and verbal acknowledgement that you are interested and repeat back (paraphrasing) that you understand. Be congruent in actions and words. Silence can allow a person time to clarify their thoughts.	*"You said that you want...?"* or *"Am I correct in saying...?"*
Display empathy	Demonstrate empathy in verbal and non-verbal communication. Listen and offer understanding (not sympathy) while acknowledging the person's feelings/ situation.	*"That would frustrate me, too"* or *"I can appreciate how this is affecting you."*
Be concise	A person's ability to concentrate is compromised when in an emotionally aroused state. Avoid jargon or medical terminology. Speak clearly and slowly; information may have to be repeated several times.	*"Let's sit down and discuss your pain"* or *"We're concerned about your health and your safety."*
Agree or accept	Validate concerns where relevant and accept that concerns are distressing for the person (even if you may not agree with them). Concentrate on opportunities for agreement.	*"I'm sorry this has happened to you, it's unacceptable"* or *"I would feel angry too if I had to wait this long."*
Offer choices and optimism	Offering choice, where relevant, is empowering and can enable a sense of internal control while providing an acceptable "out" from challenging behaviour. Also offer things perceived as acts of kindness, where relevant, such as food/drink or pain relief. Be honest and don't make promises that can't be kept or that compromise others.	*"Can I get you some water and medication for your pain? Then we can discuss this"* or *"I'm sorry, but I'm unable to do that. What I can do is help you with..."*
Self-regulation		
Self-control/remain calm	Appearing fearful may make someone feel unsafe or may escalate behaviour in the context of manipulation. Maintain emotional regulation, self-control and confidence. Concentrate on your breathing; count to three before engaging. Having positive inner dialogues that you can successfully negotiate and de-escalate can contribute to effective self-control plans.	Say to yourself: *"I'm confident I can connect with [person's name] and successfully de-escalate the situation"* or *"This will resolve with everyone safe."*
Non-judgemental approach	Separate your feelings about the person and the problem. Avoid making judgements about the person and don't personalise any challenging behaviour.	*"I don't think that of you at all"* or *"I'm sorry you think that of me"* or *"I didn't mean to give you the wrong impression."*
Self-reflection	Personal reflection following an incident allows you to consider and make sense of what went well or not so well. This enables consistency or modification of engagement/intervention strategies.	Ask your colleague: *"How did I do?"* or *"Could I have done anything differently?"*
Assessment		
Is it safe to intervene?	Assess the risks associated with any intervention. Early intervention is always recommended for escalating behaviour, but patience and caution, if safe, may be more prudent when assessing benefit–harm ratio. Ask yourself what would happen if you did nothing or waited for support.	*"Can we take a minute, then I'll attend to that?"* or *"I need you to put that blade down before I can treat that."* or *"Do you mind if we wait for my colleague? He has something that can help with your pain."*
Here and now	Assess the person's emotional state or the immediate situation in relation to safety for all. Other aspects of assessment and intervention can wait.	*"You look distressed (or angry). Can you talk to me about it?"*
Escalating aggression	Observe for and recognise known early-warning signs of violence such as pacing, clenched-fists, kicking objects, loud voice, staring, tense facial expressions, posturing or ignoring requests.	*"I need you to sit down so I can attend to your..."*
Actions		
Positional imitation	Stand if the person is standing (personal safety); sit if they are sitting. This reflects a sense of equity required for successful de-escalation.	*"Do you mind if I sit down?"* or *"Do you mind if I join you?"*

TABLE 4.3 De-escalation, Themes, Principles, Attributes and Interventions—cont'd

Themes and Principles	How You Could Do This	What You Could Say
Reduce stimuli; create a safe space	Decrease environmental stimuli and encourage private interaction free from any potential triggers or antagonists. Attempt to remove the person, or others, from the situation, thus creating a safe space for engagement and intervention.	*"Can we move over here and talk in private?"* or *"Can we sit in the ambulance so we can attend to...?"*
Distraction	Redirect the person's attention from escalating behaviour. Bringing in a different person to interact with the individual may change the dynamic of unsuccessful de-escalation.	*"Is there anyone you'd like me to call to let them know you're safe or where you are going?"* or *"This is my colleague, Jane. Do you mind if she attends to you while I get you something for the pain?"*
Set limits	Be clear about what you would like to happen and that you want to help, in a non-confrontational and respectful way. A discussion of behavioural expectations may help if safe to do so. Acknowledge if you are feeling uncomfortable – humility is a very powerful tool!	*"When you're shouting, I find it hard to understand how I can help you"* or *"I can't attend to your needs while you're threatening me."*
Therapeutic treatment	Identifying and alleviating causes of escalating behaviour such as pain or confusion can quickly inform de-escalation strategies and required treatments.	*"Can I give you something to help with the pain?"* or *"Can I give you some medication to help take your mind off it?"*
Maintaining Safety		
Situational awareness	Situational awareness is being aware of what is happening around you in terms of where you are, whether anyone or anything around you is a threat, and what supports may be available. It is essential to remain vigilant. Awareness of the environment in terms of isolation, quick egress and exit routes and removal or moderation of potential weapons, dangers and triggers is paramount.	*"Can we talk somewhere else?"* or *"Do you mind if I sit here?"* or *"If you could put the syringe down I'll attend to that."*
Situational support	Communication with colleagues is essential. Identify availability of backup should it be needed while being mindful that an excessive show of force can escalate a person's behaviour.	*"No one's in trouble. The police are here for everyone's safety"* or *"I need to contact someone to let them know we'll be longer than expected"*
Approach with caution	Approach in a measured way, careful to avoid sudden movements. Avoid being too close to someone fearful or confused (this may appear threatening) while maintaining a distance that protects from a potential punch or kick until you feel it safe for close proximity.	*"Can we take a look at that injury?"* or *"Someone phoned because they are concerned about your safety."*
Respect personal space	Acknowledge that more personal space than usual may be required while being mindful not to appear fearful or disinterested.	*"Do you mind if I have a look at that?"* or *"I won't come any closer, I just want to chat."*
Debrief all involved	Debriefing helps maintain therapeutic aspects of a relationship. It is important that a person does not feel isolated following resolution, irrespective of how this is achieved. Debriefing with colleagues ensures that psychological first aid can be administered. Bystanders may also require debriefing if witnessing potentially traumatic events. Debriefing allows learning from situations that may prove useful in future crises.	To the patient: *"I'm sorry we did that, I know you didn't want to. We did this because..."* To a bystander: *"That must have been very difficult to witness. Are you okay? Can I contact someone to take you home?"* To a colleague: *"How do you think that went? Should we do anything differently next time?"*

Adapted from Lamont & Brunero 2021

BOX 4.1 Guiding Principles for Safe Restraint

1. Restraint is the option of last resort; it is to be used when other less coercive interventions are unsuccessful or inappropriate.
2. Any restriction to a consumer's liberty and interference with their rights, dignity and self-respect should be kept to a minimum and should cease as soon as the consumer has regained self-control.
3. Restraint and seclusion should never be used as a method of punishment. All actions undertaken by staff must be justifiable and proportional to the consumer's behaviour, with the least amount of force necessary.
4. Staff must exercise reasonable care and skill to ensure the safety, comfort and humane treatment of consumers in restraint or seclusion.
5. Communication and engagement with the consumer should be maintained at all times, with all opportunities taken to de-escalate the situation.
6. Pain compliance should never be used when restraining someone, and any direct pressure on the neck, abdomen, thorax, back or joints is to be voided.
7. The consumer's physical condition should be continuously monitored, with any deterioration, in particular to the airway, noted and managed promptly.
8. All episodes of restraint should have an appointed leader throughout the restraint to maintain safety.
9. Face-up restraint (supine) should be used where it is safe to do so. Face-down restraint (prone) should be used only if it is the safest way to protect the consumer and staff. Prone restraint should be used for only the minimum amount of time necessary to administer medication and/or move the person to a safer environment.
10. A post-restraint/seclusion debrief for the consumer, staff and any relevant others should be undertaken in all situations.

Adapted from NSW Health 2020.

PERSPECTIVES IN PRACTICE

Nurse's Story 4.1: Natalie Cutler

I've been a nurse for more than 20 years, specialising in mental health. Two things drew me to mental health: firstly, that it was a "frontier" with little research happening and lots waiting to be discovered. Secondly, and most importantly, I could see "mental health" everywhere. From my previous experience as a dental nurse, I was familiar with the fear and anxiety people experienced. I became aware of how powerful human interactions could be in making people feel safe. I'd say that was my beginning as a mental health nurse, well before I'd completed any training.

Something that resonated powerfully with me when I was undertaking nurse training was the concept of the nurse as advocate. The more I learnt about this, the more determined I became to actively advocate for people with mental health problems wherever I could. As a clinician, and later as an educator and manager, this has been my most valued role.

To be an effective advocate, it is important to understand one's own motivations and be vigilant to the fine balance between seeking to build another's strength versus disempowering them by seeking to "rescue". Continuous reflection on whose needs are being met is the key. Advocacy requires being a resource for the other person to help them achieve their goals. If assertive advocacy is required, this should ideally be activated on the request or with the consent of another person. In addition to considering the needs of people with lived experience of mental illness, mental health nursing also encompasses an awareness of one's own needs. Self-advocacy and peer advocacy thus provide the foundation for safe and sustainable practice.

Being an advocate is not always easy. This is reflected in a scenario from my early career. As a new graduate nurse, my very first placement was in an acute mental health inpatient unit. Returning from a meeting on my second day, I walked into the lounge area in time to see a large male being held on the ground by several of my colleagues. Other consumers in the area looked frightened. I did not have time to process what was happening before I was commanded to "hold his foot". For the next 25 minutes, I was part of a team involved in restraining, medicating and ultimately secluding this man. I had no idea what had happened, why we were doing this or what I was expected to do. None of my university training had prepared me for this. I was shocked and inwardly distressed.

Shortly after, my colleagues resumed their usual activities and not much was said about the incident. What appeared to be routine to my colleagues left me completely bewildered. Nothing in my private life or training had prepared me to be involved in holding another person on the ground against their will. I found it hard to reconcile this "security" function with my beginning identity as a nurse and an advocate. This confusion has stayed with me to this day. However, it also started a career-long reflection on questions, such as "What is a nurse?" and "Who am I as a nurse?" It also made me determined never to see restraint and seclusion as "normal" parts of being a nurse. Consequently, I have moved towards roles that allow me to engage with consumers as equals. Wherever possible, I try to challenge "the way we do things round here". For me, being a nurse means being brave and self-aware, and providing a platform for others to have a voice.

---

early beginnings in mental health nursing, the story depicts a powerful representation of trauma associated with human interaction within the mental health specialty.

DELIBERATE SELF-HARM AND SUICIDE

Deliberate self-harm can be extremely confronting and challenging. Consumers who harm themselves often do so in the context of a situational crisis or in relation to their lived experience of trauma, and consumers often describe how deliberate self-harm is a means of managing distressing emotions. Self-harming behaviour can include injury that is either external or internal. External behaviours such as cutting, scratching, burning, picking and head banging are more common. However, internal behaviours, such as swallowing objects and substances, may also be seen in clinical practice. Trying to understand someone's motivations, emotional state and/or triggers for self-harming behaviour is essential. Assessing impulsiveness, the wish to control oneself or the effort to stop oneself is also important.

Traumatic Experiences

Physical and sexual trauma histories strongly predict and underpin self-injury. Dissociative states or feelings of detachment from physical and emotional experience are commonly described by consumers who self-harm. There may be several mediating factors in consumers who self-harm, including the type of trauma, affective dysregulation, dissociation, poor modulation of aggression and/or poor impulse control. Confusion may arise when differentiating between deliberate self-harm and suicidal behaviour. Deliberate self-harm or non-suicidal self-injury is not necessarily suicidal behaviour, as there is rarely an intention to die. The behaviour may be intended as a relief from anxiety or tension or as an escape from distressing emotions rather than an attempt at suicide. The complexity is that people with self-harming behaviour may also be suicidal. Assessing suicidality in a consumer who also self-harms is difficult, because people often feel dysphoric

with depressed mood. An issue of concern when managing deliberate self-harm is not being complacent about it; this behaviour carries extensive risks, even when there is no intention to die or when a consumer may have been engaging in this type of behaviour for many years (Staniland et al 2021).

Interventions in Self-Harm

As with most of the focus in this chapter, having empathy in exploring meanings of behaviour for the consumer is the best place to start. Understanding the pain experienced during the act of self-harm and what this means to the person may help you to engage them in a therapeutic relationship with you. Going beyond what is in front of you (i.e. the wound or cut on the arm) and exploring the meaning and significance of the act will help you to engage the consumer therapeutically. Obtaining details of incidents, thoughts, feelings, precipitating events and other ideas that occur during the self-harming behaviour demonstrates a willingness to work collaboratively with the consumer. Intolerant or dismissive approaches by nursing staff often cause an increase in self-harming behaviours because the emotional distress that underpins them is not being engaged or validated.

General strategies include the consumer learning distress management techniques, including relaxation and other distraction strategies, such as pinging rubber bands on the wrist when distressed, ice cubes, throwing or hitting soft objects and/or exercising when thoughts of self-harm occur. Consumers may learn about their early warning signs and make plans for potentially stressful or difficult situations they may encounter. Encouraging consumers to articulate these experiences into words, drawings or stories may help them to understand how they are relating to the world around them. An ongoing emphasis should be placed on developing alternatives to self-harm. Deliberate self-harm is a complex issue and treatment processes can be prolonged and unpredictable. Generally, psychotherapy is the most common treatment, with dialectical behaviour therapy having dominance in this area more recently (Toms et al 2019).

MANIPULATION

Manipulation generally refers to behaviours that someone exhibits to get their needs met. This may include the following types of behaviours and actions: attempting to maintain control and power over others; playing one staff member off against another ("splitting"); evoking guilt and shame in others; attempting to get others to take responsibility for one's actions; and attempting to gain an advantage in interactions. Manipulation can be used by both nurses and consumers. The meaning behind the word "manipulative" is negative, suggesting that the consumer is bad or difficult rather than just the individual behaviour. As nurses we need to be careful how we label behaviour and the meanings that arise out of those labels (Tyerman et al 2021).

Influence Versus Manipulation

Generally speaking, as a nurse, you hold the power in the therapeutic relationship. As such, you need to be aware of how you exercise that responsibility. Consumer–nurse collaboration and positive outcomes are more likely to be achieved by using influence rather than manipulation. The goal is encouragement and negotiation rather than coercion or manipulation, and consumer involvement in decision-making will provide the best opportunity for engaging someone in safe care. Provide balanced rather than biased information and consider the needs and concerns of the consumer, not just your own needs and concerns. Identify the manipulative behaviour and communicate this with your colleagues. It is important to maintain communication and consistency. Comprehensive documentation is important, and minimising the number of staff involved with the consumer may help. Be clear and direct when setting limits on behaviour; enforce the limits, but also reward and praise positive behaviour. Collaborative care plans should communicate clearly what you expect from the consumer and what the consumer can expect from you. A written plan may contain a set of simple statements of what you will do and what the consumer will do. It may even be signed by both parties to demonstrate an agreement, but it should not be considered as a contract. It is simply a negotiated agreement with another person (Hartley et al 2020).

❓ CRITICAL THINKING EXERCISE 4.3

A consumer is displaying "splitting" behaviour, describing one staff member as their favourite while others are the worst they have met.
1. What would you say to the consumer?
2. What would you say to the team?
3. How would you behave with the consumer and the clinical team?
4. What would be your safety plan?

UNDERSTANDING SAFETY RISKS IN CARE AND AT WORK

There is increasing pressure on nurses and other professionals to assess, predict and manage the risk of adverse events. It is unfortunate that high-profile, yet rare, events involving staff and consumers and subsequent media interest lead to heightened community concern around the safety of consumers and others, often laying the blame on inadequate or ineffective mental health care. This has led to the expectation that nurses become proficient in assessing and managing risk and in justifying their actions in terms of their risk implications and preventing adverse events. Risk therefore pervades the research literature, health service policy and practice, media and public debate, and even healthcare legislation (Hawton et al 2022; Whiting et al 2021).

As a nurse, you will be expected to provide assessment in relation to some specific forms of risk. Typically, this may involve, but is not limited to:
- aggression and violence
- suicide and self-harm (risk of further attempts and death)
- severe self-neglect (risk of poor physical health, infectious disease)
- sexual safety (risk of sexually transmitted infection, assault and trauma)
- exploitation/reputation (risk of harm to reputation, financial loss)
- fire safety (risk to personal safety and belongings)
- absconding (risk of further harm, prolonging hospital admission)
- non-compliance with medications (risk of relapse).

Risk has become an integral component of mental health care; however, there remains much controversy and debate around minimum expectations in practice, how best to facilitate risk assessment and management processes, and even whether the outcomes of processes are commensurate with our time and efforts. Box 4.2 lists the principles for working with safety risks.

The Risk Assessment Processes

The search for reliable methods of risk assessment has led to a plethora of risk tools, instruments and algorithms that attempt to measure or predict risk behaviours. It is estimated that more than 150 structured tools exist for assessing the risk of violence alone, yet these instruments have a reported low reliability in determining a consumer's risk level (Hawton et al 2022; Whiting et al 2021). Other instruments focus on suicide and self-harm. Notwithstanding, three methods of risk assessment have been prominent throughout:

- **Unstructured clinical judgement** involves a subjective clinician assessment on what factors the individual assessor believes are relevant or important in relation to a risk. Critics of this unstructured approach relate the lack of consistency and inter-rater reliability of such assessments, as individual assessors have different levels of experience, exposure to risk, values and interpersonal skills. These factors may influence the overestimation or underestimation of risk, which is obviously suboptimal to care provision.
- **Actuarial risk assessment methods** are known variously as mathematical, mechanical or statistical prediction, where individual factors that have been statistically associated with specific risks are measured. Therefore, individual clinical judgement is replaced by a score based on a formulaic equation, but this ignores the dynamic factors that are associated with risks eventuating (e.g. staff wellbeing, consumers' experiences, ward environment). Another limitation is that actuarial methods stop at prediction and ultimately fail to

---

BOX 4.2 Principles for Working with Safety Risks

- Risk is an everyday experience.
- Risk is dynamic and constantly changing in response to varying circumstances.
- Assessment of risk is enhanced by accessing multiple sources of information.
- Sources of information may be incomplete.
- Some sources of information may be inaccurate.
- Identification of risk carries a responsibility to do something about it – that is, risk management.
- An integral component of good risk management is risk-taking.
- Decision-making can be enhanced through positive collaboration.
- Risk can be minimised but not eliminated.
- Organisations carry a responsibility to meet reasonable expectations for encouraging a no-blame culture while not condoning poor practice.

Adapted from Morgan 2004.

inform prevention and management. It must be noted also that any statistical significance attached to actuarial methods may be associated with specific validation samples and identified risks.

- **Structured professional judgement** essentially integrates clinical and actuarial methods in an attempt to minimise the limitations of both methods. This approach combines empirically validated risk factors, professional experience/judgement and contemporary knowledge of a particular consumer. As this approach incorporates idiosyncratic and dynamic risk factors, it is argued to have transferability across different populations and offers provisions within the framework for prevention and management.

Positive Risk-Taking

The term "positive risk-taking" is used in this context to represent professional readiness to respect and respond to service users' own recovery goals or preferences for care. Such opportunities are perceived to be under-realised in practice, exacerbating existing power differentials between service users and professionals, and sanctioning professionals to have the "final say" (Just et al 2021; van Weeghel et al 2019).

Recovery-oriented practices adopt a position where consumers take ownership of their own personal journey and, with it, ownership of associated risks. Top-down, risk-averse cultures challenge the integrity of consumer engagement, involvement and empowerment (van Weeghel et al 2019). As such, cultures that do not embrace consumer ownership and empowerment via philosophical frameworks and practices such as positive risk-taking will probably experience challenges to safe care and work as a result of consumer disempowerment and a lack of hope.

Consequently, the concept of positive risk-taking has been catapulted to the forefront of our decision-making. Positive risk-taking involves a process of reasoning within a framework of weighing up potential benefits and harms of one choice over another. It is argued that positive risk-taking is not a negligent practice where risks are ignored; rather, situations and their potential consequences are logically and carefully considered in the context of any course of action.

A pervasive negative focus on risk can lead to defensive practices that in turn lead to often costly unnecessary interventions and care, for fear of legal recourse. By contrast, positive risk-taking involves accepting risk as part of everyday life and health care. Examples of positive risk-taking include discharging consumers from supervised inpatient care to community follow-up; unescorted leave from inpatient stays previously perceived to be too risky; pharmacology-free trials as a result of severe side effects; non-admission following presentation in crisis to an ED; or a crisis team visit at home. These are all examples of everyday positive risk-taking, where, as nurses, we accept that risks are omnipresent.

Ultimately, we take risks and utilise the knowledge gained following successes or mistakes for growth and empowerment. Consumer engagement, partnership and co-planning of care will enable better, safer outcomes when positively taking risks. The ability to flourish is a fundamental human right, and should be supported and advocated for by nurses, as opposed to legislation, policy and practice where fear of failure and adverse events pervades.

Community Settings – Safety and Situational Awareness

Creating a safe care and work environment in community settings poses different challenges to those encountered in inpatient settings. The community setting can be dynamic, requiring quick assessment of safety, with limited information and resources compared with the inpatient setting. As a result, it is an expectation that community nurses become situationally aware of risks and safety and are proficient at assessing risk. This will require you to:

- look for hazards
- consider retreat options and exits
- approach situations cautiously
- avoid placing yourself or others (consumer and families) at risk (e.g. intervening in a violent incident)
- observe for potential weapons
- consider additional resources required to safely assess and/or treat.

Table 4.4 outlines some specific safety and risk mitigation factors you should consider before arrival, upon arrival, during assessment/treatment and following your return to a community health centre.

TABLE 4.4 Safety and Situational Awareness During Community Visits

Prior To Community Visit	Arrival at Community Visit	Assessment/Treatment	Other Issues
• Recognise that risk is dynamic and that a low-risk person or situation can change at any time • Obtain as much information as possible about the patient and others (where relevant) • Obtain information about the location: Is it in a high crime area? Isolated? Does it have reduced accessibility to or availability of police? Some addresses may be listed as "no go" or "locations of interest". If so, consider police backup. • Gather specific information about the premises (if relevant): Is there security access? Stairs? External lighting? Hiding places? Are the premises modern? In good repair?	• Park the car facing the way you will be exiting and make sure you cannot be blocked in • Do not attempt to enter premises if there are any potentially aggressive animals and they are not restrained • When entering buildings check lighting and stairwells where no lift is available • If you are concerned about location or access to premises ask a family member to meet you and escort you to the client • Always check the locking mechanism on the gate so you can leave quickly if necessary • Before knocking or ringing the doorbell, listen for any arguments or other unexpected voices or anything that may make the situation unsafe (these are reasons to reassess the situation)	• Be cautious when entering a person's home • If at any time your professional instinct tells you something is wrong, leave immediately (even if you cannot work out what is wrong) • Leave immediately if you see any firearms or weapons (police need to be informed) • Be aware of all exits • Do not sit in deep-seated chairs because it is difficult to get out of some chairs in a hurry (ask for an upright chair) • Always sit between the client and the door but without blocking the client's way out • Keep your keys handy so you do not waste time searching for them at the bottom of your bag • Only take in what you need	• Always report to base at regular intervals • Always report "near misses" where aggression became a present risk but did not eventuate • Ensure your workplace has a policy and response if you do not return on time such as activating a police response • Ensure you attend all workplace violence prevention and personal safety training offered by your service

Adapted from Lamont & Brunero 2021.

Summary of Risk in Mental Health Settings

The assessment and management of risk are inextricably linked to providing mental health care. While exact predictions are not possible, this area of practice is not one in which nurses should become complacent. There is no doubt that a sense of perspective and realistic expectation is required among legislators, administrators, health professionals and the wider community. However, despite ongoing debate, there remains a community, professional and moral expectation that we engage with consumers around identified needs and potential risks, and attempt to mitigate against these. A collaborative, dynamic and continuous process of engagement and planning can support nurses when there is increased risk of adverse events, thus removing the perceived or actual burden of individual scrutiny. Box 4.2 summarises principles for working with risk as described in seminal work by Morgan (2004), which remains contemporary (van Weeghel et al 2019).

THE LEGAL CONTEXT

Nurses need to be aware of the ethical and legal contexts in which subsequent actions and interventions are considered. Some fundamental human rights underpin our ethical conduct, common law and relevant statutes within this context (see also Chapter 10).

Human Rights

Several United Nations treaties have shaped domestic and international law in relation to healthcare rights. The *Universal Declaration of Human Rights* (United Nations 1948) is an international document that states basic rights and fundamental freedoms to which all human beings are entitled. It consists of 30 Articles, some of which have direct relevance to healthcare provision:

- Article 3: Everyone has the right to life, liberty and security of person
- Article 9: No-one shall be subjected to arbitrary arrest, detention or exile
- Article 13: Everyone has the right to freedom of movement and residence within the borders of each state.

Australia and New Zealand are signatories to the Principles for the Protection of Persons with Mental Illness and for the Improvement of Mental Health Care (United Nations General Assembly 1991), which were adopted by the UN General Assembly in 1991. With the underpinning aim to provide a framework for improving mental health care globally, UN91 (as it became known) sets out basic rights-based standards for providing care for people with mental illness. Since its inception, UN91 principles have received criticism for not influencing the suboptimal standards of mental health care provision enough, with some principles offering more protection than others. Consequently, UN91 should now be read and understood in the context of the United Nations *Convention on the Rights of Persons with Disabilities* (United Nations 2022).

These frameworks set in place obligations on member states within common and legislative law for protecting others and act as a reflective guide for actions. When engaging consumers in any course of action that may impinge on these rights, nurses must be aware of where the law positions itself in relation to any subsequent interventions (Mezzina et al 2019).

Common Law Issues

Failure in duty of care and negligence are common law torts (civil wrongs) that nurses need to familiarise themselves with. All health professionals must be aware that they owe a duty of care to consumers and that this involves acting in a manner that accords with competent professional practice. Negligence arises when health professionals are deemed negligent in fulfilling their duty and where such a breach directly causes damage to a consumer. This duty pervades throughout all care provision and is not something that is invoked by specific consumer behaviours. Duty of care within this context involves maintaining safety for all, and, in doing so, being aware that other torts are not being committed (Lamont et al 2020).

The common law tort of trespass comprises three potential trespasses to the person: assault – an intentional act by someone that creates fear in another of an imminent harm; battery – a harmful or offensive touching of another (thus a distinction is created whereby assault is associated with no contact whereas battery requires contact); and false imprisonment – the illegal confinement of an individual against their will that impinges on the individual's right to freedom of movement (Staunton & Chiarella 2020). Nurses may be open to scrutiny and sometimes litigation in the course of their work, particularly when engaging in restrictive or coercive care that is unsolicited or not consented to by the consumer and when the consumer has a voluntary status. Involuntary status under the relevant mental health statute or substitute consent under the guardianship statute in general offers protection to nurses. However, this protection is not absolute, and the above torts may still apply if the nurse's actions are outside the relevant legal framework.

The common law doctrine of necessity, sometimes referred to as "emergency powers", allows nurses to act and administer care/treatment in any situation where a consumer lacks capacity and the provision of treatment is immediately necessary to prevent serious injury or even death: see *Re T (adult: refusal of medical treatment)* [1992] 4 All ER 649. Again, such practice is potentially challengeable and should be used in emergencies only, not in a consistent or planned way. When assessing capacity, the CARD approach (Comprehend, Appreciate, Reason, Decide) developed by Stewart and colleagues (2020a) can be used by clinicians to undertake brief and timely decision-making capacity assessments (see Box 4.3).

Legislative Frameworks

Mental health legislative frameworks, irrespective of geographical location, will generally be underpinned by similar philosophies and principles. These may include least restrictive care or minimising any restrictions on civil liberty, rights, dignity and self-respect, and the right

---

BOX 4.3 The CARD Approach

Comprehend (Understand)

"Please tell me what you understand about your condition."

"What do you think is wrong with you?"

"What have you been told about treatment?"

Appreciate (Retain)

"What is the treatment likely to do for you? Why do you think it will have that effect?"

"What do you believe will happen if you are not treated?"

"Why do you think we have recommended this treatment for you?"

"Can you recall what you were told about the risks and benefits of treatment?"

Reason (Weigh)

"Tell me how you reached the decision to accept (reject) treatment."

"What things were important to you in reaching the decision?"

"How do you balance those things?"

Decide (Communicate)

"Have you decided whether to go along with our suggested treatment?"

"Can you tell me what your treatment decision is?"

Stewart et al 2020a.

to appeal (Davis et al 2019). If engaging in non-consensual, restrictive or coercive management of consumers, mental health legislation may have to be applied to do so lawfully. This not only offers protection for care and treatment that consumers may not agree with, but more importantly also affords consumers a right to appeal via independent arbitration (e.g. mental health review tribunals). Relevant guardianship and public health (during a pandemic) legislation can also be used in this manner when protecting the health rights of consumers with disabilities (Stewart et al 2020b). Again, similar procedural requirements and criteria must be met within the various geographical jurisdictions. These procedures are essential if engaging in processes that effectively impinge on a consumer's freedom of movement. Without wishing to single out any particular intervention, one such intervention that becomes prominent and requires attention within a legal context is consumer restraint.

Reasonable Force

Nurses often ask what constitutes the legal definition of reasonable force in situations of consumer safety. There is no simple explanation for this. Reasonable force is essentially context-specific and is the amount of force deemed necessary at the time in relation to the risk presented. A unique set of conditions exists in each situation and essentially requires a professional judgement to be made. This judgement is quite rightly open to challenge and scrutiny by consumers and therefore any actions pursued by you as a nurse must be commensurate with the perceived risk. Potential alternative courses of action may be put forward when considering whether any force was reasonable and justified, in keeping with least restrictive principles of human rights and mental health legislation.

Notwithstanding the above, there will be occasions when, as a nurse, you feel there is no other option but to engage in restrictive practices (person-to-person, mechanical or chemical restraint), either because the perceived risk is too great for verbal engagement or when this is unsuccessful. However, you must be aware of the principles outlined above when using restrictive practices, as this practice should always be considered a last resort because of the danger to both the consumer and staff (Finch et al 2022).

CHAPTER SUMMARY

What differentiates mental health nursing from other areas of nursing is caring for consumers who at times in their lives are unable to see the need for care. The skills you develop will take you beyond seeing these challenges to safe care and work as being difficult or deliberate. Being aware of your own emotional responses to your work will allow you to de-personalise the effects that workplace challenges bring. Being able to stand back and see the wider picture of the social context that someone is in and seeing past the behaviours you are confronted with will enable you to see the person within. Achieving this level of engagement with someone indicates that you are heading towards mastery of the skills outlined in this chapter.

REVIEW QUESTIONS

In your class group, recall a situation where a risk was identified with a consumer. Complete the safety in care and safety at work plan below from a group discussion (Morgan 2004).

Safety in Care, Safety at Work Plan

Categories of safety risk identified (single or multiple – tick relevant boxes):
- Aggression and violence
- Severe self-neglect
- Exploitation/reputation
- Absconding
- Suicide and self-harm
- Sexual safety
- Fire
- Other (specify)

Detail any historical information that may indicate the potential for a safety risk (e.g. previous history of risk behaviours/threats/ ideation).

_____

_____

Detail any health-related factors that may contribute to the potential for a safety risk (e.g. mental health symptoms, personality factors, physical disabilities, substance abuse).

_____

_____

What environmental safety factors may contribute to risk (e.g. arousal in official professional settings, access to drugs/alcohol, rejection by others, access to weapons)?

_____

_____

Is there any current evidence to suggest "planned intent" to engage in risk-related behaviour?

_____

_____

Are there any safety risk factors that indicate preferred staff allocation (e.g. danger to women, intimidated by men, need for two workers)?

_____

_____

What strengths and opportunities can you identify, from the consumer and/or services, as resources to support this plan?

_____

_____

What barriers may hinder the implementation of this plan?

_____

_____

State specifically the identified risk:

_____

_____

Presents a risk of:

_____

_____

Through (behaviours/cognitions/affect):

_____

_____

In the context of (situations):

_____

_____

Early intervention signs are:

_____

_____

Interventions for the above circumstances:

_____

_____

Has this plan been discussed with the consumer?

_____

_____

Has this plan been discussed with the multidisciplinary team?

_____

_____

Frequency of review:

_____

_____

Additional comments (if discontinuing, specify reasons):

_____

_____

USEFUL WEBSITES AND RESOURCES

Safewards: www.facebook.com/groups/safewards/; www.safewards.net/
SICSAW – Safe in Care, Safe at Work: www.mentalhealthcommission.gov.au/
getmedia/aec947de-3c06-462e-bb73-51e37e810180/Safe-in-Care-Safe-at-Work-Full-version

REFERENCES

Al-Maraira, O.A., Hayajneh, F.A., 2018. Use of restraint and seclusion in psychiatric settings: A literature review. J Psychosoc Nurs Ment Health Serv, 57(4), 32–39.

Barker, P., 2001. The Tidal Model: Developing an empowering, person centred approach to recovery within psychiatric and mental health nursing. J Psychiatr Ment Health Nurs, 8(3), 233–240.

Barr, L., Heslop, K., Wynaden, D., & Albrecht, M. 2022. Nursing staff composition and its influence on seclusion in an adult forensic mental health inpatient setting: The truth about numbers. Arch Psychiat Nurs, 41, 333–340.

Beattie, J., Griffiths, D., Innes, K., & Morphet, J. 2019. Workplace violence perpetrated by clients of health care: A need for safety and trauma-informed care. J Clin Nurs, 28(1–2), 116–124.

Bowers, L. 2014. Safewards: a new model of conflict and containment on psychiatric wards. J Psychiatr Ment Health Nurs, 21(6), 499–508.

Brunero, S., Dunn, S., & Lamont, S. 2021a. Development and effectiveness of tabletop exercises in preparing health practitioners in violence prevention management: A sequential explanatory mixed methods study. Nurse Ed Today, 103, 104976.

Brunero, S., Lamont, S., Dunn, S., Varndell, W., & Dickens, G.L. 2021b. Examining the utility of the Violence Prevention Climate scale: In a metropolitan Australian general hospital. J Clin Nurs, 30(15–16), 2399–2408.

Cutler, N.A., Halcomb, E., Sim, J., Stephens, M., & Moxham, L. 2021. How does the environment influence consumers' perceptions of safety in acute mental health units? A qualitative study. J Clin Nurs, 30(5–6), 765–772.

Cutler, N.A., Sim, J., Halcomb, E., Moxham, L., & Stephens, M. 2020. Nurses' influence on consumers' experience of safety in acute mental health units: A qualitative study. J Clin Nurs, 29(21–22), 4379–4386.

Davis, M., Juratowitch, R., Brunero, S., Lamont, S. 2019. Mind the gaps: Identifying opportunities in mental health assessment and mental health certificate completion in rural and remote NSW, Australia. Australas Emerg Care, 23(3), 137–141.

Delgado, C., Roche, M., Fethney, J., & Foster, K. 2020. Workplace resilience and emotional labour of Australian mental health nurses: Results of a national survey. Int J Ment Health Nurs, 29(1), 35–46.

Finch, K., Lawrence, D., Williams, M. O., Thompson, A. R., & Hartwright, C. 2022. A systematic review of the effectiveness of safewards: Has enthusiasm exceeded evidence? Issues Ment Health Nurs, 43(2), 119–136.

Foster, K., Withers, E., Blanco, T., Lupson, C., Steele, M., Giandinoto, J.A., et al., 2019. Undergraduate nursing students' stigma and recovery attitudes during mental health clinical placement: A pre/post-test survey study. Int J Ment Health Nurs, 28(5), 1068–1080.

Gerace, A. 2020. Roses by other names? Empathy, sympathy, and compassion in mental health nursing. Int J Ment Health Nurs, 29(4), 736–744.

Gyamfi, N., Bhullar, N., Islam, M.S., & Usher, K. 2020. Knowledge and attitudes of mental health professionals and students regarding recovery: A systematic review. Int J Ment Health Nurs, 29(3), 322–347.

Haefner, J., Dunn, I., & McFarland, M. 2021. A quality improvement project using verbal de-escalation to reduce seclusion and patient aggression in an inpatient psychiatric unit. Issues Ment Health Nurs, 42(2), 138–144.

Hallett, N., Dickens, G.L., 2017. De-escalation of aggressive behaviour in healthcare settings: Concept analysis. Int J Nurs Stud, 75, 10–20.

Hartley, S., Raphael, J., Lovell, K., & Berry, K. 2020. Effective nurse–patient relationships in mental health care: A systematic review of interventions to improve the therapeutic alliance. Int J Nurs Stud, 102, 103490.

Hawton, K., Lascelles, K., Pitman, A., Gilbert, S., & Silverman, M. 2022. Assessment of suicide risk in mental health practice: Shifting from prediction to therapeutic assessment, formulation, and risk management. The Lancet Psychiatry, 9(11), 922–928.

Horgan, A., O Donovan, M., Manning, F., Doody, R., Savage, E., et al., 2021. "Meet me where I am": Mental health service users' perspectives on the desirable qualities of a mental health nurse. Int J Ment Health Nurs, 30(1), 136–147.

Just, D., Palmier-Claus, J. E., & Tai, S., 2021. Positive risk management: Staff perspectives in acute mental health inpatient settings. J Adv Nurs, 77(4), 1899–1910.

Kaihlanen, AM., Hietapakka, L. & Heponiemi, T. 2019. Increasing cultural awareness: qualitative study of nurses' perceptions about cultural competence training. BMC Nurs, 18, 38, doi.org/10.1186/s12912-019-0363-x.

Kennedy, H., Roper, C., Randall, R., et al., 2019. Consumer recommendations for enhancing the Safewards model and interventions. Int J Ment Health Nurs, 28(2), 616–626.

Kwame, A., & Petrucka, P. M. 2020. Communication in nurse–patient interaction in healthcare settings in sub-Saharan Africa: A scoping review. Int J Africa Nurs Sci, 12, 100198.

Lamont, S., Brunero, S., 2021. Managing challenging behaviour and workplace violence. In: Roberts, L., & Hains, D. (eds), Mental Health and Mental Illness in Paramedic Practice. Elsevier, Sydney.

Lamont S, Brunero S 2018. The effect of a workplace violence training program for generalist nurses in the acute hospital setting: A quasi-experimental study. Nurse Educ Today, Sept, 68, 45–52.

Lamont, S., Stewart, C., & Chiarella, M. 2020. The misuse of "duty of care" as justification for non-consensual coercive treatment. Int J Law Psychiatry, 71, 101598.

López-López, I. M., Gómez-Urquiza, J. L., Cañadas, G. R., De la Fuente, E. I., Albendín-García, L., et al., 2019. Prevalence of burnout in mental health nurses and related factors: A systematic review and meta-analysis. Int J Ment Health Nurs, 28(5), 1035–1044.

McAllister, S., Robert, G., Tsianakas, V., et al., 2019. Conceptualising nurse–patient therapeutic engagement on acute mental health wards: An integrative review. Int J Nurs Stud, 93, 106–118.

Mezzina, R., Rosen, A., Amering, M., et al., 2019. The practice of freedom: human rights and the global mental health agenda. In: Javed, A., Fountoulakis, K.N. (eds), Advances in Psychiatry. Springer International, Cham.

Morgan, S., 2004. Positive risk-taking: An idea whose time has come. Health Care Risk Rep, 10, 18–19.

Mullen, A., Browne, G., Hamilton, B., Skinner, S., & Happell, B. 2022. Safewards: An integrative review of the literature within inpatient and forensic mental health units. Int J Ment Health Nurs, 31(5), 1090–1108.

New South Wales Health 2020. Guideline: Management of patients with acute severe behavioural disturbance in emergency departments. Online. Available at: www1.health.nsw.gov.au/pds/ActivePDSDocuments/GL2015_007.pdf

Palfrey, N., Reay, R.E., Aplin, V., Cubis, J.C., McAndrew, V., et al., 2019. Achieving service change through the implementation of a trauma-informed care training program within a mental health service. Commun Ment Health J, 55(3), 467–475.

SICSAW, 2019. Safe in Care, Safe at Work: Ensuring safety in care and safety for staff in Australian mental health services. Australian College of Mental Health Nurses, Canberra. Online. Available at: www.mentalhealthcommission.gov.au/getmedia/1871cc65-e51d-43fb-b2d5-7346a17248a9/Safe-in-Care-Safe-at-Work-Abridged-version

Simpson, M.-C.G., & Sawatzky, J.-A.V. 2020. Clinical placement anxiety in undergraduate nursing students: A concept analysis. Nurse Ed Today, 87, 104329.

Smith, S., Macduff, C. 2017. A thematic analysis of the experience of UK mental health nurses who have trained in Solution Focused Brief Therapy. J Psychiatr Ment Health Nurs, 24(2–3), 105–113.

Staniland, L., Hasking, P., Boyes, M., & Lewis, S. 2021. Stigma and nonsuicidal self-injury: Application of a conceptual framework. Stigma and Health, 6(3), 312.

Staunton, P., Chiarella, M., 2020. Law for Nurses and Midwives. Elsevier, Sydney.

Stein-Parbury, J., 2021. Patient and Person: Interpersonal Skills in Nursing, 7th ed, Elsevier, Sydney.

Stewart, C., Biegler, P., Brunero, S., Lamont, S., & Tomossy, G.F. 2020a. Mental capacity assessments for COVID-19 patients: Emergency admissions and the CARD approach. J Bioeth Inq, 17(4), 803–808.

Stewart, C., Brunero, S., & Lamont, S. 2020b. COVID-19: Restrictive practices and the law during a global pandemic – an Australian perspective. Int J Ment Health Nurs, 29(5), 753–755.

Toms, G., Williams, L., Rycroft-Malone, J., et al., 2019. The development and theoretical application of an implementation framework for dialectical behaviour therapy: a critical literature review. Borderline Personal. Disord Emot Dysregul 6(1), 2.

Turgut, E.Ö., & Çam, M.O. 2020. The effect of tidal model-based psychiatric nursing approach on the resilience of women survivors of violence. Issues Ment Health Nurs, 41(5), 429–437.

Tyerman, J., Patovirta, A.-L., & Celestini, A. 2021. How stigma and discrimination influences nursing care of persons diagnosed with mental illness: A systematic review. Issues Ment Health Nurs, 42(2), 153–163.

United Nations General Assembly, 1991. Principles for the protection of persons with mental illness and for the improvement of mental health care. Online. Available at: www.ohchr.org/en/instruments-mechanisms/instruments/principles-protection-persons-mental-illness-and-improvement

United Nations, 1948. The Universal Declaration of Human Rights. Online. Available at: www.un.org/en/documents/udhr/

United Nations, 2022. Convention on the Rights of Persons with Disabilities. Online. Available at: www.un.org/development/desa/disabilities/convention-on-the-rights-of-persons-with-disabilities.html

van Weeghel, J., van Zelst, C., Boertien, D., & Hasson-Ohayon, I. 2019. Conceptualizations, assessments, and implications of personal recovery in mental illness: A scoping review of systematic reviews and meta-analyses. Psychiat Rehab J, 42(2), 169.

Volkow, N.D., Gordon, J.A., & Koob, G. F. 2021. Choosing appropriate language to reduce the stigma around mental illness and substance use disorders. Neuropsychopharmacology, 46(13), 2230–2232.

Whiting, D., Lichtenstein, P., & Fazel, S. 2021. Violence and mental disorders: A structured review of associations by individual diagnoses, risk factors, and risk assessment. The Lancet Psychiatry, 8(2), 150–161.

Wright, L., Bennett, S., & Meredith, P. 2020. "Why didn't you just give them PRN?": A qualitative study investigating the factors influencing implementation of sensory modulation approaches in inpatient mental health units. Int J Ment Health Nurs, 29(4), 608–621.

5

Working with Families in Mental Health

Sophie Isobel and Chantel Jurcevic

KEY POINTS

- Experiences of mental illness and distress can affect all members of a family.
- Supporting consumers in their personal recovery includes recognising the importance and role of families.
- Nurses have a responsibility for improving wellbeing and outcomes for families through partnering with and supporting families in the processes of family and relational recovery.
- Family-focused practices in mental health include identifying the family system, providing information and support, and providing specific strategies and interventions to strengthen family capacity, build family resilience and support family recovery.

KEY TERMS

Carers

Family-focused practice

Family of choice

Family of origin

Family recovery

Family resilience

Relational recovery

Strengths-based approach

LEARNING OUTCOMES

The material in this chapter will assist you to:
- define the key terms related to working with families in mental health
- outline a strengths-based approach to working with families when a person has mental illness
- describe family-focused practices when working with families in mental health
- understand the family and relational recovery process when a family member has mental illness
- identify how nurses can support family wellbeing, resilience and recovery in trauma-informed ways.

INTRODUCTION

We live within the context of our relationships with others, particularly our family and friends. When a person develops an illness or experiences life-interrupting distress, their experiences of the illness, recovery and treatment will inevitably affect, and be affected by, the people with whom they are most connected. Mental illness and distress affect the entire family. Recognising the vital importance of relationships for wellbeing, this chapter focuses on how nurses can provide effective mental health care that is inclusive of the needs of the whole family – the consumer and their children or their parents and/or others with whom they live or love.

DEFINING "FAMILY"

For the purposes of this chapter, the notion of "family" is understood to be defined by its members. That is, the family themselves determine who is family. This approach acknowledges the many types of family relationships that may not resemble traditional assumptions of family. Family may include people joined through relationships, circumstance or genetics, and be inclusive of close friends, kinship groups or extended family members. Family relationships can be culturally or socially defined or assumed, but family relationships can also be complicated and nuanced. As a nurse, it is important to reflect on your understanding and assumptions of what constitutes a "family", and to be open to other ways of structuring family.

In this chapter we consider two broad types of family. The first is "family of origin". This refers to the family a person is born into, where the family commonly includes parents and siblings of a child or an adult with mental illness. We all have a family of origin, even if relationships have broken down. The second is "family of choice", where the family involves relationships chosen as an adult (such as romantic partners or kinship relationships). Many of us have a family of choice. For people who have strained relationships with their family of origin, or who have been ostracised from their community, cultural group or family, family of choice can be particularly important. Both family of origin and family of choice can include other family members, such as grandparents, extended family, caregivers, and others who are considered family by the members.

In mental health services, and in the literature, families of people who experience mental illness are also commonly referred to as "family carers", "carers", or "caregivers". The terms "family" and "carer" are often used interchangeably, and young people in families are often called "young carers". The term "carer" recognises the crucial role that many family members play in providing informal or unpaid care for their loved one. However, not all family members play a caregiving role, consider themselves caregivers, or wish to be identified as carers, and not all carers are family members. The term "carer" emerged from policy and legislation that required clear distinction of these roles; however, the term "family" is used throughout this chapter to emphasise the relationships and reciprocity, rather than centralising the caring role. To focus only on the caring role minimises that most relationships within families of choice or origin involve partnership and reciprocity, alongside caring for and being cared for (Wyder & Bland 2014). Throughout the chapter we discuss the practical and emotional caregiving that many family members provide, as well as the complexity of such relationships.

In respect to formal recognition of their roles, individual states in Australia have carer recognition legislation; there is a National Carer Recognition Act and there are carer-specific standards in the National Mental Health Standards to guide the identification, collaboration with, and support of carers of people who access mental health services. Mental health legislation in many states mandates the identification and inclusion of "primary carers" or "designated carers"; however, there are differences in the language and specifics of these requirements. Similarly, Mental Health Legislation in Aotearoa New Zealand includes recognising "principal caregivers" in care, defined as friends, family or whānau most directly involved in care. The *New Zealand Mental Health Act* requires that a principal caregiver is present at points of care, including when mental health assessments may occur. The Mahi Aroha Carers' Strategy Action Plan guides government strategy in Aotearoa New Zealand to recognise and support family groups and whānau within services. It is important to familiarise yourself with local policies, legislation and procedures in the settings within which you work, related to your obligations in relation to families. Also important are local policy and procedures in relation to the identification of children and parenting roles, privacy and confidentiality, and family engagement in care planning.

Family as a Social and Ecological System

Family systems theory (Bowen 1966) is one way of understanding families. Conceptualising family as one "system" embedded within other larger social and ecological systems can be helpful for understanding why families function and interact in the ways they do. In family systems theory, it is recognised that families develop and sustain their own ways of maintaining homeostasis in the same way a biological system (such as the human body or a microclimate) does. Families develop their own ways of being, roles, patterns, behaviours and norms to sustain functioning. An example is that some families may not express or talk about certain emotions, such as anger or sadness. While this may seem problematic for expression and processing of emotional states of individuals, it may serve a purpose of sustaining the family peace. When illness occurs in a family, it can disrupt the family system, altering roles and patterns. Over time, however, the system can adjust to cope with illness and the illness may also become woven into the family system, with people assuming roles and ways of interacting that maintain the system around the illness. Imagining a "system" also helps in understanding why initiating change in the behaviours, roles and ways of relating within families can be disruptive and have sustained effects. This can include the process of developing illness, responding to distress and the process of recovery. Family systems theory theorises that families have meaning to those within them. Beyond the connections between the individuals within them, families often have an identity, expectations, pride and responsibilities of their own.

The family as a system exists within a wider context. In Chapter 2, a socio-ecological model of health and illness for mental health nursing was introduced. In the same way that understandings of individual health, illness and wellbeing can be understood as being influenced by dynamic interactions between a person and their environment, to understand families and their ways of being requires consideration of factors such as community, neighbourhood, systems and social institutions, connection to culture, membership of subcultures, and political, economic, environmental, social and historical factors that influence them.

Within any system, there are subsystems. This is true for families also. For example, siblings, couple relationships or any number of relationships of origin or choice may exist as separate subsystems, with their own roles and dynamics, within the whole. Change in any subsystem or individual affects the whole system and can have impacts beyond the immediate. For example, the birth of a baby can alter the subsystem of the parents' relationship, while also having ripple effects on other children and their relationships with their parents, as well as the functioning of the system as a whole. Many families have extended networks of members and complexity, making it difficult to anticipate what impact changes may have on a family system. For nurses, it is important to recognise that things that affect an individual may also impact the wider system, and that each individual is impacted by the dynamics of the wider systems in which they exist. Through this lens, recognising and including families in the delivery of mental health care is essential.

A family's socio-ecological context will influence how they define, identify and respond to illness, what resources they have to cope and care, how accessible appropriate services and supports are, how much caring is considered possible or reasonable, the expected roles and responses of generational groups, the pre-existing stressors and distress absorbed within the system. It is therefore also important to not make assumptions about families and to be open to and curious about people's contexts.

DEFINING RELATIONAL AND FAMILY RECOVERY

Relational Recovery

In Chapter 2, the concept of "Personal recovery" was introduced. Personal recovery differs from clinical recovery and relates to an individual process of living a meaningful life, with or without symptoms of illness. Relational recovery describes the *relational context* of recovery. Relational recovery acknowledges the ways in which personal recovery is commonly relational in nature as people, including those living with mental illness and distress, exist as part of complex interdependent networks. Relational recovery is influenced by the formal and informal presence and availability of support, companionship, reciprocity, emotional involvement with others and communication (Lauzier-Jobin & Houle 2022). Relational recovery is also commonly linked to "seeing yourself through the eyes of others". Relational recovery emphasises that people are interdependent, that their lives can't be separated from the social context within which they live, and that recovery occurs in the context of relationships. Relationships, including those with families, can therefore be understood as being at the heart of personal recovery and affect all aspects of a person's recovery from mental illness (Price-Robertson et al 2017). As nurses, understanding that recovery is grounded in relationships is important for our practice. It means that to support a person's recovery from mental illness, we need to be aware of their social context, inclusive of their chosen family and supportive of family relationships and connections.

Family Recovery

Family recovery refers to the recovery processes which family members and carers, and the family system as a whole, experience, alongside individuals' personal recovery experiences. Family recovery may involve relational recovery, but it encompasses the recovery of the family as a whole, rather than its individual members. Frequently in mental health, families are positioned as supporting a person's personal recovery; however, just as a person with mental illness can experience recovery, so too can family members. Families often experience distress, stress, confusion, fear and many other emotions and impacts when a member experiences mental illness or distress. Family recovery draws on the strengths of all members of the family, is informed by an understanding of life events and the impact of trauma, and is driven by the family, their goals and needs (Nicholson et al 2014). Family recovery is a process of finding shared connection, hope, identity, meaning and power while supporting a family member who experiences mental illness and reconciling expectations around roles, responsibilities and purpose.

Expanding recovery-oriented practice to be inclusive of both family and relational recovery provides an opportunity for clinicians to consider the family as a whole, not just those in caring roles, and to understand the strengths of the family system. Through recognising the family as a system, there is space to see that the relationships within them are important to recovery, and that the family as a whole can also adjust and recover. Relational recovery affords "a set of ideas around hope and empowerment which can shape assessments and interventions" (Price-Robertson et al 2017, p. 9) which will support clinicians understanding the person, family system, and how to best shape care and support to facilitate both personal and family recovery.

DIVERSE FAMILIES AND PERSPECTIVES

Families may have varying ways of understanding or conceptualising their loved one's distress or illness. For many families, their understanding may be nuanced and include recognition of the many ways that families can live with experiences of illness or distress. Consider this quote from a participant in a study by Chesla in 1988: *It's been devastating, on the whole family. It's a terrible thing; I wouldn't want anybody to have to go through with an illness like that ... If there was any way to avoid it. But it's done some wonderful things in our lives, too. It's brought out love that maybe just would have been buried. We've become a more giving, loving family, who's not afraid to show it* (p. 153). The participant highlights how among challenges, there can also be family growth and transformation. Often the experiences of families are more complex than can be assumed.

At times, the understandings and experiences of families may conflict with those of the person experiencing illness or distress. Rather than aligning to binaries of who is "right" and who is "wrong", nurses can support families and individuals to be able to express their perceptions and navigate tensions, while also supporting individuals within families to maintain their autonomy and individuality. Frequently, recovery from mental illness involves regaining agency and control over one's life, shifting the relationship that people may have with services and family members who provide care. Risk-taking can be central to recovery (Wyder & Boland 2014), yet many families may be fearful of a loss of control or decreased contact with services. At times, it may be family members who advocate for more coercive and intensive approaches to care than services or clinicians perceive as necessary. This can be difficult for nurses to navigate, but requires reflective practice, engaging in peer and clinical supervision and support and a willingness to engage in conversations about recovery, treatment, care and power with families and individuals. It also requires sensitivity, empathy, patience, and respect for difference of opinion (Wyder & Bland 2014).

For queer families, families of choice or non-heteronormative families, challenges in having approaches to caregiving or needs recognised within services can be amplified. The dominant culture in mental health nursing remains hetero and cis-normative (Rees et al 2021), leading to unconscious and conscious stigmatisation of LGBTIQA+ individuals and their families, as well as families with non-nuclear structures. Families from Indigenous or culturally diverse backgrounds may also experience intersectional challenges within services. Page and colleagues (2022) engaged an expert panel to model mental health services needs for Aboriginal and Torres Strait Islander peoples in Australia and determined that individual approaches to mental health treatment are particularly inappropriate for many Indigenous peoples due to a lack of understanding of the importance of the positioning of individuals within a family and community context. They describe that Indigenous kinship relationships and responsibilities are complex and dynamic and not aligned with non-Indigenous assumptions about family. Subsequently, active engagement of families and kinship systems is essential for effective and appropriate care delivery. Many services have identified Indigenous or Aboriginal mental health workers who can provide guidance in what constitutes effective care for local communities and their members.

Almost a quarter of Australia's population is born overseas and over 40% of people have at least one overseas-born parent (Population Australia 2019). In Aotearoa New Zealand, more than a quarter of the population are born overseas (EHINZ 2023). Families from diverse cultural backgrounds are likely to experience unique challenges in engaging with mental health services and it is not possible to assume sameness among groups of people, even from similar cultural groups. Nurses need to practise with cultural sensitivity and humility (Bennett & Gates 2019). Cultural humility requires openness to alternative perspectives and ways of understanding the world. Cultural humility requires nurses to apply multicultural and intersectional approaches to practice that allow for recognition of diversity, attention to life experiences, resources and needs, and openness to people's relationships and worldviews. This means recognising awareness that many cultural groups have strong expectations to care for their relatives with mental illness (Poon & Lee 2019), differing understandings of distress, or may have differing expectations of when services should be engaged, how much information should be shared and what services should provide. Communication can facilitate this space. Family members from diverse cultural backgrounds have identified that they want mental health clinicians to demonstrate acceptance, to listen, be credible, be open, show respect for cultural differences, provide culturally appropriate resources and attempt to develop cultural understanding (Cross & Bloomer 2010). Cultural humility is an approach that can inform all aspects of family sensitive practice.

WHY WORK WITH FAMILIES? INTRODUCING A STRENGTHS-BASED APPROACH

As discussed, a person's illness often affects not only them as an individual, but also those who love and support them. Family members require information and support to be able to best provide care to their loved one, and to look after themselves. Family recovery often requires a shuffling and reconsideration of how involved members are in their loved one's illness and what needs, energy and capacity all members have.

Despite their pivotal roles, families have consistently reported difficulty in gaining information about their loved one's mental illness. Families report that often mental health professionals, including nurses, are either not aware of their needs or are preoccupied with addressing the needs of the consumer. Families report being dismissed by clinicians, feeling unacknowledged, worrying about their family member, and being excluded from decisions about care (Abou Seif et al 2022). Families often report not receiving information about care and treatment, while also not being asked for their input despite their knowledge and roles in providing care (Cleary et al 2005; Martin et al 2017). At times, these decisions may occur because of clinician fears about compromising consumer privacy and confidentiality. While it is important to respect people's privacy and confidentiality, it is also important to understand local policies and procedures, so that you can feel confident in talking to families and providing information and support, even when you can't share personal or medical information. For example, a person in an inpatient mental health unit may not want you to tell their parent about their current treatment plan. As an adult, this is a choice they can make; however, if they live with their parent, the parent may still need to know information such as their planned discharge date. Similarly, a person in a mental health unit may request that staff do not talk to their family about their care, but as a nurse you can still provide general information about mental health distress and information about carer services available, without compromising confidentiality.

Fear of saying the wrong thing or breaching confidentiality can stop nurses from engaging with families. Nurses have reported being unsure of their roles with families, having limited confidence in interacting with families and being preoccupied with managing risks (Foster & Isobel 2017). These fears can lead to a breakdown of communication and result in decreased quality of care for individuals, while also leaving family members feeling dismissed or disrespected. Families express a need for health professionals to listen to them with non-judgemental attitudes, respect their concerns, recognise their needs, acknowledge their strengths and include them when appropriate in decisions made about the care of their family member or loved one (Foster et al 2019). When families communicate or interact in unexpected ways, it can be helpful for nurses to make generous assumptions about why this may be.

Many services now work from a strengths-based approach. A strengths-based approach with families requires focusing on what is working well in a family and can be further enhanced (Francis 2014). Being strengths-based with families includes recognising the positive attributes and resources of families. A strengths-based approach acknowledges that, while problems exist, families are the best judges of their circumstances and can be supported by health professionals to find their own solutions and ways of coping. Importantly, this approach does not dismiss the consumer's and family's problems, but focuses on the capacities and resources they have that can be fostered to support them in addressing their challenges. A strengths-based approach should not dismiss challenges; it is important to recognise and acknowledge the adversity that individuals and families experience, while validating the things that families have done to help them get through and manage. There is a risk that in focusing only on strengths, families may feel further invalidated and dismissed. However, nurses can support families to recognise strengths within challenges and adversity, and to reflect back to families observed strengths that they may not be aware of.

A strengths-based approach is based on understanding that:
- all families have strengths and the capacity to be resilient
- the family, as well as the consumer, goes through a process of recovery associated with mental illness, the process of which looks different for every member of a family
- as mental health professionals, we need to attend to the diversity of individual and family responses to the challenges of living with mental illness.

A strengths-based approach can assist nurses to work with families, by listening to experiences and validating challenges, while also focusing on perceived strengths, competencies and resources that families identify they have and need. Using a strengths-based framework moves us away from the idea of trying to "fix" individual or family deficits and towards recognising their existing protective attributes and abilities. Considering strengths through a family systems lens also requires less focus on problems as discrete entities, redirecting attention to the structures and dynamics that contribute to and sustain them. Even in individually focused care delivery, a strengths focus requires attention to the wider context of an individual, to ensure supports and strengths within a family and community context are recognised and supported (see Historical anecdote 5.1).

✳ HISTORICAL ANECDOTE 5.1
Know your Carer Movement History!

Since the 1960s and amplified by formal "deinstutionalisation" in the 1980s, there have been efforts to shift the care of people living with mental illness or distress out of institutions and into the community. These important efforts have been driven by advocacy by consumer groups, awareness of human rights violations occurring within institutions and increased use of psychotropic medications. However, a lack of community-based services to support deinstitutionalisation led to families and friends being required to take on significant carer roles without support and formed the context for the development of the carer movement.

In 1975, the Association of Relatives And Friends of the Mentally Ill (ARAFMI) group was formed in New South Wales to address concerns about a lack of recognition, support and information for carers, family and friends within mental health services. It was the first of its kind in Australia. Around the same time, The Schizophrenia Fellowship in Victoria pioneered family support groups to enable families to share their experiences, information and knowledge. Significant advocacy stemmed from these groups, leading to successful lobbying for changes to be made in the structure of mental health services. Carer groups have also provided the foundation from which "family peer work" has developed with family peer workers and consultants now integrated into mental health services across Australia, providing their lived experience expertise to support families and enhance family-focused practice. While historically there has been some tension between carer and consumer movements, they have also worked together to advocate for, and collectively drive, significant change in the way mental health care is delivered.

Read More About It
Mental Health Carers Australia: www.mentalhealthcarersaustralia.org.au/

POTENTIAL CHALLENGES FOR FAMILIES WHEN A PERSON HAS MENTAL ILLNESS

Families can be a major source of support for people during periods of illness and distress. For many families, they have access to existing mechanisms of support and coping that help them support their loved ones through acute or sustained illness. However, families are affected by the experiences of their members, and families can face a number of challenges when a family member has mental illness. For example, family members of people with mental illness often provide a significant amount of daily care to their relatives, which can impact upon their social, financial, psychological and physical wellbeing. In 2020, over 294,000 people aged 16 and over in Australia received a Carer Payment in recognition of their caretaking roles; however, almost 2.7 million Australians identified as unpaid carers for family members, representing around 10% of the population (Australian Bureau of Statistics 2022).

At times, the challenges of caregiving can impact on family members' own health and wellbeing. Family members who provide informal care to their loved ones who experience illness have been found to have worse physical health than the general population, with health impacts increasing alongside the length of the caregiving experience, intensity of care provision and competing responsibilities (Kenny et al 2014). The experience of caregiving in families has been linked to a concept referred to as "burden of care". Many family members would not describe their experiences of caregiving as a "burden", but this is not to say it doesn't impact upon their lives. The "burden" of care relates to all the ways that caring for someone who experiences illness can impact upon family wellbeing, as well as impacting upon life choices such as career decisions, where to live and whether to have children (Von Kardorff et al 2016). Despite the "burden", many families value their roles in caregiving and are committed to ongoing support of their loved ones. The extent of the "burden" is individual to each family and each of its members and can change over time.

Family members can experience financial hardship, relationship problems, social isolation, stigmatising attitudes from others, altered daily routines, frustration and exhaustion (Richardson et al 2013). Caregiving can markedly reduce the time available for socialising with others and in engaging in hobbies and self-care, such as movement and spending time alone. Many family members report feeling isolated from others, including within families (McCann et al 2015), leaving them without others to discuss concerns with (Digiacomo et al 2013). McCann and colleagues (2015) found that the stress of caregiving can have a serious negative impact on family relationships, especially where other family members are critical of the care delivered. Family members may feel guilty about discussing their own challenges related to caregiving out of loyalty to their loved one, not wanting to add to the family burden and taking pride in their caring role. But at the same time, they may be experiencing a lack of opportunities to access support and/or fear of others misinterpreting their experiences as an unwillingness to continue in their caring role. Caring itself may not always impact on wellbeing, although it may increase stress levels.

Young people living within a family where there is mental illness or distress, often referred to as "young carers", also experience difficulties and impacts on their social, economic and educational lives. Despite the difficulties and social, economic and educational impacts of being a young person living in a family where there is mental illness or distress, it is also important to know that young carers can experience concurrent positive effects of caregiving, such as connection and purpose (Wepf & Leu 2022). Young carers may also be overlooked in services or encounter simplistic or patronising recognition of their roles through clinicians making assumptions about the extent of their "burden" of care.

Some of the burden of caring comes from difficulty with services. Families have clearly articulated that their own wellbeing is linked to being able to access appropriate, safe and inclusive care for their family member (Walters & Petrakis 2022). When they can access such services, they require recognition of their expertise and roles, as well as inclusion in care.

Family members report concerns about accessing mental health services, often attempting to "manage" without them for as long as possible. They also describe frustration that when accessing services they have to convince clinicians that their loved one requires help and then subsequently feel ignored, dismissed and not taken seriously despite their familiarity, understanding and knowledge about their loved one (Lavoie 2018). Services are identified to be both difficult to

access, difficult to navigate and difficult to cope without. At times, family members perceive they are treated as burdens or the source of irritation within services, despite their expertise, care and relationships (Yin et al 2020). After ongoing negative experiences with services, families can develop distrust and even animosity towards services, and this can impact upon both personal and family recovery (see Perspectives in practice: Nurse's story 5.1: Felicity).

PERSPECTIVES IN PRACTICE

Nurse's Story 5.1: Felicity

As a nurse, I've always worked with families. Everyone comes from a family and I think I've always been aware of the importance of connection and relationships. Currently I work with families within an adult mental health service, promoting awareness of families and offering support to families when someone is unwell. When one person has a mental illness, there's a ripple effect; it doesn't just affect them, but it affects the people around them and everybody feels it.

Families can be understood a bit like a baby's mobile. Mental illness can cause a lot of anxiety within the family. When one bit of the mobile shakes, the whole thing shakes. The mobile can shake from any change, a change of role or a move or sickness. A mental illness in the family can cause the mobile to vigorously shake and we are often working with families to find some calm and balance again. When mental illness happens, families can feel grief, sadness, guilt or fear. There is still so much stigma and shame. Some families can be very supportive and get into patterns that work for them. Other times, the mental illness can dominate the whole family and people forget to look after themselves. I remind people that in an aeroplane you have to put your own oxygen mask on first before you help others. Sometimes people don't know they are allowed to do that.

Other people may not want their family involved or their family might be disconnected or live far away. Mental illness can cause tension within a family and conflicts within relationships. Sometimes the tension was there already, and everything gets attributed to the person with the illness. But illness in any family is a stressor. You see so much more about people when you see them with their family or you see them in their home – the environment, the dynamics – things that we don't see if we just see someone in the clinic or hospital. People are different around their family; we all are, because of the emotional investment.

As a mental health nurse, if we go to someone's home, we are always a guest and we have to be respectful of people's lives and spaces. I try to be curious, ask people about their family, and make time to listen and talk to them about what help they may want. I show kindness and empathy, which helps build trust. I also ask families what brings them joy and satisfaction, and I tell them what I observe as their strengths. Sometimes they can't see the strengths they have. There is usually a lot of love in families, even if they are having trouble showing it. In mental health, we see so many different families; there is no "usual" family. Every family is different, every family has struggles. We need to offer hope for families that things will get better than they are right now; it might take some time, but they will. Sometimes families feel stuck or feel like things won't ever change. Families are very attuned to judgement from services and clinicians. We have to be very aware of this and focus on strengths and help them find a way forward. It's a privilege to see into people's everyday lives.

Experiences of Children and Parents

Relationships between parents and children are often a component of families. Children and young people can be overlooked when considering the impacts of mental illness on families. Approximately 12–45% of people accessing adult mental health services have children under the age of 18 years (Maybery & Reupert 2018); however, adult mental health services primarily focus on treating the parent's illness and often do not consider children's needs unless there are child protection risks or children present with their own health difficulties (Reupert et al 2022).

Children of Parents with Mental Illness

Children and young people in families where there is mental illness are often required to provide care, including for their parents. Even if they don't provide direct care, mental illness in families can impact on children and young people in varying ways. Children and young people can experience unpredictability, fear, shame, confusion, heightened responsibility and worry (Patrick et al 2019); they may also be more socially isolated, be required to provide physical and psychological care for their parent and may have disrupted schooling. Children and young people may experience a lack of attunement from their parents, reduced self-worth and lack of opportunities for self-differentiation (Murphy et al 2014), as well as disruption to the cohesion of their sense of self, life and memories (Boström & Strand 2021). For many children and young people, parental mental illness becomes woven into their everyday lives. Things that can be protective for children and young people include access to accurate information about their parents' illness, social activities and belonging, housing and educational stability, as well as access to supportive adults. Children and young people may also be burdened by an excessive clinical and research focus on "risk". This focus on risk may itself be harmful across the lifespan as it can permeate self-concept and social-identity (Gladstone et al 2011), and lead to hyper-vigilance to usual experiences of distress (Trondsen 2012). While children and young people may experience social, psychological and practical challenges across their lives as a direct result of their family member's illness and will benefit from support, it is important to also note that the experiences of children and adults within families can be varied.

Parenting with Mental Illness

For parents who experience mental illness or distress, the task of parenting can become more challenging (Boström & Strand 2021). Low mood, fatigue or other symptoms may interfere in their ability to consistently provide protection, reciprocity, routine and structure. Side effects of medications and treatment may also impede upon everyday parenting capacity. Parents also commonly worry about the effects of their illness upon their children and may experience self-stigmatisation or decreased parenting confidence (Yates & Gatsou 2021). Fear of judgement and scrutiny by clinicians may impede on talking openly about parenting challenges. Parent–child relationships may be disrupted by parental mental illness, but they are also commonly embedded in mutual caring. Parenting can also form a critical component of personal recovery; for example, a parent may identify parenting goals as an important aspect to work towards or a key motivation in their recovery process. For nurses, roles may include listening to people's worries and ideas about parenting, linking people into parenting support services and supporting parents to talk to children about the illness and the child's experience.

Parents of Children with Mental Illness

Parents caring for a child or young person with mental illness can experience unique challenges. Many parents worry for their children's future and experience guilt or fear. Many also experience numerous losses. Parents have reported losses associated with their perceptions of the child's lost expectations, uncertainty for the future, loss of financial stability and loss of social and career opportunities (Richardson et al 2013). Parents have reported experiences such as anger, disappointment, hopelessness, sadness, shock, worry and denial related to the diagnosis of mental illness, and the many challenges faced in the caregiver role.

Practically, parents may lose income and social connection through increased time spent caring for, or facilitating care for, their child. Parents may experience discrimination and stigma, as well as isolation. For many parents, the wellbeing and happiness of their children is intrinsically linked to their own, meaning that when their child (even when that child is an adult) is experiencing illness or distress, they also experience distress and require support. Consistency, trusting therapeutic relationships, empathic clinicians and access to information about care and treatment options are known to be beneficial, alongside information about accessing services, what to expect and support groups (Coyne et al 2015). It is also important to identify the support needs of siblings in families where a child or young person experiences mental illness. Siblings may desire information, inclusion or respite, as well as time and space to express their own experiences, emotions and needs.

Stigma and Families

While the challenges for children, parents, adults and families associated with mental illness are often related to their own experiences and social impacts, many also experience stigma associated with having a relative with mental illness. This involves prejudice or discrimination from others. This form of stigma has been referred to as associative or family stigma (Campbell & Patrick 2022). It can include, for example, blaming mental illness in a child or young person on poor parenting or blaming family members for not helping their relative take medications as prescribed (Corrigan et al 2014). Stigma may make it harder for family members to accept their relative's illness, and, in some cases, they may experience guilt related to the shame they feel about their relative's illness or behaviour. This can be understood as "self-stigma", where family members endorse negative social views of people with mental illness (Corrigan et al 2014).

Families of people with mental illness report being subjected to daily discrimination and stigma; this stigma may come from the community, extended family members or health professionals (van der Sanden et al 2016). As a result, families may withdraw from wider social situations and connections (Murphy et al 2014). Sustained exposure to family stigma is linked to social isolation and lower quality of life for family members, as well as weakened sense of self (Campbell & Patrick 2022). Family stigma is also known to affect siblings and other extended family members (Liegghio 2017) (see Historical anecdote 5.2).

✳ HISTORICAL ANECDOTE 5.2
Families Blamed

In the past, families were often blamed for causing mental disorder. In 1948, American psychiatrist Frieda Fromm-Reichmann even went so far as to define a so-called "schizophrenogenic mother", who she asserted could cause schizophrenia. This type of mother was described as being emotionally cold, rejecting and emotionally disturbed; a perfectionist, domineering and lacking in sensitivity; rigidly moral but seductive; and overprotective of the child who she kept in a dependent state so she could exert control. This parent would, in theory, confuse the child with contradictory standards and expectations, or "double-binds", to the extent that the child grew up bewildered by society's demands and unable to decipher reality, or how to react to it.

While the "schizophrenogenic mother" concept is no longer accepted, families still experience blame and judgement within services, particularly when their family member meets criteria for a personality disorder, experiences complex trauma or distress, or when a person presents repeatedly to services.

Read More About It
Johnston, J. 2013. The ghost of the schizophrenogenic mother. AMA J Ethics 15(9), 801–805.

ADDRESSING CHALLENGES AND BUILDING STRENGTHS – FAMILY RESILIENCE

While it is apparent that family members can face many challenges when a relative has mental illness, there is also evidence that many families develop strengths that can enable them to address these challenges effectively. Overcoming these challenges or adversities can be understood through the lens of resilience.

At times, families may be the source of trauma and adversity and it is important for nurses to be aware of, engage in screening for, and engage in conversations about difficult topics such as domestic violence and child protection. There are times when families will be excluded from care or when people's choices to not have family involved in their lives are intentional and protective. Sensitivity to importance and complexity of family relationships and their individual cultural contexts does not mean accepting or witnessing harm, disrespect or abuses of power.

At other times, families can be both a place where trauma has occurred, and a place of healing and recovery. Families can experience collective trauma or interpersonal traumas and many families are also impacted by intergenerational trauma. Intergenerational trauma occurs when traumatic effects are passed on through generations in families via interactional patterns, genetic pathways, family dynamics, culture or continued exposure to disadvantage and structural inequalities (Isobel et al 2021). When nurses have contact with families and their members, there are opportunities to support shared understandings of family experiences, as well as link families to services that may be able to provide specialised interventions and support for trauma (Isobel et al 2019).

Many families and individuals who experience trauma, including intergenerational trauma, also develop collective and transgenerational resilience. It is possible to be "trauma-informed" when working with families and foster the processes that support personal and family resilience and strength in the face of adversity, alongside recognition of risks and vulnerability (Isobel et al 2019).

Family Resilience

Resilience has been variously defined, but in this context it refers to adaption to challenges. Resilience is a dynamic process that involves adapting or responding to stress or using internal and external resources to sustain wellbeing. Individual resilience is often linked to protective factors such as personal mastery, self-efficacy and positive coping strategies. Family resilience is a separate but linked process by which shared protective factors give the entire family and its individual members the ability to recover from adversity, while becoming stronger and more resourceful. Protective factors that facilitate family resilience are linked to relationships, processes such as family communication, problem-solving strategies, and access to external social and economic resources. Other factors associated with family resilience include shared values, routines, traditions and embedded activities that promote family closeness and culture. Self-efficacy, cohesion, nurturance, collaborative problem-solving, consistent support, open emotional expressions and appropriate use of humour are also linked to family resilience (Smith & Bailey 2017).

Family resilience allows families to adapt to health challenges in ways that are in synchrony with their background and practices, and to develop a pattern of response to illness that allows family members to maintain their values and concerns and find meaning in their caregiving, while at the same time responding effectively to the demands of illness (Chesla & Leonard 2017). Individuals within families can have resilience, and that may benefit the family unit; however, other intrafamilial resources, such as warm and positive relationships and connections between family members, are integral resilience factors in maintaining the family unit's ability to recover from adversity (Harrist et al 2019; Walsh 2006).

Family resilience can be distinguished from individual resilience because it refers to the wellbeing of multiple individuals within a family system and the relationships between them, as well as the key family processes that support their resilience (Power et al 2015). From a family resilience perspective, families are viewed as a unit with fundamental strengths and resources and potential for growth (Zauszniewski et al 2015). In families living with mental illness, resilience has been found to involve keeping a balance between stress and distress and maintaining family members' strength and optimism (Power et al 2015).

Nurses can recognise existing family resilience, including during periods of challenge and distress, and use strengths-focused approaches to help families identify their own protective factors. Nurses can also support families and individuals to develop their own shared narrative of illness and events, facilitate positive family communication, map resources and identify needs, and engage additional community supports or services.

Theories of Family Recovery

There are a number of emerging theories about the tasks, processes and framework of family recovery. Wyder and Bland (2014) propose that potential key tasks of family recovery include maintaining hope, reconnecting, overcoming secondary trauma and journeying from carer to family. Each task is described in detail in Table 5.1.

More recently, Wyder and colleagues (2022) used the CHIME model of personal recovery to consider the process of families supporting their relative's recovery, as well as undertaking their own (see Table 5.2). The CHIME model (Leamy et al 2011) identifies the

TABLE 5.1	Tasks for Families in Recovery
Maintaining hope	Maintaining hope for themselves as individuals and their own dreams and aspirations. Holding hope is complex. Families may need to hold hope for their loved one. As they find ways to maintain hope for themselves, they can continue their caring responsibilities while leading their own fulfilling lives.
Reconnecting	Mental illness emerges within the complex network of close relationships that includes family and friends. Reconnecting includes maintaining or re-establishing relationships and support from others, being part of peer support and support groups, and being part of the community.
Overcoming secondary trauma	Families can experience secondary traumatisation and share the trauma, isolation and stigma associated with mental illness. This can include feeling powerless to control their lives, feeling abused by the treatment system, experiencing guilt, feeling traumatised when their loved one is subjected to trauma and experiencing chronic grief and loss.
Journeying from carer to family	Families are often defined by their carer role. A family's journey is also an integral part in recovery. When families can let go of their caring role to achieve a mutually supportive role with their loved one, this ultimately enables not only their own but also their loved one's recovery.

Adapted from Wyder & Bland 2014.

TABLE 5.2   CHIME-D: A Framework of Family Recovery

Principle of Recovery	Individual Recovery	Family Tasks	Family Recovery
Connectedness	Finding genuine connection to self, others and community	Supporting, facilitating and maintaining connection to loved one	Remaining connected to each other, community and selves
Hope and optimism	Belief in the possibility of recovery and a meaningful life	Holding hope and finding ways to foster hope for loved one	Maintaining hope for future of family unit and individual members
Identity	Redefinition of self and integration of experiences into sustained narrative of self	Adapting to changes and redefining relationships, while reflecting back the person's identity	Redefinition of caring within family life and shared narrative of family roles and values
Meaning	Finding meaning within the experience of mental illness and integrating illness into wider meaning of existence	Balancing limitations incurred by distress or illness while maintaining reflection on strengths and capabilities	Regaining a sense of family cohesion and reciprocity beyond caring or illness
Empowerment	Discovering a sense of personal power and capability for controlling own life and recovery	Supporting control, agency and choice, alongside dignity of risk	Assuming control and agency over own lives and choices. Sharing power among members
Difficulty and distress	Expressing and acknowledging the challenges that come along with and may at times set back, recovery	Allowing space to recognise and validate the challenges without dismissing through constant positivity	Weaving experiences of grief, distress and challenges into the narrative of family experiences

Adapted from Wyder et al 2022.

elements of Connectedness, Hope and optimism, Identity, Meaning and Purpose, and Empowerment as crucial to individual processes of recovery. In consulting with families, Wyder and colleagues identified a limitation of the CHIME framework for family recovery as it fails to acknowledge the distress, grief and difficulties of caregiving. Subsequently, they proposed the addition of "D" to stand for difficulties and distress. Including difficulties and distress in their CHIME-D recovery framework reminds us of the need to acknowledge and validate challenges, and to consider the social, systemic and structural challenges which impact upon individual and family capacity to enact CHIME.

Focusing more on the stages of family recovery, Spaniol (2010) identifies four phases: Shock, discovery and denial; Recognition and acceptance; Coping; Personal and political advocacy. Fig. 5.1 provides a visual framework of this process. In Spaniol's process, after an initial period of shock, families develop shared understandings of distress, grieve what is lost, and develop hope, varying ways of coping, and develop a synchronous rhythm. In time, families may develop new understandings of themselves leading to confidence and advocacy for others. These stages are not linear and people may move through them at different paces. Like all models, the stages are generalisations and may not reflect all families' experiences. See Family-focused care: Carer's story 5.1.

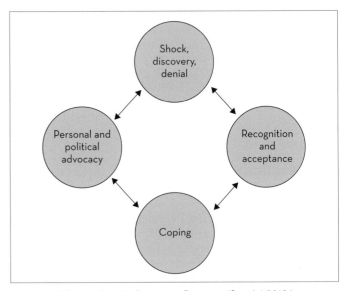

FIG. 5.1 Family Recovery Process. (Spaniol 2010.)

ⓘ CRITICAL THINKING EXERCISE 5.1

1. Consider the personal recovery processes (CHIME) (Leamy et al 2011) and the tasks for families in recovery (Wyder et al 2022). What are the similarities and differences between them? How can nurses support individuals and families in their recovery processes?

2. For each of the tasks for families in recovery outlined in Table 5.1, consider how nurses can support families in working through these tasks. Identify at least one strategy that nurses can use in supporting families in each family task.

✚ FAMILY-FOCUSED CARE

Carer's Story 5.1: Jane

My daughter has had a mental illness for nearly 20 years now. We've had a lot of contact with services and have always been very involved in her care. It's been very stressful and hard, but she's our daughter and we love her. Experiences with services are so varied. People can't really imagine what it's like to

have your daughter in a psychiatric ward and how that feels. I visit every day when she is in hospital. I had a really brilliant experience a couple of years ago in an inpatient unit. My daughter was very sick. It was very late at night when she was admitted. This really nice nurse welcomed us properly and didn't rush

FAMILY-FOCUSED CARE—cont'd

Carer's Story 5.1: Jane

me out, even though it was late, and was happy to settle both of us and make sure my daughter was comfortable, and then she even rang me later when I had gone home to let me know how my daughter was. It's unusual to get that follow-up. She really cared for us all the way through the admission. It was like she was our guardian angel. It changed my experience and my daughter's experience. It affected my daughter enormously because she didn't feel patronised; it felt like an equal relationship, and that she and the nurses were partners in her recovery.

Nurses can really affect the whole experience of care for families. Sometimes in hospital there are no nurses out on the floor. I know there's a lot of paperwork to be done, but it feels to me as a family member like they might be hiding in the office. Sometimes I've felt like the nurses aren't engaged with us as a family or even with my daughter. How people treat my daughter affects me. It's been great when nurses have shared information with me, told me how my daughter is doing

and even spoken to me on my own to see how I am. It makes me feel like she is being looked after properly and it's easier to go home and feel less worried.

There are always going to be some staff who are better than others. You get quite good at recognising who is going to be good. I've probably become one of those parents who are really pushy, but in a way, you have to be. I've learnt that because it can be the only way to make sure she gets the right care. I will ring as many times as I have to because I know her, and I know when she's not well. I know about her medication and what works, but sometimes staff don't listen to me or believe me. Staff think they are the experts, but I've known her for her whole life. In hospital, all the parents and carers you meet know a lot, but we are often dismissed. I've called before and told the mental health worker that my daughter was getting unwell and they didn't believe me and then things got a lot worse and we had to manage it at home. It's simple really, you just want staff to listen and care and have respect for our expertise as family.

CRITICAL THINKING EXERCISE 5.2

Read Carer's story 5.1: Jane.

1. Using the frameworks of family recovery discussed, identify relevant aspects of the family recovery process in Jane's story, and how they may, or may not, fit within these frameworks.
2. What elements of mental health service delivery were effective and ineffective in supporting this family's recovery?
3. In what ways can mental health service delivery be changed or improved to provide greater support for family recovery for all family members?

WORKING WITH FAMILIES: FAMILY-FOCUSED PRACTICES

Often in mental health care the focus is on caring for the individual consumer and managing their symptoms. While family are often considered through the lens of how they can assist and support the person in their recovery, family-focused practices require a perspective of seeing the family as intertwined with the individual and their experience of illness, and as a crucial context for recovery. An approach that focuses only on the individual and does not take into account the perspectives and needs of the people who love and care for them may fail to address the crucial family context of the lived experience of mental illness.

Family-focused practices include family care planning and goal setting; liaising between families and services; providing emotional

and social support to family members; assessment of family functioning; providing psychoeducation; and establishing a coordinated system of care between family members and services (Foster et al 2016). See Table 5.3 for more detail about each of these practices.

For nurses, this can include providing information for families about key issues such as confidentiality, consent and treatment, and carers' own needs for information about care, support and treatments (Foster et al 2019; Rowe 2012). It may also include acknowledging and respecting the right of people to choose not to have their families involved in their care or diverse non-traditional definitions or structures of family.

While psychoeducation is often recommended and nurses will often be providing information to families about pathways through care, the meaning of language and terms used and the effects of treatments and medications, it is also crucial that nurses feel comfortable to support individuals to talk to their families about their experiences and understandings of illness. People with lived experiences of mental health care have described that while it can be helpful for clinicians to talk directly to families, they also desire support to talk to their families about their illness in their own way (Waller et al 2019). Supporting families to develop their own narratives and understandings of events, with recognition of lived expertise and innate strengths, can be an effective component of family-focused practice. To do this requires first identifying families through asking people about their family members and roles, ensuring key relationships are documented and that the context of people's lives is considered right from the start of care and treatment planning. This can be enacted through asking questions such as

TABLE 5.3 Family-Focused Practices

Core Practice	Examples of Practice
Assessment of family members and family functioning	Asking people about their family upon intake to service, enquiring about family strengths, resources and worries, documenting parenting roles or other family responsibilities and enquiring about family understandings of mental illness
Psychoeducation	Asking families what information may be helpful to them about diagnoses, treatment and supports. Psychoeducation should not involve delivering facts or positioning clinicians as experts. Psychoeducation can include transparent discussions about treatments and plans, as well as linking family members up to support groups and sources of information that they can engage with in their own time
Family care planning and goal setting	Care planning with families includes developing individual care plans that are inclusive of family responsibilities and roles, as well as collaborating with families to develop their own crisis and recovery plans
Liaising between the family and services	Identifying services which may be of practical or psychological support to family members and supporting families to engage or make contact

"Can you tell me about the important people in your life?" and through curiosity about who people live with, love or care for. When encountering family members in care settings, it is helpful for nurses to be welcoming, to introduce yourself and your role, enquire about how they are and what support needs they may have, and to be knowledgeable about information, services and supports within your local area. Be aware of using specialist and assumed knowledge; it may be the first time this family has ever come into contact with mental health services and it can help to check that the family understands the meaning of certain words or processes. It is helpful to always check whether families have any questions or if there are things that aren't clear to them.

In ongoing care, family-focused practice requires nurses to support family members to have input into care and treatment planning (e.g. through passing information from families to treating teams, inviting families to care reviews and ensuring timely information about any change to care), to facilitate contact between parents and children during inpatient admissions (e.g. through supporting access to mobile phones, displaying photos and drawings and using family-friendly visiting spaces), to ensure family roles are considered in treatment planning (e.g. through considering how side effects of medications may impact upon caring responsibilities). Rather than be reliant on specific tasks, family-focused practice requires a lens of viewing the focus of nursing care as broader than the individual, and a constant recognition of and curiosity about the relational context of people's lives and recovery.

A Hierarchy of Family-Focused Practice

When working with families, nurses may feel they lack specific knowledge about the needs of children, parenting or the family as a whole. While there are a range of practices that are important for supporting families, it is not always feasible or necessary for nurses to provide all of them. Family-focused practice can be understood as comprising a range of practices that move from fundamental strategies through to more advanced or intensive approaches, including family therapy. See Fig. 5.2 for a visual diagram of a hierarchy of family-focused nursing practice.

When working with adults who are parents, Foster and colleagues (2012) recommend a minimum level of practice of identifying people's parental status when they enter a service, identifying the number, age, wellbeing and location of children, providing relevant mental health information and resources, including parenting information to consumers, children and family members and referring children and family members to family workers or services as appropriate. Foster and colleagues (2019) propose a framework for brief low-intensity family-focused practice known as "EASE": Engage (build rapport), Assess (strengths, worries, needs and vulnerabilities), Support (and mobilise existing supports), Educate (provide information and resources for parents and children).

When the consumer is the child, minimum levels of practice include identifying all members of the family and their roles, supporting family communication, providing relevant information and resources to all members of immediate family, including siblings, and referring parents and family members to appropriate services. For families without children, practices are similar and include identifying family members and roles, supporting communication, providing information and resources and referring to appropriate services. Sometimes pets are considered important family members and families may require support in ensuring pets are cared for during periods of hospitalisation or distress.

For all families, there is a range of practices that nurses and other health professionals can engage in to address the needs of all family members.

Many nurses feel nervous when talking to families, and this can contribute to interactions being simplistic or concrete rather than supportive. One example is that often family members are encouraged to engage in self-care. Nurses may, with good intention, encourage families to establish boundaries with the person they care for or engage in self-care, both important concepts in navigating caregiving and family relationships. However, this requires attention to the practicalities of family life and the resources available. If nurses position themselves as experts or make assumptions about what a family may need, it is likely that the family will not listen or find advice beneficial. It may be more beneficial to ask people about what things or moments in their life give them comfort or enhance their sense of coping, to collaboratively identify ways to increase even very small amounts of these activities or circumstances into their everyday lives, rather than making sweeping statements about self-care. Encouraging family members to engage in self-care can be very beneficial. However, self-care is an individual experience and families should be supported to find the self-care activities that work for them, rather than having them prescribed.

Supporting families to find strategies that work for them to enhance coping methods and reduce stress is an important practice. Nurses may find opportunities to talk with families about what support needs they have, whether they feel adequately supported and what gets in the way of them being supported. This also requires recognition of actual stressors and what feels within their control. It also requires observation and engagement with all members of a family, including children, to ensure that those who are quiet or seem resilient, also have space to share worries and seek support.

Family Therapy

On a continuum of family-focused practices, family therapy is considered a more intensive family approach and is not commonly accessible within public mental health services. Family therapy is based on the fundamental premise that when a person has a problem, it usually involves the whole family. Family interactions might be impacting the situation or prolonging the problem, or may be affecting other members of the family. Family therapists aim to effect change in the entire family system.

Family therapy usually involves multiple family members, but can also be undertaken with individual members. Even when therapy involves a single individual, its impact will be experienced by the wider family. This might be demonstrated through shifts in family functioning or communication, and/or through alleviating symptoms. The role of family therapists is to understand the dynamics that occur within families and to help the family members reconsider the ways in which

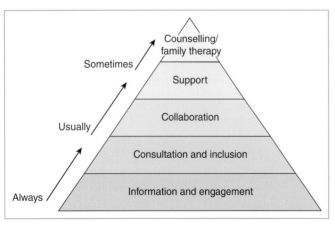

FIG. 5.2 A hierarchy of Nursing Family-Focused Practice.

they interact with each other. The therapist then supports family members to make changes.

When working with families in therapy, "problems" are viewed as emerging from, or being maintained within, the relationship between family members. The relationship therefore becomes the focus of attention. Sometimes people in families play roles, where problems exist to hold the family together. For example, consider a child whose behaviour escalates when their parents are fighting. The child's behaviour distracts the parents from their conflict and so further fighting is averted. The parents subsequently work together to manage the child's "problem" behaviour. While the focus may be on the child, ultimately the problem is not with the child but within the family relationships.

Families have their own ways of coping. But if ways of coping are causing conflict or secondary challenges, or don't suit all members of the family, support may be needed to become aware of dynamics, to consider ways to change patterns of behaviour, to facilitate collaborative planning, to advocate for those with less power, or to deepen empathic understanding. Family therapy can often aid with identifying and altering long-held patterns of communication, and for supporting differentiation.

Differentiation in Families

Differentiation refers to the conscious separating of experiences of individuals from the whole and separating the complex nuance of each individual from any possible diagnosis. This means that somebody in a family may experience illness, but they also have other strengths, challenges, characteristics and difficulties which make them who they are and contribute to the family. Galimidi and Shamai (2022) found that therapies that support family differentiation are beneficial for both family and individual recovery. The process of differentiation within families may not mean that caregiving roles are reduced or that members become less reliant upon the family unit. Differentiation is about members becoming aware of the separation between the emotions of their family members, and their own emotions; the stressors in their family members' lives and their own stressors. Differentiation is a systemic process that requires shifts in family dynamics, rather than alterations in the roles or responses of individuals (Galimidi & Shamai 2022). Differentiation can also relate to carers ensuring they take time to replenish themselves, such that they have the energy and capacity to continue to provide care for others.

Applying Family Therapy in Practice

While family therapy can be a great intervention, keep in mind that access can be limited. Nurses do not usually undertake family therapy within public mental health services, but they may often find themselves involved in family meetings or therapeutic interactions with multiple family members. Principles of family therapy still apply in these settings, namely, ensuring everyone has a chance to speak, ensuring that professionals remain as balanced as possible (i.e. don't "side" with someone in the family), that space is made to advocate for family members who may be less able to express themselves, and that interactions are safe. Safe in this context means that people don't feel overly exposed or ambushed, that attention is paid to dynamics of power and that all participants have an opportunity to express their needs from the session at the start and have opportunities to "check in" about any unresolved thoughts prior to ending the conversation.

Open Dialogue

In some mental health services across the world, open dialogue (OD) is being used. OD is an approach to implementing systemic family therapy within existing services, bringing together familial, social and professional networks to explore mental health crises (Freeman et al 2019). The aim of OD is to generate dialogue with a person in distress and the important people in their social network (Kemp et al 2020), including family members. In OD, care decisions are made in a genuinely collaborative way, with clinicians or therapists required to tolerate their own uncertainties about care decisions and not rush towards resolution. Rather than focusing on a problem with an individual, in OD there is a focus on interactional aspects of experiences across networks, with individualised plans for recovery developed with an emphasis on psychotherapeutic treatments that occur within the context of existing support networks. OD is inherently family focused. OD has seven core principles: immediate help, a social network perspective, flexibility, mobility, responsibility, tolerance of uncertainty and dialogism (Hartnett 2019). These principles are aspirational, rather than directive (Bellingham et al 2018), and enacted through network meetings, which occur as soon as possible in treatment. The purpose of the network meetings is to gather information about the "problem", build a treatment plan, and generate therapeutic dialogue. Dialogue enables development of a shared language through which individuals and networks can make sense of their experiences. In network meetings, each person is given space to talk, with open-ended questions facilitating exploration of events and perceived meaning. OD facilitators also openly "reflect" throughout the process, transparently discussing their thoughts, feelings and impressions about what is being discussed by the network and the implications for possible treatment plans.

Often in mental health settings, when family therapy or OD are not accessible, families may benefit from simple approaches. Families may need practical things, support, listening, validation and information. Consider a young person living with a parent who engages in hoarding behaviours and their household is subsequently very chaotic and cluttered. Recommending family therapy may be less useful to this young person than organising practical support for cleaning and housing. Or consider a parent who cares for their young adult child and feels very frustrated by the lack of support they experience from services. In this case the response of a nurse may be to immediately spring into action trying to set up more supports when in fact the parent wants the nurse to listen to their experiences and provide validation for the feeling of frustration and the challenges they face in caring for their child (see Perspectives in practice: Nurse's story 5.2).

PERSPECTIVES IN PRACTICE

Nurse's Story 5.2: Sophie

Everybody comes from a family and many people hold roles in families, including parenting, which form an integral part of their self. In adult mental health services, there is an increasing push to recognise the relationship between these family roles and mental health and recovery. When a parent has a mental illness, children are often not provided with any information or support to make sense of their world and are usually not included in care planning or delivery. Advocating for family-focused practice in mental health services is hard work, yet the opportunity to work with children and families has provided me with endless inspiration and motivation to continue. Many mental health services have dedicated positions such as mine that exist to improve the inclusion of families in care. A big part of my role is promoting awareness of children and families at the systems level and educating clinicians about ways to work with families in the care they provide to individuals. But the role has also included running parenting programs for parents with mental illness, organising children's activity

Continued

programs, running support groups and coordinating playgroups specifically for families affected by mental illness, as well as large amounts of conversations, family sessions and support provided to many children, parents and families.

My role varies on a day-to-day basis. You never quite know what might happen, what projects might be started or what a referral might entail. Most referrals come from mental health clinicians, but often schools, families, early childhood and other services also seek advice or resources. There are increasing amounts of good resources and books about mental illness for families, but none of them replaces a conversation with someone exploring your experiences and questions. Conversations about mental illness can occur with parents, children, young people and family members during home visits or in hospitals or health centres. Parents can often be understandably reluctant to engage in conversations about their parenting or refuse to have a professional talk to their children about their illness, so a lot of time and thought needs to be spent building rapport and including all family members in discussions where possible. While all parents have worries about their parenting roles and can benefit from parenting support, mental illness is an additional challenge that can be stressful for all members of a family.

No two days are the same in this work. One day you may find yourself walking with a teenager discussing what mental illness is, how it affects their parent and answering questions about how to tell their friends or whether they will get it too. The next you might be advocating for a parent in a family meeting in an inpatient mental health unit or navigating complex family dynamics on a home visit. Some days you might find yourself colouring in with a child and talking to them about what makes them feel worried or talking with schools or other agencies about how they can support a child or family. A lot of time is spent supporting mental health clinicians to address the needs of all family members within their care planning.

Conversations with parents might focus on what their illness stops them from being able to do as a parent, what they think their children may have noticed when they were unwell, how they can explain their mental illness to their child and what children need to feel safe and secure. Often parents are concerned that they are being judged as a bad parent or may find it difficult to engage in wider parenting supports. Conversations with children need to be appropriate to their age and circumstance and context. Sometimes children want lots of information, and other times conversations may focus on other stressors, supports and worries. Conversations may include who the child can talk to if they need to, what understanding they have of their parent's illness and reassurance about the future. Children often think their parent's illness is their fault. It is also important to make plans for periods of separation or hospitalisation and offer truthful and simple explanations. Both children and adults are open to detailed discussions about the brain and what is known and understood about mental illness, including treatment and prognosis.

Children often notice more than adults realise, and their questions can be quite poignant and challenging. I generally just try to be honest and thoughtful in my answers and admit what I don't know. Children can also be very accepting, so often something I am worried about talking about is not such a big deal once I start. I always remind myself that an awkward conversation is always better than no attempt at all. Educating other nurses on how to talk to children and families can be rewarding as they realise how much of it is about being willing to put aside their own fears and have a go at tricky conversations about topics like distress, self-harm or suicide that may make us as adults feel uncomfortable. There is a privilege in stepping into the lives of families and looking at mental illness as a part of a wider structure that affects and is affected by all its members.

RECOVERY-ORIENTED AND TRAUMA-INFORMED FAMILY INCLUSIVE CARE

As introduced in Chapter 2, mental health services are moving towards delivering recovery-oriented and trauma-informed care. It is important to consider how families fit within these often individually focused (or "person-centred") frameworks.

As noted earlier, while relationships and connection to others are considered important within personal recovery frameworks, the main emphasis remains on autonomy and self-determination (Wyder & Bland 2014). Recovery-oriented practice often does not mention the social determinants of recovery, and the onus of responsibility is usually placed on the individual, while the familial, social, material, educational, economic and political contexts of mental health distress are often not considered. This focus on autonomy and agency within the concept of personal recovery is embedded within recognition that people with lived experience can, and should, define their own experiences in meaningful ways, and on their own terms. The emphasis on self-determination and autonomy is a legacy of the consumer advocacy movement, and is important to respect, however, recovery-oriented practice can at times exclude, or fail to recognise, families. To be family inclusive in recovery-oriented practice requires overt recognition that the needs of the individual and the needs of the family are inextricably linked, and that a person with lived experience often has multiple relational identities within their own complex networks of interdependence – for example, they may be a mother, friend, neighbour, sibling, colleague, aunty, and so on. All of these relational identities are linked to their recovery. Expanding recovery-oriented practice to recognise

relational and family recovery creates an opportunity for nurses to consider the family as a whole, beyond their caring roles, and to understand the strengths of the family system.

Similarly, trauma-informed care can be a primarily individually focused approach. Trauma-informed care requires awareness of the prevalence of trauma in the lives of many people who access mental health services, and sensitivity to how trauma affects their lives, health, experiences of illness and distress, and interactions with services. Many people who access mental health services have experienced trauma in their lives, and for some this has occurred in their family unit. There is therefore a risk that increased awareness of trauma in mental health services could lead to assumptions about families, and further stigmatisation of families within care. Nurses often have to navigate how to be inclusive of families, while also being sensitive to dynamics of trauma. To do so requires duality of holding the principles of trauma-informed care in mind, while also applying these to interactions about, and with, families. Table 5.4 applies the principles of trauma-informed care to working with families.

Domestic and Family Violence

A component of being aware of families and the relational context of distress, illness and recovery is competence and confidence in identifying and responding to concerns about domestic and family violence. Domestic and family violence refers to violence between family members, and typically involves the perpetrator exercising power and control over another person (AIHW 2018). The most common and pervasive instances of family violence occur in intimate partner relationships and are also commonly referred to as domestic violence (DV).

TABLE 5.4 Applying Trauma-Informed Care Principles to Families

Principle	Individual	Examples of Applying to Family
Safety	Incorporates physical and psychological safety Psychological safety is required to engage, communicate and trust	Fostering safety in interactions, processes and expectations of families including through ensuring families are welcomed, oriented and included in care and decisions, or provided with explanations and options when this is not possible. Listening to knowledge, showing respect and validating experiences. Recognising and being curious about the roles and dynamics of families. Supporting individuals to interact with families in ways that suit their needs.
Choice	Facilitating meaningful options and control about care and treatment	Ensuring people are asked about family inclusion and that opportunities are provided for both individuals and families to contribute to care and treatment planning.
Collaboration	Shared decision-making and power in individual treatment and organisational planning	Working with families to develop services, treatment and care. Considering people in the context of their lives.
Empowerment	Enabling agency and self-efficacy through validation, affirmation, a focus on strengths and shared power	Sharing power with family members, supporting individuals to maintain family roles and supporting family resilience.
Trustworthiness	Building and sustaining consistency, respect transparency and interpersonal boundaries	Treating families with respect, communicating with transparency and consistency. Following privacy and confidentiality processes reliably and with clear explanations.

DV includes emotional, physical or sexual violence, as well as experience of coercion, stalking and psychological aggression. DV can occur in any family and the person experiencing mental distress may be either the perpetrator, the victim or exposed to the violence of others. DV in a family affects all members, including children and young people, whether they witness the violence directly or not.

In most care settings, DV screening occurs and may be undertaken by nurses. Any screening for DV requires sensitivity and care. Screening usually is guided by universal screening tools with clear prompts for nurses on what to ask and document. However, many nurses feel uncomfortable asking about DV and may worry about offending people or not knowing how to respond. Across studies, research has shown that the overwhelming majority of people feel relieved or not bothered about being asked questions about DV as DV screening is recognised as an important step towards supporting people who are experiencing violence. In mental health services, screening for DV is important for delivering care in ways that are sensitive to the dynamics of families and relationships, accurate formulation, ensuring safety and for effective care and treatment. Engagement with mental health services can also be an important window of opportunity for families to access support services for DV.

Family and domestic violence, and its intersection with mental distress and recovery, is complex. Undertaking routine screening to identify current or previous exposure to violence is important, but after screening, steps also need to be made to ensure that support for families and individuals is followed through. In responding to disclosures of DV within mental health settings, it is important to consider the issues that people experiencing DV can face in relation to safety, cultural and social expectations, confidentiality, coercive control, parenting, custody, legal issues, immigration, social support and economic independence. It is also important to consider the role that the dynamics of DV may play in undermining mental health, impacting on engagement in treatment or recovery, and using treatment to undermine credibility. Nurses may feel uncertain about how to ascertain immediate risk and how to address dual roles often held by family members as support persons and perpetrators. Accessing support from multidisciplinary teams and engaging in reflective practice and clinical supervision is crucial. Ensuring families and individuals know where to access support when they are ready is an important nursing role, as is knowing what services exist and ensuring accurate information of pathways to care is provided. In addition, the importance of listening without judgement, gentle questioning of the situation and offers of support should not be underestimated.

Awareness and consideration of the complex dynamics of families and relationships includes recognition of understanding the complexity of dynamics of abuse and the level of support required to facilitate change. At times, people choose to stay in family or other relationships where there is violence. Choosing to remain in relationships where there is violence is often based on a strategic analysis of safety and risk, and influenced by responsibilities, culture, beliefs and hope that perpetrators may change (Heron et al 2022; Warshaw et al 2013). Mental health services can initiate interventions that focus on fostering safety, as well as providing information about DV, its causes, effects, associated dynamics and safety concerns, alongside initiating support services, social connection, and supporting self-efficacy, strengths and agency of family members. While keeping a strengths-based approach is important, it is also important to always consider the presence of children in families and be aware of possible risks to the child's wellbeing. Nurses are mandatory reporters of child protection concerns. At times when working with families, nurses will become aware of situations where children are present and are concerning. These may relate to the impacts of mental illness or distress upon children, but may also relate to other aspects of family life.

At times, nurses may feel uncomfortable about making mandatory reports for fear of compromising their therapeutic relationship with the parent or because they assume another professional will make a report. It is important to check your local reporting pathways and consult with senior staff, services or helplines that provide advice on when to make reports about child protection concerns. It is important to know that staff do not need to be certain about a risk to a child to make a report about a concern for a child's wellbeing. Seeking support for families may provide an opportunity for early intervention, family preservation or prevention of future harm occurring. Multi-agency responses and collaborative planning are the most effective ways to support safety for children and families (see Family-focused care: Carer's story 5.2: Chantel).

✚ FAMILY-FOCUSED CARE

Carer's Story 5.2: Chantel

My experience with mental health services started long before I can even remember. My father lived with lifetime experiences of trauma, struggled with substance misuse, and was intermittently institutionalised throughout his life. He had a diagnosis of schizophrenia, and/or schizo-affective disorder, and/or post-traumatic stress disorder – depending on which psychiatrist you asked. Basically, he sometimes got very distressed, scary, chaotic, confusing, and at times his stories wouldn't really make sense. And at the same time, he was very much my Dad, and he made massive efforts to try and protect me and provide me with love and care.

Schizophrenia was a very scary word for me. When I was a little baby, my father was hospitalised during a period of psychosis, and my mum had no idea what was going on. She had never heard of mental illness before. A nurse took my mum aside and told her that my dad had this thing called schizophrenia, and that she should also be really careful with me because it was an illness that could be genetic. My mum was terrified, and she passed on that terror to me. Sometimes I think that the terror of becoming crazy was almost as bad as the pain and suffering of having a parent with profound mental health distress. I think that nurse had no idea about the impact that had on our family. I wish that clinicians understood that families hang onto every word they say, particularly in moments of crisis. The stories they tell matter; they matter profoundly.

If I could turn back time, I would want that nurse to say to my mum: *"Mental health distress can be very stressful on families and children, I can imagine this is a really hard time, and I'm just so sorry this is happening. Would you like to know more about supports and resources that are available to you and your daughter?"*

The strategy of first and foremost showing compassion and empathy in moments of great distress and crisis far outweighs bombarding people with information and facts. I think it would be helpful for mental health clinicians, including nurses, to reflect on their own biases, stigma and preconceived ideas about people with mental health distress and their families. They largely work within a primarily biomedical paradigm, and that sometimes stifles the possibility of seeing other perspectives. Families require all staff working in mental health services to do the work of being open and honest with themselves about their own assumptions, and to be open to really deeply listening to people's stories and experiences.

For me, what has been most helpful in my own family recovery has been to understand my family story through the lens of trauma and resilience. I have learnt that my family holds intergenerational trauma, but my family story also holds the codes and stories to some of my healing. And that's why it has been important to have safe and generous space to share my story.

💡 CRITICAL THINKING EXERCISE 5.3

In relation to Carer's story 5.2: Chantel:

1. Chantel suggests that all nurses should reflect on their own assumptions about families. Take some time to consider what assumptions you might hold about families.
2. Consider how you could describe the diagnosis of schizophrenia to a family member. What words would you use?
3. Why do you think nurses might engage in psychoeducation rather than spending time listening to families?
4. What other things can you think of that nurses could have done to support Chantel and her mother when her father was hospitalised?

CASE STUDY 5.1: Marcia

Marcia and her husband, Michael, have two daughters: Nina, aged 7, and Rosie, aged 3. They came to Australia 6 years ago and have no other family in Australia. Marcia's parents are divorced, and Michael's father died 3 years ago. Marcia had an admission to a mental health inpatient unit following the birth of Rosie, with a diagnosis of postpartum psychosis, and a recent 2-week admission for a further psychotic episode. She was then transferred to a private hospital and after discharge has been followed up by her GP.

Michael works full-time. Nina attends Year 1 at a local primary school, while Rosie stays home with Marcia. The children did not visit their mum in hospital; Michael had explained to them that Marcia was sick and needed a break. Marcia has not returned to work since the first episode of her illness 3 years ago. She has limited social support, with few friends and no family members in Australia.

Michael has rung the community mental health team with concerns that Marcia has been keeping Nina home from school. He thinks Marcia has stopped taking her antipsychotic medication, but she does not want to see the GP. Marcia has told him that she does not need help and became angry when he told her about planning to call the mental health team.

Recent financial stress has meant Michael has been working extra hours and they have been arguing. He describes that the children are well cared for, but Nina has been teary and sleeping in their bed since Marcia was in hospital.

Planned Approach to Care

(Note: all may not be possible during an initial visit and, where possible, should occur in partnership with specialised family support clinicians/workers.)

- Home visit to assess the family (including doing a genogram – see Fig. 5.3), Marcia, the children and the environment; assessment to include family dynamics, strengths, difficulties, observation of children and parent–child interactions.
- Talk to both parents about their parenting concerns and the children.
- Talk about the impact of Marcia's hospitalisation on the children; what explanations, support and reassurance their daughters may require; what fears the children may experience; and the impact of separation and Marcia's illness; offer support services if available.
- Discuss Marcia's medication and its impact on her parenting (e.g. side effects).
- Consider making safety plans for the children and parents for managing any further episodes of separation due to Marcia's illness.
- Identify social and community supports for all members of the family, including local playgroups or preschools, social groups, teachers, family support organisations, friends.
- Link Marcia to parenting support, including local groups or services.
- If appropriate, talk to the school and develop a plan to support the family (parents may be reluctant to talk to schools, but schools can be an immense support to children; information can be provided to schools without parent consent, but supporting Marcia and Michael to engage with the school and any potential supports for their daughter would be a more desirable option).
- Talk to Marcia about liaising with her GP about medications and ongoing follow-up.
- Identify other family strengths and needs and develop a collaborative care plan with Marcia and Michael.

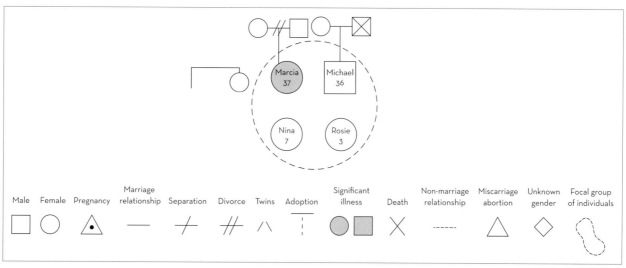

FIG. 5.3 Genogram of Marcia's Family.

CHAPTER SUMMARY

This chapter has focused on the experiences of families and the role that families may play in recovery from mental illness or distress. In addition, the roles nurses can play in supporting families through the recovery process and in building the family's resilience has been discussed. Understanding the needs of, and challenges faced by, family members when someone they love has mental illness can inform more relevant support provision from mental health nurses.

This includes the need for adequate information about mental illness and treatments, and the potential for negative impacts of care-giving upon their own physical and mental health. Focusing on building family strengths and resources, and on supporting family relationships, has potential to enable families to journey through family and relational recovery, and to foster relational resilience and wellbeing.

ACKNOWLEDGEMENT

This chapter was adapted and extended from a chapter written by Kim Foster, Sophie Isobel and Kim Usher in the 5th edition of this text.

USEFUL WEBSITES

Carers Australia: www.carersaustralia.com.au
Carers New Zealand: carers.net.nz/
Emerging Minds – training, programs and resources for health professionals, children and their families: emergingminds.com.au/our-work/
Mental Illness Fellowship of Australia (MIFA): mifa.org.au
Mind Australia – information and advocacy for mental health carers: www.mindaustralia.org.au/
Supporting Families NZ: mentalhealth.org.nz/links/link/supporting-families-new-zealand

REFERENCES

Abou Seif, N., Wood, L., & Morant, N. 2022. Invisible experts: A systematic review & thematic synthesis of informal carer experiences of inpatient mental health care. BMC Psychiatry, 22(1), 1–13.

Australian Bureau of Statistics (ABS). 2022. Unpaid work and care: Census. ABS. Online. Available at: www.abs.gov.au/statistics/people/people-and-communities/unpaid-work-and-care-census/latest-release

Australian Institute of Health and Welfare (AIHW). 2018. Family, domestic and sexual violence in Australia. AIHW, Canberra.

Bellingham, B., Buus, N., McCloughen, A., Dawson, L., Schweizer, R., et al., 2018. Peer work in Open Dialogue: A discussion paper. Int J Mental Health Nurs, 27, 1574–1583.

Bennett, B & Gates, T. 2019. Teaching cultural humility for social workers serving LGBTQI Aboriginal communities in Australia. Soc Work Ed, 38(5), 604–617.

Boström, P. K., & Strand, J. 2021. Children and parents with psychosis – balancing between relational attunement and protection from parental illness. J Child Adolesc Psych. Nurs, 34(1), 68–76.

Bowen, M. 1966. The use of family theory in clinical practice. Compr Psychiatry, 7(5), 345–374.

Campbell, C., & Patrick, P. 2022. Adult children of parents with mental illness: Family stigma and coping on sense of self. Child Fam Soc Work, 28(3), 622–634.

Chesla, C. A. 1988. Parents' caring practices and coping with schizophrenic offspring, an interpretive study. Doctoral dissertation. University of California, San Francisco, CA.

Chesla, C. A., & Leonard, V. 2017. Using a life–world approach to understand family resilience. In: Welch, G.L. & Harrist, A.W. (eds). Family Resilience and Chronic Illness. Springer, Cham.

Cleary, M., Freeman, A., Hunt, G. E., & Walter, G. 2005. What patients and carers want to know: An exploration of information and resource needs in adult mental health services. Aust NZ J Psychiatry, 39(6), 507–513.

Corrigan, P.W., Druss, B.G., Perlick, D.A. 2014. The impact of mental illness stigma on seeking and participating in mental health care. Psychol Sci Pub Int 15(2), 37–70.

Coyne, I., McNamara, N., Healy, M., Gower, C., Sarkar, M. et al., 2015. Adolescents' and parents' views of child and adolescent mental health services (CAMHS) in Ireland. J Psych Ment Health Nurs, 22(8), 561–569.

Cross, W. M., & Bloomer, M. J. 2010. Extending boundaries: Clinical communication with culturally and linguistically diverse mental health clients and carers. Int J Ment Health Nurs, 19(4), 268–277.

Digiacomo, M., Delaney, P., Abbott, P.A., et al., 2013. "Doing the hard yards': Carer and provider focus group perspectives of accessing Aboriginal childhood disability services. BMC Health Serv. Res. 13, 1–12.

EHINZ. 2023. Ethnic Profile of Aotearoa New Zealand. Environmental Health Intelligence New Zealand. Online. Available at: www.ehinz.ac.nz/indicators/population-vulnerability/ethnic-profile

Foster, K., Goodyear, M., Grant, A., Weimand, B., & Nicholson, J. 2019. Family-focused practice with EASE: A practice framework for strengthening recovery when mental health consumers are parents. Int J Ment Health Nurs, 28(1), 351–360.

Foster, K., & Isobel, S. 2018. Towards relational recovery: Nurses' practices with consumers and families with dependent children in mental health inpatient units. Int J Ment Health Nurs, 27(2), 727–736.

Foster, K., Maybery, D., Reupert, A., et al., 2016. Family focused practice in mental health care: An integrative review. Child Youth Serv, 37(2), 129–155.

Foster, K., O'Brien, L., Korhonen, T., 2012. Developing resilient children and families where parents have mental illness: A family-focused approach. Int J Ment Health Nurs, 21(1), 3–11.

Francis, A. 2014. Strengths-based assessments and recovery in mental health: Reflections from practice. Int J Social Work Human Services Prac, 2, 264–271.

Freeman, A.M., Tribe, R.H., Stott, J.C., & Pilling, S. 2019. Open dialogue: A review of the evidence. Psych Services, 70(1), 46–59.

Galimidi, N. & Shamai, M. 2022. Interactions between mental illness recovery processes in the family. Fam Relat, 71(1), 408–425.

Gladstone, B.M., Boydell, K. M., Seeman, M.V., & McKeever, P.D. 2011. Children's experiences of parental mental illness: A literature review. Early Interv Psychiatry, 5(4), 271–289.

Harrist, A.W., Henry, C.S., Liu, C., & Morris, A.S. 2019. Family resilience: The power of rituals and routines in family adaptive systems. In: Fiese, B.H., Celano, M., Deater-Deckard, K., Jouriles, E.N. & Whisman, M.A. (eds), APA Handbook of Contemporary Family Psychology: Foundations, Methods, and Contemporary Issues Across the Lifespan, vol. 1. American Psychological Association. doi.org/10.1037/0000099-013

Hartnett, D. 2019. The open dialogue approach to mental health care. Doctoral dissertation, University College, Cork.

Heron, R. L., Eisma, M., & Browne, K. 2022. Why do female domestic violence victims remain in or leave abusive relationships? A qualitative study. J Aggression, Maltreat Trauma, 31(5), 677–694.

Isobel, S., Goodyear, M., & Foster, K. 2019. Psychological trauma in the context of familial relationships: A concept analysis. TVA, 20(4), 549–559.

Isobel, S., McCloughen, A., Goodyear, M., & Foster, K. 2021. Intergenerational trauma and its relationship to mental health care: A qualitative inquiry. Community Ment Health J, 57, 631–643.

Johnston, J. 2013. The ghost of the schizophrenogenic mother. Virtual Mentor 15(9), 801–805.

Kemp, H., Bellingham, B., Gill, K., McCloughen, A., Roper, et al., 2020. Peer support and open dialogue: Possibilities for transformation and resistance in mental health services. In: Rhodes, P. (ed.). Beyond the Psychology Industry: How Else Might We Heal?, Springer, Switzerland.

Kenny, P., King, M. T., & Hall, J. 2014. The physical functioning and mental health of informal carers: Evidence of care-giving impacts from an Australian population-based cohort. Health Soc Care Comm, 22(6), 646–659.

Lauzier-Jobin, F., & Houle, J. 2022. A comparison of formal and informal help in the context of mental health recovery. Int J Soc Psychiatry, 68(4), 729–737.

Lavoie, J. A. 2018. Relative invisibility: an integrative review of carers' lived experiences of a family member's emergency mental health crisis. Soc Work Ment Health, 16(5), 601–626.

Leamy, M., Bird, V., Le Boutillier, C., et al., 2011. Conceptual framework for personal recovery in mental health: Systematic review and narrative synthesis. Br J Psychiatry 199, 445–452.

Liegghio, M. 2017. "Not a good person": Family stigma of mental illness from the perspectives of young siblings. Child Fam Social Work, 22(3), 1237–1245.

Martin, R.M., Ridley, S.C., & Gillieatt, S.J. 2017. Family inclusion in mental health services: Reality or rhetoric? Int J Social Psych, 63(6), 480–487.

Maybery, D., Reupert, A.E. 2018. The number of parents who are patients attending adult psychiatric services. Curr Opin Psych, 31, 358–362.

McCann, T.V., Bamberg, J., McCann, F. 2015. Family carers' experience of caring for an older parent with severe and persistent mental illness. Int J Ment Health, 24, 203–212.

Murphy, G., Peters, K., Jackson, D. 2014. A dynamic cycle of familial mental illness. Issues Ment Health Nurs, 35, 948–953.

Nicholson, J., Wolf, T., Wilder, C., et al., 2014. Creating options for family recovery: A providers' guide to promoting parental mental health. Online. Available at: www.employmentoptions.org

Page, I. S., Leitch, E., Gossip, K., Charlson, F., Comben, C., et al., 2022. Modelling mental health service needs of Aboriginal and Torres Strait Islander peoples: a review of existing evidence and expert consensus. ANZ J Pub Health, 46(2), 177–185.

Patrick, P. M., Reupert, A. E., & McLean, L. A. 2019. "We are more than our parents' mental illness": Narratives from adult children. Int J Environ Res Pub Health, 16(5), 839.

Poon, A. W. C., & Lee, J. S. 2019. Carers of people with mental illness from culturally and linguistically diverse communities. Aust Soc Work, 72(3), 312–324.

Population Australia. 2019. Population of Victoria 2019. Online. Available at: www.population.net.au/population-of-victoria/

Power, J., Goodyear, M., Maybery, D., et al., 2015. Family resilience in families where a parent has mental illness. J Soc Work, 16(1), doi: 10.1177/1468017314568081.

Price-Robertson, R., Obradovic, A., Morgan, B. 2017. Relational recovery: Beyond individualism in the recovery approach. Adv Ment Health 15(2), 108–120.

Rees, S. N., Crowe, M., & Harris, S. 2021. The lesbian, gay, bisexual and transgender communities' mental health care needs and experiences of mental health services: An integrative review of qualitative studies. J Psychiatric Ment Health Nurs, 28(4), 578–589.

Reupert, A., Bee, P., Hosman, C., van Doesum, K., Drost, L. M., et al., 2022. Editorial Perspective: Prato Research Collaborative for change in parent and child mental health–principles and recommendations for working with children and parents living with parental mental illness. J Child Psychol Psychiatry, 63(3), 350–353.

Richardson, M., Cobham, V., McDermott, B., et al., 2013. Youth mental illness and the family: Parents' loss and grief. J Child Fam Stud, 22, 719–736.

Rowe, J. 2012. Great expectations: a systematic review of the literature on the role of family carers in severe mental illness, and their relationships and engagement with professionals. J Psychiatr Ment Health Nurs 19, 70–82.

Smith, B.J. & Bailey, W.A. 2017. Fostering resilience among older adults living with osteoporosis and osteoarthritis. In: Welch, G. & Harrist A.W. (eds), Family Resilience and Chronic Illness. Springer, Cham.

Spaniol, L. 2010. The pain and the possibility: The family recovery process. Comm Ment Health J, 46, 482–485.

Trondsen, M.V. 2012. Living with a mentally ill parent: Exploring adolescents' experiences and perspectives. Qual Health Res, 22(2), 174–188.

van der Sanden, L.M., Pryor, J.B., Stutterheim, S.E., et al., 2016. Stigma by association and family burden among family members of people with mental illness: The mediating role of coping. Soc Psychiatry Psychiatr Epidemiol 51(9), 1233–1245.

Von Kardorff, E., Soltaninejad, A., Kamali, M., et al., 2016. Family caregiver burden in mental illnesses: The case of affective disorders and schizophrenia – a qualitative exploratory study. Nord J Psychiatry 70(4), 248–254.

Waller, S., Reupert, A., Ward, B., McCormick, F., & Kidd, S. 2019. Family-focused recovery: Perspectives from individuals with a mental illness. Int J Ment Health Nurs, 28(1), 247–255.

Walsh, F. 2006. Strengthening Family Resilience, 2nd ed. Guilford Press, New York.

Walters, C., & Petrakis, M. 2022. A systematic mapping review of family perspectives about received mental health interventions. Res Social Work Prac, 32(1), 61–72.

Wepf, H., & Leu, A. 2022. Well-being and perceived stress of adolescent young carers: A cross-sectional comparative study. J Child Fam Stud, 31(4), 934–948.

Wyder, M., Barratt, J., Jonas, R., & Bland, R. 2022. Relational recovery for mental health carers and family: Relationships, complexity and possibilities. Br J Soc Work, 52(3), 1325–1340.

Wyder, M., Bland, R. 2014. The recovery framework as a way of understanding families' responses to mental illness: Balancing different needs and recovery journeys. Aust Soc Work 67(2), 179–196.

Yates, S., & Gatsou, L. 2021. Idealisation and stigmatisation of parenting in families with parental mental illness. SSM-Qualitat Res Health, 1, 100020.

Yin, M., Li, Z., & Zhou, C. 2020. Experience of stigma among family members of people with severe mental illness: A qualitative systematic review. Int J Ment Health Nurs, 29(2), 141–160.

Zauszniewski, J.A., Bekhet, A.K., Suresky, J. 2015. Indicators of resilience in family members of adults with serious mental illness. Psychiatr Clin North Am, 38(1), 131–146.

6

Aboriginal and Torres Strait Islander Mental Health

Matthew Scott, Monica Guha and Luke Molloy

KEY POINTS

- Understanding the history and social context behind Aboriginal and Torres Strait Islander mental health presentations makes us better equipped to provide sensitive and culturally safe interactions and environments for both consumers and our colleagues.
- An ongoing reflection of our cultural values, beliefs and attitudes is essential, for within the nurse–consumer relationship an opportunity exists for a significant difference to be made in the health outcomes of Aboriginal and Torres Strait Islander consumers.
- By being trauma-informed, we are in a better position to understand the impact of trauma on the wellbeing of families and

communities and understand how it appears in the behaviour of the Aboriginal and Torres Strait Islander consumer, enabling us to develop strategies which help to reduce re-traumatisation and increase positive engagement and care.
- Being open to ongoing learning and seeking support, and having an attitude of openness, curiosity and respect are the foundations for positive and effective therapeutic relationships with the Aboriginal and Torres Strait Islander consumer and their families.

KEY TERMS

Aboriginal and Torres Strait Islander mental health
Social and emotional wellbeing

Cultural safety
Trauma-informed care
Strength and resilience

Truth-telling
Self-determination

LEARNING OUTCOMES

The material in this chapter will assist you to:
- analyse the impact of Australia's history on the mental health outcomes of Aboriginal and Torres Strait Islander people, and how this relates to the person requiring mental health care today
- discuss the context of social and emotional wellbeing, and how Aboriginal and Torres Strait Islander culture, values and social practices influence access and engagement with health services

- describe the nurse's role in promoting a recovery-oriented, trauma-informed care and culturally safe practice for Aboriginal and Torres Strait Islander people
- analyse the role of culturally safe communication and reflexivity, and the value this has in the building of therapeutic relationships with Aboriginal and Torres Strait Islander people
- understand the impacts of government policies on Aboriginal and Torres Strait Islander health care and explore what more could be done to improve mental health outcomes in the future.

INTRODUCTION

In this chapter the term "Indigenous" is used respectfully and interchangeably with the terms Aboriginal or Aboriginal and Torres Strait Islander people. These terms are used to describe and acknowledge the original inhabitants and traditional owners of Australia and their descendants. Aboriginal and Torres Strait Islander people belong to an ancient culture that thrived for over 65,000 years prior to colonisation (Australian Institute of Aboriginal and Torres Strait Islander Studies (AIATSIS) 2022). Sustainable land management and custodianship, connection to family and community, traditional medicine and healing, traditional astronomy and law, are just a few examples of the proud heritage of Aboriginal and Torres Strait Islander people. It is important to note that prior to colonisation mental illness and suicide were rare in Aboriginal and Torres Strait Islander culture. Aboriginal people had developed systems that ensured the survival, wellbeing and harmony of

their communities, as well as their ecosystems. These systems were deeply connected to their spiritual beliefs and were refined over thousands of years of practice. Despite the large expanse of land, inhabited by many different clans and nations, disputes were settled in relative harmony and governed by "lore", children were kept safe through "kinship" social structures, and ailments were treated through natural medicine.

However, post-colonisation mental health data highlights the impact that colonisation has had on Indigenous mental wellbeing and the vital importance for nurses to offer culturally appropriate services. Levels of psychological distress are more than twice as high for Indigenous Australians than non-Indigenous Australians, and there is a higher overall level of mental health issues. Over the last 10 years, the rate of suicide among Aboriginal and Torres Strait Islander peoples has been more than twice that of non-Indigenous Australians (Australian Institute of Health and Welfare (AIHW) 2022a). In 2022, suicide accounted for 4.6% of all deaths of Aboriginal and Torres Strait Islander people while the comparable proportion for non-Indigenous Australians was 1.7% (AIHW 2022a). Indigenous males have higher rates than females, with the younger populations of those aged 0–24 and 25–44 being at highest risk. Suicide is now the leading cause of death for Aboriginal and Torres Strait Islander children (AIHW 2022a), and the rates of suicide are more than twice as high among Indigenous children compared to non-Indigenous children (AIHW 2022a). These statistics highlight why improving the wellbeing of Aboriginal and Torres Strait Islander people and communities is an urgent health priority. While health policy has attempted to address the unequal risk factors to health and life expectancy between Aboriginal and Torres Strait Islander peoples and non-Indigenous Australians, a significant health inequality continues to exist. The 10-year review of "Closing The Gap" revealed that the targets to close the gap on life expectancy by 2023 were not on track (AHRC 2018). In 2021, the Productivity Commission's first annual data report revealed in fact there were increased rates of suicide, incarceration for Aboriginal and Torres Strait Islander people, and children in out-of-home care (Productivity Commission 2021).

This chapter aims to illustrate how colonisation continues to impact on the health and social outcomes of the Aboriginal and Torres Strait Islander population. The strength and resilience of the Aboriginal and Torres Strait Islander population in the face of centuries of adversity is palpable, yet it is important to acknowledge there are many inaccurate beliefs about Aboriginal and Torres Strait Islander peoples that exists today. This chapter also aims to dispel them, as it is important that nurses are equipped with accurate, trauma-informed understanding of the people and their culture. This accurate understanding provides vital context on how historical events impact the person presenting to a mental health service today. For example, by considering how government policies led to the disconnection of Indigenous people from their families and communities, their land, language, identity and culture, we are able to understand the lack of trust that Aboriginal and Torres Strait Islander peoples have for government services, including mental health services.

The purpose of the information provided here is not to induce feelings of guilt for being a non-Indigenous person living on Indigenous land, but about becoming aware of your own ways of viewing the world. This chapter aims to equip you with the knowledge, skills and confidence required to create clinical environments which are trauma-informed and culturally safe for Indigenous Australians. Consequently, you will contribute to creating culturally safe organisations, which ultimately leads to better health outcomes and community healing. Each encounter that a nurse has with an Indigenous person provides an opportunity for faith and trust in health services to be restored. As nurses form the largest cohort of staff in many health services, they are well positioned to make a significant difference in the health outcomes of Aboriginal and Torres Strait Islander consumers through their nurse–consumer relationships, and this should not be underestimated.

HISTORICAL CONTEXT

A deeper understanding of the influences of history on contemporary Australian culture is essential if we are to better understand the current experiences of Aboriginal and Torres Strait Islander people. This section will help to illustrate these cultural influences through truth-telling, the definition of which is "telling the facts openly, honestly, and unambiguously" (Law & Martin 2020). Until recent times, Australian history was predominantly told through the European settler or explorer perspectives. Truth-telling with respect to Aboriginal and Torres Strait Islander history is focused on bringing previously untold

parts of their history to the foreground, as well as being told from their perspectives. Having this wider perspective equips us with a full historical account of post-colonial Australia, giving us a deeper understanding of Aboriginal and Torres Strait Islander people. It is especially important to take note of how "health" and other "government" organisations played a part in this history, in order to understand the relationship that Aboriginal and Torres Strait Islander people have with them today.

The colonisation of Australia brought with it a set of events, policies and a culture that led to the decimation and ongoing marginalisation of the Aboriginal and Torres Strait Islander population (George et al 2019). Government policies implemented soon after colonisation involved atrocities such as the forced removal of children from their families, leaving a devastating legacy of trauma that has been passed down through generations of Aboriginal and Torres Strait Islander people (Menzies 2019). When considered along with the fatal impact of unfamiliar diseases, and the devastating introduction of alcohol and other substances, we can begin to understand why Aboriginal and Torres Strait Islander people have issues of mistrust, fear and suspicion of government-operated services. However, it is also important for us to understand how the consequent burden of mental health issues have transcended not only communities, but generations. This section will illustrate how the impact of these historical traumas presents in the Indigenous mental health consumer we see today through intergenerational trauma.

> ### ❓ CRITICAL THINKING EXERCISE 6.1
>
> As you read the information presented here, we encourage you to explore and reflect on the following:
> 1. What information here is new to you?
> 2. What did you know already?
> 3. What reaction, if any, does this information bring up in you?
> 4. Where might you think this reaction/emotion originates?

Terra Nullius

The Indigenous people of Australia consist of two distinct cultural groups – the Aboriginal and the Torres Strait Islander peoples. Aboriginal people are the first inhabitants of mainland Australia, including Tasmania and many of the country's offshore islands. There are numerous diverse nations among Aboriginal people, each with their own language and traditions. Torres Strait Islander people are the original inhabitants of the 274 islands between the tip of Cape York in Queensland and Papua New Guinea, collectively called the Torres Strait. They too have their own languages and traditions. There were between 300,000 and 1 million Aboriginal people living on the mainland at the time of colonisation (Dudgeon et al 2014).

From a settler perspective, when the British landed on 26 January 1788 they assumed they could claim the land as their own. As the land didn't look like the European model of large permanent structures and razed and farmed land, they termed it "*Terra Nullius*", the Latin term for "not inhabited" or "empty land". However, Indigenous perspectives are strikingly different. Contrary to popular and long-standing colonial beliefs, Indigenous knowledge and evidence from written records show that Aboriginal people had cultivated land and had developed sustainable and complex systems of farming and living (Lynch et al 2018). Similarly, prior to making contact with British settlers, Torres Strait Islanders were fishermen, hunters and agriculturalists, who associated themselves with the land, the sea and the sky, which had strong connections to their spiritual beliefs. Aboriginal people identify themselves as either Saltwater people or Freshwater people depending on their location of origin and have a deep spiritual connection to the land, signified by an attitude of respect and non-ownership. Core to the Aboriginal person's identity is being a "custodian" of the land, meaning they have a specific role to "look after" it. Hence its appearance at the time as looking largely "untouched".

Impacts of Colonisation

Contrasting perspectives are also evident around colonisation. From the perspectives of the settler nation, colonialism is the entitled practice by which a powerful country directly controls less powerful countries, and uses their resources to increase its own power and wealth (Collins English Dictionary 2020). Aboriginal people did not claim the land in the sense of "ownership", which colonisers interpreted as meaning it was there to be taken. Colonisation from the perspective of Indigenous peoples meant the loss of their land, the introduction of new diseases and violence being directed towards them. As settlement expanded and more land was taken away, Aboriginal people began resisting, as protectors of the land that was now being razed for settler farming, which led to violence.

As land was seized and destroyed, so were traditional ways of being connected to the land. Loss of land also meant a lack of access to a community's traditional food and water supply causing further de-population through diet-related disease. British colonisation also brought with it previously unknown European diseases. While the British colonists had developed some disease immunity through exposure, the Aboriginal population had none. In the year after the arrival of the First Fleet smallpox killed up to 70% of the Aboriginal population living in the Sydney Basin before spreading across the rest of the country, and affecting entire generations of Indigenous populations (Silverstein 2020). Influenza, measles, tuberculosis and sexually transmitted diseases shortly followed, causing further devastation to communities, which were left without leaders, and family (Campbell 2022).

Conflicts between settlers and Aboriginal people as they attempted to resist British settlement, and the devastation caused by introduced diseases and alcohol, reduced the Aboriginal population during the first 100 years of settlement to 60,000 (Department of Aboriginal

HISTORICAL ANECDOTE 6.1

Lock Hospitals and the Myall Creek Massacre

In an attempt to control the spread of venereal disease, "lock hospitals" were established on the islands of Bernier and Dorre in Queensland in the early 1900s. Several hundred Aboriginal people were forcibly sent to be separated from their family and country. Lock hospitals were just one way in which Aboriginal and Torres Strait Islander people were treated differently medically from the non-Indigenous population. There was a separate system for non-Indigenous carriers of disease, which involved free medical treatment and education and release from quarantine once clear of infection. Aboriginal and Torres Strait Islander people were treated with quarantine only, with minimal testing, diagnosis or treatment. They were rarely released, even if they became disease-free (Stewart et al 2016).

The most notable Aboriginal massacre was the "Myall Massacre" in Northern New South Wales, because of the justice brought by the Supreme Court. In 1838 at Myall Creek near Inverell in New South Wales, 28 Aboriginal people were killed. They were mainly women and children. The first non-Indigenous to ever be charged for the killing of Aboriginal people were the stockmen who committed this crime, and they were hung for murder.

Read More About It
National Museum of Australia 2023. Defining moments: Myall Creek massacre. Online. Available at: www.nma.gov.au/defining-moments/resources/myall-creek-massacre

Affairs 1981). As land continued to be taken over and communities were treated with violence, including rape and massacre by settlers, Aboriginal clans were forced to relocate far from their traditional lands. They were often forced to reside in reserves or missions where policies dictated punishment for speaking in their language or practising traditional ways, with a resultant loss of culture and identity. Torres Strait Islanders suffered from a similar but less brutal impact of colonisation. It wasn't until 1873 that the first British settlement was established on Albany Island. The discovery of large amounts of pearl shell attracted thousands of foreigners in the years following. Christian missionaries also arrived with the intent of teaching Aboriginal and Torres Strait Islander people how to conform to westernised ways (Torres Strait Islands Regional Authority n.d.).

Protectionism and Assimilation

From settler perspectives, as the Aboriginal and Torres Strait Islander population declined they became thought of as a "dying race" and the idea to assimilate Aboriginal people into the wider community began. Protection boards were established throughout Australia to prevent the spread of disease to Indigenous people (Silverstein 2020). The Board also had the power to take away Aboriginal children from their families and communities. However, alongside this an awareness of the general mistreatment of Aboriginal and Torres Strait Islander people grew. As Aboriginal and Torres Strait Islander people were being largely used for labour in missions and reserves, the need for more effective regulation brought about policy with the initial aim to "protect" Aboriginal people from abuse, consequently heralding a loss of rights for Indigenous peoples in Australia (Attwood 2020). "Protectors" were commonly policemen or pastoralists who were appointed to provide populations with basic rations and medicine. However, from an Indigenous perspective this was not an experience of being protected. Those left in Aboriginal communities were made to relocate to missions or reserves, where they were forbidden to use traditional language or customs. As families were divided, cultural traditions and lore were lost. "Protectors" also monitored all movements and were usually hostile in the way they "managed" Aboriginal communities. Use of traditional ways and food were met with hostility, there was widespread physical and sexual abuse, and Aboriginal and Torres Strait Islander people were forced to eat a diet mainly of flour and tea. Protectors restricted contact between "full-blood" Aboriginal people from "part-Aboriginal" people and their children for the purpose of assimilating those who weren't "full-blood", especially children who were "half-caste" (Dudgeon et al 2014).

Due to ongoing concerns about Aboriginal and Torres Strait Islander communities, in 1936 the Commonwealth Government declared that Aboriginal and Torres Strait Islander peoples not of "full blood" needed to be absorbed into the wider populations. The Assimilation policy was defined as:

… in the view of all Australian governments that all aborigines and part-aborigines are expected eventually to attain the same manner of living as other Australians and to live as members of a single Australian community enjoying the same rights and privileges, accepting the same responsibilities, observing the same customs and influenced by the same beliefs, hopes and loyalties as other Australians. Thus, any special measures taken for aborigines and part-aborigines are regarded as temporary measures not based on colour but intended to meet their need for special care and assistance to protect them from any ill effects of sudden change and to assist them to make the transition from one stage to another in such a way as will be favourable to their future social, economic and political advancement.

(AIATSIS 2008)

From Indigenous perspectives the ultimate aim of assimilation was to make Aboriginal and Torres Strait Islander people gradually lose their cultural identity fully, by effectively "breeding out" Aboriginality. This was carried out by stepping up the forcible removal of Indigenous children from their families and their placement in white institutions or foster homes.

✳ HISTORICAL ANECDOTE 6.2

Stolen Generations

Between 1910 and 1972, approximately 20,000 to 30,000 children were forcibly removed from their families and communities and sent to institutions or adopted by non-Indigenous families. A National Inquiry into the Separation of Aboriginal and Torres Strait Islander Children from their Families in 1996 preceded the *Bringing them Home* report (HREOC 1997), which estimated that between 1 in 10 and 1 in 3 Indigenous children, approximately 50,000 children, were "stolen", and that many were abused, neglected or exploited for labour. In 2018–19, there were an estimated 33,600 Stolen Generations survivors across Australia, although this is likely to be an underestimation. Around 1 in 3 Indigenous Australian adults were estimated to be descendants of the Stolen Generations (AIHW 2021). The term "Stolen Generations" was coined, as what occurred could have been described as stealing or kidnapping. It has also been described as genocide (Bailey 2020).

Exemption

A less widely known but equally harmful policy to "assimilate" Aboriginal people into the wider populations was the Aboriginal Exemption policy. Aboriginal people were offered access to education, health services, housing, employment and citizenship, things which they would have otherwise been denied for being Aboriginal, in exchange for giving up their cultural identity. This was a way to escape the oppression described above, allowing Aboriginal people to live independently. However, this meant walking past and ignoring family members in public, and not speaking the language of their ancestors for fear of being gaoled. While many took up this offer to keep themselves and their families safe, others derisively called the certificate of exemption a "dog licence" or "beer tickets" and refused to apply for one (Aberdeen & Jones 2021)

Read More About It

AIATSIS 2023. Exemption: the high price of freedom. Online. Available at: aiatsis.gov.au/explore/exemption-high-price-freedom

---

At this point it is quite natural to question how nurses could possibly resolve this prolonged mistreatment. Acknowledging Aboriginal and Torres Strait Islander history is a first step to understanding a person's mental health needs while being culturally sensitive. It is important to note that throughout post-colonisation history there have been non-Indigenous people who have advocated for the better treatment of Indigenous Australians. Advocates who, alongside the strength, resilience, will and activism of Aboriginal and Torres Strait Islander people, have supported the slow and incremental improvements that have enabled the continuance of culture and community that we see today. Advocates are required in current times no less than previously. Being an advocate is central to person-centred care, and even more so in the mental health setting where consumers may not have the capacity to self-advocate. Nurses improve the quality of care delivered by using their voice to help protect mental health consumers. While advocacy is a key responsibility of every nurse, it is core to the identity of the mental health nurse.

If we look at First Nations communities around the world, it has been documented that these societies were relatively healthy prior to colonisation (Axelsson et al 2016). The physical and mental health of Aboriginal and Torres Strait Islander communities were good (Wilson et al 2020), with robust child-rearing practices which contemporary research has found to be healthier than modern approaches (Narvaez & Tarsha 2021). The disproportionately high burden of mental illness compared to that of non-Indigenous populations today can be directly attributed to the impacts of colonisation (Murrup-Stewart et al 2019) and what many Aboriginal and Torres Strait Islander people see as a lack of acknowledgement for the injustices that have been made to their land, culture and people.

The next section will illustrate how these historical events have continued to impact generations of Aboriginal and Torres Strait Islander populations.

CRITICAL THINKING EXERCISE 6.2

Trauma is often associated with events which equate to grief and loss. What have you identified from Aboriginal and Torres Strait Islander history and present day that equates to grief and loss?

TRAUMA-INFORMED CARE

As outlined in Chapter 2 of this text, trauma-informed care acknowledges the high prevalence of trauma in the lives of people accessing mental health services. The growing understanding of the neurological, biological, psychological and social impact of distressing events of the past on an individual has necessitated that mental health services look at organisational culture and ensure not only that they reduce practices that cause re-traumatisation, but also that they provide care that is "personalised, holistic, creative, open and therapeutic" (Mental Health Coordinating Council (MHCC) 2013). To understand what needs to be changed in our mental health systems to ensure an experience of safety for Aboriginal and Torres Strait Islander consumers, we must first understand the different types of trauma experiences for the Aboriginal and Torres Strait Islander persons.

Across populations different types of trauma affecting different groups have been identified. These include, but are not limited to, individual trauma, the personal experience of distressing events; intergenerational trauma, historical trauma which is passed down through generations; and collective trauma, a shared community response to that group's history or loss event.

- **Individual trauma:** describes the daily experience of racism, micro-aggression, stigma and socio-economic disadvantage (Dudgeon et al 2022), as well as the individual's personal experiences of traumatic events, such as sexual abuse or domestic violence. Increasing evidence recognises racism as a significant determinant of health that contributes to negative mental and general health outcomes among Aboriginal and Torres Strait Islander peoples (Kairuz et al 2021).
- **Intergenerational trauma:** a term used to describe how the trauma from the events described earlier on in this chapter have been passed down through generations. There are still many Aboriginal and Torres Strait Islander families and communities that are working on healing the psychological and emotional damage from the past injustices, and most are affected by the ongoing impacts of colonisation, such as the loss of family members through early mortality, family dysfunction, community violence and ill health (Menzies 2019). In their final report, the Royal Commission into Childhood Sexual Abuse in Institutions recognised

the psychological and emotional damage to victims and their families, and the intergenerational impact that Aboriginal and Torres Strait Islander children have inherited today (Commonwealth of Australia 2017b).

- **Collective trauma:** This term helps us to understand how the traumatic experience of child removal continues to impact Aboriginal and Torres Strait Islander people as a group (Menzies 2019). Such an event impacts the foundation of a culture and is captured in a "collective memory" which impacts people beyond the direct survivors of the events and is remembered by group members who were not present at the time of the event.

A Common Misconception and a Deep Wound

Having some knowledge of the circumstances that lead to child removal with the child protection systems we have today, such as parental abuse and neglect, we often mistakenly associate similar factors as causes for the removal of Aboriginal families in the past. When the first child protection systems were established, a separate system was set up for Aboriginal and Torres Strait Islander children, one that would allow children to be forcibly removed solely on the basis of their race. Often Aboriginal children were taken away from their families for reasons that were not to do with the welfare of the child. Families did all they could to hide their children from police and "protectors", usually moving from mission to mission, but were eventually found and torn apart. Children were ripped from the arms of their parents and a deep wound, the pain of which still reverberates strongly in communities today, was opened. The profoundly negative impacts of childhood trauma on physical health and social outcomes across all populations have been discussed in Chapter 5 of this text. However, for the Aboriginal and Torres Strait Islander consumer specifically, a deep mistrust of self and others, fear and anticipation of betrayal, shame and humiliation, losing traditional values, violence against women, suicide and risk-taking behaviour, and substance abuse, are just some of the behaviours that show up as a result of collective and intergenerational trauma (Menzies 2019). Nurses were sometimes involved in such removals of Aboriginal and Torres Strait Islander children, a practice which denied Aboriginal and Torres Strait Islander children of the fundamental human right of being able to grow up in a loving family. In 2022 the Council of Deans of Nursing and Midwifery (CDNM) offered a formal national apology (CDNM 2022).

> **LIVED EXPERIENCE COMMENT BY MATTHEW SCOTT, ABORIGINAL MENTAL HEALTH NURSE**
>
> *"We need to understand the injustice of this, so that we can understand the anger and pain that continues to exist today in Aboriginal communities. Every march, every fight for injustice contains the pain of children being taken from their families."*

As outlined in previous chapters, the essence of trauma-informed care is not to re-traumatise those accessing mental health services. A focus on simply reducing the use of restrictive and coercive practices for Indigenous consumers is not sufficient (Guha et al 2022). It is important to focus on the use of early intervention strategies, which increase the feeling of safety for the consumer. Promoting a person's autonomy and ability to make choices around their care, as well as creating clinical environments which feel culturally safe are important strategies that help to reduce the inherent power dynamic that exists within health institutions. A practical example is assisting the Aboriginal and Torres Strait Islander consumer to make contact with their families and carers and involving them wherever possible, especially if people are "off country" (not on their traditional lands).

Elsewhere in this book you will find trauma-informed strategies that apply to every mental health consumer which are no less relevant for the Aboriginal and Torres Strait Islander consumer. Some other points to keep in mind:

- Understand that addiction is a coping mechanism for the symptoms of trauma.
- Understand that the fear and mistrust Aboriginal and Torres Strait Islander people have of government services, hence their reluctance to engage, does not necessarily mean they don't want help.
- Understand that a person's reaction is a form of communication, usually in fear, and not to take what they say personally.

 CRITICAL THINKING EXERCISE 6.3

What are the similarities and differences of Indigenous and non-Indigenous consumers' experiences of trauma?

CULTURAL SAFETY IN MENTAL HEALTH SERVICES

A critical component of trauma-informed care is to embed culturally safe practices in mental health services. The Indigenous people of Australia are two distinct cultural groups – the Aboriginal and Torres Strait Islander peoples. As such, beliefs and practices will also differ according to location and culture. Aboriginal and Torres Strait Islander people do not expect you to be aware of all of the specific protocols, but *respecting* there are cultural beliefs and protocols that are important to the Aboriginal and Torres Strait Islander person, *understanding* that this may look different across the country and between nations, *and being open* to learning further about them, is often all that is required.

Culturally safe nursing care is about the person who is providing that care to reflect on their own assumptions and culture in order to work in a genuine partnership with Aboriginal and Torres Strait Islander peoples (Nursing and Midwifery Board of Australia 2018). Cultural safety influences nursing care through reflection; it requires you to identify and explore your assumptions surrounding your nursing care. You start by reflecting on your own culture and the way that it influences how you see the world. You reflect on how this shapes the care you provide to people. Because cultural safety aims to empower the person receiving nursing care, only that person can assess its effectiveness in relation to cultural safety. This gives the person the power to shape their nursing care by contributing to the nursing process in a meaningful way. Cultural safety challenges us to look at our practice and reflect on its consequences, questioning professional traditions, such as the ethic of treating everyone the same, regardless of their ethnicity or gender (Taylor & Guerin 2019). This process of reflection will enable you to develop a capability and ease in working with Aboriginal and Torres Strait Islander people, who will in turn feel more confident and safer to work with you.

Cultural safety enables nurses to develop an awareness of the power differences inherent in the relationships with health professionals and systems. Cultural safety provides a model for decolonising our practice and practice settings that is based on dialogue, negotiation and power-sharing. By using the concept to guide practice, the mental health nurse can provide care that is focused on the person receiving care, and their personal recovery. Culturally safe nursing care demands a move beyond health professional-controlled, biomedical-dominated approaches to mental health, and promotes ways of caring that have the potential to promote reconciliation within the experience of mental health service use (Molloy 2019).

With its clear focus on critical reflection, cultural safety can also challenge the assumptions of Western psychiatric traditions that can limit the scope of mental health service delivery. This can challenge issues such as institutional racism. A seminal description of institutional racism outlines it as being an organisationally wide failure to provide proper service to people because of their racial or cultural background. This default position becomes manifest in attitudes and behaviour that culminate in discrimination and racist stereotyping (MacPherson 1999).

In order to effectively meet the mental health and social and emotional wellbeing needs of the Aboriginal and Torres Strait Islander population, all health services must strive to become more culturally safe and responsive to the needs of Aboriginal people. It is also the responsibility of every nurse to be culturally safe in their practice, as stipulated by the Code of Conduct for nurses (Nursing and Midwifery Board of Australia 2018).

Code of Conduct for Nurses

The Code of Conduct (Nursing and Midwifery Board of Australia 2018) identifies that nurses practising in Australia must:

- acknowledge that Australia has always been a culturally and linguistically diverse nation. Aboriginal and/or Torres Strait Islander peoples have inhabited and cared for the land as the First Peoples of Australia for millennia, and their histories and cultures have uniquely shaped our nation
- require nurses and midwives to understand and acknowledge the historical factors, such as colonisation and its impact on Aboriginal and/or Torres Strait Islander peoples' health, which help to inform care. In particular, Aboriginal and/or Torres Strait Islander peoples bear the burden of gross social, cultural and health inequality
- provide clear guidance and set expectations for nurses and midwives in supporting the health of Aboriginal and/or Torres Strait Islander peoples
- provide care that is holistic, free of bias and racism, challenges beliefs based upon assumption and is culturally safe and respectful for Aboriginal and/or Torres Strait Islander peoples
- advocate for, and act to facilitate, access to quality and culturally safe health services for Aboriginal and/or Torres Strait Islander peoples, and

- recognise the importance of family, community, partnership and collaboration in the healthcare decision-making of Aboriginal and/or Torres Strait Islander peoples, for both prevention strategies and care delivery.

CULTURALLY APPROPRIATE CARE

Nurses have historically reported difficulty in developing culturally appropriate care for Aboriginal and Torres Strait Islander people while working within a largely biomedical paradigm of mental health nursing care (Molloy et al 2019). An absence of accurate history telling in mainstream education and the maintenance of stigmatising attitudes towards Aboriginal and Torres Strait Islander People have contributed to many nurses having little understanding or often a misunderstanding of Aboriginal and Torres Strait Islander people and their culture. Aboriginal and Torres Strait Islander identities are also often spoken about in a narrative of negativity, deficiency and failure throughout health policies and practices. It is important to acknowledge the impact that these negative beliefs have on the therapeutic relationship between the nurse and the consumer, which is shaped by the knowledge and attitudes the nurse brings to the encounter (see Chapter 2). Often it is a paucity of reliable information and feeling ill equipped that leads to our falling short of providing an effective and positive encounter, resulting in our inability to form a therapeutic relationship.

This section aims to provide guidance around Aboriginal and Torres Strait Islander cultural perspectives and some protocols that will help you understand the behaviours that a consumer might present with. By understanding what is behind certain behaviours, we are less likely to misinterpret, misunderstand and misdiagnose, all of which have critical consequences for the consumer. Hence, it is important to appreciate that learning about Aboriginal and Torres Strait Islander culture doesn't end here and we strongly recommend that you take opportunities for further learning and reflection that are offered to you, such as cultural safety training, and clinical supervision. Again, developing an attitude of *openness*, *curiosity* and *respect* goes a long way.

⊕ CULTURAL CONSIDERATIONS 6.1

Scenario: Anthony

When I first came over to work in Australia, I began working on an acute inpatient unit for a busy metropolitan hospital. It was easy for me to form assumptions about Aboriginal and Torres Strait Islander people. As a non-Australian I knew little about Australian culture in general. Aboriginal and Torres Strait Islander consumers presented with a wide range of mental health issues, often coupled with a drug or alcohol issue and physical health complications. I felt that I didn't fully understand Aboriginal and Torres Strait Islander issues and their issues seemed too complex. I found myself restricting my interactions for fear I would do or say something wrong, and felt ill equipped to talk with families and carers.

My curiosity and sense that "I can do better than this" led me to approach an Aboriginal mental health nurse colleague and tell them about my experiences of feeling ill equipped. I asked whether there were some skills or knowledge that could help me engage with Aboriginal and Torres Strait Islander people better, but was almost disappointed with his response, "You just treat us like human beings". "But what if I say something wrong?" I asked. Surely there were other protocols aside from being aware of eye contact that I needed to know? "No, just be genuine, be yourself."

One afternoon, Anthony – a 32-year-old Aboriginal male – self-presented to the Emergency Department (ED) in a disorganised state, which led to a decision

for security to hold him down so he could be sedated. By the time Anthony got to the ward it was late at night and he was heavily sedated, although I was able to pick up that he had an engaging personality. It was his first mental health inpatient stay. While he could answer some of the questions I needed for the admission paperwork, I could see that he just needed to get to sleep. He told me he hadn't eaten, so I managed to get some food from the kitchen and showed him to his room. The next day was the Thursday before a long Easter weekend, which I happened to be working right through. Anthony was up talking to some other consumers when I walked in and he greeted me pleasantly. As his admitting nurse, I sat in on his psychiatric assessments. A urine drug test had come up positive for amphetamine and concerns were raised that he had been expressing delusional and paranoid thoughts in the ED the night before. He had not displayed any further psychotic symptoms the next day, but his treating team decided to keep him in as an involuntary patient for further observation until he was reviewed again.

The next day was Good Friday and it was relatively quiet on the ward. I spent most of my shift out in the day area and observed how Anthony used his bright personality and humour to brighten the spirits of the other consumers. Later Anthony approached me to have a chat. He was confused as to why he had been kept in hospital, even though he felt well. I explained the reasons why he had

CULTURAL CONSIDERATIONS 6.1—cont'd

Scenario: Anthony

been admitted and for the continued stay. He explained that he had brought himself to hospital due to feeling strange after taking some flu tablets the day before. The tablets had caused him to stay awake all night and while he was at work he knew that something else was wrong, so took himself to hospital. He couldn't remember the events clearly after this. I reminded him about the positive drug test. He told me he had never taken amphetamine-based substances before, "Maybe a little pot in my youth, but that's it, Miss". While frustrated at himself for bringing himself to hospital in the first place, he was otherwise accepting of the fact that as it was now going into a public holiday weekend there would be a scarcity of medical staff to review him and the day continued with no apparent issues.

On Saturday I could see that despite his attempts at keeping his spirits up by talking to the other consumers and being involved in ward activities, being on a locked ward with no leave was starting to wear on him. He hadn't displayed any overt psychotic symptoms and had been sleeping well every night despite refusing the antipsychotic medication the doctors had prescribed him. However, it was clear that being held in a locked ward was impacting his mood. By Sunday his mood was visibly low and he was showing signs of anxiety – restlessness, spending longer periods in his room and low appetite. He told me that he would have been at home with his family right now watching the footy, probably over a BBQ. It occurred to me that seeing as Monday was also a public holiday he wouldn't be reviewed for discharge until Tuesday. I tried to keep his spirits up and reassured him that he would be discharged in a few days. Tuesday eventually came and I greeted his family, who had travelled a few hours to make sure

they got to speak to his medical team. I got them comfortable in the family room and spoke to them while I waited for the medical team to make their rounds. They corroborated for me much of what Anthony had told me and were as confused, if not a little annoyed, as to why he had been kept locked in hospital for so many days, as they too didn't believe he had taken any drugs. Fortunately, I bumped into the ward pharmacist that morning who confirmed that the urine drug test may have picked up on the pseudoephedrine in the flu tablets he had mentioned taking. She printed out this information for me and I kept it in my uniform pocket. Finally, it was Anthony's turn to see the psychiatrist.

Following a brief assessment, the psychiatrist made the decision to keep Anthony in for another week. I saw the devastation on Anthony's face, but more than this, based on my clinical judgement I couldn't comprehend the decision. The treating team had been informed of his lack of psychotic presentation over the long weekend, but were still concerned that he had not been taking the prescribed medication. It didn't make sense. I asked Anthony to step outside the room so I could talk to the doctors. I presented them with the information I had received off the pharmacist, reiterated his presentation over the last 4 days and argued that by keeping him in against his will they were going to cause further harm. Despite being told that it wasn't my decision to make, I advocated that they at least discuss the decision with the family who they hadn't yet spoken with. Fortunately, they agreed and reversed their decision. Anthony left the ward with his family, relieved and grateful for the support. However, I couldn't shake a feeling of unease that if it wasn't for my advocacy this person would be spending another week in hospital and be at risk of serious psychological harm.

CRITICAL THINKING EXERCISE 6.4

Answer the following questions after reading Scenario: Anthony.
1. Can you identify anything the treating team could have done which may have better informed their decision-making?
2. What in this scenario demonstrates the absence of cultural safety?
3. What in this scenario demonstrates the presence of cultural safety?
4. Where in this story/case study can you identify institutional racism?

Engaging with Aboriginal and Torres Strait Islander Consumers

Interpretation of Cultural Differences

A significant challenge that mental health clinicians often identify is to know whether or not a behaviour that a consumer is presenting with is an indicator of deteriorating mental health or would otherwise be how they would normally respond to a situation. This is particularly an issue when people are displaying ways that can be interpreted as a potential risk to themselves or others, such as displaying emotional escalation, when in fact the behaviours are simply a response to social disadvantage, racism and discrimination. There are also cultural differences in the interpretation of certain experiences, such as seeing spirits or hearing the voices of deceased relatives, that non-Indigenous people may misinterpret as the symptoms of mental illness. This can have severe implications for the care of the person, such as inappropriate treatment and wrongful detainment under the Mental Health Act. Calling on family members, carers, members of the community, or Aboriginal health staff to help interpret and provide information is imperative in such circumstances to help guide decision-making.

Like other cultures that differ from our own, what you might perceive as culturally appropriate behaviour may be different for an Indigenous person. For example, for a non-Indigenous person, avoiding eye

contact may be read as being dismissive or rude when speaking to someone. A mental health assessment characterises it as an indicator of low mood or being distracted. However, maintaining eye contact is often a sign of disrespect in many Aboriginal communities. To the Aboriginal person, not making eye contact is not being disrespectful, in fact, looking away and turning your "ear" to someone is a sign that you are in fact "listening". As is the nature of such protocols in regards to body language and the use of certain words, they differ from region to region. The key is just to be aware that such differences exist to stop us from making unhelpful assumptions (Leckning et al 2019).

Fear and Lack of Trust

Based on our current understanding of Aboriginal and Torres Strait Islander history, we can appreciate why they may be guarded and reluctant to engage with government services. Government policies, such as assimilation and forced removal from their families and communities, have meant that many Aboriginal and Torres Strait Islander people do not trust government agencies. To the Aboriginal and Torres Strait Islander person, health services are often unwelcoming and alienating, due to discriminatory attitudes from staff, being misunderstood, and being in an unfamiliar environment. However, there is an even greater issue with mental health services that employ restrictive interventions, such as detainment under the Mental Health Act, restriction of freedom of movement, and coercive practices, such as forced medication, seclusion and restraint. For Aboriginal and Torres Strait Islander people, seclusion and restraint can be a humiliating, degrading and dehumanising experience as it mirrors the discriminatory and degrading treatment that many have experienced by governments, police and health services since colonisation began (Molloy et al 2021). A mental health establishment will be intimidating enough for anyone suffering from a mental health issue. For a Aboriginal and Torres Strait Islander person, this is then compounded with the expectation that they will be treated differently, the historical trauma of forced removal from families and communities, and the fear and lack of trust they have of service providers.

Use of Community and Family Support

As mentioned above, all health staff are encouraged to call on family members, carers or members of the community to provide information that will help guide decision-making. However, often mental health services will have access to an Aboriginal or Torres Strait Islander mental health team, clinician, liaison officer or health worker. While this is becoming increasingly common, there is still a paucity of trained Indigenous staff working in mental health services, so they may not always be available.

Yarning

Many Aboriginal and Torres Strait Islander people prefer to begin a conversation with general talk about where someone might be from, who their family is, and other questions that help them get to know you before sensitive topics are explored. This allows time for the person to become relaxed and for a feeling of trust to build. It is also important to use plain language instead of clinical terminology – as it is with anyone in the mental health space. Taking the time to get to know the person, and for them to get to know you is an important tool to aid engagement. Matthew Scott says: "Be genuine, be yourself, and if able, use humour!"

Deep Listening

Openness, curiosity and respect are most effective when partnered with *dadirri*. Dadirri is the state of deep listening and connection to oneself and others (Ungunmerr-Baumann et al 2022). Elements of dadirri that can be employed by the clinician are non-judgemental listening and communication, providing space for someone to tell their story, listening carefully with respect and not doing or saying something that might make them feel ashamed (Ungunmerr-Baumann et al 2022) (see Perspectives in practice: Nurse's story 6.1: Lim). Using elements of dadirri can enable the practitioner to really hear what is being said, without being clouded by their own assumptions.

PERSPECTIVES IN PRACTICE

Nurse's Story 6.1: Lim

The Experience of a Non-Indigenous Nurse in the Aboriginal and Torres Strait Islander Mental Health Space

Lim is a mental health nurse, originally from Cambodia, who has worked in a range of mental health settings for over a decade. He completed a Post Graduate Certificate in Clinical Redesign, which involved creating a project that would improve the overall quality of the healthcare experience for Aboriginal and Torres Strait Islander peoples. This was done by developing interventions to improve the length of stay and reduce incomplete treatment rates. The project team gained national and international recognition, which led to Lim working with the Aboriginal Health Unit to implement a "Flexi Clinic", which consisted of a team dedicated to responding to Aboriginal and Torres Strait Islander consumers who present to the ED within a short space of time of arriving and reduce extended waiting periods.

Q: What drew you to work closely with Aboriginal and Torres Strait Islander consumers?

I could see the gaps in health outcomes and how closely the trauma experienced by Aboriginal and Torres Strait Islander people and Cambodian people are relatable. Cambodian people also experienced land dispossession, and their culture was wiped out, as well as the people. The histories were so similar and there are also parallels between our cultures, such as our respect for elders.

Growing up in Australia, I remember having preconceived judgements; it was just the way I was taught. Society made you feel like Aboriginal people were bad, but as I grew up and understood more, I realised I was wrong. I could see the ongoing disparities and challenges faced by Aboriginal and Torres Strait Islander people such as institutionalised racism in the health service. It made me want to contribute to improving health outcomes more.

Q: What helped you to feel comfortable in your approach with Aboriginal and Torres Strait Islander consumers?

Guidance from the Aboriginal people I work with, including my colleagues at the Aboriginal Health Unit. Also just drawing on my communication skills in general, like being able to read body language and being sensitive to someone's responses by adapting my own. And it's the same with everyone. There's no special way for any one culture or group of people, because even within cultures people are all different. People from the same country are different because they are just different people. There are no algorithms. You adapt your approach to the individual you are working with. It's on an emotional human level. It's not prescriptive. And it's based on a genuine "seeking to connect" before you can start unpacking the clinical problem and coming at them with your intervention. If there is no connection established first, you may as well forget good outcomes.

But in saying that, there are some things that I draw from my experience with my own culture like the ability to connect with elders was informed by my own culture. I remember a time when I was speaking to an Aboriginal female elder. She said, "So what, you done a course on Aboriginal health and now you think you're an expert?" I replied, "I have never claimed to be an expert, but I am here to learn and make sure you get everything you need." A simple interaction about tea broke things down further and helped us to connect.

Q: What would be the main advice you would provide to anyone working with Aboriginal and Torres Strait Islander consumers?

When you greet someone, introduce yourself, say why you are there to see them and reassure them that you are there to help, you are not an expert and that you are guided by what they need. Learning from them is an important point. Learning which country people come from, "What's your country?"; this displays an interest in their Aboriginality and is a good ice breaker.

Read their body language. If someone is uncomfortable with how you are talking to them, then change your approach. Employ your therapeutic use of self. Be able to connect on a human level, irrespective of the differences between your respective cultures. It's not about knowing particularly about the culture or the country – it is about connecting on a personal level – a human and emotional level. Sometimes this looks like connecting over similarities instead of differences; not seeing the person as "other" but as "us".

HEALING

As Aboriginal and Torres Strait Islander people were pulled away from their traditional ways of living, beliefs and identity, a system of dominance and control over their lives grew in its place. We see the dominance continue today as biomedical models of diagnosis and treatment of mental health issues are more readily available than traditional models of healing. Prior to the British landing over 200 years ago, Aboriginal and Torres Strait Islander people had holistic methods of maintaining health and wellbeing, which covered mental, physical, cultural and spiritual health and enabled them to thrive for tens of thousands of years. Since then, many of these practices were lost as Aboriginal and Torres Strait Islander people were forced to relinquish their culture and identity in order to keep their families and themselves safe.

The events that Aboriginal and Torres Strait Islander people suffered were carried out based on the assumption that their culture was primitive and needed to be assimilated into westernised culture. However, in recent times there has been increasing recognition that incorporating Aboriginal and Torres Strait Islander understandings of health and wellbeing into ways of responding to mental health needs is required to close the gap in health.

Social and Emotional Wellbeing

Over the past 30 years there has been a policy agenda for the mental health of Indigenous Australians that recognises Aboriginal and Torres Strait Islander people's mental health and wellbeing are intrinsically connected within a holistic concept of health. This holistic concept recognises the importance of the connection Aboriginal and Torres Strait Islanders have to country, culture, spirituality, ancestry, and the health of their family and community. This experience of social and emotional wellbeing varies across different cultural groups and individuals. The *National Strategic Framework for Aboriginal and Torres Strait Islander Peoples' Mental Health and Social and Emotional Wellbeing 2017–2023* proposed a model of social and emotional wellbeing with seven overlapping domains as illustrated in Fig. 6.1 (Commonwealth of Australia 2017a).

The *National Strategic Framework for Aboriginal and Torres Strait Islander Peoples' Mental Health and Social and Emotional Wellbeing* (Commonwealth of Australia 2017a) comprises nine principles that describe the view of "whole-of-life health" held by Aboriginal and Torres Strait Islander peoples:

1. *Aboriginal and Torres Strait Islander health is viewed in a holistic context that encompasses mental health and physical, cultural and spiritual health. Land is central to wellbeing.*

Crucially, it must be understood that when the harmony of these interruptions is disrupted, Aboriginal and Torres Strait Islander ill health will persist.
2. *Self-determination is central to the provision of Aboriginal and Torres Strait Islander health services.*
3. *Culturally valid understandings must shape the provision of services and must guide assessment, care and management of Aboriginal and Torres Strait Islander people's health problems generally, and mental health problems in particular.*
4. *It must be recognised that the experience of trauma and loss, present since European invasion, are a direct outcome of the disruption to cultural wellbeing. Trauma and loss of this magnitude continues to have inter-generational effects.*
5. *The human rights of Aboriginal and Torres Strait Islander people must be recognised and respected. Failure to respect these human rights constitutes continuous disruption to mental health. Human rights relevant to mental illness must be specifically addressed.*
6. *Racism, stigma, environmental adversity and social disadvantage constitute ongoing stressors and have negative impacts on Aboriginal and Torres Strait Islander people's mental health and wellbeing.*
7. *The centrality of Aboriginal and Torres Strait Islander family and kinship must be recognised, as well as the broader concepts of family and the bonds of reciprocal affection, responsibility and sharing.*
8. *There is no single Aboriginal and Torres Strait Islander culture and group, but numerous groupings, languages and kinships, and tribes, as well as ways of living. Furthermore, Aboriginal and Torres Strait Islander people may currently live in urban,*

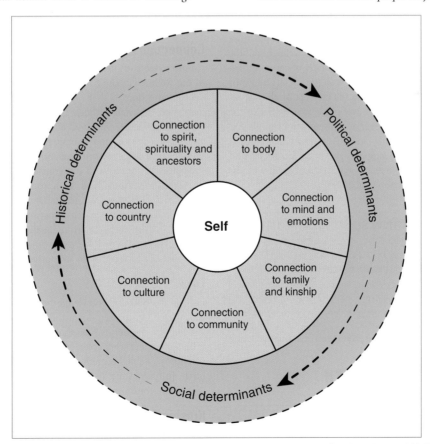

FIG. 6.1 Social and Emotional Wellbeing Model. (Source: Gee, Dudgeon, Schultz, Hart and Kelly, 2013. Artist: Tristan Schultz, RelativeCreative.)

rural or remote settings, in traditional or other lifestyles, and frequently move between these ways of living.

9. *It must be recognised that Aboriginal and Torres Strait Islander people have great strengths, creativity and endurance, and a deep understanding of the relationships between human beings and their environment.*

(Commonwealth of Australia 2017a, p. 3)

Social and Emotional Wellbeing Versus Mental Health

As Aboriginal and Torres Strait Islander people continue to present with a disproportionately high burden of mental illness compared to that of non-Indigenous populations, it has become increasingly recognised that the implementation of mental health programs has not been successful (Ketheeson et al 2020). The biomedical model of care and its concept of "clinical recovery" that presides in mental health services focuses on the elimination of symptoms from the individual, but fails to attend to Aboriginal and Torres Strait Islander mental health and wellbeing perspectives, as well as their needs (Bailie et al 2019). It has been recognised that closing the Aboriginal and Torres Strait Islander health gap will require challenging the dominant models of care within mental health services, which assume that psychological wellbeing can be treated as a separate entity, and will need to incorporate Aboriginal and Torres Strait Islander understandings of healing. The Social and Emotional Wellbeing framework is a more collective and holistic concept of mental health from western concepts, and extends beyond the idea of mental health being an individual journey. It takes into account factors such as education, unemployment, and a broader range of problems resulting from colonisation and its intergenerational legacies of grief, trauma and cultural dislocation, as well as discrimination and social disadvantage (Dudgeon et al 2022). The Social and Emotional Wellbeing framework recognises that these factors, also known as the "social determinants of health", currently have a disproportionate impact on Indigenous communities compared to the non-Indigenous population, and have a significant impact on the overall health and wellbeing of the individual. It is worth noting that the recovery model of care outlined in Chapter 2 of this text is partially congruent with the Social and Emotional Wellbeing framework by challenging the concept of clinical recovery and considering a journey of recovery that is personal to the individual (Winsper et al 2020). However, it too tends to propose that recovery is dependent on the individual and does not take into account how social aspects, such as external supports and other factors beyond the individual, affect the onset, course and outcomes of mental illness and substance use disorder (Davidson et al 2021).

LIVED EXPERIENCE BY MATHEW SCOTT, MENTAL HEALTH NURSE Aboriginal people don't believe that mental illness is a physiological disease with a diagnostic label and symptoms that are to be managed through medication. They are fully aware that what they are experiencing is the outcome of deeper issues from their childhood, the past and the present via the ongoing marginalisation and discrimination they face. It is a symptom of the loss of connection to the land and each other. It feels like we are aliens on our own country.

SOCIAL DETERMINANTS OF HEALTH AND PROTECTIVE FACTORS

The social factors that impact on mental health, such as education, employment, housing, transport, food and financial security, are recognised internationally as the "social determinants of health" (Brodie et al 2021). They are estimated to contribute to one-third (34%) of the overall burden of disease experienced by Aboriginal and Torres Strait Islander people (AIHW 2022). Government consultations have highlighted the importance of incorporating a coordinated, culturally appropriate and strengths-based approach to tackling this gap. While there are challenges associated with ensuring that care is coordinated across health and social services, frontline clinical workers, such as nurses, can clearly play a crucial part in tackling this issue by ensuring the early identification and management of needs.

Attending to the social determinants of health is an essential component of the factors that strengthen social and emotional wellbeing. These are collectively known as "protective factors", and include cultural and spiritual practices such as storytelling, traditional healing, and spending time in nature, as well as cultural traits, such as creativity, kinship and respecting elders (AIHW 2022). A survey by the Australian Bureau of Statistics (ABS) demonstrated the impact of these determinants, showing that Aboriginal and Torres Strait Islander people who lived on their homelands or traditional country were more likely to assess their own health as between excellent and good (78%) compared to those who were not allowed to visit their homelands or traditional country (47%) (ABS 2019). Culture and connection to family and community has been well documented as a strength and protective factor for good mental health and wellbeing for Aboriginal and Torres Strait Islander people in Australia (Hunter et al 2021). Elements of these are discussed below.

Traditional Healing

Cultural knowledge and practices are now being acknowledged and incorporated into mainstream health services. An example is the Ngangkari healers of the APY lands in South Australia, who visit communities, health services and jails to provide ancient therapeutic techniques that are said to cure depression and other forms of mental illness (Dudgeon & Bray 2018).

Connection to Country

Country refers to everything including the land, air and water. Central to the wellness of the Aboriginal or Torres Strait Islander person is a deep connection to their ancestral country. A person's country is a place that they can withdraw to, to regain a sense of wellbeing. This connection has been fostered over thousands of years of responsibility and knowledge of land management passed down through generations, as well as a deep spiritual connection explained through Dreamtime stories. Loss of land can equate to a sense of loss of one's self as disconnection from land compromises cultural connections and causes distress and powerlessness. The health and wellbeing benefits of Aboriginal land management programs have been acknowledged as a method of addressing health inequalities. Horticulture and gardening have been shown to have psychological benefits, but simply being outdoors can be effective in strengthening wellbeing.

Lore

Lore is the body of knowledge held by tribal elders who contained, interpreted and passed down the knowledge that defined the culture. Customary law defined responsibilities to the land, nature and each other, and there were consequences if they were not kept. Traditional ceremony enabled a method of dealing with life's transitions through birth, initiation and death, and men and women had defined roles within the community.

Kinship Structures

Aboriginal and Torres Strait Islander kinship structures define where a person fits into their family and community. They are complex and sophisticated systems which determine behaviour, responsibilities, obligations, roles and relationships, and are reflected in the fact that Aboriginal and Torres Strait Islander families are much larger than western "nuclear" families, as they have a closer relationship with a wider circle of people, whom non-Indigenous Australians would regard as "extended" family. Children are well protected within the group with a range of aunties and older siblings able to take over the child care role if the mother is fulfilling other communal responsibilities or is stressed.

Truth-telling

Telling the truth about Aboriginal and Torres Strait Islander history allows for their perspective to be acknowledged, which in turn assists health and wellbeing services in accurately identifying the areas for healing. Truth-telling is recognised by Indigenous cultures around the world as central to the process of healing. Truth-telling also acknowledges the strength and resilience of Aboriginal and Torres Strait Islander peoples and cultures, and is crucial to the ongoing recovery of communities (Butler et al 2019; Menzies 2019).

SOCIAL AND EMOTIONAL WELLBEING AS A STRENGTHS-BASED FRAMEWORK FOR SELF-DETERMINATION

Assisting Aboriginal and Torres Strait Islander people to strengthen protective factors is a strengths-based and person-centred approach that serves to empower Aboriginal and Torres Strait Islander people to take control over their own lives. Culturally relevant approaches enable this, known as "self-determination". Self-determination is in direct contrast with the powerlessness felt by the Aboriginal and Torres Strait Islander population as a result of colonisation, and is being recognised as critical to closing the health gap between the Indigenous and non-Indigenous population. Some basic principles include living in accordance with values, adopting a collective Aboriginal identity and having broad societal representation (Dudgeon 2020).

Nursing staff once more have a key role in fostering self-determination by utilising a strengths-based approach to focus on clients' abilities, talents and resources, which will then help them to develop resilience, improving the person's ability to respond or navigate similar situations in the future (Dudgeon et al 2022). Self-determination also recognises the ability of community-led solutions to be able to innovatively respond to the health needs of Aboriginal and Torres Strait Islander consumers in a holistic way, helping to improve health and wellbeing outcomes and maintain it through periods of crisis such as the pandemic (Lowitja Institute 2022).

✴ HISTORICAL ANECDOTE 6.3

The Emergence of Community-Controlled Health Services Through Self-Determination and Advocacy

In the 1960s, both Indigenous and non-Indigenous advocates for health began a rights-based movement to drive change in healthcare due to increasing concerns about the health outcomes of Aboriginal and Torres Strait Islander peoples. Their determination led to the development of Aboriginal community-controlled health services (ACCHSs), which are now commonly known as Aboriginal Medical Services (AMS). AMS respond to the needs of Aboriginal and Torres Strait Islander communities all over Australia by attending to the common barriers associated with accessing mainstream health services, such as cost, cultural sensitivity and trust.

Read All About It

Aboriginal Medical Services (AMS) 2021. Our history and future. Online. Available at: https://amsredfern.org.au/our-history-future/

❓ CRITICAL THINKING EXERCISE 6.5

1. What type of things do you need in your own lives to maintain a sense of balance and security?
2. What do you incorporate into your lives to help you attain a sense of peace and balance?
3. How do these things help you deal with life's inevitable stressors?
4. What activities for an overall sense of health and wellbeing do you come across in mainstream culture that are also foundational to the wellbeing of Aboriginal and Torres Strait Islander people?

Social and emotional wellbeing for self-determination is enhanced through building partnerships with Aboriginal and Torres Strait Islander colleagues, communities and organisations. This includes co-design, a process of meaningfully engaging with people who use mental health services, including their family, carers and support persons, to ensure that delivered care reflects both best practice and the needs of those who access services. Co-design also ensures that mental health service provision is shaped not only by understandings of Aboriginal and Torres Strait Islander culture, but that the interventions developed suit the specific needs of the communities. When providing nursing care, it is equally important to build strong working therapeutic relationships with Aboriginal and Torres Strait Islander colleagues, communities and organisations. These relationships will strengthen your ability to deliver a higher standard of care and expand your understanding of Indigenous culture and health.

Aboriginal Health Workforce

Building a workforce valued for its specialist expertise and cultural capability is a crucial factor in improving the health and wellbeing of Aboriginal people accessing mental health services (CATSINaM 2017). It is recognised by both the Department of Health's (2022) *Aboriginal and Torres Strait Islander Health Workforce Strategic Framework and Implementation Plan 2021–2031* and the Australian Health Practitioner Regulation Agency's (2019) *National Scheme's Aboriginal and Torres Strait Islander Health and Cultural Safety Strategy 2020–2025* that an increase in the Indigenous workforce is required to ensure the cultural safety of both patients and staff.

It is important to note that while the presence of Aboriginal health staff is incredibly beneficial, the roles come with specific challenges. Aboriginal health staff are often members of the local community, and while this assists in bridging communications between the health service and the community, it can also mean that work life and personal life are not easily separated, and they continue to perform their role outside of work hours. The experience of trauma, grief and loss and other impacts of colonisation, which they often have to deal with in work, is often reflected outside of work. Aboriginal health staff may also have to endure workplaces that are culturally unsafe, experience institutionalised racism, and work with staff and colleagues who are not culturally informed, while often being called on to be the ones to rectify this by providing education. The Aboriginal health staff role can also come with excessive workloads, pressure, lack of support, stress, and a lack of recognition for their work, leading to burnout and high rates of staff turnover (Deroy & Schütze 2019). (See Cultural considerations 6.2: Jess.)

Key points that have been identified as important to the retention of Aboriginal health and wellbeing staff are:
- feeling culturally safe and secure within the workplace
- teamwork and collaboration
- supervision and strong managerial leadership and support from peers (to debrief, reflect, receive emotional support and strengthen coping mechanisms)

- professional development (the opportunity for skill development and role progression)
- recognition (of work load, quality of work performed, being trusted to work autonomously, and financial remuneration that reflects the high pressure of the role) (Deroy & Schütze 2019).

🌐 CULTURAL CONSIDERATIONS 6.2
Aboriginal Mental Health Trainee's Story: Jess

As an Aboriginal mental health student, I was frequently asked how to "properly" engage with Aboriginal and Torres Strait Islander consumers. I recognised that there was a very unconscious but overt "othering" of Aboriginal and Torres Strait Islander consumers and an incredibly overcautious approach towards engagement. Aboriginal and Torres Strait Islander people are incredibly relational, and our cultural practices transmit via word of mouth. Aboriginal and Torres Strait Islander people establish safety in conversations by facilitating conversations with questions around identity, for example, where are you from, and who is your mob? In the context of therapeutic alliance with Aboriginal and Torres Strait Islander peoples, sharing identity is integral to establishing safety and trust. Regularly check in on your own racial bias towards Aboriginal and Torres Strait Islander people. It is also necessary to remember that one person's cultural experience may be different to another's.

Healthcare is also not necessarily a space that attracts a large number of Aboriginal and Torres Strait Islander professionals due to the cultural genocide that occurred historically in these institutions. Additionally, bearing the burden of working in a mainstream system that places ownership on Aboriginal and Torres Strait islander staff to be culturally responsive places Aboriginal and Torres Strait Islander staff at the risk of higher rates of burnout and cultural fatigue.

My experience as a Wiradjuri Kalari woman within the mental health care space felt both odd and political. As an Aboriginal woman with fair skin, I was unfortunately exposed to micro and macro aggressions, which impacted my sense of identity. My experience of both racism and discrimination impacted on my emotional, cultural and physical safety within this work environment and was detrimental to the care I provided to consumers. I also recognised that what I was experiencing as an Aboriginal mental health student was reflective of the overarching systemic racism that permeates healthcare systems and other institutions. The by-product of this is an incredibly entrenched culture of distrust and contributes to poor mental health outcomes for my mob. This was an environment where I felt culturally restricted and culturally silenced. In addition, it felt hypocritical for me to promise Aboriginal and Torres Strait Islander consumers a safe environment and encourage families to re-access services if they required ongoing mental health support, when I was directly experiencing overt racism and discrimination as a staff member.

REFLECTIONS ON SOCIAL AND EMOTIONAL WELLBEING FOR A FUTURE OF BEST PRACTICE

When we acknowledge Aboriginal and Torres Strait Islander history, we can acknowledge the strength and spirit of Aboriginal and Torres Strait Islander people which has helped them survive and withstand the devastating and ongoing impact of colonisation. Having an understanding of Aboriginal and Torres Strait Islander culture helps us to assist Aboriginal and Torres Strait Islander individuals and communities to build on the existing strengths to promote social and emotional wellbeing. We invite you to understand the simplicity of the social and emotional wellbeing concept and how it might translate to the things you might need to maintain a sense of balance in your own lives. You may be able to see the parallels between Aboriginal and Torres Strait Islander concepts of healing and things that you may try yourself to achieve balance – ancient understandings of healing that hold weight today, which would be good for any of us.

Nurses play an ongoing pivotal role in improving the quality of care experienced by Aboriginal and Torres Strait Islander consumers. This includes ongoing quality improvement in consultation with the Aboriginal and Torres Strait Islander community, creating culturally welcoming environments, communicating effectively with Aboriginal and Torres Strait Islander people and building collaborative partnerships with Aboriginal and Torres Strait Islander communities, colleagues and organisations (McGough et al 2018). Most importantly, it will be your own ongoing reflection of the attitudes and beliefs that you bring to the nurse–consumer encounter that is most necessary, as this will not only have an impact on the person's experience of the health service, but will have an impact on the culture of the service. See Personal perspectives: Consumer's story: Ernie.

👤 PERSONAL PERSPECTIVES
Consumer's Story 6.1: Ernie

Ernie has been in a mental health inpatient unit in a hospital off country for 6 months. This stay has been longer than usual due to his having lost housing prior to coming into hospital through no fault of his own. Due to miscommunications between staff, who told his family (who are 5 hours away) he had been discharged and the Aboriginal liaison worker who left their position soon after Ernie's arrival, he had no visitors and consequently has not been able to have any leave off the ward. However, Ernie had free access to a phone, which he used to contact the Aboriginal mental health liaison nurse from another hospital where he had an inpatient stay previously, and developed a good relationship with. Ernie explained to the Aboriginal mental health liaison nurse his experiences of what factors made him feel culturally vulnerable or conversely, safe, when he was in hospital:

"It's not easy to be in hospital. There are a lot of people going through a lot here – it's not easy to be around. I've been in the same clothes for 6 months; I've felt like an animal for 6 months. I miss my family and I miss you my brother. It's boring here, no DVDs, no games, no activities, they got nothing here. They don't take you outside for fresh air or a smoke, being told what time to go to bed. It's not a place to come.

Good staff make me feel safe when they listen, and tell me the truth about what's happening with my discharge plan. I feel safe when my family are able to visit me, or I can do some activities or go outside, and connect with someone. Being able to ring you when I've had a bad day helps, just to have a yarn, have a cry, and knowing that my ancestors are watching over me, keeping me safe."

CHAPTER SUMMARY

The colonial history of Australia had, and continues to have, a significant impact on the mental wellbeing of Indigenous Australians. Often, we get trapped in a perception that the needs of Aboriginal and Torres Strait Islander consumers are too great or too different from other consumers to be able to apply an effective intervention or support. The negative assumptions that are often applied to mental health consumers in general, including that they are aggressive, attention-seeking or uncooperative, are in addition to the stigma and discrimination that Aboriginal and Torres Strait Islander people already face.

We acknowledge the rich diversity of traditions, languages and protocols within these cultural groups, and while it is not possible, nor expected, that everything about these two cultures is known, we hope that this chapter has illustrated that the experience of the Indigenous consumer and the non-Indigenous consumer should not be so different, and that the impact of past trauma has the same effect on an individual no matter what your background is. Therefore, the approach to healing and recovery is very much similar too. The universal mental health nursing skills of getting to know the person who has presented to your service, listening to them, and providing a space that is both physically and psychologically safe, are key and core to the nurse–consumer therapeutic relationship for anyone. An approach of openness, respect and curiosity as you work with people from these communities, as well as the information provided in this chapter, will support you to understand the experience of the Aboriginal and Torres Strait Islander person, free from misperceptions, and assist you to create a workplace that is culturally safe for both the consumer and your colleagues. We hope that this information will also help you to develop therapeutic relationships in which you are able to listen and understand more deeply, as it is from this space – between nurse and consumer – that healing can occur.

ACKNOWLEDGEMENT

We would like to acknowledge the strength and resilience of the Aboriginal and Torres Strait Islander consumers and staff who we have had the privilege of working alongside, and who have generously shared their experiences and perspectives which have guided this chapter. The authors pay their respect to all Aboriginal and Torres Strait Islander people, who are the traditional custodians of the land, their ancestors and elders past and present, and the future young leaders of the sacred land we work, walk, and live on, whose connection and belonging to the land has never and will never cease.

USEFUL WEBSITES AND RESOURCES

AIATIS: https://aiatsis.gov.au/
Australian Indigenous Health InfoNet: www.healthinfonet.ecu.edu.au
Indigenous Mental Health and Suicide Prevention Clearing House: www.indigenousmhspc.gov.au/
Transforming Indigenous Mental Health and Wellbeing: timhwb.org.au/
Working with Aboriginal People: Enhancing Clinical Practice in Mental Health Care: www.youtube.com/watch?v=2mrz8p4t-qo

REFERENCES

Aberdeen, L. & Jones, J. A. (eds) 2021. Black, White and Exempt: Aboriginal and Torres Strait Islander Lives Under Exemption. Aboriginal Studies Press, Acton, ACT.

AIATSIS 2022. Australia's First Peoples. Online. Available at: https://aiatsis.gov.au/explore/australias-first-peoples

AIATSIS 2008. To remove and protect: Laws that changed Aboriginal lives. Online. Available at: aiatsis.gov.au/collection/featured-collections/remove-and-protect

Attwood, B. (ed.) 2020. The Struggle for Aboriginal Rights: A Documentary History. Routledge, New York.

Australian Bureau of Statistics (ABS) 2019. National Aboriginal and Torres Strait Islander Health Survey. Online. Available at: www.abs.gov.au/statistics/people/aboriginal-and-torres-strait-islander-peoples/national-aboriginal-and-torres-strait-islander-health-survey/latest-release

Australian Health Practitioner Regulation Agency (Ahpra) 2019. National Scheme's Aboriginal and Torres Strait Islander Health and Cultural Safety Strategy 2020–2025. Online. Available at: www.ahpra.gov.au/About-Ahpra/Aboriginal-and-Torres-Strait-Islander-Health-Strategy/health-and-cultural-safety-strategy.aspx

Australian Human Rights Commission (AHRC) 2018. Close the Gap – 10-year review. Online. Available at: https://humanrights.gov.au/our-work/aboriginal-and-torres-strait-islander-social-justice/publications/close-gap-10-year-review

Australian Institute of Health and Welfare (AIHW) 2022a. 'Death by suicide among First Nations people. Online. Available at: www.aihw.gov.au/suicide-self-harm-monitoring/data/populations-age-groups/suicide-indigenous-australians

Australian Institute of Health and Welfare (AIHW) 2022b. Determinants of health for Indigenous Australians. Determinants of Health. Online. Available at: www.aihw.gov.au/reports/australias-health/social-determinants-and-indigenous-health

Axelsson, P., Kukutai, T., & Kippen, R. 2016. The field of Indigenous health and the role of colonisation and history. J Population Res, 33, 1–7.

Bailey, M. 2020. "You betray your country": Remembering and forgetting the stolen generations in the metropolitan press. J Aust Stud, 44(1), 114–126.

Bailie J., Laycock, A., Matthews, V., Peiris, D., & Bailie, R. 2019. Emerging evidence of the value of health assessments for Aboriginal and Torres Strait Islander people in the primary healthcare setting. Aust J Prim Health, 25(1), 1–5.

Brodie, T., Pearson, O., Cantley, L., Cooper, P., Westhead, S., 2021. Strengthening approaches to respond to the social and emotional well-being needs of Aboriginal and Torres Strait Islander people: The cultural pathways program. Prim Health Care Res Dev, 22, e35.

Butler, T. L., Anderson, K., Garvey, G., Cunningham, J., Ratcliffe, J., 2019. Aboriginal and Torres Strait islander people's domains of wellbeing: A comprehensive literature review. Soc Sci Med, 233, 138–157.

Campbell, J. 2002. Invisible Invaders: Smallpox and Other Diseases in Aboriginal Australia, 1780–1880, Melbourne University Press, Carlton.

Collins English Dictionary. 2020. Online. Available at: www.collinsdictionary.com/english/creative

Commonwealth of Australia 2017a. National Strategic Framework for Aboriginal and Torres Strait Islander Peoples' Mental Health and Social and Emotional Wellbeing. Department of the Prime Minister and Cabinet, Canberra. Online. Available at: www.niaa.gov.au/sites/default/files/publications/mhsewb-framework_0.pdf

Commonwealth of Australia 2017b. Royal Commission into Institutional Responses to Child Sexual Abuse, Final Report, Vol. 3. Impacts. Commonwealth of Australia. Canberra. Online. Available at: www.childabuseroyalcommission.gov.au/impacts

Congress of Aboriginal and Torres Strait Islander Nurses and Midwives (CATSINaM) 2017. The Nursing and Midwifery Aboriginal and Torres Strait Islander Health Curriculum Framework: An adaptation of and complementary document to the 2014 Aboriginal and Torres Strait Islander Health Curriculum Framework. CATSINaM, Canberra.

Council of Deans of Nursing and Midwifery (CDNM) 2022. CDNM National Apology at CATSINaM Conference. Online. Available at: www.cdnm.edu.au/cdnm-national-apology-at-catsinam-conference

Davidson, L., Rowe, M., DiLeo, P., Bellamy, C., & Delphin-Rittmon, M. 2021. Recovery-oriented systems of care: A perspective on the past, present, and future. ARCR, 41(1).

Department of Health 2022. Aboriginal and Torres Strait Islander Health Workforce Strategic Framework and Implementation Plan 2021–2031. Commonwealth of Australia, Canberra.

Deroy, S., & Schütze, H. 2019. Factors supporting retention of aboriginal health and wellbeing staff in Aboriginal health services: A comprehensive review of the literature. Int J Equity Health, 18(1), 1–11.

Dudgeon, P. 2020. Decolonising psychology: Self-determination and social and emotional well-being. In: Hokowhitu, B., Moreton-Robinson, A., Tuhiwai-Smith, L., Andersen, C., Larkin S. (eds), Routledge Handbook of Critical Indigenous Studies. Routledge, New York.

Dudgeon, P. & Bray, A. 2018. Indigenous healing practices in Australia. Women Ther, 41 (1–2), 97–113.

Dudgeon, P., Derry, K.L., Mascall, C., Ryder, A. 2022. Understanding Aboriginal models of selfhood: The National Empowerment Project's Cultural, Social, and Emotional Wellbeing Program in Western Australia. Int J Environ Res Pub Health, 19(7), doi.org/10.3390/ijerph19074078

Dudgeon, P., Walker, R., Scrine, C., Shepherd, C., Calma, T., et al., 2014. Effective strategies to strengthen the mental health and wellbeing of Aboriginal and Torres Strait Islander people. Closing the Gap Clearing House. Australian Government, AIHW, Australian Institute of Family Studies, Canberra. Online. Available at: www.aihw.gov.au/getmedia/6d50a4d2-d4da-4c53-8aeb-9ec22b856dc5/ctgc-ip12-4nov2014.pdf.aspx?inline=true

Gee, G., Dudgeon, P., Schultz, C., Hart, A., & Kelly, K. 2014. Social and emotional wellbeing and mental health: An Aboriginal perspective. In: Dudgeon, P., Milroy, H., & Walker, R. (eds), Working Together: Aboriginal and Torres Strait Islander Mental Health and Wellbeing Principles and Practice, 2nd edn. Department of the Prime Minister and Cabinet, Australian Government, Canberra.

George, E., Mackean, T., Baum, F., & Fisher, M. 2019. Social determinants of Indigenous health and Indigenous rights in policy: A scoping review and analysis of problem representation. Int Indig Policy J, 10(2), doi.org/10.18584/iipj.2019.10.2.4.

Guha, M.D., Cutler, N., Heffernan, T., Davis, M. 2022. Developing a trauma-informed and recovery-oriented alternative to aggression management training for a metropolitan and rural mental health service. Iss Ment Health Nurs, 43(12), doi.org/10.1080/01612840.2022.2095471.

Hunter, SA., Skouteris, H., & Morris, H. 2021. A conceptual model of protective factors within Aboriginal and Torres Strait Islander culture that build strength. J Cross-Cult Psych, 52(8–9), doi.org/10.1177/00220221211046310.

Kairuz, C.A., Casanelia, L.M., Bennett-Brook, K., Coombes, J., & Yadav, U.N. 2021. Impact of racism and discrimination on physical and mental health among Aboriginal and Torres Strait Islander peoples living in Australia: A systematic scoping review. BMC Public Health, 21(1), 1–16.

Ketheesan, S., Rinaudo, M., Berger, M., Wenitong, M., Juster, R. P., et al., 2020. Stress, allostatic load and mental health in Indigenous Australians. Stress, 23(5), 509–518.

Law, J. & Martin, E. 2020. Oxford Medical Dictionary. Oxford University Press, Oxford.

Leckning, B., Ringbauer, A., Robinson, G., Carey, T. A., Hirvonen, T. et al., 2019. Guidelines for best practice psychosocial assessment of Aboriginal and Torres Strait Islander people presenting to hospital with self-harm and suicidal thoughts. Menzies School of Health Research, Darwin.

Lowitja Institute 2022. Close the Gap Campaign Report 2022 – Transforming Power: Voices for Generational Change, The Close the Gap Campaign Steering Committee. Online. Available at: www.lowitja.org.au/page/services/resources/Cultural-and-social-determinants/culture-for-health-and-wellbeing/close-the-gap-campaign-report-2022—-transforming-power-voices-for-generational-change

Lynch, J., Ross, H., & Carter, R.W. 2018. Indigenous guidance in Australian environmental management. Australas J Environ Manage, 25(3), 253–257.

MacPherson, W. 1999. The Stephen Lawrence Inquiry. Stationery Office, London.

McGough, S., Wynaden, D., & Wright, M. 2018. Experience of providing cultural safety in mental health to Aboriginal patients: A grounded theory study. Int J Ment Health Nurs, 27(1), 204–213.

Mental Health Coordinating Council (MHCC) 2013. Trauma-informed care and practice: Towards a cultural shift in policy reform across mental health and human services in Australia. A National Strategic Direction, Position Paper and Recommendations of the National Trauma-Informed Care and Practice Advisory Working Group. Authors: Bateman, J & Henderson, C (MHCC) Kezelman, C (Adults Surviving Child Abuse, ASCA). Online. Available at: mhcc.org.au/publication/trauma-informed-care-and-practice-ticp/

Menzies, K. 2019. Understanding the Australian Aboriginal experience of collective, historical and intergenerational trauma. Int Soc Work, 62(6), 1522–1534.

Molloy, L. 2019. The ideas of Frantz Fanon and practices of cultural safety with Australia's First Peoples. In: Turner, L., Neville, H. (eds), Frantz Fanon's Psychotherapeutic Approaches to Clinical Work. Routledge, New York.

Molloy, L., Guha, M.D., Scott, M.P., Beckett, P., Merrick, T.T., et al., 2021. Mental health nursing practice and Aboriginal and Torres Strait Islander people: An integrative review. Contemp Nurse, 57(1–2), 140–156.

Molloy, L., Walker, K., Lakeman, R., & Lees, D. 2019. Encounters with difference: Mental health nurses and Indigenous Australian users of mental health services. Int J Ment Health Nurs, 28(4), 922–929.

Murrup-Stewart, C., Searle, A.K., Jobson, L., & Adams, K. 2019. Aboriginal perceptions of social and emotional wellbeing programs: A systematic review of literature assessing social and emotional wellbeing programs for Aboriginal and Torres Strait Islander Australians perspectives. Aust Psychologist, 54(3), 171–186.

Narvaez, D., & Tarsha, M. 2021. The missing mind: Contrasting civilization with non-civilization development and functioning. In: T. Henley & M. Rossano (eds), Psychology and Cognitive Archaeology: An Interdisciplinary Approach to the Study of the Human Mind. Routledge, London.

Nursing and Midwifery Board of Australia (NMBA) 2018. Code of Conduct. NMBA, Melbourne. Online. Available at: www.nursingmidwiferyboard.gov.au/Codes-Guidelines-Statements/Professional-standards.aspx

Productivity Commission 2021. Closing the Gap Annual Data Compilation Report. Online. Available at: www.pc.gov.au/closing-the-gap-data/annual-data-report/2021/report/closing-the-gap-annual-data-compilation-report-july2021.pdf

Silverstein, B. 2020. Aboriginal Australians: A history since 1788. Australian Aboriginal Studies (Canberra), (1), 85–87.

Stewart, M., McCallum, K., Geia, L., Musulin, K. 2016, What do the newspapers *really* tell us about the lock hospital histories? The Conversation. 23 Sept. Online. Available at: theconversation.com/what-do-the-newspapers-really-tell-us-about-the-lock-hospital-histories-65713

Taylor, K., & Guerin, P.T. 2019. Health Care and Indigenous Australians: Cultural Safety in Practice. Bloomsbury, Sydney.

Torres Strait Islands Regional Authority n.d. General history. Online. Available at: www.tsra.gov.au/the-torres-strait/general-history

Ungunmerr-Baumann, M.R., Groom, R.A., Schuberg, E.L., Atkinson, J., Atkinson, C., et al., 2022. Dadirri: An Indigenous place-based research methodology. AlterNative, 18(1), 94–103.

Wilson, A., Wilson, R., Delbridge, R., Tonkin, E., Palermo, C. et al., 2020. Resetting the narrative in Australian Aboriginal and Torres Strait Islander nutrition research. Curr Dev Nutr, 4(5), nzaa080.

Winsper, C., Crawford-Docherty, A., Weich, S., Fenton, S.J., & Singh, S.P. 2020. How do recovery-oriented interventions contribute to personal mental health recovery? A systematic review and logic model. Clin Psych Rev, 76, 101815.

7

Kua Takoto Te Manuka

(The leaves of the manuka tree have been laid down.[1])

Andrea E. Donaldson and Bryce Taiata Samuel

Ko Pirongia te maunga,
Ko Waipa te awa
Ko Tainui te waka,
Ko Ngati Maniapoto te iwi,
Ko Parewaeono te hapuu
Ko Otorohanga te wahi
Ko Te Keeti Marae.
Ko Knapp/Rowan te ingoa whānau o toku kuia whaea
Ko Andrea Evelyn Donaldson toku ingoa

Ko Maungatautari me Maungakawa nga maunga
Ko Topehaehae me Piako-Iti nga awa
Ko Tainui te waka
Ko Ngaati Hauaa te iwi
Ko Ngaati Werewere te hapuu
Ko Rukumoana me Kai-a-te-mata nga marae
Ko Hamiora/Samuels te ingoa whaanau o tooku tupuna papa
Ko Bryce Taiata Samuel ahau

KEY POINTS

- Māori mental health disparities are due to colonisation, urbanisation, social economic and western paradigms of mental health service delivery.
- There are five principles of Te Tiriti o Waitangi to provide deeper clarity and guidance around nursing and health care.
- Culturally safe mental health care for Māori is based on the Māori principle of whakawhānaungatanga, which reflects a recovery-oriented model of care where the needs of tangata whāiora (service users) are the focus.

- Māori models of health create an environment for increased engagement and duration of care for Māori whānau.
- Māori health professionals enable Māori tangata whāiora to reach a greater understanding of their own experiences through mātauranga Māori, whereby they feel empowered to use their knowledge within to heal themselves, their whānau, hapū and iwi.

KEY TERMS

Cultural safety	Māori mental health nurses	Te Tiriti o Waitangi
Kaupapa Māori service	Māori models of health	Whakawhānaungatanga
Kawa Whakaruruhau	Mātauranga Māori	
Māori mental health	Prevalence of Māori mental illness	

---

[1]The chapter title, "Kua Takoto Te Manuka" is a form of wero, which is performed in very formal situations on the marae. This proverb is used when being challenged, or when you have a challenge ahead of you. The title of this chapter was chosen because it represents the challenges faced by nurses in learning, understanding, and showing commitment to the importance of Māori mental health history, Te Tiriti, kawa whakaruruhau and mātauranga Māori, and why priority and demonstration of this knowledge is needed in mental health nursing practice today.

LEARNING OUTCOMES

The material in this chapter will assist you to:
- explore Māori views on health and understand how colonisation has affected Māori mental health today
- understand the importance of Te Tiriti o Waitangi, kawa whakaruruhau and mātauranga Māori and how they guide nursing practice
- explore what it means to be a Māori nurse working in mental health today
- identify why Kaupapa Māori services are important to facilitate and develop culturally safe practice through whānaungatanga, Māori models of health and Māori mental health interventions.

INTRODUCTION

The sense of belonging and strength that whānau provides is one of the key foundations of Māori health. Thoughts, feelings and emotions are invariably linked to physical and spiritual wellbeing. Māori health and culture are linked, so if a person identifies as Māori there are aspects of Te Ao Māori (Māori worldview) that must be understood to provide safe and effective mental health care. In this chapter we discuss the pre-colonisation view of Māori health, the impact that colonisation had on Māori health and mental health, as well as why mental health problems are common in Māori today. This chapter will also discuss how, despite Māori mental health problems being common, there is an unmet need for treatment and how the current health reforms are rising to the challenge of addressing this disparity. We also discuss Māori nurses, racism, institutional racist rhetoric, kawa whakaruruhau (cultural safety), including Te Tiriti o Waitangi and how these things influence and guide nurses' ability to care for Māori. We explore different Māori models of health, Kaupapa Māori services and current Māori mental health interventions.

We hope that this chapter will inspire and educate you to carefully consider and engage with the issues raised and apply them to your own nursing care in whatever setting you may practise during your nursing career. To assist your reading, an explanation of Māori terms is provided in Box 7.1, below.

BOX 7.1 Glossary of Māori Terms

aroha	to love, compassion	ngakau	relationships that influence the way we live
atua	god or gods	ngaro	hidden, the subconscious
awa	river	noa	neutral or relaxed state with no restrictions
hā a koro mā a kui mā	the "breath of life" that comes from ancestors	oranga	wellbeing
hangi	traditional cooking	pae ora	healthy futures
hapū	subtribe(s)	pākehā	European/colonial settlers
hauora	health and wellbeing	pepeha	introducing yourself and your connections in Te Reo
hinengaro	emotional and mental wellbeing	pono	true and genuine
iho matua	spiritual connection	poorewarewa	be insane, mentally unwell
iwi	tribe(s)	pooteetee	be insane, mentally unwell
iwi katoa	services and systems that provide support for patients/whānau within the health environment	porangi	be insane, mentally unwell
		powhiri	formal welcome ceremony
kai	food, meal, to eat	pumanawa	the skills taught to us throughout our lives from parents
kaiwhakahaere	director/manager	pūrākau	story, myth, ancient legend
karakia	prayer	rangatahi	youth/adolescents
kaumātua	elders	rangatiratanga	chief
kaupapa	philosophy	rongoā	Māori medicinal system
kaupapa Māori	Māori research methods	roopu	organisation, group, or collective.
kawa	customs	taiao	physical environment
kawa whakaruruhau	cultural safety	tamariki	children
kawanatanga	good governance	tangata	people, men, emergent concepts
kotahi	unity	tangata whāiora	service user
kōwhiringa	options	tangata whenua	Indigenous people of the land
kupu	concepts or themes	taonga	treasure, anything prized
mana	prestige and authority	tapu	sacred state or condition
mana ake	uniqueness of individual and family	Te Ao Māori	Māori society
manākitanga	hospitality, kindness, process of showing respect	Te Reo	Māori language
Māori	Indigenous people of Aotearoa New Zealand	Te Tiriti o Waitangi	The Treaty of Waitangi
Māoritanga	Māori way of life	tiakitanga	to watch for
marae	the courtyard of a Māori meeting house	tikanga	Māori customary values and practices
mātauranga Māori	Māori knowledge systems	tinana	physical wellbeing
maunga	mountain	tino rangatiratanga	self-determination
mauri	life force	tohunga	to be proficient, a chosen expert, priest, healer
mirimiri	therapeutic massage	waiata	song

BOX 7.1 Glossary of Māori Terms—cont'd

waihanga	physical make-up	whakapapa	genealogical tables
wairangi	to be beside oneself, suffering from mental illness	whakaruruhau	to protect, shield, shelter
wairua	spirituality	whakatauki	proverbial expressions
wānanga	cultural forum and knowledge	whakawhānaungatanga	process of establishing relationships
whaikorero	formal speeches	whānau	family, or the individual as part of the collective
whakamoemiti	to praise, express thanks	whatumanawa	deep-seated emotions

MĀORI MENTAL HEALTH HISTORY

It is important to understand how Māori viewed health prior to colonisation and how colonisation impacted Māori understanding of health and therefore how these views on health have led to the current mental health problems recognised today. As discussed in Chapter 2, this book encourages a "social ecological" understanding of mental health nursing practice, which views mental health as an interactive process that occurs between people and their environment/ecology. The following section discusses the history of Māori mental health pre- and post-colonisation and is an important place to begin learning how to address the current Māori mental health disparities.

Pre-Colonisation

Before the arrival of western medicine, understandings of health/wellness/illness for the Māori population were integrated and inseparable from the wider system of beliefs, customs, myths and practices of the whānau (family or immediate community) and iwi (tribe). Each marae and hapū had a tohunga (priest) whose role was to ensure wellbeing of the whānau, and hapū governed by the laws of tapu (sacred state or condition). Tapu could be applied to people, places, animals, plants, events and social relationships. The tohunga kept the balance of tapu and noa (neutral or relaxed state with no restrictions) (Durie 1998). In terms of health, breaking tapu was seen as the cause of sickness and earnt ridicule or intense mental suffering, as well as physical symptoms, including death (Durie 1998). Therefore, the understanding of health was a holistic one.

Mental illness (as defined by western criteria) is likely to have existed within Māori communities before European contact. Concepts such as "porangi, wairangi, poorewarewa, haurangi, and pooteetee" (Kingi 2017, p. 17) describe whānau who were mad, or losing their mind, and inferred behaviours that deviated from community and cultural norms. Kingi (2017) considered how diseases of the mind may have been perceived by Māori and referred to historian Ernest Beaglehole's research of the 1940s, which suggested that prior to colonisation Māori would have been unaware of mental illness. According to Beaglehole, these types of issues would have been explained within cultural and spiritual paradigms as "transgression of sanctity" (Kingi 2017, p. 8), where transgressions were the root cause of the person's unwellness and manifested as deterioration in one's "state of mind", as opposed to an "illness of the mind".

Colonisation

During the 1800s, Māori mental health was literally unheard of. At that time, Māori experienced low prevalence of mental illness in comparison to non-Māori (Kingi 2017). Furthermore, Māori were described by settlers as having considerable mental determination and strength, with strong cultural identity. This positive view of Māori mental health is significant, as recent research has identified parallels between "Māori cultural identity" and "positive mental health" (Kingi 2005).

At the same time, New Zealand Crown authorities were confining people (mainly non-Māori) referred to as "lunatics" (people who were drunks, socially deviant, disorderly, homeless, who threatened public safety, or could not look after or care for themselves) in jails and prisons, with custodial care provided by untrained non-clinical staff (Brunton 2011). In response to this early colonial experience of mental illness, the first asylums were built in 1844 and attached to Wellington and Auckland jails. These purpose-built asylum facilities were established on the outside of city borders and were based on the British model of institutional care (Cohen 2014). Due to demand and changes in service delivery, larger asylums evolved on rural farms, and by the late 19th century, asylums collectively housed both children and adults, and those rejected by society, such as confused elderly (Cohen 2014). The emphasis of care was on confinement and custody rather than treatment and care.

During the early period of colonisation, rates of Māori mental illness remained consistently low, with Māori mental disorders about one-third that of the non-Māori population. Major psychotic episodes for Māori were about half that for non-Māori (Kingi 2005). One factor that may have contributed to low reported rates of Māori mental illness was the Māori preference for care at home. Māori whānau who suffered with mental illness or trauma were "given special status" and were historically cared for by whānau members at home and in their communities, not in isolated rural hospitals removed from society. Non-Māori had little to no knowledge or understanding of Māori cultural norms, or the way seemingly bizarre behaviours were accepted and supported within Māori society.

The evolving processes of colonisation and non-Māori influences have led to Māori experiencing "cultural decay" arising from the demise and separation from their own identity as Māori. This process caused rates of Māori mental illness to increase and align "more and more to those of the Pākehā population" (Kingi 2005). Māori approaches to mental health were strikingly different to those of non-Māori. The Western mental health system was designed to purposefully remove and segregate those suffering with mental illness from their family and society, by placing them in hospitals located in remote isolated areas, thus drastically limiting access or support from family or other outsiders. It is no surprise that this form of treatment did not appeal to Māori (Kingi 2005).

Post Colonisation

There is little evidence precisely pinpointing why or when serious Māori mental health problems first emerged; however, there is sufficient evidence to identify a surge in Māori rates of mental illness over the latter part of the 20th century. During the 1950s Māori experienced 'urban drift' where Māori migrated from their familiar protective supports and norms of whanau, culture and land to the foreignness of big urban towns and cities in search of employment and the benefits of economic and social opportunities. Geographical separation and isolation made it increasingly difficult (if not impossible) for many Māori to maintain meaningful whānau or cultural connections. The rise in unemployment and financial stress from the 1970s' economic crisis further impacted on Māoris' "increased susceptibility to mental health problems" (Kingi 2005, p. 7).

The cultural, economic and social stresses of urbanisation added to the consumption of alcohol and other mind-altering (psychoactive) substances by Māori, which were traditionally and culturally unknown to Māori. Over the years, alcohol became an entrenched cultural norm for urban Māori, who (like non-Māori) adopted unhealthy consumption practices (e.g. binge drinking). This often occurred in conjunction with other substance abuse, such as drugs, and led to an increase in social problems and a rise in rates of Māori mental illness (Kingi 2005).

What is clear is that a combination of factors, including colonisation, cultural, environmental, socioeconomic and behavioural factors, resulted in urban Māori no longer being able to care of and support whānau with mental illness, as they were traditionally accustomed to. By the 1970s, many Māori felt they had little choice but to surrender their responsibility for whānau with mental illness to non-Māori psychiatric hospitals (institutionalisation), resulting in a considerable increase in Māori hospital admissions (Kingi 2005). By the mid-1980s, Māori mental health hospital rates of admissions began to outnumber those of non-Māori by two to three times.

From the 1960s onwards, there was an increase in public acceptance of people with mental illness as Aotearoa New Zealand health services followed a policy of deinstitutionalisation, the closure of psychiatric hospitals, in favour of community care. In 1963 planning for further psychiatric hospitals ceased, and by the 1970s the development of non-government organisations assisted in the transferring of mental health services from inpatient to community-based treatment services. This transition was messy and disorganised, and during the 1990s considerable attention was given to Māori mental health, as they were significantly overrepresented in mental health services. This led to the 1996 Mason Inquiry's investigation into mental health services (Committee of Inquiry into Mental Health Services 1996) and the subsequent formation of the Mental Health Commission as the government's watchdog over mental health services. The Mental Health Commission published two "blueprints" for improving services *How things need to be*, in 1998 and 2012, which also identified the specific needs of Māori.

Since the early 2000s, community-based mental health care has become the primary focus of mental health service treatment and delivery via government and non-government organisations. During the 2010s, mental health services evolved into more specific specialist areas to meet mental health needs and now include services directed towards crisis and emergency response, alcohol and other drugs, child and adolescent, adult, and forensic services, as well as the addition of Kaupapa Māori mental health services, which are explained later in this chapter (Ramalho et al 2022).

DEMOGRAPHICS

Māori in Aotearoa New Zealand continue to be subjected to the consequences of colonisation and the impact of urbanisation and this is seen in the high levels of socio-economic deprivation and poor health for Māori. This section discusses these statistics in terms of Māori mental health to highlight why nurses need to address the needs of Māori they care for in practice.

Between 1960 and 1990 there was a 200% increase in hospital admissions for Māori (Kingi 2017). From 1984 to 1994 Māori rates of hospital re-admissions were double the rate for non-Māori males, and three times higher than the rates for Pacific Islanders. Drug and alcohol use was prevalent (particularly among young Māori) and accounted for close to a third of first-time Māori hospital admissions. Māori had the highest suicide rates (1980–91), particularly Māori men, where numbers soared by 162% (Kingi 2017).

Māori mental health statistics have remained disproportionately high in recent years. In 2010–12 Māori suicide rates were almost twice as high as those of non-Māori, with Māori females more than twice as likely to commit suicide than non-Māori. Overall, Māori were more likely than non-Māori to be hospitalised for intentional self-harm, with Māori males being one-and-a-half times as likely as non-Māori males to be hospitalised for intentional self-harm (Ministry of Health 2015).

Seclusion is also disproportionately used with Māori tangata whāiora (service users). In 2015, Māori were almost five times more likely than other ethnic groups to be secluded in adult inpatient services, meaning out of all seclusions 44% of tangata whāiora secluded were Māori. In the same year, Māori were four times more likely to be subjected to community treatment orders compared to non-Māori (Ministry of Health 2016). Similar trends have been noted in the use of mental health services. Regarding hospital care, Māori have more acute admissions to mental health facilities than others and are re-admitted more often after discharge. Māori with psychotic illnesses are also disproportionately incarcerated in prison forensic units (Ministry of Health 2016).

These statistics show a disturbing picture of Māori mental health. Effective mental health care requires nurses to understand the experience of Māori people, and Māori practices, and to take a holistic and culturally safe approach to care.

In the following sections, we discuss the ways in which nurses can respond to the needs of Māori to address these statistics.

Te Tiriti o Waitangi

Te Tiriti o Waitangi[2] is the founding document of Aotearoa which underpins the relationship between Māori and the British Crown. Te Tiriti o Waitangi consists of four articles which outline obligations, and which are also expressed through principles. The principles have evolved over time, with the most recent addition arising from the Waitangi Tribunal Claim – Wai 2575: the Health Services and Outcomes Inquiry (Waitangi Tribunal 2023), in which the three historic principles of partnership, participation and protection were expanded to five principles to provide deeper clarity and guidance around nursing and health care. The five principles are listed alongside Te Tiriti o Waitangi articles described in Table 7.1, with examples of their application to mental health care.

Article One of Te Tiriti o Waitangi requires the Crown to consult and collaborate with iwi (tribes) and hapū (subtribes) in regards to functions and operations of kawanatanga ("good governance"). This includes functions and operations of health services. This article is the basis of the principles of **partnership** (working together) and **tino rangatiratanga**, or **self-determination**, in the design, delivery of the care and treatments we provide.

Article Two guarantees Māori tino rangatiratanga "self-determination, autonomy and ownership" of land possession and taonga (treasures) such as Te Reo and health. This article underpins the principles of **active protection** through culturally safe practice and **equity** through achieving equitable health outcomes.

Article Three guarantees Māori the same rights and privileges as the British subjects, which includes the right to good mental health and wellbeing and equal access to mental health support services. This article describes the principle of **participation** and **kōwhiringa**, or **options**, to ensure that all health services are provided in a culturally

---

[2]Te Tiriti o Waitangi/The Treaty of Waitangi has two texts: one in Te Reo Māori and one in English. They are not exact translations of each other. Most māori chiefs signed the Te Reo version which differs from the English version around the understanding of sovereignty. The Waitangi Tribunal has exclusive authority to determine the meaning of Te Tiriti as embodied in the English and Māori texts.

TABLE 7.1   Principles of Te Tiriti o Waitangi

Principle	Meaning	Example
Partnership	Māori and non-Māori working together to develop mental health services	More Māori in leadership and decision-making roles alongside non-Māori in the development of new mental health initiatives and in the delivery of mental health services.
Active protection	Māori health and culture are protected, to achieve equitable health outcomes for Māori	Māori have adequate mental health services or resources, and cultural safety is applied in treatment to address health disparities.
Equity	Recognises that Māori and non-Māori have different mental health needs, so is about allocating mental health resources and services differently to reach an equal outcome	Māori to have access to kaupapa Māori mental health services or treatments, including rongoā Māori (traditional medicine), which are also afforded equitable funding to prevent discrimination.
Tino Rangatiratanga	A Te Ao Māori term referring to self-determination, sovereignty, independence, autonomy and ownership	Māori to make their own decisions and choices around the type of care that they wish to have, such as inclusion of tikanga Māori in mainstream mental health services.
Kōwhiringa (options)	Māori to have options to choose their social and culturally safe treatment path	Māori can choose a kaupapa or mainstream mental health service provider to seek treatment from or to have the inclusion of Te Ao Māori practices/Māori models and/or Māori staff providing treatment.

appropriate way that recognises and supports the expression of Te Ao Māori models of care and nursing.

Article Four is a verbal addition to Te Tiriti and guarantees **religious freedom**.

In 1985, the Department of Health recommended that Te Tiriti o Waitangi be integrated into health services due to breaches of Te Tiriti and the growing discontent coming from Māori leaders of its failure to meet Treaty obligations in terms of Māori health (NiaNia et al 2017). Today, Te Tiriti o Waitangi has been incorporated into health governance frameworks and Māori models of health, including Te Whare Tapa Whā, the Meihana model and Te Wheke. These models are well utilised today and reinforce that Māori concepts and epistemologies of healthcare matter and have a place in today's health system.

For mental health, the articles and principles of Te Tiriti highlight the need to work with Māori to improve health outcomes, recognise that health is a taonga and worthy of protection and to facilitate equal access to health and health care through mātauranga Māori, whereby they feel empowered to use traditional knowledge within to heal themselves, their whānau, hapū and iwi.

❓ CRITICAL THINKING EXERCISE 7.1

Thinking about the five principles listed above, identify how you would apply the principles of Te Tiriti o Waitangi to your nursing practice. Identify the barriers to applying these principles in nursing practice and in the health services you have practised in.

Waitangi Tribunal – Wai 2757

The Waitangi Tribunal was established in 1975 to research, investigate, hear and settle alleged breaches of Te Tiriti o Waitangi. These include breaches of Article Three, "guarantee all the Rights and Privileges of British Subjects", which is inclusive of health. The Tribunal's 2019 Health Services and Outcomes report, known as WAI 2757 (Waitangi Tribunal 2023), identified Treaty breaches within the health sector around health equity, healthcare, disability and substance use and the government, undermining Māori efforts to exercise tino rangatiratanga (self-determination and autonomy) over their own health. This undermining by the government of health has been longstanding, beginning with colonisation and using legislation to undermine Māori health. For example, the *Tohunga Suppression Act*, passed in 1907, criminalised Indigenous health practices, including the use of tohunga. This Act forced Māori to use western medicine or face imprisonment. The consequences of this were detrimental to mātauranga Māori (Māori knowledge) through loss of intergenerational knowledge and it was detrimental to the sustainability and future of rongoā Māori (Ahuriri-Driscoll et al 2008).

WAI 2757 is primarily focused on Māori having (on average) the poorest health status of any ethnic group in Aotearoa New Zealand. The Tribunal received statistical evidence demonstrating that Māori health inequities have persisted despite reform of the health sector over the last 20 or 30 years. The government and all parties involved in the WAI 2757 claim acknowledge that the poor state of Māori health (including Māori mental health) outcomes is unacceptable. As nurses, it is important that we acknowledge our responsibilities and obligations under Te Tiriti o Waitangi in our nursing practice.

Cultural safety has been developed as one means of honouring Te Tiriti and is discussed in the following section.

Cultural Safety/Kawa Whakaruruhau

Over 30 years ago, Dr Irihapeti Ramsden, along with others, pioneered and championed "kawa whakaruruhau", or cultural safety, as a revolutionary Indigenous response to longstanding inequitable health outcomes for Māori (Papps & Ramsden 1996; Ramsden 2002).

Kawa whakaruruhau initially related to the "protection" of Māori nurses, midwives, students and whānau interacting within an "unsafe" healthcare system in Aotearoa. Kawa whakaruruhau sought to integrate the principles of Te Tiriti o Waitangi into nursing education, and promoted recruitment and retention of Māori nurses (Ramsden 2002).

In 1992, nursing's governing body the Nursing Council of New Zealand (NCNZ) formally adopted the concept of Kawa Whakaruruhau and guidelines for cultural safety into the education of nurses (Papps & Ramsden 1996). This was met with resistance from nurses, the media and public alike, as it was perceived by some as "separatism". The ensuing public debate resulted in an external parliamentary review in 1995. Findings from the review led to the Nursing Council developing guidelines for cultural safety in nursing education.

To placate the critics of Kawa Whakaruruhau, or cultural safety, the concept would be retained in nursing education, albeit in a revised, more acceptable definition. "Cultural safety" would now include *all* people encountered by the nurse who differed in any way from the nurse's own culture or ethnicity, as opposed to just the relationship between "the nurse and Māori, as originally championed, thereby improving health outcomes for *all* people in Aotearoa" (Ramsden 2002). The new definition of culture, as defined by NCNZ states,

The effective nursing practice of a person or family from another culture and is determined by that person or family. It includes but is not restricted to, age or generation; gender; sexual orientation; occupation and socioeconomic status; ethnic origin or migrant experience; religious or spiritual belief; and disability.

(Nursing Council of New Zealand 2011)

Despite cultural safety now having a broader definition, the concept remains pivotal in the nursing care of Māori. The NCNZ (2020) makes it clear that *all* nurses need to be "culturally safe; that is, to understand the Te Ao Māori worldview, work biculturally and practise in ways that are responsive to Te Tiriti o Waitangi and that promote equity of health outcomes. It is also important here to realise that when working with Māori some western concepts that form the basis of therapies in Aotearoa New Zealand can conflict with Māori worldviews. Therefore, it is important that, as nurses, you first examine your own personal assumptions and recognise that your own culture can impact on that of the tangata whāiora. Additionally, it is important to recognise that Māori are not a homogenous group, and individual values, beliefs and ways of seeing the world will differ among Māori.

Culturally safe mental health care for Māori is based on the Māori principle of whakawhānaungatanga, which reflects a recovery-oriented model of care where the needs of tangata whāiora are the focus. The person and their culture, rather than the clinical diagnosis, are crucial to providing effective care to Māori. Whakawhānaungatanga (Māori worldview, tikanga Māori, whakarongo, understanding the whānau context, clear boundaries and communication) needs to be central to all aspects of mental health care. Whakawhānaungatanga should include the whole care team and the whānau of the tangata whāiora. Whakawhānaungatanga usually begins with a karakia to bless the space and the people involved before a pepeha (introductions and connections) are made. It is a caring, nurturing process which demonstrates the willingness of the health professional to work in culturally safe ways. Therefore, Kawa Whakaruruhau provides for a holistic model of Māori health care that moves beyond an individual's treatment and acknowledges the interaction between physical, mental, spiritual and whānau wellbeing. See Cultural considerations: Nurse's story 7.1: Ola, which discusses cultural safety.

CULTURAL CONSIDERATIONS 7.1: OLA'S STORY
The Importance of Cultural Safety as a Nurse

My journey into the area of mental health began when I decided to train as mental health nurse, and later went on to train as a psychotherapist. Over the years, I have been privileged to experience two different countries outside where I was raised and have learnt to appreciate the significance of culture in the field of mental health, having worked with people from various backgrounds across forensic and adult mental health inpatient and community settings.

Almost 14 years ago, I decided to settle in Aotearoa New Zealand. I remember being struck by how the concept of culture and identity was valued and appreciated among the people. Suffice to say, I felt safe. As a professional, when I think of cultural safety, and what might be integral to practising in a culturally safe way, what first arises for me are the meanings I and others give to the concept of culture. In essence, what does culture mean? How do we understand the concept of culture? I think of culture not as a static concept, but one that evolves over time, is dynamic, individual, but also collective, and to some degree complex; a complexity which, in my view, is revealed in several aspects of our humanity both at a conscious level and at an unconscious level.

The second thought that arises for me is considering whether we seek to understand a tāngata whaiora's culture. Do we have a desire to *really* know the tāngata whaiora's culture and way of life, and not presume we know it based on their name, or where they are from, or what ethnicity they belong to, or what the colour of their skin is and so on?

Thirdly, I think of the importance of continually reflecting on one's own culture and background. My culture includes everything I am, my ethnicity, my race, my gender, where I grew up, my professions, my spirituality, my religion, the influences in my life journey, and so on. All of which evoke values, ideas, attitudes, expectations, identities and traditions, some of which I agree with and some which I do not agree with but am able to accept.

So, what does it mean to me to be a culturally safe mental health nurse? It means to be open, to be curious, to be empathic, to be thoughtful, to seek knowledge and understanding, to share, to have flexibility of thought, to be respectful, to be accepting, to be tolerant, to be observant, to minimise presumptions, to be open to being challenged, and, importantly, to know that you will get it wrong sometimes and be humble enough to acknowledge and apologise when you get it wrong.

To work in a culturally safe way is to work in a therapeutic way, where a tāngata whāiora feels comfortable, are seen, heard, understood, and validated and have their needs met whoever they are. In my practice over the years, I have worked with several tāngata whāiora of mixed heritage, born to Māori and Pākehā parents. A number of these tāngata whāiora struggled with their identity and belonging. Some expressed how they felt they were not accepted by the Pākehā side of their family because the colour of their skin was not white enough, and not accepted by their Māori side of their family because the colour of their skin was not dark enough.

In a few cases, the tāngata whāiora were raised by their Pākehā side, and felt more aligned with their Pākehā identity as they did not grow up learning Māori history, tikanga and values. In one case, the tāngata whāiora felt disempowered and disrespected by the pressure he felt from staff to claim his Māori identity. This man was hoping to gradually grow into his Māori identity, but had felt pressure by requests and expectations placed on him, and consequently began to feel culturally unsafe.

Working therapeutically creates a milieu and an experience of cultural safety where a tāngata whāiora can feel safe in who they are and, in their identity, feel respected and not have to feel ashamed. This is possible when mental health nurses practise in a way that is open-minded and reflective, and where implicit biases can be identified and examined thoroughly. Lastly, in our bicultural Aotearoa New Zealand, where Māori are tangata whenua, it is also important that we continually seek cultural support and guidance towards fostering care that is culturally safe.

CRITICAL THINKING EXERCISE 7.2

Explore your own cultural identity and list any values and beliefs or practices that you consider important for inclusion within your practice to create a culturally safe nursing environment. Explore your own biases, whether conscious or unconscious, and how you will address these to ensure you are providing culturally safe care.

MĀORI MENTAL HEALTH NURSES

One of the ways of addressing the mental health needs of Māori and to improve outcomes for Māori is to expand the Māori mental health nursing workforce capacity and capability, as the New Zealand Government has tried to do over the last four decades. Today Māori registered nurses tend to choose mental health nursing over other specialty areas of practice (NCNZ 2019). However, Māori nurses only comprise

7.5% of the practising registered nursing workforce (NCNZ 2019), and that proportion has remained static over the decades (Wilson et al 2022), despite Māori making up 15% of the Aotearoa New Zealand population. Racism and racist rhetoric in healthcare have been described as factors for Māori nursing numbers remaining static (Wilson et al 2022). Additionally, expectations on Māori mental health nurses to meet the cultural needs of their non-Māori colleagues' tangata whāiora require the Māori nurse to have dual competencies in both Māori culture and nursing (Wilson & Barker 2012). This expectation can result in stress, especially if the Māori nurse has lost cultural connections and therefore cultural knowledge due to colonisation and/or upbringing. In addition, most Māori nurses complete their nursing training in mainstream programs using western models rather than Māori models, creating further difficulties in achieving this expectation. Furthermore, Māori nurses are often burdened with unrecognised workloads (i.e. educating their non-Māori colleagues, undertaking powhiri, karakia, waiata and other cultural requirements, and acting as unofficial spokespersons for Māori tangata whāiora and whānau) (Komene et al 2023). Finally, Māori tangata whāiora and whānau have much higher expectations of Māori health professionals to get it right. All these extra expectations and demands, including identifying and responding to racism, eventually lead to loss of job dissatisfaction while increasing the desire to leave the profession.

Te Ao Māramatanga, the New Zealand College of Mental Health Nurses, is the professional body for practising mental health nurses in Aotearoa New Zealand. Te Ao Māramatanga supports a bicultural governance and operational model and includes a kaiwhakahaere (director/manager) who, supported by a Māori Caucus, provides professional support and guidance to Māori mental health nurses via projects that aim to enhance Māori mental health nursing practice. This organisation is a way for Māori nurses to gain support through supervision or mentors, as well as providing opportunities to continuously develop their practice both culturally and professionally.

One of the ways in which Māori nurses can have this extra work recognised and be supported is though the Huarahi Whakatū Professional Development and Recognition Programme (PDRP). Huarahi Whakatū is a PDRP program delivered by Te Rau Ora (formally Te Rau Matatini) and Te Ao Māramatanga, which promotes the philosophy of dual competency; that is, clinical and cultural competencies. Clinical competencies are drawn from the Nursing Council of New Zealand, whereas cultural competencies are informed by Te Ao Māori. The program has been running since 2009, and in 2019 was reaccredited by the NZNC for a further five years (Te Rau Ora 2023).

To truly address the health needs of Māori and to improve their health outcomes, nurses need to recognise this reality of being a Māori nurse and extend culturally safe practice to their Māori colleagues, as well as to tangata whāiora. A way of demonstrating this is by non-Māori nurses learning Māori customs and practices, so as not to burden their Māori colleagues. For example, Te Rau Ora have two education programs: He Puna Whakaata and Kaitiaki Ahurea (Te Rau Ora 2023). These education programs are focused on educating nurses about Māori culture, Māori concepts and a Māori worldview, unconscious bias and how these impact on the design or delivery of health and social services, as well as how to use elements of mātauranga Māori in a therapeutic context.

Furthermore, Māori mental health nurses need to embody self-care and become role models for tangata whāiora to prevent burnout and to continue doing a job which they choose over other specialty areas. Self-care includes protected personal time, peer support at times of difficulty, debriefing with a trusted colleague, and clinical and cultural supervision. It also includes eating well, sleeping well and getting adequate exercise, as well as taking regular leave. See Perspectives in practice: Nurse's story 7.1: Carlee.

PERSPECTIVES IN PRACTICE

Nurse's story 7.1: Carlee

Being A Māori Mental Health Nurse

I fell into nursing, you could say, by default. My intent was to become New Zealand's first female prime minister. To do this I was going to become a lawyer, but I'm not sure exactly what direction of law was going to lead to this. However, I ended up doing my nursing training and becoming a mental health nurse. Who would have thought that a career in nursing could open so many doors and provide so many opportunities?

I applied to complete my nursing with a friend. I was accepted and I think she went into law. At any rate she now manages restaurants and I'm a Principal Clinical Advisor within Te Aka Whai Ora, the Māori Health Authority. I guess it helps that I was fortunate to grow up with a whānau who worked in acute mental health services, before successfully running a mental health NGO service for 34 years. The sadness when my safe space closed and residents were moved to a new whare was huge. Most of the residents have not had positive outcomes and this I can understand. When residents call your father Dad, and long-standing staff Mum or Aunty, you see that these residents were whānau. We were lucky we had an amazing group of staff; the GP and his practice were phenomenal, and the community support was incredible. I guess we were one of the largest employers, and our staff, some on a recovery journey, and some who had not previously been employable, found an accepting environment where they were able to be their authentic selves. To be fair, we had a low re-admission rate, easy when you know each individual and how they think and communicate when they are in distress or faced with uncertainty. There are so many examples of what I now know is excellent interpersonal therapeutic relationships, not just the authenticity of the staff. I think Māori nurses have a lot of interpersonal therapeutic relationship skills since oral communication and whakawhānaungatanga is so easy and normal for us.

The year I qualified as a nurse, placement within hospitals was scarce and most of my roopu ventured overseas or into NGO services. The local District Health Board offered six spaces for new graduates. Now they need every new graduate nurse they can get. How times change. A two-year OE and three years in various acute medical spaces, where – wait for it – I was allocated the mental health whāiora, which saw me move to the "dark side" on a six-month secondment in community mental health and a post graduate qualification. Who knew I would spend the next 15 years in this space and eventually specialise in child and adolescent mental health? Each encounter with these tamariki and rangatahi has shown me how resilient and resourceful our young can be and how detached as adults we can be. So often we are consumed by our own emotions without realising the impact this is having on our children. This almost put me off having children. Post childbirth you realise that at times your own mental wellbeing impacts parenting and decision-making. It also softens you and makes you aware that what was a harmless idea or plan can have disastrous consequences. We are only human and to err is to learn.

As a Māori nurse in a rural environment, you become the jack of all trades and the master of none, taking in by default the whānau no one wants to deal with. Or that could be my non-PC manner or the fact that I get it with a look, or an eyebrow raise, a kai. I have learnt that at times, the non-verbal responses speak volumes. So does listening, not talking, just listening. It's no wonder that at the end of the week you want to go home and hide away. Lucky that you have colleagues who become mentors, whānau and a safe space to just be. Clinical supervision and looking after yourself as a Māori mental health nurse is important to ensure that you are well and can continue to support whānau and your colleagues.

MENTAL HEALTH CARE IN AOTEAROA NEW ZEALAND

There is no single and distinct Aotearoa New Zealand mental health system. Rather, mental health services are delivered in a variety of ways throughout the broader health system, as well as in a range of specialist mental health services. Services are designed to cater to the needs of those with mental health problems of varying degrees of severity and include everything from primary treatment by a general practitioner (GP) through online self-help services and inpatient specialist mental health services. This range of services is designed to form part of a stepped-care approach, covering self-help, primary and specialist services that are appropriate, timely and involve intervening in the least intrusive way to provide a seamless, integrated response. However, this model of healthcare responds to people as individuals in isolation from their families, communities and social contexts, with an emphasis on the assessment of individual pathology and deficits. This mainstream framework does not work for Māori and is responsible for maintaining Māori–non-Māori disparities rather than working actively to address them.

Some individuals can be compelled to undergo compulsory mental health care and treatment. The *Mental Health (Compulsory Assessment and Treatment) Act 1992* sets out the circumstances in which individuals may be ordered to undergo assessment and treatment for a mental disorder, where they pose a serious danger to the health and safety of themselves or others, or have a diminished capacity to take care of themselves (see also Chapter 10). While Māori have higher recorded rates of mental illness and use of mental health services than the general population, the rates of compulsory treatment for Māori compared to non-Māori are even more disproportionate. In 2016, Māori were 3.6 times more likely to be under a community treatment order than non-Māori and 3.4 times more likely to be under an inpatient treatment order (Ministry of Health 2017a). These health disparities are the reason the government has decided to repeal and replace the *Mental Health (Compulsory Assessment and Treatment) Act 1992* legislation.

Elevated rates of Māori accessing services for mental health issues do not, however, necessarily indicate that Māori needs for appropriate services are being met, or even that they are being met to the same extent as non-Māori, as discussed in the section above on WAI 2757. The ways in which these disparities are being addressed is discussed below.

Te Aka Whai Ora and Te Whatu Ora

To be able to meet the Treaty obligations and reduce health disparities including in mental health, a significant cultural shift in the health system is required. This significant cultural shift came about in 2022 with the development of a new national health system to replace the 20 District Health Boards (DHBs). Te Whatu Ora (Health New Zealand) and Te Aka Whai Ora (Māori Health Authority) were established to address inequities in healthcare and to support the development of health services to Māori. In addition, the *Pae Ora (Healthy Futures) Act (2022)* is designed to embed Te Tiriti principles and equity for all in the health sector by focusing on what people need rather than on where they live or who they are, as occurred under the old District Health Board system (Te Whatu Ora 2022). This will mean that more choice is offered in terms of culturally appropriate health services. One approach to providing culturally appropriate services to Māori is the development of Kaupapa Māori services, described in the following section.

Kaupapa Māori Mental Health Services

Kaupapa Māori mental health services are delivered both directly by Te Whatu Ora providers, which operate them in addition to their mainstream services, and by a multitude of Māori-led non-government organisations (NGOs) located around the country. Kaupapa Māori mental health and addiction services are an indigenous response to effectively meeting the mental health and/or addiction needs of tangata whāiora (people who use mental health services). They are Māori mental health services run by Māori, for Māori, which provide assessment and treatment grounded in mātauranga Māori (Māori knowledge) using holistic Māori models of health and wellbeing inclusive of whānau, hapū and iwi. Kaupapa Māori services receive funding from both Te Aka Whaiora and Te Whatu Ora.

Mātauranga Māori is about a Māori way of being and engaging in the world. Simply, it uses kawa (cultural practices) and tikanga (cultural principles) to critique, examine, analyse and understand the world. It is based on the spiritual realm of Te Ao Mārama (the cosmic natural world of life and light) and is constantly evolving as Māori find their place within it.

Kaupapa Māori units and services were first developed in the mid 1980s and early 1990s as a response to addressing Māori mental health needs (Durie 1998). Today, there is a range of different Kaupapa Māori mental health services, from crisis intervention services to hospital inpatient wards through to community-based counselling, respite beds, drug and alcohol rehab and the provision and expansion of rongoā Māori (traditional Māori medicine) services. See Cultural consideration: Bryce's story 7.2 and Personal perspectives 7.1: Consumer's story: Arana.

⊕ CULTURAL CONSIDERATIONS 7.2: BRYCE'S STORY

Working in a Kaupapa Māori Service

For the last five years I have been nursing at a Kaupapa Māori forensic psychiatric community mental health hospital. The 23-bed facility was founded over 20 years ago (as a result of the governmental move from institutional to community care); it is well resourced, and is a mere 15-minute commute from the main city. The low security inpatient service is situated on 10 acres of rural land with well-established manicured grounds and modern high-end, meticulously maintained, marae-style accommodation, which has often been described by whānau and visitors as "five-star".

The hospital is a mid-transition point from acute and semi-acute inpatient services to community. The whānau are all male, predominantly Māori, and are all under some form of inpatient treatment order, with a significant number of whānau being treated under ministerial "special patient" orders, due to being assessed as clinically insane at the time of their index offence, or unfit to stand trial.

The hospital staff vary in ethnicities (English, Australian, African, South African, Indian, Pakistani, Arab, Pacific Islander, New Zealanders and Māori). This diversity in ethnicity brings a wealth of knowledge, experience and sentiments regarding cultural practice. However, the cultural philosophy of whānau (family), ensures continuity of care is followed and fundamentally adhered to from a Te Ao Māori worldview.

The Māori concept of whānau extends well beyond the academic definition of a nuclear family. We refer to the tangata whāiora or service user as whānau — our whānau — and we deliver our nursing care with the same consideration and respect we would to our own personal family members. The kaupapa concept of whānau extends to include my colleagues (both Māori and non-Māori), manuhiri (visitors), or essentially anyone I encounter, and I am obligated to demonstrate the same respect as I would give my own whānau. Regardless of the position held within the organisation, cleaners, grounds people, psychologists, psychiatrists

CULTURAL CONSIDERATIONS 7.2: BRYCE'S STORY—cont'd
Working in a Kaupapa Māori Service

and management all endeavour to give and receive the same level of courtesy and respect. This reciprocating kaupapa value is essential in the establishment and preservation of a harmonious therapeutic environment conducive of cultural healing and wellness.

A large proportion of the whānau we nurse are victims of historical trauma, violence and abuse, and have come from dysfunctional families or social welfare care. Consequently, they have been estranged from any healthy form of Māoritanga (Māori way of life). For many, this is the first time they have experienced Māori kaupapa processes or had the support and positive influence of social and culturally sensitive role models. During the initial hospital admission, whānau are generally guarded and suspicious; however, over time (in some cases, years), whānau eventually come to the realisation they are residing in a protective and unconditionally loving environment. This setting allows whānau to develop trust, feel holistically safe and subsequently expose their sense of vulnerability to others. It is during this time of their journey that I have frequently witnessed a genuine sense of healing and recovery occurring.

Māori-focused educational programs take place daily and are considered to be a valuable indispensable taonga (cultural treasure) in the whānau's recovery. Every effort is made to ensure all other therapeutic interventions do not dilute or interfere with the integrity and daily procession and delivery of the kaupapa Māori programs and this is stringently enforced by the kaumātua. Consequently, all psychiatrist appointments, allied health or legal appointments, community and home leaves and formal or informal functions are strictly organised outside the daily program hours of 8.30 am – 2.30 pm.

Every day starts and ends with whakamoemiti, which is a dedicated time for all to gather and give thanks and appreciation to Atua (the gods) for the new day. This daily custom unifies whānau, clinicians and health workers as one people. Karakia (prayer) and waiata (singing) enhance the ability for all to collectively centre themselves mentally and spiritually for the day. In the evening, the process of whakamoemiti is a means of ending the day together and grounding oneself mentally and spiritually in preparation for rest and sleep.

Daily structured group and individualised habilitation and rehabilitation programs are based on kaupapa Māori values and practices, and delivered in accordance with Māori models of service delivery; for example, Te Whare Tapa Wha. Whānau actively participate in learning te reo Māori (language), whakapapa (genealogy), Mātauranga Māori (traditional knowledge and teachings), waiata, karakia, tikanga, traditional cooking (hangi), and Māori arts and crafts, to name a few. These cultural experiences contribute significantly to a whānau's mental and spiritual wellness and overall recovery, as they gradually develop their own sense of belonging and cultural identity, which gives homage to their tupuna (ancestors) and whenua (ancestral land). Whānau often experience a sense of revelation, particularly towards the later stages of their recovery when they are supported and accompanied back to reconnect with their whānau, whenua, maunga (ancestral mountain) and awa (ancestral waters).

Although kaupapa Māori cultural processes are directed at whānau, they are positively imparted to anyone who is privileged to be part of this cultural environment. I am a Māori male registered nurse raised in a non-Māori (European) family and am nearing 60 years of age. I have only recently started to venture through my own journey of cultural identity since I started working at the hospital. Consequently, I am limited in cultural knowledge and experience and have naively made many mistakes through the process of learning. However, I have done so with the ongoing encouragement and guidance of my colleagues.

There are many individuals at the hospital who are culturally positioned similarly to me. To mitigate the risk of cultural malpractice, kaumātua (elders) simplified the kaupapa into three trains of thought: respect for self, respect for others and respect for the environment and everything within it. These three principles are embedded within the cultural aspects of Maoridom, and accordingly are religiously adhered to by all whanau and staff at the hospital. As we all aspire to live and move within these principles, it guarantees both cultural and social law and order are achieved in various degrees and are pivotal in guiding kawa-whakaruruhau (cultural safety) in my nursing practice. My nursing practice and cultural interventions are embedded with various tikanga and kawa, which are too numerous to mention in this article. However basic tikanga and kawa are included throughout Aotearoa New Zealand hospital's guidelines, *The Tikanga Māori Best Practice*, and are a reliable resource for mental health nurses working in partnership with Māori to reference.

I recall as a nursing student the lecturers and literature denoting whānau as the priority and centre of their own recovery ("bottom-up" approach to service delivery). After many years of working in community and public health settings, it became apparent that many organisations implement a "top-down" approach to service delivery; that is, where management agendas heavily influence the distribution of health resources and, ultimately, the direction and quality of whānau recovery.

My involvement with the Māori kaupapa service has provided me with the opportunity to experience (for the first time as a registered nurse) a truly devoted and committed implementation of a "bottom-up" approach to service delivery; that is, where decisions and distribution of health resources are allocated in accordance with individualised whānau-centred recovery goals and needs, which have been collaboratively determined by the whānau and their clinical team. This ideology in service delivery is vital to me as a mental health nurse, as I genuinely feel I have a voice, can advocate on behalf of whānau and access various resources in a timely manner, with minimal political or bureaucratic barriers, in the best interests of whānau recovery and rehabilitation.

The aroha (love) and manākitanga (the process of giving respect, generosity and caring for people) I witnessed being implemented by the Māori mental health service resonates in the following infamous Māori whakatauki (proverb).

He aha te mea nui? Māku e kii atu, he tāngata, he tāngata, he tāngata.

What is the most important thing in the world? Well, let me tell you, it is people, it is people, it is people.

PERSONAL PERSPECTIVES
Consumer's Story 7.1: Arana

My Journey as a Tangata Whāiora
I spent over a year in institutional mental health care in the 1980s. I lost my job through living in the hospital and not being able to turn up. My strained relationship then became estranged through the long absence. We trialled a time of me living back at home. I appeared to decompensate further. My wife subsequently dropped me off at a mental health clinic and announced our marriage was over. I was driven back to the institution in the country with no clear pathway out of

that service at the time. I knew what the back wards were about, and I was frightened. I had become "a mental patient". "Mental patient" was my whole identity now. I made an escape. That escape was my first positive choice to act for myself in a long time. And because of my choice to escape, the outcome was that I never went back to institutional care again.

Three years later I chose to attend residential rehab. There was a kaupapa space there. I attended that kaupapa service. I lay on the floor and cried much

Continued

Consumer's Story 7.1: Arana

of the time. My tears were not pathologised. The group, the karakia, the waiata, and being present to other healing narratives were restorative for me. Even though I am non-Māori, they suggested my name might be Arana. I adopted that new name and made a firm commitment to my recovery. This was the second major event in my "career" as a mental patient. Later, I chose to work in mental health services. That was over 30 years ago.

Over the past eight years I have worked as a peer support within an iwi-based mental health service. I started a peer support group. Our peer group always opened each session with karakia, waiata and mihi. We all learnt together about our pepeha and how to mihi. This process was itself connecting, and connection is healing. People who were hard to connect with heard about the group from other clients, and they were attracted to attend. They would just turn up on the day of the group. There have been positive outcomes.

Some from our peer group went from homelessness with recurring admissions to working full-time and living in a house. I have been particularly touched by the story of a young woman in her 20s. She had been in a pattern of multiple abusive relationships after her children were taken out of her care. She chose to make changes. She placed her children into the care of their fathers. She then agreed to live in a supported accommodation service. She is now working part-time, while maintaining her antipsychotic medication and mental health appointments. Her children visit her regularly.

I have played a small part in the national quality process to end seclusion in mental health services. One thing we have learnt about zero seclusion quality projects in New Zealand is that when cultural participation welcomes people into the ward, then most often, people settle into the ward with a positive therapeutic outcome.

Māori Models of Health and Nursing

Low engagement of mental health and addiction services with Māori in mainstream services is associated with barriers that are directly related to Māori beliefs, perceptions and understandings of health and mental health, coupled with lack of shared decision-making and experiences of institutional racism and neglect, which have led to distrust of the system (Durie 1998). Research has shown that for Māori, successful models of engagement and intervention are based in Māori cultural world views and processes (Bennett 2009; Durie 1998). Māori health is often described as holistic due to the integration of mind, body and spirit within a context of social and cultural collectiveness (Durie 1998). Western medical models have historically separated these areas. For mental health nurses, it means incorporating holistic

Māori models and perspectives into practice, and using interventions that optimise physical, social, cultural, spiritual and mental aspects of health to help address the Māori mental health disparities.

Sir Mason Durie, a psychiatrist and academic who was instrumental in promoting understanding of Māori health and higher academic learning, not only led the transition of the current health reforms, such as the Māori Health Authority (Te Aka Whai Ora) and Te Whatu Ora, but also developed the Māori health model, Te Whare Tapa Whā, represented in Fig. 7.1 (Durie 1998). This model consists of four components (wairua (spirituality), whānau (family and relational values), tinana (physical wellbeing), hinengaro (emotional and mental wellbeing)), each of which is essential to the wellbeing of the whole person, underlined by values such as manākitanga (taking care

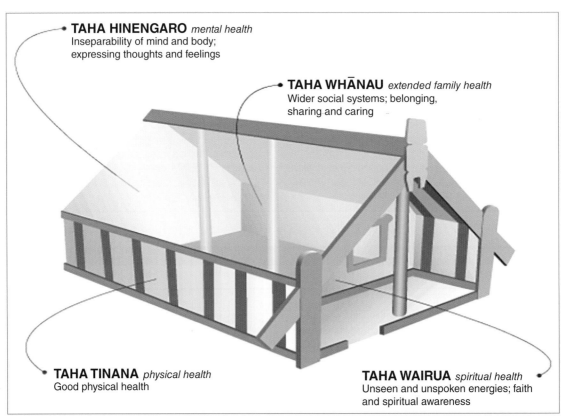

TAHA HINENGARO *mental health*
Inseparability of mind and body;
expressing thoughts and feelings

TAHA WHĀNAU *extended family health*
Wider social systems; belonging,
sharing and caring

TAHA TINANA *physical health*
Good physical health

TAHA WAIRUA *spiritual health*
Unseen and unspoken energies; faith
and spiritual awareness

FIG. 7.1 Te Whare Tapa Wha.

TABLE 7.2 Te Wheke (the Octopus)	
Tentacles	**Represent**
Hinengaro (emotional and mental wellbeing)	Whānau (family/relationships/ connections)
Tinana (physical wellbeing)	Wairua (spirituality)
Mana ake (uniqueness of individual and family)	Mauri (life force)
Hā a koro mā a kui mā (the "breath of life" that comes from ancestors)	Whatumanawa (open and healthy expressions of emotions, deep-seated emotions)

TABLE 7.3 Components of the Te Kapunga Putohe Model	
Left Hand	**Right Hand**
Tikanga (cultural principles/rules)	Whānaungatanga (relationships/ connections)
Pono (true and genuine)	Wairua (spirituality)
Aroha (compassion and love)	Oranga (wellbeing)
Manaakitanga (respect and kindness)	Mana Tangata (personal authority, power)
Tiakitanga (to watch for)	Tikanga Māori (Māori customs and practices)

of family) or whakawhānaungatanga (relationships). The essential point of this model is that all dimensions are considered necessary, are balanced and are strengthened to achieve wellbeing. This model has been incorporated into government frameworks and health service delivery.

Another holistic Māori model, Te Wheke (the octopus) has been articulated by Rosemary Pere, and is used to define family health. The head of the octopus represents te whānau, the eyes of the octopus represent waiora (total wellbeing for the individual and family), and each of the eight tentacles represents a specific dimension of health, as described in Table 7.2. The model proposes that sustenance is required for each tentacle/dimension if the organism is to attain waiora or total wellbeing (Ministry of Health 2017b). This model is also widely endorsed by Māori.

Suzanne Pitama's Meihana model, represented in Fig. 7.2, encompasses Durie's Te Whare Tapa Wha, but inserts two additional elements – taiao (physical environment) and iwi katoa (societal context). The Meihana practice model (alongside Māori beliefs, values and experiences) is used to guide clinical assessment and intervention with Māori clients and whānau accessing mental health services

(Pitama et al 2014). The Meihana model is also discussed in Chapter 9, Mental Health Assessment.

Pipi Barton and Denise Wilson's Te Kapunga Putohe (the restless hands) model is designed to guide Māori-centred nursing practice within a Māori cultural context. It is designed to aid nurses by being guided by Māori values, beliefs and practices, promoting positive relationships between nurses and Māori clients and whānau (Barton & Wilson 2008). It consists of 10 components of wellbeing, which are listed in Table 7.3.

There are many more Māori models of health, each with a core philosophy of creating an environment for increased engagement and duration of care for Māori whanau while in health services, particularly mental health and addictions.

❓ CRITICAL THINKING EXERCISE 7.3

From the different Māori models listed above, choose one model that you would use in your practice and describe how you would use this model with both Māori and Non-Māori, and whether this model would be applicable to other non-Indigenous cultures.

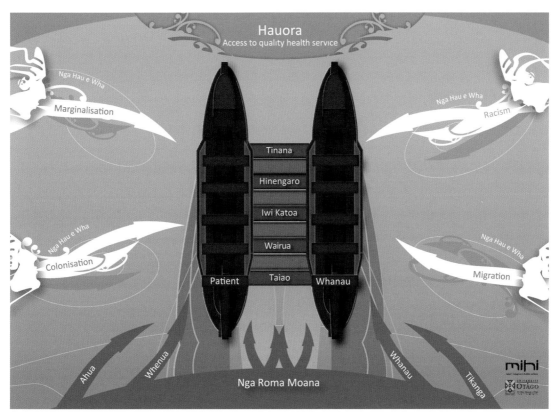

FIG. 7.2 The Meihana Model.

MĀORI MENTAL HEALTH INTERVENTIONS

In 2017, a wānanga called Tūmata kōkiritia (shifting the paradigm) was held with people who had lived experience of mental distress and/or addiction, mental health providers, addiction support, community workers and whānau representing 25 iwi. The purpose of this wānanga was to capture the richness of mātauranga Māori (Māori knowledge) and to find solutions to increase self-sufficiency for Māori health and wellbeing (Butler & Te Kiwai Rangahau 2017). What this wānanga identified was four concepts that are critical to health and wellbeing for Māori. These concepts are mātauranga Māori (Māori knowledge), mana-enhancing practices, tino rangatiratanga (self-determination, autonomy) and kotahitanga (unity) (Butler & Te Kiwai Rangahau 2017).

The mental health interventions below are all examples of Māori practices delivered by Māori health professionals to enable Māori tangata whāiora to reach a greater understanding of their own experiences through mātauranga Māori, whereby they feel empowered to use their knowledge within to heal themselves, their whānau, hapū and iwi. The challenge for health professionals is to recognise that these interventions are legitimate, with their own epistemology, rationality and validity.

Pūrākau—Māori Creation Narratives

The role of oratory healing in Māori society is well founded in the traditions of whānau and hapū (Lee 2009). For Māori, karakia (prayers), waiata (songs), whakataukī (proverbial expressions), whakapapa (genealogical tables) and whaikōrero (formal speeches) are all examples of how the use of oral traditions has an active and meaningful role in supporting, protecting, informing and healing within Māori society. Today in mental health, talking therapies are a natural fit for Māori, providing a modern approach to what was a traditional and familiar way of communicating. In particular, pūrākau (Māori creation and custom narratives) are now becoming commonly used in mental health practice (Standing & Kahu 2021). These narratives allow Māori to better understand and interpret their experience(s) according to cultural understandings, as well as providing culturally safe assessment and Mental health interventions (Kopua et al 2020).

Te Tuakiri o te Ora – Art Therapy

Te Tuakiri o te Ora is a form of Māori-based art therapy that makes use of creation theories and links the characteristics of the atua (gods) to

TABLE 7.4 Nine Kupu of Te Tuakiri o te Ora	
Nine Kupu (Concepts)	**Mana (Spiritual Strength)**
Hinengaro (Hine (female) is the conscious and Ngaro (hidden) the subconscious)	Waihanga (Physical make-up)
Tapu (sacred, restricted or forbidden)	Pumanawa (The skills taught to us throughout our lives from parents, whānau)
Iho Matua (spiritual connection)	Mauri (life force)
Ngakau (relationships – the bonds that influence the way we live and react with one another)	Whatumanawa (Deep-seated emotions)

that of the whānau. It is centred on the exploration of nine significant Māori concepts (Table 7.4), in which a person is encouraged to consider their sense of identity, including cultural identity and reflect on these nine themes (NiaNia et al 2017).

Te Tuakiri o te Ora art-based therapy is currently being used more frequently in practice as an effective therapeutic process to strengthen identity with cultural values and beliefs, explore issues and challenges, build self-confidence and develop self-esteem in a way that is distinctly Māori (Manaia 2017).

Rongoā – Traditional Māori Healing Practices

Rongoā are healing practices that use native plants to create medicines that can prevent sickness or provide remedies where sickness has already occurred or fail to respond to standard medical treatment (Jones 2007). Rongoā also includes physical therapies such as massage and manipulation, including spiritual healing using traditional Māori practices, to support health and wellbeing (Jones 2007).

Mirimiri (Therapeutic Massage)

Mirimiri provides physical and spiritual healing using touch and connection to the elements. Mirimiri practitioners are spiritual mediators, seen as a vessel for communication between client and tūpuna, and known as spiritual guides or protectors who guide the healing process (Mark & Lyons 2010). Mirimiri has been shown to help manage stress and provide a better emotional and spiritual balance (Mark & Lyons 2010). It utilises a holistic approach to restoring wellness to the mind, spirit, body and emotional wellbeing.

▋ CHAPTER SUMMARY

We hope that this chapter has inspired and deepened your understanding of the issues raised, such as the impact that colonisation had on Māori health, as well as why mental health problems are common among Māori today. This chapter also discussed Māori nurses, racism, kawa whakaruruhau, including Te Tiriti o Waitangi, and how these things influence and guide nurses' ability to care for Māori. We explored different Māori models of health, kaupapa Māori services and current Māori mental health interventions used to support tangata whāiora, so that you can have knowledge of these services and health interventions to apply them to your own nursing practice during your nursing career.

The ability to transform mental health care for Māori and achieve equity is enormously overdue but welcomed, and will require significant

thought and action so that we can ensure that the opportunity to achieve oranga (wellbeing) for all Māori is realised. This is our societal opportunity to get this right. We finish with this karakia:

Mā te whakapono – By believing and trusting
Mā te tumanako – By having faith and hope
Mā te titiro – By looking and searching
Mā te whakarongo – By listening and hearing
Mā te mahitahi – By working and striving together
Mā te manawanui – By patience and perseverance
Mā te aroha – By all being done with love
Ka taea e tātou – We will succeed

REVIEW QUESTIONS

1. Culturally safe mental health care for Māori is based on the Māori principle of whakawhānaungatanga. Discuss how you would demonstrate whakawhānaungatanga in practice.
2. The principle of tino rangatiratanga, involving self-determination, sovereignty, independence, autonomy and ownership, can be shown in good mental health practice. Discuss how this would be shown.
3. Kawa whakaruruhau (cultural safety) was revolutionary when it was first proposed as a way of practising in nursing in the 1990s. How would you explain it to a nursing colleague or student who has never heard of cultural safety and for whom English is a second language? Why is cultural safety so important in Aotearoa New Zealand?

USEFUL WEBSITES/RESOURCES

Frame. The Spinoff. Under the Korowai: A look at Māori mental health practice: youtu.be/odo_-Vh2-fI

Rhys Jones, "Rongoā – medicinal use of plants", Te Ara – the Encyclopaedia of New Zealand, www.TeAra.govt.nz/en/rongoa-medicinal-use-of-plants

Rongoā Māori: Finding medicine in the bush: www.youtube.com/watch?v=F4C5A7hIXOw&t=109s

Te Pou o Te Whakaaro Nui (2010) He rongoā kei te kōrero. Talking therapies for Māori: Wise practice guide for mental health and addiction services. Auckland: Te Pou o Te Whakaaro Nui: www.tepou.co.nz/resources/talking-therapies-for-māori

Te Reo Hāpai – a glossary of Te Reo Māori in the mental health, addiction and disability sectors: www.tereohapai.nz

Tuia te ao Mārama – Oral history of Māori mental health nurses. From Te Ao Māramatanga New Zealand College of Mental Health Nurses: www.maorinursinghistory.com/themes/mental-health-nursing

REFERENCES

Ahuriri-Driscoll, A., Baker, V., Hepi, M., Hudson, M., Mika, C., et al., 2008. The future of rongoā Māori: Wellbeing and sustainability. University of Canterbury, Health Sciences Centre, Canterbury.

Barton P, Wilson D. 2008. Te Kapunga Putohe (the restless hands): A Māori-centred nursing practice model. Nurs Praxis NZ, 24(2), 6–15.

Bennett, S. 2009. Te huanga o te ao Māori: Cognitive behavioural therapy for Māori clients with depression: Development and evaluation of a culturally adapted treatment programme. Massey University, Wellington.

Brunton, W. 2011 "Mental health services", Te Ara: The Encyclopaedia of New Zealand. Online. Available at: teara.govt.nz/en

Butler, K., & Te Kīwai Rangahau. 2017. Tūmata Kōkiritia –shifting the paradigm. Te Rau Matatini. Online. Available at: terauora.com/tumata-kokiritia-shifting-paradigm/

Cohen, B. 2014. Passive-aggressive: Māori resistance and the continuance of colonial psychiatry in Aotearoa New Zealand. Disability Global South, 1(2), 319–339.

Committee of Inquiry into Mental Health Services. 1996. Inquiry under Section 47 of the Health and Disability Services Act 1993 in Respect of Certain Mental Health Services: Report of the Ministerial Inquiry to the Minister of Health Hon. Jenny Shipley. Ministry of Health, Wellington.

Durie, M. 1998. Whaiora: Māori Health Development. 2nd ed. Oxford University Press, Auckland.

Jones, R. 2007 "Rongoā – medicinal use of plants", Te Ara: the Encyclopedia of New Zealand, Online. Available at: www.TeAra.govt.nz/en/rongoa-medicinal-use-of-plants

Kingi, T. 2005 Cultural interventions and the treatment of Māori mental health consumers. Massey University, Wellington. Online. Available at: www.massey.ac.nz/documents/499/T_Kingi_Cultural_intervention_and_the_treatment_of_Māori_mental_health_consumers.pdf

Kingi, T., Durie, M., Elder, H., Tapsell, R., Lawrence, M., et al 2017. Maea te toi ora: Māori health transformations. Huia, Wellington.

Komene, E., Gerrard, D., Pene, B., Parr, J., Aspinall, C. et al., 2023. A tohu (sign) to open our eyes to the realities of Indigenous Māori registered nurses: A qualitative study. J Adv Nurs, 79, 2585–2596.

Kopua, D. M., Kopua M.A., Bracken, P.J. 2020 Mahi a Atua: A Māori approach to mental health. Transcult Psychiatry, 57(2), 375–383.

Lee, J. 2009 Decolonising Māori narratives: Pūrākau as a method. MAI Review. 2(3), Natlib.govt.nz/records/20915864.

Manaia, A.V. (2017) Kaupapa Māori arts therapy: The application of arts therapy in a Kaupapa Māori setting. ANZ J Arts Ther 12(1), 29–39.

Mark, G.T. and Lyons, A.C. 2010 Māori healers' views on wellbeing: The importance of mind, body, spirit, family and land. Soc Sci Med, 70(11), 1756–1764.

Mental Health (Compulsory Assessment and Treatment) Act, 1992 (sec. 2). Wellington. Ministry of Health. Online. Available at: www.legislation.govt.nz/act/public/1992/0046/latest/DLM262181.html

Mental Health Commission 2012. Blueprint II: Improving mental health and wellbeing for all New Zealanders. How things need to be. Mental Health Commission, Wellington.

Mental Health Commission 1998. Blueprint: Improving mental health and wellbeing for all New Zealanders. How things need to be. Mental Health Commission, Wellington.

Ministry of Health 2017a. Office of the Director of Mental Health Annual Report 2016. Ministry of Health, Wellington. Online. Available at: www.health.govt.nz/publication/office-director-mental-health-annual-report-2016

Ministry of Health 2017b. Māori Health models – Te Wheke. Ministry of Health, Wellington. Online. Available at: www.health.govt.nz/our-work/populations/maori-health/maori-health-models/maori-health-models-te-wheke

Ministry of Health 2016. Office of the Director of Mental Health Annual Report 2015. Ministry of Health, Wellington.

Ministry of Health 2015. Tatau Kahukura: Māori Health Chart Book 2015, 3rd ed. Ministry of Health, Wellington.

NiaNia, W., Bush, A., & Epston, D. 2017. Collaborative and Indigenous Mental Health Therapy: Tataihono – Stories of Māori Healing and Psychiatry. Routledge, Taylor & Francis, New York.

Nursing Council of New Zealand 2020. Te Tiriti o Waitangi Policy Statement. Te Kaunihera Tapuhi o Aotearoa Nursing Council of New Zealand, Wellington.

Nursing Council of New Zealand (NCNZ) 2019. Te Ohu Mahi Tapuhi o Aotearoa/The New Zealand nursing workforce: A profile of nurse practitioners, registered nurses and enrolled nurses 2018–2019. Workforce Statistics. NCNZ, Wellington.

Nursing Council of New Zealand (NCNZ) 2011. Guidelines for cultural safety, the Treaty of Waitangi and Māori Health in nursing education and practice. Te Kaunihera Tapuhi o Aotearoa Nursing Council of New Zealand, Wellington.

Papps, E., & Ramsden, I. 1996. Cultural safety in nursing: The New Zealand experience. Int J Qual Health Care, 8(5), 491–497.

Pitama, S., Huria, T., and Lacey, C. 2014. Improving Māori health through clinical assessment: Waikare o te Waka o Meihana. NZ Med J, 127(1393), 107–119.

Ramalho R., Groot S., Adams P.J. 2022 Community mental health care in Aotearoa New Zealand: Past, present, and the road ahead. Consortium Psychiatricum, 3(4), 53–62.

Ramsden, I.M. 2002. Cultural Safety and Nursing Education in Aotearoa and Te Waipounamu. Doctoral thesis. Victoria University of Wellington, Wellington.

Standing, M., & Kahu, E.R. 2021. Story, myth, and Purakau: An exploration of the use of narrative in the therapeutic setting in Aotearoa New Zealand. NZ J Psychol, 50(3), 29–38.

Te Rau Ora 2023. Huarahi Whakatū PDRP. Te Rau Ora. Online. Available at: teraumatatau.com/courses/huarahi-whakatu-pdrp/

Te Whatu Ora 2022. Te Pae Tata: Interim New Zealand Health Plan 2022. New Zealand Government, Wellington. Online. Available at: www.tewhatuora.govt.nz/publications/te-pae-tata-interim-new-zealand-health-plan-2022/

Wilson, D., Barton, P., & Tipa, Z. 2022. Rhetoric, racism, and the reality for the Indigenous Māori nursing workforce in Aotearoa New Zealand. Online J Issues Nurs, 27, 1–2.

Waitangi Tribunal 2023. Hauora: Report on Stage One of the Health Services and Outcomes Kaupapa Inquiry. Lower Hutt, New Zealand. Online. Available at: forms.justice.govt.nz/search/Documents/WT/wt_DOC_195476216/Hauora%202023%20W.pdf

Wilson, D., & Baker, M. 2012. Bridging two worlds: Māori mental health nursing. Qual Health Res, 22(8), 1073–1082.

8

Professional Self-Care

Julie Sharrock

KEY POINTS

- Self-awareness and holistic self-care are essential for mental health nurses to provide compassionate care to consumers and carers, to maintain productive working relationships with colleagues, to manage the demands of mental health nursing practice and to sustain a rewarding career.
- Holistic self-care includes physical, psychological, social and spiritual strategies.

- Lifelong learning and ongoing professional development are essential to maintaining skills and knowledge in the ever-changing world of healthcare.
- There are a multitude of career opportunities for mental health nurses in clinical, education, managerial and/or research roles.

KEY TERMS

Burnout

Clinical supervision

Compassion fatigue

Emotional labour

Holistic self-care

Professional development

Resilience

Workplace stress

LEARNING OUTCOMES

The material in this chapter will assist you to:

- understand the challenges, workplace stressors and health risks associated with mental health nursing
- understand how self-awareness and holistic self-care can help maintain your wellbeing in mental health nursing
- review your own self-care and health maintenance strategies to lay the groundwork for a sustainable career in mental health nursing

- develop awareness of different professional development strategies, in particular the role clinical supervision plays in maintaining practice
- consider strategies for professional development and career choices within mental health nursing.

INTRODUCTION

All nurses need to have strategies for self-care in place throughout their careers to maintain their health and wellbeing, provide compassionate care to consumers and carers, maintain productive working relationships with colleagues, and manage the demands of nursing practice. Applying the social ecological lens described in Chapter 2 to our own health and wellbeing, we need to consider the interaction between ourselves and our environment, and to understand ourselves from physical, psychological, social and spiritual perspectives. To maintain our therapeutic selves and sustain our therapeutic work without sacrificing our own health, we need to care for ourselves holistically. While self-care is an individual responsibility, both employees and the organisations we work for have a responsibility to contribute to healthy workplaces that support the wellbeing of all staff.

The focus of this chapter is on the importance of caring for ourselves as nurses in the context of the rewards and demands of nursing, with particular attention to mental health nursing. Ongoing learning and professional development are essential elements of career progression and work satisfaction, and contribute to professional self-care. This chapter also presents information on the multiple career options for nurses who are planning to go into mental health.

THERAPEUTIC USE OF SELF

As discussed in Chapter 2, the therapeutic relationship is the central activity of mental health nursing practice and is the foundation upon which all other nursing interventions are based. In mental health, actively participating in therapeutic relationships requires cognitive, emotional and behavioural work on the part of the nurse. This is done through intentionally and consciously drawing on our personality, background and life skills, as well as interpersonal skills and professional knowledge as a way of establishing human connection with another person. The aim of this connection is to alleviate that person's distress and suffering in the moment and to support their healing and recovery in the long term.

The therapeutic relationship is a privileged one for both the consumer and the mental health nurse, but it is the responsibility of the nurse to maintain professional boundaries (Zugai et al 2018). Maintaining professional boundaries within the nurse–consumer relationship is essential for it to be therapeutic and is a skill that cannot be underestimated (Thomson et al 2022). Of particular importance is maintaining boundaries and being able to regulate one's emotional state (Hofmeyer et al 2020) through self-monitoring and self-awareness in order to minimise reactivity when working closely with consumers. Being self-aware is essential if the mental health nurse is to intentionally use their self to develop therapeutic and safe relationships with consumers.

Self-Awareness

As discussed in Chapter 2, understanding others begins with understanding oneself. The concept of self is a complex one that has been widely studied as we try to understand human psychology and behaviour. The self is our uniqueness as a human being and consists of attributes that pervade the way we live in and experience the world (Leary & Price Tangney 2012). When we pay attention to ourselves (reflect, think, see ourselves in the mirror or on video, hear our voice), we recognise our self and this helps us to distinguish our self from others. It is through the process of self-reflection and examination of experiences that nurses can learn and enhance the ways in which they understand and relate to others. In addition, self-awareness. or being an "expert of self" (Prosser et al 2017) and having a strong understanding of our own personal experience, skills, knowledge, strengths and limitations (Foster et al 2019a), has been associated with increased resilience (Foster et al 2023).

Reflection

A key component of self-awareness is the ability to reflect. Reflection in clinical practice supports learning from experience in that it includes critically reviewing practice so it can be learnt from, and then positively informs future practice. It assists in integrating theory and practice, generates knowledge from practice, increases self-awareness and confidence in decision-making, and is essential for autonomous and accountable practice (Patel & Metersky 2022; Sweet et al 2019).

It is particularly important that nurses reflect on what brings us to a helping role. Hawkins and Shohet (2012) argue that it is essential that those who enter the helping professions to honestly reflect on the complex motives that have led us to our current profession and role. To do this they suggest considering the "positive" motives as well as the "shadow" motives. The shadow motives are how we get our own needs met through helping others. For example, when we fix things or reduce suffering we feel a strong sense of satisfaction; or when we help others, we feel useful or worthwhile. These motivations are not wrong, but if we are not aware of them they may affect not only the way we relate to consumers but also our ability to self-care. Exploring these aspects of our professional selves can be challenging, but it is essential to help us maintain our capacity to be a functional helper. Clinical supervision is one of the areas where such exploration can be undertaken in a safe and trusting relationship (Hawkins & Shohet 2012).

Self-awareness needs to take place in tandem with self-compassion. Self-compassion involves accepting our common humanity, including our own suffering, frailties and wisdom. It is about being kind to ourselves in a mindful, caring and non-judgemental way (Biber 2022). Self-compassion is a necessary element of being able to demonstrate empathy and compassion to others (Hofmeyer et al 2020; Mills et al 2018a). Accepting our own humanness, frailties and strengths enhances our ability to be with others in their own humanness, living with their frailties and strengths. Self-awareness also supports us when we experience workplace challenges.

PROFESSIONAL CHALLENGES

Prior to the COVID-19 pandemic, it was recognised that working in healthcare could be challenging (Safe Work Australia 2018), and that despite working within the health industry, the health of nurses was generally not good (Kelly et al 2016). It has been said that many nurses would fail their own health checks with diabetes, arthritis

(Larter 2014), obesity (Ross et al 2019a), poor sleep (Keller et al 2023) and musculoskeletal conditions (Kox et al 2020) commonly experienced. The already lower health of nurses was compounded by the COVID-19 pandemic and projected nursing workforce shortages further exacerbated (ICN 2021). Out of all healthcare workers, nurses were the most frequently infected with the virus (Gómez-Ochoa et al 2021). Health and wellbeing issues identified in nurses pre-pandemic, such as depression, anxiety (Chiang & Chang 2012) and substance misuse (Searby et al 2023), have been exacerbated since the COVID-19 pandemic (Dragioti et al 2022; Mercer et al 2023; Sun et al 2021). In a report published in 2016, the suicide rate in male nurses was found to be higher than for their non-nursing counterparts, while the suicide rate for female nurses was significantly higher than for the general female population (Milner et al 2016). Suicidality among nurses increased though the pandemic, along with post-traumatic symptoms, depression, anxiety, compassion fatigue and burnout, as reported in multiple papers (see Dragioti et al 2022; Hur et al 2022). Some of the complex factors associated with the poor health of our workforce are discussed in the following section.

Workplace Stress

Stress is when we feel that the demands placed upon us exceed the resources needed to respond to those demands. When someone experiences stress, their sense of balance is disturbed. Physiologically, a stress response is activated within the body. Any foundational anatomy and physiology textbook can provide details of the stress response, but for the purposes of this chapter it is enough to understand that the response involves the release of stress hormones into the blood that cause a range of physiological changes, including changes to heart rate, blood pressure and the gastrointestinal tract. Prolonged stress can be harmful and have a negative effect on physical and mental health. It is important to learn to monitor and manage our own stress because unchecked stress can become chronic and result in burnout (Giannakakis et al 2017; Kunzler et al 2022). Stress is often thought of as a negative experience with negative impacts. However, stress can also have positive effects, as seen later in the chapter when we discuss career transitions, as it can be a catalyst for a person to make changes or a stimulant to positive action.

Nursing can involve long periods of working in intensely stressful situations, which can be exacerbated by shift work (Badu et al 2020). In mental health nursing, stress arises from the interpersonal work with consumers, carers and colleagues within the demanding organisational context of the health system (Cranage & Foster 2022; Foster et al 2019b). The nature of nursing work involves a high level of close contact with people at the extremes of human experience when a person or a loved one is experiencing life-changing health crises. Nurses are in contact with the best and worst of human nature, and everything in between.

Consumers with acute or chronic mental health conditions have complex and sometimes long-term needs and can have frequent and regular encounters with the healthcare system. The long-term and cyclical nature of some mental health conditions means that the therapeutic relationships between mental health nurses and consumers can last for long periods. They can also vary in intensity as consumers move along a continuum between periods of high dependence at one end (in acute phases when they are experiencing symptoms of their illness) and independence at the other (when their symptoms are less troublesome or their mental health condition has resolved). Ethical concerns (Salzmann-Erikson 2018) and the legal aspects of mental health care (Johnson et al 2018) add a further layer of complexity, where compulsory treatment presents additional challenges for mental health nurses (Muir-Cochrane et al 2018).

Two Australian studies grouped challenging workplace stressors for mental health nurses as:

1. *consumer/carer issues*, in terms of addressing the needs of consumers and carers, challenging or confrontational behaviours and nursing interactions
2. *organisational and role challenges*, such as practice-related concerns in performing the nursing role and maintaining standards of practice, shift work, inadequacies in organisational policy, staffing and work environment, lack of managerial support, organisational responses to critical incidents and consumer throughput and management
3. *colleague-related stressors*, such as negative staff interactions, poor communication, conflict, challenging behaviours and negative team culture (Cranage & Foster 2022; Foster et al 2019b).

Some or all of these stressors are likely to be experienced by nurses throughout their career. The COVID-19 pandemic has added another layer of challenge to the wellbeing of nurses. Managing the personal and professional impacts of the pandemic, negotiating the unknown and relentless nature of the infections surges has been stressful, and learning about the disease and infection controls have been demanding (Dragioti et al 2022; Gómez-Ochoa et al 2021; Hur et al 2022). However, one of the positive outcomes from the pandemic is that a spotlight has been cast on the nursing workforce and their wellbeing, with an avalanche of research being conducted on the impacts of the pandemic on nurses, and recommendations made for strategies to support their health and wellbeing (Dragioti et al 2022; Hur et al 2022). In addition, benefits and "new ways of working", such as the increased use of technology and clinical skill development, have emerged (Whiteing et al 2022).

In the following sections, some specific forms of psychological stress and their potential impacts on nurses are described: emotional labour, compassion fatigue, burnout and exposure to trauma.

Emotional Labour

The concept of emotional labour was initially developed in relation to flight attendants (Hochschild 1983), and refers to managing emotions to meet the expectations of the work environment. It is the requirement of a worker to suppress or create feelings so they can present an outward appearance that will give another person (e.g. a consumer) a sense of being cared for. Emotions and emotional expression are managed through facial and body language. The emotional expression considered appropriate to a situation is guided by "feeling rules", which are the personal and professional norms to which we are socialised. Hochschild (1983) described "surface acting" and "deep acting" as strategies for emotional self-management. Surface acting occurs when workers actively suppress their felt emotion or simulate an emotion that is considered appropriate. The worker does not genuinely experience the emotion, but is seen to. Deep acting involves invoking and genuinely feeling emotions that are appropriate to the situation (Hochschild 1983).

Emotional labour is considered a form of workplace stress for nurses (Theodosius 2008) and is increasingly part of nursing discourse (Christensen et al 2022; Delgado et al 2017; Edward et al 2017; Yilmaz et al 2022; Yu et al 2022). Theodosius (2008) identified three types of emotional labour in nursing work:

- **therapeutic** – arising from interactions between nurses and recipients of services
- **instrumental** – arising from nurses' levels of confidence in their ability to perform clinical work to reduce consumer/carer discomfort
- **collegial** – arising from interpersonal interactions with colleagues.

Aspects and realities of mental health nursing work that have been identified as emotionally labour-intensive include:

- witnessing human distress and suffering
- feeling and expressing compassion
- managing one's emotions at the same time as managing others' emotions (particularly anxiety, distress, frustration and anger)
- engaging in consumer interactions that are intense and that trigger a range of emotions
- interactions that require a significant degree of effort on the part of the nurse, such as working with consumers who are difficult to engage
- interactions where the nurse perceives higher levels of stress and a strong sense of responsibility for consumer outcomes
- managing crisis situations, promoting compliance with treatment and navigating the power structure within the therapeutic relationship
- conflict between professional identity (professionalism) and personal identity (authenticity) of nurses, such as in ethical dilemmas or threats that challenge the physical or psychological safety of the nurse
- feeling blamed by the organisation or service-users
- feeling burdened by or unprepared for what is expected
- interpersonal difficulties and conflict with other staff (Delgado et al 2017; Edward et al 2017).

Paradoxically, emotional labour in nursing work is also experienced as a source of satisfaction. The emotional work of nursing has been described as "emotionful" work and a "gift" (Bolton 2000). Demonstrating compassion, using oneself as the therapeutic tool and dealing with emotionally charged interpersonal interactions are all sources of both satisfaction and labour (Edward et al 2017). This view is consistent with the evidence that there is a "bright side of emotional labour" (Humphrey et al 2015), in that deep acting, as well as the expression of naturally felt emotions, have positive impacts on workers. It is surface acting that is associated with negative impacts on worker health and wellbeing (Delgado et al 2017). The associated emotional discomfort and loss of the "authentic self" (Humphrey et al 2015) can result in stress, emotional exhaustion and burnout (Delgado et al 2017).

To make sense of this, mental health nursing requires emotional work, which is part of its rewards, but also its challenges. In my own practice, to be with people during life-changing or life-threatening experiences and to bear witness to their vulnerability and their resilience has been precious and rewarding, albeit not easy at times. I recognise that much of the emotional labour of my work was not only deep acting, but also genuinely experiencing emotions towards consumers, carers and my work. It is possible that this nourished me and potentially protected me against the negative impacts of surface acting and other workplace stressors.

As nurses, we make a choice to be in an occupation that involves emotional labour, and we have a responsibility to undertake activities that help us manage this. Some of these are outlined later in this chapter. However, this responsibility does not rest solely with the nurse (Delgado et al 2022). The organisation must also contribute to a practice environment that is ethical and healthy, that eliminates avoidable harm to staff and that mitigates against the detrimental impacts of emotional labour on workers (Maslach 2017). Some of the services you can expect from your workplace are outlined later in the chapter.

Compassion (Empathic Distress) Fatigue

The concept of compassion fatigue entered healthcare discourse in 1992 and was initially seen as a particular form of burnout in caregivers (Joinson 1992). Since then, the concept has evolved and is now seen as an individualised, progressive process resulting from prolonged exposure to the suffering, distress and pain of others (Hofmeyer et al 2020; Sabery et al 2018). Hofmeyer and colleagues (2020) have challenged the term "compassion fatigue" in light of neuroscientific findings that demonstrate that fatigue is not caused by showing compassion; "empathic distress fatigue" has been proposed as being a more accurate description (Hofmeyer et al 2020). *Empathic distress fatigue* is linked with prolonged expression of empathy where the distress of those suffering is absorbed by the caregiver, which leads to a loss of capacity to care for others (consumers, carers, colleagues and the organisation), and this also flows on to an inability to care for self and family (Hofmeyer et al 2020). Further to this, if it is not addressed it can lead to disinterest, lack of concern for others' suffering, moral distress and burnout (Cross 2019). Burnout is a related concept, but it is more likely to be associated with the cumulative effects of workplace stressors more broadly and can happen to any worker (Hofmeyer et al 2020; Sabery et al 2018).

Burnout

Burnout research began in the 1970s and those working in caregiving occupations were identified as being at risk (Maslach 2017). The phenomenon that we now know as burnout initially had no name and it was rarely discussed or acknowledged (Maslach 2017). The literature is now replete with attention to burnout, and it continues to be of concern in the nursing workforce (Laker et al 2019), and even more-so since the COVID-19 pandemic (Hur et al 2022). Burnout is included in the International Classification of Diseases (World Health Organization 2018) as an occupational phenomenon in the chapter titled "Factors influencing health status or contact with health services".

The psychological syndrome of burnout is a response to chronic occupational interpersonal stressors and has three key dimensions:

- feelings of overwhelming physical and emotional **exhaustion** and depletion, lacking the energy to face another day and over-extended by the demands of work without seeing any source of replenishment and recovery
- feelings of cynicism and **detachment**, negative, harsh or disinterested responses, a loss of idealism and doing the bare minimum of work
- a sense of **ineffectiveness** and lack of accomplishment, lowered sense of confidence, competence, self-efficacy and self-regard, regret about career choice and decreased productivity (Maslach & Leiter 2017).

The words "burnout" and "stress" often appear together because stress is seen as a precursor to burnout. However, stress is a feature of life and, when managed properly, does not lead to burnout. Unlike stress, which has some positive features (e.g. it can be a catalyst for effecting positive change such as learning a new skill), burnout has no positive aspects for the person experiencing it or for those around them.

Burnout can lead to significant problems for those experiencing it, including poor professional and personal relationships, poor physical health and worsening mental health (Maslach & Leiter 2017), such as depression, substance misuse and suicidal ideation. Fulfilment and identification with the work role are lost. Work becomes a burden without joy or satisfaction, which results in a desire to avoid it to the point of leaving the profession (Maslach & Leiter 2017).

From the perspective of the affected person, there is nothing worse than going to work when feeling unhappy and distressed. Working with colleagues who are irritable, depressed and exhausted adds to everyone's stress. It is not difficult to imagine how distressing it would be for a consumer to be nursed by someone who responds to them and their situation in a cold and unfeeling way rather than with the warmth, caring, empathy and respect we ourselves would wish for if we were sick and needing care.

Burnout comes at significant cost to the employing organisation in terms of poor quality of care provided by that person. This has been demonstrated through decreased consumer satisfaction, increased consumer mortality and increased errors (Maslach & Leiter 2017). It is important to note that burnout is not a personal failing or the sole responsibility of the individual nurse to prevent. Given the high rates of burnout among health professionals, it is more accurate to consider it as an organisational and systemic issue that develops as a response of the employee to demands in the workplace (Maslach & Leiter 2017). Therefore, the organisation also has a responsibility for supporting the physical and mental health of employees and to adopt policies and practices that support nurses rather than contribute to stress and burnout. Stress and burnout need to be considered within the organisation as a whole, within teams, and at the individual employee level (Maslach 2017). See Perspectives in practice: Nurse's story 8.1.

PERSPECTIVES IN PRACTICE

Nurse's Story 8.1: James Houghton

Sometimes I find it hard to believe that almost 40 years have passed since I first decided to be a nurse. It's been a challenging and sometimes confronting journey, and I've worked in several different clinical settings as a mental health nurse, including a long period in child and youth services.

When I reflect on resilience and how I've managed to stay passionate about mental health nursing and engaged in this work for so long, I can identify several factors that have been really important. I am part of a team who are kind, supportive, generous with their time and typically very positive in their outlook. We regularly and intentionally celebrate each other's strengths. Over the years I have developed and strengthened my ability to use thought processes, such as reframing, depersonalising and not catastrophising situations or events. More recently, I have come to identify strongly with the neuroplastic approach (the brain's capacity to change in response to learning) to managing my inner dialogue, which is not always my "best friend". And this has proven to be highly effective for me. These skills have enabled me to challenge my thinking, so that when I encounter sometimes serious difficulties (which we all do from time to time), I see them as challenges or barriers to be negotiated rather than devastating or insurmountable roadblocks.

Another very important factor is my clinical supervision, which has become an essential component of my practice. The people I have had as clinical supervisors have provided me with excellent guidance and support for my practice and encouraged me to become more involved in professional organisations like the Australian College of Mental Health Nurses and the Australian Clinical Supervision Association. This has contributed positively to my professional identity, which contributes to my self-esteem.

Outside of work I have quite a large group of friends and acquaintances, with a smaller group of really close friends, all of whom are prepared to spend time with me doing the things we all enjoy – be that sport, dancing, live music, movies, theatre or just having dinner and "hanging out". Having fun and being able to completely forget about work for a while are really important factors in not burning out.

I'm proud that when anyone asks me what I do for work or when I spend time with early career nurses, I can say that I enjoy being a nurse more now than I did when I began my nursing career.

Exposure to Trauma

Mental health nurses are very likely to be exposed to traumatic events within the workplace. Traumatic events are those that are usually unexpected and may involve threats of or actual serious injury, death or sexual violence (Phoenix Australia 2022). In mental health nursing, exposure to actual or threatened aggression, self-harming behaviour, attempted or completed suicide or inappropriate sexual behaviour (Cranage & Foster 2022) are some situations that can be experienced as traumatic.

While people identify and respond to traumatic events differently, there are common physical, emotional, cognitive, behavioural and social reactions that occur. A sense of shock, disbelief, being over-whelmed and loss of the world as one knew it before the event, are common. Most people recover within the first week or two with the help of colleagues, family and friends, but for a few, trauma can have long-term effects. Immediate practical and emotional support goes a long way to alleviating the distress of such events. The Centre for Post-traumatic Mental Health, based at the University of Melbourne, has resources available to the public on helping yourself and helping others after traumatic events (see Useful websites at the end of this chapter).

Mental health nurses are also exposed to trauma through caring for consumers who have had traumatic experiences, which puts them at risk of "vicarious traumatisation". Vicarious traumatisation is a change that occurs within a worker who engages with people who have had traumatic experiences, hears their stories and sees the effects of their trauma experiences. The worker may begin to re-experience the trauma stories with hyperarousal and intrusive images and thoughts. They may develop a depressed mood, anxiety and avoid exposure to further traumatic material (Benuto et al 2018). Conversely, positive effects and personal growth can occur as a result of exposure to trauma. This growth, which has been called "post-traumatic growth", is experienced as a greater appreciation for one's own life, improved rela-tionships with others and increased spirituality. Growth following trauma can occur if the trauma is not overwhelming, if there is support available and if the person exposed to the trauma has a sense of efficacy to get through it, the ability to reflect, to change core beliefs and to make meaning of the experience (Chen et al 2021). The capacity to make meaning from challenging or traumatic experiences is also important when we look at resilience.

While the challenges of stress, emotional labour, compassion fatigue, potential burnout and exposure to trauma exist for nurses, there are many approaches that can successfully mitigate their impact on nurses' health and wellbeing. Mental health nurses can learn and develop skills and strategies that will support their health and well-being. In addition, a range of services is available to mental health nurses from within and outside their employing organisation that support them to maintain their health and wellbeing. Some key approaches are described in the next section.

HOLISTIC SELF-CARE

Given the challenges and potential stressors in mental health nursing, it is vital that we extend the same care to ourselves that we offer our consumers. As mentioned previously, developing awareness and un-derstanding of what brings us to take up a helping role is important. If we do not do this, we can fall into the trap of compulsive helping, which results in metaphorically "giving ourselves away" with nothing left for ourselves or anyone else. Self-care is vital for nurses to mitigate against workplace stressors and challenges, and to maintain our health and wellbeing. Self-care is also essential to provide compassionate care and should be included as a "professional expectation inherent to the role of nurses" (Mills et al 2015, p. 792).

As a student, you may have had education in relation to self-care (Flatekval 2023; Jenkins et al 2019). Maintaining a self-care program is important for wellbeing, but can be a challenge, especially for shift workers. Nurses are generally not good at prioritising their own care (Christie et al 2017; Perry et al 2018; Ross et al 2019b). Challenges

include being busy, lack of planning and prioritising self-care, the stigma associated with putting yourself first, a work environment that is not supportive of self-care, inadequate boundaries between work and home, self-criticism and low self-worth (Mills et al 2018b).

These challenges can be addressed by having a commitment to and belief in the need for self-care (Mills et al 2018b). Self-care goes beyond developing skills to cope with and manage the workplace challenges and stressors. Self-care needs to be consciously prioritised, practised deliberately, be personalised and ongoing (Mills et al 2018b). Self-care strategies and behaviours need to be in place within and external to the workplace and include work–life balance, adequate sleep, rest and exercise, a healthy diet and general health maintenance.

Work–Life Balance

Increasingly, the community is recognising the importance of main-taining a balance between our work lives and our personal lives. As a society we have borne the brunt of focusing on work, money and pos-sessions, at the expense of family, community, the environment, and what gives meaning to our lives. Maintaining a work–life balance is particularly important for nurses who have the additional challenge of working unsociable hours through shift work (Badu et al 2020). The work–life boundary was even more blurred for nurses during the pandemic due to anxiety about spreading the virus to relatives (Sahay & Wei 2023).

In a study of nurses and doctors, the participants described that finding harmony between personal and work lives was an effective self-care strategy (Mills et al 2018b). They described some approaches to creating a boundary between work and home. These included the mode of travel to and from work used as a strategy to ensure they were not overworking, and the commute itself was an opportunity to un-wind from work. Taking a bath at home was described as a way of metaphorically washing away the workplace stressors. When work–life harmony or balance is achieved, people have enough energy for work and non-work life (Köse et al 2021), and this has been associated with increased resilience (Foster et al 2019a).

Sleep, Rest, Exercise and Diet

Restful and restorative sleep is an important self-care strategy for both the mind and the body. Sleep is essential to health and vitality, and as-sists us to approach stressful situations more calmly (Chopra 2023). Sleep hygiene is something we teach consumers, but as nurses we often do not practise it ourselves. Some key principles of sleep hygiene are to obey your body clock, improve your sleeping environment, limit elec-tronic devices (e.g. phones and computers) at bedtime and avoid drugs/alcohol, stimulants (e.g. coffee), stimulating activity and heavy meals before sleep (Chopra 2023).

Of course, obeying your body clock poses challenges for shiftwork-ers, especially working overnight and grabbing a meal whenever you can on a busy shift. However, given that shiftwork impacts negatively on health, it essential that shiftworkers pay attention to their sleep practices, diet and exercise (Wilson & Brooks 2018). Ensuring ade-quate intake of all food groups, especially fruit and vegetables, avoiding obesity and maintaining enough exercise (especially if the nursing work undertaken involves less activity) are key areas for nurses to pay attention to (Torquati et al 2018).

Psychological Strategies
Meaning-Making

Making meaning of our work and our lives can also support our energy and passion for our work. It has been postulated that to make meaning out of the experiences of life is central to survival and impor-tant in understanding human responses to adversity (Park 2010).

The cognitive process of trying to make sense of stressful events, suffering and death is an important one for nurses. Giving meaning to our work, why we do it and how we evaluate whether our input makes a difference are important areas to reflect on. When the meanings made lead to adaptive behaviours (Park 2010), then a cognitive system is developed that supports us in the work we do. The ability to reframe adverse situations into those that are meaningful (Prosser et al 2017), having the capacity to make sense of challenging situations through placing them in a context or structure and identifying a given situation or action in terms of making a potentially positive contribution (Foster et al 2019a), are examples of meanings that lead to adaptive behaviours. Meaning-making that leads to adaptive behaviours helps us to manage our expectations, sit with the suffering of others and maintain the passion of our work, and is also a key part of resilience.

Self-Compassion

As mentioned earlier, having self-compassion is an important part of being self-aware. Self-compassion includes self-kindness, mindfulness and recognising our common humanity and wisdom. Demonstrating self-compassion results in increasing our capacity to self-care, to relate and demonstrate compassion to others, to be autonomous and to develop a sturdier sense of self (Biber 2022; Hofmeyer et al 2020; Mills et al 2018b).

Spiritual Care

For some nurses, holding sustaining belief systems that include cultural and religious dimensions (Prosser et al 2017) supports practice and forms part of self-care. Nurturing our spirit does not solely refer to religious practice, but also to "our life force that gives us the will to live, love and endure" (Lloyd 2019, p. 23). You may have met consumers whose spirit is shattered, but this can also happen to health professionals who overwork or burn out. Ensuring we have work–life balance that includes spiritually nurturing experiences, with attention to energising our life force, is essential. Mind–body practices and being among nature are effective energisers of our life force. A wise mother once said to me, "Food nurtures our body, but gardening nurtures our spirit". While gardening is not everybody's thing, going outside, seeing the light and the sky and the wonders of nature is good for us and can have a revitalising effect.

Mind–Body Practices

In the workplace, nurses cognitively focus on the issues confronting them at work, continually assessing and considering how to respond and intervene with consumers, carers and colleagues. The body can easily be forgotten and considered a vehicle through which nursing work is delivered. The risk that we treat ourselves as objects is exacerbated by a reductionistic approach to health care. It is a curious thing that the idea of the mind and the body as separate entities has dominated western thinking for centuries. This contrasts with Eastern philosophies which have a long history of understanding the mind and body as an indivisible whole.

A range of practices that bring the mind and body together have been reported by nurses and other health professionals as useful in managing workplace stress and promoting health (Bonamer & Aquino-Russell 2019; Di Mario et al 2023; Mills et al 2018b). Mind–body practices, such as mindfulness, yoga, meditation, qi gong and tai chi, come from Eastern cultures and are centuries old. These practices involve gentle movements, specific postures and breathing coupled with mental focus that engages the whole person and enhances a sense of wellbeing. A common theme in these practices is they are thought to reduce the physiological and psychological stress response.

Meditation is a simple yet powerful tool that takes us to a state of profound relaxation that dissolves fatigue and the accumulated stress that accelerates the ageing process. During meditation, our breathing slows, our blood pressure and heart rate decrease, and stress hormone levels fall. By its very nature, meditation calms the mind, and when the mind is in a state of restful awareness, the body relaxes too. Research shows that people who meditate regularly develop less hypertension, heart disease, insomnia, anxiety and other stress-related illnesses (Chopra 2023).

Massage is another ancient practice where soft tissue is rubbed or manipulated to enhance relaxation and, sometimes, to relieve pain. Jon Kabat-Zinn (2023) has been credited for bringing mindfulness from the ancient Eastern practices into medicine and western society. As a student of Zen Buddhism, he integrated these teachings into mainstream science. There has been a significant amount of research into mindfulness that has found physical and mental health benefits (Di Mario et al 2023; Khazan 2019; La Torre et al 2022). You can incorporate mindfulness into your daily work through routine activities such as mindful handwashing (see Box 8.1).

Resilience

As has been discussed in this chapter, working in healthcare is very rewarding, but it can be challenging. Resilience is a process of positively adapting to adversity and regaining personal wellbeing after stressful situations or difficult events. Resilience has been associated with nurses' improved wellbeing by mitigating against the potentially

---

BOX 8.1　Mindful Handwashing

Handwashing is an essential part of health care and must be done for long enough to be effective. McNamara (2016) suggests:

*. . . if you're going to do hand hygiene dozens of times a day anyway, don't just do it for your patients: do it for your***self*** *too. We're not cold callous reptilian clinicians, we're educated warm-blooded mammals who do emotional labour. We need to nurture ourselves if we are to safely continue to nurture others.*

So why not wash mindfully and clear the grime out of your head as well as off your hands? Here are some tips:

1. Step towards the sink with intent and remind yourself you are taking a break.
2. Let the water flow.
3. Feel the water flowing over both hands. Notice the temperature of the water and savour the feeling.
4. Add soap. Notice the frictionless feelings it adds.
5. Start with cleaning. Think about washing stuff away. Let the stuff you need to get rid of flow down the drain. Let it flow away.
6. Move on to restoration, healing. Rub in resilience and health. Let the stuff that sustains you seep into your skin.
7. Check in on the breathing. The slower and deeper the better. If the breathing or the brain are running too fast, slow down and repeat the last two steps.
8. There's no rush. Slowly scan the surroundings. With any luck someone from infection control is watching.
9. Smile.
10. Breathe slowly, thinking: It is time to rinse both hands.
11. Then, again breathing slowly, think: "It is time to thoroughly dry both hands together".
12. Throw the towel in the bin.
13. Take another slow breath: It is time to get back to work.
   Clean hands save lives. Clear heads save lives too!

Adapted from McNamara 2016.

harmful aspects of nursing work (Delgado et al 2017; Foster et al 2018b; Wu et al 2023). Like burnout, resilience can be constructed as a process and interaction between an individual and their environment (Maslach 2017). This understanding of resilience recognises not only the capacity of the individual to find the resources in their environment to sustain their wellbeing, but also the capacity of their environment (family, community and workplace) to provide the resources in a culturally meaningful way (Ungar 2008). Considering resilience in this way provides balance, in that the individual nurse has some responsibility, but so too does the employer.

Resilience involves our own resources and skills; that is, managing our thoughts, emotions and responses to challenging situations. Emotional intelligence supports mental health nurses to do this and is an aspect of personal resilience (Foster et al 2018a). Emotional intelligence is the ability to recognise others' emotions, to experience and recognise our own emotions, connect our thoughts and emotions to assist in our thinking and behaviour and manage our emotions (Mayer et al 2004). The capacity to reflect on and regulate emotions is not only central to emotional intelligence, but also an important aspect of being a resilient and well-functioning mental health nurse. Understanding and managing emotions is essential for mental health nurses to be able to effectively work with consumers and carers who are often distressed. The skills of reflection, self-awareness, emotional regulation, social awareness and skilled relationship management (Delgado et al 2022) support the therapeutic use of self. Self-awareness and a strong sense of self, as described earlier in this chapter, support mental health nurses to develop resilience in dealing with the difficulties and complexities of human communication and experiences.

However, resilience also involves using the emotional and practical support we get from others and from our workplace. Universities are paying attention to developing emotional intelligence in students (Cleary et al 2018), and employers are beginning to offer programs aimed at building staff resilience (Foster et al 2018a). There is promising evidence that these programs support the development of resilience through strengthening skills to manage adversity and stress (Foster et al 2019a; Kunzler et al 2022). See Perspectives in practice: Nurse's story 8.2 on p. 107 for an example of how a nurse has maintained their resilience during their career.

Mental health nursing–specific resilience programs have been found to have an impact on the health and wellbeing of mental health nurses (Foster et al 2018a; Foster et al 2018b) through harnessing the strengths of participants, developing their cognitive, emotional, behavioural and interpersonal skills with the aim of promoting "self and affect/emotion regulation in the face of stress" (Foster et al 2018b, p. 1472). A nurse in this study described resilience as:

> ... where you grow and you learn and excel through hardship. That doesn't mean that you can't be affected by something, but that in time you use that positively, or to improve yourself, or improve your practice in some way as you go on.
>
> **(Foster et al 2018b, p. 342)**

General Health Care

As noted earlier in this chapter, nurses can neglect their own health needs. Maintaining a healthy diet, getting adequate sleep, rest and relaxation, moderating alcohol intake and maintaining exercise and fitness (Mills et al 2018b) are all important aspects of health care. Engaging in health-screening programs as appropriate, such as Pap smears and breast and prostate checks, as well as visiting a general practitioner regularly, are part of maintaining our health. Many organisations offer health programs, such as staff clinics and immunisation programs that are easily accessible to employees.

Having worked as a nurse, and with nurses, I know that asking for help with mental health issues can be particularly challenging. Organisations often offer confidential psychological services to staff to support the emotional, mental and general psychological wellbeing of their employees and immediate family members, such as the Employee Assistance Program (EAP). Services may include educative services on self-care generally or specific programs, such as resilience or mindfulness training. They also offer critical incident stress debriefing to help staff regain their equilibrium after disturbing experiences or traumatic events.

The nursing profession also offers confidential services to nurses through programs such as the Nursing and Midwifery Health Program Victoria, and the national Nurse and Midwife Support service (see Useful websites). Whether you choose to make use of the services offered by your organisation or utilise community services, attending to your own psychological and physical health is essential to keeping yourself in the best shape to engage in your professional practice.

LIFELONG LEARNING AND PROFESSIONAL DEVELOPMENT

In addition to self-care, mental health nurses need to engage in lifelong learning through professional development and further academic pursuits to maintain and develop practice throughout their careers. As you know, healthcare is an ever-changing world. The developments in technology and treatments, in understanding and preventing the causes of illness, are growing rapidly. To do our job competently as health professionals we need to be willing to continually learn and develop our knowledge and skills; to grow as clinicians.

A Growth Mindset

An important predictor of achievement is when learners have a "growth mindset". This is holding a belief that intelligence can be developed; that it is not fixed (Dweck 2015). Carol Dweck (2015) coined the term and says that people who believe their talents and abilities can be developed (i.e. that they can get smarter) through hard work, good strategies and input from others, have a growth mindset. Her research has demonstrated that people with a growth mindset achieve more than those with a fixed mindset (i.e. people who believe their talents are innate). She says this is because people with a growth mindset worry less about looking smart and put more of their energy into learning. Having a growth mindset is not just about putting effort into learning, but having a range of approaches to learning and skill development. For example, if you become stuck in the learning process, try out new strategies or seek out others to assist. Instead of looking for praise in your efforts and remaining stuck, ask for help, discuss what you have tried and what you can try next (Dweck 2015). A growth mindset is not only important to learning but also to nurses' practice and maintaining a positive sense of professional self. Engaging actively with practice, holding a positive approach to practice challenges, seeking alternatives and solutions to practice, and taking up learning opportunities in practice have been associated with mental health nurses' wellbeing and resilience (Foster et al 2023). In your graduate year you will have access to a range of supports and education that will help you maintain a passion for learning and develop a growth mindset.

Early Graduate Programs

Early graduate (or transition) programs support nurses in the transition from academic learning at university into their first experience of professional nursing practice, generally over the first year of employment and usually in a hospital setting. They have at their foundation a high level of structure and support with the aim to assist new graduates to consolidate skills and knowledge, develop confidence in practice

(Tuckett et al 2017), and assist with socialisation into the healthcare setting (Bakon et al 2018). Programs can include:
- orientation, supernumerary and study days
- preceptorship
- clinical skills and theory-based learning
- clinical exemplars and skills labs
- professional transition sessions
- feedback, reflection and debriefing (Bakon et al 2018).

Graduate programs have a positive impact on work satisfaction and intention to stay in the profession (Bakon et al 2018; Tuckett et al 2017). Strategies that can maximise your experiences in a graduate program include the following:
- Choose your hospital or health service carefully.
- Make the most of your orientation, professional development and practical support.
- Work at becoming part of the team and utilise their support.
- Give it time, but don't stay if you are really unhappy.
- Find out about your work schedule and speak out if you have difficulties (Yu & Kang 2016).
- Identify and use your team supports and clinical supervision (Hussein et al 2016).

Professional Development

In addition to graduate programs, during your career you will have opportunities to use a range of professional development resources.

Point-of-Care Learning

You have already experienced point-of-care learning when on clinical placements in your undergraduate program, where you learn and apply practice skills in the clinical setting. Point-of-care learning includes clinical teaching, clinical facilitation, buddying and preceptorship (Health Education and Training Institute 2013). You may have had the added experience of working in paid employment in a healthcare setting during your undergraduate program where you would have had the opportunity to learn more about nursing work in the clinical setting, build confidence and consolidate clinical skills (Kenny et al 2021; Willetts et al 2022). These professional development supports form part of graduate programs, but may also be available to you throughout your career, especially when joining a new team or transitioning into a new role or specialty area.

Clinical teaching is when a more experienced nurse shares professional knowledge with a less experienced nurse in the workplace.

Clinical facilitation is part of the practice development approach and has a strong focus on collaborating with teams and individuals to influence positive cultural change within a workplace. Practice development mental health nurses may be available in your workplace, and, if so, these nurses can be a valuable resource to help you develop specific skills and knowledge.

Buddying is often used for students, but also for staff starting in a new work environment. The buddy is usually a skilled and effective team member and resource who can support and engage the new team member into the workplace.

Preceptorship is a formalised relationship with an allocated preceptor who is usually a nurse with considerable experience in a specific clinical environment, and who has completed a specialised preceptor training program. The aim of preceptorship is to support the orientation and integration of the nurse into the new roles and responsibilities.

Structured Reflective Practice Relationships

Once you graduate or transition into mental health, there are other formal relationships where you engage with a colleague or group of colleagues to reflect on your practice and role. As already discussed, managing the often intense emotional work of caring for people facing life-threatening or life-changing health problems within the complex health system poses unique and often perplexing challenges for nurses. The importance of reflection in developing self-awareness has been described earlier. Participating in forums that are designed to support reflection on practice contribute to the mental health nurse making meaning of these unique and perplexing challenges.

Through reflecting *on* practice, the supervisee becomes more skilled at reflecting *in* practice and *before* practice. This increases their ability to make choices of how to respond to others (consumers, carers or staff) in the moment. This decreases reactivity and the risk of impulsive reactions, which results in the increased possibility of helpful communications, less emotional drain on the nurse and the ability for the nurse to practise with increased awareness (Freshwater 2008).

Clinical supervision is a professional development opportunity and an effective forum to reflect on practice after the event, as opposed to point-of-care learning, which is in the clinical area and very likely to occur at the time of a practice event.

Clinical Supervision is a formally structured professional arrangement between a supervisor and one or more supervisees. It is a purposely constructed regular meeting that provides for critical reflection on the work issues brought to that space by the supervisee(s). It is a confidential relationship within the ethical and legal parameters of practice. Clinical Supervision facilitates development of reflective practice and the professional skills of the supervisee(s) through increased awareness and understanding of the complex human and ethical issues within their workplace.

(Australian College of Mental Health Nurses et al 2019, p. 2)

The material discussed in clinical supervision relates to the work of the supervisee. This includes clinical care, therapeutic relationships and interactions between the nurse and consumers. Clinical supervision can also provide an opportunity for nurses to reflect on the subjective experience of their work. To develop the nurse's capacity for empathy, acceptance, nurturing and honest reflection, the clinical supervisor needs to be able to model these capacities in their relationship with the supervisee. Clinical supervision can occur in one-to-one sessions or in groups. In both settings, establishing a safe, confidential, non-blaming environment in which nurses feel able to share their clinical experiences is paramount (Australian College of Mental Health Nurses et al 2019).

HISTORICAL ANECDOTE 8.1
Origins of Clinical Supervision

The origins of clinical supervision for nurses can be traced back to Florence Nightingale, who had her own experience of depression as a young woman that she related to the intense boredom she experienced as a consequence of her privileged upbringing. After developing an interest in caring for others as a way out of her depression, Nightingale trained as a nurse at a Lutheran community in Kaiserwerth, Germany, before returning to England and gaining experience through managing a hospital for upper-class women. In 1854, the British Secretary of War, Sidney Herbert, whom she had met as part of her wealthy social circles, recruited Nightingale as chief nurse for the armed forces during the Crimean War (1853–56). During the war, Nightingale achieved fame for influential work on sanitation, introduced the concept of senior nurses guiding junior nurses in their clinical practice, and organised frequent group meetings for all grades of nursing staff, in which, through democratic process, ideas could be pooled for the general welfare of patients and staff.

Read More About It
Russell, L. 1990. Clinical supervision: History 23. Nightingale to now: nurse education in Australia. Churchill Livingstone, Sydney.

More information about clinical supervision can be found in the joint position statement for Australian nurses and midwives (Australian College of Mental Health Nurses et al 2019) and the suite of supervision documents developed for the New Zealand mental health and addiction workforce (Te Pou o te Whakaaro Nui 2023). While the New Zealand documents use the term "professional supervision", it is one and the same as clinical supervision. These documents outline what your role is as a supervisee, what to expect from a clinical supervisor and what your organisation should provide. The Australian Clinical Supervision Association is also a great resource and, in particular, offers guidance on how to choose your clinical supervisor.

Mentoring is a relationship where an experienced and knowledgeable professional (mentor) is chosen by a less experienced professional (mentee) to nurture professional growth (Olaolorunpo 2019). Mentors are usually chosen because of their personal qualities and achievements. An effective mentor invests time, effort, knowledge and expertise to nurture the professional expertise of the mentee. Mentoring is particularly useful when transitioning into a more advanced role – for example, from a registered nurse to nurse practitioner. Mentor relationships can be short term or lifelong, formal or informal, and are not mediated through employment in a particular ward or unit.

Coaching is a professional relationship that can be used for specific knowledge and skill development (Health Education and Training Institute 2013), particularly for advanced practice (Waldrop & Derouin 2019). Coaching relationships are usually over a shorter timeframe than clinical supervision or mentorship and involve a collaborative teaching, training or development process (Health Education and Training Institute 2013).

Peer review is more commonplace in medicine, but can also be utilised by nurses. It involves monitoring and improving practice, and by purposefully observing, evaluating and discussing our own work with peers, usually within a group (Health Education and Training Institute 2013). See Perspectives in practice: Nurse's story 8.2.

PERSPECTIVES IN PRACTICE

Nurse's Story 8.2: Nicola

Nicola is working in an acute inpatient unit. She has two years' experience. She arrives at clinical supervision saying she feels angry with one of her consumers, a young woman with a diagnosis of depression who self-harms. Nicola had spent considerable time with the consumer in the preceding days and felt that she had developed a good relationship with her. Last night, after she had gone home, the consumer cut her arms with a razor blade, and today she is belligerent, appearing to take delight in having "fooled" the nurses. Nicola says that the other staff have reinforced her belief that she was "sucked in" and she is now confused about how to proceed with this consumer.

The supervisor asks Nicola to tell in detail the story of what happened. She then asks Nicola to outline her feelings about, and knowledge of, the consumer before and after the incident. The supervisor listens attentively and empathically, encouraging further exploration of the incident and Nicola's feelings about it. Nicola admits to feeling guilty and is concerned that she may have said or done something to provoke the incident. Together, they consider how the consumer might have been feeling and what possible triggers to self-harm might have existed. They then consider what Nicola saw as important in developing the relationship with the consumer. The supervisor suggests some reading that Nicola could undertake to increase her understanding of self-harm-related behaviours. Together they identify what might be the goals of nursing interventions with this consumer. Nicola resolves to talk to the consumer about how the consumer was feeling on the previous night and what provoked the self-harm incident.

Ongoing Education and Training

There are numerous education and training opportunities within and external to your organisation. In addition to mandatory training (e.g. management of clinical aggression, handwashing and emergency procedures), you will have the opportunity to access a range of knowledge and skill development opportunities, so make the most of these. Also, remain open to the idea of engaging in postgraduate education. Explore options for support from within your organisation and to external scholarship providers to assist yourself in your endeavours.

Professional Supports and Organisations

As has been highlighted throughout this chapter, building positive and nurturing professional relationships has been linked to work satisfaction and resilience (Foster et al 2019a). Joining professional groups is a very effective way to do this. Te Ao Māramatanga New Zealand College of Mental Health Nursing is the professional body for practising mental health nurses in Aotearoa New Zealand. The Australian College of Mental Health Nurses is the peak professional mental health nursing organisation and the recognised credentialling body for mental health nurses in Australia. Such organisations offer conferences, professional development activities and networking opportunities. In addition to the professional knowledge that can be gained through professional organisations, many nurses have made lifelong colleagues and personal friendships through participating in their professional body throughout their career.

MAINTAINING A SATISFYING CAREER

There are many factors that contribute to work satisfaction during our careers, and some have already been described. We spend a large part of our day at work, so it is important we enjoy it. In addition, work satisfaction has been linked to increased resilience (Foster et al 2019a) and mitigates against burnout (Maslach 2017). It is important to make choices about where to work and who to work with. Carefully consider who you want as your role models, mentors and clinical supervisors. Watch how others work and ask them questions about their practice. Make choices about your professional standards and work environments. You will have many transitions throughout your career, so make sure you support yourself during these times.

Career Transitions

Life is full of transitions and stages where we move into new roles. You may remember the mixed feelings you had when finishing secondary school, moving to university or transitioning from the student role into the graduate nurse role. Role transition can be exciting, in that it precipitates many opportunities. Simultaneously there may be feelings of vulnerability and uncertainty (Bridges & Bridges 2017). Taking up a new role is a process of change from "what was" to "what is" (Duchscher 2009). There are losses and gains in that we need to let go of old ways and develop new ways; we need to adapt old skills and learn new ones (Bridges & Bridges 2017) and we need to build new role identities and self-images. The discomfort that comes with role transition is inevitable and necessary for growth to occur (Bridges & Bridges 2017).

Graduation and moving into the role of a registered nurse can be accompanied by feelings of anxiety, depression and stress (Chernomas & Shapiro 2013), with feelings of doubt, inadequacy and insecurity, a phenomenon that has been called "transition shock" (Duchscher 2009). Graduates can believe that they will be expected to know everything and doubt their capacities to fulfil the responsibilities of a registered nurse. This sense of doubt has been termed "imposter syndrome", where there is a sense of inadequacy, anxiety, lack of self-confidence, frustration and depression. It is accompanied by a tendency to question our sense of belonging to the profession and being up to the task (Christensen et al 2016).

Thankfully, transition shock and imposter syndrome are transient and, as mentioned previously, discomfort during stages of transition is a necessary part of growth and development (Bridges & Bridges 2017). If you ask most registered nurses, they will be able to recount many tales of challenging transitions, recalling the discomfort and sometimes the hilarity of what it feels like to be so unsure and excited at the same time. The beauty of nursing as a career is that there can be many of these transitions because we have so many choices about where we work and who we work with.

Work Environments

The importance of safe and healthy workplaces is being increasingly recognised and promoted (Safe Work Australia 2023). Workplaces with a positive culture are more likely to have satisfied staff, consumers and carers. The key characteristics of safe and healthy workplaces (Hart 2017) are:

- open, effective, respectful and democratic communication where there are opportunities for "speaking up" and "speaking out"
- support of the wellbeing of staff where there is access to resources, professional development and staff support programs
- strong leadership where values and professional standards are embedded
- commitment to quality care with clinical review, practice audits, open disclosure and a "no blame" culture.

Management Processes

It is important for organisations to have clear and effective management processes. These processes are organisationally driven and aim to ensure the goals, standards, procedures and guidelines of the organisation are being maintained and that the service outcomes are being achieved. They include managerial supervision, disciplinary processes, performance review, professional development planning and operational team meetings. Organisations with positive cultures engage in these processes consistently and respectfully.

Managerial supervision is usually undertaken by the nurse's line manager, who reviews both the quality and the quantity of the work and can include instruction, direction and evaluation. More senior staff may tend to have individual meetings with their line manager, whereas teams tend to meet in operational team meetings. These meetings should be regular and are a forum for reviewing team functioning and addressing team issues.

Performance review is part of managerial supervision and is where the nurse's work performance is evaluated and goals are set for the following period. Having access to open and respectful performance reviews can be invaluable in skill and career development.

In addition, use your educators, buddies, preceptors, mentors and clinical supervisors to gather feedback on your performance. Interact with them to explore your successes and failures in an honest and curious way. Not all colleagues will be able to engage in this way, so find those who can. Clarify feedback from others if it is vague or general, ask for specific examples where improvements can be made and use what you have learnt from your successes to help approach the things you find more challenging.

Clinical Management Processes

Robust clinical management processes also support nurses and are characteristic of positive work cultures. Processes such as handovers, case reviews, case presentations and grand rounds are examples of clinical management processes that provide clinicians with a place to review clinical work and to gather direct and indirect feedback on their practice.

Job–Person Fit

A key finding from research into burnout is the misfit or misalignment between the worker and the work environment (Maslach 2017). This chapter has offered a range of strategies nurses can use to reduce the risk of burnout. Maslach (2017) also highlighted the importance of getting the right "job–person fit" in reducing the risk of burnout. She identifies the following areas as important when considering how well a job is right for you:

- **Workload**: is it manageable and sustainable?
- **Control**: Do you feel heard and understood when you discuss your work issues? Do you feel you can influence decision-making that relates to your work?
- **Reward**: Do you feel valued and recognised for the contribution you make?
- **Community**: Are the relationships within the workplace supportive and safe? Are conflicts addressed?
- **Fairness**: Are the approaches taken to decision-making fair and equitable?
- **Values**: Do the values of the workplace match your professional and personal values?

Maslach (2017, p. 150) describes the "areas-of-work-life model", which has "six positive 'fits' that promote engagement and well-being can be defined as: (a) a sustainable workload; (b) choice and control; (c) recognition and reward; (d) a supportive work community; (e) fairness, respect and social justice; and (f) clear values and meaningful work".

Clinical Practice Settings

In addition to consciously considering the quality of your work environment, exercise choice about the practice settings that suit you. As has been described in other chapters of this book, mental health nurses work in a wide range of settings and practise with a variety of consumers of all ages using different models of service delivery. Gaining experience in a range of practice settings adds a depth and breadth to your practice (see Table 8.1). There are also multiple options for mental health nurses further afield. An observant father once said to me, "As a nurse you can get a job anywhere in the world". Nurses can travel the world and work in the most amazing places in developed and developing nations. The experiences and insights gained enhance your career and your life.

Expertise Development

The seminal work of Patricia Benner (1984) offered the profession an understanding of the development of nursing expertise. Her book provides numerous exemplars of nursing development through the stages of novice, advanced beginner, competent, proficient and expert practice. She shows how nurses with little or no experience draw on sets of steps and rules to practise, and as experience is gathered and reflected on, expertise in nursing practice becomes more imbedded and flexible (Benner 1984).

Expert mental health nursing practice has been demonstrated in a study that explored the nature and impact of mental health nursing (Santangelo et al 2018a; 2018b). The expert mental health nurses in this study drew on a range of experiences to develop meaningful recovery-oriented relationships with consumers and demonstrated the ability and willingness to be with consumers in the here-and-now, in both the extreme and the mundane moments of the consumer's existence. This placed the mental health nurse in a position where they could be alert to disruptions in health, and from those observations be able to gauge what needed to be done and when it needed to be done.

TABLE 8.1 Practice Settings

Setting	Description
Inpatient mental health units	Part of the nursing team that provides around-the-clock care to consumers
	Work closely with consumers and as a multidisciplinary team
	Has opportunities for increased support and professional development
Generalist inpatient settings and emergency departments	Work directly with consumers and carers
	Work alongside hospital staff
	Work with staff to increase their capacity to recognise and attend to the mental health needs of consumers in their care
	Work with organisations on mental health-related projects, education, policy development and research
Residential community care	Focus on the day-to-day functioning of consumers, supporting them to develop skills for recovery
Community	A range of options available in community services including care coordination, crisis and intensive or early intervention
	Can be clinic-based where consumers attend
	Can be outreach where the consumers are met in their own environments
Primary health care	Opportunities for early intervention
	Work alongside general practitioners and community health services
	Work with staff to increase their capacity to recognise and attend to the mental health needs of the community
	Provide assessment and counselling to consumers
Maternal and child health	Work closely with pregnant women, new mothers and their families
	Working alongside midwives and other health professionals
	Can be inpatient such as mother–baby units or community-based maternal and child health services
Alcohol and other drugs services	Can be inpatient and community settings along a continuum of care from detoxification to rehabilitation services
Forensic mental health	Range of settings including custody centres, courts, custodial diversion services, prisons and specialised forensic mental health services
Schools and tertiary education	Work with public or private and secondary or tertiary education settings
	Provide assessment and counselling services
	Address health and wellbeing of students and the school community
	Work with teachers and other staff
Asylum seekers and refugees	Work with refugees and asylum seekers
	A range of settings including onshore and offshore immigration detention centres and post-release/resettlement support and trauma services
e-mental health	Opportunity to develop web-based education and treatment programs
	Provide assessment and counselling over the internet

Advanced Practice

As discussed earlier, career transitions are necessarily uncomfortable. Often when we become proficient in one area of practice, we move to another and can feel like a novice again. Stepping into an advanced practice role for the first time is another one of those transitions. The concept of advanced practice recognises that nurses seeking career progression may wish to retain their clinical focus while incorporating aspects of research, education and leadership into their roles. Advanced practice nursing is "firmly grounded in the unique body of knowledge that is nursing" (New Zealand Nurses Organisation 2020, p. 1). Advanced practice nurses are expected to be prepared to Masters level and are able to draw on nursing and other relevant theories, critically analyse current research and provide a solid understanding and rationale for nursing interventions. Their clinical reasoning, problem-solving skills, judgement and decision-making are well developed (New Zealand Nurses Organisation 2020; Nursing and Midwifery Board of Australia 2020). It is important to note that: "*Advanced practice in nursing is demonstrated by a level of practice and is not by a job title or level of remuneration*" (Nursing and Midwifery Board of Australia 2020, p. 1).

In the past two decades, nurses in Australia and New Zealand have developed advanced practice roles that reflect contemporary clinical practice within each country. In some cases, advanced practitioners extend their practice to become a nurse practitioner, which is a protected title in Aotearoa New Zealand and Australia requiring licensing by a nursing regulatory body. The growth of advanced practice roles is part of a global development in nursing recognising the contribution that experienced clinicians make to consumer outcomes and are aimed at maximising the nursing contribution to healthcare and improving health outcomes (New Zealand Nurses Organisation 2020; Nursing and Midwifery Board of Australia 2020).

Advanced practice mental health nurses can choose to go into private practice, providing counselling and psychotherapy to individuals, families and/or groups and, if a nurse practitioner, use their expanded scope of practice to cease, initiate and monitor treatments. Mental health nurses also work as mental health nurse consultants, clinical supervisors and educators in private practice. Nurses choosing to take this path need to identify the client groups that are appropriate to their scope of practice and consider their practice location, fees charged, indemnity insurance and leave coverage.

Management

Progressing along a managerial career path is a popular option for mental health nurses. Nurse unit managers are critical to establishing and maintaining the culture and emotional climate of the unit and the quality of consumer care (Siren & Gehrs 2018). Not only has the nurse unit manager role evolved in diversity and complexity, there are also many more opportunities for management roles in health organisations. Managers have opportunities to collaborate with a range of staff and groups within and external to the organisation. As managers of clinical services, it is important to demonstrate clinical (Ennis et al 2016) and managerial (Johnson & Smith 2018) leadership. There are opportunities for ongoing formal education in management through professional development programs and tertiary institutions. In addition, mentoring, coaching and clinical supervision are invaluable supports if you choose this career path.

Education

Moving into education is another potential career path. If you are interested in educating others, look for opportunities to buddy and precept nurses coming into your practice setting. Learn how to be a good preceptor through the many programs that are available. Keep your skills up to date and develop your clinical leadership abilities (Ennis et al 2015). Within health organisations there will be opportunities for formal education positions in the clinical area and/or in professional development programs. Make use of mentors and clinical supervisors as you endeavour to understand education work and develop skills.

Consider opportunities within the academic sector, including with universities and training providers. Take up opportunities that might arise when students are on placement and liaise with the academic staff that are involved with the students. It is not uncommon that mental health nurses working clinically can take up clinical education roles with the students and have input in the classroom.

Research

Undertaking research is often seen as the domain of academics, but it is possible to be involved in research and maintain a clinical role. If opportunities arise in your practice setting, consider becoming involved to find out if it is an area you are interested in. A great way to start is to take up the role of participant when researchers are requesting a nursing perspective. You not only learn about research, but also add to the professional body of knowledge. Mental health nurses can also be part of research teams as co-investigators or as research assistants or research leads. Mental health nurses can conduct research through postgraduate study on issues of clinical significance through a research Masters (commonly referred to as a Master of Philosophy or MPhil) or a PhD (Doctor of Philosophy). Mental health nurses in New Zealand and Australia continue to make a significant contribution to research on the international stage. It is a terrific buzz when you receive feedback from colleagues that your research work has made a difference.

CHAPTER SUMMARY

This chapter has described self-awareness and self-care as essential strategies to maintain wellbeing, to be able to provide compassionate care to consumers and carers, to maintain productive working relationships with colleagues, to manage the demands of mental health nursing practice and to sustain a rewarding career. Mental health nursing is a rich and rewarding career with its own challenges and workplace stressors. This chapter has provided information on these challenges and introduced concepts such as emotional labour, vicarious trauma and, as the process of positive adaptation to stressors, resilience. Individual nurses, organisations and the mental health nursing profession all play a part in supporting nurses' professional self-care and development. Understanding the impact of nursing work and developing strategies for addressing workforce health and stress management is an encouraging and developing body of knowledge. Systems of support for mental health nursing are emerging all the time. A nursing career provides an opportunity to work in a range of environments with diverse people and communities. It is also a career of lifelong learning and ongoing professional development. Reflecting on the information in this chapter will assist you to establish healthy self-care and professional development practices early in your career, which will serve you well as you progress through your work in nursing.

PERSPECTIVES IN PRACTICE

Nurse's Story 8.3: Julie Sharrock

I have been a nurse for a long time, at least four decades in fact. And like most older people, I say things like: "It feels like yesterday that I was a young woman starting out as a nurse". I have always been interested in working with people and I also wanted to travel; nursing gave me both.

Nursing gave me the opportunity to understand the dimensions of the human condition. I witnessed the polarities of resilience and vulnerability co-existing in the people I cared for. I was exposed to the absolute mystery of suffering and death. To be with people at the extreme times of their existence has been a privilege, but it has not been without its challenges. In my early years as an intensive care nurse I was close to burnout. Thankfully I had access to staff counselling, which helped me avoid completely imploding. I realised that I was using a lot of energy being angry at the health system and its shortcomings. I also learnt that I had choices about what causes to fight for and which jobs to take. These have proved to be important lessons and have helped me to stay in the public health system for most of my working life.

I knew I wanted to be a mental health nurse when I had my first mental health placement. This was after a classmate and I overcame our overwhelming feelings when confronted by a locked women's ward in an old psychiatric institution. By lunchtime on my first day I knew one day I would do my psychiatric nurse training. When I did, I knew I had found my niche and I really found my passion when I became a consultation-liaison nurse in a general hospital. I particularly loved the combination of clinical and education work, as well as contributing to quality improvement and becoming involved in research.

The challenges of working with people (consumers, relatives and staff) are ever-present. I have often been asked how I do the work I do and, without doubt, a key component of my survival in health care is good clinical supervision. I continue to enjoy travel and I have had the opportunity to combine travel with my work through conference attendances. In addition, I have maintained my interests outside of work, including the surf and the snow, the arts, creative pursuits and of course family and friends. I used my cycling commute (incorporating mindful practices) to bookend my working day. I have engaged in lifelong learning through academic and professional development programs, as well as personal growth. Professional associations have always formed part of my support system, and spending time with like-minded colleagues is always energising. I have loved the opportunity to write this chapter and share with you some ideas about how to get the most out of your nursing career. I want you to love nursing as much as I have.

EXERCISES FOR CLASS ENGAGEMENT

An effective way of developing self-awareness is to use questioning. To raise your awareness of some important issues, ask yourself the following questions, and then discuss your responses with other members of your group or class.

1. What kinds of values do I hold important as a framework for living? Where do these values come from? How do they inform my understanding of what it is to be a person in this world?
2. How has my family of origin influenced how I view the world? What values did my family hold as important? What do I see as important in family life?
3. What do I know about why I chose to be a nurse? Does this still hold true or have my ideas changed over time?
4. What are the pervading social attitudes towards people in mental distress or with mental illness? What are my beliefs about people in mental distress or with mental illness?
5. What experiences have I had that influence how I feel about people with mental illness?

? CRITICAL THINKING EXERCISE 8.1

Reflect on your personality style and unique characteristics:
• How can these characteristics support you in your work?
• How might these characteristics increase your vulnerability in your work?
Reflect on your supports within and outside of work:
• What energises you?

• What calms you?
• Who or what would you turn to if you did not feel you were coping?
How can you use these insights to support yourself during your nursing career?

ACKNOWLEDGEMENT

This chapter includes some information adapted from chapters in previous editions of this book by Debra Jackson and Louise O'Brien.

USEFUL WEBSITES

Australian Clinical Supervision Association: clinicalsupervision.org.au/
Australian College of Mental Health Nurses: acmhn.org/
Centre for Post-traumatic Mental Health: www.phoenixaustralia.org/your-recovery/
Health Direct: www.healthdirect.gov.au/
Manatū Hauroa Ministry of Health: www.health.govt.nz/
Nurse and Midwife Support Program: www.nmsupport.org.au/
Nursing Health and Midwifery Program Victoria: www.nmhp.org.au/
Te Ao Māramatanga New Zealand College of Mental Health Nursing: www.nzcmhn.org.nz/
Te Pou o te Whakaaro Nui: www.tepou.co.nz/

REFERENCES

Australian College of Mental Health Nurses, Australian College of Midwives & Australian College of Nursing, 2019. Position statement: Clinical supervision for nurses and midwives Online. Available at: www.acn.edu.au/wp-content/uploads/clinical-supervision-nurses-midwives-position-statement-background-paper.pdf

Badu, E., O'Brien, A. P., Mitchell, R., Rubin, M. James, C. et al., 2020. Workplace stress and resilience in the Australian nursing workforce: A comprehensive integrative review. Int J Ment Health Nurs, 29(1), 5–34.

Bakon, S., Craft, J., Wirihana, L., Christensen, M., Barr, J. et al., 2018. An integrative review of graduate transition programmes: Developmental considerations for nursing management. Nurse Educ Pract, 28(1), 80–85.

Benner, P., 1984. From Novice to Expert. Addison-Wesley, Menlo Park.

Benuto, L., Singer, J., Cummings, C., Ahrendt, A. 2018. The Vicarious Trauma Scale: Confirmatory factor analysis and psychometric properties with a sample of victim advocates. Health Soc Care Comm, 26(4), 564–571.

Biber, D. 2022. Mindful self-compassion for nurses: A systematic review. Nurs Manage, 29(3), 18–24.

Bolton, S.C., 2000. Who cares? Offering emotion work as a "gift" in the nursing labour process. J Adv Nurs, 32(3), 580–586.

Bonamer, J., Aquino-Russell, C., 2019. Self-care strategies for professional development: Transcendental meditation reduces compassion fatigue and improves resilience for nurses. J Nurses Prof Dev, 35(2), 93–97.

Bridges, W., Bridges, S., 2017. Managing Transitions: Making the Most of Change, 4th ed. Nicholas Brealey Publishing, London.

Chen, R., Sun, C., Chen, J.J., Jen, H-J, Kang X.L. et al., 2021. A large-scale survey on trauma, burnout, and posttraumatic growth among nurses during the COVID-19 pandemic. Int J Ment Health Nurs, 30(1), 102–116.

Chernomas, W.M., Shapiro, C., 2013. Stress, depression, and anxiety among undergraduate nursing students. Int J Nurs Educ Scholarsh, 10(1), 255–266.

Chiang, Y.M., Chang, Y., 2012. Stress, depression, and intention to leave among nurses in different medical units: Implications for healthcare management/nursing practice. Health Policy, 108(2–3), 149–157.

Chopra, D., 2023. 7 mind-body practices to transform your relationship with stress. Online. Available at: chopra.com/articles/7-mind-body-practices-to-transform-your-relationship-with-stress

Christensen, M., Aubeeluck, A., Fergusson, D., Craft, J., Knight, J. et al., 2016. Do student nurses experience Imposter Phenomenon? An international comparison of final year undergraduate nursing students readiness for registration. J Adv Nurs, 72(11), 2784–2793.

Christensen, S.S., Wilson, B.L. Hansen, S.D. 2022. Using affective events theory to conceptualise nurses' emotional behaviour: A scoping review. Collegian, 1(30), 147–153.

Christie, C., Bidwell, S., Copeland, A., Hudson, B. 2017. Self-care of Canterbury general practitioners, nurse practitioners, practice nurses and community pharmacists. J Prim Health Care, 9(4), 286–291.

Cleary, M., Visentin, D., West, S., Lopez, V., Kornhaber, R. 2018. Promoting emotional intelligence and resilience in undergraduate nursing students: An integrative review. Nurse Educ Today, 68(9), 112–120.

Cranage, K., Foster, K., 2022. Mental health nurses' experience of challenging workplace situations: A qualitative descriptive study. Int J Ment Health Nurs, 31(3), 665–676.

Cross, L.A., 2019. Compassion fatigue in palliative care nursing: A concept analysis. J Hosp Palliat Nurs, 21(1), 21–28.

Delgado, C., Evans, A., Roche, M., et al., 2022. Mental health nurses' resilience in the context of emotional labour: An interpretive qualitative study. Int J Ment Health Nurs, 31(5), 1260–1275.

Delgado, C., Upton, D., Ranse, K., Furness, T., Foster, K. 2017. Nurses' resilience and the emotional labour of nursing work: an integrative review of empirical literature. Int J Nurs Stud, 70(5), 71–88.

Di Mario, S., Cocchiara, R.A., Torre, G L., 2023. The use of yoga and mindfulness-based interventions to reduce stress and burnout in healthcare workers: An umbrella review. Altern Ther Health Med, 29(1), 29–35.

Dragioti, E., Tsartsalis, D., Mentis, M., Mantzoukas, S., Gouva, M. 2022. Impact of the COVID-19 pandemic on the mental health of hospital staff: An umbrella review of 44 meta-analyses. Int J Nurs Stud, 131(7), 104272.

Duchscher, J.E.B., 2009. Transition shock: The initial stage of role adaptation for newly graduated registered nurses. J Adv Nurs, 65(5), 1103–1113.

Dweck, C., 2015. Carol Dweck revisits the growth mindset. Education Week, 22 Sept, 35, 20–24.

Edward, K.L., Hercelinskyj, G., Giandinoto, J.A., 2017. Emotional labour in mental health nursing: An integrative systematic review. Int J Ment Health Nurs, 26(3), 215–225.

Ennis, G., Happell, B., Reid-Searl, K., 2016. Intentional modelling: A process for clinical leadership development in mental health nursing. Issues Ment Health Nurs, 37(5), 353–359.

Ennis, G., Happell, B., Reid-Searl, K., 2015. Enabling professional development in mental health nursing: The role of clinical leadership. J Psychiatr Ment Health Nurs, 22(8), 616–622.

Flatekval, A. M. 2023. Utilizing a mindfulness application in the nursing classroom. Reflective Pract, 24(1), 113–123.

Foster, K., Evans, A., Alexander, L., 2023. Grace under pressure: Mental health nurses' stories of resilience in practice. Int J Ment Health Nurs, 32(3), 866–874.

Foster, K., Roche, M., Delgado, C., Cuzzillo, C., Giandinoto, J.A., et al., 2019a. Resilience and mental health nursing: An integrative review of international literature. Int J Ment Health Nurs, 28(1), 71–85.

Foster, K., Roche, M., Giandinoto, J.A., Furness, T., 2019b. Workplace stressors, psychological well-being, resilience, and caring behaviours of mental health nurses: A descriptive correlational study. Int J Ment Health Nurs, 29(1), 56–68.

Foster, K., Cuzzillo, C., Furness, T., 2018a. Strengthening mental health nurses' resilience through a workplace resilience programme: A qualitative inquiry. J Psychiatr Ment Health Nurs, 25(5–6), 338–348.

Foster, K., Shochet, I., Wurfl, A., et al., 2018b. On PAR: A feasibility study of the Promoting Adult Resilience programme with mental health nurses. Int J Ment Health Nurs, 27(5), 1470–1480.

Freshwater, D., 2008. Reflective practice: The state of the art. In: Freshwater, D., Taylor, B., Sherwood, G. (eds), International Textbook of Reflective Practice in Nursing. Wiley-Blackwell, Oxford.

Giannakakis, G., Pediaditis, M., Manousos, D., Kazantzaki, E., Chiarugi, F., et al., 2017. Stress and anxiety detection using facial cues from videos. Biomed Signal Process Control, 31(1), 89–101.

Gómez-Ochoa, S.A., Franco, O.H., Rojas, L.Z., et al., 2021. COVID-19 in health-care workers: A living systematic review and meta-analysis of prevalence, risk factors, clinical characteristics, and outcomes. Am J Epidemiol, 190(1), 161–175.

Hart, B., 2017. Identify barriers to best practice. Lamp 74, 18–19.

Hawkins, P., Shohet, R., 2012. Supervision in the Helping Professions. Open University Press, Maidenhead, UK.

Health Education and Training Institute, 2013. The Superguide: A Supervision Continuum for Nurses and Midwives. Health Education and Training Institute, Sydney.

Hochschild, A.R., 1983. The Managed Heart: Commercialization of Human Feeling. University of California Press, Berkeley.

Hofmeyer, A., Kennedy, K., Taylor., R. 2020. Contesting the term "compassion fatigue": Integrating findings from social neuroscience and self-care research. Collegian, 232–237.

Humphrey, R.H., Ashforth, B.E., Diefendorff, J.M., 2015. The bright side of emotional labor. J Organ Behav, 36(6), 749–769.

Hur, G., Cinar, N. & Suzan, O.K. 2022. Impact of COVID-19 pandemic on nurses' burnout and related factors: A rapid systematic review. Arch Psychiatr Nurs, 41(12), 248–263.

Hussein, R., Everett, B., Hu, W., et al., 2016. Predictors of new graduate nurses' satisfaction with their transitional support programme. J Nurs Manag, 24(3), 319–326.

International Council of Nurses (ICN), 2021. International Council of Nurses COVID-19 update. Online. Available at: www.icn.ch/news/covid-19-effect-worlds-nurses-facing-mass-trauma-immediate-danger-profession-and-future-our

Jenkins, E.K., Slemon, A., O'Flynn-Magee, K., Mahy, J. 2019. Exploring the implications of a self-care assignment to foster undergraduate nursing student mental health: Findings from a survey research study. Nurse Educ Today, 81, 13–18.

Johnson, C.S., Smith, C.M., 2018. Preparing nursing professional development practitioners in their leadership role: Management and leadership skills. J Nurses Prof Dev, 34(2), 99–100.

Johnson, J., Hall, L.H., Berzins, K., Baker, J, Melling, K. et al., 2018. Mental healthcare staff well-being and burnout: A narrative review of trends, causes, implications, and recommendations for future interventions. Int J Ment Health Nurs, 27(1), 20–32.

Joinson, C., 1992. Coping with compassion fatigue. Nursing, 22(4), 116–121.

Kabat-Zinn, J., 2023. Guided mindfulness meditation with Jon Kabat-Zinn. Online. Available at: www.mindfulnesscds.com/.

Keller, E., Hittle, B.M., Smith, C.R. 2023. Tiredness takes its toll: An integrative review on sleep and occupational outcomes for long-term care workers. J Gerontol Nurs, 49(10, 27–33.

Kelly, E.L., Fenwick, K., Brekke, J.S., Novaco, R.W. 2016. Well-being and safety among inpatient psychiatric staff: The impact of conflict, assault, and stress reactivity. Admin Policy Ment Health 43(5), 703–716.

Kenny, A., Dickson-Swift, V., DeVecchi, N., Phillips, C. Hodge, B. et al., 2021. Evaluation of a rural undergraduate nursing student employment model. Collegian, 28(2), 197–205.

Khazan, I. 2019. Biofeedback and mindfulness in everyday life: Practical solutions for improving your health and performance. WW Norton & Company, New York.

Köse, S., Baykal, B., Bayat, İ.K. 2021. Mediator role of resilience in the relationship between social support and work life balance. Aust J Psychol, 73(3), 316–325.

Kox, J.H.A.M., Bakker, E.J.M., Bierma-Zeinstra, S., Runhaar, J., Miedema, H.S., et al., 2020. Effective interventions for preventing work related physical health complaints in nursing students and novice nurses: A systematic review. Nurse Educ Pract, 44, 102772.

Kunzler, A. M., Chmitorz, A., Röthke, N., Staginnus, M, Schäfer, S.K., et al., 2022. Interventions to foster resilience in nursing staff: A systematic review and meta-analyses of pre-pandemic evidence. Int J Nurs Stud, 134, 104312.

La Torre, G., Leggieri, P.F., Cocchiara, Dorelli, B., Mannocci, A. et al., 2022. Mindfulness as a tool for reducing stress in healthcare professionals: An umbrella review. Work, 73(3), 819–829.

Laker, C., Cella, M., Callard, F., Wykes, T. 2019. Why is change a challenge in acute mental health wards? A cross-sectional investigation of the relationships between burnout, occupational status and nurses' perceptions of barriers to change. Int J Ment Health Nurs, 28(1), 190–198.

Larter, A., 2014. Nurses need healing. Nurs Rev, 3, 4.

Leary, M.R., Price Tangney, J. (eds), 2012. Handbook of Self and Identity. Guilford Press, New York.

Lloyd, J., 2019. A hospital is the place to heal a ravaged body, but what about a wounded spirit? Aust Nurs Midwifery J, 26(6), 23.

Maslach, C., 2017. Finding solutions to the problem of burnout. Consult Psychol J Pract Res, 69(2), 143–152.

Maslach, C., Leiter, M.P., 2017. New insights into burnout and health care: strategies for improving civility and alleviating burnout. Med Teach 39(2), 160–163.

Mayer, J.D., Salovey, P., Caruso, D.R., 2004. Emotional intelligence: Theory, findings, and implications. Psychol Inq 15(3), 197–215.

McNamara, P., 2016. Hand hygiene and mindful moments. Online. Available at: web.archive.org/web/20220925023523/

Mercer, M., Stimpfel, A.W. Dickson, V.V., 2023. Psychosocial factors associated with alcohol use among nurses: An integrative review. JNR, 13(4), 5–20.

Mills, J., Wand, T, Fraser, J.A. 2018a. Examining self-care, self-compassion and compassion for others: A cross-sectional survey of palliative care nurses and doctors. Int J Palliat Nurs, 24(1), 4–11.

Mills, J., Wand, T., Fraser, J.A., 2018b. Exploring the meaning and practice of self-care among palliative care nurses and doctors: A qualitative study. BMC Palliat Care, 17, 1–12.

Mills, J., Wand, T., Fraser, J.A., 2015. On self-compassion and self-care in nursing: Selfish or essential for compassionate care? Int J Nurs Stud, 52(4), 791–793.

Milner, A.J., Maheen, H., Bismark, M.M., Spittal, M.J. 2016. Suicide by health professionals: A retrospective mortality study in Australia 2001–2012. MJA, 205(6), 260–265.

Muir-Cochrane, E., O'Kane, D., Oster, C., 2018. Fear and blame in mental health nurses' accounts of restrictive practices: Implications for the elimination of seclusion and restraint. Int J Ment Health Nurs, 27(5), 1511–1521.

New Zealand Nurses Organisation, 2020. Position Statement: Advanced Nursing Practice, 2020. Online. Available at: www.nzno.org.nz/resources/nzno_publications

Nursing and Midwifery Board of Australia, 2020. Fact sheet: Advanced nursing practice and specialty areas within nursing. Online. Available at: www.nursingmidwiferyboard.gov.au/Codes-Guidelines-Statements/FAQ.aspx

Olaolorunpo, O. 2019. Mentoring in nursing: A concept analysis. Int J Car Sci, 12(1), 142–148.

Park, C.L., 2010. Making sense of the meaning literature: An integrative review of meaning making and its effects on adjustment to stressful life events. Psychol Bull, 136(2), 257.

Patel, K.M., Metersky, K., 2022. Reflective practice in nursing: A concept analysis. Int J Nurs Knowl, 33(3), 180–187.

Perry, L., Xu, X., Gallagher, R., et al., 2018. Lifestyle health behaviors of nurses and midwives: The "fit for the future" study. Int J Environ Res Public Health 15(5), 945.

Phoenix Australia, 2022. What is trauma? Centre for Posttraumatic Mental Health, University of Melbourne. Online. Available at: phoenixaustralia.org/recovery/fact-sheets-and-booklets/

Prosser, S.J., Metzger, M., Gulbransen, K., 2017. Don't just survive, thrive: Understanding how acute psychiatric nurses develop resilience. Arch Psychiatr Nurs, 31(2), 171–176.

Ross, A., Touchton-Leonard, K., Perez, A., Wehrlen, L., Kazmi, N., et al., 2019a. Factors that influence health-promoting self-care in registered nurses: Barriers and facilitators. ANS Adv Nurs Sci, 42(4), 358.

Ross, A., Yang, L., Wehrlen, L., et al., 2019b. Nurses and health-promoting self-care: Do we practice what we preach? J Nurs Manage, 27(3), 599–608.

Russell, L., 1990. Clinical Supervision: History 23. Nightingale to Now: Nurse Education in Australia. Churchill Livingstone, Sydney.

Sabery, M., Tafreshi, M.Z., Hosseini, M., et al., 2018. Compassion fatigue in clinical nurses: An evolutionary concept analysis. J Nurs Midwifery, 27(3), 7–14.

Safe Work Australia, 2023. Australian Work Health and Safety (WHS) Strategy 2023–2033. Australian Government, Canberra.

Safe Work Australia, 2018. Australian Work Health and Safety Strategy 2012–2022: Healthy, Safe and Productive Working Lives. Safe Work Australia, Canberra.

Sahay, S., Wei, W. 2023. Work–family balance and managing spillover effects communicatively during COVID-19: Nurses' perspectives. Health Commun 38(1), 1–10.

Salzmann-Erikson, M., 2018. Moral mindfulness: the ethical concerns of healthcare professionals working in a psychiatric intensive care unit. Int J Ment Health Nurs, 27(6), 1851–1860.

Santangelo, P., Procter, N., Fassett, D., 2018a. Mental health nursing: Daring to be different, special and leading recovery-focused care? Int J Ment Health Nurs, 27(1), 258–266.

Santangelo, P., Procter, N., Fassett, D., 2018b. Seeking and defining the "special" in specialist mental health nursing: a theoretical construct. Int J Ment Health Nurs, 27(1), 267–275.

Searby, A., Burr, D., Taylor, G., et al., 2023. Alcohol consumption among Australian nurses: A cross-sectional national survey study. Collegian. 30(3), 440–448.

Siren, A., Gehrs, M., 2018. Engaging nurses in future management careers: Perspectives on leadership and management competency development through an internship initiative. Nurs Leadersh, 31(4), 36–49.

Sun, P., Wang, M., Song, T., et al., 2021. The psychological impact of COVID-19 pandemic on health care workers: A systematic review and meta-analysis. Front Psychol 12(7), 626547.

Sweet, L., Bass, J., Sidebotham, M., et al., 2019. Developing reflective capacities in midwifery students: enhancing learning through reflective writing. Women Birth 32(2), 119–126.

Te Pou O Te Whakaaro Nui, 2023. Supervision. Online. Available at: www.tepou.co.nz/initiatives/supervision

Theodosius, C., 2008. Emotional Labour in Health Care: The Unmanaged Heart of Nursing. Routledge, New York.

Thomson, A.F., Smith, N., Karpa., J. 2022. Strategies used to teach professional boundaries psychiatric nursing education. Iss Ment Health Nurs, 43(10), 895–902.

Torquati, L., Kolbe-Alexander, T., Pavey, T., et al., 2018. Changing diet and physical activity in nurses: a pilot study and process evaluation highlighting challenges in workplace health promotion. J Nutr Educ Behav, 50(10), 1015–1025.

Tuckett, A., Eley, R., Ng, L. 2017. Transition to practice programs: What Australian and New Zealand nursing and midwifery graduates said. A Graduate eCohort Sub-Study. Collegian, 24(2), 101–108.

Ungar, M., 2008. Resilience across cultures. Br J Soc Work, 38, 218–235.

Waldrop, J., Derouin, A., 2019. The coaching experience of advanced practice nurses in a national leadership program. J Contin Educ Nurs, 50(4), 170–175.

Whiteing, N., Massey, D., Rafferty, R., et al., 2022. Australian nurses' and midwives' perceptions of their workplace environment during the COVID-19 pandemic. Collegian, 30(1), 39–46.

Willetts, G., Nieuwoudt, L., Olasoji, M., et al., 2022. Implementation of a Registered Undergraduate Student of Nursing (RUSON) program: The nurses' perspective. Collegian, 29(1), 70–77.

Wilson, D.R., Brooks, E.J., 2018. Sleep and immune function: nurse self-care and teaching sleep hygiene. Beginnings, 38, 6–23.

World Health Organization (WHO), 2018. International Classification of Diseases – revision for mortality and morbidity statistics (11th rev,). Online. Available at: www.who.int/classifications/icd/en/

Wu, C.F., Liu, T.H., Cheng, C.H. et al., 2023. Relationship between nurses' resilience and depression, anxiety and stress during the 2021 COVID-19 outbreak in Taiwan. Nurs Open, 10(3), 1592–1600.

Yilmaz, A.N., Derya, Y.A., Altiparmak, S., et al., 2022. Investigating the relationship between the depression levels of midwives and nurses and their emotional labor and secondary traumatic stress levels in the COVID-19 pandemic period with structural equation modelling. Arch Psychiatr Nurs, 40, 60–67.

Yu, J.F., Ding, Y.M., Jia, R.Y., Liang, D-D., Wu, Z. et al., 2022. Professional identity and emotional labour affect the relationship between perceived organisational justice and job performance among Chinese hospital nurses. J Nurs Manag, 30(5), 1252–1262.

Yu, M., Kang, K.J., 2016. Factors affecting turnover intention for new graduate nurses in three transition periods for job and work environment satisfaction. J Contin Educ Nurs, 47(3), 120–131.

Zugai, J.S., Stein-Parbury, J., Roche, M., 2018. The nature of the therapeutic alliance between nurses and consumers with anorexia nervosa in the inpatient setting: A mixed-methods study. J Clin Nurs, 27(1–2), 416–426.

PART 2

Knowledge for Practice

9

Mental Health Assessment

Graham Holman and Michelle Cameron

KEY POINTS

- Assessment, the consideration of facts and the collection and processing of information, is integral to clinical reasoning, and is ongoing throughout each episode of care.
- The primary focus purpose of mental health nursing assessment is to understand the mental health distress and problems the person is experiencing and what nurses can do to help.
- Mental health reflects a person's physical, mental, spiritual and emotional characteristics, the dynamic interaction with family, community and environment, and is strongly influenced by social determinants of health.

- Mental health nursing assessment can involve both conversational and structured interviews, in addition to nursing observation and information from third parties.
- Clinical formulation is the process of developing, with the consumer, a summary of the various influences on the consumer's current problems, and how the consumer and clinician can work towards resolving those problems.

KEY TERMS

- Assessment
- Case formulation
- Clinical reasoning
- Cultural assessment
- Diagnosis
- Differential diagnosis
- Documentation
- DSM-5
- Holistic
- ICD-11
- Integrated health assessment
- Interviewing
- Mental state assessment
- Physical health assessment
- Risk assessment
- Screening
- Spiritual assessment
- Standardised assessment
- Strengths assessment
- Triage

LEARNING OUTCOMES

The material in this chapter will assist you to:

- understand the purpose and process of mental health nursing assessment
- utilise a model of comprehensive mental health nursing assessment in clinical practice

- discuss the place of holistic health assessment within comprehensive mental health nursing assessment
- conduct and document a mental state assessment
- discuss the relationship between assessment and clinical decision-making.

INTRODUCTION

Assessment is one of the most important and fundamental skills of the mental health nurse. Through assessment we can develop an understanding of consumers, collaborate with them and their families on a plan of care, and contribute to the decision-making of multidisciplinary teams. A comprehensive assessment encompasses multiple aspects of consumers' lives, including current and past mental health problems, physical health, family and social history, use of alcohol and other drugs, and cultural and spiritual influences on mental health. Assessment focuses on problems in the consumer's life, as well as the strengths and capabilities available to the person to respond to those challenges. As the consumer's recovery progresses, assessment will reflect the developing understanding between the consumer and the nurse, new issues in response to support and treatment, and the

consumer's development of new coping skills and strategies for maintaining wellbeing.

This chapter outlines the process of mental health nursing assessment. Assessment is explained both as a structured process in which the nurse seeks to gather important information about the consumer's history and functioning, and as an exploratory process in which the nurse and the consumer review their understandings of the nature of the consumer's problems, and the care and treatment the consumer is receiving. The aim is always one of clarifying the shared understanding that provides the basis of nursing care. The chapter also introduces current models of assessment and the various skills of mental health nursing assessment, such as taking a history, assessing mental state, using standardised assessment instruments, clinical formulation and diagnosis.

ASSESSMENT AND NURSING

Assessment is fundamental to mental health nursing and provides the platform on which nursing care is delivered (Coombs et al 2011; Wand et al 2019). Nurses are the single largest group of professionals in mental health care and are well positioned throughout the continuum of care to make significant contributions to care delivery. Nursing assessment is carried out in a variety of settings, throughout each episode of care and at key transition points, such as discharge and admission. Assessment makes a significant contribution to diagnosis and treatment planning. Mental health nursing assessment adds to the decisions about the care provided by nurses and other members of the multidisciplinary team. As such, nursing assessment is both an independent activity and is interdependent with the treating team.

Despite the potential strengths of mental health nursing assessment, there is a lack of clarity over what this entails in practice (Coombs et al 2013a). The published research literature does little to help here. There is evidence that nurses often gather assessment information in the course of other "simple social activities", such as making a cup of tea (Coombs et al 2013b). However, nurses also have difficulty in articulating a model of mental health nursing assessment, and current models do not always reflect nursing's commitment to person-focused care (Wand et al 2019; Wand et al 2022). Nurses rely on the eclectic nature of nursing, their own intuition and a "tacit, experiential model of assessment" (MacNeela et al 2010, p. 1298) when assessing consumers. The lack of a clear description and demonstration of what constitutes a nursing mental health assessment has historically contributed to this essential activity being viewed as less than substantial and less reliable than assessment by other team members (MacNeela et al 2010). This chapter provides a clear way through this maze and offers both a framework for mental health nursing assessment and a description of the key tasks of assessment.

Professional Standards and Mental Health Nursing Assessment

In addition to being a set of clinical skills, assessment is also a professional obligation of mental health nurses. All nurses are expected to be able to conduct a comprehensive assessment, and this core skill is reflected in nursing standards for practice. Standard 5 of the Nursing and Midwifery Board of Australia (NMBA) competency standards states that nurses can "conduct a comprehensive and systematic assessment" (NMBA 2016), while Competency 2.2 of the Nursing Council of New Zealand (NCNZ) competencies for registered nurses states that the registered nurse "undertakes a comprehensive and accurate assessment of health consumers in a variety of settings" (NCNZ 2007). The New Zealand College of Mental Health Nurses standards expect mental health nurses to have knowledge of "contemporary models of assessment and clinical decision making" (Te Ao Maramatanga New Zealand College of Mental Health Nurses 2012). Professional standards, together with the skills to articulate the findings to others, contribute to sound mental health nursing assessment.

CRITICAL THINKING EXERCISE 9.1

Why is assessment considered fundamental to nursing practice? Why is it important to develop skills in assessment as a basis for any nursing intervention?

Trauma

Trauma is a major contributor to developing mental illness and is a common experience among people in health care settings, and especially in people with mental illness (Duhig et al 2015; Loewy et al 2019).

Approaches to assessment conversations require an appreciation that trauma may not be visible, and of the intersectionality of social, cultural and historical trauma (Sweeney et al 2018). Experiences of trauma may emerge in any clinical interaction. In many cases you will not need to make a specific inquiry about trauma, but you do need to be prepared to respond empathically to disclosures about trauma and to offer any further intervention or referral, if necessary. Consumers commonly feel their experience of trauma is discounted in healthcare services, so any disclosure should be validated, together with the opportunity for further exploration. Trauma can take many forms, including bullying, physical violence, sexual assault, intimate partner violence, neglect, exposure to traumatic events such as war or military conflict, torture or refugee experiences. Trauma should be approached with tact and sensitivity. Clinicians need to be alert for indications that the consumer does not currently feel safe to discuss experiences of trauma and in such cases should leave exploration of trauma until a more appropriate time. This decision needs to be communicated to the consumer, together with an explanation of how the consumer can seek further help.

Approaches to an Integrated Health Assessment

In Chapter 2, a socio-ecological approach to mental health nursing practice was identified as supporting effective practice. Health assessment requires a whole-person view and has the consumer and their family at the centre of their care (Cameron et al 2022). Person-centred care in the assessment context includes consideration of physical comfort, the involvement of family and friends and respect for the person's preferences and values (Brown & Jeon 2021). In order to achieve the latter, the nurse will need to spend time in connecting with the person, establishing a mutual understanding that the consumer, as an active participant in their own care, has expertise in their own experience of health (Brown & Jeon 2021).

Integrated health assessment encompasses a comprehensive consideration of needs, and additionally encourages equal consideration of the different, interrelated domains of holistic health and wellbeing. Robust evidence highlights that stress and distress can have significant impacts on physical health and on the resilience and identity of individuals, families and communities (Doan et al 2022; Te Pou 2020). Likewise, poor physical health, social isolation, or challenges with cultural, spiritual and personal identity, can adversely affect mental health and wellbeing (Doan et al 2022). An assessment approach that reflects this clinical reality offers opportunities to directly address what the consumer experiences as their priorities, itself key to engaging people in care. Additionally, holistic health assessment can be an opportunity to offer health promotion advice, part of the role of the registered nurse (NCNZ 2007; NMBA 2016).

In an example from Aotearoa New Zealand, integration is inclusive of how an assessment interview is structured to support culturally responsive practice, an aspect of the socio-ecological approach to nursing. In this example, integration is facilitated by the Hui Process as part of the Meihana model (Fig. 9.1). This underpins the establishment of a trusting and responsive "nurse–patient"/whānau relationship (Minton et al 2022; Pitama 2014). Within the Meihana model, understanding and implementation of the Hui Process is essential for relationship-building with health consumers. Literature from Australia also highlights the connection between cultural safety in nursing practice and holistic approaches to assessment and health promotion (Molloy et al 2021).

CRITICAL THINKING EXERCISE 9.2

What methods of nursing assessment are you familiar with? How can they be used in a mental health clinical setting?

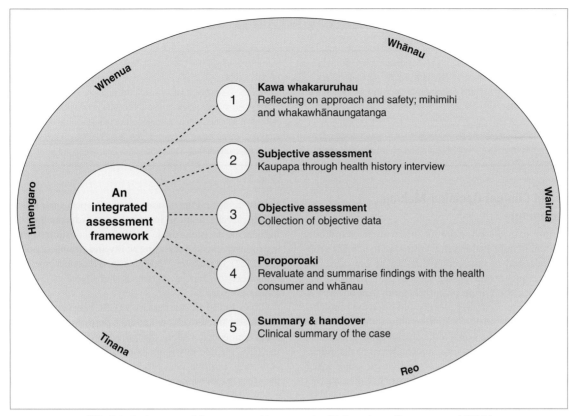

FIG. 9.1 An Integrated Assessment Framework – Mahere hau. (Cameron et al 2023.)

Assessing Strengths

Assessment of strengths considers the personal resources that consumers can access to manage their mental health concerns (Rapp & Goscha 2012). Strengths-based assessment provides an opportunity to understand the context of a consumer's situation and their life beyond their current distress or challenge. This narrative is integral to providing balance to an assessment process that may be structured to highlight pathology and problems (Wand et al 2020). Many consumers have had years of experience of adversity and self-management, and have developed individual and interpersonal strategies for preventing and responding to their issues. Consumers who are newly presenting to mental health services will also have developed life skills that will be valuable to them in coping with their mental health challenges. As in all areas of mental health nursing assessment, developing a therapeutic rapport is essential for understanding the strengths a consumer may have. At times of crisis, consumers may feel they have no available strategies, so it is important initially to respond to the consumer's current concerns and distress before exploring strengths. Assessing strengths involves inviting the consumer to identify their individual strategies and how they have responded to life challenges in the past. Rather than being the expert, the nurse needs to ask what they can learn from the consumer. Examples of individual strengths that consumers may identify include pleasurable activities that provide distraction and reduce stress, the availability of family members and friends, spiritual beliefs, and skills learnt in stress management and problem-solving.

■ PERSONAL PERSPECTIVES

Consumer's Story 9.1: Gareth Edwards

I'd never been in a police cell before. Without a comparison, or a *Lonely Planet* guide to incarceration, I assumed it was your bog-standard police cell. Concrete block walls painted institutional grey with hint of drab, a formidable steel door and a thin bench and/or bed next to a half-wall discreetly housing a metal toilet. So at least I got an en suite. It was very much like a room at an airport hotel, though with possibly a little more charm. Not exactly what most people would think of as an ideal environment for a "health assessment". But then assessment is different in mental health than physical health. There are no blood tests, MRI scans or even an old man in a leather-elbowed jacket tapping your knee with a fairy hammer. Sometimes you might get a questionnaire, like those Facebook games that tell you if you are "an extrovert who likes to stay home" or "an introvert who likes to go out". But mostly my assessment in-

volved a psychiatrist looking at the way I talked and behaved and deciding if I was fit for society.

In the cell, the assessment took less than a minute. Though all it actually did was buy the system some time by sectioning me for 28 days for further assessment. Assessment then became a 24/7 activity. It's hard enough being paranoid without knowing that your every moment is under close scrutiny by people who are writing secret notes about you.

Then every week there was "the day" when you were formally assessed. My most vivid memory was sitting in the ward lounge with over a dozen strangers with clipboards and being asked, "How are you today?". "Er ... intimidated and overwhelmed" would have been an accurate answer. However, assessment in mental health once you are sectioned is less about "How are you?" and more

Continued

Consumer's Story 9.1: Gareth Edwards

about "Will this end up in the headlines if you are discharged?" So, when asked "How are you?" the right answer is "Not a threat to myself or others". Once you have found a way to say and demonstrate that, you are rewarded with your freedom. And then you can really start answering the question "How am I?"

"Health assessment" in mental health is mostly "risk assessment". The small "health" portion is more like those shape-matching toys toddlers have.

If it looks enough like depression, you go through the antidepressants-shaped hole. If it looks enough like mania or psychosis, you go through the antipsychotics-shaped hole. And if you don't fit the holes neatly, you are called "complex" and pushed through anyway, like a frustrated child pushing a star-shaped block through a square-shaped hole. And if all this sounds pretty bleak, it is. But the worst part is no-one ever does a "final assessment" to say you are no longer ill. Like a puppy bought at Christmas time, assessment is for life.

Assessment and Clinical Decision-Making (Clinical Reasoning)

Assessment is more than the extraction of information (Wand et al 2022). The collection of information is for a purpose; to identify problems, establish goals, and to take action that can be evaluated and reflected upon. Assessment is the pulling together and analysis of different sources of information, from potentially more than one assessment moment, in order to accurately identify and prioritise problems. Effective engagement with consumers and families about their needs and circumstances requires the nurse to be able to think critically in their decision-making and clinical judgements. Mental health nurses need to have an awareness of how the personal lens through which they gather information, observe people and experience the care they

are providing and the response to it influences their practice. Engaging in critical reflection can include acknowledgement of the nurse's bias influencing decisions made in relation to consumers, who are presenting to services with increasing acuity and complexity of need (Maguire et al 2022). In Chapter 2, it is identified that nursing practice is directly influenced by nurses' personal characteristics, which makes self-awareness essential.

The Clinical Reasoning Cycle (CRC) (Levett-Jones et al 2010) is a systematic framework for guiding person-centred care with assessment embedded within the process (Fig. 9.2). The eight steps of the CRC include intentionally considering the context and situation, collecting information, processing information, identifying needs or issues, establishing goals, taking action, evaluating outcomes and

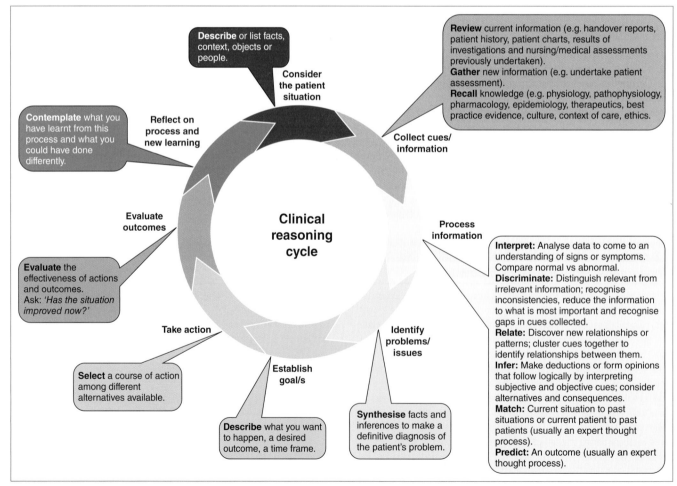

FIG. 9.2 Clinical Reasoning Cycle. (Levett-Jones 2010.)

reflecting on the process. The CRC offers a non-linear framework, enabling assessment, analysis and discussion that encourages critical thinking and reflection (Maguire et al 2022). Assessment tells us about the effectiveness and acceptability of mental health nursing care.

Effective comprehensive health assessment uses a recognised nursing assessment framework to clarify the purpose of the encounter, strengths, health history and risks, and to formulate goals for care. Clinical reasoning supports nursing practice that brings together the threads of mental health nursing assessment; the weaving together by the clinical practitioner of process, content, interpretation and communication (see Box 9.1, Fig. 9.3). The completion of a robust comprehensive assessment requires the interplay of complex skills, including those of critical thinking and reasoning, and ultimately leads to a sound nursing formulation and care planning.

A suggestion for new graduates is to focus on developing competency in each thread of assessment. While the threads are interdependent, each also has its own skills. Focusing on individual threads will provide a transparent pathway for skill acquisition. Perspectives in practice: Nurse's Story 9.1 looks at how assessment works in community mental health nursing.

BOX 9.1 The Threads of Mental Health Nursing Assessment

Assessment comprises several main threads woven together:
- **process:** *the way* information is gathered, including the therapeutic relationship, observation, rating instruments and informal/formal methods
- **content:** *what* information is gathered, such as defining the presenting problem, mental health history, mental state, physical health review and substance use
- **interpretation:** the *meaning* ascribed to the above content that is jointly understood by the consumer, the nurse and the treating team and informs treatment planning (nursing and other theories help the nurse in the process of interpretation)
- **communication:** the *articulation* of the assessment – formulation, sharing of assessment information, presentation of assessment at handover, multidisciplinary team meetings and clinical review, and documentation (the written record of assessment findings).

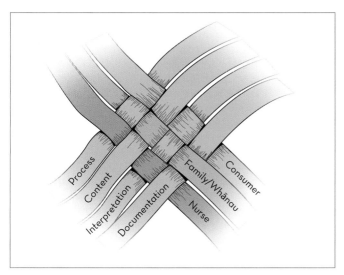

FIG. 9.3 The Threads of Mental Health Nursing Assessment. (Adapted from the Ministry of Education New Zealand, CC BY 3.0 NZ.)

Nurse's Story 9.1: Tania Smith

As a new graduate on the New Entry to Specialty Practice (Mental Health and Addiction) (NESP) program, assessment and diagnosis are utilised daily within my role as a community mental health nurse case manager. This is an autonomous role where I am required to be proactive within a variety of settings from multidisciplinary meetings to liaising with non-government organisations to seek guidance and support regarding my assigned caseload. First and foremost, both professional and therapeutic relationships need to be established to ensure that my assessment and nursing diagnosis is at a consistent level of professionalism to be an advocate and support person for service users on my assigned caseload. I have an affinity with Dr Mason Durie's Te Whare Tapa Wha framework (Māori model of health assessment) (Pitama et al 2014), and with the utilisation of biopsychosocial comprehensive assessment and relapse prevention plan documentation. I am able to obtain an all-encompassing view of not only the service user's mental and physical health, but also a comprehensive history and their understanding of their situation. I utilise this information to assist service users' journeys to wellness, along with being able to monitor their individual progress.

On completion of my "supernumerary" 6-week period with my preceptor, I was effectively "let loose". Not surprisingly, around this time the enormity of "I was now it!" struck, and I found myself doubting my ability to work within the community on my own. After in-depth discussions with my colleagues and other NESP graduates, I found I was not alone in feeling this way and this was considered a normal reaction. Personal acknowledgement and processing of the huge leap across a seemingly endless chasm from a third-year nursing student to registered nurse, responsible for my own caseload, was a lot to decipher.

There are several factors that need to be taken into account when working within the community environment and developing the skill to identify the nuances of when service users are experiencing increased problems. I incorporate a mental state assessment within my notes, which assists in identifying specific issues in a service user's presentation. No one expects me to be an expert as a new grad, but I am expected to build on my core assessment skills and, as time goes on, my individual practice and professional development reflect my learning and growth. Initially, the hardest questions I found to ask were along the lines of: "Have you cut yourself since I saw you last?", "Do you want to harm others?", "Are you having thoughts of suicide?" When the answer is yes to any or all of the above, then your questioning for your assessment teases out the risk component. As my own practice continually develops, it is apparent that a core understanding of not only the nursing process but also a holistic health model assists to form a "whole picture" of service users, along with input from identified key support people and agencies. Working within a supportive environment is invaluable, and this has assisted my learning and growth immensely. This is reflected in my personal growth and confidence as a community mental health nurse case manager.

Assessment is Ancient

One of the earliest known methods of mental health assessment was invented by the Roman politician and lawyer Cicero (c. 63 BC). He invented an interview schedule that sought to collect the following information: (1) nomen (clan/tribe, region); (2) natura (sex, nationality, family status, age, physique); (3) victus (education, habits/lifestyle); (4) fortuna (rich/poor, free/slave, social class); (5) habitus (appearance); (6) affectio (passions, emotions, temperament); (7) studium (interests); (8) consilium (motivation); (9) factum (working history); (10) casus (significant life events); and (11) orationes (form and content of discourse). Use of similar interview schedules for mental health assessment spread throughout the Roman Empire.

Read More About It
King, H. (ed.) 2004. Health in Antiquity. Routledge, New York.

INFORMATION GATHERING

Mental health nursing assessment can be thought of as comprising two key tasks: developing an understanding of each consumer and their perspectives of their current situation, and collecting and interpreting assessment information (which can be assessed using standard tools and templates). The tasks of assessment should not determine the process of assessment, which can include a variety of methods from conversational interviewing, with its focus on the individual narrative to completing consumer- or clinician-rated assessment instruments (Barker 2004). Skilled mental health nurses combine the tasks in any assessment and can move between the more descriptive approach of seeking specific information and the exploratory approach of narrative inquiry. Both approaches have an important place in comprehensive assessment, and together they yield a fuller understanding of each consumer and contribute to developing rapport and a therapeutic relationship.

Mental health nursing assessment uses formal and semi-formal tools, as well as a range of interpersonal processes. It can sometimes seem that the tools of nursing assessment, such as the assessment templates provided by clinical services, dominate the assessment process, due to their requirement to collect a large amount of detailed information. Services usually require clinicians, often nurses, to complete risk assessment forms in which assessment information is used to establish levels of risk. In addition, standardised assessment tools such as mood rating scales, risk scales, symptom scales and measures of cognitive functioning may appear to reduce assessment to eliciting answers to a "tick box" rather than exploring with consumers the meaning of their experiences. The essence of mental health assessment lies in understanding a person's experience through developing rapport and trust in a way that is collaborative and strength focused. This is key to gathering subjective information (see Box 9.2). The collection of objective information, such as vital signs or laboratory tests, can be equally important in formulating an understanding of what is happening for a person and then planning care, and also relies on positive interpersonal engagement.

METHODS OF SUBJECTIVE INFORMATION GATHERING

Mental health nursing assessment uses a range of methods, including structured and conversational interviews, standardised assessment instruments, diaries, direct observation and information from third parties including friends and family and clinical records. All these methods have a common purpose: to enhance our understanding of the person seeking mental health care and to help with the problems that led them to seek mental health care. In this section we describe the assessment methods of interviews, mnemonics, standardised assessment tools, diaries, direct observation and information from third parties. Box 9.3 provides an overview of the differences between screening, assessment and diagnostic tools.

Preparation for Assessment

Before undertaking a comprehensive assessment interview, the nurse needs to consider several factors in order to provide person-centred care, be trauma-responsive, as well as engage with the CRC. This includes preparation of the assessment space and any equipment, as well as active consideration of physical, emotional and psychological safety for everyone. Once the interview commences, time needs to be taken to connect and build rapport in a way that meets the needs of the consumer and their family (Australian College of Mental Health Nurses 2010). The nurse should clarify and document that the consumer gives informed consent for the assessment to continue, allowing time to answer specific questions. If consent is not able to be obtained and yet the consumer remains in the assessment space and engages with the interview in some way, this should also be documented.

Time-Critical Needs

It is important not to assume that the referral or triage information the nurse takes into the assessment identifies the most acute issue for the consumer. Nurses should not assume that a person will tell you if they are experiencing pain or physical discomfort that may be symptoms requiring urgent investigation. Therefore, it is important to clarify early on in the process of engaging with someone if they are experiencing time-critical concerns. Clarifying time-critical needs can be explored through specific prompts with closed-ended questions or an open-ended approach by inquiring about an individual's comfort. Such concerns may include physical discomfort, safety concerns or immediate health risks. These need to be managed first, with an individual's safety and comfort prioritised before the assessment process continues.

BOX 9.2   Subjective and Objective Information Gathering

A comprehensive nursing assessment includes the collection and synthesis of subjective and objective information, the latter of which may include physical assessment/examination techniques.

Subjective Information Examples	Objective Information Examples
• Personal information	• Aspects of mental state assessment/examination
• Preferences	• Vital signs
• Experiences	• Laboratory results
• Beliefs and ideas	• Data related to nutritional status
• Values	• Data related to metabolic health
• Perceptions	
• Feelings	
• Thoughts	
• Desires	
• Sensations or symptoms	

Adapted from Lewis & Foley 2020.

BOX 9.3   Defining Screening Tools, Assessment Tools, and Diagnostic Tests

Screening tools are brief questionnaires or rating tools that may be part of routine ward or service procedures to examine potential unrecognised health and social risk factors or asymptomatic disease. This will determine whether further, more in-depth assessment is needed on a specific area of concern, such as family harm, mental health, trauma, substance use. Some screening tools have been empirically developed and are statistically validated and reliable. Screening is part of a preventative health approach that can mitigate symptoms or adverse events, or prevent serious illness or loss of function. Examples include the Kessler Psychological Distress Scale and the Depression Anxiety Stress Scale (DASS). Screening tools alert the clinician to the presence of symptoms and do not diagnose consumers.

Assessment tools support systematic inquiry of a particular issue or offer a structure for approaching history taking. Examples include the Camberwell Assessment of Need (CAN) and the Mental State Assessment.

Diagnostic tests and tools are tests, procedures or criteria that can clarify a clinical impression gained from subjective or other objective data collection. Examples include the *Diagnostic and Statistical Manual of Mental Disorders, 5th Edition* (DSM-5), and performing an electrocardiogram (ECG).

Interviews

An assessment interview can be thought of as a relatively structured conversation that has specific goals: to elicit information about the consumer, to help the nurse understand the consumer's problems and to develop a plan of care. While it is possible to describe a structured assessment interview as a logical series of topics – such as the consumer's reason for presentation, history of mental health problems and social history – in practice, assessment interviews rarely follow a prescribed course. Interviewing is a core skill of mental health nursing and requires a range of nursing skills. Interviews may be brief or lengthy, depending on the demands of the situation and the needs of the consumer. Interviews may also be formal or informal, and in practice a combination of formal and informal approaches may be necessary. Nurses need to be flexible in their approach to interviews and be ready to change their planned approach as the interview progresses. In particular, at times it may be necessary to stop an interview – for example, if it proves to be too distressing for the consumer, or if the consumer is not able to concentrate on the interview process. In developing their interview skills, nurses should take opportunities to work with different colleagues from the multidisciplinary team and to observe how colleagues conduct interviews, manage the complex issues that arise, and engage with consumers around difficult and sensitive issues, such as experiences of trauma, identity, thoughts of self-harm and risk to self and others.

Interviews are more manageable if the nurse and the consumer have a clear idea of the purpose and goals of the interview, the time available and the possible outcomes of the interview. Because the outcomes of an interview depend on the problems identified, their severity and the support available, outcomes should initially be stated in general terms, such as clarifying current problems and planning future care rather than, for example, deciding on whether hospital admission is necessary. Although the nurse should always have a plan for an interview, and should be clear about its purpose, the interview should begin informally. The nurse should briefly explain the purpose of the interview and provide an opportunity for the consumer to make opening comments about their current concerns. This may include discussing any concerns the consumer has about the interview, such as privacy or confidentiality, what will happen to the information collected and possible outcomes of the interview. From there, the interview can either focus on the concerns expressed by the consumer or begin with background discussion that will provide a wider context for understanding the presenting issues.

It is not possible to prescribe the exact order of an interview – that will largely depend on the needs of the consumer at the time. The interview should begin with general questions and proceed to more specific questions as rapport develops and the consumer's concerns become clearer. In this way, the more sensitive areas of assessment can be included naturally in the interview and will seem less intrusive. Some consumers will freely discuss their concerns and may need to be provided with structure to manage issues one at a time. Others may be withdrawn or less forthcoming and may need more prompting with specific questions. The flow of the interview can be determined by the consumer's responses, although the nurse has to be aware of the need to achieve the aims of the interview. An unstructured interview that simply follows its own course, unguided by a sense of purpose, is of little use to the consumer. It will not help to clarify problems or to decide on an appropriate plan of care.

As the interview progresses, the nurse should be attentive to the verbal and non-verbal responses of the consumer and to any changes in those responses as the areas of discussion change. A consumer who begins with good eye contact and an open body posture may close up when discussing distressing events, giving valuable clues to the intensity of the feelings involved. The nurse carries responsibility for keeping the interview "on track" and avoiding digressions that do not help the assessment process. It may be necessary at some points to comment when an interview is losing focus and to gently redirect the focus to the main issues. If friends or family members are present, the nurse will need to manage their participation, sometimes by encouraging comments and at other times asking that comments be limited until a more appropriate point in the interview. Interviews are designed to elicit sensitive issues from consumers/clients, and it is critical that the nurse acknowledges these issues and validates the consumer's experience. A skilled interviewer will provide opportunities to discuss important issues, but will also move the interview on so all important aspects can be covered.

Interview Settings

Interviews take place in a range of locations, and nurses need to be able to adapt their interview skills according to the setting. These settings include primary care offices, community clinics, consumers' homes, emergency departments (EDs), in-patient wards, general hospital wards, courts, prisons and police stations. In planning an interview, the nurse needs to consider the safety of the consumer and themselves, privacy, adequate seating (especially if multiple family members are to be involved), and the availability of the interview room. Some settings, such as general hospital wards or consumers' homes, may present difficulties in ensuring privacy, and, whenever possible, an area separate from the consumer's bed space should be sought. The ideal setting is a separate room that is close to other work areas and that provides adequate space and privacy.

Safety in Conducting Interviews

In arranging an interview, the nurse needs to be mindful of the consumer's safety and their own. An interview can be a challenging experience for a consumer, who may feel vulnerable in the presence of health professionals. Gender, ethnicity and age differences may also contribute to a consumer's feeling of vulnerability. Family members or friends may be present at the interview, although the support they provide needs to be balanced against their potentially inhibiting effect on the interview process. The consumer also needs to consent to the family member or friend being present and should be asked about this confidentially, so they are able to express their preference free of any sense of obligation or coercion.

Another safety consideration is the mental state of the consumer. Before the interview begins the nurse will have some indication of the consumer's level of distress, ability to tolerate the nurse's questions and willingness to participate in the interview. It is often advisable for a second clinician to be present, both as a means of supporting the first clinician and to respond to any difficulties that may arise. In conducting the interview, the nurse needs to continuously assess the consumer's mental state and take steps if the consumer becomes too distressed. If the nurse feels threatened by the consumer's attitude or behaviour (e.g. the emergence of paranoid ideas or anger directed at the nurse), consider abandoning the interview. The nurse should always advise other team members where they will be conducting an interview and how long they expect to take. This allows colleagues to be aware of the consumer and nurse's whereabouts and to be available if additional support is needed.

Managing Potential Problems in the Interview Process

With the best possible plan, and the best attempt to develop rapport, it is still possible that an interview may become "bogged down" with limited dialogue. There may be interpersonal tension between the nurse and the consumer, or the consumer may have difficulty answering questions or be reluctant to discuss certain topics. There can be many reasons for problems in the interview process, and the nurse should not assume that the source of the problems is the consumer. Problems may arise from cultural, age or ethnicity differences, the nurse's attitude or non-verbal behaviours, as well as factors to do with the interview setting, such as noise, limited time and an uncongenial environment. As in any therapeutic interaction, difficulties in the interview process should be acknowledged and discussed as part of the process. Methods to help an interview progress include deferring topics until later, asking questions in different ways, exploring reasons for a consumer's discomfort with specific topics, and acknowledging that some issues are hard to discuss. It may be necessary to defer some areas of assessment to a later time, once rapport has been firmly established. This can be acknowledged at the time of the interview, so the consumer is not left feeling that these issues cannot be addressed. Finally, if the consumer becomes too distressed to continue with the interview, this can be acknowledged and the interview terminated with a plan for further assessment later.

Summarising and Concluding

As the interview concludes, the nurse should begin to move the discussion towards a shared understanding of what has been achieved, clarification of presenting problems and discussion of possible interventions and further care. This can involve the nurse offering a summary or asking the consumer to provide a summary. This phase of the interview provides an opportunity to engage the consumer in a plan of care that recognises unresolved problems and draws on the consumer's strengths and supports. The nurse should indicate when the allotted time for the interview is almost up, so the consumer is able to introduce any issues not previously discussed. Friends or family members can also be invited to ask final questions at this stage. It can be helpful for the nurse to ask if there are any questions the consumer wishes to raise about the assessment information, further care and so on. Summarising can provide an opportunity to further validate the consumer's concerns. If the nurse feels unsure about the best course of action following an interview, they should openly discuss this with a co-interviewer and include the consumer in that discussion. Acknowledging uncertainty does not need to undermine confidence in the nurse or the clinical service, but can be an opportunity for the nurse to share different perspectives on the assessment and future plan. It is important at the end of an interview to establish what has been agreed upon, as well as where there may be differences between the nurse and the consumer. The interview should terminate with discussion of the next step in terms of further care and confirmation of contact details. While an assessment interview is designed to establish a broad understanding of a consumer and the problems they seek help with, it is not the only assessment tool available to nurses. Even the best interviews provide only a limited range of information, and the interview needs to be supplemented with other sources of information.

Direct Observation

Of all the professionals involved in mental health care, nurses have the most direct contact with consumers. In inpatient settings this can include contact in the context of activities of daily living, such as care of the bed area, meals and social activities. Other forms of contact are in providing medication, running therapeutic activities such as groups or teaching sessions, and discussing issues such as leave requests. In community settings, nurses may have contact with consumers in their homes, in community clinics or at a consumer's workplace. Any contact with a consumer is an opportunity to make direct observations of mental state, physical health, socialisation patterns, side effects of medication and other areas. Direct observations can be "triangulated" with the consumer's self-reports, the observations of other nurses or clinicians and observations of third parties, such as friends or family members. Nurses can gain a great deal of information from other clinicians and from clinical notes, but there is no substitute for seeing, talking to and interacting with the consumer. Your assessment and experience of engaging with a person may seem very different from the picture suggested from other sources, or from your past understanding.

Interviews should be seen as a form of nursing intervention, thus requiring the interpersonal skills of attending, empathy, listening, reflection, paraphrasing and responding, which are inherent in mental health nursing practice. In an interview, the nurse is inviting the consumer to share sensitive and personal information, so it is essential that the nurse approaches the interview with an attitude of respect and a genuine interest in what the consumer has to say. The nurse needs to be available to the consumer, which means not being distracted by other commitments or obligations, and responding to the concerns the consumer expresses. Establishing rapport is essential to conducting an interview. The nurse needs to spend the initial part of the interview developing rapport and then maintain that rapport as the interview progresses. Any issues of cultural or language differences need to be acknowledged as they would in any therapeutic interaction. In considering the development of interview skills, it is helpful to review the principles of therapeutic communication outlined in Chapter 3. Some questions and responses that can be used in interviews are listed in Table 9.1.

Diaries

Diaries are records of important experiences that are kept by consumers for their personal use or in collaboration with clinicians. A diary might record feelings, thoughts, activity levels, interpersonal interactions, food intake or other self-observations. They can help to actively engage the person in their care, contributing to assessment and increasing the consumer's self-awareness of important areas of functioning. Diaries can be helpful in developing your understanding of consumers because they contain information that might not be accurately remembered. They have been shown to help intensive care unit (ICU) patients recover psychologically from what can be a traumatising experience, with the numbers of people who have been exposed to ICU care and mechanical ventilation increasing exponentially with the spread of COVID-19 (Lomax 2021). If you are going to use a diary as part of an assessment, you need to explain its purpose to the consumer, clarify what is to be recorded and discuss how the diary will contribute to care.

Third Party Information

In addition to information obtained directly from the consumer, nurses use information from friends and family members, other clinical services and clinical records. In obtaining information from family members you need to be mindful of confidentiality and potential conflicts between family members. Some consumers welcome the involvement of their family; others prefer not to have family involved (Cameron et al 2022). By using a collaborative approach, nurses can explore the potential contribution of family members to care and the important role played by families in supporting their loved one. Families have a unique perspective on the care of their loved one and often remind mental health clinicians that it is they who know the consumer best. From the above description of the methods of mental health nursing assessment, note that information contributing to an understanding of the consumer as a person comes from a variety of sources. These include consumers, nurses' subjective and objective

TABLE 9.1 Questions and Responses for Assessment Interviews

Consumer's Statement	Nurse's Response	Comment
"I don't know where to start."	"Perhaps if we begin by talking about what brought you into the (clinic/hospital/service) today?"	At the beginning of the interview the consumer may feel overwhelmed by the issues they are facing. A concrete question or statement can help in initiating dialogue.
"I've been seeing my GP for depression, but it's not getting better."	"Can you tell me more about the depression? How bad has it been?"	By using the term "depression" the nurse communicates that they are listening and are aware of the significance of the problem.
"The voices are there all the time. They never leave me alone."	"That sounds very difficult for you. Tell me more about the voices. What sorts of things do they say?"	The nurse's responses are designed to validate the consumer's experience and to encourage dialogue about the voices.
"I feel so hopeless; I can't seem to do anything right."	"It can feel really bad when nothing is going right for you."	This response focuses on the consumer's emotional state and need to have their distress recognised.
"I sometimes wish it was all over."	"Are you saying that you don't want to be alive any longer?"	Consumers may talk indirectly about suicidal thoughts. A direct question can help the consumer to acknowledge suicidal thoughts and can be followed up with further exploration of these thoughts, including intent, available means, etc.

observations, interviews, information from rating scales and information from a range of other people and clinical records. No one source of information is enough on its own, and some of the information from various sources may appear to conflict with each other. The skill of mental health nursing assessment is to use the range of information available to build a picture of the consumer as a person, to develop a shared understanding of what problems the consumer is seeking help with and a plan of how the nurse and other members of the multidisciplinary team can help with the identified problems. Perspectives in practice: Nurse's story 9.2 illustrates how the scope and purpose of nursing assessment can be expanded.

Mnemonics

Mnemonics (or acronyms) are aids to memory that prompt the nurse to ask specific questions or consider specific areas of assessment. Mnemonics are non-standardised structured assessment tools that provide a convenient reminder when undertaking an assessment.

For example:

- OLDCART can be used for assessing pain, where the letters stand for Onset, Location, Duration, Characteristics, Aggravating factors, Radiation and Timing (Chase 2015).
- The HEADSS assessment is used in youth services, where the letters stand for Home, Education, Activities, Drug and alcohol use, Sexuality and Suicide (Eade & Henning 2013). There are many variations of the HEADSS assessment format, and HEADSS can be adapted for your own practice.
- The SAD PERSONS mnemonic (Sex, Age, Depression, Prior suicidality, Ethanol (alcohol) abuse, Rational thinking, Support systems, Organised support system, No significant other, Sickness) can be used to assess suicidality (Patterson et al 1983). This mnemonic should be used only as a prompt to memory, not as a rating instrument, as the scoring system of SAD PERSONS has no validity in predicting future self-harm (Warden et al 2014).

Mnemonics remind clinicians of important areas of inquiry, but do not result in a numerical score. Because they are not standardised, mnemonics may be used differently by different clinicians. Important assessment findings resulting from use of mnemonics identify areas for further assessment.

Standardised Assessment Tools

In some areas of mental health nursing assessment, standardised instruments are used to gain a quantified measure of some aspect of

PERSPECTIVES IN PRACTICE

Nurse's Story 9.2: Antony Abbey

Reflecting on my early exposure to assessment as a student mental health nurse in 1981, I observed it initially as a linear and two-dimensional procedure. It appeared at the time to sit definitively within the context of gathering information. Clients were on the receiving end of this activity. They (or others who knew of them) would provide information in accordance with a set of questions and observations. Nursing care, although linked to the assessment, was a discrete and subsequent step within an overall process.

I discovered along the way that assessment becomes buoyant and three-dimensional when it allows the client to explore the less familiar and sometimes unknown corridors of his psyche. When this occurs, there is an opportunity for discovery, catharsis and positive change. In this sense, assessment becomes a therapy in its own right. Good questions are enabling, as are the variety of standardised assessment tools that are available. It is also useful to approach the assessment with a comprehensive framework in mind. But we should not be restricted and contained by these tools. We should stop, open up and listen to the client's story, picking up on cues and gently guiding, much like the style that is eloquently described by Brown (1995) in her conversational approach to the assessment interview.

Take the example of Mr C, a man in his 40s who was admitted to the general hospital with severe headache, left-sided weakness and paraesthesia. After medical causes were ruled out, I was asked, within the context of my psychiatric liaison nurse role, if I could help to unravel the mystery of this presentation. Mr C's personal story was one of hard work, stoicism and battling along in the face of any adversity. Emotional expression was not a language that he knew. His narrative was also one of significant recent stressors. It was a story of loss, redundancy and housing and financial struggles. Within the safety of a confidential and non-judgemental setting, and enabled by a conversational approach, Mr C discovered a dialectic side to his story. He discovered that he had been caged in by his emotional illiteracy and "stiff upper lip" rule. He realised that it didn't have to be that way. Supported with a further three or four sessions, with a focus on learning the language of emotion, Mr C was freed from his rule. He was supported also with developing new tools to help him accept and deal with emotional distress so that he could perhaps be liberated from his somatic manifestation.

Mr C is now free of his neurological symptoms and is working successfully through many of the stressors that he struggled with. So, for this clinician, assessment and intervention work together in partnership, but also have interchangeable properties. Assessment as a therapy is one of the most satisfying interventions that a psychiatric nurse can deliver.

psychological or social functioning – for example, mood, cognitive functioning, risk or alcohol problems. Wood and Gupta (2017) provide an overview of some useful rating scales. Of the many instruments available, nurses will use only a small number, but it is helpful to be aware of the range of instruments available and their application to clinical practice. A list of commonly used standardised assessments that nurses can incorporate into their practice is shown in Table 9.2. All the instruments listed in the table can be used by nurses in their clinical practice, although in each case training is required to ensure reliable administration of the instrument. Training can occur in formal staff development sessions or as part of supervised clinical practice. Some instruments are subject to licensing, so before using any instrument check whether your service holds the necessary licence.

Standardisation refers to the statistical evaluation of instruments aimed at ensuring their reliability and validity. Standardised instruments can be regarded as screening tools that alert clinicians to a problematic area of mental health and signal the need for further assessment. An important consideration in using standardised instruments is that they should not be regarded as complete assessments: they do not replace comprehensive assessment. Instead, they augment clinical assessment by providing a uniform means of measuring one aspect of functioning. Most instruments have cut-off scores; that is, scores that indicate levels of severity, need for treatment or need for further assessment. Standardised instruments contribute to assessment in several ways. They provide a benchmark – for example, of mood or cognitive functioning – and a basis for comparing the same area of functioning at some future time. Comparing scores over time allows the clinician to determine any improvement or deterioration in the area measured. This can be very helpful in assessing the response to medication or other interventions, or to determine whether the consumer's problems are escalating, indicating a need for a review of the treatment plan. Standardised measures also allow teams of clinicians to communicate about the extent of a problem, knowing that each is using the same criteria to estimate the level of severity. Another advantage is that they remind clinicians of questions they should ask in assessment. For example, the Alcohol Use Disorder Inventory Test (AUDIT) asks 10 specific questions about alcohol use; without this tool, clinicians may not remember all 10 questions in the course of an interview.

Instruments can be either clinician- or consumer-rated. Self-rated instruments enable consumers to report various experiences to the nurse that they might find hard to express in words. For example, someone who is very depressed might find it difficult to verbalise their low mood, but might be able to indicate low mood on a rating form that requires only a tick. If you are using a standardised instrument, take the opportunity to discuss the instrument with the consumer and use the findings to develop collaborative means of addressing significant problems. As clinical problems improve, the changes measured on a standardised instrument can provide the consumer with reassurance of their improvement. On a cautionary note, it is important to consider the conditions under which a standardised instrument is used. We all feel anxious if we feel we are being assessed, and consumers may feel that the findings of an instrument will be used to show there is something wrong with them, or that a "score" does not sufficiently describe their experience.

TABLE 9.2   Standardised Assessment Instruments

Test	Purpose	Description
Cognitive Functioning		
MMSE (Mini-Mental State Examination) (Folstein et al 1975)	Measure cognitive impairment	An 11-item test that provides a cut-off score indicating significant cognitive impairment
ACE-R (Addenbrooke's Cognitive Examination—Revised) (So et al 2018).	Measure cognitive impairment	A 26-item test that provides cut-off scores for severity of cognitive impairment; ACE-R incorporates the 11 items of the MMSE
CAM (Confusion Assessment Method) (Inouye et al 1990)	Screen for delirium	An 11-item instrument to detect delirium; CAM measures four different areas of cognitive functioning
Substance Use		
AUDIT (Alcohol Use Disorder Inventory Test) (Babor et al 2001)	Detect the presence of alcohol problems	A 10-item test available in clinician- or consumer-rated formats; AUDIT provides cut-off scores for four levels of clinical intervention
Mood		
BDI (Beck Depression Inventory) (McPherson & Martin 2010)	Screen for clinically significant depression	A 21-item self-report of experiences of low mood, with cut-off scores for levels of depression severity; subscales can be used to assess suicidality
GDS (Geriatric Depression Scale short form) (Burke et al 1991)	Screen for clinically significant depression in older adults	A 15-item clinician-administered instrument with three cut-off scores representing different levels of depression severity
Medication Side Effects		
LUNSERS (Liverpool University Neuroleptic Side Effect Rating Scale) (Day et al 1995)	Identify the presence of side effects of antipsychotic medication	A 51-item clinician- or consumer-administered instrument that rates areas of medication side effects on a five-point Likert scale; provides scores for seven different areas of medication side effects
Risk of Violence		
HCR-20 (Historical Clinical Risk Management Scale) (Jaber & Mahmoud 2015)	Assess risk of violence	A 20-item clinician-rated instrument that combines historical, current clinical and future risk factors
Non-Specific Mental Health Problems		
GHQ 12 (General Health Questionnaire) (Tseliou et al 2018)	Detect risk of developing mental illness in primary care populations	A 12-item clinician-rated instrument that provides a single cut-off score indicating possible mental illness

Anxiety about completing a rating instrument will adversely affect the results, so it is important that the nurse creates optimal conditions for using the instrument and takes account of factors, such as age, literacy level, sensory deficits, pain and discomfort, and the explanation provided for using the test.

 CRITICAL THINKING EXERCISE 9.3

Read the list of standardised assessment instruments included in Table 9.2 and consider the areas of psychological and social functioning they address. How could one of these instruments help you in performing a comprehensive nursing assessment?

TYPES OF ASSESSMENT

Triage

Triage refers to the assessment that takes place when a consumer first contacts a health service. A consumer may present with self-harm, hearing voices, self-neglect or suicidal thoughts. Presentations may involve use of alcohol or other substances. Triage assessments may occur in the ED, at community mental health clinics, at ambulance callouts, in primary care settings or in private homes. Triage may also be conducted by telephone. The aims of triage are to establish how urgent the problem is, any immediate safety issues and the immediate priorities for health service response.

In an ED setting, clinicians may use an instrument such as the Australasian Triage Scale (see Useful websites), which has five categories of increasing urgency of response, with a response time associated with each category. A modified version of the Australasian Triage Scale has been found to have the strongest evidence for use in an emergency setting, although supportive evidence for use of such instruments in general is very limited (Watson et al 2022). Questions to be addressed in mental health triage are outlined in Box 9.4. Triage is usually followed by comprehensive assessment, once immediate issues of safety have been addressed.

Comprehensive Assessment

This section explains the components of the comprehensive assessment process. Most services will have a template for initial assessment and may have an additional template for risk assessment. The content of these templates will vary between services, so you will need to be familiar with the models used in your own service, as well as with more general assessment issues. A comprehensive mental health assessment involves collecting a wide range of information from the consumer and from other sources.

Identifying Information

This is the first part of the comprehensive assessment and includes key demographic information about the consumer, including their name,

BOX 9.4 Important Questions for Mental Health Triage

- Does the consumer feel safe in their current situation?
- Is the consumer at imminent risk of self-harm?
- Is the consumer at risk of harming others?
- If there are risks of harm to self or others, does the consumer have the means in their possession to carry out that harm?
- Is the consumer likely to stay where they are or are they likely to leave?
- How soon does the consumer need to be seen?
- Are there physical health problems that may be contributing to the presentation?

age, gender, employment, ethnicity, main support persons, living situation, address and contact details. Although some of these details will previously have been recorded, the nurse needs to ensure they are accurate.

Presenting Need

The presenting need is the issue that causes the person to present for mental health care. The presenting need, also termed presenting problem or concern, should always be expressed from the consumer's perspective, not from the perspective or assumptions of the health professional. For example, a consumer may seem to be very depressed when first seen, but their reason for presenting might be expressed as "I'm desperate. I can't go on." In the case of a consumer who does not agree that they need mental health care, their presenting problem might be: "They forced me to come here. I don't need to see anyone." Likewise, when documenting the presenting need it can be beneficial to include the quoted description from the individual, as this guides healthcare professionals towards the priority of needs and supports a person-centred approach. It is important to note that pragmatically, when working with people clinically, there is often more than one presenting need. Therefore, through the process of inquiry and exploring the history of each presenting need, it is essential to prioritise the needs and have a shared understanding of needs as a basis for providing care.

History of Presenting Need

The history of the presenting need is a process of subjective inquiry that focuses specifically on the identified need and explores the events leading up to the assessment. It can include establishing the onset, duration, course and severity of the identified area of concern. Mnemonics can provide structure to asking about the history of the presenting need(s). Suggested mnemonics can include OLDCARTS (Onset, Location, Duration, Characteristics, Aggravating/Associated factors, Relieving factors, Treatment, Severity), or similarly, COLDSPA (Character, Onset, Location, Duration, Severity, Pattern, Associated Factors). The additional inclusion of the mnemonic ICE (Impact on Activities of Daily Living, Coping strategies, Emotional response), after a primary framework, can provide insight into the chronic impact of the presenting need. If such frameworks are employed to guide history-taking it is essential to adapt the questions in response to the presenting need (see Box 9.5).

Once again, throughout the assessment process it is important to try to get an understanding of the history as the consumer has experienced it and not only as the health professional sees it. Factors that have led to the presentation will be varied and may be positive (e.g. winning the lottery) or negative (e.g. losing a job) because both positive and negative events can trigger mental health presentations. It is also important to focus on recent precipitants as triggers; for example, the context of a presenting problem may be long-standing relationship discord, but the cause for presentation may be that the spouse has left recently. In documenting the history of the presenting problem, pay attention to the chronological order of events. Consumers may relate events in order of their significance, rather than in chronological order, and while the meaning and significance of events are very important, the order of events is also important in understanding how the presenting problem has developed. Exploring the history of the presenting problem should include a review of symptoms of the most common mental illnesses, such as mood disorder, anxiety, psychosis or disorders of cognition. Some symptoms will be obvious, but others might need to be elicited by asking probing questions. As much as possible, these questions should be incorporated into an interview; however, you might also need to make a direct inquiry about some symptoms, such as unusual perceptions. Factors of significance will not be limited

BOX 9.5 Use of I.C.E Mnemonic in Taking a Health History

	Example Question	Example Response
Impact on daily living	"You've described that your low mood is affecting you every day. What particular activities is this experience impacting on?"	"I find that it takes all of my energy just to concentrate at work. I have no energy for tidying the house or cooking proper meals."
Coping strategies	"What coping strategies have you found helpful for those moments in the day when you feel overwhelmed?"	"I don't know if I am coping. I just try to avoid conversations when I'm feeling like that."
Emotional response	"In those moments of not feeling like you're coping, how would you describe those feelings? How would you describe your response? What is your physical response? How might others observe your response?"* *These would be asked as separate questions if the consumer's initial description of their experiences does not provide this information.	"I can feel hopeless. I imagine that I look scared or frightened or something ... my chest tightens. I just want to get away from people."

to clinical factors (mood, thoughts, perceptions), but will also include personal factors such as changes in relationships, interests and activities. The nurse should consider the consumer's self-help and support strategies, and how effective these have been. Consumers may have used previously learnt methods of stress management and distress tolerance and may have sought support from friends and family members. Other responses can include increased use of prescribed medication, use of non-prescribed medication, and use of alcohol or other drugs.

Health History

Mental health. Information gathered for the mental health history is concerned with the consumer's previous mental health concerns. It is important to ask about past attempts the consumer has made to receive help for their mental health. This information should be documented chronologically. Most people will have sought help from various sources at some point in their life; it is important to be aware of this because it helps to better comprehend the nature, longevity and understanding that the person has given their concerns. People may ask a pharmacy or health-food shop for assistance with symptoms relating to mental health. Some may have been to a naturopath, chiropractor or massage therapist, others to their general practitioner (GP), church minister or school or university counsellor. For some people, the main source of help will be family, extended family or their own cultural advisers. All this information is valid and adds to our understanding. It is important to ask what treatment the consumer has tried and what the results were. If the consumer has had psychological therapy or has been prescribed medication such as antidepressants, this should be recorded along with the response. A helpful way to explore past treatment is to inquire whether the consumer found it helpful, how long they had the treatment for and, if relevant, their reasons for discontinuing. Hospital admissions and contacts with community mental health services should also be documented in this part of the assessment. If the consumer has had previous admissions or periods of community care, their legal status should be recorded during these episodes of care. Areas of risk should be explored, including history of self-harm or suicidality, history of violence towards others and any history of victimisation such as exposure to domestic violence or assault from others.

❓ CRITICAL THINKING EXERCISE 9.4

Mental health assessment involves asking consumers about areas of their lives usually considered private and personal such as questions about sexuality, use of drugs and experiences of trauma. How comfortable do you feel about exploring these areas with consumers? Why is it important that nurses can overcome discomfort about asking very personal questions? What are some of the risks of asking very personal questions and how can those risks be managed?

Substance use history. Taking a comprehensive substance use history is essential because all substances influence mental health. Some issues of substance use may have been discussed in relation to past mental health experiences and these areas should be explored in more detail (see Chapter 13). Rates of co-existing mental illness and substance use are very high (Reilly et al 2019), and substance use will complicate recovery from a mental illness. In some cases, substance use may have precipitated mental illness, or may be a factor in perpetuating mental illness. In taking a substance use history, you will need to name the specific substances the consumer has used. Consumers may be concerned that information about use of illegal substances will be passed onto the police, so the assessment should include reassurance that the information is sought for the purposes of health care and will remain confidential. In exploring substance use, consumers should be asked for specific information about the level of use; for example, the statement, "I don't drink much" could have different meanings for different people. Ask clarifying questions to establish the level and pattern of alcohol or other drug consumption. There are many useful screening tools for assisting with this assessment. Consumers can be asked to complete a brief questionnaire such as the AUDIT (Babor et al 2001). Assessing substance use provides an opportunity to explore readiness to change using a model such as motivational interviewing (DiClemente et al 2017) and to discuss whether referral to a substance use agency might be helpful.

Family history. It is important to ask about the mental health history of the family, particularly close relatives such as parents, grandparents, siblings, aunts, uncles and cousins. We are interested in knowing this for two reasons. First, some of the major mental health conditions are known to have familial patterns (e.g. schizophrenia, bipolar disorder and depression). These conditions are more common in people who have close relatives with the disorder (Rasic et al 2013). Second, we know that the environment a person grows up and lives in affects their health generally and their mental health specifically. As we grow, we all role-model to significant others around us our ways of living, behaving and coping. For example, a child raised in a family with a depressed parent who has taken to their bed for prolonged periods may replicate this behaviour as their way of coping with the world, and this may lead to a mental health presentation. Inquiring about family history can begin with a question such as, "Has anyone else in your family had problems like these?" The consumer's answers can be explored to gain more detailed information and to gain an understanding of the consumer's past and current relationships with family members.

Developmental and social history. This area of assessment considers the stages of the consumer's life and their possible influence on personality, coping style and the current problem. Understanding experiences at various life stages is an important component of comprehensive assessment. The developmental history can take a chronological approach, although some social stressors may relate to early life

HISTORICAL ANECDOTE 9.2

Freud and Psychoanalysis

One of the most influential paradigms of the 20th century was psychoanalysis, developed by the Austrian neurologist Sigmund Freud (1856–1939). Psychoanalysis was one of the first attempts to assess mental health from a developmental perspective. Although Freud noticed that several of his clients had experienced trauma, he rejected the idea that trauma might be a source of distress and mental ill health. Instead, Freud proposed that a person's mental health is heavily influenced by unconscious motivating forces. This premise suggests that all behaviour has meaning and may therefore be understood. According to psychoanalysis, human personality can be understood as comprising three parts: the id, the ego and the superego. These components are thought to develop within the personality by the age of 5 years and often includes inner turmoil, giving rise to anxiety. In response, psychological defence mechanisms are unconsciously created by the personality to deal with such anxiety, which can lead to episodes of mental ill health.

Read More About It

Westen, D. 1998. The scientific legacy of Sigmund Freud: Toward a psychodynamically informed psychological science. Psycholog Bull 124(3), 333.

experiences and so may have been discussed at other stages of the comprehensive assessment process. Areas of assessment include infancy and early childhood, early family experiences, past relationships with siblings, developmental milestones, peer relationships and friendships, experiences of schooling, academic achievements and relationships with parents and caregivers. Following the life course will lead to discussions about employment, university or other study, intimate relationships and sexuality. Adult relationships are important, especially any pattern of difficulty in maintaining long-term relationships, and relationships with children. For older adults, the nurse should discuss later life milestones such as retirement, socialisation patterns, relationships and illnesses, especially those that limit mobility or social functioning or that cause sensory deficits.

Cultural beliefs and views. Cultural beliefs can have a major impact on the expression of mental distress and illness and on consumers' engagement with mental health care (McKenna 2020). The populations of Australia and New Zealand have increasingly culturally diverse populations, comprising Indigenous peoples, descendants of early immigrants and significant populations of new immigrants. Assessment should identify consumers' cultural experiences and seek to understand how these issues might impact on the expression of distress and on care and treatment. Cultural difference between clinicians and consumers can be a barrier to assessment, and clinicians should consider whether the presence of a translator or cultural support person will help facilitate engagement. It is an expectation that the nurse demonstrates cultural safety in a way that is acceptable to the health consumer (Nursing Council of New Zealand 2011). Clinicians should work in partnership to identify consumers' cultural needs during assessment, and seek advice if unsure. Cultural issues in mental health nursing are also discussed in Chapters 6 and 7.

CRITICAL THINKING EXERCISE 9.5

Consider your own cultural beliefs and practices. How comfortable would you feel discussing these beliefs with a mental health professional? How can you help consumers to feel comfortable discussing these areas as part of their mental health care?

Spirituality. As with culture, spirituality is an important aspect of mental health and should be considered in every comprehensive assessment (Barber 2018). Spirituality can include membership or identification with organised religions or faith communities, or non-religious spiritual beliefs. Spiritual beliefs are important in helping consumers give meaning to their experiences of mental distress and illness. Faith communities are also significant sources of informal support. Consideration of spirituality in assessment can include the consumer's developmental experience of religion, current engagement with religious practices and personal belief systems. Some consumers may say they do not have spiritual beliefs, and this expression should be respected and recorded.

Forensic history. It is not unusual for people with mental illness to have had contact with the police or the legal system and possibly contact with forensic mental health services. These aspects of the personal history may emerge spontaneously or may need to be the subject of specific assessment questions. In the context of an assessment interview, it may become clear from responses to more general questions that the consumer has no history of police involvement, in which case no specific inquiry is needed. In addition to noting specific events, such as any arrests, convictions and sentencing, it is important to know the consumer's current perceptions of events involving legal issues and whether there are any outstanding charges, as these may be sources of significant stress. Forensic history can help in documenting any events involving interpersonal violence and form part of risk assessment. See Chapter 29 for further discussion of forensic mental health issues.

General health history. The interrelationship between mental and physical health is not a new concept to nursing practice. Nurses have a role to play in breaking down barriers between physical and mental health care in all practice settings (Bhugra & Ventriglio 2017). It is essential to gather the consumer's medical history to check for health problems and medical comorbidities that might be impacting on their mental health. Thorough questioning may uncover health problems that you might not have considered; for example, pain is an often-overlooked problem, which, unless specifically asked about, can go undetected. As you develop your assessment interview skills, having a systematic approach to taking a medical history will help avoid missing important findings. Key themes of inquiry within a general health history can include:

- childhood health conditions and surgeries
- medical and surgical history, including current or chronic health conditions
- known allergies
- history of loss of consciousness (including general anaesthetics) or head injury
- medications and supplements; prescribed or over-the-counter medication.

Mental health consumers are frequently prescribed second-generation antipsychotic agents, which are associated with higher risk of metabolic syndrome (Wand 2019). Other medications such as clozapine, lithium and sodium valproate require skills of physical health assessment to ensure safe monitoring (see Chapter 20).

Taking a health history is also an opportunity for discussion about physical issues that might not directly affect the person's mental health, but may require attention. Uncovering this information will add to your clinical picture and help the team to decide if seeking additional historical medical information is pertinent to treatment planning. It may also indicate the need for diagnostic tests such as computed tomography (CT) imaging of the head or psychometric assessments.

At the end of a discussion about general health history, the nurse should capture a snapshot of the consumer's whole health through a review of body systems. This involves the nurse systematically asking specific questions related to each body system to draw out information that might be relevant or that highlights additional areas of health needs.

Screening and Health Promotion Opportunities

The assessment process also provides the nurse with an opportunity to inquire about lifestyle and choices that promote mental and physical wellbeing, and potentially offer brief advice based on evidence-based recommendations and guidelines related to modifiable risk factors. Health promotion can include discussing whether the consumer is enrolled in a primary care practice and is receiving regular primary health care.

People with serious mental illness have high rates of physical disorders (Scott et al 2016), so this part of the comprehensive assessment is an opportunity to reinforce important health promotion messages. This may not be appropriate in all assessment contexts, or it may only be appropriate to explore a few topics. Where helpful, information can be shared about sleep, nutrition, physical activity, alcohol, tobacco and substance use, sexual health, metabolic and cardiovascular risk screening. Chapter 20 provides an extensive discussion of physical health issues experienced by people with mental illness.

Risk Assessment

Risk assessment is not a separate form of assessment: it is a process that selectively draws on information obtained in the comprehensive assessment to identify the existence of risk, the level of risk and a plan to manage risk. Risk assessment is a requirement of most mental health service providers and it is therefore important that nurses understand the language and limitations of risk assessment. However, there is controversy about the value of risk assessment (Wand 2015) and about the ability of clinicians to accurately identify consumers at high risk and to predict the likelihood of adverse events. The most commonly identified areas of risk are risk to self through self-harm or neglect, risk of violence to others and risk of victimisation. In in-patient settings, nurses also need to assess risk of absconding.

A very good summary of risk assessment and management, including the limitations of risk assessment, is provided by Flewett (2010). Flewett makes the important point that risk assessment and management are not about eliminating risk or about predicting the occurrence of adverse events. Rather, they are about understanding the factors that contribute to risk and working with consumers to manage that risk. Nurses also need to balance awareness of risk with the positive value of risk in the lives of consumers and of the value of learning from the consequences of decisions (Morgan & Andrews 2016). Risk assessment is further discussed in Chapter 4.

Mental State Assessment

In this chapter the term "mental state assessment" is used in preference to "mental state examination", as the latter implies an objectified evaluation of the consumer's mental state, whereas we wish to promote an understanding based on an engaged relationship. Mental state assessment is part of every comprehensive assessment and provides a statement of the consumer's emotional and cognitive functioning at a single point in time (Assadi 2020; Soltan & Girguis 2017). The importance of focusing the mental state assessment on a single point in time is that it can provide a point of comparison for future assessments. Other elements of the consumer's presentation, such as social functioning, history and risk, are excluded from the mental state assessment. Many elements of a mental state assessment can be integrated into routine nursing interactions, such as the initial assessment interview, reviewing a plan of care or discussing recovery goals. During these interactions the nurse will be able to observe the consumer's behaviour, appearance and mood, and will gain a good understanding of thought content. However, some elements of mental state assessment require specific inquiry on the part of the nurse. For example, the nurse may need to ask direct questions to test their impression that a consumer is disoriented or has problems with memory.

Mental state assessment requires both objective observation and empathic communication. Appearance and behaviour can be objectively observed, while to assess the consumer's mood the nurse will need to establish rapport and enter the consumer's emotional world. Many situational variables affect mental state (e.g. an unfamiliar environment, anxiety or pain), and these can be considered when the findings of the mental state assessment are interpreted.

The structured format used for recording a mental state assessment does not mean that the mental state assessment requires a question-and-answer interview. In fact, the opposite is true: a supportive therapeutic conversation will probably provide most of the information required for a mental state assessment. Additional information can be elicited, if necessary, by direct questions, but these should flow naturally from the interaction with the consumer. A standardised measure of cognitive functioning can be used to augment a mental state assessment (refer to Table 9.2 for standardised assessments of cognitive functioning).

There is no set format for recording a mental state assessment, but we suggest the BATOMI mnemonic as a useful means of organising the findings (Behaviour and appearance; Affect and mood; Thought and speech; Orientation, cognition and sensorium; Memory; Insight and judgement). An example of a documented mental state assessment using this mnemonic is provided in Box 9.6. The following sections outline the types of observations that can contribute to a mental state assessment.

Behaviour and Appearance

Behaviour and appearance refer to the consumer's general appearance and activity. Begin with the most obvious aspects of behaviour such as clothing, grooming and hygiene, evidence of self-care or neglect and distinguishing marks, such as tattoos, piercings and notable physical features, such as scars. This section also includes observations of motor activity and behaviour, such as posture, eye contact, restlessness, tearfulness, nervous mannerisms (e.g. tremors and shaking), and behaviour indicating level of interest in the interaction. The consumer's attitude towards the assessment process can be seen in their appearance, responses, body language and facial expressions. Consider not only what you are observing, but how appropriate it is, considering the setting of the assessment. For example, in an assessment in an ED you might expect someone to look dishevelled and perhaps sleepy (at least initially). Anxiety about the assessment process will also influence behaviour.

Affect and Mood

Affect and mood have various definitions that sometimes conflict with each other. Both refer to emotional state, with mood referring to sustained emotional state (especially because it is experienced by the individual) and affect referring to expressed emotion – something that the clinician can observe. A skilled clinician can often gauge a consumer's mood, especially if a good rapport has been developed and the consumer feels safe to communicate their emotional state. However, it is important that consumers are given the opportunity to describe their mood. Because this may be difficult for people who are depressed, consumers can be asked to rate their mood on a scale of 1 to 10, where 1 is the lowest it has ever been and 10 is the highest. Emotional state can be appropriate or inappropriate to the assessment context – for example, a consumer who is elated and buoyant despite an objectively formal context such as a clinical review. Terms sometimes used to describe affect and mood are dysphoric, flat, elevated, depressed, anxious, labile (fluctuating without obvious reason) and restricted. The

BOX 9.6 Documentation of Mental State Assessment

The following assessment records the mental state of a woman assessed following an overdose of prescribed medication and medical treatment in an emergency department.

Behaviour and Appearance
54-year-old European woman who is attentive to interview, although a little sleepy from lingering effects of overdose. Looks older than her chronological age. Dressed in jeans and T-shirt. Is well groomed and appears well cared for. No unusual movements or mannerisms. Maintains good eye contact. Tearful at times.

Affect and Mood
Affect sad. Intermittently brighter in response to interview. Mood is objectively depressed. She describes her mood as low, rates it at 4 on a 1–10 scale, where 1 is the lowest it has been. Not irritable.

Thought and Speech
Thoughts focus on recent events, and her perception that she is not well supported by family members. Returns to the theme of past long-term relationship that ended 12 months ago. Ruminates about abandonment. Limited ability to focus on problem-solving in relation to current stressors. Depressive themes: loneliness, undeserving of help, lack of confidence in future. Slow rate of thought and talk. No delusional ideas expressed. No unusual perceptions. Has occasional thoughts of suicide, but stresses she would not act on these. Has no specific plan. Gives involvement with grandchildren as a protective factor.

Orientation, Cognition and Sensorium
Alert and oriented to time, place and person. Knows her whereabouts, and the date and time of day. Accurately identifies staff by role or name. Able to perform "serial sevens" (subtracting in sevens starting from 100).

Memory
Both short- and long-term memory are intact. She remembers events of the past few days, and more distant. Able to recall three objects after 5 minutes.

Insight and Judgement
Identifies that her mood is currently low and has been low for several weeks. Is aware that alcohol has a disinhibiting role when her mood is low and increases suicidal thoughts. Accepts referral to mental health service and the need to review current antidepressant medication. Judgement is unimpaired when not intoxicated.

---

term "euthymic" is often used if the consumer's mood is neither happy nor sad. In assessing mood, you are using your own emotional state as a means of understanding the emotional state of the consumer. Nurses who have established an empathic understanding of a consumer will be best able to assess that consumer's emotional state.

Thought and Speech

Thought and speech are usually described together (sometimes called "thought and talk") and focus on the rate, form and content of thought, and the nature of the consumer's verbal communications. It is not possible to assess thoughts directly, so thought is assessed through the indirect medium of speech. Speech is more easily observed because it is the major medium of communication. Aspects of speech are rate (speed of speech), volume, amount of speech, tone and content. Speech that is rapid or slowed, very quiet or loud, hesitant or limited may be significant in assessing mental state and should be recorded. For

example, rapid or pressured speech might indicate mania or anxiety; quiet or hesitant speech might indicate low mood or anxiety; and loud speech might indicate anger or suspicion. It is important to note whether speech is goal-directed or circumstantial and tangential. This part of the mental state assessment (sometimes called "perception") also records any delusional ideas, such as ideas of being influenced by others, paranoid ideas, thoughts that radio or television news are referring to the individual, and other forms of disordered thinking. Auditory or other hallucinations are noted in this section of the assessment. It is helpful to describe the nature of voices, whether the consumer feels threatened by them or whether they perform an important function for the consumer, such as providing company.

Orientation, Cognition and Sensorium

Orientation is easily assessed and may not require direct questioning. Orientation refers to understanding of time, place and person, and can be assessed by asking questions about time of day and place. Because these might seem odd questions to some consumers, it is important to explain that these are part of routine assessment. Cognition refers to the ability to recognise and manipulate information and to perform tasks of reasoning. General interview questions will give some evidence of cognitive functioning. Cognition can also be tested by asking the consumer to perform individual tasks from standardised assessments such as spelling "world" backwards, or naming different common objects (e.g. pen, book, watch). Disturbances in sensorium are likely to be evident in many interactions, especially in structured interviews. Sensorium can be assessed by observing the consumer's attentiveness and ability to stay focused on tasks. Consumers with an altered level of consciousness may show limited ability to attend and fluctuation in attention and awareness.

Memory

Memory involves the capacity to recall information and extends from initial registration of information to recall of information that is years old. Registration can be assessed by asking the consumer to repeat back to the nurse the names of three unrelated common objects (e.g. pen, clock, tree). Short-term memory can be assessed by asking for recall of the same three objects after 5 minutes, during which time other discussion takes place. Finally, long-term (or remote) memory involves recall of years-old information, such as events from childhood or adolescence.

Insight and Judgement

Insight can be a controversial area of assessment because it is sometimes interpreted as a test of whether the consumer agrees with the clinician's opinion about what is happening, in particular whether or not the consumer is mentally ill (Fiorillo et al 2020; Lysaker et al 2018). Insight is best understood as a consumer's perception of their current situation. It is not always helpful to simply record "lacks insight" because this does not tell us what the consumer believes about their problems. Judgement refers to the person's ability to act safely and with understanding of the possible consequences of their actions. A confused person may have markedly impaired judgement and hence be unsafe unless in a situation where they can be observed.

Focused Assessment

Initial assessment occurs when the consumer first accesses mental health care and has the aim of developing a shared understanding of what problems the person seeks help with, their strengths and resources, and what the mental health service can do to assist with those problems. As the nurse and the consumer develop their relationship, and as initial problems are resolved, the shared understanding of the goals of care will change. Ongoing focused assessment helps review goals, redefine problems and strengths, and develop new strategies to assist in the consumer's recovery.

Some ongoing assessment interviews are unplanned; for example, when a consumer experiences acute distress or sudden deterioration in their mental state. Assessment in these contexts might not be undertaken by a clinician who knows the person. The ability to build rapport quickly, access previous clinical notes, gather third party information and engage in the critical reflection cycle will be important. Alternatively, the focus of assessment might change during different phases of care and treatment. At the beginning of an episode of care, information gathering and verification of its reliability and accuracy may have primacy, whereas after a period of time, the assessment focus may be in understanding a consumer's motivation to remain engaged in care and treatment (Todd 2010). Additionally, a focus of assessment may include identifying physical health concerns and whether a consumer needs to be supported to access other services.

Methods of Objective Information Gathering

Information gathered from the subjective history-taking process may lead to the need of further objective data being collected by the nurse (see Box 9.2). The process extends beyond the gathering of information and also includes the interpretation of findings and clinical reasoning (Lewis & Foley 2020). If we consider that subjective information is generally gathered by listening to the health consumer and their family, objective data is then collected by observing the consumer and physically collecting further information. Objective data can include making specific observations during an assessment (general appearance), physical examination techniques and diagnostic values. When there are time-critical or urgent concerns for the individual, examination techniques and diagnostic tests can be performed earlier in the assessment process; for example, undertaking an ECG and vital signs for someone who develops chest pain during the assessment who has historically experienced anxiety with similar somatic experiences.

Some observations take place before the face-to-face interview commences and can continue alongside the interview dialogue. There can be a distinct point in the engagement where the interaction moves from talking with people, to a more "hands-on" approach. Therefore, before the assessment continues it is vital that the nurse prepares for the examination and reconsiders the safety of themselves and the individual, as described earlier in this chapter. During this step it is essential that the process is explained to the consumer and that consent is gained before physical contact.

Physical Examination Techniques and Diagnostic Tests

Objective data collected from examination techniques and diagnostic tests provides further knowledge to inform care and guide formulation. Information collected in assessment is informed by the presenting need, the history and what the consumer describes they are experiencing in aspects of their wellbeing. This may elicit the need to undertake a focused assessment on another system (cardiac assessment for example), or a broader approach using a head-to-toe framework. During the process, four assessment techniques are utilised by the nurse to collect information; these include inspection, palpation, percussion and auscultation (Lewis & Foley 2020).

Laboratory investigations are part of any comprehensive assessment and have several purposes, including to understand the role of physical illness in the current presentation; establish adherence to prescribed medication; assess organ functioning and how it might be impacted by prescribed medication (e.g. the effect of liver functioning on the half-life of benzodiazepines); identify potentially toxic blood levels of prescribed medication (e.g. lithium carbonate); and identify

HISTORICAL ANECDOTE 9.3

Assessment and the Clinical Gaze

In the 18th century, clinical work involved doctors listening to patients' stories of symptoms and illness. Diagnoses were made based on indirect evidence rather than direct observation of pathological changes. The advent of new technologies and the proliferation of hospitals as the major site of medical practice meant that assessment shifted in focus from the patient to the disease. Historian Michel Foucault has referred to the new focus on pathology as the "clinical gaze". The clinical gaze made the patient's story less important because the "truth" of their illness was seen to lie inside the patient's body, in diseased organs and tissues, not in their experience of symptoms. Psychiatry has long struggled with this notion of the clinical gaze. While there have been many attempts to provide biological understandings of mental illness, clinical practice in assessment still relies on listening to the patient's story and understanding symptoms in the context of the patient's life and culture. Comment is frequently made that psychiatry is unlike other branches of medicine because there are no objective phenomena (blood tests, laboratory studies) that can be observed to support a diagnosis. In nursing we focus first on the patient as a person. Disease, even where it is present, is not the primary focus of nursing. The clinical gaze of the 18th century helps us to understand diseases, but it is not the basis of nursing assessment.

Read More About It
Foucault, M. 1994. The birth of the clinic: An archaeology of medical perception. Vintage Books, New York.

any use of non-prescribed drugs. Laboratory tests are used in initial assessment and to monitor the impact of new and ongoing prescribed medication (e.g. the development of markers of metabolic syndrome). Nurses should be familiar with the most commonly used laboratory tests and be able to interpret the results of tests using knowledge of the consumer's general health status and the accepted range of values for the particular test. Most results are reported along with the normal range. For full lists of reference ranges see Laboratory values in Useful websites at the end of the chapter.

In addition to laboratory tests, there are a range of investigations that may be considered as part of a comprehensive assessment. For example, every consumer should have an electrocardiogram (ECG), both to assess their baseline cardiac functioning and to identify any vulnerability to the effects of prescribed medication. Other tests that might be considered are a CT scan to exclude space-occupying lesions or other pathology, magnetic resonance imaging (MRI) for more detailed imaging of organs, and an electroencephalogram (EEG) to assess possible abnormalities of brain function.

CLINICAL FORMULATION

Once all assessment information has been gathered you will have both a subjective impression of the consumer as a person and a set of objective data about the consumer. You will also understand the consumer's perceptions of their current problems and how those problems relate to the consumer's life history. Clinical formulation is the process of bringing this information together to develop an individualised explanatory account of the consumer. Different models of psychological therapy often have their own model of formulation – for example, the cognitive formulation used in cognitive therapy (Johnstone 2018). In this section we discuss a more general model of formulation, but one that can incorporate psychological understandings of the person.

Clinical formulation is a potentially complex process, but fortunately there are several models available to assist nurses in writing clinical formulations and developing skills in this aspect of assessment. Biological, psychological and social theories help explain the relationships between the various aspects of the consumer's history and presentation. Clinical formulation is not undertaken by the clinician alone, although in some literature (e.g. Selzer & Ellen 2014) this is how formulation is described. However, as Crowe and colleagues (2008) explain, clinical formulation is an opportunity for the nurse and the consumer to discuss their different perspectives and negotiate both common understandings and differences in understandings. If the assessment has been a collaborative process throughout, there will be a strong enough relationship between the nurse and the consumer to allow this negotiation to occur.

A useful model for developing clinical formulation is the 4 P's model described by Selzer and Ellen (2010; 2014) and shown in Table 9.3. In this model the 4 P's (predisposing, precipitating, perpetuating and protective) are used to describe factors that contributed to the current problems, factors that contribute to the persistence of the problem and those that protect the person from the effects of the problem. In addition to the 4 P's, this model allows for consideration of biological, psychological and social factors. Theoretical and philosophical understandings, such as learning theory, adaptation theory and recovery philosophy, can be used to interpret the contribution of the various factors. Using this model, the clinician can focus on factors in any cell of the matrix, depending on what the significant factors are for the individual consumer. With some consumers there will be a greater emphasis on social factors, while for others, psychological or biological factors will be more important.

Clinical formulation is written in narrative form. The clinician and the consumer work together to reach agreement regarding how different aspects of the consumer's history affect the current presentation. It

may not always be possible to reach agreement. In such cases, the formulation is written to reflect the different perspectives of the clinician and the consumer (Baird et al 2017). The written formulation concludes with a statement about the possible future for the consumer and focuses on how strengths and protective factors can be enhanced by support from clinical services. Writing clear, clinical formulations takes practice. A typical difficulty encountered by clinicians is attempting to include too much information. Remember, the clinical history contains all the relevant information about the consumer. The formulation is a selective summary: only the most pertinent information should be included, and the emphasis is on how the various factors interact.

Diagnosis

A diagnosis is a definition of a problem once all available information has been considered (Zanotti & Chiffi 2015). A diagnosis is, first, identifying diseases via signs and symptoms and by other investigations, and second, developing an opinion or conclusion based on those investigations. The current model of psychiatric diagnosis most employed in Australia and New Zealand is the *Diagnostic and Statistical Manual of Mental Disorders* (DSM), now in its fifth edition (American Psychiatric Association 2013). In most clinical practice settings, psychiatric diagnoses are assigned by medical practitioners, not always by psychiatrists, especially in primary care. Nurses need to be familiar with the diagnostic criteria of the more common mental illnesses and of the diagnostic reasoning process applied to making these diagnoses. A full list of DSM-5 diagnoses and criteria is available on the American Psychiatric Association website (see Useful websites).

> ### ❓ CRITICAL THINKING EXERCISE 9.6
>
> Psychiatric diagnosis is a process of assigning a category to a consumer's unique subjective experiences and problems in living. How can you work with consumers to help them understand the process of diagnosis and to consider whether their diagnosis accurately reflects their experiences?

Classification in Psychiatry

There have been many attempts at developing systems of psychiatric classification. One notable early example is that of psychiatrist Emil Kraepelin in the late 19th century. Kraepelin's system, which included just 13 diagnoses, assumed that each mental illness is distinct rather than comprising clusters of symptoms with a significant degree of overlap. The most common system of psychiatric diagnosis in current use, the DSM-5, is also based on the assumption of distinct illnesses, although such categorical systems do not reflect the human experience of distress and illness. For a full analysis of these issues, see Zachar and colleagues (2014). There are two manuals of diagnoses in psychiatry: the *International Classification of Diseases and Health Related Problems* (ICD) (World Health Organization 1989) and the DSM. Since their initial establishment, both manuals have undergone numerous revisions. The most current versions are the ICD-11 and the DSM-5. The ICD-11 is a comprehensive manual of all known diseases, with its fifth chapter being devoted to mental and behavioural disorders, while the DSM-5 exclusively catalogues mental illnesses. The two systems are broadly similar and have become more so in their most recent editions. In Australia and New Zealand, the ICD AM (Australasian Modification) is more commonly used for collecting administrative health information, while the DSM is more commonly used in clinical practice.

Psychiatric diagnosis is not formally part of the practice of most mental health nurses, but it is important for nurses to understand the diagnostic process and the criteria for the most commonly used

TABLE 9.3 Clinical Formulation – The 4 P's Model

Factor	Biological	Psychological	Social
Predisposing	Genetic Birth trauma Brain injury Illness – psychiatric, physical Medication Drugs/alcohol	Pain Personality Modelling defences (unconscious) Coping strategies Self-esteem Body image Cognition Trauma	Socioeconomic status Culture/spirituality
Precipitating	Medication Drugs/alcohol Trauma Acute illness	Pain Stage of life Grief Loss Treatment Stressors	Work Finances Connections Relationships
Perpetuating	Any of the above factors that are continuing	Any of the above factors that are continuing	Any of the above factors that are continuing
Protective	Physical health	Engagement Insight Adherence Coping strategies Intelligence	Group belonging and affiliations Family and social relationships

Adapted from Selzer & Ellen 2010.

diagnostic categories. Consumers may have questions about their diagnoses, and nurses need to be able to respond knowledgeably to these questions. Nurses may at times question the diagnosis assigned to a consumer in their care, and it is important that such questioning is well informed. Understanding diagnoses does not mean that nurses are practising within a biomedical model. Diagnostic models are only one of many frameworks for practice, but they are important because they form part of the common language of mental health care. The purpose of diagnosis is to accurately group people whose clinical symptoms are sufficiently similar, with the aim of optimising treatment and clinical outcomes for each group. Accurate diagnosis is essential to identifying optimal treatment. To assist clinicians in making diagnoses, the DSM-5 provides lists of criteria and decision rules about applying those criteria in individual cases.

Despite the statement of explicit criteria and rules in the DSM-5, a diagnosis may not be clear, especially for consumers new to a mental health service or with complex histories. For those reasons, clinicians may defer diagnosis, assign a provisional diagnosis or make a list of differential diagnoses. A differential diagnosis is a list of possible diagnoses, any of which may eventually prove to be the final diagnosis (Baid 2006). Diagnosis should always be regarded as open to revision as clinicians' understanding of the consumer develops. Clinicians should also discuss the diagnosis with the consumer and should be prepared to share their uncertainty about the diagnosis and the role of diagnosis in clinical care.

CHAPTER SUMMARY

Assessment is one of the foundational skills of mental health nursing and is integral to clinical reasoning. Assessment begins with the person's first contact with a health service and continues throughout the episode of care. The aim of assessment is to develop an understanding of the person and the problems that have led them to seek mental health care. It is through assessment that nurses can ensure a consumer's needs are met, their preferences respected, and that care is planned which reflects the circumstances of their life. Assessment is based on developing rapport and a therapeutic relationship. It is both a structured process in which the nurse seeks information about many aspects of the life of the consumer and a process of exploration in which consumers are encouraged and supported to share their experiences with the nurse. Assessment methods include structured and conversational interviews, standardised assessment instruments and diaries recording aspects of functioning such as thoughts, feelings, activities and social interactions. A range of tools is available to assist in the process, including standard assessment templates and standardised assessment instruments. In conducting assessments, nurses need to use the standard tools available as well as engage in dialogue in which consumers feel safe to share significant aspects of their lives. The tools of mental health nursing assessment provide the structure for the assessment to occur, while the process of assessment allows the nurse to integrate philosophical and theoretical frameworks into the assessment.

REVIEW QUESTIONS

You are a newly registered nurse working in a community mental health clinic. One of your roles in the service is to take phone calls from health practitioners and members of the public who are considering whether someone they know has a mental illness and would benefit from assessment and treatment. You receive a call from Donna, who describes her 19-year-old son, Matthew, as moody and irritable for the past 6 months after losing his job as a shop assistant. Soon after the loss of his job, Matthew ended a 12-month relationship with his girlfriend. During the past 6 months he has been drinking excessively, but will not discuss his problems with anyone in the family.

1. In mental health telephone triage, it is quite common to have limited information, and rapport with the caller may be tenuous. Refer to the "Triage" section of this chapter where mental health triage is discussed. Discuss the triage nurse's phone call with Donna with members of your class and make a list of six questions you would want to ask at some point during the telephone interview. List the questions in order of priority. What interview skills would you use to ensure you have the opportunity to ask these questions?

2. Donna tells you that Matthew does not know she is calling as he is currently out of the house. During the telephone interview, how would you work with Donna to help her in discussing her concerns with Matthew and supporting him to accept a face to-face assessment?

3. Two days later Matthew presents at the mental health clinic for a face-to-face assessment. Reflecting on the narrative and descriptive approaches to mental health assessment, how could you use each approach in your assessment of Matthew?

4. The face-to-face assessment involves Matthew, his mother and several members of the multidisciplinary team. The assessment interview takes an hour and the team works with Matthew to develop a collaborative understanding of what is happening for him and what the service can do to help. A plan is agreed that you will visit Matthew at home in a week's time. After Matthew has left, the team discusses psychiatric diagnosis. Most agree that Matthew is experiencing an adjustment disorder with depressed mood. In small groups, discuss the place of diagnosis in Matthew's care. The groups should consider:
   a. Is a diagnosis necessary for Matthew to receive appropriate care?
   b. What problems could a diagnosis of adjustment disorder with depressed mood cause for Matthew?
   c. On your visit next week, how will you discuss Matthew's diagnosis with him? What questions might he have and how will you respond to those questions?

USEFUL WEBSITES

American Psychiatric Association: www.psychiatry.org
   Diagnostic and Statistical Manual of Mental Disorders, 5th Edition, Text Revision (DSM-5-TR): www.psychiatry.org/dsm5
Australasian Triage scale: acem.org.au/Content-Sources/Advancing-Emergency-Medicine/Better-Outcomes-for-Patients/Triage

Clinical guideline for mental state assessment: www.rch.org.au/clinicalguide/guideline_index/Mental_state_examination/
HEADSS assessment: headspace.org.au/health-professionals/clinical-toolkit/psychosocial-assessment/
Head-to-toe assessment: nurse.org/articles/how-to-conduct-head-to-toe-assessment/
International Classification of Diseases (ICD): icd.who.int/en

Laboratory values: www.labtests.co.nz (New Zealand); www.mps.com.au/ (Australia)
Risk assessment (information about the HCR-20 instrument): hcr-20.com
Strengths-based assessment: www.iriss.org.uk/resources/insights/strengths-based-approaches-working-individuals
Suicide risk assessment: www.psychiatryadvisor.com/home/topics/suicide-and-self-harm/is-this-patient-suicidal-tips-for-effective-assessment/
Trauma-informed mental health assessment: www.samhsa.gov/resource/dbhis/screening-assessment

REFERENCES

American Psychiatric Association (APA), 2013. Diagnostic and Statistical Manual of Mental Disorders, 5th ed. APA, Washington.

Assadi, G., 2020. The Mental State Examination. Br J Nurs, 29(22), 1328–1332.

Australian College of Mental Health Nurses, 2010. Standards of Practice for Australian Mental Health Nurses. Australian College of Mental Health Nurses, Canberra.

Babor, T.F., Higgins-Biddle, J.C., Saunders, J.B., et al., 2001. AUDIT: The Alcohol Use Disorders Identification Test guidelines for use in primary care. World Health Organization, Geneva.

Baid, H., 2006. Differential diagnosis in advanced nursing practice. Br J Nurs, 15(18), 1007–1011.

Baird, J., Hyslop, A., Macfie, M., Stocks, R. & Van der Kleij, T., 2017. Clinical formulation: Where it came from, what it is and why it matters. BJ Psych Adv, 23(2), 95–103.

Barber, C.F., 2018. Mental health and spirituality. BJMHN 7(3), 124–128.

Barker, P.J., 2004. Assessment in Psychiatric and Mental Health Nursing: In Search of the Whole Person. Nelson Thornes, Cheltenham, UK.

Bhugra, D., Ventriglio, A., 2017. Mind and body: Physical health needs of individuals with mental illness in the 21st century. World Psychiatry 16(1), 47.

Brown, N. & Jeon, Y-H. 2021. Partnership in care. In: Crisp, J., Douglas, C., Reberio, G. & Waters, D. (eds), Potter and Perry's Fundamentals of Nursing. 6th ed. Elsevier, Sydney.

Brown, S.J., 1995. An interviewing style for nursing assessment. J Adv Nurs, 21, 340–343.

Burke, W.J., Roccaforte, W.H., & Wengel, S.P., 1991. The short form of the Geriatric Depression Scale: A comparison with the 30-item form. J Geriatr Psychiatry Neurol 4(3), 173–178.

Cameron, M., Foxall, D., & Holman, G. 2023. Mahere hau – an integrated bicultural nursing assessment framework. Kaitiaki, Nursing New Zealand, 1–8. Online. Available at: kaitiaki.org.nz/article/mahere-hau-an-integrated-bicultural-nursing-assessment-framework/

Cameron, S.L., Tchernegovski, P. & Maybery, D. 2022. Mental health service users' experiences and perspectives of family involvement in their care: A systematic literature review. J Ment Health, 1–17.

Chase S.K. 2015. The art of diagnosis and treatment. In: Dunphy L.M., Winland-Brown J., & Porter B. (eds): Primary Care: The Art and Science of Advanced Practice, 4th ed. FA Davis, Philadelphia.

Coombs, T., Crookes, P., Curtis, J., 2013a. A comprehensive mental health nursing assessment: Variability of content in practice. J Psychiatr Ment Health Nurs, 20(2), 150–155.

Coombs, T., Curtis, J., Crookes, P., 2013b. What is the process of a comprehensive mental health nursing assessment? Results from a qualitative study. Int Nurs Rev, 60 (1), 96–102.

Coombs, T., Curtis, J., Crookes, P., 2011. What is a comprehensive mental health nursing assessment? A review of the literature. Int J Ment Health Nurs, 20(5), 364–370.

Crowe, M., Carlyle, D., Farmar, R., 2008. Clinical formulation for mental health nursing practice. J Psychiatr Ment Health Nurs, 15(10), 800–807.

Day, J.C., Wood, G., Dewey, M., et al., 1995. A self-rating scale for measuring neuroleptic side-effects. Validation in a group of schizophrenic patients. Br J Psychiatry, 166(5), 650–653.

DiClemente, C.C., Corno, C.M., Graydon, M.M., et al., 2017. Motivational interviewing, enhancement, and brief interventions over the last decade: A review of reviews of efficacy and effectiveness. Psychol Addict Behav, 31(8), 862.

Doan, T., Ha, V., Strazdins, L., & Chateau, D. 2022. Healthy minds live in healthy bodies – effect of physical health on mental health: Evidence from Australian longitudinal data. Curr Psychol (New Brunswick, N.J.). doi.org/10.1007/s12144-022-03053-7.

Duhig, M., Patterson, S., Connell, M., et al., 2015. The prevalence and correlates of childhood trauma in patients with early psychosis. Aust N Z J Psychiatry, 49(7), 651–659.

Eade, D.M., Henning, D., 2013. Chlamydia screening in young people as an outcome of a HEADSS; Home, Education, Activities, Drug and alcohol use, Sexuality and Suicide youth psychosocial assessment tool. J Clin Nurs, 22(23–24), 3280–3288.

Fiorillo, A., Barlati, S., Bellomo, A., Corrivetti, G., Nicolò, G. et al., 2020. The role of shared decision-making in improving adherence to pharmacological treatments in patients with schizophrenia: A clinical review. Ann Gen Psychiatry, 19(1), 1–12.

Flewett, T., 2010. Clinical Risk Management: An Introductory Text for Mental Health Clinicians. Elsevier, Sydney.

Folstein, M.F., Folstein, S.E., McHugh, P.R., 1975. "Mini-Mental State": A practical method for grading the cognitive state of patients for the clinician. J Psychiatr Res, 12(3), 189–198.

Foucault, M., 1994. The Birth of the Clinic: An Archaeology of Medical Perception. Vintage Books, New York.

Inouye, S.K., van Dyck, C.H., Alessi, C.A., et al., 1990. Clarifying confusion: The Confusion Assessment Method. A new method for detection of delirium. Ann Intern Med, 113, 941–948.

Jaber, F.S., Mahmoud, K.F., 2015. Risk tools for the prediction of violence: VRAG, HCR–20, PCL-R. J Psychiatr Ment Health Nurs, 22(2), 133–141.

Johnstone, L., 2018. Psychological formulation as an alternative to psychiatric diagnosis. J Humanist Psychol, 58(1), 30–46.

King, H. (ed.), 2004. Health in Antiquity. Routledge, New York.

Levett-Jones, T., Hoffman, K., Dempsey, J., Jeong, S.Y.S., Noble, D., et al., 2010. The "five rights" of clinical reasoning: An educational model to enhance nursing students' ability to identify and manage clinically "at risk" patients. Nurse Ed Today, 30(6), 515–520.

Lewis, P. & Foley, D. 2020. Health Assessment in Nursing, 3rd ed. Wolters Kluwer, Australia.

Loewy, R.L., Corey, S., Amirfathi, F., Dabit, S., Fulford, D. et al., 2019. Childhood trauma and clinical high risk for psychosis. Schizophrenia Research, 205, 10–14.

Lomax, J., 2021. How diaries help ICU patients recover. Kaitaki, Nursing New Zealand, 27(7), 40–41.

Lysaker, P.H., Pattison, M.L., Leonhardt, B.L., et al., 2018. Insight in schizophrenia spectrum disorders: Relationship with behavior, mood and perceived quality of life, underlying causes and emerging treatments. World Psychiatry 17(1), 12–23.

MacNeela, P., Scott, A., Treacy, P., et al., 2010. In the know: Cognitive and social factors in mental health nursing assessment. J Clin Nurs, 19 (9–10), 1298–1306.

Maguire, T., Garvey, L., Ryan, J., Willetts, G. & Olasoji, M., 2022. Exploration of the utility of the Nursing Process and the Clinical Reasoning Cycle as a framework for forensic mental health nurses: A qualitative study. Int J Ment Health Nurs, 31(2), 358–368.

McKenna, B. 2020. Cultural safety: There is no turning back! J Psychiatric Ment Health Nurs, 27(5), 495–496.

McPherson, A., Martin, C.R., 2010. A narrative review of the Beck Depression Inventory (BDI) and implications for its use in an alcohol–dependent population. J Psychiatr Ment Health Nurs, 17(1), 19–30.

Minton, C., Burrow, M., Manning, C. & van der Krogt, S., 2022. Cultural safety and patient trust: The Hui process to initiate the nurse–patient relationship. Contemp Nurse, 58(2–3), 228–236.

Molloy, L., Guha, M.D., Scott, M.P., Beckett, P., Merrick, T.T. et al., 2021. Mental health nursing practice and Aboriginal and Torres Strait Islander people: An integrative review. Contemp Nurse, 57(1–2), 140–156.

Morgan, S., Andrews, N., 2016. Positive risk-taking: From rhetoric to reality. J Ment Health Train Educ Pract, 11(2), 122–132.

Nursing and Midwifery Board of Australia (NMBA), 2016. National Competency Standards for the Registered Nurse. Nursing and Midwifery Board of Australia, Melbourne.

Nursing Council of New Zealand (NCNZ), 2011. Guidelines for Cultural Safety, the Treaty of Waitangi and Māori Health in Nursing Education and Practice. Nursing NCNZ, Wellington.

Nursing Council of New Zealand (NCNZ), 2007. Competencies for Registered Nurses. Nursing NCNZ, Wellington.

Patterson, W.M., Dohn, H.H., Bird, J., et al., 1983. Evaluation of suicidal patients: the SAD PERSONS scale. Psychosomatics, 24(4), 343–349.

Pitama, S., Huria, T., Lacey, C., 2014. Improving Māori health through clinical assessment: Waikare o te Waka o Meihana. N Z Med J, 127(1393), journal. nzma.org.nz/journal-articles/improving-maori-health-through-clinical-assessment-waikare-o-te-waka-o-meihana

Rapp, C.A., Goscha, R.J., 2012. The Strengths Model. A Recovery-Oriented Approach to Mental Health Services, 3rd ed. Oxford University Press, New York.

Rasic, D., Hajek, T., Alda, M., et al., 2013. Risk of mental illness in offspring of parents with schizophrenia, bipolar disorder, and major depressive disorder: A meta-analysis of family high-risk studies. Schizophr Bull, 40(1), 28–38.

Reilly, J., McDermott, B., & Dillon, J. 2019. Standardized drug and alcohol questions at admission to an acute adult mental health unit: Clarifying the burden of dual diagnoses across a five-year period. Australas Psychiatry, 27(3), 270–274.

Scott, K.M., Lim, C., Al-Hamzawi, A., et al., 2016. Association of mental disorders with subsequent chronic physical conditions: World mental health surveys from 17 countries. JAMA Psychiatry, 73(2), 150–158.

Selzer, R., Ellen, S., 2014. Formulation for beginners. Australasian. Psychiatry, 22(4), 397–401.

Selzer, R., Ellen, S., 2010. Psych-Lite: Psychiatry That's Easy to Read. McGraw-Hill, Sydney.

So, M., Foxe, D., Kumfor, F., et al., 2018. Addenbrooke's cognitive examination III: Psychometric characteristics and relations to functional ability in dementia. J Int Neuropsychol Soc, 24(8), 854–863.

Soltan, M., & Girguis, J. 2017. How to approach the mental state examination. BMJ, 357.

Sweeney, A., Filson, B., Kennedy, A., Collinson, L., Gillard, S., 2018. A paradigm shift: Relationships in trauma-informed mental health services. BJ Psych Adv, 24(5), 319–333.

Te Ao Maramatanga New Zealand College of Mental Health Nurses, 2012. Standards of Practice for Mental Health Nursing in Aotearoa New Zealand, 3rd ed. Te Ao Maramatanga New Zealand College of Mental Health Nurses, Auckland.

Te Pou, 2020. Achieving physical health equity for people with experience of mental health and addiction issues: Evidence update. Online. Available at: www.tepou.co.nz/resources/achieving-physical-health-equity-for-people-with-experience-of-mental-health-and-addiction-issues—evidence-update-july-2020

Todd, F.C, 2010. Te Ariari o te Oranga: The Assessment and Management of People with Co-Existing Mental Health and Substance Use Problems. Ministry of Health, Wellington.

Tseliou, F., Donnelly, M., O'Reilly, D., 2018. Screening for psychiatric morbidity in the population – a comparison of the GHQ-12 and self-reported medication use. Int J Popul Data Sci, 3(1), 5.

Wand, T., 2019. Is it time to end our complicity with pharmacocentricity? Int J Ment Health Nurs, 28(1), 3–6.

Wand, T., 2015. Recovery is about a focus on resilience and wellness, not a fixation with risk and illness. Aust N Z J Psychiatry, 49(12), 1083–1084.

Wand, T., Buchanan-Hagen, S., Derrick, K. & Harris, M., 2020. Are current mental health assessment formats consistent with contemporary thinking and practice? Int J Ment Health Nurs, 29(2), 171–176.

Wand, T., Glover, S. & Paul, D., 2022. What should be the future focus of mental health nursing? Exploring the perspectives of mental health nurses, consumers, and allied health staff. Int J Ment Health Nurs, 31(1), 179–188.

Warden, S., Spiwak, R., Sareen, J., et al., 2014. The SAD PERSONS scale for suicide risk assessment: A systematic review. Arch Suicide Res, 18(4), 313–326.

Watson, T., Tindall, R., Patrick, A. & Moylan, S., 2022. Mental health triage tools: A narrative review. Int J Ment Health Nurs, 32(2), 352–364.

Westen, D., 1998. The scientific legacy of Sigmund Freud: Toward a psychodynamically informed psychological science. Psychol Bul,l 124(3), 333.

Wood, J.M., Gupta, S., 2017. Using rating scales in a clinical setting: A guide for psychiatrists. Curr Psychiatr, 16(2), 21–25.

World Health Organization (WHO), 1989. ICD-10: International Statistical Classification of Diseases and Related Health Problems, 10th rev. WHO, Geneva.

Zachar, P., Stoyanov, D.S., Aragona, M., et al., (eds), 2014. Alternative Perspectives on Psychiatric Validation: DSM, IDC, RDoC, and Beyond. Oxford University Press, Oxford.

Zanotti, R., Chiffi, D., 2015. Diagnostic frameworks and nursing diagnoses: A normative stance. Nurs Philos, 16(1), 64–73.

10

Legal and Ethical Issues

Anthony J. O'Brien

KEY POINTS

- Mental health care involves reflecting on ethical issues and applying principles of ethical reasoning.
- Codes of ethics guide members of the professions as to the nature of proper conduct and their obligations to the public.
- Ethical principles provide nurses with guidelines for ethical practice.
- A sound knowledge of legal issues is critical to contemporary mental health nursing.
- Mental health legislation is the legal framework that informs the involuntary treatment of individuals, defines their legal rights and ensures appropriate treatment.
- Australia and New Zealand have high rates of use of community treatment orders, raising questions about coercion and human rights.

KEY TERMS

- Autonomy
- Beneficence
- Code of ethics
- Community treatment orders
- Confidentiality
- Consent
- Duty of care
- Ethics
- Human rights
- Involuntary treatment
- Justice
- Least restrictive alternative
- Mental health legislation
- Non-maleficence

LEARNING OUTCOMES

The material in this chapter will assist you to:
- identify common ethical issues in mental health nursing
- apply ethical principles to the analysis of ethical issues in mental health nursing
- understand the importance of health legislation in mental health care
- identify issues related to privacy and confidentiality
- discuss the issue of informed consent in relation to compulsory mental health care
- understand the significance of the United Nations Convention on the Rights of Persons with Disabilities
- identify how the concept of duty of care applies in the mental health setting.

INTRODUCTION

Mental health nursing is practised within an ethical and legal context and within a framework of ethical principles. This chapter outlines the ethical and legal context of mental health nursing and provides guidance to assist nurses in maintaining professional practice that meets professional, legal and ethical standards. Mental health nurses are legally mandated to practise nursing in accordance with professional competencies and societal expectations. As professionals, mental health nurses must be aware of health-related legislation, including legislation specific to the domain of mental health. Ethical principles and theories assist nurses to make decisions on issues of conflict and to maintain clear and safe boundaries around their practice. In addition to the ethical issues inherent in every practice setting, the mental health context presents unique issues of coercion and treatment without consent.

The mental health context presents unique challenges for nurses because the use of compulsory treatment under mental health legislation involves significant departures from normally accepted human and healthcare rights. The United Nations Convention on the Rights of Persons with Disabilities is an international instrument aimed at protecting the human rights of people with mental illness. In recent years, Australia and Aotearoa New Zealand have been challenged under the Convention to rethink how they protect the rights of mental health consumers. In particular, the basis for compulsory treatment under mental health legislation has been challenged. Mental health legislation provides a legal framework for treatment without consent and specific guidelines for procedures such as electroconvulsive therapy (ECT), psychosurgery and seclusion. Rates of compulsory treatment in Australia and Aotearoa New Zealand are high by international standards.

This chapter explores the ethical and legal context of practice. It outlines the principles of ethical conduct and discusses some ethical issues commonly encountered in mental health nursing. It also outlines the use of mental health legislation and rights issues raised by compulsory treatment. Capacity-based legislation, advance directives and supported decision-making are explored as responses to the challenges of the Convention on the Rights of Persons with Disabilities.

A Fairer Society Can Improve Mental Health

The French Revolution (1789–99) heavily influenced understanding of how to manage mental disorders, emphasising principles such as individual rights and equality. As a consequence of the revolution, people in France who experienced mental illness began to be considered victims of a poorly ordered society. This attitude shifted the focus of blame for mental ill health away from the individual concerned and onto the ills of society. It also supported the idea that mental health care should take a social form and prompted hope for recovery if their environment could be more supportive. As introduced in Chapter 3, the ideals of the revolution emboldened French psychiatrist Phillippe Pinel and asylum superintendent Jean Baptise Pussin, who led the development of a kinder, more humane approach to mental health care, which came to be referred to as "moral therapy".

Read More About It
Pinel, P. 1806. A treatise on insanity. Messers Cadell & Davies, Strand.

ETHICS AND PROFESSIONAL PRACTICE

A profession is a collective with a clear definition of its roles and responsibilities to ensure the quality of professional practice provided by its members. The right of a group of practitioners such as nurses to call itself a profession arises through the trust between the group of practitioners and the people to whom the group provides a service. Nursing and nursing practice are guided by the law, ethical principles and the public trust in the nurse as an ethical practitioner. As a professional group, nurses must practise within the law and adhere to a code of professional conduct.

Internationally, professional nursing organisations have identified the need for codes of ethics to guide practice. A code of ethics provides a formalised set of expectations that reflects the ideals and values of a group. Codes of ethics are not a set of rules, they are a guide to professional conduct and decision-making. A nurse remains a moral agent in every situation. The first international code of ethics for nurses was developed by the International Council of Nurses (ICN) in 1953, with the most recent revision published in 2012 (International Council of Nurses 2021). The ICN code has been adopted by the Nursing and Midwifery Board of Australia as the guiding document for ethical decision-making for nurses in Australia, replacing the ANMC code of 2008. A New Zealand code of ethics was first developed in 1988 and has been redeveloped to reflect a Māori worldview (New Zealand Nurses Organisation 2019). The redeveloped code includes a guideline for ethical reflection and decision-making. Codes of ethics are informed by conventionalised ethical principles. The four most commonly adopted principles (Beauchamp & Childress 2019) – autonomy, beneficence, non-maleficence and justice – are explained in Box 10.1.

Ethical Theories

Ethical theories are formalised statements that attempt to provide a unifying framework for ethical decision-making. These theories give expression to ethical principles, although different ethical theories can lead to different decisions depending on the significance given to the different principles. While ethical theories are helpful in providing broad frameworks, each has its own limitations. Nurses need to consider the various theories, and also reflect on the effect of any decision on an individual consumer. The following section outlines the three major ethical theories that inform professional practice.

Utilitarianism

According to the theory of utilitarianism, an action is right if it produces the best or most desirable consequences compared with other action(s). Actions are right if they *maximise* happiness, pleasure, interests or preferences, and simultaneously minimise unhappiness, pain or harm. This requires one to do the "greatest good for the greatest number". A weakness of utilitarianism is that it can seem to provide a justification for acting against the interests of vulnerable individuals because they are a smaller group, because this will serve the interests

---

BOX 10.1   Seven Areas That Need to be Considered When Thinking About Clinical Scenarios and Applying Ethical Reasoning

1. **Rights:** Rights form the basis of most professional codes and legal judgements and consider ideas such as self-determination rights, rights and cultural relativism, the right to health care and rights to privacy and confidentiality.

2. **Autonomy:** Autonomy involves the right of self-determination, independence and freedom. Autonomy promotes the right of an individual to make their own decisions and implies that the person will also take responsibility for decisions made. Respect for autonomy means that nurses recognise the individual's uniqueness, right to lead a life they want and right to set personal goals. Nurses who follow the principle of autonomy respect a client's right to make choices, even if they are not always the best options in the opinion of the nurse.

3. **Beneficence** and **non-maleficence:** Beneficence means "doing good". Nurses should work towards actions that support and benefit clients and their family members. However, in an increasingly technological healthcare system, doing the best by a person can also do harm by potentially putting that person at risk (e.g. intensive therapy programs). Non-maleficence means the duty to do no harm. Harm can be caused deliberately, or it may involve actions that put the person at risk of harm, even if this was unintentional. In nursing, intentional harm is always unacceptable. The risk for potential to cause harm is not always clear. For example, a nursing intervention that is implemented to be helpful may cause harm (e.g. medication administration).

4. **Justice:** Justice can also be considered as fairness. Nurses frequently face decisions in which a sense of justice should prevail. For example, a person may be detained under mental health legislation, but justice requires this to be the case only while that person is at risk to themselves or other people and unable to self-assess and manage their own risk.

5. **Fidelity:** Fidelity means to be faithful to agreements and responsibilities one has undertaken. Nurses have responsibilities to clients, employers, government, society, the profession and themselves. Circumstances often affect which responsibilities take precedence at a particular time.

6. **Veracity:** Veracity means telling the truth. Consumers expect nurses to be truthful in matters such as planned treatment and any limits on autonomy. Veracity also applies to information about medication, where the nurse has the obligation to be truthful about risks and side effects as well as the benefits of medication.

7. **Trust and reciprocity:** We trust that colleagues will act in ways that are mutually supportive and do no harm to each other. The principle of reciprocity is essential for nurses to build trust in working relationships between professionals, as well as their clients. Consumers also rely on trust and the principle of reciprocity to ensure health practitioners do their best to do no harm and promote recovery.

of a larger number of people. However, in mental health care we sometimes want to prioritise the needs of an individual over a group; for example, in providing subsidised access to primary health services for mental health consumers.

Deontology

Deontological theory guides the duty to perform acts that are considered intrinsically good or inherently good. We have a duty to refrain from acts that are considered intrinsically bad or intrinsically wrong. Deontology is sometimes referred to as a rule-based approach to ethics, because of the concept that certain acts are morally obligatory regardless of their human consequences. Deontology is also associated with the "categorical imperative", the idea that individuals should only act towards others in ways that apply to all moral actions. A weakness of deontology is that it appears to limit room for moral agency. For example, if it is a rule that we prevent self-harm in all circumstances, there is no freedom to consider self-harm as something consumers can learn to manage autonomously.

Virtue Ethics

In contrast to the emphasis of utilitarianism on action based on its consequences and the emphasis of deontology on the right action with reference to one's duty to fulfil moral obligation(s), virtue ethics emphasises the moral character of the agent, in this context the nurse. Some consider virtue ethics to be especially pertinent to nursing because of nursing's concern with the moral character of the nurse (Varagona et al 2022). However, even a nurse who has a strong moral character will need to consider the ethical challenges of specific issues, and cannot rely on character alone to make those decisions.

Ethical concepts guide us in our everyday work as health professionals. Although ethical theory provides frameworks to help in making ethical decisions, nurses sometimes feel that the context of practice – for example, institutional rules and culture – places limits on nurses' ethical decision-making, resulting in "moral distress" (Morley 2018). Discussion with nursing colleagues and supervisors can help with difficult ethical decisions. The seven areas shown in Box 10.1 need to be considered when thinking about clinical scenarios and applying ethical reasoning.

 CRITICAL THINKING EXERCISE 10.1

Consider the current diagnostic label of borderline personality disorder (BPD) and the clinical signs and symptoms of BPD (see Chapter 16). People with BPD often present in states of high arousal with varying degrees of self-harm, and clinicians can find these presentations stressful and difficult. People with BPD are seen as providing major challenges to the healthcare service, and the label "BPD" often invokes feelings of helplessness in clinicians, who may respond by attempting to dissuade the person from accessing the health service. However, many people labelled with BPD have experienced sexual or physical abuse and have been invalidated in their lives. If this consideration persuaded us to view BPD as post-traumatic stress disorder, would this change our attitudes to working with people who are given this diagnostic label?

Ethical Principles

Ethical principles represent the view that ethical decision-making requires adhering to reliable ethical standards, sometimes described as "imperatives". The four principles explained below, identified by Beauchamp and Childress (2019), and universally adopted in healthcare, specify actions or conduct that is either prohibited, permitted or required in the circumstances. In addition, the practice of paternalism in mental health nursing is discussed.

Autonomy

Autonomy means that people are free to choose, make decisions and act on their own preferences, so long as they do not unreasonably impinge on the freedoms of others. Hence, consumers' decisions are to be respected concerning what is "in their best interests". Accordingly, in providing care and treatment a consumer's *consent* is usually required. Some exceptions to this requirement are outlined later in this chapter.

Beneficence

Beneficence mandates a positive obligation on nurses to act for the benefit of others. Beneficence embraces such virtuous acts as compassion, empathy, kindness, altruism, care, charity, friendship and mercy in providing care. An important qualification is that a nurse is not obliged to act for the benefit of others if to do so would compromise their own moral interests.

Non-Maleficence

Non-maleficence prescribes the view that nurses should "above all, do no harm". Indeed, the principle of doing no harm underpins nearly all health practice. Accordingly, in providing care, non-maleficence obliges nurses to refrain from acts that unnecessarily cause injury, harm or suffering. "Harm" includes violating a consumer's wellbeing or interests. Importantly, if there is a conflict between beneficence and non-maleficence concerning a nurse's proposed action, the latter is usually more stringently applied.

Justice

In the context of providing health care, "justice" usually means facilitating what is due and owed to a consumer. Within the limited resources available, this often means making decisions about rationing resources to ensure an equal distribution of benefits and harms – distributive justice. To make such a decision requires impartiality and objectivity on the part of the nurse to ensure fairness for all consumers.

Paternalism

While not among the frequently cited principles of ethics, paternalism is a common feature of mental health nursing practice (Bladon 2019). Actions which involve acting against the autonomy of consumers, with the intention of providing benefit, are paternalistic (Beauchamp & Childress 2019). While such actions are usually justified as being in the best interests of consumers (Paradis-Gagné 2021), they nevertheless involve a conflict with otherwise accepted ethical standards, especially autonomy. Mental health nursing has a long history of paternalism, beginning in the times when nursing was located in the asylums of the 19th century. Current practice still reflects paternalism; for example, in nurses' decisions to limit the choices available to consumers, to withhold full explanations of the side effects of medication, and in contributing to decisions to detain consumers under mental health legislation.

 CRITICAL THINKING EXERCISE 10.2

Using the four most commonly cited principles of ethical conduct (autonomy, beneficence, non-maleficence and justice), consider when and if it is appropriate to administer an intramuscular injection of medication against a consumer's will.

Ethical Issues in Mental Health Practice

Nurses will encounter many ethical issues in clinical practice in mental health. The ethical theories and principles outlined above are intended to assist in ethical reflection and decision-making and to guide nurses towards actions that meet the ethical standards of the profession. Five ethical issues that are unique to mental health care are discussed below. These are psychiatric diagnosis, psychological therapy, psychopharmacology, coercive practices and electroconvulsive therapy.

Psychiatric Diagnosis

Psychiatric diagnosis is a fundamental issue in mental health care, and requires ethical reflection by nurses. Stigma surrounding mental illness means that people who receive a psychiatric diagnosis may feel labelled, and marginalised from their friends, family and community (Flaskeraud 2018). There is also a perception that a psychiatric diagnosis is lifelong. Personal consequences of a psychiatric diagnosis may include discrimination in employment, housing and healthcare, all of which can impact social functioning and recovery. Complicating this picture is the observation that some people find diagnosis helpful, because it seems to offer an explanation for experiences that they have found concerning, confusing and distressing (O'Connor et al 2018).

A further ethical issue with psychiatric diagnosis arises from questions about the reliability and validity of the diagnosis. Reliability refers to the consistency with which a diagnosis can be made, while validity refers to whether constructs such as "schizophrenia" refer to real diseases. The process of psychiatric diagnosis has been reported as being of poor or questionable reliability (Paris 2020; Zachar et al 2014), while schizophrenia has been referred to as a "scientific delusion" (Guloksuz et al 2021). Recent research has emphasised the contribution of trauma to development of psychosis (Popovic et al 2019), raising questions about the continued use of terms such as "schizophrenia", which are often taken to imply a biologically-based disease. In addition, it is not always easy for consumers to relate experiences of trauma to a clinician. Consumers may not have enough trust in professionals to tell their story, and some aspects of their history may be too painful to recount in full. Clinicians will therefore not always have a full understanding of what may have contributed to their problems. Given the potential harms that diagnosis might cause, continued use of diagnostic concepts, especially to the exclusion of more helpful alternatives, raises ethical questions of a nurse's role in contributing to harm (*maleficence*). A different perspective on the benefits of diagnosis is provided by Campbell and colleagues (2020). These authors argue that diagnosis of borderline personality disorder, along with psychological formulation (see below) can be helpful in legitimising access to mental health care and facilitating recovery.

Diagnosis is often justified on the basis of the need for a common language to describe the experiences of people believed to be mentally ill. The most commonly used system of classification, the *Diagnostic and Statistical Manual of Mental Disorders* (DSM) (American Psychiatric Association (APA) 2013) provides a list of psychiatric diagnoses, and sets of criteria for applying diagnostic labels. However, the DSM has been criticised for creating an ever-expanding catalogue of mental illnesses, even beyond the boundaries of psychiatry (Harbusch 2022), resulting in more people being labelled with mental illness. Expansion of the practice of diagnosis constructs general problems in living or traits of personality as psychiatric disorders that are then treated with pharmaceuticals. Furthermore, once a diagnosis is made, future behaviours and actions may be attributed to the diagnosis and hence used as evidence of its validity.

Psychological formulation is an alternative to psychiatric diagnosis suggested by psychologist Lucy Johnstone (Johnstone 2018). Johnstone argues that psychological formulation can assist consumers to gain an understanding of their problems without the loss of meaning that can occur with psychiatric diagnosis. From an ethical perspective, psychological formulation offers the benefits of the consumer understanding what is happening for them (*beneficence*) without the potentially harmful effects of being labelled mentally ill (*non-maleficence*). Formulation is further discussed below, and is also discussed in Chapter 9.

✴ HISTORICAL ANECDOTE 10.2

Psychiatric Diagnosis Used to Justify Breaches of Human Rights

Psychiatric diagnoses reflect contemporary concerns about behaviour that is considered concerning. A late as 1973 homosexuality was classified as a mental illness. Less known is that an early 19th-century American physician and medical writer, Samuel A Cartwright, developed a number of diagnoses to describe the behaviour of enslaved African-Americans. Diagnoses included "drapetomania" – a disease that caused slaves to run away; "rascality" – a disease that led to slaves committing petty crimes; and "dysaesthesia ethiopica"– which made slaves indifferent to punishment. Cartwright was not alone in inventing psychiatric diagnoses that embodied the racist views of the times. Racialised views of medicine were prevalent throughout the western world during Cartwright's time. This historical example gives us cause to contemplate how our current models of mental health and mental health care reflect the views and interests of dominant groups, and can potentially marginalise the experience of minorities.

Read More About It

Willoughby, C.D. 2018. Running away from drapetomania: Samuel A. Cartwright, medicine, and race in the Antebellum South. J South Hist, 84(3), 579–614.

Psychiatric Treatment

The intention of all health care is to provide benefits to consumers (beneficence), and to avoid harm (non-maleficence). Health care should also involve consent and respect the *autonomy* of consumers. From an ethical perspective then, it is concerning if psychiatric treatment falls short of these ethical ideals. Mental health consumers are critical of the use of coercive practices (e.g. overuse of pharmaceuticals, restraint and seclusion, and treatment orders) and perceive their use by nurses as punishment (Hawsawi et al 2020; Muir-Cochrane et al 2021). Interestingly, nurses are more likely than consumers to view coercive practices as providing benefits to consumers. Worldwide, lengths of stay in hospital have decreased, while admission rates have increased. This has resulted in changes to the overall environment of in-patient units where the predominant use of medication and containment reflect a paternalistic medical model of care with little opportunity for recovery-focused practice. Similarly, community mental health services often have high case numbers which limit the opportunities for nurses and other practitioners to engage in non-pharmacological treatments such as psychological therapy and family-focused therapy. In some services, many consumers are subject to community treatment orders (CTO), raising ethical issues of consent, reduced autonomy, paternalism and coercion. Use of CTOs raise further issues concerning the human rights of a person diagnosed with a mental illness compared with members of the general public (Brophy et al 2018). Further discussion of CTOs is provided later in this chapter.

Some initiatives that seek to improve care provided in mental health services are seclusion reduction initiatives, which have been successful in Australia and Aotearoa New Zealand (Boulton et al 2022; Jury et al 2019), Safewards, a set of interventions designed to reduce incidents of conflict and containment (Dickens et al 2020) and trauma-informed care (Isobel et al 2021), an approach to care that recognises that many consumers have experienced trauma in their lives and may experience aspects of mental health care as traumatic. The impetus to reduce use of restrictive practices and to accord greater respect for autonomy is grounded in ethical awareness, illustrating the need for nurses to critically reflect on ethical issues in mental health nursing.

Psychopharmacology

The drugs prescribed for mental illness can cause major side effects and problems with toxicity. Second generation antipsychotic agents, such as clozapine and olanzapine, can cause cardiac complications and metabolic disorders (Pillinger et al 2020). Psychotropic medications can also interact with other therapeutic agents and so need to be monitored closely. Side effects, such as metabolic syndrome and dependence, raise ethical issues of non-maleficence, while administration of medication without consent, as frequently occurs in mental health nursing, compromises the consumer's autonomy. People who have been taking psychotropic medication may find it difficult to stop or reduce their medication due to discontinuation syndrome (Massabki & Abi-Jaoude 2020; Watts et al 2021), which carries further ethical implications. As with other psychiatric treatments, nurses may adopt a paternalistic position, arguing that their practice in this area is motivated by beneficence, but issues of non-maleficence and compromised autonomy also need to be considered. The benefits of the medication must outweigh the hazards.

With respect to drug treatment, a question that needs to be considered is: What are a person's rights when placed on psychopharmacological agents? These rights include access to effective non-pharmacological treatment and information concerning the drug prescribed (desired effects, side effects, contraindications, complications) and the freedom to accept or refuse treatment. These rights may be limited if the person is an involuntary patient under mental health legislation, although involuntary patients retain the right to informed consent to the maximum extent possible. All consumers should have a voice in treatment decisions, including medication. Benefits and risks should be explained. If the side effects of a particular drug are difficult to live with, the person should be offered a medication review and change of treatment, including a non-pharmacological alternative. Psychopharmacology is further discussed in Chapter 21.

Electroconvulsive Therapy

Electroconvulsive therapy (ECT) is a treatment that attracts considerable controversy (Lonergan et al 2021) and stigma (de Anta et al 2023), in part due its past indiscriminate and sometimes punitive use (Royal Commission of Inquiry 2022). Currently, ECT is used mainly for major depressive disorder (Griffiths & O'Neill-Kerr 2019). A significant ethical conflict occurs when a psychiatrist prescribes ECT in order to reduce a consumer's risk of self-harm or harm through neglect, but the individual does not give consent for the therapy (Surya et al 2019). The thought of having ECT can be traumatic to consumers and families due to the negative perceptions about this form of treatment and the potential for memory loss. Porter and colleagues (2020) outline issues of choice and effectiveness related to ECT and urge nurses to carefully consider their views on this form of treatment. As with all treatments, consent for ECT needs to be negotiated with consumers to prevent medical paternalism. For depressed people, lowered mood and pessimistic outlook may mean they are unable to see any solution to their depression. In the case of refusal to consent, doctors in Aotearoa New Zealand and in some Australian states have the power under mental health legislation to administer ECT without the consumer's consent, but require a second psychiatric opinion to do so. Treatment without consent involves a significant limitation on the consumer's autonomy and so needs sound ethical justification. Nurses need to ensure that consumers and their families are informed of the nature of the procedure and why substituted consent has been provided by treating psychiatrists. ECT is also discussed in Chapter 12.

PERSPECTIVES IN PRACTICE

Nurse's Story 10.1: Simon

I have worked in many areas of nursing, but found my way into mental health about 15 years ago. All clinical areas have their challenges, and the challenges are often about the legal requirements, as well as ethical issues about practice and treatment options for consumers. Nurses make a big difference in consumer advocacy and are often the person who checks the legal requirements and thinks about ethical decision-making. It is an essential part of reflective practice for a nurse. Thinking how the benefits of treatment outweigh the harm of treatment is often difficult in mental health. We have mental health legislation that governs our practice. That gives us a lot of power, but it also places a greater amount of responsibility and decision-making on the nurse working in mental health with people who are detained and prescribed treatment without their consent. We work in partnership when we can with consumers and their carers, but often when a person is severely depressed or psychotic it is difficult to engage. That doesn't mean you don't try.

One of my main roles is ECT nurse coordinator. This means I work with the medical staff, the psychiatrist and the anaesthetist to administer ECT. I'm responsible for the consumer's care once they come to the ECT suite and during the procedure, and I manage and support the nurses who are escorting people and providing after-treatment care in the recovery suite. We also have a lot of students come through as it is a teaching hospital.

ECT is a controversial topic. I have care-coordinated ECT for years and seen good outcomes, but there is a lot of stigma and misunderstanding about ECT as a treatment. The *Mental Health Act* provides direction for the procedure and states that the person needs to have given voluntary consent. If they are unable to do this, then there are provisions to provide the prescribed ECT treatment against the consumer's wishes. So, this may be legal to do but it reduces the person's autonomy in decision-making, and you have to ensure the benefits outweigh the potential harms. ECT is a safe treatment and it is conducted within guidelines and standards directed by the Chief Psychiatrist's Office.

Consumers are often quite frightened by the thought of having ECT, and this has been influenced by the media. Consumers can also be passive in their treatment, especially if the psychiatrists have prescribed and consented to it for them. What we try to do here is bring the person down to the ECT suite and take them through. I think this really helps them to be more at ease and also to have a better recovery. The idea to do an orientation came from the number of events we had with people becoming distressed and disoriented in recovery. So, we take them to a room and say this is where you will come and wait for the treatment, explain the procedure and that they need to fast and encourage questions. Then they go into the suite and we say this is where you will lie down and be given a short-acting anaesthetic and how they will be hooked up to some monitors. We then show them the recovery area and say you will wake up here and once you are ready you can go back to the ward area and have breakfast. I try to include student nurses in this orientation as well and always ask the consumer if it would be OK to have students in the room during the procedure. It is very rare that they have a problem with students.

I like to have student nurses. They don't just observe, they can have supervised but hands-on experience with the care of the consumer, placing on the monitoring equipment, turning them, taking vital signs and recovering them. They also get to see the Mental Health Act in practice and how we check the consent and that it is the correct consumer and the prescription is correct and current. The whole team takes an interest in students and we encourage them to ask questions and speak to the consumer after the treatment once they are recovered.

Seclusion and Restraint

Seclusion is the involuntary supervised isolation of a person in a locked, non-stimulating room (Haugom et al 2019). Seclusion rooms are usually spartan, containing only a mattress with a blanket and a bed pan. Limited furniture is aimed at preventing consumers from hurting themselves or others. Although some Australian courts have interpreted mental health legislation to determine that seclusion is deemed to be treatment and not a management action, nursing literature is clear that seclusion should not be regarded as a therapeutic intervention (Jackson et al 2019).

Under current legislation, seclusion is generally deemed lawful when it is necessary to protect the mental health consumer's health and welfare or to protect another person from imminent risk to their health or safety. However, although seclusion is legal, ethical issues remain.

Consumers and some clinicians and researchers have been influential in raising awareness about the negative impact of seclusion for consumers (see Chapter 4 for further discussion about seclusion).

Consumers have expressed dissatisfaction with seclusion, finding the experience negative, frightening, cold, drab and untherapeutic, while increasing their feelings of distress or agitation (Askew et al 2019; Allikmets et al 2020). And the World Health Organization (WHO) (2019) has suggested that authorities should pursue the elimination of isolation rooms and prohibit the provision of new ones. Because of the ethical and human rights issues associated with seclusion, in recent years both Australia and Aotearoa New Zealand have followed policies of reducing or eliminating seclusion (Australian College of Mental Health Nurses 2019; Te Pou o te Whakaaro Nui 2018; Wilson et al 2023); however, the goal of elimination has not yet been achieved. The Safewards program mentioned above aims to reduce the use of seclusion and has now been implemented in many countries internationally (Ward-Stockholm 2022).

PERSPECTIVES IN PRACTICE

Nurse's Story 10.2: Rachael

I was educated to believe that we should have shared male/female wards. The end of the 1970s was when they had segregated wards and that was before my time. After that, wards only had beds, and nurses would care for consumers, be they male or female. We always tried to allocate a female with a female nurse and a male with a male nurse when personal care was required, but largely we based the ward bed allocation not on gender but on consumers' need for safety. And when I went into the community you had to go to people's homes and give injections, be they either gender.

On reflection, this has caused a lot of concern for consumers coming into the ward environment and I am glad to say it has been identified as a major need by the Department of Health. Our ward has had funding to develop a female-only area. This provides a space for meeting and also a separate corridor for female-only beds and bathrooms. It was controversial at first, but it is part of everyday practice now.

Women feel more comfortable having a separate space to go to and an area where they can rest and shower without the fear of males coming in. Doors on bathrooms don't lock in mental health facilities, and that can make many women feel uncomfortable and unsafe. No matter how hard we try to make this a welcoming and home-like environment, it is still a public space. We don't want women coming into mental health facilities and feeling uncomfortable when there is no need for them to feel this way.

Management obtained the funding and a committee of clinicians and the carer and consumer consultant guided the development of policy, as well as the spending to redesign the ward. A great outcome! It was also an example of how you can work with consumers, listen to them and develop ways to provide the least restrictive environment possible as per the Mental Health Act. So, in this case an environment could be created where women can move freely and attend to their ablutions in a safe-feeling environment. Where we aim to care but do no harm.

We did also plan for transgender consumers. There is a room with an ensuite bathroom so anyone who identifies as transgender can have the option to stay here if their risk assessment upon admission allows for this plan of care. If they need closer monitoring, then we consider this as part of their care plan.

It is important to think about the restrictive environments we work in within mental health. There has been a lot of work done on reducing the use of seclusion, but we often find that this means the person is within a high dependency area that has secure doors and a quite rigid routine. Nurses need to ensure that consumers feel comfortable in this environment and monitor this. When they need less observation and care, we transfer people to the open ward as soon as we can. But sometimes the doors to these units are locked as well, as there are many people on the ward who are a danger to themselves. The locked ward resolves a lot of the problems that you would experience with consumers in a general ward where you don't have this facility, but it poses human rights and ethical issues. Legally the wards can be locked if even one consumer at the time poses a danger to themselves or to others. For example, if they were actively wanting to harm themselves. But the guidelines of the Mental Health Act do not take away from the ethical decision-making we must do to always place the consumer in the least restrictive environment, promote their self-advocacy and choice. We must ensure that the benefits of a locked ward area are clear and that the need for this is conveyed to the consumer and their family. We must also make provision for others to have leave from the ward to go about their business without restriction. This can be time-consuming to do, but it is very much part of the day-to-day work of a mental health nurse to ensure we provide the best care we can.

Suicidal Behaviour

Caring for suicidal people is one of the most challenging clinical situations that mental health professionals face. The topic of suicide is well documented, but few realise that the number of unsuccessful attempts at suicide is eight to ten times the figure for actual suicide (Ministry of Health 2019). The high incidence of suicide and suicidal behaviour makes this a significant issue for mental health nurses. The ethical debate about suicide largely centres on the justification for intervening in a person's choice to live or die. Clearly, intervention to prevent suicide contravenes the autonomy of the consumer. Clinicians commonly invoke a paternalistic justification of benefit to the consumer. The benefit of maintaining life is considered to outweigh the harm of supporting autonomy where that would lead to the death of the consumer and would be in contravention of nursing ethics and duty of care. Compounding this ethical dilemma is that a suicidal person may not be suffering from a mental illness and may have decision-making capacity. In addition, although a suicide attempt increases the likelihood of suicide in the future, it is not possible to predict a suicide attempt by an individual consumer. Researchers suggest that instead of prediction, the aim of care should be engagement and collaborative safety planning (Hawton et al 2022). In clinical settings, nurses have a duty of care to prevent suicide but must weigh up what the limits of that duty are, and when a consumer should retain autonomy to make and take responsibility for their own decisions. A key consideration is the imminence of suicide. If a consumer is on the phone to a nurse from a crisis team and has taken a potentially lethal overdose of medication, intervention, even involuntary intervention, could be considered ethically justifiable. However, if the risk is some time in the future, then immediate intervention to prevent suicide may be neither necessary nor justifiable.

HISTORICAL ANECDOTE 10.3

Australian Mental Health Care Began in a Jail

In the early days of Aotearoa New Zealand and Australia, the colonial governments of both countries were unable to afford the cost of establishing stand-alone mental health facilities, which meant people who became mentally ill were kept in jails alongside criminals. Australia's first "lunatic asylum" was opened in 1811 when Governor Macquarie and his wife, Elizabeth, inspected Parramatta Gaol and were so moved with compassion for people in the jail who were experiencing mental ill health that he gave orders to open Australia's first asylum at Castle Hill. Macquarie's empathy was linked to his older brother Donald's experience of mental illness following his return from the Napoleonic wars. Aotearoa New Zealand's first asylum was opened some years later in 1844 for remarkably similar reasons, when Wellington Jail became overcrowded.

Read More About It

Raeburn, T., Liston, C., Hickmott, J., Cleary, M. 2018. Life of Martha Entwistle: Australia's first convict mental health nurse. Int J Ment Health Nurs, 27(1), 455–463.

Involuntary Treatment

Involuntary (or compulsory) treatment refers to treatment provided under mental health legislation without the consent of the consumer. Because treatment without consent contravenes the ethical principle of autonomy, it requires a strong ethical justification. The justification for involuntary treatment is usually one of paternalism, based on assessment of risk. Treatment without consent is considered justified if there is a significant risk that without treatment severe harm would occur to the consumer or to another person. Consumers frequently find this restriction of autonomy depersonalising and demeaning (Hawsawi et al 2020), creating the further ethical issue of a breach of the principle of non-maleficence. Further harm can result from the limitations that involuntary treatment places on the therapeutic nurse–consumer relationship. Consumers who feel they have few rights and are restricted by legislation may be less likely to engage in a working relationship with a mental health nurse.

When a person is committed to a mental health facility, or placed under a CTO, a major ethical debate centres on the tension between the state's legal responsibilities (parens patriae – the state's duty to act as a parent) versus individual human rights (liberty, autonomy). When should a person be admitted involuntarily under mental health legislation? Under current legislation, the answer is usually about when the person is a danger to themselves or others *and* suffering from a mental illness (McSherry 2021). However, consider whether you would feel comfortable committing a person to a mental health facility if the person was a member of your family or a close friend.

A consumer voluntarily seeking treatment for a mental illness should be treated as having decision-making capacity and retains the right to give or withhold consent to treatment, unless assessed otherwise. Conversely, an involuntary consumer admitted to hospital under mental health legislation may be deemed to have limited legal capacity to refuse or consent to treatment (Mandarelli et al 2018). As nurses, we should advocate for such disempowered consumers; for example, by creating opportunities to maximise the choices available, however limited they may be. However, we must advocate in collaboration with consumers or else we risk being paternalistic by assuming our actions are in their best interests and that we are qualified to speak on the consumer's behalf. Although the intention is to provide benefit, consumer autonomy is at risk. All consumers should be treated with the same degree of respect that you would require for yourself and, whenever practicable, their autonomy should be maintained. This ensures consumers maintain their integrity and do not feel so vulnerable and powerless.

CRITICAL THINKING EXERCISE 10.3

Beth is 23 years old and is admitted to an acute mental health in-patient unit as an involuntary patient. She has been diagnosed with a drug-induced relapse of psychosis and it is expected that she will have a short admission. Beth remembers a past admission where a male consumer came into her room at night and rummaged through her belongings. Because of that experience, she is having problems sleeping on the ward this time. Should Beth be prescribed prn (pro re nata) sedatives? Considering contemporary beliefs concerning gender equality and mixed-sex wards, is allocating beds on a needs basis always appropriate? What gender issues arise from having integrated ward environments with involuntary consumers, and what can we do about them?

Interpersonal Therapy

Interpersonal therapy involves a consumer working with a clinician in the context of a relationship of trust. This may be individual or group therapy. In therapy, the clinician (or therapist) attempts to help the consumer make changes in their thinking, behaviour, emotional responses and social relationships. Consumers place trust in their therapist, expecting that the therapist will not exploit it. This places the therapist in a position of considerable power. Nurses practising as therapists, or using methods of interpersonal therapy in their clinical practice need to ensure that their practice is focused on what benefits the consumer, not what is comfortable to the nurse. In particular, it is important that therapists do not foster dependence in consumers, as this limits the consumer's autonomy.

In general, the ethical guidelines for one-on-one and group therapy are threefold: (1) to protect the consumer from exploitation, incompetence and coercive pressure; (2) to uphold the right of the consumer to make informed decisions concerning their life; and (3) to foster personal growth and wellness (Adshead 2021). The first two goals protect and promote the consumer's autonomy, while the third outlines the expected benefits of therapy. It is often taken for granted that therapy is beneficial for the consumer. After all, looking at oneself or sharing beliefs during group or individual therapy should help consumers to grow and understand why their lives have evolved as they have. This aim is compromised when the therapy is focused on the needs of the therapist, rather than on those of the consumer. In extreme cases, this can lead to unprofessional conduct, including sexual exploitation of the consumer.

Professional Boundaries

The therapeutic relationship is a privileged relationship for both the consumer and the clinician. Courts often refer to the relationship as a "fiduciary relationship" – one in which the consumer is asked to place trust in the clinician. Responsibility for maintaining the required professional boundaries rests with the clinician, who needs to have safeguards in place that will enable issues involving professional boundaries to be identified and appropriately managed (Daigle 2020). Without adequate professional boundaries there is a risk that consumers may suffer emotional harm, which would be a breach of the ethical principle of non-maleficence. Safeguards include reflective practice, especially use of a colleague or supervisor to discuss consumer care confidentially. You may notice at times when you are working closely with a consumer that you have feelings of friendship, wanting to save the consumer from reckless behaviour, frustration with their lack of progress or a sense of knowing better than the consumer what their needs are. Consumers may disclose personal issues that are not related to their care, or may invite you to social events. These are all indications that the boundary between nurse and consumer, which is intended to keep both nurse and consumer safe, is at risk.

You should be aware of the boundaries needed to keep nursing care therapeutic and consumer-centred. When a nurse moves outside the therapeutic relationship and establishes a friendship or social relationship with a consumer, the professional boundaries between the nurse and the consumer become confused. When professional boundaries are blurred, the relationship can become non-therapeutic and potentially harmful to both the consumer and the nurse. Utilising ethical decision-making principles is especially important to ensure that professional boundaries are not transgressed.

❓ CRITICAL THINKING EXERCISE 10.4

Kirsty has been employed in an in-patient ward for 3 months and has been working with her clinical supervisor on developing interpersonal skills and maintaining professional boundaries. One of the consumers Kirsty is caring for is Marissa, a young woman close to Kirsty's age. In talking with Marissa, Kirsty becomes aware that they share certain life issues. These are to do with trust, forming intimate relationships and a fear of being abandoned if they let anyone get too close to them. Because they have so much in common Kirsty feels able to help Marissa more than the other nurses on the ward. Kirsty's friends are having a party next weekend and she decides to invite Marissa so that Marissa can meet some new people and perhaps form some friendships. Kirsty decides to discuss this with her supervisor after the party, when she will be able to report on how the intervention has worked. Do you think Kirsty is at risk of breaking professional boundaries? What suggestions can you make that would help Kirsty to develop safe and positive interpersonal relationships?

Confidentiality

Confidentiality is essential to health care. It is a primary principle of the therapeutic relationship and is based on the ethical principle of autonomy. For nurses to engage in professional practice, consumers need to be able to trust that their personal information will not be disclosed to others. This means that information should only be shared with others who are responsible for the care of the consumer. However, there are some limitations to confidentiality. In some cases, ethical principles of non-maleficence and justice might dictate that confidential information should be disclosed to a third party. For example, if a consumer reveals information about an intention to harm others, that information must be shared with the rest of the team. In this case, the principle of justice might override that of autonomy. There might also be occasions where it is necessary to share a consumer's health information with another practitioner, such as a general practitioner, to ensure that harm does not result from the GP being unaware of prescribed treatments. Most health services have policies for these situations, and these policies guide professional practice within the law and within codes of ethics. Nurses should seek guidance in cases where they are unsure. Another issue that can arise is that of secrecy. Consumers sometimes ask nurses to keep secrets. Secrets are appropriate within a friendship, but never within a therapeutic relationship. It is paramount that the consumer is made aware that information will be shared with the team and that this information will remain within the team. Hence, confidentiality in such circumstances is a *prima facie moral principle* and not an *absolute obligation*. This is reflected in the common law and also in nursing codes of conduct and professional practice.

LAW AND MENTAL HEALTH

Like other areas of nursing, mental health nursing occurs within a framework of legislation and the common law. Every jurisdiction has professional regulations legislation that govern professional practice. Legislation covers such issues as privacy, guardianship and healthcare rights. In addition to these various legal frameworks, mental health care is unique compared with other areas of nursing because mental health is the only specialty in which a significant proportion of services are provided under a framework of legal compulsion and without consent. This section outlines the major areas of law that impact on the care of mental health consumers and the practice of mental health nurses.

Professional Regulation

In Australia, nursing and other health practitioners, including students, are registered with and regulated by, the Australian Health Practitioner Regulation Authority (Ahpra) and through boards such as the Nursing and Midwifery Board of Australia (NMBA). Ahpra and the NMBA operate under what is known as statutory law – that is, an Act of Parliament. In Australia, there is uniform regulation of nurses through the *Health Practitioner Regulation National Law Act*, also known as the National Law, passed by all Australian state and territory parliaments. This mandates registration of health practitioners annually, certification and reporting of any relevant events (e.g. a charge or finding of guilt relating to serious criminal offences).

Aotearoa New Zealand nurses' practice is governed by Te Kaunihera Tapuhi o Aotearoa/The Nursing Council of New Zealand (NCNZ). This is a statutory body authorised under the *Health Practitioners Competence Assurance Act 2003*. Both the Aotearoa New Zealand and Australian Acts are primarily concerned with protecting the safety of the public. The nursing regulatory boards are therefore authorised to make judgements about individual nurses' eligibility for registered and fitness to practise. Decisions made by regulatory boards are subject to court rulings on appeal. The National Law (Australia) defines professional misconduct, unprofessional conduct and notifiable conduct and the relevant board (e.g. the NMBA) may investigate nurses whose practice or conduct is or may be unsatisfactory. For example, the board may assess a nurse's knowledge, skill, judgement or care, and evaluate this in relation to the standard reasonably expected of a nurse of an equivalent level of training or experience. Additionally, the Act authorises boards to intervene if nurses or students have an impairment (e.g. a physical or mental health impairment) that affects patients' safety. Furthermore, there is a mandatory requirement for nurses, employers, and (in the case of students) educators to report such an impairment; that is, impairment is one ground for "notifiable conduct". The other grounds for notifiable conduct (and hence mandatory reporting) are when a nurse:

- provides care while affected by alcohol or drugs
- engages in sexual misconduct in connection with practice
- places consumers at risk of harm by significantly departing from professional standards.

The NMBA has adopted codes and competency standards to articulate minimum standards – including compliance with relevant law (NMBA 2008; 2016) – and the values that should inform practice. Similarly, the NCNZ (2012) refers to Acts that impose legal obligations on Aotearoa New Zealand nurses, as well as the council's expectations about the values nurses are expected to demonstrate. Failure by nurses to practise according to the standards of conduct and values could lead to disciplinary proceedings, with the form of investigation, hearing and outcome outlined in the regulatory legislation regimes.

Privacy Legislation

Privacy is important to health consumers in any setting, and especially in mental health where consumers may be subject to stigma or discrimination if their mental health history is known. In clinical practice, nurses have many therapeutic encounters with consumers in which sensitive, deeply personal information is discussed. There may also be conflict within families that accentuates the need for privacy in consumers' relationships with mental health professionals. Legislation has been introduced to address these issues, although privacy also remains an ethical obligation on the part of nurses.

At common law, medical and nursing notes, whether in paper, electronic or other form, belong to the health service, although the information is owned by the consumer. For clarity, the Commonwealth created a legislative scheme in relation to the issues of privacy and confidentiality including health records and data. The Australian Information Commissioner is responsible for administering the *Privacy Act 1988*. The 13 Australian Privacy Principles (APPs), which are contained in Schedule 1 of the Privacy Act, outline how most Australian government agencies (e.g. Medicare, health services and hospitals) and all private health service providers must handle, use and manage personal information. The APPs are not prescriptive; each agency needs to consider how the principles apply to its own situation. The principles cover:

- the open and transparent management of personal information, including having a privacy policy
- rules for collecting solicited personal information and receiving unsolicited personal information, including giving notice about collection
- how personal information can be used and disclosed (including overseas)
- maintaining the quality of personal information
- keeping personal information secure
- access to personal information
- the right for individuals to access and correct their personal information.

APP 12 requires agencies that hold personal information about an individual (e.g. a consumer) to give the individual access to that information on request, although there are limits. APP 12.3 lists 10 grounds on which an organisation can refuse to give access to personal information, including:

- the organisation reasonably believes that giving access would pose a serious threat to the life, health or safety of any individual (consumer), or to public health or public safety (APP 12.3(a))
- giving access would have an unreasonable impact on the privacy of other individuals (APP 12.3(b))
- the request for access is frivolous or vexatious (APP 12.3(c)).

Some mental health legislation contains laws about confidentiality and when information can be disclosed. For example, where the consumer does not consent, information may be disclosed to carers under the *Mental Health Act 2014* (Victoria) if the information is reasonably required for the ongoing care of the person and the carer will be involved in providing that care. Conversely, where a consumer does not consent to the disclosure of information to a carer, this must be respected (such as s. 288 (2)(a) of the *Mental Health Act 2016* (Queensland)). However, there is some tension between carers' requests to be lawfully provided with more information and consumers' concern about protecting their rights to privacy and confidentiality.

The New Zealand Privacy Commissioner's website provides information about the New Zealand *Privacy Act 1993*, which applies to all health agencies (see Useful websites). A Health Information Privacy Code sets out specific rules for agencies in the health sector and covers health information collected, used, held and disclosed by health agencies. The code requires that health information is kept confidential, but also allows information to be passed on to third parties under certain circumstances, such as to other health professionals involved in the consumer's care, or where other legislation requires it. Within the health sector, health information can only be disclosed if the reason for the disclosure is the same reason the information was collected (i.e. for providing health care). Other legislation with implications for consumers' privacy includes the *Mental Health (Compulsory Assessment and Treatment) Act 1992* and the *Health and Disability Commissioner Act 1996*.

Finally, codes of conduct and ethics for nurses require nurses to respect the privacy of consumers. The NMBA Code of Conduct for Nurses in Australia (2018) and the International Council of Nurses Code of Ethics for Nurses (2021) outline the requirement for nurses to observe confidentiality in the course of their practice. Privacy is one of the principles of the NCNZ's Code of Conduct for Nurses.

Guardianship Legislation

Issues of guardianship arise when an adult lacks legal capacity and is therefore deemed to be unable to provide a valid consent (Chesterman 2018). Each jurisdiction has guardianship legislation that facilitates consent for treatment on behalf of adults who have been assessed as lacking capacity. In Australian jurisdictions (except the Australian Capital Territory and the Northern Territory), the consent of a relative or carer may be lawful where no other legal guardian has been appointed. For example, the Victorian *Guardianship and Administration Act 2019* regulates the appointment of guardians by the Victorian Civil and Administrative Tribunal, and determines whether the consumer's spouse or domestic partner and primary carer can act as a guardian.

Depending on the circumstances of the consumer for whom an order is made, a guardian's authority may be full or limited (e.g. in decision-making scope or period of authorisation). Typically, the legislation refers to the guardian acting in the consumer's best interests or the consumer's health and wellbeing, along with acting according to the consumer's wishes if these are known. Mental health (or sometimes guardianship) legislation may limit the capacity of guardians to consent to or refuse some psychiatric treatments (e.g. ECT and psychosurgery); it may be necessary to obtain authorisation from a guardianship authority or mental health tribunal. This highlights the need for nurses to become familiar with both the relevant mental health and the guardianship legislation in their jurisdiction.

In New Zealand, guardianship for adults is provided for in the *Protection of Personal and Property Rights Act 1988* (Douglass et al 2020). Under that legislation a person can assign an enduring power of attorney (EPOA) to a trusted individual, as long as they are competent to do so. The Act provides two forms of guardianship – one for personal affairs (financial affairs, personal business, etc.) and another for welfare (including decisions about health care). If an EPOA has been assigned it must be "activated" to become effective. Activation requires a health professional to determine that the individual now lacks decision-making capacity. Once activated the power of attorney allows the nominated person to make decisions on behalf of the incompetent individual. Most mental health consumers, including compulsory patients under the *Mental Health (Compulsory Assessment and Treatment) Act*, retain the legal capacity to make decisions, including about health care, although compulsory patients may be treated without consent subject to assessment by a second clinician. If the individual has not named an EPOA, this role can be assigned by the Family Court.

TABLE 10.1	Mental Health Legislation and Related Guidelines in Australia and New Zealand	
Jurisdiction	**Legislation**	**Guidelines**
Australian Capital Territory	*Mental Health Act 2015*	Information about the Act www.health.act.gov.au
New South Wales	*Mental Health Act 2007*	*Mental Health Act 2007:* guide book www.health.nsw.gov.au
Northern Territory	*Mental Health and Related Services Act 1998*	Mental health information for health professionals https://health.nt.gov.au/professionals/mental-health-information-for-health-professional
Queensland	*Mental Health Act 2016*	*Mental Health Act 2016:* Chief Psychiatrist policies and guidelines www.health.qld.gov.au
South Australia	*Mental Health Act 2009*	Clinicians' guide and code of practice www.sahealth.sa.gov.au
Tasmania	*Mental Health Act 2013*	*Mental Health Act 2013:* a guide for clinicians www.dhhs.tas.gov.au
Victoria	*Mental Health Act 2014*	*Mental Health Act 2014:* handbook www.health.vic.gov.au
Western Australia	*Mental Health Act 2014*	Clinicians' practice guide to the *Mental Health Act 2014* www.mentalhealth.wa.gov.au
Aotearoa New Zealand	*Mental Health (Compulsory Assessment and Treatment) Act 1992*	Guideline to the *Mental Health (Compulsory Assessment and Treatment) Act 1992* www.health.govt.nz

Mental Health Legislation

Compulsory treatment under mental health legislation carries significant human right implications for consumers and presents unique clinical, ethical and professional issues for mental health nurses. This section on law and mental health provides an outline of the rationale for mental health legislation, the process of enacting civil commitment, discussion of the rights of people subject to compulsory treatment, ethical issues for mental health nurses, and human rights issues related to mental health legislation. Several Australian states have passed new legislation in recent years, and a full list of current legislation is provided in Table 10.1. The 1992 mental health legislation of Aotearoa New Zealand is described, although that legislation is scheduled for replacement. Information about new legislation will be available on the Ministry of Health website (see Useful websites). Some aspects of the legislation of the State of Victoria are outlined as an example of Australian legislation. A detailed comparison of Australian and Aotearoa New Zealand mental health legislation has been provided by the Royal Australian and New Zealand College of Psychiatrists (see Useful websites at the end of this chapter). Discussion of mental health legislation is followed by a section discussing the human rights implications of mental health legislation, with special reference to the UN Convention on the Rights of Persons with Disabilities. Many jurisdictions provide separate legislation for the compulsory treatment of alcohol and other addictions. That legislation is not covered in this chapter, and readers are referred to more specialised resources and the websites of each jurisdiction. A list of key concepts related to mental health legislation is provided in Box 10.2.

Rationale for Mental Health Legislation

Legal powers to protect individuals from the consequences of their behaviour resulting from mental illness, or to protect others from such behaviour, have a long tradition in western societies (Wilson 2021). In Australia and Aotearoa New Zealand, these provisions are contained in mental health legislation by a process known as "committal" or "civil commitment". These two terms are used interchangeably in the discussion that follows. The term "civil commitment" indicates that the legal procedure is a civil rather than a criminal process. Civil commitment provides states with two powers to restrain an individual and hence

breach their autonomy. The first is the "parens patriae" (Latin; "parent of the state"), a doctrine that grants courts and the government inherent powers and authority to protect individuals who are unable to act on their own behalf and in their best interests. The second is the public policy powers of the state to empower certain persons or services (e.g. police, ambulance officers, medical and authorised mental health practitioners) to breach the autonomy of individuals if their behaviour is considered a significant risk to themselves or others. An example of this power would be the case of an individual who might harm another person because of a delusional belief that that person means to harm them.

Two consequences of civil commitment are that the individual is either physically restrained by being forcibly hospitalised or has conditions placed on their freedoms as a member of society. Conditions typically include accepting mental health care (e.g. medication) or living at a particular location (usually the consumer's home). From an ethical perspective, civil commitment is usually based on an ethical justification of paternalism, which means that the harm of breaching a consumer's autonomy is justified by being in the best interests of the person restrained. Justification is vexed, but paternalism is considered part of the state's obligations to individuals. Mental health legislation provides clinicians with a legal framework within which to provide involuntary treatment for people who meet the criteria of that legislation. It will be apparent that civil commitment involves significant departures from the normally accepted rights of citizens and health consumers, especially the right to personal freedom and the right to consent to treatment.

The Process of Civil Commitment

The procedures of civil commitment vary from one jurisdiction to another, and the section below is intended as an overview of the main steps of the process. In most Australian and Aotearoa New Zealand jurisdictions legislation requires that the individual concerned has a mental illness (sometimes termed "mental disorder") *and* that a degree of risk is present. It is not enough that the person has a mental illness and in the opinion of professionals would benefit from treatment that they refuse. Mental illness must also coexist with a significant degree of risk. An example would be a person who hears voices commanding

BOX 10.2 Key Concepts Related to Mental Health Legislation and Compulsory Mental Health Care

Advance directive: A document in which a person specifies what actions should be taken for their health if they are no longer able to make decisions for themselves because of acute distress and lack of decision-making capacity.

Assessment: For the purposes of mental health legislation, assessment is a clinical assessment with the specific purpose of determining whether the consumer meets the criteria of the legislation for civil commitment.

Capacity: There are two uses of capacity in health care.
1. The cognitive ability of a consumer to make informed healthcare decisions.
2. The legal right of the person to make decisions about their health care. In some cases if a person is assessed as lacking decision-making capacity a court may rule that they do not have the legal capacity to make their own decisions.

Case law: Rulings (judgments) of courts that create precedents about how legislation is interpreted and the law is to be applied.

Civil commitment or committal: The process being made subject to mental health legislation.

Committed: The legal status of a person under mental health legislation.

Coercion: Care or treatment in which a consumer's autonomous decision-making is limited. Coercion may be formal or informal and is not limited to consumers subject to mental health legislation.

Community treatment order (CTO): A determination for compulsory treatment applying to consumers living in the community.

Compulsory treatment or involuntary treatment: Treatment provided under mental health legislation that does not involve informed consent.

Convention on the Rights of Persons with Disabilities: A United Nations Convention that outlines the rights of people with disabilities, including people with mental illness.

Dangerousness: The assessed degree of risk concerning the level (amount) and likelihood of self-harm, self-neglect or harm to others occurring as a result of mental illness.

Duty of care: The legal obligation owed by nurses to consumers to take all reasonable actions (both positive and negative) to provide the standard of care necessary to avoid foreseeable harm or injury to a consumer. Failure to meet the standard of care can result in a case of negligence.

Forced treatment: Compulsory treatment (usually medication and hospitalisation) provided when a consumer is not consenting and usually when physically restrained.

Informed consent: The process of making healthcare choices based on full information about alternatives and free from coercion or undue influence. Informed consent is an ethical and legal obligation on health practitioners.

In-patient order: A form of compulsory treatment provision applying to consumers admitted to hospital.

Judicial review: A review by a judge of a consumer's legal status under mental health legislation.

Least restrictive alternative: The legal and general principle that requires clinicians to use the least possible restrictive measures in providing care and treatment.

Mental health legislation: Legislation (Acts of parliament) that are specific to mental health that govern the provision of mental health services and treatment whether with or without consent.

Parens patriae power: Power invested in the state to protect individuals who are mentally unwell and who are considered to be at risk as a result of mental illness. Use of parens patriae power may involve a restraint on individual autonomy.

Police power: Power invested by the state in the police to restrain or breach the autonomy of individuals who are mentally unwell and considered to represent a risk to themselves or others.

Review tribunal (Mental Health Review Tribunal): A panel established under mental health legislation to review the legal status of consumers and/or appeals brought by consumers seeking judicial review.

Statutory officials: Nurses, doctors, lawyers and others (e.g. ambulance officers) who are assigned specific roles and powers under mental health legislation.

Substitute decision-making: A process that allows clinicians to make decisions for involuntary consumers on the basis of the clinician's perception of the consumer's best interests.

Supported decision-making: A process that allows people with disabilities to exercise decision-making capacity by choosing supporters to help them make choices.

Voluntary treatment: Treatment that involves informed consent and is provided voluntarily and freely – for example, without inducement, threat or sanction.

them to harm others, where it seems likely that the person will act on those voices if not prevented from doing so. Note that this example includes features of mental illness (hearing voices) *and* risk (risk of harm to others). It is important to note that hearing voices is not always associated with mental illness and that most people with mental illness are not at risk of harming others. Mental health legislation therefore only applies to a small minority of people with mental illness, and only when their symptoms are assessed as sufficiently severe. An additional criterion of capacity is included in the legislation of the Northern Territory, Queensland, South Australia, Tasmania and Western Australia (McSherry 2021). "Capacity" is a legal concept requiring an individual to demonstrate the cognitive ability to understand, consider and make rational choices. Under an assessment of capacity, the focus is on the consumer's capacity for decision-making, not on mental illness and risk.

If a person becomes acutely mentally unwell, a clinician or family member may feel that they represent a significant risk to themselves or others and may begin the process of civil commitment. Civil commitment may be initiated in a variety of settings, including consumers'

homes, primary care, court hearings, police custody, emergency departments (EDs) and community or in-patient mental health services. The initial step is usually an application whereby a concerned person requests that the individual with signs of a mental illness be assessed with a view to civil commitment. Applications may be completed by family members, GPs or other authorised health professionals (e.g. mental health nurses). There may be a need for a supporting certificate written by a nurse as part of the application. Next, the individual will be formally assessed by a health practitioner, who will decide whether there is a need for the person to be committed. If this assessment demonstrates there is a need, a "committal order" will be made. Committal will initially be to an in-patient setting, although in some regions involuntary treatment can be provided out of hospital. The initial period of involuntary treatment is from one day or up to two weeks, depending on the jurisdiction, usually with a proviso that if the consumer's mental state improves, the period of compulsory treatment can cease. Once a consumer is subject to committal, the period of compulsory treatment can be extended. In some jurisdictions the extension may be indefinite.

Although the initial process of committal is undertaken by clinicians, including nurses, committal is a legal procedure and so is subject to appeal and review by a mental health tribunal or a judge in a court of law. The judge will ultimately determine whether the clinician's assessment is consistent with the requirements of legislation and/or whether the consumer continues to require involuntary treatment. Mental health legislation includes various support and appeal processes that allow the consumer to question decisions and to have legal representation in the decision-making process. If an application for civil commitment has been made, the consumer will need to be informed of their rights, and about the possible decision to make an order for compulsory treatment. Other processes include the right to have a family member or a nominated support person involved in care and decision-making, the right to consult a lawyer, the right to seek review by a judge and the right to have their legal status considered by a review tribunal.

Assessment Under Mental Health Legislation

An assessment under mental health legislation involves a clinical assessment that follows the standard process of a comprehensive assessment (see Chapter 9), but with a focus on whether the consumer meets the legislative criteria for committal. Assessments under mental health legislation are usually conducted by psychiatrists and include careful consideration of current and historical risk issues. Nurses may also be involved and, in some cases, may have initiated the process by raising concerns about the consumer and their safety. Although the psychiatrist will complete and sign the assessment document, nurses often contribute important observations and information to the assessment. Nurses may also be able to advocate for alternatives to committal – for example, by exploring additional community and home support, utilising respite care and negotiating the consumer's voluntary engagement with the mental health team. These considerations are important to ensure the care provided involves the least restrictions for the consumer. Care should be voluntary whenever possible and compulsory only if options for voluntary care cannot be safely employed. It is important to understand that in most cases assessment under mental health legislation is not an assessment of the consumer's capacity for informed decision-making. Rather, assessment is one of mental state in the context of the person's social and clinical history, thoughts, behaviours and level of risk. The issue of assessing capacity is addressed in a separate section below.

Compulsory Treatment

Once subject to civil commitment a consumer can be treated without their consent, although as discussed below there is still a continuing obligation on clinicians to seek consent and in some cases a second clinical opinion may be required. Clinicians should also consult an advance directive if the consumer has one (see further discussion below). People made subject to civil commitment have very often refused to consent to voluntary treatment – that is one of the reasons for seeking an order for compulsory treatment. The plan of compulsory treatment will include ensuring safety by providing a safe and secure environment, ongoing clinical assessment, medication aimed at reducing acute symptoms, personal care for those consumers unable to care for themselves (hygiene, hydration, nutrition) and supportive psychological care (being with the person, psychotherapeutic support, safe socialisation, visits or contact with friends or family members).

Although the power to treat without consent is provided by legislation, nurses should always attempt to obtain consent rather than simply exercise the legal right to treat without it. Compulsory treatment does not override nurses' ethical and professional obligation to work collaboratively with consumers. For example, a consumer may have

medication prescribed but might refuse to accept that medication when it is first offered. The nurse should then work with the consumer to negotiate consent by explaining the intended benefits of the medication, validating any concerns the consumer has about the medication and providing the consumer with choices about how the medication is administered and any acceptable alternatives. An option might be to provide as much explanation as possible and give the consumer time to reconsider their refusal. In these situations, nurses should always be honest in disclosing whether administering the medication by force is a possibility. In cases where medication does need to be administered by force, safety of the consumer and the nurse is paramount. This includes psychological and physical safety. Every service has policies and procedures relating to the use of force and these should be followed carefully. In addition, these policies will outline the explanations to provide to consumers, how to offer reassurance to consumers about the nurse's actions and use of the least possible force necessary in the situation. Remember that the law only permits reasonable and proportionate force in the circumstances. Consumers should be provided with subsequent opportunities to review their experience of forced medication, and nurses should have an opportunity to debrief with colleagues.

Protective Mechanisms in Mental Health Legislation

Because mental health legislation involves significant limitations on normally accepted health care and human rights, mental health Acts include a range of measures aimed at counterbalancing the legislative power to detain consumers and impose compulsory treatment. Protective mechanisms include the right to advocacy (legal or otherwise), processes of appeal and review by tribunals and courts, appointment of statutory officials (e.g. district inspectors) to oversee the operation of legislation and complaints procedures. Readers should consult the legislation for their own jurisdiction, as well as the guidelines for applying mental health legislation listed in Table 10.1.

As with other legislation, actions taken under mental health laws may be subject to challenge in the courts, where decisions of clinicians can be tested and may be legally overturned. Decisions arising from legal challenges create a body of case law that instructs and provides guidance concerning legal actions, decision-making and procedures implemented by clinicians pursuant to mental health legislation. Case law precedents can affect clinical practice because clinicians are obliged to work within the precedents. One set of cases in Aotearoa New Zealand involved mental health nurses acting as duly authorised officers under the legislation. This role includes arranging assessments under mental health legislation, which in Aotearoa New Zealand requires a person subject to an assessment to be advised of the assessment in the presence of a member of their family, a caregiver or a person concerned with their welfare. Three cases were heard where the consumers, through their lawyer, argued that an appropriate third party was not present. As a result of these cases, nurses acting in the duly authorised officer role must now be vigilant that the third party is an appropriate person. A full discussion of these cases is provided by Thom and colleagues (2009).

Working with Coercion and Compulsion: The Role of Procedural Justice

The legal concept of the doctrine of procedural fairness and due process (procedural justice) provides a template for working with consumers whose autonomy is restricted by their legal status or by any imposed limiting conditions (Martinez et al 2022). Procedural justice is a branch of natural justice and can be defined as the fairness with which decisions are made. Fairness relates to both decision-making processes and their outcome for the consumer. Procedural justice includes nursing skills such as listening, treating consumers with respect, offering choices, being open and transparent, and availing the consumer time to consider their position and how to respond when their autonomy is limited. Because these skills are inherent in therapeutic relationships, nurses do not need to develop a new set of skills. It is therefore especially important for nurses to be aware of any coercive actions and how they affect consumers. When interactions are legally coercive, the principles of procedural justice demand limitations on the use and impact of those interactions such as undue influence and duress.

An example of procedural justice is provided by Maguire and colleagues (2014), who studied the coercive practice of limit-setting in a mental health in-patient setting. Limit-setting can be important to the safety of in-patient setting and can help consumers by providing clear boundaries for their behaviour. At the same time, limit-setting can constrain a consumer's autonomy. In Maguire and colleagues' (2014) study, nurses and consumers were interviewed about their experience of limit-setting and reported that empathic engagement helped in maintaining therapeutic relationships. The researchers also found that treating consumers in a fair, respectful, consistent and knowledgeable way enhanced positive outcomes compared with interactive styles that were controlling and indifferent. This example from an in-patient setting has application in many situations when nurses are working with consumers who are subject to the restraints of mental health legislation or other forms of coercion. In community settings, where nurses are working with consumers under compulsory community treatment, researchers have reported that procedural justice is associated with a reduced experience of coercion (Nakhost et al 2018). Procedural justice is not a substitute for ensuring that consumers' rights are respected and upheld, but it does help to guide interactions towards being less coercive.

Aotearoa New Zealand Mental Health Legislation

Aotearoa New Zealand's *Mental Health (Compulsory Assessment and Treatment) Act* was introduced towards the end of the period of deinstitutionalisation and reflected a shift from a therapeutic (need for treatment) standard to a legal standard based on dangerousness in decisions about involuntary treatment. This shift influenced mental health legislation in many western countries in the late 20th century (Hudson 2019). Consumers have access to legal counsel, appeal processes and reviews of their status under legislation by courts of law (Dawson & Gledhill 2013). In addition to establishing criteria for civil commitment, the Act contains provisions for ECT, psychosurgery and seclusion. For nurses, the Act introduced changes in their responsibilities by creating a range of new roles, from providing advice to the public to the exercise of temporary holding powers (McKenna & O'Brien 2013).

A decision to place a person under involuntary status does not mean the person needs to be admitted to hospital. Treatment can occur in a hospital or in any other place deemed suitable by the treating clinician. The intent and wording of the Act allow clinicians to explore less-restrictive alternatives such as care in a community respite facility or care at home. Criteria for invoking mental health legislation involve two components: "abnormal state of mind" and "serious danger to self or others" (Dawson & Gledhill 2013). Section 2 of the Act defines mental disorder as:

> *an abnormal state of mind (whether of a continuous or intermittent nature), characterised by delusions, or by disorders of mood or perception or volition or cognition, of such a degree that it:*
> *(a) Poses a serious danger to the health or safety of that person or of others; or*
> *(b) Seriously diminishes the capacity of that person to take care of himself or herself.*

There are certain exclusions to the application of the New Zealand legislation. Section 4 of the Act specifies that the Act cannot be invoked solely by reason of the person's:

- political, religious or personal beliefs
- sexual preferences
- criminal or delinquent behaviour
- substance abuse, or
- intellectual disability.

In keeping with recognition of Te Tiriti o Waitangi, s. 5 of the Act requires that powers be exercised under the Act with respect for the cultural identity of consumers.

For an individual to be placed under mental health legislation, there first needs to be an application by a person over 18 years of age and an accompanying certificate of assessment. Following an initial assessment examination, the person may be required to undergo further periods of assessment and treatment, coordinated by a "responsible clinician" appointed under the Act. During this time, the individual can apply under s. 16 of the Act for a review of their condition by a judge. At the conclusion of the assessment, if the individual is thought to meet the criteria for compulsory treatment, the responsible clinician applies to the court for a compulsory treatment order. Compulsory treatment orders can be either in-patient orders or community treatment orders (CTO) and are for an initial period of six months. Other provisions of the Act apply to consumers following the issue of a CTO. These include the right to seek a review by a judge, regular clinical review, access to a review tribunal and specific rights under the Act. A detailed outline of the process of compulsory assessment and treatment, including definitions of key concepts, is provided by the Ministry of Health (2020).

Nurses are involved, through several statutory roles, in facilitating assessment and treatment under the Mental Health Act. The role of duly authorised officer involves aiding members of the public who may be concerned that a person is mentally disordered and in need of treatment under the Act. Although the legislation does not specify the professional background of individuals acting as duly authorised officers, in most cases this role has been assigned to nurses.

As discussed above, consumers with involuntary status may, under s. 16 of the Act, seek a review of their condition by a District Court judge. In most s. 16 reviews, the second health professional providing an opinion to the court is a nurse. Acting as second health professional can cause a sense of conflict between a custodial and a therapeutic role, but with specific training nurses have demonstrated an increased sense of confidence and competence in the role (Muir et al 2023).

Australian Mental Health Legislation

Each Australian state and territory has mental health legislation (mental health Acts) designed to protect individuals with mental illness from inappropriate treatment; direct the provision of mental health care and the facilities in which it is provided; and instruct mental health professionals' practice in providing treatment and care (McSherry 2021). For example, mental health Acts detail physical treatments involving "prescribed" actions such as ECT, psychosurgery and some invasive medical interventions such as seclusion practices. While the Acts vary regarding the requirements of psychiatrists and mental health nurses, core issues such as a definition of mental illness and basic criteria for the admission and detention of voluntary and involuntary consumers reflect UN human rights principles and are purposively present in all Acts.

Like Aotearoa New Zealand legislation, several Australian mental health Acts identify behaviours and personal characteristics that are *not* indicative of mental illness. For example, the *Victorian Mental Health Act* stipulates:

- particular political views or activities
- particular religious views or activities

- particular philosophies
- particular sexual preferences or sexual orientation
- particular illegal conduct or use of drugs and/or alcohol
- an antisocial personality
- having an intellectual disability.

This is expressly included to ensure that mental health Acts are not used perniciously and unconscionably against the individual as a form of social control.

Australian mental health Acts provide for the care and treatment of both voluntary and involuntary consumers. In amendments made to the Acts in recent years, caution has been taken to consider consumers' perspectives on issues such as providing appropriate and timely responses to complaints about care during treatment (in the hospital and the community). As in other international jurisdictions, detained consumers are more likely than ever before to receive care in the community, and the Acts facilitate this via CTOs. In cases where consumers under CTOs are prescribed depot medication, they may be forcibly transported to hospital for treatment.

Australian mental health Acts have a stronger treatment focus than in other Commonwealth countries such as Canada. An involuntary admission will only occur if a person requires treatment and all other alternatives have been considered. For example, a person will be admitted if they are assessed to be a danger to themselves or others and there is no other less restrictive alternative available to manage that risk and provide treatment. Conversely, where the consumer is voluntary (i.e. with informed consent), two criteria common to Australian mental health Acts are that: (1) the severity of the mental illness requires treatment in an "approved mental health facility"; and (2) the individual is suffering from an acute episode of a mental illness. Mental health Acts generally include statements about the need to involve consumers in all appropriate aspects of their care and treatment regardless of their status (voluntary or detained). Consumer advocates and advance directives are examples of this. Circumstances may occur where a consumer is admitted voluntarily and then asks to leave but is deemed too unwell and is therefore detained against their will. For a consumer to be detained in such circumstances, they must be mentally ill and in need of immediate treatment that can only be provided in an approved mental health facility. In such circumstances the detention is lawful.

Australian mental health Acts vary in the time for which they specify that consumers can be detained involuntarily when first admitted to a mental health unit. Generally, a person may be detained against their will for an initial period of 24 hours by a medical practitioner, but then must be reviewed by a psychiatrist as soon as is practicable. The consumer may be further detained for 21 days, or the detention may be revoked, and the consumer will assume voluntary status. Under a continuing detention order, consumers have a right of appeal, which is heard through a sitting of the state or territory mental health tribunal. For consumers, there is an uneasy tension between self-determination and the determinations made by mental health authorities "in their best interests".

Although all Australian mental health Acts have adopted the tenets of least-restrictive and consumer-focused practice in relation to the law, an issue facing Australian consumers and mental health nurses is the variation in language and provisions contained in the various state and territory Acts (Tosson et al 2022). In different jurisdictions, various terms are used for "compulsory detention" (e.g. "section" is used in one state; "schedule" or "order" in another), the length of time for which a person may be detained varies, and there are contrasting conditions surrounding the use of seclusion and restraint. In addition, the protective provisions of the various mental health Acts are different across regions, and there are different processes for obtaining legal advocacy.

Community Treatment Orders in Australia and New Zealand

For the past three decades compulsory mental health care in the community has been implemented through CTOs. CTOs are recommended as an alternative to hospitalisation (Barnett et al 2018)) and as a means of providing care in the least restrictive environment. There are, however, concerns that CTOs represent part of an increasing preoccupation with minimising "risk" (McMillan et al 2019) and contribute to stigmatisation of consumers by reinforcing a perception of dangerousness.

CTOs vary in their conditions, but generally require consumers to attend and consent to treatment or be sanctioned with the possibility of re-hospitalisation. Hence, CTOs are legally enforceable against a consumer's consent, but are subject to judicial review on appeal by consumers. Justifications for CTOs are that they reduce rates of hospitalisation, improve access to services, reduce relapse rates and improve the consumer's social functioning by assisting them to remain in the community.

A consumer who is subject to a CTO will live in their own home, whether a private residence, boarding house or some form of supported community accommodation. CTO conditions may specify the residential address where they must live and that they must refrain from using alcohol and other recreational drugs. Consumers under CTOs will usually receive follow-up care from a community-based mental health service, which will provide coordination of wraparound care, such as social support, psychological treatment, medication and support to navigate health and social services. Services are delivered in the consumer's home or at a community mental health centre, or some combination of both, often by community mental health nurses. Another frequent CTO condition stipulates compliance with prescribed medications, usually an antipsychotic in depot (long-acting) form. Part of the community mental health nurse's role will be to monitor the consumer's physical health and ensure they receive primary healthcare. This last function is important to address the health disparities experienced by people with severe mental illness, particularly those who have been prescribed second-generation antipsychotic medication for long periods of time (see Chapter 20 for further discussion of physical health). Despite the more intensive care provided to people on CTOs, mortality rates from medical and non-medical causes are higher than for people in comparison groups (Beaglehole et al 2023), which may be a reflection of the overall poorer health of this group.

CTO rates are high in Australia and New Zealand. Light and colleagues (2012a; 2012b) surveyed Australian mental health tribunals and health district providers concerning the frequency of CTOs and the number of consumers subject to them. The lowest rate was in Tasmania, with 30.2 per 100,000 population, and the highest was in Victoria, with 98.8 per 100,000. These rates are high by world standards. New Zealand's rate of 84 per 100,000 is also high by world standards (O'Brien 2014).

Although CTOs are now an established and frequent treatment option facilitated by mental health legislation in Australasia, debate about their human rights implications and effectiveness continues (Barnett et al 2018; Kisely et al 2021). Critics have argued that the CTO represents an unnecessary extension of coercion into community settings and that this coercion and compulsory care/treatment is likely to lead to consumer resistance by disengaging from services. As a nurse you need to be aware of your legal obligations for consumers subject to CTOs and of their potential to negatively affect your therapeutic relationships.

CRITICAL THINKING EXERCISE 10.6

1. How would you feel if a friend or a member of your family was discharged from hospital under a CTO?
2. What rights should apply to consumers subject to CTOs?
3. Why is it important that countries commit to international treaties such as the UN Convention on the Rights of Persons with Disabilities?
4. What domestic legislation is aimed at protecting the rights of mental health consumers?

Human Rights and Mental Health Legislation

People with mental illness have historically been subject to specific discriminatory laws and systemic denial of rights has been enshrined in mental health legislation. Much of this denial of rights stemmed from medical ignorance, few treatment options and stigma. With greater awareness, various international instruments have been drafted and ratified to help protect the rights of individuals with mental illness. Until 2008, human rights protections under mental health legislation were protected mainly by three instruments: the 1966 International Covenant on Civil and Political Rights; the 1966 International Covenant on Economic, Social and Cultural Rights; and the 1991 United Nations Principles for the Protection of Persons with Mental Illness and the Improvement of Mental Health Care. Australia and Aotearoa New Zealand are signatories to all three instruments. However, because international conventions are not binding or mandatory on Australian and Aotearoa New Zealand domestic laws, people with mental illness continued to experience discrimination, often reflected in and perpetrated by mental health legislation.

The Convention on the Rights of Persons with Disabilities was adopted in 2006 and entered into force in May 2008, and has considerable implications for mental health care, and especially mental health legislation (Gill 2019; McBride 2021). The Convention has been ratified by both Australia and Aotearoa New Zealand, and is now considered to be the most internationally authoritative document articulating the rights of people with mental illness. The Convention does not create new rights for people with disabilities but clarifies existing rights under other instruments, such as those mentioned above. Unlike some other rights instruments, the Convention does not focus solely on one issue, in this case mental illness. Instead, it focuses on the concept of disability and provides a wide definition, which includes mental illness alongside other disabilities. A foundation principle of the Convention is equality; that is, not only should people with disabilities enjoy the rights to be free from prejudice and discrimination, but also barriers to social inclusion should be removed so that people with disabilities are able to enjoy the full range of opportunities available to other members of society. The 50 Articles of the Convention make this a wide-ranging instrument, covering issues such as equal access to justice, gender issues, housing, rights of children and older people, and mobility. The full text of the Convention can be downloaded from the United Nations website (see Useful websites).

One of the major implications of the Convention is the Article 12 requirement for equality before the law. Internationally, this requirement has been interpreted to mean that any legislation that limits rights based on an individual's membership of a "status group" (e.g. people with disabilities) is considered discriminatory (Dawson 2015). As noted in the discussion of mental health legislation above, most Australian and Aotearoa New Zealand mental health legislation limits the rights of people with mental illness and is therefore considered discriminatory under the terms of Article 12 (Szmukler et al 2014). The argument is that this legislation is discriminatory because it only applies to people with mental illness.

Recent reforms in mental health legislation have attempted to give effect to concerns raised under the Convention. Tasmania and Victoria amended their mental health legislation to respond to the Convention and have adopted a capacity-based standard for treatment without consent (Callaghan & Ryan 2012). An argument has been made for adopting the same standard in Aotearoa New Zealand (Gordon & O'Brien 2014), and legislative reform is now underway in Aotearoa New Zealand (Ministry of Health 2021). In light of the Convention, understandings of the rights of people with mental illness and how legislation should address the issue of treatment without consent continues to evolve.

Substituted and Supported Decision-Making

When consumers are subject to mental health legislation, traditional approaches to decision-making have seen health professionals, usually doctors, replacing the individual's usual autonomous decision-making with a decision made by the health professional. This is known as substitute decision-making and is frequently used when adults are considered to lack capacity (White et al 2018; Szmukler 2019), sometimes with some form of legal guardianship. Substitute decision-making has been challenged under Article 12 the Convention on the Rights of Persons with Disabilities, which has been interpreted to require that health consumers should always make their own decisions, even when they lack capacity. The argument is that with adequate support the individual will be able to articulate their preferences and make the decision they would have made if they had capacity. This is an argument for supported decision-making: providing consumers with the support they need to make their own decisions, rather than have another person make that decision for them (Brophy et al 2019). Supported decision-making helps professionals meet their ethical obligations to respect consumers' autonomy and is also likely to promote consumers' recovery (Kokanović et al 2018). Barriers to supported decision-making include clinicians' lack of skills in this area and the lack of legal requirements for it. Although supported decision-making does not need to be legally mandated, changing legislation to require supported rather than substitute decision-making would help to promote this practice and is likely to address some of the coercion experienced by people on CTOs (Brophy et al 2019). Some arguments have been made that rejection of any form of substitute decision-making is likely to have adverse effects on consumers and instead efforts should be made to improve the quality of substitute decision-making; for example, by promoting the use of advance directives (Scholten & Gather 2018). Although legislation is changing to require supported decision-making, under current legislation nurses can work with consumers to assist them to make their own decisions rather than impose decisions under the guise of paternalism.

DUTY OF CARE AND DECISION-MAKING CAPACITY

This section considers emergency situations arising in nursing when a nurse needs to act urgently, sometimes without consumer consent, to prevent significant harm to a consumer or others. In these situations, nurses act under a duty of care. In emergency situations of a threat to life or a serious threat to health and injury, restraint, hospitalisation and treatment without consent is a common-law protected duty of clinicians. Emergency situations might arise in mental health settings or general health settings, including community settings, mental health in-patient units, EDs and general hospital wards. In EDs, individuals may temporarily lose capacity because of the impact of physical trauma causing physiological shock and impaired consciousness, the toxic effects of recreational drugs or the high emotional arousal associated with acute anxiety. A common example of impaired decision-making capacity in a general health setting is where an individual has developed delirium and become acutely confused. There are many causes of delirium, which is characterised by a rapid deterioration in mental state that can fluctuate rapidly. This may be secondary to medical illness, anaesthesia, high temperature or other causes. In some cases, the precise cause of delirium is not known, and the diagnosis is based on the clinical history. However, in delirium there is often severe impairment of cognitive functioning, with loss of decision-making capacity.

In people displaying acute confusional states such as delirium, clinicians commonly apply a test of capacity. Capacity refers to the mental or cognitive ability to understand the nature and effects of one's actions. Note that legally an individual is presumed to have capacity unless otherwise demonstrated. Although it is not a standardised test, the applied test contains four criteria:

- **Comprehension:** Does the person understand the information provided by a health professional?
- **Expressing a choice:** Is the person capable of weighing alternatives and stating their preferences?
- **Appreciation:** Does the person appreciate their situation and its consequences?
- **Reasoning:** Is the person able to think rationally about the situation?

In most situations it is necessary for the person to meet all four criteria in order to have decision-making capacity. Additional assessment may involve using standardised assessment instruments that can be repeated to detect improvement or deterioration in mental state (Cheung et al 2015), as capacity can change over time.

Assessment of capacity is dependent on the seriousness of the situation the person faces. For example, deciding to leave hospital while confused is clearly more serious than making a decision about whether or not to have a shower. Each situation must be assessed individually, and clinicians should consult with colleagues if they are unsure. Family members should also be consulted to establish what the person's normal preferences would be. Factors such as cultural and language differences, sensory impairment, pain and an unfamiliar environment need to be considered to contextualise a capacity assessment. If an individual's decision-making capacity is thought to be permanently impaired (e.g. in dementia), clinicians should consider provisions for legal guardianship. This normally involves a court process to appoint a "substitute decision-maker". This can be a family member, lawyer or the Guardianship Board, who will make decisions on the individual's behalf and in their best interests. Again, if the person regains capacity the guardianship order on application may be discharged.

Advance Directives

Mental health advance directives are statements of preferences for mental health care if a mental health crisis leaves the person unable to express their preferences. The aim is to increase consumer autonomy in mental health crises. Many mental health consumers experience crisis events when they may be too distressed or cognitively impaired to state their preferences. In such cases, a statement of preferences, prepared in advance at a time when the consumer is well, can act as a guide to clinicians as to what the consumer's preferences are.

Various models of advance instructions have been developed, including psychiatric advance directives, joint crisis plans, wellness recovery action plans, advance statements and mental health advance preference statements (Lenagh-Glue et al 2018). An advance directive can include treatment preferences, such as which medication to use or avoid, preferences about use of seclusion and restraint, involvement of particular clinicians, treatment setting and methods of calming and de-escalation (Thom et al 2019). They can also include preferences for personal affairs, such as care of the consumer's house or flat, care of pets, who to contact in the event of a crisis, and who the consumer would prefer not to have involved. Research has shown that consumers value the opportunity to make an advance directive, although in practice many are not given that opportunity. Mental health advance directives help to meet obligations under the Convention on the Rights of Persons with Disabilities (Szmukler 2019), and several Australian states have recognised advance directives in their mental health legislation (Ouliaris & Kealy-Bateman 2017). Advance directives have been proposed for inclusion in revised legislation in Aotearoa New Zealand (Lenagh-Glue et al 2020).

A mental health advance directive does not override mental health legislation, although even for consumers subject to mental health legislation, clinicians have an ethical and legal obligation to attempt to work with consumers' competently expressed preferences. A mental health advance directive can only be effective if clinicians take the trouble to access it from the consumer's clinical records and then work with the consumer towards meeting the preferences expressed. This presents a key advocacy role to mental health nurses within multidisciplinary teams in helping ensure the advance directive is used to negotiate care and treatment with consumers.

CHAPTER SUMMARY

This chapter has explored ethical and legal issues associated with mental health nursing practice in Australia and Aotearoa New Zealand. Mental health nursing is fraught with ethical issues arising from the classification of mental illness, diagnoses, treatment and working within the constraints of mental health legislation and guidance provided by professional codes of ethics. The mental health setting poses unique challenges to nurses in the form of treatment without consent under mental health legislation. In addition, nurses must practise within legislation governing consumer rights, privacy and guardianship. The UN Convention on the Rights of Persons with Disabilities provides challenges to current legislation and practice. Capacity-based legislation, advance directives and supported decision-making provide some responses to these challenges.

REVIEW QUESTIONS

Read the four scenarios below and consider appropriate responses to the questions that follow. You can either split into discussion groups or work individually.

Scenario 1

A 33-year-old woman under a CTO is refusing to have her regular antipsychotic medication, although she does agree that her symptoms were lessened when taking the medication. She is concerned about her increase in weight as a result of taking the medication and tells you that you do not understand what it is like taking medication with such side effects.

Scenario 2

Henry is a 19-year-old consumer who was admitted to the mental health unit for the first time two weeks ago. At the time of admission Henry was hearing voices, but these have now diminished. Henry has told the staff that the voices began soon after he began smoking cannabis. Henry's father visits the ward and tells you he is aware of Henry's cannabis use. He asks you if Henry has informed the staff about this. How would you respond to Henry's father while respecting Henry's confidentiality?

Scenario 3

A 15-year-old girl presented at an emergency department after ingesting 24 paracetamol tablets. She had been struggling with anorexia nervosa since she was 11 and felt that her life was heading nowhere. She was transferred as an involuntary consumer to the local mental health hospital and prescribed nasogastric tube feeding, which was given without her consent. Three weeks later she remains suicidal and is still being tube fed. She wants to be left alone as she cannot face the pain of life anymore.

Scenario 4

In a discussion with a colleague you learn that the colleague has developed a personal relationship with a consumer on the ward. The colleague tells you that they and the consumer have romantic feelings for each other, and that when they are together the consumer really opens up about their past life and the problems they have experienced. The colleague asks you to keep this information private, because the consumer becomes distressed at the thought that the relationship may not be able to continue. What ethical principles would guide your response to this situation?

Questions

1. Considering the above four scenarios:
   - Are there any circumstances in which you would keep information about a personal relationship between a colleague and a consumer secret?
   - What are our responsibilities in each case as a health professional?
   - How does the principle of autonomy apply in each scenario
2. Discuss contemporary developments in mental health services globally and in Australia or Aotearoa New Zealand, and their impact on how people with mental illness are cared for in the community.
3. Think about some recent clinical experiences you have had with consumers with a mental health problem or illness and discuss your responses to the following questions with your group or class members.
   - Identify some coercive interventions you have been involved with or have observed. If you were involved, how did you feel about being involved?
   - Were there alternatives that could have been less restrictive?
   - What are your own beliefs about how and where people with mental illness should be cared for?
   - Should legislation have the power to contain or control people with a mental illness to protect them from themselves and/or other people?

USEFUL WEBSITES

Australian Commission on Quality and Safety in Health Care: www.safetyandquality.gov.au/
Australian Health Practitioner Regulatory Agency: www.ahpra.gov.au/
Australian Human Rights Commission: www.humanrights.gov.au/
Australian Nursing and Midwifery Accreditation Council: www.anmac.org.au/
Clinical Excellence Queensland, Queensland Government 2016. Guide to Informed Decision-making in Health Care. Interim update 2.2. www.health.qld.gov.au/__data/assets/pdf_file/0019/143074/ic-guide.pdf
Community Law (New Zealand): communitylaw.org.nz
Health and Disability Commissioner (New Zealand): www.hdc.org.nz/
Involuntary commitment and treatment (ICT) criteria in Australian and New Zealand Mental Health Acts: acem.org.au/getmedia/df3f33f9-49bd-414a-a6ec-73ce9f15fc5b/Mental-Health-Acts-Comparative-Tables-all
Mental Health Coordinating Council (New South Wales) – online Manual of legal and human rights related to the mental health system: mhrm.mhcc.org.au/home
MindFreedom – ethics and mental health page: mindfreedom.org/
Ministry of Disabled People (New Zealand): www.whaikaha.govt.nz
Ministry of Health (New Zealand) for information on mental health legislation updates: www.health.govt.nz/
Nursing and Midwifery Board of Australia: www.nursingmidwiferyboard.gov.au/

Nursing Council of New Zealand: www.nursingcouncil.org.nz/
Office of the Public Advocate (South Australia): www.opa.sa.gov.au/information-service/your-rights/mental-health-treatment-and-your-rights
Privacy Commissioner (New Zealand) for information on New Zealand *Privacy Act 1993* www.privacy.org.nz
United Nations Convention on the Rights of Persons with Disabilities: www.un.org/development/desa/disabilities/

REFERENCES

Abuse in Care Royal Commission of Inquiry 2022. He Purapura Ora, he Māra Tipu. From edress to puretumu torowhānui, vol. 1. Royal Commission of Inquiry, Wellington.
Adshead, G. 2021. The psychotherapies. In: Bloch, S., Green, S. (eds), Psychiatric Ethics, 5th ed. Oxford University Press, Oxford.
Allikmets, S., Marshall, C., Murad, O., & Gupta, K. 2020. Seclusion: A patient perspective. Iss Ment Health Nurs, 41(8), 723–735.
American Psychiatric Association (APA) 2013. Diagnostic and Statistical Manual of Mental Disorders, 5th ed., text rev. APA, Washington.
Askew, L., Fisher, P., & Beazley, P. 2019. What are adult psychiatric inpatients' experience of seclusion: A systematic review of qualitative studies. J Psychiatr Ment Health Nurs, 26 (7–8), 274–285.

Australian College of Mental Health Nurses (ACMHN) 2019. Safe in Care, Safe at Work (SICSAW): Ensuring safety in care and safety for staff in Australian mental health services. ACMHN, Canberra, ACT.

Barnett, P., Matthews, H., Lloyd-Evans, B., Mackay, E., Pilling, S., et al., 2018. Compulsory community treatment to reduce readmission to hospital and increase engagement with community care in people with mental illness: A systematic review and meta-analysis. The Lancet Psychiatry, 5(12), 1013–1022.

Beaglehole, B., Newton-Howes, G., Porter, R., & Frampton, C. 2023. The association between compulsory community treatment order status and mortality in New Zealand. B J Psych Open, 9(1), e15.

Beauchamp, T.L., Childress, J.F. 2019. Principles of Biomedical Ethics, 8th ed. Oxford University Press, New York.

Bladon, H. 2019. Avoiding paternalism. Issues Ment Health Nurs, 40(7), 579–584.

Boulton, K.A., Raghupathy, V., Guastella, A.J., & Bowden, M.R. 2022. Reducing seclusion use in an Australian child and adolescent psychiatric inpatient unit. J Affect Disord, 305, 1–7.

Brophy, L., Ryan, C.J., & Weller, P. 2018. Community treatment orders: The evidence and the ethical implications. In: Spivakovsky, C., Seear, K., Carter, A. (eds), Critical Perspectives on Coercive Interventions: Law, Medicine and Society. Routledge, New York.

Brophy, L.M., Kokanović, R., Flore, J. et al., 2019. Community treatment orders and supported decision making. Front Psychiatry, 10, 414.

Callaghan, S. & Ryan, C.J. 2012. Rising to the human rights challenge in compulsory treatment: New approaches to mental health law in Australia. Aust N Z J Psychiatry, 46(7), 611–620.

Campbell, K., Clarke, K. A., Massey, D. & Lakeman, R. 2020. Borderline personality disorder: To diagnose or not to diagnose? That is the question. Int J Ment Health Nurs, 29(5), 972–981.

Chesterman, J. 2018. Adult guardianship and its alternatives in Australia. In: Spivakovsky, C., Seear, K., Carter, A. (eds), Critical Perspectives on Coercive Interventions: Law, Medicine and Society. Routledge, New York.

Cheung, G., Clugston, A., Croucher, M., et al., 2015. Performance of three cognitive screening tools in a sample of older New Zealanders. Int Psychogeriatr 27(06), 981–989.

Daigle, A. 2020. Social media and professional boundaries in undergraduate nursing students. J Prof Nurs, 36(2), 20–23.

Dawson, J. 2015. A realistic approach to assessing mental health laws' compliance with the UNCRPD. Int J Law Psychiatry, 40, 70–79.

Dawson, J., Gledhill, K. 2013. The complex meaning of "mental disorder". In: Dawson, J., Gledhill, K. (eds), New Zealand's Mental Health Act in Practice. Victoria University Press, Wellington.

de Anta, L., Alvarez-Mon, M.A., Donat-Vargas, C., Lara-Abelanda, F.J., Pereira-Sanchez, V., et al., 2023. Assessment of beliefs and attitudes about electroconvulsive therapy posted on Twitter: An observational study. Europ Psychiatry, 66(1), e11.

Dickens, G.L., Tabvuma, T., Frost, S.A., & SWSLHD Safewards Steering Group, 2020. Safewards: Changes in conflict, containment, and violence prevention climate during implementation. Int J Ment Health Nurs, 29(6), 1230–1240.

Douglass, A., Young, G. & McMillan, J. 2020. Assessment of mental capacity. A New Zealand guide for doctors and lawyers. Victoria University Press, Wellington.

Flaskeraud, J.H. 2018. Stigma and psychiatric/mental health nursing. Iss Ment Health Nurs, 39(2), 188–191.

Gill, N.S. 2019. Human rights framework: An ethical imperative for psychiatry. A N Z J Psychiatry, 53(1), 8–10.

Gordon, S., O'Brien, A. 2014. New Zealand's mental health legislation needs reform to avoid discrimination. N Z Med J 127 (1403), 55.

Griffiths, C., O'Neill-Kerr, A. 2019. Patients', carers' and the public's perspectives on electroconvulsive therapy. Front Psychiatry 10, 304.

Guloksuz, S., van Os, J. 2021. En attendant Godot: Waiting for the funeral of "schizophrenia" and the baby shower of the psychosis spectrum. Frontiers Psychiatry, 12, 618842.

Harbusch, M. (ed.) 2022. Troubled Persons Industries: The Expansion Of Psychiatric Categories Beyond Psychiatry. Springer Nature.

Haugom, E., Ruud, T., & Hynnekliev, T. 2019. Ethical challenges of seclusion in psychiatric inpatient wards: A qualitative study of the experiences of Norwegian mental health professionals. BMC Health Serv Res, 19, 1–12.

Hawsawi, T., Power, T., Zugai, J., & Jackson, D. 2020. Nurses' and consumers' shared experiences of seclusion and restraint: A qualitative literature review. Int J Ment Health Nurs, 29(5), 831–845.

Hawton, K., Lascelles, K., Pitman, A., Gilbert, S. & Silverman, M. 2022. Assessment of suicide risk in mental health practice: Shifting from prediction to therapeutic assessment, formulation, and risk management. The Lancet Psychiatry, 9(11), 922–928.

Hudson, C.G. 2019. Deinstitutionalization of mental hospitals and rates of psychiatric disability: An international study. Health & Place, 56, 70–79.

International Council of Nurses (ICN), 2021. The ICN Code of Ethics for Nurses. ICN, Geneva.

Isobel, S., Wilson, A., Gill, K., & Howe, D. 2021. "What would a trauma-informed mental health service look like?" Perspectives of people who access services. Int J Ment Health Nurs, 30(2), 495–505.

Jackson, H., Baker, J., & Berzins, K. 2019. Factors influencing decisions of mental health professionals to release service users from seclusion: A qualitative study. J Adv Nurs, 75(10), 2178–2188.

Johnstone, L. 2018. Psychological formulation as an alternative to psychiatric diagnosis. J Humanistic Psychol, 58(1), 30–46.

Jury, A., Lai, J., Tuason, C., Koning, A., Smith, M., et al., 2019. People who experience seclusion in adult mental health inpatient services: An examination of health of the nation outcome scales scores. Int J Ment Health Nurs, 28(1), 199–208.

Kisely, S., Yu, D., Maehashi, S. & Siskind, D. 2021. A systematic review and meta-analysis of predictors and outcomes of community treatment orders in Australia and New Zealand. A N Z J Psychiatry, 55(7), 650–665.

Kokanović, R., Brophy, L., McSherry, B., et al., 2018. Supported decision-making from the perspectives of mental health service users, family members supporting them and mental health practitioners. Aust N Z J Psychiatry, 52(9), 826–833.

Lenagh-Glue, J., O'Brien, A., Dawson, J., et al., 2018. A MAP to mental health: The process of creating a collaborative advance preferences instrument. N Z Med J, 131(1486), 18–26.

Lenagh-Glue, J., Potiki, J., O'Brien, A.J., et al., 2020. The content of mental health advance preference statements (MAPS): A qualitative assessment of completed advance directives in the Southern District Health Board. Int J Law Psychiatry 68, 101537.

Light, E., Kerridge, I., Ryan, C., et al., 2012a. Community treatment orders in Australia: Rates and patterns of use. Australas Psychiatry 20(6), 478–482.

Light, E., Kerrige, I., Ryan, C., et al., 2012b. Out of sight, out of mind: Making involuntary community treatment visible in the mental health system. Med J Aust, 196(9), 591–593.

Lonergan, A., Timmins, F. & Donohue, G. 2021. Mental health nurse experiences of delivering care to severely depressed adults receiving electroconvulsive therapy. J Psychiat Ment Health Nurs, 28(3), 309–316.

Maguire, T., Daffern, M., Martin, T. 2014. Exploring nurses' and patients' perspectives of limit setting in a forensic mental health setting. Int J Ment Health Nurs, 23 (2), 153–160.

Mandarelli, G., Carabellese, F., Parmigiani, G., et al., 2018. Treatment decision-making capacity in non-consensual psychiatric treatment: A multicentre study. Epidemiol Psychiatr Sci, 27(5), 492–499.

Martinez, D., Brodard, A., Silva, B., Diringer, O., Bonsack, C., et al., 2022. Satisfaction and perceived coercion in voluntary hospitalisations: Impact of past coercive experiences. Psychiatric Quart, 1–14.

Massabki, I., Abi-Jaoude, E. 2020. Selective serotonin reuptake inhibitor "discontinuation syndrome" or withdrawal. Br J Psychiatry, 1–4.

McKenna, B.G., O'Brien, A.J. 2013. Mental health nursing and the Mental Health Act. In: Dawson, J., Gledhill, K. (eds), New Zealand's Mental Health Act in Practice. Victoria University Press, Wellington.

McMillan, J., Lawn, S., Delany-Crowe, T. 2019. Trust and community treatment orders. Front. Psychiatry 10, 349.

McSherry, B., 2021. Australian mental health laws and human rights. In: Paula Gerber and Melissa Castan (eds), Critical Perspectives on Human Rights Law in Australia, vol 1. Thomson Reuters, Sydney.

Ministry of Health 2021. Transforming our Mental Health Law: A public discussion document. Ministry of Health, Wellington.

Ministry of Health 2020. Guideline to the Mental Health (Compulsory Assessment and Treatment) Act (1992). Ministry of Health, Wellington.

Ministry of Health 2019. Every life matters – He Tapu te Oranga o ia Tangata: Suicide Prevention Strategy 2019–2029 and Suicide Prevention Action Plan 2019–2024 for Aotearoa New Zealand. Ministry of Health, Wellington.

Morley, G. 2018. What is "moral distress" in nursing? How, can and should we respond to it?. J Clin Nurs, 27(19–20), 3443–3445.

Muir-Cochrane, E., & Oster, C. 2021. Chemical restraint: A qualitative synthesis review of adult service user and staff experiences in mental health settings. Nurs Health Sci, 23(2), 325–336

Muir, R., O'Brien, A., Butler, H., & Diamond, D. 2023. Are mental health nurses meeting the requirements of second health professionals in presenting opinions to the court? J Psychiatr Ment Health Nurs, 30(4), 813–821.

Nakhost, A., Sirotich, F., Pridham, K.M.F., Stergiopoulos, V. & Simpson, A.I. 2018. Coercion in outpatients under community treatment orders: A matched comparison study. Canad J Psychiatry, 63(11), 757–765.

New Zealand Nurses Organisation 2019. Guideline – Code of Ethics. NZNO, Auckland.

Nursing and Midwifery Board of Australia, 2018. Code of conduct for nurses. Online. Available at: www.nursingmidwiferyboard.gov.au/Codes-Guidelines-Statements/Professional-standards.aspx

Nursing and Midwifery Board of Australia 2016. Registered Nurse Standards for Practice for Nurses in Australia. NMBA, Canberra.

Nursing Council of New Zealand, 2012. Code of Conduct for Nurses. NCNZ, Wellington.

O'Brien, A.J. 2014. Community treatment orders in New Zealand: Regional variability and international comparisons. Australas Psychiatry 22(4), 352–356.

O'Connor, C., Kadianaki, I., Maunder, K., & McNicholas, F. 2018. How does psychiatric diagnosis affect young people's self-concept and social identity? A systematic review and synthesis of the qualitative literature. Soc Sci Med, 212, 94–119.

Ouliaris, C., Kealy-Bateman, W. 2017. Psychiatric advance directives in Australian mental-health legislation. Australas Psychiatry 25 (6), 574–577.

Paradis-Gagné, E., Pariseau-Legault, P., Goulet, M.H., Jacob, J.D., & Lessard-Deschênes, C. 2021. Coercion in psychiatric and mental health nursing: A conceptual analysis. Int J Ment Health Nurs, 30(3), 590–609.

Paris, J. 2020. Overdiagnosis in psychiatry: How modern psychiatry lost its way while creating a diagnosis for almost all of life's misfortunes. Oxford University Press.

Pillinger, T., McCutcheon, R.A., Vano, L., Mizuno, Y., Arumuham, A., et al., 2020. Comparative effects of 18 antipsychotics on metabolic function in patients with schizophrenia, predictors of metabolic dysregulation, and association with psychopathology: A systematic review and network meta-analysis. The Lancet Psychiatry, 7(1), 64–77.

Pinel, P., 1806. A Treatise on Insanity. Strand, Messers Cadell & Davies.

Popovic, D., Schmitt, A., Kaurani, L., Senner, F., Papiol, S., et al., 2019. Childhood trauma in schizophrenia: Current findings and research perspectives. Frontiers in Neuroscience, 13, 274.

Porter, R.J., Baune, B.T., Morris, G., Hamilton, A., Bassett, D., et al., 2020. Cognitive side–effects of electroconvulsive therapy: What are they, how to monitor them and what to tell patients. B J Psych Open, 6(3), e40.

Raeburn, T., Liston, C., Hickmott, J., et al., 2018. Life of Martha Entwistle: Australia's first convict mental health nurse. Int J Ment Health Nurs, 27(1), 455–463.

Scholten, M., Gather, J. 2018. Adverse consequences of article 12 of the UN Convention on the Rights of Persons with Disabilities for persons with mental disabilities and an alternative way forward. J Med Ethics, 44(4), 226–233.

Surya S., Bishnoi, R.J., & Shashank, R.B. 2019. Balancing medical ethics to consider involuntary administration of electroconvulsive therapy. J ECT, 35(3), 150–151.

Szmukler, G. 2019. "Capacity", "best interests", "will and preferences" and the UN Convention on the Rights of Persons with Disabilities. World Psychiatry, 18(1), 34–41.

Szmukler, G., Daw, R., Callard, F. 2014. Mental health law and the UN Convention on the Rights of Persons with Disabilities. Int J Law Psychiatry, 37(3), 245–252.

Te Pou o te Whakaaro Nui 2018, Reducing and eliminating seclusion in mental health inpatient services: An evidence review for the Health Quality and Safety Commission New Zealand, Te Pou o te Whakaaro Nui, Auckland.

Thom, K., Lenagh-Glue, J., O'Brien, A.J., et al., 2019. Service user, whānau and peer support workers' perceptions of advance directives for mental health. Int J Ment Health Nurs, 28(6), 1296–1305.

Thom, K.A., O'Brien, A.J., McKenna, B.G., et al., 2009. Judging nursing practice: Implications of habeas corpus rulings for mental health nurses in New Zealand. Psychiatr Psychol Law, 15(1), 31–39.

Tosson, D., Lam, D., & Raeburn, T. 2022. Why Australia should move towards nationally consistent mental health legislation? Australas Psychiatry, 30(6), 743–745.

Varagona, L., Ballard, N.M., & Hedenstrom, M. 2022. Virtue ethics in health care teams; its time has come: Review of the nursing virtue ethics literature. J Nurs Manage, 30(7), 2394–2402.

Ward-Stockham, K., Kapp, S., Jarden, R., Gerdtz, M., & Daniel, C. 2022. Effect of Safewards on reducing conflict and containment and the experiences of staff and consumers: A mixed-methods systematic review. Int J Ment Health Nurs, 31(1), 199–221.

Watts, M., Murphy, E., Keogh, B., Downes, C., Doyle, L., et al., 2021. Deciding to discontinue prescribed psychotropic medication: A qualitative study of service users' experiences. Int J Ment Health Nurs, 30, 1395–1406.

White, B., Then, S.N., Willmott, L. 2018. Adults Who Lack Capacity: Substitute Decision-Making. Health Law in Australia, 3rd ed. Thomson Reuters, Pyrmont, NSW.

Wilson, A., Hurley, J., Hutchinson, M., & Lakeman, R. 2023. Trauma-informed care in acute mental health units through the lifeworld of mental health nurses: A phenomenological study. Int J Ment Health Nurs, doi.org/10.1111/inm.13120

Wilson, K. 2021. The history, justification, and purpose of mental health law. In: Wilson. K. Mental Health Law. Reform or Abolish? Oxford University Press, Melbourne.

World Health Organization (WHO), 2019. Strategies to end seclusion and restraint: WHO quality rights specialized training: Course slides. WHO, Geneva. https://apps.who.int/iris/handle/10665/329747

Zachar, P., Stoyanov, D.S., Aragona, M., et al., (eds), 2014. Alternative perspectives on psychiatric validation: DSM, IDC, RDoC and beyond. Oxford University Press, Oxford.

11

Anxiety

Anna Elders

Anna Elders

KEY POINTS

- Anxiety is a necessary, protective emotion that functions to stimulate several adaptive responses in the face of a stressor or threat. Anxiety can become problematic when excessively and/or unnecessarily triggered, causing significant impacts on functioning and quality of life.
- Most people experiencing anxiety disorders present to primary care settings for help; however, treatment can often be complex due to the severity of presenting symptoms, and comorbidity with substance use, depressive disorders and suicidality.
- Therapies such as cognitive behaviour therapy, and acceptance and commitment therapy are evidence-based treatments for anxiety,
- trauma and stress-related disorders. Combined psychological and pharmacological treatment may be warranted in more severe and complex presentations.
- Nurses are in a good position to provide support and treatment for people experiencing anxiety disorders due to our ability to develop collaborative, therapeutic relationships, undertake holistic assessments and offer psychoeducation, socioeconomic support and psychological interventions.

KEY TERMS

Avoidance behaviours
Chronic stress
Cognitions
Hyperarousal
Hypervigilance

Hypothalamus–pituitary–adrenal (HPA) axis
Intrusive anxious thoughts
Post-traumatic stress disorder
Psychological interventions

Rumination
Stress response
Stressor
Trauma-informed care

LEARNING OUTCOMES

The material in this chapter will assist you to:
- understand anxiety from an evolutionary, adaptive and functional perspective
- consider the aetiology of stress and anxiety and their mechanisms of action
- be aware of the demarcation between anxiety as a normal stress response and a diagnosable anxiety disorder

- be aware of the diagnostic symptoms and characteristics of specific anxiety disorders
- understand the considerations in assessing a person presenting with anxiety and identify effective interventions for alleviating the distress and symptoms of anxiety disorders.

INTRODUCTION

To clinically define and understand what an anxiety disorder is, we must first understand the basis for fear and anxiety as they naturally occur within our human experience. Fear is a conscious emotion experienced in the face of threat or impending danger. Anxiety is helpfully defined as a future-oriented mood state, designed to support cognitive, physiological and behavioural reactions to reduce the level of perceived danger within a future, anticipated, real or imagined threat (Penninx 2021). Anxiety is therefore an evolutionary survival trait that allows for the identification and initiation of necessary responses to potentially dangerous stimuli, including the body's fight/flight/freeze response, to ensure survival in the face of the numerous life-threatening situations that human beings can experience over a lifetime.

However, anxiety can change from a response that ensures survival to one that significantly reduces quality of life, causing ongoing levels of distress and day-to-day functional impairment.

Considering anxiety and fear responses on a continuum and within a functional framework helps us to both objectively assess anxiety, and work alongside consumers to make better assessments as to whether an anxiety disorder may be present or not.

This chapter examines the complex interactions that occur during an anxiety response and the different anxiety, trauma and stress-related disorders we can encounter in practice, their common symptoms and the current evidence-based treatments available. A concise overview of symptoms is provided in Table 11.1 later in the chapter.

Anxiety can originate from survival responses to early adverse life experiences, such as abuse, attachment difficulties and family or environmental stressors, which often leave indelible psychological and

TABLE 11.1 Key Features of Specific Anxiety, Trauma- and Stress-Related Disorders

Disorder	Key Features
Generalised Anxiety Disorder (GAD)	• Excessive, difficult-to-control anxiety and worry (apprehensive expectation) about multiple events or activities (e.g. school/work difficulties) • Accompanied by symptoms such as restlessness/feeling on edge or muscle tension
Obsessive-Compulsive Disorder (OCD)	• Obsessions: Recurrent and persistent thoughts, urges or images that are experienced as intrusive and unwanted and that cause marked anxiety or distress • Compulsions: Repetitive behaviours (e.g. handwashing) or mental acts (e.g. counting) that the individual feels driven to perform to reduce the anxiety generated by the obsessions
Panic Disorder (PD)	• Recurrent unexpected panic attacks, in the absence of triggers • Persistent concern about additional panic attacks and/or maladaptive change in behaviour related to the attacks
Agoraphobia	• Marked, unreasonable fear or anxiety about a situation • Active avoidance of feared situation due to thinking that escape might be difficult or help unavailable if panic-like symptoms occur
Social Anxiety Disorder (SAD)	• Marked, excessive or unrealistic fear or anxiety about social situations in which there is possible exposure to scrutiny by others • Active avoidance of feared situation
Specific Phobia	• Marked, unreasonable fear or anxiety about a specific object or situation, which is actively avoided (e.g. flying, heights, animals, receiving an injection, seeing blood)
Post-Traumatic Stress Disorder (PTSD) and Acute Stress Disorder (ASD)	• Exposure to actual or threatened death, serious injury or sexual violation • Intrusion symptoms (e.g. distressing memories or dreams, flashbacks, intense distress) and avoidance of stimuli associated with the event • Negative alterations in cognitions and mood (e.g. negative beliefs and emotions, detachment), as well as marked alterations in arousal and reactivity (e.g. irritable behaviour, hypervigilance)
Adjustment Disorder (AD)	• Development of emotional or behavioural symptoms occurring within 3 months of the onset of a stressor (not including normal bereavement) • Distress is noted to be out of proportion to the severity or intensity of the stressor

biological marks. The chapter will explore some of the internal triggers and reinforcing elements of anxiety shaped by past experiences and significant life events. Using a trauma-informed approach to care allows nurses to establish an essential historical context for anxiety, making the care and treatment we provide for people more meaningful, supportive and effective.

AETIOLOGY OF STRESS, FEAR AND ANXIETY

Stress, fear and anxiety are normal internal experiences that occur in response to a stressor. A stressor can be defined as any internal or external stimulus that promotes physical or emotional stress. Historically, humans have been exposed to numerous life-threatening situations, from tribal warfare to environmental disasters such as famine. When we study the role that stress, fear and anxiety play in human evolution, we see a system containing inbuilt mechanisms that allow for early recognition, physiological priming and behavioural adaptation in the face of danger. For the purposes of survival, the human brain developed the capability to learn and store information to aid timely responses in the face of threats. Human behaviour is shaped by our stress response system, and it is this system that is implicated in the development of anxiety disorders and most other mental health conditions.

The physiological response to stress is a complex myriad of feedback mechanisms involving nearly every system of the body. Our stress response commences in the amygdala, a key part of our brain's limbic system. When we encounter a potential threat, our eyes and ears send sensory information to the amygdala, which interprets the information, looking for signs of danger. When danger is detected, the amygdala signals the hypothalamus to create a rapid preparatory response, activating the sympathetic nervous system, and our body's fight, flight

or freeze response through a cascade of hormonal signals, including epinephrine (adrenaline). At the same time, the sensory information is processed against stored memories in the hippocampus, allowing us to ascertain the level of risk and prepare for further physiological and behavioural responses. The system that collates these responses is known as the hypothalamic–pituitary–adrenal axis, or HPA axis (see Fig. 11.1). The HPA axis plays other important roles, such as being part of our immune response in the face of infection and assisting in the regulation of glucose levels during times of stress.

Exposure to high levels of stress during childhood in response to significant adversity, such as childhood abuse, is associated with heightened stress responses in later life (King 2021). Early trauma has been identified as a significant contributor to a range of mental health conditions that can subsequentially develop (King 2021).

Chronic stress, such as that experienced during an enduring, traumatic stressor like an abusive relationship, also leads to hypersecretion of cortisol and sustained sympathetic nervous system response. Sustained sympathetic nervous system activity and excessive systemic exposure to cortisol have been shown to result in both physical illness and psychopathology in both anxiety and depression due to the production of an ever-increasing and difficult-to-manage allostatic load (see Fig. 11.2), causing detrimental effects on key systems in the body, such as the central nervous and cardiovascular systems (James et al 2023).

Differing responses to stressful life experiences can be understood as a combination of individual genetic (nature) and environmental (nurture) differences. Genetic vulnerability has been shown to greatly contribute to the presence of depression and anxiety symptoms in children up until age seven. However, environmental factors (positive or negative) are known to be important predictors of the presence and stability of symptoms throughout adolescence and adulthood (James et al 2023).

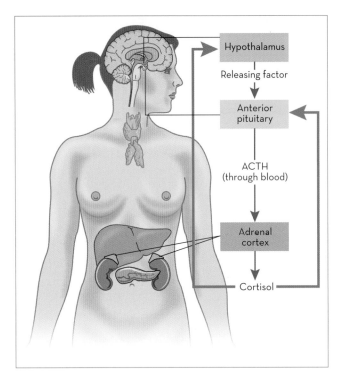

FIG 11.1 The Hypothalamic–Pituitary–Adrenal Axis. (Adapted from Simon 2015.)

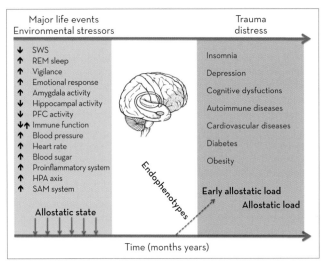

FIG 11.2 The Effects of Allostatic State and Allostatic Load on the Brain. Major life events and environmental stressors can create an allostatic state (imbalance) within pivotal centres of the brain, such as the hypothalamus, the prefrontal cortex and the amygdala due to increased adaptive responses to stress (indicated in the blue column). If maintained over months or years, this can create an allostatic load (wear and tear), increasing susceptibility to insomnia, mental health disorders, cardiovascular disease, diabetes and so on. SWS: Slow wave sleep; HPA axis: Hypothalamic–pituitary–adrenal axis; REM: Rapid eye movement; SAM system: Sympatho–adreno–medullary system. (Palagini et al 2013. Copyright © 2012 Elsevier Ltd.)

Chronic stress is both a predisposing and a perpetuating factor for a range of difficulties in mental health and general wellbeing over the lifespan. Stress is initially activated in the face of real-life crises and adversity; however, it can continue long after these events have ceased through the fear generalisation process. The fear generalisation process

is thought to support survival in the face of previously faced danger, through the utilisation of retained fear information and fear responses. In chronic stress, however, the limbic system becomes hypersensitive and hyperreactive, risking the misinterpretation of benign information in a person's environment as threatening, thus creating multiple unhelpful and unnecessary anxiety responses.

Over the course of our lives, each of us develops belief systems and associated cognitive or thinking styles based on our early environments and experiences that help us to make sense of ourselves, others, the world and our future. These cognitions help to guide decision-making and event processing as we move through life. They play an important role in the generation of stress and development of reactive mood states or affects when they become violated and negatively biased through the experience of traumatic events (Milman et al 2020). Hammen's (1991) stress generation effect refers to the contribution that our cognitive vulnerabilities (depressive thinking styles, hopelessness and rumination) make towards increasing the likelihood of experiencing challenging life events negatively and often catastrophically, thereby generating further stress and anxiety. And so develops a potentially vicious cycle of anxious physiological reactions, anxious thinking, anxious feeling and anxious doing, all perpetuating each other and creating an increased risk to our mental and physical wellbeing.

ANXIETY DISORDERS

Anxiety commonly presents in the face of a trigger, as high levels of experienced fear and thoughts of imminent danger and perception of risk, accompanied by a range of safety behaviours and significant physiological arousal. The term "anxiety disorder" refers to a level of symptoms of anxiety and related distress that cause significant impairment in functioning and quality of life. Anxiety disorders are diagnosed following the application of a diagnostic reasoning process in which specific symptoms of an anxiety disorder are identified during an assessment.

Most people experiencing anxiety disorders receive treatment within the primary care setting. Symptoms of anxiety disorders can be missed in people presenting with features of major depressive disorder, which commonly co-occurs with anxiety and has much higher rates of detection (NICE 2014). This presents a huge barrier for treatment and burden for people living with anxiety disorders, as well as significant resource implications for healthcare systems, due to the high service usage of services that often arise due to the chronically disabling nature of anxiety disorders (Penninx et al 2021).

People with anxiety disorders often delay seeking treatment, due in part to self-stigma and fear of judgement from others, but also a tendency to utilise a more avoidant coping style in the face of distress. The resulting delay means the person has to live with often high ongoing levels of distress, impairment in functioning and considerable reduction in quality of life.

Anxiety disorders contribute significantly to a higher risk of self-harm and suicide (De La Vega et al 2018). Anxiety as an emotion can distort perceptions, leading to feelings of hopelessness with a sense of not having the ability to cope, and believing that things won't work out.

Although there are no fail-safe treatments for anxiety disorders, there are many options available that provide hope and relief of symptoms. Due to the prevalence of anxiety disorders, screening and assessment to detect problematic anxiety, alongside other mental health conditions, is an essential part of all nursing assessments.

The demarcation between "normal" anxiety and that which may be considered "disordered" can be difficult to make if we fail to obtain all

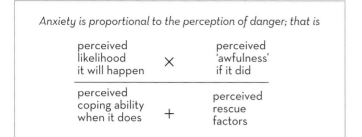

FIG 11.3 Anxiety and Perceptions of Danger. (Salkovskis 1996.)

Anxiety is proportional to the perception of danger; that is

$$\frac{\text{perceived likelihood it will happen} \times \text{perceived 'awfulness' if it did}}{\text{perceived coping ability when it does} + \text{perceived rescue factors}}$$

the information required to make an informed assessment. Collaboration and a good therapeutic rapport are therefore imperative to ensure all necessary information, including trauma histories, are collected as early as possible to inform care. The context or environment a person is living in provides a basis on which to formulate possible precipitating and perpetuating factors that we must consider in the care we decide upon. Anxiety disorders can lead to misinterpretations of presenting triggers; for example, a person's catastrophic response to noticing a change in their heart rate may lead them to believe that they are going to die of a heart attack. On the other hand, symptoms of anxiety disorders can appear in response to dangerous external stimuli, such as generalised anxiety in relation to emotional or physical abuse from a violent partner. Identifying if there is current risk of danger is essential to ensure safety and attempt to help the person escape further trauma.

Salkovskis (1996) provides a helpful illustration for understanding the role that perception of danger plays in the development and intensity of anxiety (see Fig. 11.3). Our interpretation of the world, others and ourselves dictates our emotional, physiological, cognitive and behavioural responses. Many symptoms of anxiety can be understood in relation to the level of threat perceived by the individual. Any potential threat is processed through an estimation of the likelihood that such an event will occur and, if it seems likely, how catastrophic it would be for the person. Internal coping resources are considered alongside any external support/rescue that may be available. When the likelihood of catastrophic danger seems high without a sense of protection from self and others, we experience high levels of anxiety and fear, resulting in a cascade of survival-focused responses until a sense of safety returns.

Salkovskis' model (1996) provides a way of understanding how previous trauma and the associated impact on our cognitions affects our processes of threat assessment. Trauma can negatively change our perception and responses to future situations. If we no longer feel capable of protecting ourselves and we do not trust others to come to our aid, we feel less in control and therefore more vulnerable. These factors are often at play in the experiences of those living with high levels of anxiety. They can wreak havoc on a person's functioning, reducing their behaviours to those that appear to reduce the sense of immediate risk and avoid further anxiety-triggering situations, rather than behaviours that provide engagement in meaningful, valued life activities. The same safety behaviours utilised to give a sense of safety and certainty end up perpetuating later anxiety, as the person continuously acts as if there is danger in the present and/or future, triggering continued physiological stress activation and reinforcing an unhelpful and inaccurate sense of threat. It is these physiological, behavioural, emotional and cognitive experiences that form the basis for the diagnostic symptoms of anxiety and other mental health disorders, including significant predisposition to depression.

EPIDEMIOLOGY OF ANXIETY DISORDERS

Data describing the prevalence of anxiety disorders was last collected in Australia by the Australian Bureau of Statistics (ABS) in 2020–21 and in Aotearoa New Zealand in 2003–04 (Wells 2006). The Australian study focused on Australians aged between 16 and 85, showing that over two in five people (43.7%) had experienced a mental disorder at some time in their life, with 21.4% experiencing symptoms in the 12 months prior to data collection (ABS 2023). Anxiety disorders were found to be the most prevalent of all disorders, with 16.8% of participants reporting symptoms in the preceding 12 months. The most commonly experienced anxiety disorder was social anxiety disorder (SAD) (7%), with 5.7% of people experiencing post-traumatic stress disorder (PTSD). People identifying as female reported higher rates of anxiety disorders than people identifying as male (21% compared to 12.4%); however, rates were much higher, at 44.7%, in people identifying as gay, lesbian, bisexual, asexual, pansexual or queer within the survey. Specific data on Indigenous Australians was not reported in the 2020–21 survey; however, a separate survey on Aboriginal and Torres Strait Islander health was conducted by the ABS between 2018 and 2019, which found that 17% of Indigenous persons experienced an anxiety disorder.

Aotearoa New Zealand survey results indicated a 46.6% lifetime prevalence rate of mental health disorders in the general population, with 20.7% of respondents indicating prevalence in the 12 months prior to data collection (Wells 2006). At the time of the study, prevalence estimates indicated that 24.9% of the population would experience an anxiety disorder over their lifetime. Specific phobia (7.3%) and SAD (5.1%) were the most commonly experienced of the anxiety disorders, while other disorders were found at lower rates: PTSD, 3%; generalised anxiety disorder (GAD), 2%; panic disorder, 1.7%; agoraphobia, 0.6%; and obsessive-compulsive disorder (OCD) 0.6%. The survey found a higher lifetime prevalence of mental health disorders for Māori (50.7%, with a 29.5% 12-month prevalence). Anxiety disorders for Māori were found to be most prevalent, at 19.4% in the 12 months prior to the study, with an estimated lifetime prevalence of 31.3%. Māori not only experienced higher rates of mental health disorders compared with non-Māori, but also experienced greater levels of severity (Wells 2006), further highlighting how essential it is to focus on addressing these inequalities within Aotearoa New Zealand's health system and wider society.

Pacific peoples living in Aotearoa New Zealand were shown to have slightly higher 12-month prevalence rates (23.9%) than non-Pacific peoples (not including Māori), but lower rates of service utilisation for severe mental health disorders. An important finding for Aotearoa New Zealand's health sector to consider was an increased vulnerability to mental health disorders for Pacific peoples who were born in Aotearoa New Zealand versus those born in Pacific Island countries (Wells 2006).

Aotearoa New Zealand has not conducted a further survey directly related to levels of mental health since 2003–04; however, the Ministry of Health's annual Aotearoa New Zealand Health Survey reported a 13.7% prevalence rate for anxiety disorders in 2021–22, which is an increase from 6.1% reported in the 2011–12 survey (Ministry of Health 2022).

Collective Australasian survey findings show that anxiety disorders are the most commonly occurring mental health problems within our populations. Females experience higher rates of anxiety disorders than males, and younger people (16–24 and 25–44) generally experience higher rates than older groups within the surveys (ABS 2023; Wells 2006; Ministry of Health 2022).

Mental health statistics for Māori and Pacific peoples highlight the importance of considering the impact that loss of culture and connection to land through acculturation and colonisation can have on a person's mental wellbeing and sense of self. Although there is no breakdown by ethnicity of prevalence of mental health conditions in the 2020–21 Australian survey, it is well known that colonisation has created a significant loss of land and culture for Aboriginal and Torres Strait Islander peoples, with associated major impacts on their mental health. These issues are further discussed in Chapters 6 and 7.

> ### ❓ CRITICAL THINKING EXERCISE 11.1
>
> How do you currently deal with stress and anxiety in your own life? What thoughts do you notice you experience regularly during these times and what behaviours do you engage in? What things do you do that provide the most effective support for yourself? Do you have any responses that are not so helpful? What would be the most helpful way to think and act towards stress and anxiety when it shows up? How could you use this learning in your practice?

COMORBIDITY

Comorbidity in anxiety disorders is so prevalent that it is often considered the rule, rather than the exception. Lifetime prevalence rates of comorbidity within anxiety disorders are high, particularly alongside depressive disorders, and 46–68% of adults with an anxiety disorder meet the criteria for a concurrent anxiety disorder with a strong correlation with depressive disorders (Katzman et al 2014; Penninx 2021).

It is important to consider that people presenting with other types of mental health conditions often experience heightened anxiety as well, and to plan interventions focused on reducing problematic anxiety as a key part of treatment. There is strong evidence suggesting an important link between anxiety disorders and schizophrenia, with heightened anxiety a potential precursor to psychosis and a potential risk factor for relapse (Hall 2017). Research shows high levels of comorbid anxiety disorders such as social anxiety, PTSD, GAD and OCD in people with a diagnosis of schizophrenia (Hall 2017), with strong correlations between positive symptoms of schizophrenia (social avoidance, suspiciousness of other's intentions and judgements) and symptoms of conditions such as social anxiety. Anxiety disorders are also known to occur with other mental health conditions, such as bipolar disorder, personality disorders and substance dependence (Penninx 2021).

These findings support the essential need to deliver therapeutic interventions for anxiety for people who have a primary diagnosis of schizophrenia, or other mental health conditions.

> ### BOX 11.1 Recommendations for Increased Awareness of Anxiety Disorders
>
> - Become familiar with the main features of anxiety disorders, PTSD and OCD and the main symptoms that distinguish them from each other.
> - Develop systematic questions to ask about the nature, severity, duration, distress and associated impairment in people presenting with anxiety symptoms to decide whether an anxiety disorder, PTSD or OCD is present.
> - Become familiar with the fluctuating nature of symptoms in patients with anxiety disorders, and with the tendency for symptoms to change in nature over time

Baldwin et al 2014.

Box 11.1 provides recommendations for increasing awareness of anxiety disorders.

ASSESSMENT AND DIAGNOSIS

Engaging with services can initially heighten a person's anxiety due to uncertainty regarding outcomes, experience of self-stigma and feared judgement from others, as well as exposure to fear-inducing experiences through the initial assessment and treatment processes. Becoming adept with the skills of engagement and conveying a sense of unconditional positive regard supports consumers to feel safer and develop a sense of trust (for further discussion of assessment, see Chapter 9), allowing people to begin to open up about their current and historical experiences.

Due to the high prevalence of trauma and childhood adversity, trauma screening should be incorporated into assessment to help identify important past experiences that play a significant role in present-day challenges. This is particularly pertinent for refugee communities who experience extremely high rates of trauma. Trauma screening does not assess exactly what happened to the person, but rather gathers enough information to ascertain that trauma has occurred, and whether there is present-day danger. When trauma is disclosed, screening should be conducted for symptoms of PTSD (see information on PTSD later in this chapter).

In Perspectives in practice: Nurse's story 11.1, Karen Jones describes her use of assessment skills to develop an understanding of a consumer's anxiety and to plan effective intervention.

Conducting a thorough nursing assessment includes reviewing relevant psychosocial information, enabling exploration of current stressors that may be producing an understandable anxiety response, such as major financial challenges, physical danger or significant losses (employment, relationships, health status, acculturative stress).

General screening questions have been recommended to support consumers to disclose any aspects of anxiety that are becoming problematic (see Box 11.2). Questioning relating to anxiety needs to be simple, time-specific and able to capture both a change in levels of anxiety and anxious thinking, as well as associated behavioural changes such as avoidance.

Exploring the impact of anxiety symptoms on quality of life and functioning helps to consider whether a clinically significant level of anxiety is being experienced. New migrants and refugees often experience major stress adapting to a new country, and culture and language barriers may affect engagement. There may also be misunderstandings about what services can and cannot provide if the person has little experience of local healthcare systems. Integrating care with other social and healthcare providers can be hugely beneficial if it can enhance assistance in gaining access to essential needs such as housing, allowing the person to then better focus on their wellbeing.

PERSPECTIVES IN PRACTICE

Nurse's Story 11.1: Karen Jones

I recall working with a man in his 40s who was so anxious he wasn't sleeping or eating at all and couldn't sit still. He described walking around with earmuffs on his head to try to block noise, which he felt was worsening his anxiety. The man took a year off work and felt unable to drive or participate in his usual daily life, including caring for his two young children due to his hyperanxious state and lack of concentration. This took a real toll on his family, as his wife was required to take over running the household. His children did not understand what had happened but noticed their father had completely withdrawn into himself. Through thorough assessment and ongoing support from his GP, practice nurses and primary mental health services it was established that certain changes occurring within his workplace were the cause of his anxiety. A combination of medication and cognitive behaviour therapy assisted him in identifying coping strategies, enabling him to recover and regain the ability to get back into his life. A variety of further resources were also accessed to support the patient and his family, including help from a social worker, financial support and guidance in accessing educational and self-help websites.

Karen Jones is a designated nurse prescriber and practice nurse working in a marae-based health clinic.

BOX 11.2 General Screening Questions

During the past 2 weeks, how much have you been bothered by the following problems:
- Feeling nervous, anxious, frightened, worried or on edge?
- Feeling panicked or being frightened?
- Avoiding situations that make you anxious?

APA 2022

Pervasiveness of anxiety across roles and life domains should be assessed to help identify whether anxiety is generalised, or more in the face of a particular stress-inducing trigger, such as flying on a plane or starting a new job. Scaling questions (0–10) can assist with identifying the intensity of experienced anxiety. Questions assessing the presence of physiological arousal (e.g. tachycardia, sweating, hyperventilation) and behavioural responses (avoidance of triggers or other described behaviours to reduce anxiety and promote sense of safety) assist in determining functional and physical levels of impact of anxiety.

Assessing other presenting issues or difficulties – such as depressive mood states, alcohol and drug use, psychotic symptoms or mood lability – helps ascertain the presence of possible comorbid disorders. Equally, anxiety should be assessed if people present with another disorder, due to both the detrimental impacts of excessive anxiety on other conditions, and the rates of comorbidity.

Assessment should include special consideration of the consumer's health history, particularly conditions known to cause anxiety (e.g. Graves' disease) and those that are negatively affected by anxiety (e.g. hypertension).

It is important to be aware of different cultural presentations and beliefs about anxiety present within our communities. In some cultures, people may present with more somatic symptoms, such as physical sensations experienced throughout the body (e.g. pain), or intrusive thoughts may be believed to be caused or linked to spiritual or supernatural experiences. It is important to gain the perspectives of the consumer and family, and attempt to understand the cultural context from which people come, so as to support an effective, shared understanding and approach to treatment to aid engagement and outcomes. Cultural experts can be extremely helpful in bridging the cultural–clinical gap, helping to ensure care remains acceptable, culturally inclusive and safe for the consumer. Assessment should also consider the specific cultural aspects of wellbeing of Indigenous peoples to identify pathways to support them to regain their wellbeing, connection to important aspects of self and overall health. See chapters 6 and 7 for further discussion of cultural safety in mental health nursing.

Finally, the high prevalence of self-harm and suicidal ideation and behaviours in anxiety disorders has previously been discussed. It is imperative that nurses become comfortable asking about these issues in order to assess any risk of harm that may be present.

Assessment Tools

There are several helpful assessment tools available that can assist nurses to screen for anxiety disorders. Below are a few examples, many of which are self-administered and available for free use via the internet. Most of the tools mentioned below can be used within any health setting and are helpful for detecting anxiety disorders, although in themselves don't determine a diagnosis. Outcomes from such assessments need to be viewed together with historical and current information to ensure a thorough diagnostic reasoning process. Experienced nurses, particularly those in autonomous roles, such as clinical nurse specialists and nurse practitioners, can diagnose anxiety disorders. Less experienced nurses can provide essential contributions to diagnostic processes by gathering information that may help clarify any eventual diagnoses made.

Social Phobia Inventory (SPIN)

The SPIN (Connor et al 2000) is a 17-item self-rating questionnaire assessing each of the three symptom domains of social anxiety: fear, avoidance and psychological arousal. A score of 19 or more indicates the presence of symptoms of social anxiety.

GAD-7

The GAD-7 (Spitzer et al 2006) is a seven-question self-report assessment tool designed to screen and measure the severity of any presenting symptoms of excessive worry and generalised anxiety. Scores of 5, 10 and 15 are considered cut-off points for mild, moderate and severe anxiety, respectively. Scores above 10 indicate that further assessment is required to enable exploration as to whether a diagnosis of GAD may be present.

Yale-Brown Obsessive-Compulsive Scale (Y-BOCS)

The Y-BOCS (Goodman et al 1989) is a lengthy, comprehensive measure of the severity, impact and type of symptoms of OCD. The Y-BOCS requires a reasonable degree of experience to administer as it is carried out as a semi-structured interview.

Impact of Event Scale – Revised (IES-R)

The IES-R (Weiss & Marmar 1996) is a 22-item short self-report tool designed to measure symptoms following exposure to a trauma that may indicate the presence of PTSD. Questions aim to measure the presence of the major cluster of symptoms of PTSD: Intrusive re-experiencing, hyperarousal and persistent avoidance (see later information on PTSD within this chapter).

In the following section, symptoms of the different anxiety disorders are outlined. A summary of key features is provided in Table 11.1.

Anxiety Disorders

Generalised Anxiety Disorder (GAD)

GAD is a condition that can be debilitating due to the constant, excessive and consuming worry about numerous everyday situations that people experience. People experiencing GAD often find their worry is difficult to control and highly disruptive to their day-to-day functioning due to the intrusive nature of the thoughts and physical symptoms of anxiety they experience. For people experiencing GAD, worry is often a double-edged sword – on the one hand it is a perceived helpful aid to reduce uncertainty and manage the numerous risks in life, and on the other hand, it is a loathed and consuming worry in and of itself.

GAD is often accompanied by somatic complaints including fatigue, and a sense of restlessness, irritability, insomnia and hyperarousal that arises out of the constant state of anxiety-induced alertness that people can experience (APA 2022).

GAD can become chronic in nature due to its exacerbation by life stressors (Andrews et al 2018). It is thought to cause the most interference with life compared with other anxiety disorders, with almost half (48%) of responders in one study stating that it impacted considerably in at least four domains of their life (McEvoy et al 2011). GAD may go undetected and therefore untreated as people may present with more complaints about their physical health and mood than anxiety (Andrews et al 2018).

Lifetime prevalence of GAD in Australasia is around 6% of the general population (Andrews et al 2018) and mean age of onset is around 33 years of age (McEvoy et al 2011; Wells 2006). Having an anxious temperament is considered a vulnerability factor, with people often reporting that they have always been a worrier (Penninx 2021). There are noted inherent genetic risks (Penninx 2021), increasing the prevalence of comorbidity with other anxiety and depressive disorders that share similar predisposing risk factors. Major depressive disorder commonly occurs alongside GAD (Shin 2019), causing a more severe range of symptoms and complications for treatment.

It is important to note that cultural differences can equate to different expressions of anxiety symptoms, with some people experiencing more somatic complaints while other people may report more cognitive symptoms.

Recent guidelines developed by the Royal Australian and New Zealand College of Psychiatrists identify psychoeducation and active monitoring as an important first step, with delivery of either face-to-face cognitive behaviour therapy (CBT) or supported e-CBT as a second step, and consideration of a pharmacological treatment, such as a selective serotonin reuptake inhibitor (SSRI), specifically sertraline, in combination with psychological intervention as a third step (Andrews et al 2018). Personal perspectives: Consumer's story 11.1 provides an account of how one consumer developed strategies to help manage an anxiety disorder.

HISTORICAL ANECDOTE 11.2

Socratic Questioning

In modern times, CBT has become well known as a first-line treatment for several types of anxiety disorder. CBT has historical links to the stoic philosophy of ancient Greece, which observed that because life perpetually changes, people need to strive to maintain clear thinking. In particular, a key tenant of CBT is the ancient technique skill known as "Socratic questioning". This refers to a method of learning named after the ancient Greek philosopher Socrates (470–399 BC). He believed that rather than teaching people information laid out as facts people learnt more when they were taught how to ask thoughtful questions to examine ideas and determine their validity.

Read More About It
Brickhouse, T.C., Smith, N.D. 2009 Socratic teaching and Socratic method. In: Siegel H (ed). The Oxford handbook of philosophy of education. Oxford University Press, New York.

PERSONAL PERSPECTIVES

Consumer's Story 11.1: Thomas

Quite often I don't know when anxiety is going to hit as it can creep up or come on suddenly; however, I know the warning signs: Feeling more tense and on edge, getting irritable with my family, feeling something just isn't right and having a sense of urgency to everything. I notice my thoughts begin to race and it is harder to enjoy things or be as present in the moment because I'm either thinking about something I have to do or worrying about something I've done and whether it was right or not.

My anxiety comes partly from my temperament (I've always been a worrier), partly from my lifestyle (I don't always get a good balance between work and life) and from experiences in my childhood. I grew up with a parent who worried a lot. The older I get, the more I can see my parent's worries in the way that I see the world when anxiety descends.

Learning about how anxiety works and what goes on in my body, how to identify anxious thinking and focus on slowing down and looking after myself have been the most helpful approaches to anxiety. Quite often, stopping and paying attention to my distress, being willing to feel it and not fight with it, and being kinder to myself really helps. The next step is making lifestyle changes to ensure I protect my sleep, keep a balance in diet and activity and do things I enjoy with people I love. I know it is important to keep these important wellbeing behaviours in my everyday life to maintain balance.

Obsessive-Compulsive Disorder (OCD)

OCD involves a recurring experience of anxiety-creating intrusive cognitions (thoughts, impulses or images) that become obsessive in nature, and risk dominating a person's internal world over time. Obsessive cognitions often involve themes of risk of harm to self or others, such as developing a life-threatening disease or harm coming to family members. These cognitions are experienced with significant accompanying physiological symptoms of anxiety, increasing the person's perception of heightened danger. In response to obsessive cognitions and anxious bodily sensations, compulsive behaviours develop that serve the purpose of reducing the perception of harm and creating a sense of safety. Compulsive behaviours may be directly related to obsessions, such as washing hands to prevent acquisition or transmission of disease, or totally unrelated, such as tapping surfaces a particular number of times to reduce the risk of an unwanted outcome. The relief provided and sense the compulsive behaviours have successfully averted catastrophe work to "fuse" the compulsive behaviours to the obsessions. Thus, the more the obsessions are experienced, the more the compulsions are carried out.

Despite attempts to reduce anxiety by carrying out compulsions or attempting to suppress intrusions, both recur. This leads into a very disruptive and often distressing reinforcing cycle as compulsions take up more time and obsessive thinking disrupts usual day-to-day cognitive processes.

OCD is not a particularly common anxiety disorder. Twelve-month prevalence rates in Aotearoa New Zealand were last recorded at about 0.6% and lifetime rates at 1.2%; however, Māori rates were higher, with 12-month prevalence at 1% and lifetime rates at 2.6% (Wells 2006). The Australian survey noted higher 12-month prevalence at 3.1% (ABS 2023).

Despite lower rates of OCD, symptoms are often more severe compared with other anxiety disorders, with higher rates of suicidal ideation, plans and suicide attempts (Wells 2006) indicating necessity to ensure prompt treatment and close monitoring of risk.

Treatment commonly involves a combination of medication and concurrent talking therapies due to the severity of symptoms; however, a stepped care approach is common, with low intensity psychological treatment identified as a first-line approach with the addition of an SSRI medication as a second step for either more severe presentations or where improvement is not achieved (Nezgovorova et al 2022). Exposure and response prevention, a specific type of CBT developed for OCD, has good evidence for efficacy; however, it is often difficult to access due to a lack of trained specialist therapists available (Nezgovorova et al 2022).

Panic Disorder

Panic disorder (PD) is characterised by unpredictable experiences of intense, episodic surges of anxiety that occur in the form of panic attacks. Intense physiological anxiety symptoms are experienced (tachycardia, sweating, shaking, dyspnoea, chest pain, dizziness, nausea, tingling), along with a sense of depersonalisation (feeling detached from oneself). Panic attacks can occur outside of PD in relation to other presentations of anxiety; however, the higher frequency, non-selective triggering environments and anticipatory anxiety helps differentiate PD from other diagnoses.

Panic attacks reach a peak of severity within approximately 10 minutes and can last up to 45 minutes. It is common to experience catastrophic cognitions during panic attacks due to the surge of physiological symptoms. These can include a sense of imminent death ("I'm going to have a heart attack and die"), mental health deterioration ("I'm going to lose my mind") or a negative outcome regarding fear of losing consciousness ("I'll pass out and something will happen to me when I'm unconscious"). As a result, people engage in rapid safety behaviours during panic attacks in order to seek help (e.g. phoning emergency services), lessen the attack (e.g. sit down) and further monitor symptoms (e.g. body scanning, taking one's pulse).

As the panic attack begins to abate, the person obtains a false impression that: (a) they were on the brink of a catastrophic event; and (b) their safety behaviours prevented the imminent catastrophe that was occurring during the attack. This signals a major misinterpretation of anxiety symptoms (e.g. "I could have a panic attack and die"), leading to scanning for a further attack and greater anticipatory anxiety. A number of preventive safety behaviours develop to avoid future attacks and reduce perceived risk, such as becoming dependent on others to go out, body hypervigilance (body scanning for symptoms) and avoiding potential triggering or perceived high-risk situations. These safety behaviours can lead to agoraphobia (see later description) in approximately one-third to one-half of cases (Andrews et al 2018) and vicious cycles of panic attacks, anxiety and ever-increasing safety behaviours – see Fig. 11.4, which illustrates Clark's cognitive model of panic disorder (PD).

PD is one of the less common anxiety disorders, with a 12-month prevalence rate of 1.7% in Aotearoa New Zealand and 3.7% in Australia (ABS 2023; Wells 2006). However, PD often presents with high levels of severity, with 44.9% of cases within the Aotearoa New Zealand survey being classified as serious (Wells 2006).

PD has a high comorbidity rate with conditions such as depression (Baldwin et al 2014) and is strongly correlated with suicidal ideation, planning and completed suicide (Wells 2006). PD is linked to higher rates of help-seeking (Wells 2006) due to both the accompanied fear of medical illness-linked attacks causing high rates of presentation to medical services during and after attacks.

Treatment for PD largely centres on brief psychological interventions such as CBT, which can be delivered through online CBT courses or in face-to-face sessions (Andrews et al 2018). Selective serotonin reuptake inhibitor (SSRIs), selective noradrenaline reuptake inhibitor (SNRIs), tricyclic antidepressants and benzodiazepines have been shown to be effective for PD (Andrews et al 2018); however, it is

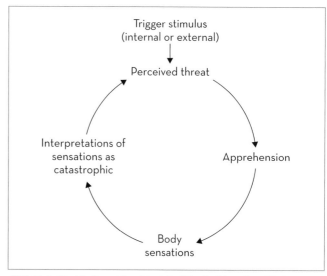

FIG 11.4 Clark's Cognitive Model of Panic Disorder. (Clark 1986.)

important to note that benzodiazepines should not be used long term and use of exposure through a psychological approach like CBT should always be incorporated throughout treatment so that people can build skills and experience to manage PD in the long term.

Agoraphobia

Agoraphobia is characterised by generalised, consistent and significant unrealistic fear responses to exposure or anticipated exposure to public spaces such as shopping centres, crowded areas or open spaces. Common associated anxious cognitions relate to fears that help may not be available or escape possible should the person begin to panic or experience considerable symptoms of distress. Avoidance is commonly used as a safety behaviour, thereby causing impairment in day-to-day functioning. Techniques such as distraction and dependency on others to go out are used regularly in order to enter situations that trigger anxiety.

Agoraphobia is highly comorbid with panic disorder and functional impairment can be significant, although panic attacks are not always experienced.

Agoraphobia has been found to occur at 12-month prevalence rates of 4.6% within the Australian population (ABS 2023) and 0.6% within the Aotearoa New Zealand population, with the highest age representation being between 25 and 44 years old (Wells 2006). Despite its lower prevalence rate compared with other anxiety disorders, agoraphobia is highly correlated with suicidal ideation, plans and suicide attempts (Wells 2006), highlighting the significance of screening for suicide risk in assessment.

Social Anxiety Disorder (SAD)

SAD is poorly recognised in primary health care (Baldwin et al 2014) and may be misconstrued as shyness and introversion. People with SAD experience high levels of socially induced distress and impairment in day-to-day functioning due to persistent and objectively unreasonable fears of embarrassment, humiliation and negative judgement by others during social situations, particularly where there may be performance expectations, such as within a classroom or at a party. Negative and inflexible beliefs about self, commonly precipitated by internalised past or present emotional abuse (I'm stupid, I'm boring, I'm unlikeable) often drive social anxiety, with a sense of fear that others may "discover" these perceived personal flaws. This fear results in an intensely negative and distorted over-monitoring of the self in social situations, which then perpetuates the held negative core beliefs and, in turn, the associated social anxiety through further social avoidance and other developed safety behaviours. Developed safety behaviours may include conversation rehearsal, conversation redirection towards others (away from self), avoidance of interactions during social events and negatively focused post event-analysis (thinking back on self and others' behaviours during recent social situations). Safety behaviours further fuel social anxiety as the person acts, and therefore continues to feel as if they are socially incompetent and unacceptable to others.

It is common for people with SAD to have considerable fear of losing control of their bodies due to physiological responses to anxiety (incontinence, vomiting, blushing or shaking) in social situations, causing further fear of social humiliation and negative evaluation by others.

SAD can have serious impacts on a person's family and romantic relationships, occupational opportunities and day-to-day functioning as it becomes both harder to make and maintain relationships and present oneself for educational and career development opportunities.

SAD was found to be the second most common anxiety disorder in Aotearoa New Zealand after GAD in terms of lifetime prevalence (5.1%) in the 2003–04 survey, with prevalence rates higher for Māori (6.2%) and Pacific peoples (5.8%) (Wells 2006). Australian prevalence rates for SAD were found to be at 7% over a 12-month period (ABS 2023). Aotearoa New Zealand youth (16–24 years) were found to have the highest rates of SAD, with a median age of onset of 12 years of age (Wells 2006). There is an estimated 28-year delay in treatment from age of onset, with only 4.9% of affected youth seeking help at the start of symptoms (Wells 2006), indicating a lack of screening within primary care youth services and reluctance to engage, no doubt due to feared negative appraisals by clinicians. While SAD shows greater comparability of rates between the sexes in youth (males 4.5%, females 5.6%), in contrast with other anxiety disorders, females have higher rates of SAD in adult populations (Wells 2006).

SAD is strongly correlated with comorbid depression and drug and alcohol abuse. These issues often lead to engagement in services, rather than symptoms of SAD itself (Baldwin et al 2014).

Treatment for SAD depends on the severity of symptoms and whether comorbid conditions, such as depression or another anxiety disorder, are present. Research indicates that a combination treatment of CBT with administration of either an SSRI or an SNRI may be a helpful approach to treatment, with CBT showing greater enduring effects than pharmacotherapy (Andrews et al 2018). Other medications, such as benzodiazepines, are not suggested due to the risk of developing dependence. Case study 11.1 describes the experience of social anxiety.

CASE STUDY 11.1: Jenny

Jenny is a 21-year-old woman with a diagnosis of dyslexia and marked anxiety in social situations. Jenny constantly fears the judgement of others and believes that when she speaks to others they can "hear her dyslexia" and will think she is stupid. Jenny regularly avoids social situations and, when she has to attend, has a number of safety behaviours to protect her from making a fool of herself, such as practising her replies to discussions in her head and deflecting attention by asking other people a lot of questions.

Jenny very much believes that her problem lies in her level of intellect and that her low perceived intelligence will mean that people won't want to know her when they discover this about her. Jenny is unsure how she can make any changes and is beginning to experience low moods as a result of her lack of social contact and constant anxiety.

Specific Phobia

It is common to experience transient fears of situations, animals or natural environments. However, a fear that becomes disproportionate to the actual level of risk posed and causes distress and functional impairment can be considered a specific phobia. Specific phobias involve a persistent, irrational (out of proportion), intense fear reaction in the face of triggers that are generally clustered into animal, situational, natural environment or blood-injection-injury subtypes.

The major criterion for diagnosis involves a consistently elevated anxiety response in the face of the phobic trigger for a period of 6 months or more, with considerable avoidance or intense fear being endured during exposure to the phobic trigger, causing impacts on general life functioning and elevated levels of distress.

Fear of phobic objects can be experienced through direct or distant contact, or anticipation of contact with the phobic trigger, and can produce a continuum of anxiety responses, including panic attacks at the more severe end. The degree of anxiety experienced may be reduced by certain elements of safety that may be present during exposure to the phobic trigger, such as having others around or situations that seem to create less perceived danger (e.g. for a person with a dog phobia, seeing a smaller dog versus seeing a bigger dog or seeing a dog on a lead across the street versus seeing a dog off the lead on the same side of the road).

Specific phobia is one of the most prevalent mental health conditions; however, many people often do not seek treatment (Eaton 2018).

Phobias seem to be interrelated, with up to 75% of people with a diagnosis of specific phobia having multiple phobias of certain objects or situations (APA 2022; Baldwin et al 2014).

The 12-month prevalence rates of specific phobia in Aotearoa New Zealand are around 7.3% within the general population (Wells 2006). Although specific phobias were found to produce the least interference with life in the most recent Aotearoa New Zealand mental health survey (Wells 2006), severity and impact need to be considered on an individual basis. In some instances, phobias can produce life-threatening dangers, such as a person with a serious medical illness refusing treatment via needles because of a blood-injury-injection phobia.

Specific phobias typically develop between 7 and 11 years of age, although situational or natural environment subtypes have a later age of onset (APA 2022). Some phobias spontaneously remit during childhood and adolescence; however, they can persist into adulthood. It is important to assess factors around the development of phobias as they can occur secondary to trauma; for example, fear of the dark may develop following childhood sexual abuse or fear of dogs may develop after witnessing or being attacked by a dog. Phobias can also develop secondary to vicarious trauma, such as watching media coverage of plane crashes or natural disasters or witnessing, hearing about or losing a significant person in a car accident.

Avoidance behaviours can have a major influence on day-to-day functioning, dictating choice of home and work locations and routines. It may be a change in circumstances that leads to help-seeking, such as a move that increases the person's direct contact with their phobic trigger.

Treatment of phobic disorders has been relatively under-researched in comparison with other anxiety disorders (Eaton et al 2018). Current treatment indications depend on the level of severity and impairment in functioning. In the case of subclinical or mild symptoms, monitoring and face-to-face or online psychoeducation through CBT tools are recommended to assist in normalising distress and assisting people to begin to identify their triggers for anxiety. Pharmacotherapy is an uncommon and largely unsupported treatment for specific phobia, with exposure therapy through either a prolonged duration single-session or multiple-sessions considered the treatment of course (Eaton et al 2018).

CRITICAL THINKING EXERCISE 11.2

Many people experience mild symptoms of anxiety disorders throughout life due to the number of significant life stressors that come their way. What are the benefits of making a diagnosis of an anxiety disorder versus using a more normalising approach for mild presentations? When can a diagnosis be helpful and when might it not be?

Trauma- and Stressor-Related Disorders

Post-traumatic stress disorder (PTSD), acute stress disorder (ASD) and adjustment disorder (AD) were previously categorised as anxiety disorders. Their current classification as trauma and stress-related disorders reflects an identification of the significance of trauma both in itself, and as a cause of mental health distress and other developmental lifespan challenges.

Exposure to potentially traumatising events is common, with up to 75% of people reporting at least one traumatic event over their lifetime (Phelps et al 2022). A variety of distress responses are normal following trauma, from experiencing insomnia to heightened fear and anxiety; however, some people may go on to develop ASD, PTSD or other anxiety or affective disorders.

Post-Traumatic Stress Disorder (PTSD)

PTSD can develop following direct exposure to one or more traumatic events, either by first-hand experience or by vicarious traumatisation (witnessing a trauma, hearing about a loved one's trauma or extreme/repeated exposure to details of trauma). The types of trauma considered for the purposes of diagnosis include threatened or actual physical or sexual harm, personal violence, war, serious accidents, natural disasters and sudden, catastrophic medical events.

PTSD is characterised by symptoms located within four distinct symptom clusters (APA 2022): intrusive re-experiencing (nightmares, dissociative flashbacks, recurrent memories), hyperarousal (heightened startle response, intense physiological response to trauma recall, hypervigilance), persistent avoidance of trauma stimuli (avoiding external reminders and internal trauma-related experiences such as memories), and mood and cognitive alterations (emotional numbing, anhedonia, fear, low mood, impartial trauma memory recall, poor concentration, generalised thoughts about danger). Behavioural changes occur such as avoidance of associated triggers, increased interpersonal irritability, violence, recklessness or behaviours, such as substance abuse to try to escape distress. Individuals may experience more severity of symptoms such as dysphoric mood states, dissociation or constant hyperarousal (APA 2022).

Symptoms typically develop within 3 months of the trauma; however, it is possible for a delayed expression of symptoms to occur months or years later (APA 2022). A diagnosis of PTSD is not made in the first month after the trauma as approximately 50% of people fully "recover" from traumatic events within 3 months, although some still experience distressing responses to trauma years or even decades later (APA 2022).

Associative learning processes (making connections between different life experiences to produce similar responses) help us to survive in the face of new dangers, allowing us to recall previously processed threat triggers, and respond accordingly in novel situations. During trauma, various types of sensory information are collected (e.g. certain sounds, sensations, smells, sights). These can later become triggers to the trauma memory, for example, the smell of petrol triggering the memory of a car accident. When trauma memories are properly "processed" at the time of the event and in the days, weeks and years following, the memories are recalled giving an accurate sense of time, place and person. In PTSD, however, there is thought to be a fault in processing of the event both during and after the trauma, resulting in the development of "broken trauma memories" that are incomplete, inappropriately stored with a range of sensory trauma triggers and a generalised sense of danger that become easily identified with non-dangerous sensory stimuli. These broken, unprocessed trauma memories are hypothesised to contribute to an inaccurate sense of placement of the memory in time, leading to a perceived sense (physiologically and cognitively) of current danger and associated and behaviour responses when the memory is triggered. As a result, traumas are re-experienced rather than simply remembered. Significant avoidance strategies develop due to the emotional load and sense of danger created through the continual trauma re-experiencing that people can have, leading to significant functional impairment in day-to-day life. The trauma, alongside other predisposing generic, cognitive and temperamental vulnerabilities, is thought to create a heightened fear response within the person (Zoellner et al 2014), leaving them feeling overwhelmed and struggling to function under the weight of their symptoms, while expending considerable effort in an attempt to avoid the memories and reduce the likelihood of the trauma recurring.

The 12-month prevalence rates for PTSD in Aotearoa New Zealand and Australia are similar, with 4.4–5.7% of the general population receiving a diagnosis within a year (Wells 2006; ABS 2023); however, prevalence rates for Māori are significantly higher at 9.7% (Wells 2006). The rate of PTSD in Aboriginal and Torres Strait Islander peoples is also considerably higher than non-Indigenous Australians. A study of PTSD in Aboriginal people living in remote Western Australia showed concerningly high lifetime prevalence rates of 55.2% in the sample of 221 people, while 91% of the sample with PTSD had comorbid alcohol-related disorders (Nadew 2012). The authors cite this as the highest ever recorded PTSD rate found within a sample when compared with other studies around the world. The comorbidity of substance abuse within this sample points to a link between use of substances as a way of self-medicating for symptoms of PTSD. This is supported by the high rates of comorbid substance use disorder among people diagnosed with PTSD, with prevalence rates shown to be around 46% in Western countries (Lortye et al 2021).

Rates of PTSD are shown to be much higher after exposure to specific types of interpersonal trauma; for example, in one study 50% of rape survivors were noted to have PTSD (Cooper et al 2014).

Many people diagnosed with PTSD report multiple trauma events (Phelps et al 2022), leading to the concept of complex PTSD. Complex PTSD symptoms relate to the impact of the enduring and/or compounding nature of multiple traumas, causing commonly experienced ongoing interpersonal difficulties, emotional dysregulation, prolonged dissociative states, somatic distress/symptoms and fixed, distorted belief systems.

It is important to note that prevalence of PTSD has been found to be much higher for health consumers accessing specialist mental health services. A historical, large multi-site US study found that 84% of its sample of 782 reported experience of lifetime interpersonal violence, while 52% of the sample reported lifetime sexual assault. When the sexual assault was reported to occur in childhood, higher rates of further traumas into adulthood were found (Mueser et al 2004). In addition, 34.8% of the sample met the criteria for PTSD, with high comorbidity of mood disorders and current substance abuse. Those identified with PTSD had higher rates of psychiatric re-admission over the past year, poorer physical health and higher rates of hospitalisation for physical health issues in the past 6 months. These findings highlight the widespread and disabling effects of trauma over a lifetime.

An important consideration is the rate at which PTSD is screened for in relation to other diagnoses in clinical settings. One early study identified an alarming rate of under-diagnosis within a multi-site study containing a sample of 275 service users. Of the sample, 98% reported exposure to at least one traumatic event, with 43% (119) meeting criteria for a diagnosis of PTSD. Of these 119 service users, only three had the diagnosis documented in their clinical notes (Mueser et al 1998). A later study containing 70 participants with schizophrenia (Newman et al 2010) noted a significant effect on severity of symptoms and increased chronicity of illness when participants had a comorbid diagnosis of PTSD. It was noted that none of the 70 participants had been diagnosed with PTSD before the study (Newman et al 2010). A more recent study undertaken with a sample of adults engaging in an outpatient mental health service found that 20.5% of people met criteria for PTSD; however, only 2.4% had been formally diagnosed (de Silva et al 2019). These findings highlight a concerning, ongoing inability within mental health services to successfully screen for, detect and treat PTSD.

PTSD has high rates of comorbidity, particularly with anxiety and affective disorders and substance abuse (APA 2022; Phelps et al 2022). Screening for risk of harm to self is essential because trauma is a known risk factor for suicide, particularly when a person has experienced violence or trauma in childhood (APA 2022). Due to the potential for current trauma, assessment should also cover risk of harm from others so that necessary protective measures can be considered.

Current Australasian and international guidelines for treating PTSD advise offering trauma-focused psychological interventions such as eye movement desensitisation reprocessing (EMDR) and trauma-focused CBT (Cooper et al 2014; NICE 2018; Phelps et al 2022). These specialist psychological interventions are offered by experienced health professionals (including nurses) who have undertaken training in trauma-focused talking therapies and engage in ongoing supervision. There is little evidence to show benefit from use of pharmacological treatments, although SSRIs can be used if a consumer does not wish to engage in or is not finding benefit from psychological therapies alone and may be supportive if there is a comorbid moderate-to-severe affective or anxiety disorder (Phelps et al 2022).

CRITICAL THINKING EXERCISE 11.3

How does anxiety operate as part of different mental health diagnoses such as schizophrenia, depression or eating disorders? What challenges does anxiety pose to people experiencing these conditions? Which interventions for anxiety might be helpful within these different presentations?

Acute Stress Disorder (ASD)

ASD is clinically very similar to PTSD; however, ASD can be diagnosed within a month of exposure to a traumatic event, whereas PTSD is not diagnosed until after one month. It is important to note that people who receive a diagnosis of ASD do not necessarily go on to develop PTSD – therefore, one is not predictive of the other. Similarly, those who receive a diagnosis of PTSD may not have had symptoms of ASD within the first month of exposure (Phelps et al 2022).

The evidence and guidelines for treatment of ASD are similar to those of PTSD, with trauma-focused CBT recommended as a first-line treatment (Phelps et al 2022).

Adjustment Disorder (AD)

AD is characterised by an objectively determined, significant, enduring and atypical stress response to one or more life stressors, such as a potential or an actual significant event like a relationship ending, job loss, socioeconomic difficulties, developmental events (retirement) or ongoing illness or disability. Symptoms typically involve emotional or behavioural changes such as low mood, worry, a sense of inability to cope and withdrawal from activities, which often impairs social or occupational functioning (APA 2022). Symptoms often develop within 3 months and remit within 6 months of cessation of the stressor. Diagnosis of AD following bereavement is complicated and only considered if grief symptoms occur at a level of intensity and persistence considered outside of expected grief responses (APA 2022).

AD is fairly common, particularly in people who have experienced recent unemployment or serious medical conditions (O'Donnell et al 2019), although it is relatively under-researched, with few validated diagnostic tools available. Delineation from other disorders, such as major depressive disorder, is difficult, therefore recognition of AD in primary care services can be very difficult.

There are few epidemiological studies of AD, particularly in Australasia. Worldwide prevalence has found to be around 2% in the general population, with rates as high as 12% in samples of patients engaging in consultation liaison settings (O'Donnell et al 2019). An Australian study found AD with features of depressive and anxiety symptoms was the most prevalent mental health condition (13.4%) in a sample of 172 postpartum couples (Wynter et al 2013). This identifies a need to assess for AD in populations entering significant life transition (parenthood, retirement) due to increased vulnerability and potential significant impact on individual and family functioning.

AD is found across all cultures (Patra & Sarkar 2013); however, cultural responses to life stressors differ. Careful consideration and input from cultural advisers is recommended during assessment.

There is little evidence to support the use of pharmacological treatments for AD, with psychological interventions delivered either in person or digitally considered best practice (O'Donnell et al 2019). Psychological treatment focuses largely on enhancing individual coping mechanisms through cognitive behavioural, mindfulness-based and solution-focused therapies.

IMPACTS OF COVID-19 AND CLIMATE CHANGE ON ANXIETY

Recent global crises such as the COVID-19 pandemic and the undeniable realities of climate change and the increase in associated natural disasters, are creating ongoing significant psychosocial, environmental and financial impacts on populations around the world, including an increase in presentations of anxiety disorders and other mental health conditions (COVID-19 Mental Disorders Collaborators 2021; Cianconi et al 2020; Mahoney et al 2021). These challenges have placed additional pressures on already-stretched mental health systems around the world. COVID-19 produced an estimated 25.6% increase in the global prevalence of anxiety disorders in 2020 alone (COVID-19 Mental Disorders Collaborators 2012), with emerging research showing a clear association between climate anxiety and risk of development of depression and anxiety disorders (O'Brien & Elders 2021).

While it is important to ensure we don't pathologise all distress responses to the life-changing, catastrophic experiences attached to these crises, we must also consider how we support people, families and communities most at risk.

Digital technology is one potential way to disseminate accessible psychological tools, education and interventions to wide groups of people experiencing climate anxiety, trauma from associated natural disasters or continued distress following COVID-19. Studies regarding digital tools built during COVID-19 show that uptake of tools by the public has been high (Mahoney et al 2021), with particularly nimble and adaptable delivery of support to a range of people experiencing different levels of distress across a continuum.

TREATMENT AND NURSING INTERVENTIONS

Nurses play a significant role in supporting people who experience anxiety and have a history of trauma. Being present for people with openness, compassion and a sense of hope is essential. Providing unconditional support, respect, and validating people's challenges and attempts to cope are the first and perhaps most helpful interventions we can provide. Conducting a thorough assessment allows us to assist in making sense of the origins of anxiety and its impacts on a person's life. This cannot be achieved unless we seek to develop a partnership with the people and families we work with. Working together in partnership along the care journey allows for the gathering of a much richer depth of information, providing a greater range of potential solutions and significantly better outcomes for people. This requires not only an awareness of the impacts that social, cultural, environmental and historical factors can have on people's experiences and life trajectories, but also the skills and attitudes required to ensure their discovery, apply helpful meaning and incorporate these factors into the care we provide. The interventions we provide should always work to ensure people can become empowered through developing hope for their future and an improved sense of self that will help them achieve greater levels of functioning and quality of life. Chapter 2 discusses a supportive framework to support nurses to provide a holistic and person-centred social ecological approach within their practice.

For an account of how a consumer made use of interventions for anxiety, see Personal perspectives: Consumer's story 11.2.

👤 PERSONAL PERSPECTIVES

Consumer's Story 11.2: Amy

I think one thing that is misunderstood about anxiety is its physical nature. It is often uncomfortable but can become quite painful at times. At my worst, my physical anxiety was at or near a panic attack level for most of the day and night for the final 2 months of my last pregnancy. My thought processes were rational, but I was unable to shut down the adrenaline and cortisol pumping through my body by trying to use calming, rational thoughts. From the moment I woke, I was acutely aware of my body and how it was feeling. It was in overdrive and hyped up to such a level of discomfort that focusing on anything else was difficult. Medication helped me sleep for 4 hours at a time, but the only time I could find peace during the day was if I was deeply engaged in an activity. Even then these moments were fleeting. My psychiatrist described me as being minute to minute and there were many times throughout this that I was not sure I would survive until the next minute.

Several things helped me through. I had to be busy, constantly and without question. I asked for tasks and my family kindly made jobs up if they needed to. Looking back, the tasks needed to be both physical and productive for them to distract my mind and allow some moments of peace. Puzzles were a failure as my panic easily broke through the level of distraction they provided, but actively playing with my son worked for a few minutes at a time. On one of my worst days, my psychologist told me to drive to a park on my way home and walk barefoot in the grass while focusing on nature and the feeling of the grass underneath me. I thought he was the crazy one, but I also knew I had to do it. It worked. I survived that day and all the other days using medication, therapy, mindfulness techniques, active distraction and family support. Three years later and after EMDR (eye movement desensitisation reprocessing) therapy, I use only one medication instead of the six I needed at delivery, I run and practise Pilates, and try every day to look at one thing in nature very closely. I try to analyse it in detail and remind myself that the moment I am in is actually all there is.

Psychoeducation

"Psychoeducation" refers to knowledge that is provided to increase a person's mental health literacy and self-awareness in order to inform future decision-making. Poor mental health literacy and self-stigma have been associated with low levels of help-seeking behaviours in people struggling with their mental wellbeing (Taylor-Rodgers & Batterham 2014). Psychoeducation is therefore a powerful therapeutic tool in alleviating the distress caused by anxiety, helping improve consumer engagement, treatment outcomes and psychosocial functioning.

Psychoeducation involves teaching people about the function and purpose of anxiety as an emotion, so that it can be viewed as a normal, necessary and shared human experience that does not necessarily have to be avoided or feared. Heightened anxiety responses can be explored by talking through real-life scenarios to help raise insight and reflection regarding mechanisms in which anxiety is perpetuated.

Psychoeducation should always be provided free from unnecessary jargon and delivered in a well-paced, collaborative manner, allowing time for processing of information and questions. Self-directed learning through websites, handouts and self-help books provides flexibility and choice for learning, therefore it is invaluable to identify and carry helpful resources for use in clinical settings.

Social Support

Social support has consistently been found to protect individuals against the potential long-term negative effects of trauma and distress (Kazantzis et al 2012). Social support provides multiple benefits, such as companionship, a sense of connection and increased access to resources and opportunities for engaging in activities that provide enjoyment. Identifying and enhancing a person's current level of social support can have a powerful impact on recovery.

Unmet socioeconomic needs (e.g. housing, poverty, social isolation) can be huge barriers to wellbeing and engagement in treatment, therefore it is essential that these factors are considered alongside other interventions, with referrals made to other agencies as required.

Trauma-Informed Care and Psychological Formulations

A trauma-informed approach to care places a strong emphasis on attempting to understand what has happened in people's lives, rather than what is wrong with them. Diagnosis may be a part of the care process; however, the diagnostic process centres around trauma screening and understanding any presenting issues through a trauma lens, rather than a solely pathological one. Trauma-informed care is person-centred, delivered in a respectful, sensitive and collaborative manner throughout all aspects of service provision. In the case of presenting anxiety, consideration must be given to any trauma-based experiences that may predispose and perpetuate current heightened states of anxiety, such as bullying, any type of abuse, significant loss, disaster or exposure to parental mental health difficulties. See the assessment section of this chapter for more information on trauma screening.

Psychological formulations are essential in the delivery of trauma-informed care and when done well, become therapeutic interventions in themselves, providing an opportunity for people to understand the reasons they may be struggling as they are. In this sense, psychological formulations are very much about making meaning, providing insight to both clinicians and consumers and assisting in the careful process of intervention selection.

Collaborative formulations provide the potential to deepen the therapeutic alliance, align the wider clinical team and assist in empowering consumers through gaining a deeper understanding of themselves.

Psychological formulations have previously been considered a tool of psychologists, yet their application is becoming more and more essential as we continue to shift away from a sole biomedical focus in mental health, towards more holistic models of care.

Psychological Interventions

Psychological interventions help to modify feelings, cognitions, attitudes and behaviours using a variety of resources such as cognitive or thought challenging, behavioural experiments, psychoeducation, psychotherapy, skills training, taught relaxation or written activities.

Psychological interventions are considered efficacious, evidence-based and often preferable treatment options for anxiety and trauma-related disorders (Baldwin et al 2014; Peters 2007; Phelps et al 2022). They can be provided as a one-off session, over a brief to long-term package of therapy (6–20+ sessions), within group treatment settings or through the use of digital or written self-help packages. Psychological therapies, or talking therapies as they are often called, are delivered by suitably trained health professionals, including registered nurses, who adhere to evidence-based treatment protocols while engaging in specialist supervision. However, psychological interventions (which are more micro interventions than formal therapy itself) can be learnt through a range of shorter-term educational mediums, and woven into care by a range of practitioners to enhance outcomes.

Current evidence-based psychological approaches for anxiety disorders include CBT, acceptance and commitment therapy (ACT), applied relaxation and mindfulness-based stress reduction. There is consistent evidence that psychological therapies such as CBT have a general benefit for people experiencing mental health conditions such as anxiety disorders (Fordham et al 2021), with lower relapse rates than medication alone (Baldwin et al 2014).

Perspectives in practice: Nurse's story 11.2 provides an outline of a nurse using psychological interventions in nursing practice.

Cognitive Behaviour Therapy (CBT)

CBT is an effective, evidence-based talking therapy used to treat a multitude of mental health conditions, including the full range of anxiety disorders (Penninx et al 2021; Fordham et al 2021). Originally developed in the 1960s by US psychiatrist Dr Aaron Beck, as a short-term treatment for depression, CBT has been extensively modified and enhanced for a range of mental and physical health disorders, including anxiety and trauma-related disorders. Table 11.2 provides a summary of cognitive behavioural interventions, which are further discussed below.

PERSPECTIVES IN PRACTICE

Nurse's Story 11.2: Katie Waite

Jerry fills his chair, his eyes wide open, eager and willing. He has been doing this with others like me, on and off, for 10 years. I quickly notice Jerry is eager to please and open to suggestions. I must tread carefully. Jerry has anxiety. We all have anxiety; with Jerry this very natural experience has been amplified, turning life into a world of fear.

Together we talk about what isn't working in his life. His anxiety is crippling. Finding joy is close to impossible when you're trapped behind your rented curtains, frightened to come out. Joy is in a bag of chips, a bottle of fizzy.

The irrational fears are everywhere. They feel as if they are closing in. A social invitation has become a threat to Jerry: "My friend invited me round . . . I was so angry. How dare he? He knows I can't go!" Any situation where he may come under scrutiny, Jerry fears. He fears he will come up short, like he always has, especially as a little boy trying to impress his unimpressed dad.

His thoughts are twisted: "I can't go . . . I won't cope . . ." – from these thoughts, a cascade is launched. Anxious emotions ping through the air. His heart races, pupils dilate, muscles tense, palms sweat. These physical sensations become so severe he could fear for his heart. All of these sensations feed an old belief: "I must stay here behind my curtain where it's safe . . . I'm not feeling good enough to leave."

In this safe room we put words to his struggles: The thoughts, feelings and fears. Jerry's fears are spoken and heard and explored objectively. The power of the fear begins to fall away. We explore anxiety, its natural rhythm and purpose. As we explore this, he begins trusting himself to manage any negative outcome. He then exposes himself to his fears one by one. Bringing these experiences to our room to discuss, critique and learn from. Now Jerry can challenge his thoughts. He uses mindfulness and relaxation to calm the physical sensations. Emotions are noticed and acknowledged.

Today, Jerry sits with a grin and an air of confidence. He was at work earlier, it wasn't easy, but it was OK. He's been visiting a friend; he'll be off soon to a family gathering and he's thinking of starting up rugby again. Today, Jerry is thoughtful about his life and the scary parts it holds, but he is not afraid.

Katie Waite works as a nurse practitioner intern for a community mental health team. She has previously completed a postgraduate paper in psychological therapies. Jerry is a pseudonym.

TABLE 11.2 Components of Cognitive Behavioural Interventions

Exposure	Encourages patients to face fears
	Patients learn corrective information through experience
	Extinction of fear occurs through repeated exposure
	Successful coping enhances self-efficacy
Safety Response Inhibition	Patients restrict their usual anxiety-reducing behaviours (e.g. escape, need for reassurance)
	Decreases negative reinforcement
	Coping with anxiety without using anxiety-reducing behaviour enhances self-efficacy
Cognitive Strategies	Cognitive restructuring, behavioural experiments and related strategies target patients' exaggerated perception of danger (e.g. fear of negative evaluation in SAD)
	Provides corrective information regarding the level of threat
	Can also target self-efficacy beliefs
Arousal Management	Relaxation and breathing control skills can help patients control increased anxiety levels
Surrender of Safety Signals	Patients relinquish safety signals (e.g. presence of a companion, knowledge of the location of the nearest toilet)
	Patients learn adaptive self-efficacy beliefs

CBT focuses on the collaborative establishment of a working formulation that attempts to make sense of the consumer's historical experiences, developed belief systems and current-day cognitions, physiological symptoms, emotional experiences and behavioural reactions within the context of their current environment. By identifying how these factors interact with each other to perpetuate distress and difficulty, the therapist and client can identify behavioural change experiments and work to restructure cognitions to allow for greater flexibility and function in life. Changes to long-held negative belief systems and often unhelpful, habitual ways of behaving towards distress and distressing experiences may explain the research findings on CBT's enhanced effectiveness for relapse prevention in comparison with pharmacological treatment for anxiety and depressive disorders (Fordham et al 2021).

CBT can be delivered as a digital intervention, within a brief package of face-to-face or virtual sessions (3–6 sessions), over a longer period of therapy for more intensive benefits (6–20+ sessions) or pared down as part of brief, one-off psychological intervention in crisis work.

CBT has been adapted into what are considered "third-wave" approaches such as dialectical behavioural therapy (DBT), acceptance and commitment therapy (ACT; see below), Schema therapy and behavioural activation.

Acceptance and Commitment Therapy

Developed by Steven Hayes, Kirk Stroshal and Kelly Wilson in the late 1980s, ACT takes quite a different approach to working with distress by changing the way we relate to internal representations of it (negative thoughts, distressing emotions, physiological manifestations) as opposed to directly challenging or trying to change the level of distress itself (Hayes et al 2012). ACT proposes that internal experiences, such as negative thoughts, distressing emotions and their accompanying physical symptoms, are normal aspects of the human experience and that rather than trying to avoid or battle to attempt to get rid of them, we can choose to accept and work with them using mindfulness and commitment to values-based actions to create greater flexibility in life and a present-moment focus. Treatment involves developing skills to improve psychological flexibility, allowing us to have a more flexible view of ourselves, being able to tolerate distress and difficult thoughts without being governed by them, and being able to be in contact with the present moment.

ACT is well evidenced, with more than 60 randomised controlled trials providing a good empirical base in working with anxiety and other mental health conditions (Hayes et al 2012).

Transdiagnostic Treatment Approaches

Despite the differences between the anxiety disorders, several shared vulnerabilities have been found, leading to the belief that single treatments targeting these commonalities could be efficacious and more cost-effective than targeting interventions at single disorders. Transdiagnostic treatments have been shown to be effective in the treatment of anxiety disorders (Carlucci et al 2021) and are often adapted to be more easily implemented across healthcare settings by different clinicians, while retaining many of the known scientifically-evidenced interventions that support their use.

Sensitivity to the experience of anxiety itself is one of the transdiagnostic vulnerabilities found within all anxiety disorders. Anxiety sensitivity is a fear of the arousal, cognitive and emotional symptoms of anxiety and is particularly problematic in PD and PTSD. ACT is a good example of a transdiagnostic treatment that aims to reduce fear of anxiety itself through promoting acceptance of anxiety as a necessary and important human experience. In this way, if such vulnerability to anxiety is noted, ACT can be utilised no matter which anxiety disorder may be diagnosed.

Digital Mental Health Resources

We are increasingly identifying the benefits of harnessing technology to deliver psychological interventions to allow us to disseminate psychological treatments in a flexible, often more accessible way across large populations with greater ease, less expense and with higher fidelity to evidence-based approaches. Digital psychological tools can often be accessed at little to no cost, without the need for a referral, and can be utilised at a time and place that works for people and their schedules. Digital psychological tools can support people with lower levels of distress, through to people with enduring and more severe challenges. They can be either accessed independently by consumers, or blended into care either alongside general interventions, or as an added resource within formal therapy. The last option helps therapists better structure sessions, administers vital psychoeducation, which allows the therapist to focus on more complex aspects of treatment, and provides an invaluable and ever-available post-therapy booster.

Most digital psychological tools are based on CBT and are commonly referred to as eCBT (electronic-based CBT) or iCBT (internet-based CBT). eCBT provides users with the opportunity to access CBT through regular structured online lessons, engage with between-lesson "homework" activities just as people would in face-to-face CBT; assess and monitor their own wellbeing; learn integral psychoeducation about different conditions; and select the time, place and pace of utilisation. Digital psychological tools can support people to seek further support and input in times of high distress through built-in prompts.

Tools such as "Just a Thought" in Aotearoa New Zealand or "THIS WAY UP" in Australia provide specialised courses to support people experiencing an array of mental health disorders and general wellbeing challenges, and can be undertaken independently or prescribed by a range of healthcare workers, including nurses. Research shows that concurrent guidance and support provided by a health worker allows for greater adherence and outcomes than non-guided forms of e-CBT (Guiney et al 2023; Andrews et al 2018).

Some websites offer free downloads of self-help treatment manuals, while others, such as SPARX (an abbreviation of Smart, Positive, Active, Realistic, X-factor thoughts; Merry et al 2012) and Quest – Te Whitianga (Christie et al 2019) incorporate learning and self-help utilising CBT through an interactive gaming program targeted at supporting young people with anxiety and depression. See Useful websites at the end of the chapter.

There is a growing number of studies that compare face-to-face with online CBT showing similar levels of effectiveness (Cuijpers et al 2014) and generally better than waiting list comparisons (Baldwin et al 2014). Therapies delivered via the internet can be considered a helpful first step for people with mild to moderate anxiety in line with stepped-care models of treatment (Earl et al 2014), while also proving effective for people with greater levels of distress (Guiney et al 2023). Digital psychological interventions provide a multitude of benefits for both consumers and services alike, particularly through opening up greater access and choice to effective treatments through the novel use of eCBT as a "prequel" treatment for people waiting for face-to-face therapy. The many benefits technology provides will see a huge growth in the future in terms of the choice of digital psychological interventions, and manner in which mental health and addiction services integrate them into service delivery.

Cultural Support

Our culture is inherently as much a part of who we are as are our mind and body, and connection to our culture is essential for wellbeing. Culture can be difficult to define, but it is commonly thought to comprise a set of collective values, practices, customs and traditions

(Gee et al 2014), and is not necessarily bound solely by ethnic identity. Connection to culture provides a multitude of protective factors and greater levels of personal, family and community resilience. Connection to our culture provides people with a greater sense of belonging, security and meaning, as well as helping people, families and communities find their place within their histories, establish a context for present-day strengths and challenges, as well as assistance to grow a future vision of themselves.

Our health systems typically originate from western models of health, bringing about potential obstacles, challenges and in built inequities for people from different cultures. The Indigenous peoples from Aotearoa New Zealand and Australia – Māori, Aboriginal and Torres Strait Islanders – have their own unique belief systems, values and health and life practices, which are essential for the achievement and maintenance of wellbeing. If we are to achieve equitable outcomes for Indigenous peoples, they must become essential partners in our healthcare systems, and we must work to identify the current barriers to equity, and widen our understanding of the determinants to health and wellbeing, including identifying connection to culture as an essential, and learning from and utilising the many indigenous models of health available to drive care, such as Sir Mason Durie's (1982) model, Te Whare Tapa Wha. Te Whare Tapa Wha diagrammatically depicts the deep connections and essential roles that taha whānau (extended family health and wider social systems), taha hinengaro (mental wellbeing and the inseparable nature of the mind and body), taha tinana (physical health) and taha wairua (spiritual health) have for Māori, as well as the importance of their connection with whenua (land), their whakapapa (genealogy) and tikanga Māori, or the Māori way. Cultural issues in mental health care are also discussed in Chapters 6 and 7.

PSYCHOPHARMACOLOGY

Generally, medication is not a first-line approach for anxiety and trauma-related disorders, given the risk of side effects and inability to target important perpetuating factors that often drive distress and which psychological interventions work with. It has also been difficult to prove the efficacy of medication in treating mild anxiety disorders because assessment and monitoring of symptoms alone have often provided high placebo responses, indicating that any sense of an intervention can lead to an improvement for people struggling with anxiety (Baldwin et al 2014).

The drivers for using pharmacological treatments for anxiety disorders are the intensity and duration of symptoms, impact on daily functioning and lack of response to non-pharmacological interventions. Psychopharmacology should always be utilised through a collaborative process assessment, and sharing of information about the medication, including its side effects and adverse risks to ensure the person can give informed consent to treatment.

Short-term use of medication can be supportive for people with more moderate to severe symptoms, assisting them to engage in psychological therapies (Baldwin et al 2014), and combined use in more severe cases of GAD, for example, has been shown to be more efficacious than either treatment alone (Andrews et al 2018).

Psychotropic medications used for anxiety (apart from benzodiazepines) often do not produce an immediate response. There can be a short-term worsening of symptoms, which the consumer should be prepared for. Choice of medication is steered by levels of evidence, safety in terms of side effects and any contraindications for the individual, as well as any prior positive responses with past use.

SSRIs are used to treat depression and affective disorders and are commonly prescribed when necessary for the treatment of anxiety disorders due to a comparable evidence base, broad-spectrum efficacy and high levels of tolerability in terms of side effects (Baldwin et al 2014). SNRIs are less well tolerated, with a higher side effect profile, though have proven efficacy in anxiety disorders, particularly GAD, and the acute treatment and relapse prevention phase of PD (Baldwin et al 2014). Benzodiazepines, such as lorazepam and diazepam, have some proven efficacy for short-term treatment of PD, SAD and GAD (Baldwin et al 2014), though often cause sedation and cognitive impairment and there is risk of dependence in prolonged use. They can also become an unhelpful coping mechanism for people attempting to avoid feeling anxiety, therefore becoming a perpetuating factor in the vicious cycle of anxiety many people find themselves in.

Chapter 21 contains further discussion of psychopharmacology.

CHAPTER SUMMARY

Anxiety as an emotion in itself is normal and plays a vital protective role in our day-to-day lives, helping to motivate us to achieve what we need to, and maintain our safety. However, high levels of anxiety can trigger a range of catastrophic, intrusive anxious thoughts, causing people to filter for negativity and potential danger in their environments. This can lead to the misinterpretation of a range of day-to-day events and experiences as dangerous, with accompanying adverse and unhelpful behavioural responses that can impair functioning and quality of life. Chronically high levels of anxiety can also cause significant detrimental impacts to health.

Anxiety and trauma-related disorders can develop following a range of significant life events and early experiences and are often perpetuated by the stress of day-to-day life and activation of negative belief systems, impairing functioning and connectedness with values, loved ones and essential activities and sense of meaning in life. Psychological interventions play an essential role in the treatment of anxiety disorders, and may be complemented with thoughtful pharmacological treatment.

Nurses will be well equipped to effectively work alongside people with anxiety disorders if they can enhance their assessment and formulation skills, as well as learning and incorporating into care psychological interventions that are effective across different diagnoses and problems. However, the greatest tool we have to work with is the collaborative therapeutic relationship, recognising consumers' own expertise and helping them harness this source of knowledge and experience within their own lives.

REVIEW QUESTIONS

Separate the class into two groups in order to undertake a debate on the benefits of anxiety and worrying, versus the pitfalls. Allow time for both groups to independently discuss and devise arguments on their allocated topic and then set up a debate. Ensure the major points of each argument are summarised and later discussed by the class, identifying the learning points and how they could support practice.

USEFUL WEBSITES

CALM (Computer Assisted Learning for the Mind) – online self-care package: www.calm.auckland.ac.nz/

e-Couch – free, self-help modules for depression and anxiety: ecouch.com.au

GET Self-Help – cognitive behaviour therapy self-help resources: www.getselfhelp.co.uk/

Just a Thought – free CBT tool that can be used independently or prescribed by a health worker: justathought.co.nz

MindSpot – a free service for Australian adults experiencing anxiety, stress, depression and low mood: mindspot.org.au/

National Institute for Health and Care Excellence (NICE) – guidelines for a range of mental health conditions: www.nice.org.uk/guidance

Royal Australian and New Zealand College of Psychiatrists (RANZCP): www.ranzcp.org/home

SPARX – self-help e-therapy tool for young people: www.sparx.org.nz/

This Way Up – low-cost online CBT courses: thiswayup.org.au

REFERENCES

American Psychiatric Association (APA), 2022. Diagnostic and statistical manual of mental disorders, 5th ed., text rev. APA, New York.

Andrews, G., Bell, C., Boyce, P., et al., 2018. Royal Australian and New Zealand College of Psychiatrists clinical practice guidelines for the treatment of panic disorder, social anxiety disorder and generalised anxiety disorder. Aust N Z J Psychiatry, 52 (12), 1109–1172.

Australian Bureau of Statistics (ABS) 2023. National Study of Mental Health and Wellbeing, 2020–22. ABS, Canberra. Online. Available at: www.abs.gov.au/statistics/health/mental-health/national-study-mental-health-and-wellbeing/latest-release

Australian Bureau of Statistics (ABS) 2019. National Aboriginal and Torres Strait Islander Health Survey, 2018–19. ABS, Canberra. Online. Available at: www.abs.gov.au/statistics/people/aboriginal-and-torres-strait-islander-peoples/national-aboriginal-and-torres-strait-islander-health-survey/latest-release

Baldwin, D.S., Anderson, I.M., Nutt, D.J., et al., 2014. Evidence-based pharmacological treatment of anxiety disorders, post-traumatic stress disorder and obsessive-compulsive disorder: A revision of the 2005 guidelines from the British Association for Psychopharmacology. J Psychopharmacol, 28(5), 403–439.

Brickhouse, T.C., Smith, N.D., 2009. Socratic teaching and Socratic method. In: Siegel, H. (ed), The Oxford Handbook of Philosophy of Education. Oxford University Press, New York.

Carlucci, L., Saggino, A., & Balsamo, M. 2021. On the efficacy of the unified protocol for transdiagnostic treatment of emotional disorders: A systematic review and meta-analysis. Clin Psychol Rev, 87, 101999.

Christie, G.I., Shepherd, M., Merry, S.N., et al., 2019. Gamifying CBT to deliver emotional health treatment to young people on smartphones. Internet Interv, 18, 100286.

Cianconi P, Betrò S, Janiri L, 2020. The impact of climate change on mental health: A systematic descriptive review. Front Psychiatry, Mar 6; 11, 74.

Clark, D.M., 1986. A cognitive approach to panic. Behav Res Ther, 24, 461–470.

Connor, K.M., Davidson, J.R., Churchill, L.E., Sherwood, A., Foa E., et al., 2000. Psychometric properties of the Social Phobia Inventory (SPIN). New self-rating scale. Br J Psychiatry, 176(4):379–386.

Cooper, J., Metcalf, O., Phelps, A., 2014. PTSD: An update for general practitioners [online]. Aust Fam Physician, 43(11), 754–757.

COVID-19 Mental Disorders Collaborators, 2021. Global prevalence and burden of depressive and anxiety disorders in 204 countries and territories in 2020 due to the COVID-19 pandemic. Lancet, 398(10312), 1700–1712.

Cuijpers, P., Sijbrandij, M., Koole, S., et al., 2014. Psychological treatment of generalised anxiety disorder: A meta-analysis. Clin Psychol Rev, 34, 130–140.

da Silva HC, Furtado da Rosa MM, Berger W, Luz MP, Mendlowicz M, et al., 2019. PTSD in mental health outpatient settings: Highly prevalent and under-recognized. Braz J Psychiatry, 41(3):213–217.

De La Vega, D., Giner, L. & Courtet, P., 2018. Suicidality in subjects with anxiety or obsessive-compulsive and related disorders: Recent advances. Curr Psychiatry Rep, 20, 26.

Durie, M., 1982. Whaiora: Māori Health Development. Oxford University Press, Auckland.

Earl, T., Hodgson, E., Bunting, A., et al., 2014. Talking therapies in times of change. J NZCCP 24, 5 24.

Eaton W.W., Bienvenu O.J., Miloyan B., 2018. Specific phobias. Lancet Psychiatry, 5(8), 678–686.

Fordham B, Sugavanam T, Edwards K, et al., 2021. The evidence for cognitive behavioural therapy in any condition, population or context: A meta-review of systematic reviews and panoramic meta-analysis. Psychol Med, 51(1), 21–29.

Gee, G., Dudgeon, P., Schultz, C., et al., 2014. Aboriginal and Torres Strait Islander social and emotional wellbeing. In: Dudgeon, P. et al., (eds), Working Together: Aboriginal and Torres Strait Islander Mental Health and Wellbeing Principles and Practice. Commonwealth of Australia, Canberra.

Goodman, W.K., Price, L.H., Rasmussen, S.A., et al., 1989. The Yale–Brown Obsessive–Compulsive scale. I. Development, use, and reliability. Arch Gen. Psychiatry, 46, 1006–1011.

Guiney, H., Mahoney, A., Elders, A., David, C., & Poulton, R,. 2023. Internet-based cognitive behavioural therapy in the real world: Naturalistic use and effectiveness of an evidence-based platform in New Zealand. Aust N Z J Psychiatry, online, doi.org/10.1177/0004867423118

Hall, J. 2017. Schizophrenia—an anxiety disorder?. Br J Psychiatry, 211(5), 262–263.

Hammen, C., 1991. Generation of stress in the course of unipolar depression. J Abnorm Psychol, 100, 555–561.

Hayes, S.C., Pistorello, J., Levin, M.E., 2012. Acceptance and commitment therapy as a unified model of behaviour change. Couns Psychol, 40(7), 976–1002.

James, K.A., Stromin, J.I., Steenkamp, N. et al., 2023. Understanding the relationship between physiological and psychosocial stress, cortisol and cognition. Front Endocrinol, 14, 1085950.

Katzman, M.A., Bleau, P., Blier, P., et al., 2014. Canadian clinical practice guidelines for the management of anxiety, posttraumatic stress and obsessive-compulsive disorders. BMC Psychiatry 14 (Suppl. 1), S1–S83.

Kazantzis, N., Kennedy-Moffat, J., Flett, R., et al., 2012. Predictors of chronic trauma-related symptoms in a community sample of New Zealand motor vehicle accident survivors. Cult Med Psychiatry, 36(3), 442–464.

King, A.R., 2021. Childhood adversity links to self-reported mood, anxiety, and stress-related disorders. J Affect Disorders, 292, 623–632.

Klein, D.F., 2002. Historical aspects of anxiety. Dialogues Clin Neurosci, 4(3), 295.

Lortye, S.A., Will, J.P., Marquenie, L.A. et al., 2021. Treating posttraumatic stress disorder in substance use disorder patients with co-occurring post-traumatic stress disorder: Study protocol for a randomized controlled trial to compare the effectiveness of different types and timings of treatment. BMC Psychiatry, 21, 442.

Mahoney AEJ, Elders A, Li I, David C, Haskelberg H, et al, 2021. A tale of two countries: Increased uptake of digital mental health services during the COVID-19 pandemic in Australia and New Zealand. Internet Interv, 27(7), 25, 100439.

McEvoy, P.M., Grove, R., Slade, T., 2011. Epidemiology of anxiety disorders in the Australian general population: Findings of the 2007 Australian National Survey of Mental Health and Wellbeing. Aust N Z J Psychiatry 45(11), 957–967.

Merry, S.N., Stasiak, K., Shepherd, M., et al., 2012. The effectiveness of SPARX, a computerised self-help intervention for adolescents seeking help for depression: Randomised controlled non-inferiority trial. BMJ, 344, e2598.

Milman, E., Lee, S.A., Neimeyer, R.A., Mathis, A.A., & Jobe, M.C. 2020. Modeling pandemic depression and anxiety: The mediational role of core beliefs and meaning making. J Affect Disorders Rep, 2, 100023.

Ministry of Health. 2022. Annual Data Explorer 2021/22: New Zealand Health Survey [Data File]. Online. Available at: minhealthnz.shinyapps.io/nz-health-survey-2021-22-annual-data-explorer/

Mueser, K.T., Goodman, L.B., Trumbetta, S.L., et al., 1998. Trauma and post-traumatic stress disorder in severe mental illness. J Consult Clin Psychol, 66, 493–499.

Mueser, K.T., Salyers, M.P., Rosenberg, S.D., et al., 2004. Interpersonal trauma and posttraumatic stress disorder in patients with severe mental illness: Demographic, clinical, and health correlates. Schizophr Bull 30(1), 45–57.

Nadew, G., 2012. Exposure to traumatic events, prevalence of posttraumatic stress disorder and alcohol abuse in Aboriginal communities. Rural Remote Health, 12(4), 1667.

Newman, J.M., Turnbull, A., Berman, B.A., et al., 2010. Impact of traumatic and violent victimization experiences in individuals with schizophrenia and schizoaffective disorder. J Nerv Ment Dis, 198, 798–814.

National Institute for Health and Care Excellence (NICE), 2018. Guideline for Post-traumatic stress disorder. In: NICE Quality Standard NG116. NICE, London.

National Institute for Health and Care Excellence (NICE), 2014. Anxiety disorders. In: NICE Quality Standard QS53. NICE, UK.

Nezgovorova,V., Reid, J., Fineberg, N.A., Hollander, E,. 2022. Optimizing first line treatments for adults with OCD. Comprehens Psychiatry, 115, 152305.

O'Brien, A.J. & Elders, A. 2022. Climate anxiety. When it's good to be worried. J Psychiatr Ment Health Nurs, 29, 387–389.

O'Donnell M.L., Agathos J.A., Metcalf O., Gibson K., Lau W., 2019. Adjustment disorder: Current developments and future directions. Int J Environ Res Public Health, 16(14), 2537.

Palagini, L., Baglioni, C., Ciapparelli, A., et al., 2013. REM sleep dysregulation in depression: State of the art. Sleep Med Rev, 17(5), 377–390.

Patra, B.N., Sarkar, S., 2013. Adjustment disorder: Current diagnostic status. Indian J Psychol Med, 35, 4–9.

Penninx, Brenda WJH et al., 2021. Anxiety disorders. The Lancet (Br ed.) 397(10277), 914–927.

Peters, J., 2007. We Need to Talk: Talking Therapies – a Snapshot of Issues and Activities Across Mental Health and Addiction Services in New Zealand. Te Pou O Te Whakaaro Nui, Auckland.

Phelps, A.J., Lethbridge, R., Brennan, S., Bryant, R.A., Burns, P. et al., 2022. Australian guidelines for the prevention and treatment of posttraumatic stress disorder: Updates in the third edition. A NZ J Psychiatry, 56(3), 230–247.

Salkovskis, P.M. (ed.), 1996. Frontiers of Cognitive Therapy. Guilford Press, New York.

Simon, D.P., 2015. The science of stress and addiction: A mini-review of the research, Part 1. Online. Available at: drsimonsaysscience.org/2015/03/22/the-science-of-stress-and-addiction-a-mini-review-of-the-research-part-1.

Shin, K. E., LaFreniere, L. S., & Newman, M. G., 2019. Generalized anxiety disorder. In Olatunji, B. (ed.), The Cambridge Handbook of Anxiety and Related Disorders. Cambridge University Press, Cambridge.

Spitzer, R.L., Kroenke, K., Williams, J.B., et al., 2006. A brief measure for assessing generalized anxiety disorder: The GAD-7. Arch Intern Med, 166(10), 1092–1097.

Taylor-Rodgers, E., & Batterham, P.J. 2014. Evaluation of an online psychoeducation intervention to promote mental health help seeking attitudes and intentions among young adults: Randomised controlled trial. J Affect Disord, 168, 65–71.

Weiss, D.S., Marmar, C.R., 1996. The impact of event scale: Revised. In: Wilson, J., Keane, T.M. (eds), Assessing Psychological Trauma and PTSD. Guilford Press, New York.

Wells, J.E., 2006. Twelve-month prevalence. In: Oakley Browne, M.A., Wells, J.E., Scott, K.M. (Eds), Te Rau Hinengaro: The New Zealand Mental Health Survey. Ministry of Health, Wellington.

Wynter, K., Rowe, H., Fisher, J., 2013. Common mental disorders in women and men in the first six months after the birth of their first infant: A community study in Victoria, Australia. J Affect Disord, 151(3), 980–985.

Zoellner, L.A., Pruitt, L.D., Farach, F.J., et al., 2014. Understanding heterogeneity in PTSD: Fear, dysphoria, and distress. Depress Anxiety, 31, 97–106.

12

Mood Disorders

Greg Clark and Sophie Temmhoff

KEY POINTS

- There are key nursing principles and interventions for working with people experiencing a mood disorder.
- As with all mental health disorders, establishing a therapeutic, interpersonal relationship is critical to treatment success.
- Mood disorders respond to a variety of psychological, sociocultural and biological interventions.

- Antidepressants and mood stabilisers are the major classes of medication used to treat mood disorders.
- People with depression and bipolar disorder are more likely to think about suicide, but this is not the case for everyone experiencing depression and bipolar disorder, and nurses need to assess this on an individual basis.

KEY TERMS

Bipolar disorder
Depression
Family history

Physical health and comorbidity
Psychology and medicine
Signs and symptoms

Spirituality and culture

LEARNING OUTCOMES

The material in this chapter will assist you to:
- describe behaviours associated with mood disorders
- describe cognitive (thinking) changes associated with mood disorders
- understand communication changes associated with mood disorders
- describe mood changes associated with major depressive disorder and bipolar disorder
- describe changes in physical functioning associated with mood disorders
- explain the reasons for nursing interventions and the expected client responses

- outline cognitive, social and biological theories that contribute to the understanding of the aetiology (origin) of mood disorders
- understand the use of antidepressants and mood stabilisers and examine the nature of medication collaboration
- outline psychotherapies, cognitive behaviour therapy (CBT) and other therapeutic options
- describe the therapeutic use of self and recognise some of the personal challenges arising for nurses working with people experiencing mood disorders.

INTRODUCTION

This chapter examines the nature of mood disorders. It also explores mental health assessment, interventions, knowledge and attitudes that nurses need to work effectively with people with mood disorders. A holistic view is essential because mood disorders affect all aspects of daily living.

Depression and elevated mood commonly occur in many mental disorders. This chapter considers disorders where the change in mood predominates. When a person has a mood disorder, the changes they experience are more intense and persistent than those that most people experience in their day-to-day lives, and may affect functioning both at work and at home. The person experiences a

range of disturbances in behaviour, cognition, communication and physical functioning.

This chapter addresses major depressive disorder (major depression), bipolar disorder, postpartum depression and depression associated with ageing. It also makes a distinction between major depressive disorder (major depression) and feeling sad.

The key to working effectively with someone with a mood disorder is a collaborative relationship characterised by openness and respect. This is emphasised throughout the chapter. The collaborative relationship is an essential part of counselling and pharmacotherapeutic interventions. At all times, the nurse must be a partner in the client's recovery.

✳ HISTORICAL ANECDOTE 12.1
Searching for Effective Treatments

Over much of human history and across cultures, people have recorded experiences of depression and the attempts of those trying to ameliorate the impacts of it, with varying degrees of success. A promising emergent and evidenced-based treatment is the use of psychedelic drugs such as psilocybin, in combination with supportive psychotherapy. However, the use of such treatments is not entirely new (Pearson et al 2022). Ancient indigenous cultures painted rock art depictions of mushrooms, and temples were built to honour mushroom deities. In more modern western culture, there was significant interest in the therapeutic potential of all psychedelics in the United States starting from the 1950s. Albert Hofmann (1906–2008) identified psilocybin in mushrooms in 1958, which helped trigger a wave of research into possible therapeutic benefits. However, many of these experiments were poorly controlled and by the end of the 1960s most psychedelics were made illegal.

Read More About It
Very recent research is reported here from John Hopkins Medicine Centre 2022. Psilocybin treatment for major depression effective for up to a year for most patients, study shows. John Hopkins Medicine. News and Publications Newsroom. Online. Available at: www.hopkinsmedicine.org/news/newsroom/news-releases/psilocybin-treatment-for-major-depression-effective-for-up-to-a-year-for-most-patients-study-shows

TYPES OF MOOD DISORDERS

The *Diagnostic and Statistical Manual of Mental Disorders*, *5th Edition Text Revision* (DSM-5-TR) (American Psychiatric Association (APA) 2022) lists several diagnoses relating to mood disorders. These include diagnoses related to depression and bipolar disorder, the two major categories of mood disorder.

Diagnoses relating to depression include disruptive mood dysregulation disorder, major depressive disorder (including major depressive episode), persistent depressive disorder (dysthymia), premenstrual dysphoric disorder, substance/medication-induced depressive disorder, depressive disorder due to another medical condition, other specified depressive disorder and unspecified depressive disorder (APA 2022).

Postpartum or perinatal depression are types of depression that affect women who are pregnant or who have recently given birth. Some women develop depression during their pregnancy, while other women become depressed soon after the birth of their child. This is different from the "baby blues", a relatively common phenomenon after the birth of a child (Royal Women's Hospital n.d.). Postpartum depression is more severe and enduring than the baby blues. Depression in the postpartum period can have significant consequences for the woman and her baby, and it is important to ensure help is delivered as soon as possible after the problems become evident. Depression can affect the mother's bonding with her baby and her availability as the primary carer. Attachment and early bonding are important for the welfare of the baby, both in the immediate postpartum period and throughout childhood. It is also important for the woman to feel she is doing her best in caring for her baby and providing everything her baby needs to thrive.

Bipolar disorder can also affect both the mother and the baby. Many women already have a diagnosis of bipolar disorder when they become pregnant and are taking pharmacological treatments for this. As with many medications, mood stabilisers can cause problems for the fetus, and managing a pregnant woman with bipolar disorder requires a high level of specialist knowledge. Some medications are specifically contraindicated in pregnant women, such as those in the anticonvulsant class, but lithium carbonate seems to be a safer choice (Uguz 2020). The safest choice is no medication at all, but this is rarely possible for women who

have a history of bipolar disorder. Accessing a psychiatrist with specialist knowledge in perinatal and postpartum mental illness is essential. Mental health nurses also work in this specialist field and can provide ongoing support and therapeutic interventions to overcome the problems.

Depression seems to occur more frequently in older people. This may follow on from a previous history of depression, but in many cases the consequences of ageing bring on an episode of depression (Mallett et al 2022). Common issues are loss of purpose following retirement, the death of a spouse or other close relative or friend, difficulty accepting the limitations produced by an ageing body and the effects of "ageism". Older people may feel they are no longer as valued as they were when they could be seen to be contributing members of society. Older people with a pre-existing diagnosis of bipolar disorder may also be seen in mental health services. It is extremely rare for bipolar disorder to appear for the first time in later life. Older people with bipolar disorder may also be experiencing the long-term effects of their medications, and this can affect their physical health. There are some psychiatrists who specialise in older people's mental health, and it is helpful to access this expertise when possible.

Diagnoses relating to bipolar disorder include bipolar 1 disorder, bipolar 2 disorder, cyclothymic disorder, substance/medication-induced bipolar and related disorder, bipolar and related disorder due to another medical condition, other specified bipolar disorder and unspecified bipolar disorder (APA 2022).

Although not usually classified as a mood disorder, it is useful to be aware of another condition that has a significant mood component. This is schizoaffective disorder. It is essentially a type of schizophrenia that also has a significant alteration in mood as part of the presentation. The mood can be either depressed or elevated, but the predominant problem is psychotic symptoms.

Diagnoses help to clarify the problems that people are experiencing and indicate the medical treatment options that could be used for that specific diagnosis. Some people with mental health problems can also find a diagnosis helpful in making sense of the problems they are experiencing. Knowing that the problems they are experiencing can be identified and named can be reassuring for some people. However, formal diagnosis can be more relevant to medical practitioners and psychiatrists than nurses, or indeed the consumer. While diagnosis is important, mental health nurses are well positioned to ask "What happened to you?" rather than "What is wrong with you?" Diagnosis look for deficits in the consumer. In contrast, when we ask what has happened to a person that led them to come into contact with mental health services, we are acknowledging their resilience and wider determinates of mood disorders, and other mental health challenges (Harper & Cromby 2022).

Mental health nurses have the experience and expertise to help people with their problems of daily living, however these problems are labelled.

✳ HISTORICAL ANECDOTE 12.2
Phil Barker

Phillip Barker was a leading nursing figure and nursing theorist of the 20th century. He was also a mental health nurse. He challenged mental health nurses to think beyond diagnosis alone and instead focus on the consumers' experiences of their problems, what they call those problems and what help might be of most use to them. He developed a mental health nursing model call the "Tidal Model", using the analogy of life being similar to a voyage. At times in life, we run aground and our role as a mental health nurse is to work in equal partnership with the consumer to enable them to resume that voyage.

Read More About It
Barker, P. Welcome to the Tidal Model 2015. Online. Available at: www.tidal-model.com/

PREVALENCE OF MOOD DISORDERS

In 2020–21 approximately one in five Australians had experienced some type of mental health disorder in the preceding 12 months, with double that prevalence (43.7% of Australians) over a lifetime. Twelve-month rates of reported mood disorders were 7.5% in 2020–21. The rates varied across demographics with those in the LGBTIQA+ community reporting rates at 30%, and those without stable housing at 17%. Prevalence rates for bipolar disorder were 2.2% (ABS 2022).

In New Zealand, prevalence data is reported differently. However, the most recent mental health national survey data shows a quarter of young New Zealanders reported high levels of psychological distress and rising unmet mental health need across all age groups at 8.8%. (Manatu Hauora Ministry of Health 2022). This suggests similar rates for mood disorders to that reported in Australia. Rates of bipolar affective disorder (BPAD) over a one-year period in New Zealand are 1.56 per 100,000 women and 1.20 per 100,00 men, with women being more likely to have service contact then men (Cunningham et al 2020). Interestingly, prevalence rates of BPAD are generally increasing. In the past, bipolar disorder was known as manic-depressive psychosis and this was thought to be a rare condition with a prevalence rate of 0.3% to 0.4% of the population in 1973 (Sainsbury 1973). In more recent times, and with a change of name, bipolar disorder has become a more acceptable diagnosis, and it has been suggested that psychiatrists overuse this diagnosis so they can treat problems medically rather than psychologically. There is a longstanding view that problems that may not be true bipolar disorder become medicalised and are treated with medications, even though this may not be the best or most effective treatment option (Whitaker 2010). Whatever the merits or problems with these issues, the reality is that there is a group of people who are diagnosed with bipolar disorder and treated with mood-stabilising medications. Psychological or talking therapies and psychosocial interventions are also beneficial for people with bipolar disorder, and an integrated approach using medication and other therapies is the optimal approach (Malhi et al 2021).

FACTORS CONTRIBUTING TO MOOD DISORDERS

Depression and bipolar disorder are complex phenomena that have a range of contributing factors. Malhi and colleagues (2021) suggest that we need to consider several factors when considering the origins of mood disorders. These include biological issues, psychological issues, relationship issues, family and societal issues and the worldview and spirituality of the person. Each of these factors may contribute to developing mood disorders in different ways, and not all factors will have an impact on every person, although it is worthwhile exploring all of these areas when assessing a person who presents with a mood disorder (Malhi et al 2021).

McLaren (2007) reflects longstanding views that the causes of depression can stem from different origins. Herrman and colleagues (2022) expand on this view in a robust overview of depression and its causes. Certainly, it is complex, heterogenous and interacts with events in the social world, making it the most significant mental illness in the Global Burden of Diseases (Herrman et al 2022).

It is also important to differentiate between depression that seems to appear out of the blue, for no specific reason, and depression that has an identifiable cause. People can become depressed following a major loss of some type, such as the death of a loved one, loss of employment or following some other calamity in their lives. In the past, this type of depression was known as exogenous depression – that is, depression with an identifiable, external cause. This terminology is no longer used, but it remains a helpful way of considering the factors that may lead to depression in some people.

THE EXPERIENCE OF MOOD DISORDERS

Mood disorders disrupt people's lives. This applies with both depression and bipolar disorder.

Depression saps people of their energy, their ability to think clearly and their feelings of enjoyment and pleasure in life. It can make simple tasks like shopping or cooking extremely difficult. Some people have great difficulty in leaving their house or doing the things that keep them functioning at an acceptable level, such as going to work, looking after their personal hygiene or fully participating in the important relationships in their lives (Visagie et al 2020).

People often feel guilty, frequently with no real basis for their guilt. They withdraw from those around them because they feel they are a burden or unworthy of other people's love and attention. It can be a very isolating experience, and people often feel hopeless about the possibility of feeling better and getting back to a normal level of functioning.

In the manic phase of bipolar disorder, however, the opposite happens. People may feel very happy and energetic. They may also engage in behaviours that are out of character for them, and this can lead to feelings of guilt and shame when their mood returns to normal levels. People in a manic state may also exhaust themselves physically because they feel they have boundless energy and a reduced need for sleep. Their judgement may be impaired and so they can make poor decisions that can have long-term consequences. This includes issues such as overspending, accruing debt and possibly engaging in indiscrete sexual behaviours that the person would not usually consider. Harm to their reputation is a real possibility for people in the manic phase of bipolar disorder, and this is one of the criteria for involuntary treatment due to the damaging effects of this harm.

SIGNS AND SYMPTOMS OF MOOD DISORDERS

The signs and symptoms of depression and bipolar disorder are listed in diagnostic manuals such as the DSM-5 (APA 2022) and the ICD-11 (World Health Organization 2022). In Australia and New Zealand, most doctors and other health professionals in mental health services use the DSM-5 as the main diagnostic classification system. However, health systems tend to rely more on ICD-11 as their main diagnostic system because the ICD-11 also includes diagnoses for physical health problems and this makes it more useful across all areas of a health system, particularly in the area of data collection.

The main symptoms of depression are depressed mood most of the day, nearly every day as indicated by self-report or observations made by others. The other main symptom is loss of enjoyment and pleasure in life. Either one or both of these symptoms need to occur nearly every day, for most of the day, for at least 2 weeks, before a diagnosis of depression can be considered. Other psychological symptoms include excessive feelings of inappropriate guilt, anxiety, worthlessness and hopelessness. Another symptom of depression is recurrent thoughts of death (not just fear of dying), recurrent suicidal thinking without a specific plan or a suicide attempt or a specific plan for attempting suicide (APA 2022).

There is also decreased energy or increased feelings of fatigue, psychomotor agitation or retardation nearly every day, insomnia or hypersomnia and significant weight loss when not dieting, or weight gain or changes in appetite (APA 2022).

Some people can have psychotic symptoms as part of their depressive illness. The most common psychotic symptoms are delusional beliefs. These delusional beliefs tend to be congruent with the experience of depression and include nihilistic delusions and somatic delusions. These are delusions where the person believes their internal organs have deteriorated or died or that parts of their body or their self no longer exist. This is a rare but serious type of depression that usually needs hospital treatment in the initial stages.

DSM-5 has two main diagnoses for bipolar disorder: Bipolar 1 disorder and bipolar 2 disorder. The main difference between these two diagnoses is the severity of the problems. The signs and symptoms are similar, but bipolar 2 includes the criterion that the episode is not severe enough to cause marked impairment in social or occupational function, or to necessitate hospitalisation (APA 2022).

The distinctive feature of bipolar disorder is fluctuations in mood between a depressed mood state and a manic or hypomanic mood state. A person must experience a manic mood state before a diagnosis of bipolar disorder can be made. If a person only ever has a depressive mood state, then they are diagnosed with major depressive disorder. These fluctuations in mood can be rapid in some people, with the mood fluctuating over periods of days to weeks. This is known as rapid-cycling bipolar disorder and fortunately is rare. It is more common for the mood fluctuations to occur over periods of months to years.

The main symptoms of a manic episode in bipolar disorder are a distinct period of persistently elevated, expansive or irritable mood, and abnormally and persistently increased energy or activity, present for most of the day, nearly every day and lasting at least one week (or any duration if hospitalisation is needed). The person also needs to demonstrate three or more of the following symptoms:

- inflated self-esteem or grandiosity
- decreased need for sleep
- more talkative than usual or experiences pressure to keep talking
- flight of ideas or a subjective experience that thoughts are racing
- distractibility, as reported or observed
- increase in goal-directed activity (either socially, at work/school or sexually) (APA 2022).

The mood disturbance is sufficiently severe to cause marked impairment in social or occupational functioning or to necessitate hospitalisation. This last criterion is where the main difference between bipolar 1 and bipolar 2 is noted.

DSM-5 states that in bipolar 2 the episode is associated with an unequivocal change in functioning, but the episode is not severe enough to cause marked impairment in social or occupational functioning or to necessitate hospitalisation (APA 2022). Based on this criterion, bipolar 2 is obviously a less severe form of bipolar disorder and is not as disruptive to the person's life as bipolar 1 disorder.

The depressive phase in bipolar disorder is remarkably similar to major depressive disorder. For a diagnosis of bipolar disorder to be made, a hypomanic or manic episode must occur at some point in the course of the illness.

It is important to differentiate between what might be called normal unhappiness or happiness and what might be depression or mania. It is normal for people to experience unhappiness and joy in response to the ups and downs of life. Many people experience fluctuations in their mood and there is nothing pathological in this process. It is a normal response to the vicissitudes and triumphs of life. We need to avoid the tendency to medicalise normal responses. A good understanding of the person's life story can help us determine where a person falls on the spectrum from normal to abnormal, and to distinguish between a temporary state and a longer term problem. Unnecessary and inappropriate treatment can be harmful and needs to be avoided.

PHYSICAL HEALTH AND MOOD DISORDERS

Depression and bipolar disorder both have physical symptoms that can affect a person's physical health and wellbeing. In both disorders sleep problems can manifest. In depression, insomnia is one of the

symptoms of the illness, whereas in bipolar disorder, people feel they need less sleep because of their heightened energy levels.

Decreased appetite can also cause physical health problems because of decreased nutritional input. As with sleep problems, reduced appetite manifests differently in depression and bipolar disorder. Reduced appetite is a symptom of depression, whereas people with bipolar disorder may be just too busy to eat properly.

Some physical health problems can lead to or exacerbate depression. Issues such as chronic pain or a chronic, disabling illness are examples of this (Li et al 2019). This is understandable when we think of the problems of living with chronic pain, for example. Pain relief is sometimes minimally effective, and the burden of chronic pain can affect many aspects of a person's life. Even simple tasks like washing and dressing can become difficult. Going out and doing the shopping can also be a pain-laden experience. People with chronic pain restrict their activities to reduce their level of pain and, as their world becomes more restricted, they can become depressed. There are no simple solutions to these complex issues, but some alternative approaches such as mindfulness and meditation can be helpful (Mistretta & Davis 2021).

People with other chronic illnesses such as diabetes may neglect their health care when they have depression or mania. Those with insulin-dependent diabetes may not check their blood sugar levels regularly and may neglect their diet, which can lead to deterioration in their physical health.

ASSESSMENT AREAS

Assessing people experiencing depression and bipolar disorder can be complex, with a number of issues that need to be considered and managed throughout the assessment process. These include biological issues, psychological issues, relationship issues, family and societal issues, and the worldview and spirituality of the person.

Patience is required when assessing a person with a mood disorder because there are several issues that can make the assessment process more complex. People experiencing depression may have difficulty with their thinking and concentration. Their thinking may be slower than usual and, along with reduced concentration, this can make it difficult for the person to put their thoughts and feelings into words. It is usually necessary to give the person more time to formulate answers and to think through the issues at hand. This also means that more time may need to be allocated when assessing someone with depression.

On the other hand, people experiencing the manic phase of bipolar disorder often speak too much, have racing, disorganised thoughts, and have problems with concentration because their mind is constantly racing. It is usually necessary to use strategies to help the person stay focused. This may require constant redirection to keep the person on task.

An assessment is an opportunity to undertake therapeutic work with a person, even when it is a one-off process. Engaging a person in an assessment process requires good interpersonal skills (Rice et al 2022). Engagement is a skillset that can be developed and refined. One of the most powerful tools for engagement is a respectful, courteous approach on the part of the nurse. Being respectful and courteous conveys acceptance and a preparedness to listen to the person's story and to be helpful. Being fully present and available during an assessment also has a strong therapeutic effect and is highly regarded by consumers and carers (Hurley et al 2023). If a person feels you are fully focused on them, their story and their needs, they are more likely to engage in the assessment process. Collaboration is also important. This involves promoting a sense of working with a person rather than doing things to them. We increase collaboration with a person through careful listening and encouragement to tell their story, involving them in decision-making about the therapeutic options and treating them as a partner in their care rather than us being the "expert" and provider of care.

The use of good therapeutic relational skills can have a profound impact on the person we are caring for. For many people, a well-conducted mental health assessment can provide a sense that they are being listened to and taken seriously, and that help is available to resolve the difficulties they are facing. This can promote hope, an important factor in recovery. We, as mental health nurses, have an important role to play in promoting hope.

Health History

It is important to obtain a complete history of the course of a mood disorder, including the time preceding the onset of the problems (Malhi et al 2021). Depression, in particular, rarely appears out of the blue, and it is also the case that the manic phase of bipolar disorder builds up over several weeks or months. It is therefore important to go back as far as necessary to find a time when the person was not experiencing any problems. Finding out more about the times before the person became unwell can give us a good baseline as to how the person functions when they are well. It may also indicate the existence of any precipitating factors that contributed to the person becoming unwell.

We need to know if the person has experienced a disturbance in mood in the past. This helps build a picture of the course of their illness over time and to understand what may have helped them in the past. This information is particularly relevant for medication choices and can take the guesswork out of prescribing if we know what worked for the person in previous episodes of disturbed mood.

It is also helpful to gain knowledge about any other interventions that were helpful in the person's recovery. This may include a range of therapeutic and psychosocial interventions, such as cognitive behaviour therapy (CBT), other talking therapies and assistance with work, daily activities or developing social networks.

Substance Abuse

Alcohol and other substances can have a negative impact on a person's mood, producing either depression or elevated mood (Hunt et al 2020). Alcohol is a depressant drug and can induce depression in susceptible people. Likewise, amphetamines and other stimulant drugs can induce mania in susceptible individuals.

Some people use drugs or alcohol to self-medicate in an effort to overcome their difficulties. This is seldom an effective approach and generally leads to more problems as people may then need to deal with and manage addiction. Drugs and alcohol can also lead to physical health problems that further complicate the recovery process.

Alcohol and other drugs can also interfere with pharmacological treatments used in mental health. For these reasons it is important to take a complete history of alcohol and other drug use.

Physical Health

Physical health problems can imitate mental health problems or can produce mental health problems as part of their symptomatology (Roughan et al 2021). Chronic pain or longstanding, disabling physical health problems can lead to depression. Conditions such as hyper- or hypothyroidism can mimic the manic phase of bipolar disorder or depression. It is, therefore, informative and necessary to take a full physical health history.

The other aspect of physical health that needs to be considered is any treatments the person may be taking for physical health problems. Some of these treatments can cause problems for a person, either due to side effects or effects of the medications or other treatments. We also need to consider any potential interactions that may occur with medications used to treat depression or bipolar disorder.

Psychological (Cognitive and Affective) State

A person's worldview is an important aspect of their approach to life in general and any difficult issues they might be dealing with. It is important for us to understand this worldview and how it shapes the person's perceptions of issues in their life and their responses to these issues. This is a broad description of issues that fit within the psychological realm.

Some aspects of a person's worldview that may assist or hinder their recovery are their level of optimism or pessimism and their feelings of being in control of things in their lives. If a person has a generally pessimistic view of the world and their place within the world, and also has a feeling of limited control over their life circumstances, then it is difficult for them to mobilise their internal resources and work towards recovery.

Included in this category is the person's feeling state. This is generally referred to as "mood", and assessment of mood relies on what the person tells us about how they are feeling. We can also get some idea of how the person is feeling by how they look, in terms of emotional expression. This latter aspect is known as "affect". A person's affect may, in some cases, provide a more accurate picture of their feeling state than what they tell us about how they are feeling. Some people find it difficult to acknowledge that they have a problem such as depression and they may attempt to put on a "happy face" to convince others that they are okay. They may not be able to sustain their "happy face" for prolonged periods of time and this is when we may see the "sad face" that reflects their true feeling state. It is therefore important to closely observe a person's affect during an assessment interview. Any change in affect should be noted and commented on. Gentle questioning can reveal the true emotional state of the person.

Mental health problems can also affect a person's cognitive capacities such as concentration and planning. One of the symptoms of both depression and mania is reduced capacity for concentration. This may be reflected in an inability to read or perform necessary tasks in the workplace.

Social Networks

A person's social networks can be either helpful or unhelpful in their efforts to manage a mental illness. It is, therefore, useful to understand the social networks surrounding the person we are assessing.

Do they have strong, supportive family connections or are they in conflict with or unconnected with their families? Do they have friends who are supportive? Do they have interests that help them find purpose in life and that require a commitment of time and effort? Are they part of wider social networks with people with shared interests such as sport or hobbies? Do they work and have positive relationships with their work colleagues or are there difficulties with colleagues in their workplace?

It is useful to know about these issues because people generally do better if they have good family and social networks. These networks not only provide support to the person, but can also be instrumental in the person's recovery, providing interests and activities that can help the person re-engage with the world around them. Sometimes, something as simple as going for a walk around the neighbourhood can provide connections with other members of the community, and this can be the start of a positive recovery process, particularly for people experiencing depression.

Spiritual Beliefs

Spirituality is a broad-based concept that is not only concerned with religious affiliation. Spirituality can provide a sense of meaning and purpose in a person's life. For example, many Aboriginal and Māori people have strong traditions and beliefs that do not fit within mainstream religious systems of belief, but these traditions and beliefs provide a spiritual foundation for the lives of these people.

For some people, religious affiliations provide the foundations for their understandings of life and their place and purpose in the world. There are a wide range of religions and associated belief systems, and it is important for us to gain an understanding of these issues.

This may be a sensitive issue for some people, and it is important that our inquiries about a person's spiritual beliefs are conducted in a sensitive way. It is vitally important to maintain a respectful approach when discussing a person's spiritual beliefs and to not do or say anything that may come across as critical or negative. There are several current conflicts in the world that have religious connections, such as Islamic State and its associations with the Muslim religions. People of Muslim faith have also been subjected to persecution and discrimination, and for these reasons, a person of Muslim faith may be reluctant to speak about their religious affiliations. People of other religious faiths may have similar experiences, perhaps dating back in their family for several generations, but their family culture and beliefs may still hold grievances about past treatment, so it is vital that we approach the topic of spirituality in a highly sensitive and compassionate way.

Ethnically-based spiritual associations may also generate difficulties for people, such as the issue of the "Stolen Generations" in the Aboriginal Australian population. In some parts of these communities, this may produce strong negative feelings that can affect our ability to connect with them. We need to be aware of and sensitive to these types of situations and respond in a caring and supportive way. If we show genuine interest in a person's spirituality and work from a compassionate frame of reference, we are more likely to gain an understanding of each person's spiritual frameworks.

Cultural Views

Cultural issues are also a broad concept. This not only refers to a person's ethnic background, but can include issues such as sexuality and cultural identities imposed by events. An example of this is people who become refugees when they are fleeing from difficult circumstances in their home country. Being a refugee can attract many negative experiences and interactions with others, and their refugee status takes over other aspects of the person's cultural background. Refugees are particularly prone to developing feelings of hopelessness, particularly those who are detained in processing centres. Procter and colleagues (2022) discuss the effects of isolation and trauma on the mental health of refugees, as well as the iatrogenic (medically induced) effects of the systems used to manage people seeking refugee status, such as the use of temporary protection visas. These visas create high levels of uncertainty and stress and contribute to the poor mental health of refugees.

There are many different cultural views about what we, in mainstream Australian and New Zealand culture, call mental illness. The white Anglophile view of mental illness is not universal, and it is important that we gain an understanding of an individual's cultural perspectives on mental illness. Their views may be quite different, and while it is not expected that we can be experts on all cultural views about mental illness, we are expected to be experts on discovering these differences. A sensitive, non-judgemental, non-critical inquiry into these issues can provide the perspectives we need to understand the different ways that people from other cultures think about mental illness.

It is also important to be aware of and sensitive to a person's ability and capacity to communicate in English. Australia and New Zealand have significant migrant populations whose first language is not English. Using interpreters can help facilitate good communication, but it requires some skill and experience to work effectively with interpreters. Working with interpreters increases the amount of time required to undertake assessments and clinical work, so we need to factor this into our clinical planning. It also sometimes happens that concepts that can be expressed in the person's native language cannot be easily translated into English. This

is where the use of skillful, qualified interpreters is most useful. It is always recommended that qualified interpreters be used in preference to family members. Interpreters are more likely to provide accurate interpretations of what a person is saying, and this can assist us in gaining a clear picture of the issues. One problem that can arise, however, is when working with people who come from a very small language group – for example, the Tibetan language and some African languages. In these cases, the interpreter may know the person socially, and this can influence the interpreting process. When using interpreters from small language groups it is useful to know if this is the case and whether a pre-existing relationship may affect the interpretation process.

Risk Assessment

Suicidal thinking can increase, particularly during an episode of depression, but also in the manic phase of bipolar disorder, so it is important to inquire about this. Importantly, be mindful that suicidal thinking can occur outside of the context of mood disorders, and treating depression may not successfully reduce suicide risk (Batterham et al 2019). Risk assessment requires high levels of skill and knowledge and sound clinical judgement. These skills can be developed over time with input from experienced mental health nurses. It is important not to overreact when suicidal risk is revealed, but rather to develop a clear understanding of the levels of risk and whether the person has the capacity and resources to manage their risk. It is rarely necessary to admit people to hospital due to suicide risk. With the right type and level of support from mental health workers, it is possible to maintain people with suicide risk in the community.

We need to inquire about issues such as whether the person has a plan about how they will kill themselves and, if so, whether they have access to the means to carry out this plan (Hawton et al 2022). We also need to understand their level of intent. This refers to the likelihood that the person will act on their plans. Intent is one of the more accurate predictors of suicide risk. We also need to gain an understanding about why the person thinks suicide might be an option for resolving their problems. When we understand why a person is thinking about suicide as a solution to their problems, we can then instigate interventions to address these issues. It is easy to feel overwhelmed and helpless when working with people with suicide risk, but a clear-headed, supportive, flexible approach can make all the difference. Most people move beyond suicidal thinking if they have the right levels and types of support, and this is valuable mental health nursing work. Whenever risk is present, we need to ensure that we monitor the level of risk as an ongoing process.

✳ HISTORICAL ANECDOTE 12.3

Suicide has always been with us

Experiences of mental ill health and suicide are as old as time itself. The ancient Greek document The Histories contains one of the earliest written descriptions of mental illness and suicide. Author Herodotus (490–425 BC) describes the plight of Cleomenes of Sparta who probably experienced mental illness throughout his life. In the end his state of mind deteriorated so badly that his family had him confined to stocks, bound and guarded. Cleomenes' suicide occurred when he tricked a guard who was a slave into giving him a knife. Herodotus describes how "as soon as the knife was in his hands, Cleomenes began to mutilate himself, beginning on his shins. He sliced his flesh into strips working upwards to his thighs, and from them to his hips and sides until he reached his belly and while he was cutting it into strips he died".

Read More About It

Strassler RB, Purvis AL 2009 The landmark Herodotus: The histories. Anchor Books/Random House, New York.

INTERVENTIONS

Interpersonal Interventions

The interpersonal relationship is one of the foundation principles and interventions of mental health nursing. Much has been written about this type of relationship, beginning with the work of Helena Render in 1947 (Render 1947), with further contributions from Hildegarde Peplau in 1952 (Peplau 1952) and Joyce Travelbee in 1966 (Travelbee 1966). This earlier work is reflected in contemporary mental health nursing with the utilisation of non-technical skills associated with emotional intelligence being essential to effective helping (Hurley et al 2022).

One of the essential elements of the therapeutic relationship is engagement. Engagement arises out of several attitudes and behaviours on the part of the nurse. The aim of engagement is to help the person in care to feel safe and valued as a fellow human being.

Presence is one of the most important aspects of engagement. Presence means being fully present and available to the person in care. It requires being fully conscious of the person and their needs with a minimum of unconscious behaviour (Younger 1995). Other factors that influence engagement are a respectful, non-judgemental approach combined with active listening – that is, looking beneath the surface of what is being said to detect underlying issues and themes. Listening and clarifying are two important aspects of engagement. We do not learn anything when we are speaking, but listening provides a gateway into another person's experiences. If we do not fully understand what a person is telling us, then we need to seek clarification so we are clear about what is being discussed. This can also help the person to clarify their own perceptions and thoughts.

Much has been written about the interpersonal aspects of mental health nursing. It is still, in some ways, a poorly articulated approach to helping people (Clark 2017). It can be helpful to return to the original works on interpersonal nursing, such as those by Peplau and Travelbee, mentioned above. These authors articulated the core principles and concepts of interpersonal nursing, and these principles and concepts are as relevant today as they were when they were first discussed (Clark 2017; Hurley et al 2022). Interpersonal relationships are a fundamental aspect of life and of being human and, as Travelbee (1966) stated, it is a human-to-human process that requires an educated heart and an educated mind on the part of the nurse to turn this fundamental human process into a therapeutic wonder. This capability of the nurse to form and maintain therapeutic relationships through interpersonal relating is highly regarded by consumers and carers (Lakeman et al 2022).

Establishing a good interpersonal relationship provides the foundation for the other interventions we use. If we can establish a positive, supportive relationship with the person in our care it is more likely that they will follow through with the interventions we suggest to them. They are also more likely to let us know when things are not going well, and this provides us with additional opportunities to finetune our interventions. See Perspectives in practice: Nurse's story 12.1.

PERSPECTIVES IN PRACTICE

Nurse's Story 12.1: Greg Clark

I am a registered nurse who has worked in mental health services for 40 years. Working in mental health has provided me with an enjoyable mix of challenges and rewards. When I reflect on my practice, one story that comes to mind is that of Henry. Henry was a man in his 70s who was referred to the mental health service by his general practitioner because of depression. Henry had recently returned from an overseas trip with his wife. She had inherited money from one of her relatives and so they had embarked on a lifelong dream to travel through Europe. During the trip Henry became increasingly anxious and depressed. This occurred because of the constant changes of location, time zones and accommodation during their journey. He had a long history of diabetes and he became increasingly anxious and rigid around the management of his blood sugar levels and insulin dosing, and the constant changes exacerbated his anxiety. This led to a state of deep depression, partly because he felt guilty about the effect of his behaviour on his wife and her enjoyment of the travel, and partly because he was constantly worried that he would give himself too much insulin and die. He normally had a very strict routine around his mealtimes and blood sugar testing, and this was thrown into disarray because of the travel. Anxiety and depression are frequently found together in a person and they exacerbate each other, as in this story.

When Henry returned to Australia his GP referred him to the local community mental health service. The psychiatrist started Henry on an antidepressant, venlafaxine. I arranged to see Henry at his home. I worked on helping Henry manage his anxiety and depression through talking about the issues that led to his depression and the current difficulties he was experiencing, as well as assisting him to develop skills and strategies that would help him get back to his more usual way of being. I also worked with Henry and his wife to work through the feelings of disappointment and anger that arose as a result of the difficulties in their overseas holiday. Henry was seen every week over a period of months, and I encouraged him to gradually take up some of the interests and activities that he had before the emergence of depression. Henry had worked as a motor mechanic all his adult life and, following retirement he had taken on the job of repairing and maintaining his neighbour's lawn mowers and other motorised garden equipment. Once Henry overcame his reluctance and inertia and repaired his first lawn mower since becoming depressed, he was on the road to recovery. He felt pleased with himself and his confidence returned, but most importantly, he felt useful and competent once more.

Henry and his wife began planning a cruising holiday around New Zealand, which was a very positive sign of recovery. They chose a cruising holiday because of the stable accommodation aboard the ship and the lack of disruption it would cause in Henry's diabetes routines. It was very gratifying for me to see the effects of my work with Henry and his wife as exemplified in their thinking and planning around future travel plans.

As a nurse it is important to be patient and work with the person at the pace they are comfortable with. Recovery cannot be rushed, and when working with people with depression it is important to pay attention to and acknowledge the small steps that lead to recovery. Recovery is not usually a dramatic process. It is incremental and takes time. It is a great privilege to work with people like Henry and to see positive outcomes from careful, thoughtful work over sometimes lengthy periods of time.

Pharmacological Interventions

The main pharmacological treatments for depression are antidepressants. There are many different types of antidepressant medications available and these will be described in more detail below. The main pharmacological treatments for bipolar disorder are antidepressants for the depressive phase and mood stabilisers, both for the manic phase and for maintenance.

Effective antidepressants were first developed in the 1960s. The early medications included tricyclic antidepressants and monoamine oxidase inhibitors (MAOIs). Both these groups of medications are still used, although MAOIs require dietary restrictions in their use and are now prescribed less frequently.

Since the 1970s, there has been a significant growth in the number and types of antidepressants available. These include selective serotonin reuptake inhibitors, serotonin noradrenaline reuptake inhibitors, selective noradrenaline reuptake inhibitors, alpha-2 antagonists and melatonin agonists, and others. Unfortunately, it is not possible to determine in advance the most effective antidepressant for any particular person, and so a process of trial and error is needed. Given that antidepressants usually take 2–3 weeks before their full effects become evident, this can be a difficult period for people hoping for fast relief. Ongoing support is necessary during this period of waiting, to maintain hope and to help the person manage their symptoms as best they can while waiting for the medications to provide relief (Stahl 2021). This initial few weeks is also when side effects from the medications are most prominent, and this is another area where mental health nurses can help people with strategies to manage their side effects.

One of the dangers of using antidepressants in people with bipolar disorder is that these medications can induce a manic phase, so caution and close monitoring are needed for people receiving antidepressants during the depressive phase of their illness. If a manic phase develops, the antidepressant medication needs to be stopped, following medical advice.

There is a variety of mood stabilisers available for people experiencing the manic phase of bipolar disorder. The first mood stabiliser that became available in the 1940s was lithium carbonate. This medication was discovered in 1948 by an Australian psychiatrist, John Cade (1949). Lithium carbonate is a mineral salt, similar to common table salt, but it has a strong therapeutic, stabilising effect on elevated mood. Lithium is used less commonly these days because it requires regular monitoring of blood levels to avoid the risk of toxicity and it has some significant long-term adverse effects on the kidneys and thyroid gland (Stahl 2021). It also causes a hand tremor in many people who take it.

An alternative treatment to lithium carbonate which is now used far more commonly is a group of medications that are designed as anticonvulsants – that is, treatments for epilepsy. These medications include sodium valproate (Epilim), carbamazepine (Tegretol) and lamotrigine (Lamictal). These medications are generally safe and effective, although, as with all medications, they do have side effects.

Some antipsychotic medications also have mood-stabilising effects and these can be quite effective for some people. Antipsychotics that are used as mood stabilisers include quetiapine (Seroquel), olanzapine (Zyprexa) and ziprasidone (Zeldox). These medications can be particularly helpful for women who are pregnant or breastfeeding because the other mood stabilisers cannot be used during pregnancy. Sodium valproate is particularly harmful to a developing fetus and it is recommended that this medication not be used in any woman with childbearing potential (Austin et al 2017; Ng et al 2021).

Although not a pharmacological treatment, electroconvulsive therapy (ECT) is included among the medical treatments for mood disorders. It is particularly effective for depression, but is also used very infrequently for mania. ECT involves applying electrodes to a person's head. The small electric current that is delivered via the electrodes induces an epileptic-like seizure. A course of treatment usually involves 12 episodes of ECT delivered three times a week. The person receives a general anaesthetic and a muscle relaxant before beginning each treatment, so they have no conscious experience of the treatment. The main side effects from ECT are transient memory loss and the aftereffects of the anaesthetic. For people with severe depression who need access to a faster recovery than can be achieved with medications, ECT can be a valuable addition to their treatment armamentarium. ECT is rarely used as a sole treatment option and is usually combined with antidepressant medications.

Digital/Web-Based Interventions

Organisations such as The Black Dog Institute and Beyond Blue provide information about mood disorders on their websites. Information can be a powerful tool in helping people understand what is happening in their lives. See the Useful websites section at the end of this chapter for more details.

Other Interventions

There is a range of alternative therapies that people access independently, such as chiropractic care, homeopathy, herbal medicine, acupuncture and traditional Chinese medicine. Many of these treatment approaches have a limited evidence base and their use is generally not supported by conventional medical practitioners. Nevertheless, people do use these alternative approaches and may find them helpful.

Whatever your thoughts about these alternative practices, it is important to keep an open mind and develop an understanding of why people find them helpful. It is not up to us to dissuade people from using alternative practices unless they are clearly dangerous. The alternative treatments listed above are not generally considered dangerous.

THE ROLE OF NURSING

Nurses have a range of roles in interventions for people with mood disorders. As previously mentioned, the interpersonal relationship is the foundation of mental health nursing work and has therapeutic outcomes as a result of establishing this relationship. However, and probably more importantly, the therapeutic, interpersonal relationship facilitates a range of other interventions. If people have a sense of trust in their nurse, they are more likely to accept the interventions offered by the nurse (Clark 2017).

Psychosocial issues are one area where nurses can provide helpful interventions. This covers a range of possibilities and it is helpful to think broadly about psychosocial issues. For example, helping a person to re-engage with their community in some way can facilitate recovery from depression. This may involve helping the person reconnect with activities or groups that they were previously involved with. This can also involve connecting a person with services that might help them manage their lives more easily. Accessing home help or personal care services may be very helpful for people with issues such as chronic pain and the ensuing depression. Getting help with personal hygiene and shopping can relieve some of the burden of living with depression. An added advantage with services like these is the personal contact that takes place with someone from outside the person's usual circumstances.

Walking alongside people during their recovery journey and providing the gift of time is a valuable but underappreciated aspect of mental health nursing work (Jackson & Stevenson 1998). Sometimes, just sitting with people and letting them tell whatever story is important to them at that moment in time can be a valuable intervention for people with mood disorders. Spending unfocused, unprogrammed time with someone can make a difference to their mental health, perhaps through the simple act of spending time with someone who is interested, non-judgemental and available – a rare experience in today's often busy world. Using a non-directive, sensitive approach, allowing people to focus on whatever is important to them at any moment in time is valuable nursing work that can make a positive difference to a person's mental wellbeing.

Helping people access other services such as employment assistance or government services such as Centrelink or the Department of

Housing can be a useful intervention. Many services are overly bureaucratic and require knowledge and persistence to navigate. Nurses working in community settings can help people access and successfully navigate these bureaucratic processes.

Mental health nurses can also provide a range of formal therapies, following appropriate training. Nurses are engaged in providing CBT, psychotherapy and mindfulness practices (Lakeman et al 2020); however, these therapies are also provided by other suitably qualified and trained health professionals and are not the exclusive remit of mental health nurses. The unique contribution that mental health nurses make is the person-centred, practically focused, holistic care that helps people get on with their lives and have the best

quality of life possible. Mental health nurses engage in helping people with the ordinary, small details of life that other disciplines do not have access to. In an in-patient setting, mental health nurses "inhabit the liminal space between the doctors and the patients, affecting in important ways the fate of both" (Clark 2017, p. 185). We have access to this liminal space 24 hours per day, 7 days a week, and this provides us with a unique opportunity to help people manage the difficulties they are facing. It also provides us with a unique opportunity to gain a more detailed understanding of the issues that are important for each person. This is a great privilege that should never be underestimated. See Personal perspectives: Consumer's story: Sophie Temmhoff.

PERSONAL PERSPECTIVES

Consumer's Story 12.1: Sophie Temmhoff

In my early 20s, the deep heavy depression that had come off and on since I was a child was back again, and this time it was not leaving. I had just left an abusive marriage and was rebuilding from nothing. I had lived for 6 months with family and during that time had experienced constant suicidal thoughts. By the time I moved into my own small flat, I was a complete mess, drinking heavily and self-harming daily. I didn't know where to start getting help, so I saw my GP. He prescribed me antidepressants, and that was all. They made things worse, and I ended up in the mental health unit at hospital for an extended stay.

Being on the ward was like some strange kind of holiday. I was in a bad state, the most vulnerable I had ever been. I was scared, alone and had everything taken away from me. All of a sudden, my outside responsibilities were gone. All I had to do was eat, sleep, shower and take my meds. I was forced to stop and confront just how bad things had become.

Being on the ward can feel dehumanising. You don't have your usual comfort and freedom, and you suddenly have little contact with the outside world. All of this happens while you are in an incredibly vulnerable space. It meant so much to me for the nurses to treat me in a way that respected my autonomy. A collaborative effort during treatment helped me to stay in control of myself, even though everything else was stripped away. The compassionate care of the nurses was really vital during my stay.

The nurses did their best to spend time with the patients socially, which helped foster some friendships and a sense of comfort. This was really helpful for the times when I needed to speak to a nurse about how I was feeling. For me to be able to speak freely and have a connection with the nurses meant it didn't feel like I was unloading onto a stranger. For a nurse to sit with me for an extended period of time without making me feel rushed or like I was bothering them was really important. It not only helped me, but I feel it gave the nurses a wider scope of information that would then help my treatment plan, as well as fostering an open dialogue where I felt comfortable expressing myself.

I think it's really important to have information on medications. I am the sort of person who reads as much as possible about a medication before I start taking it. This was tricky on the ward as there was no internet access. It was incredibly helpful when the nurses were able to readily give me information about my medications by giving me printouts, as well as spending time with me discussing side effects and what the medication might do for me. It helped me feel like I was still in control of my treatment. Otherwise, it would have felt really dehumanising to just be told, "here, take this!", with no information and no say on my part about whether I even wanted to try the medication. Being able to collaborate with the nurses and doctors to figure out what I wanted to do with my treatment really helped me come to terms with my diagnosis, as it wasn't just something that was happening to me, I was guiding it.

One of the worst things a nurse could do while on the ward was to treat me like a child. Thankfully, this rarely happened, but there were definitely a few nurses who thought that just because I was mentally ill and on the ward that

I must not have known what I needed. This mostly happened with a change of shift. Often the night or weekend nurses wouldn't know the patients very well and would question my requests that previous nurses had no issues with. This felt really infantilising and like my autonomy had been taken. I understand that the nurses would need to question things sometimes and say no to some requests, but to have it done in a very dismissive way, as if I had no idea what I was talking about, was extremely upsetting.

It was hard to know what was going on in the ward at times – when you were going to see the psychiatrist, if you had been written up for leave, when you were going home. It was important that the nurses kept communicating to me what was happening. When you are in the ward you don't have much control over when things were happening, so to be vaguely told you were seeing the psychiatrist and then waiting all day for nothing was really horrible. It helped for the nurses to keep me in the loop with what was going to happen, if they could.

Most nurses spoke in a positive way, where recovery was something attainable for me. They held space and listened to me while supporting me with my discharge plans. The next year or so, I was unable to work and spent most of my time in and out of the mental health unit. The nurses were compassionate every time I reappeared in the ward for another stay; they remembered me and never made me feel as if I had failed by returning. Recovery is never linear, and the open and welcoming support I received each time helped me to feel like even though I was back in hospital, I was still on my way to recovery.

I was referred to the community mental health team and started seeing a clinical psychologist weekly. I did my best to wade through my past and untangle the beliefs I had about myself while my psychologist held space and facilitated growth and resilience. It was during this time I was diagnosed with bipolar 2, and things started making more sense from a treatment point of view. The next 6 years were spent trying countless medication combinations, in therapy, and with more trips to the mental health unit. At times treatment felt pointless, but my psychiatrist and case manager never seemed to give up trying to find a way to stabilise me. I had built myself a strong support base with family and friends and eventually found myself in an incredibly supportive and healing relationship.

One of the catalysts for my healing was starting to undo my trauma with mindfulness and therapy. Thankfully, I had started a combination of desvenlafaxine and quetiapine and I was finally stable for the first time I could remember in my whole life. The stability from my psych meds allowed me to be in the right space to start understanding and applying the years of therapy, and I am ever thankful for learning how trauma works and how to move it through my body.

I know I am incredibly lucky with the experiences I have had through the public health system. Having continuous compassionate care throughout my journey has been truly priceless, and I am aware that not everyone has this same experience.

CHAPTER SUMMARY

This chapter has provided an overview of mood disorders – their symptoms and presentations, issues that need to be considered in assessment and some of the things that nurses can do that will be helpful for people with mood disorders. We have also discussed some of the treatment options such as medications, ECT and talking therapies. The importance of psychosocial interventions delivered by nurses has also been discussed.

Interpersonal relations, a foundation process in mental health nursing, have been described and the essential elements of this work have been elucidated. Mental health nursing as a person-centred, relational process is a fundamental aspect of working with people with mood disorders and any other type of mental illness or life problem, however labelled. The importance of working with people in a respectful, non-judgemental, compassionate framework is a key concern for mental health nurses. Being fully present and available to those in need of our help is a vitally important aspect of mental health nursing.

USEFUL WEBSITES

Beyond Blue: www.beyondblue.org.au/

Bipolar Australia: www.bipolaraustralia.org.au/services-directory/wpbdp_category/support-groups/

Black Dog Institute: www.blackdoginstitute.org.au/clinical-resources/bipolar-disorder/seeking-help

ReachOut: au.reachout.com/articles/support-services-for-bipolar-disorder

REFERENCES

American Psychiatric Association (APA), 2022. Diagnostic and Statistical Manual of Mental Disorders, 5th edition, Text Revision. APA, Washington DC.

Austin, M.P., Highet, N., the Expert Working Group, 2017. Mental Health Care in the Perinatal Period: Australian Clinical Practice Guidelines. Centre of Perinatal Excellence, Melbourne.

Australian Bureau of Statistics (ABS), 2022. National Study of Mental Health and Wellbeing. Online. Available at: www.abs.gov.au/statistics/health/mental-health/national-study-mental-health-and-wellbeing/latest-release

Batterham, P.J., van Spijker, B.A., Mackinnon, A.J., Calear, A.L., Wong, Q., et al., 2019. Consistency of trajectories of suicidal ideation and depression symptoms: Evidence from a randomized controlled trial. Depression and Anxiety, 36(4), 321–329.

Cade, J.F. 1949. Lithium salts in the treatment of psychotic excitement. MJA, 2(10), 349–352.

Clark, G.J. 2017. The past is not a foreign country: A history of ideas in psychiatric nursing scholarship – 1885 to 2013. PhD thesis. University of Newcastle, Newcastle.

Cunningham, R., Crowe, M., Stanley, J., Haitana, T., Pitama, S., et al., 2020. Gender and mental health service use in bipolar disorder: National cohort study. B J Psych Open, 6(6), e138.

Harper, D.J. & Cromby, J. 2022. From "what's wrong with you?" to "what's happened to you?": An introduction to the special issue on the power threat meaning framework. J Constructivist Psychol, 35(1), 1–6.

Hawton, K., Lascelles, K., Pitman, A., Gilbert, S., Silverman, M. 2022. Assessment of suicide risk in mental health practice: Shifting from prediction to therapeutic assessment, formulation, and risk management. Lancet Psychiatry, 9(11), 922–928.

Herrman, H., Patel, V., Kieling, C., Berk, M., Buchweitz, C., et al., 2022. Time for united action on depression: A Lancet–World Psychiatric Association Commission. The Lancet, 399(10328), 957–1022.

Hunt, G.E., Malhi, G.S., Lai, H.M.X., & Cleary, M. 2020. Prevalence of comorbid substance use in major depressive disorder in community and clinical settings 1990–2019: Systematic review and meta-analysis. J Affect Disord, 266, 288–304.

Hurley, J., Foster, K., Campbell, K., Edan, V., Hazelton, M., et al., 2023. Mental health nursing capability development: Perspectives of consumers and supporters. Int J Ment Health Nurs, 32(1), 172–185.

Hurley, J., Lakeman, R., Linsley, P., McKenna-Lawson, S., & Ramsay, M. 2022. Utilizing the mental health nursing workforce: A scoping review of mental health nursing clinical roles and identities. Int J Ment Health Nurs, doi.org/10.1111/inm.12983

Jackson, S., Stevenson, C. 1998. The gift of time from the friendly professional. Nurs Stand, 12(51), 31–33.

Lakeman, R., Cashin, A., Hurley, J., & Ryan, T. 2020. The psychotherapeutic practice and potential of mental health nurses: An Australian survey. Aust Health Rev, 44(6), 916–923.

Lakeman, R., Foster, K, Hazelton, M, Rope, C. & Hurley, J. 2022. Helpful encounters with mental health nurses in Australia: A survey of service users and their supporters. J Psychiatric Ment Health Nurs, doi.org/10.1111/jpm.12887

Li, H., Ge, S., Greene, B., & Dunbar-Jacob, J. 2019. Depression in the context of chronic diseases in the United States and China. Int J Nurs Sci, 6(1), 117–122.

Malhi, G.S., Bell, E., Boyce, P., Bassett, D., Berk, M., et al., 2021. The 2020 Royal Australian and New Zealand College of Psychiatrists clinical practice guidelines for mood disorders: Bipolar disorder summary. Bipol Disord, 22(8), 805–821.

Mallett, J., Redican, E., Doherty, A.S., Shevlin, M. & Adamson, G. 2022. Depression trajectories among older community dwelling adults: Results from the Irish Longitudinal Study on Ageing (TILDA). J Affect Disord, 298 (Part A, 1), 345–354.

Manatū Hauora Ministry of Health, 2022. Annual update of key results 2021/22. Online. Available at: www.health.govt.nz/publication/annual-update-key-results-2021-22-new-zealand-health-survey

McLaren, N. 2007. Humanizing madness: Psychiatry and the cognitive neurosciences. Loving Healing Press, Ann Arbor, MI.

Mistretta, E.G., & Davis, M.C. 2021. Meta-analysis of self-compassion interventions for pain and psychological symptoms among adults with chronic illness. Mindfulness, 1–18.

Ng, V.W., Man, K.K., Gao, L., Chan, E.W., Lee, E.H., et al., 2021. Bipolar disorder prevalence and psychotropic medication utilisation in Hong Kong and the United Kingdom. Pharmacoepidemiol Drug Safe, 30(11), 1588–1600.

Pearson, C., Siegel, J., & Gold, J.A. 2022. Psilocybin-assisted psychotherapy for depression: Emerging research on a psychedelic compound with a rich history. J Neurologic Sci, 434, 120096.

Peplau, H. 1952. Interpersonal Relations in Nursing. G.P. Putnam's Sons, New York.

Procter, N., Hamer, H.P., McGarry, D., et al., 2022. Mental Health: A Person-Centred Approach, 3rd ed. Cambridge University Press, Cambridge.

Render, H.W. 1947. Nurse–Patient Relationships in Psychiatry. McGraw-Hill, New York.

Rice, S.M., McKechnie, B., Cotton, S., Brooker, A., Pilkington, V., et al., 2022. Severe and complex youth depression: Clinical and historical features of young people attending a tertiary mood disorders clinic. Early Intervent Psychiatry, 16(3), 316–322.

Roughan, W.H., Campos, A.I., García-Marín, L.M., Cuéllar-Partida, G., Lupton, M.K., et al., 2021. Comorbid chronic pain and depression: Shared risk factors and differential antidepressant effectiveness. Front Psychiatry, 12, 643609.

Royal Women's Hospital, Victoria. n.d. Baby Blues. Online. Available at: www.thewomens.org.au/health-information/pregnancy-and-birth/mental-health-pregnancy/baby-blues

Sainsbury, M.J. 1973. Key to Psychiatry: A Textbook for Students. Australian and New Zealand Book Co., Sydney.

Stahl, S.M. 2021. Stahl's Essential Psychopharmacology, 5th ed. Cambridge University Press, Cambridge.

Strassler, R.B., Purvis, A.L. 2009. The Landmark Herodotus: The Histories. Anchor Books/Random House, New York.

Travelbee, J. 1966. Interpersonal Aspects of Nursing, 1st ed. F.A. Davis, Philadelphia.

Uguz, F. 2020. Pharmacological prevention of mood episodes in women with bipolar disorder during the perinatal period: A systemic review of current literature. Asian J Psychiatry, 52, 102145.

Visagie, H.M., Poggenpoel, M., & Myburgh, C. 2020. Lived experiences of psychiatric patients with mood disorders who attended group therapy facilitated by professional psychiatric nurses. Curationis, 43(1), 1–9.

Whitaker, R. 2010. Anatomy of an Epidemic. Magic Bullets, Psychiatric Drugs and the Astonishing Rise of Mental Illness in America. Crown, New York.

World Health Organization (WHO), 2022. The International Classification of Diseases, 11th rev. WHO, Geneva.

Younger, J. 1995. The alienation of the sufferer. Adv Nurs Sci, 17(4), 53–72.

13

Substance Use and Co-occurring Mental Health Disorders

Megan McKechnie

KEY POINTS

- Excessive alcohol consumption is the leading substance identified in treatment episodes within the alcohol and other drug treatment sector.
- Harmful alcohol use is the primary contributor to a wide range of health harms, including, but not limited to, the major cause of motor vehicle accidents, domestic violence, public aggression and violence, crime, chronic health conditions and brain injuries. It contributes to family breakdown and broader social dysfunction.
- There is a considerable degree of co-occurrence between substance use disorders and other mental health disorders.

- Psychoactive drugs can cause harm through acute states of intoxication, as well as the development of dependence.
- Interventions for substance use disorders may include harm reduction, intoxication management, withdrawal management, management of pharmacotherapy, early interventions, brief interventions, longer term maintenance therapies and psychosocial interventions.
- Treatment is inclusive of pharmacological, psychological and psychosocial interventions to assist with reducing the harm associated with substance use.

KEY TERMS

Co-occurring disorder	Intoxication	Substance use disorder
Dependence	Novel psychoactive substance	Synthetic cannabinoid
Detoxification	Psychoactive drug	Tolerance
Harm reduction	Psychosis	Withdrawal

LEARNING OUTCOMES

The material in this chapter will assist you to:
- discuss the incidence and impact of substance-related disorders and co-occurring disorders in Australia and Aotearoa New Zealand
- describe the pharmacokinetics and pharmacodynamics of psychoactive drugs
- identify the importance of undertaking a drug and alcohol assessment for all mental health clients

- describe a range of interventions that can be used for clients with a co-occurring substance use disorder and mental health disorder
- describe the different substance withdrawal syndromes
- describe a range of harm minimisation strategies that can be used for clients with substance use disorders
- critically analyse the range of treatment services available for clients with a co-occurring diagnosis.

INTRODUCTION

Wherever nurses work they will come across people who struggle with substance use disorders. This may involve people who use legal and illegal substances, as well as working with patients who have accidentally developed an iatrogenic (medically induced) dependence on prescribed medication. We may have experienced our own mental health or substance use problems or that of family and friends, and we need to consider the impact of this pre-existing bias on treatment. If we understand the nature of these problems, we can offer the best care possible, in a non-biased and empathetic way.

This chapter explores issues of substance use, substance use disorders and co-occurring disorders (mental health problems and substance use problems) in Australia and Aotearoa New Zealand. The pharmacology of psychoactive drugs is explored, and various terms are defined. The nursing skills needed to ask targeted questions and to provide a comprehensive drug and alcohol assessment are explained.

Specific interventions, such as early interventions, brief interventions and harm reduction strategies are discussed. The assessment and treatment of patients who are intoxicated or withdrawing from substances is described.

The final section of the chapter discusses co-occurring substance use and mental health disorders, the significance of co-occurring disorders and why people with a mental illness use alcohol and other drugs. You will find additional information and specific nursing interventions for co-occurring presentations in other relevant chapters.

TYPES OF SUBSTANCE USE DISORDERS

Substance use exists on a spectrum that ranges from abstinence to occasional use, to harmful use, to addiction. Occasional use may not cause problems or may even be therapeutic. In general, the more often the substance is used or the greater the amount used, the more severe the health consequences, psychosocial consequences and risk of dependence. Substance use disorders may be defined as disorders that develop due to the use of psychoactive substances that result in mental and behavioural changes over time (World Health Organization (WHO) 2018a).

Intoxication

Intoxication refers to a clinically significant yet transient state that develops rapidly after using alcohol or other substances, and is characterised by a range of changes to consciousness, cognition, perception, affect, behaviour or coordination (WHO 2018a). Nurses need to manage intoxication effectively because it may complicate assessment and client management and increase the risk of mortality. Intoxication can mask serious illness or injury (e.g. infections, hypoxia, head injury and cerebrovascular accidents). It can also be life threatening by directly altering physical functions (e.g. depressed respiration, temperature dysregulation) or via secondary events associated with altered mental/conscious states (e.g. aspiration when acutely intoxicated on alcohol, and motor vehicle accidents).

Dependence

Dependence can be both physical and psychological. A key feature of dependence is when withdrawal symptoms occur after abrupt cessation or reduction in use after a sustained period of time. Physiological dependence is the cluster of physiological, behavioural and cognitive symptoms that lead to an individual re-prioritising their substance use over other behaviours that were once important (WHO 2018). There are two central processes to dependence: The desire to continue taking the substance (despite a clear knowledge of the potential negative consequences of use) and the continued use to avoid symptoms of withdrawal (WHO 2018a).

"Psychological dependence" refers to the process of impaired control of alcohol or other drug use, whereas "physiological dependence" is associated with developing tolerance and withdrawal (WHO 2018a). Often, physical and psychological dependence are combined, but not always. For example, a person might be psychologically dependent on cannabis (with regular daily consumption and cravings), but demonstrate no significant withdrawal symptoms upon cessation of use.

Tolerance

Physiological tolerance occurs as a result of the brain being repeatedly exposed to a substance over time. Brain neural circuitry involving a range of neurotransmitters (e.g. dopamine and serotonin) adapts to the addition of the drug and reduces the responsiveness of those receptors. This decreased responsiveness leads to tolerance, which reduces the positive effect that the drug may have. Simply put, greater amounts of the drug are required to create the same effect as the first time it was used. This may also occur with behavioural addictions such as problem gambling.

Withdrawal

Withdrawal is the presence of a range of clinically important symptoms and behaviours, of varying intensity and duration, that occur upon cessation or reduction in alcohol or other drug use in those who have developed dependence (WHO 2018a). The different withdrawal syndromes will be discussed in more detail later in the chapter.

BEHAVIOURAL ADDICTIONS

There is increasing recognition of disorders that occur as a result of repetitive behaviours. The *International Classification of Diseases, 11th Revision* (ICD-11) (World Health Organization (WHO) 2018) and *Diagnostic and Statistical Manual of Mental Disorders, 5th Edition Text Revision* (DSM-5-TR) (American Psychiatric Association (APA) 2022),

both recognise behavioural disorders, in particular, gambling disorders (American Psychiatric Association 2022; WHO 2018a). Behavioural addictions are commonly associated with gambling, food, sexual intercourse, playing video games, exercise and shopping.

Gambling Disorders

During 2018–19 approximately $25 billon was lost by Australians on legal forms of gambling and around 41% of people were concurrently seeking treatment for mental health changes gambled (Victorian Responsible Gambling Foundation 2022; Australian Institute of Health and Welfare (AIHW) 2021b). Gambling is associated with a range of mental health disorders including alcohol and other drug use, mood disorders, impulse control disorders and personality disorders (Victorian Responsible Gambling Foundation 2020). Two categories of gambling disorders exist: Pathological gambling and problem gambling. "Problem gambling" refers to lower, or intermediate, levels of gambling pathology that result in harm but do not necessarily meet the criteria for a formal diagnosis of a gambling disorder (Chamberlain et al 2017). "Pathological gambling" refers to the more severe forms of gambling disorders where individuals experience social, financial and occupational losses due to gambling (Grant et al 2017).

Treatment for gambling disorders focus primarily on psychological and psychosocial interventions. Similar to treatment for substance use disorders, motivational interviewing, brief interventions and cognitive behaviour therapy (CBT) have been established as mainstay treatment options. Screening for gambling disorders can form the first step of a brief intervention (see Box 13.1). There is now also evidence to support using pharmacotherapy to treat pathological gambling. The opioid antagonist naltrexone has been shown to improve psychosocial functioning and support abstinence from gambling when compared with placebo (Grant et al 2014).

PREVALENCE OF SUBSTANCE USE AND CO-OCCURRING DISORDERS

Internationally, there is increasing recognition of the difficulties faced by people with substance use and co-occurring mental health disorders (Substance Abuse and Mental Health Services Administration (SAMHSA) 2023; United Nations Office on Drugs and Crime (UNODC) 2020; Alcohol and Drug Foundation (ADF) 2022). People with substance use disorders are at a heightened risk for the development of a range of primary health and chronic diseases and this is often associated with overall poorer engagement in treatment (SAMHSA 2023). The presence of co-occurring disorders is also correlated with a number of functional impairments which may manifest as difficulties in relationships, social isolation, poor education and vocational achievement and legal problems (Otasowie 2020).

During 2020, approximately 284 million people across the world had used a drug in the preceding 12-month period (UNODC 2022). In Australia, there has been a marked increase in the number of deaths associated with substance use, which peaked during 2016 at 1808 deaths (Australian Bureau of Statistics (ABS) 2017). It is important to note that more recent data has to be interpreted with caution due to the impact on reporting during the COVID-19 pandemic. Drug-related deaths are primarily associated with prescription medications such as benzodiazepines and opioids, which is consistent with increasing concern internationally about the abuse of prescription drugs (UNODC 2022).

There are also causal relationships between alcohol consumption and more than 200 types of disease and injury (WHO 2018a). It is worth noting that a significant proportion of the alcohol disease burden is due to road accidents, violence and suicides. In 2022, the harmful use of alcohol caused more than 5.1% of the total global burden of

BOX 13.1   Problem Gambling Severity Index (PGSI)

The PGSI is the standardised measure of risk associated with problem gambling. The PGSI asks participants to self-assess gambling over the preceding 12 months.

Scores
- Never = 0
- Rarely = 1
- Sometimes = 1
- Often = 2
- Always = 3

Categories
- Non-problem gambler (score: 0) – Non-problem gamblers gamble with no negative consequences.
- Low-risk gambler (score: 1–2) – Low-risk gamblers experience a low level of problems with few or no identified negative consequences (e.g. occasional spend over their limit or feel guilty for gambling).
- Moderate-risk gambler (score: 3–7) – Moderate-risk gamblers experience a moderate level of problems leading to some negative consequences (e.g. sometimes spending more than they can afford, lose track of time or feel guilty about their gambling).
- Problem gambler (score: 8 or above) – Problem gamblers gamble with negative consequences and a possible loss of control (e.g. often spending over their limit, gambling to win back money, feelings of stress associated with gambling).

- It is important to note that these categories do not reflect a diagnosis, rather an identification of risk.

Questions
1. Have you bet more than you could really afford to lose?
   Never   Sometimes   Most of the time   Always
2. Have you needed to gamble with larger amounts of money to get the same feeling of excitement?
   Never   Sometimes   Most of the time   Always
3. Have you gone back on another day to try to win back the money you lost?
   Never   Sometimes   Most of the time   Always
4. Have you borrowed money or sold anything to gamble?
   Never   Sometimes   Most of the time   Always
5. Have you felt that you might have a problem with gambling?
   Never   Sometimes   Most of the time   Always
6. Have people criticised your betting or told you that you had a gambling problem, whether or not you thought it was true?
   Never   Sometimes   Most of the time   Always
7. Have you felt guilty about the way you gamble or what happens when you gamble?
   Never   Sometimes   Most of the time   Always
8. Has gambling caused you any health problems, including stress or anxiety?
   Never   Sometimes   Most of the time   Always
9. Has your gambling caused any financial problems for you or your household?
   Never   Sometimes   Most of the time   Always

Victorian Responsible Gambling Foundation 2018.

disease (approximately 3 million deaths) (WHO 2022). Specifically, in those aged 20–39 years, around 13.5% of all deaths are associated with alcohol (WHO 2022).

Australia

The use of alcohol, tobacco and other drugs continues to be a major cause of preventable disease in Australia (AIHW 2022a). The proportion of Australians drinking in excess across their lifetime has gradually declined since 2001 (AIHW 2022a). Nevertheless, most Australians aged over 14 years continue to consume alcohol, and alcohol remains the most commonly detected substance across all states and territories in the national wastewater drug monitoring program (AIHW 2022).

Wastewater analysis in Australia provides estimates on drug use patterns by measuring concentrations of drug metabolites found in wastewater samples (Australian Criminal Intelligence Commission (ACIC) 2020). Alcohol and nicotine consistently remain the highest out of the substances tested for and substance use more broadly remains slightly higher in regional settings when compared to capital cities (ACIC 2020). Despite this, there has been a steady increase in the number of Australians who have never smoked tobacco (AIHW 2022a).

The most commonly abused drug in Australia, after alcohol and tobacco, is cannabis (AIHW 2022a). However, there has been a significant increase in the number of deaths associated with methamphetamine use despite a reduction in recent use in those aged 14 and over from 3.4% in 2001 to 1.3% in 2019 (AIHW 2022c). From 2013 to 2016 the percentage of methamphetamine users reporting mental health changes had also increased from 29% to 42% (AIHW 2017). Across Australia it has been consistently reported by those who regularly use stimulants that methamphetamine is easily accessible when compared to other illicit substances (AIHW 2022c).

Similarly, the harms associated with using illicit opioids, primarily heroin, continue to rise. There has been a gradual increase in the number of hospitalisations associated with heroin use; however, in those admitted to hospital with a principal diagnosis of opioid poisoning, it was more likely that prescription opioids were involved rather than heroin or other illicit opioids (AIHW 2022b). Importantly, the Australian market for heroin has changed dramatically since the years prior to the COVID-19 pandemic, with less stability in terms of purity and availability of heroin (AIHW 2022b).

The impact of medically supervised injecting rooms (MSIR) in supporting people who inject drugs must not be overlooked in this context. The Sydney Medically Supervised Injecting Centre (MSIC) has managed over 10,000 overdoses since opening in 2001 (Uniting Care 2022) and the Melbourne MSIR managed over 5000 overdoses from 2018 to 2021, while also providing in excess of 100,000 episodes of health and social support (North Richmond Community Health 2022).

Hospital emergency departments (EDs) across the country continue to provide front-line treatment for a range of complications associated with substance use, with 13% of ED presentations across Australia associated with alcohol use and 2.8% related to methamphetamine use (Australasian College for Emergency Medicine 2020). The nature of substance use continues to change, and it has become increasingly prevalent that people will use more than one substance concurrently. Subsequently, EDs must consider the impact of multiple substance use, rather than focusing on one substance only, and consider how those substances may interact.

Finally, prescription drug use has steadily increased in Australia over the past decade. During 2019, Australians were more likely to endorse the use of non-prescribed prescription opioids and analgesics than any other illicit substance (AIHW 2022d). From 1997 through to 2020 the rate of deaths associated with benzodiazepines continued to rise from 1.9% per 100,000 population to 3.2% per 100,000 population (AIHW 2022d). This is of particular concern for nurses because many of these prescription drug use disorders begin while people are patients in the hospital setting and as part of a therapeutic treatment regimen.

Aotearoa New Zealand

There has been an overall decline in alcohol drinking patterns across Aotearoa New Zealand; however, one in five adults still meet criteria for engaging in hazardous drinking (Ministry of Health 2018a). In 2015–16, 80% of adults reported drinking alcohol at least once in the previous year, with 31% indicating they had consumed alcohol at least twice in the previous week (Ministry of Health 2018a).

Tobacco consumption has reduced significantly across Aotearoa New Zealand when compared with Australia. Nevertheless, despite the consistent decline in cigarette smoking, Aotearoa New Zealand continues to struggle with an estimated 9% physical health loss directly attributable to tobacco use (Drug Foundation 2018). Cannabis is reported to be used by 15% of adult men and 8% of adult women (Ministry of Health 2015). Of those who regularly use cannabis, 42% report medicinal use (e.g. to treat pain), with older users (over 55 years) reporting higher rates of medicinal use (Ministry of Health 2015). Amphetamine use has not changed significantly over the past decade in Aotearoa New Zealand, remaining stable at around 1.1% of adults reporting use (Ministry of Health 2018a). For a more detailed examination of multicultural differences between Australian and Aotearoa New Zealand populations, which may in part explain some of these trends, see Chapter 1.

✳ HISTORICAL ANECDOTE 13.1

Ancient Remedies

Alcohol, cannabis and opium all have a long history of being prescribed for symptoms of mental ill health. Alcohol was a standard medical prescription up until the 1900s. In 1892 Dr Adolphus Bridger (1852–1920) wrote: "Depressed elderly should be given full bodied burgundy, high class claret, port, the better French, German and Italian wines... A suitable form of alcohol will often do more to restore nervous health in old age than any medicine."

Cannabis was regularly prescribed for patients who experienced depression or mania and was widely marketed as a medication in England and Germany up until 1940. Opium, the milky juice of the unripe poppy, has been prescribed by physicians since the days of the ancient Greeks. In the 1700 and 1800s private asylums that used opium to treat depression and anxiety became popular throughout Europe.

Read More About It
Ishizuka H 2010 Carlyle's nervous dyspepsia: Nervousness, indigestion and the experience of modernity in nineteenth-century Britain. In: Salisbury L, Shail A (eds), Neurology and modernity: A cultural history of nervous systems, 1800–1950. Palgrave Macmillan, London.

SUBSTANCE USE AND MISUSE AMONG SPECIFIC POPULATIONS

Indigenous Australians

Substance use and misuse among Indigenous Australians is a matter of the utmost concern and continues to be another area of healthcare where Indigenous Australians are over-represented. The health of Aboriginal and Torres Strait Islander people is improving in several areas; however, they continue to suffer from the results of colonisation, causing significant health inequalities (AIHW 2021a).

Alcohol use is associated with significant social disruption, and approximately nine out of ten Indigenous Australians who have had contact with the criminal justice system used alcohol which then contributed to their offence (AIHW 2021a; Brett et al 2016). Across all indicators (rates of hospitalisation, mental health disorders, physical and social harms, and drug and alcohol use), Indigenous Australians are disproportionately affected. The Goanna study was a large national survey of 2877 Indigenous participants from across all states and territories of Australia and provides the most representative data regarding illicit substance use among Indigenous Australians (Bryant et al 2016). Cannabis was found to be the most commonly used illicit substance, with around one in five reporting weekly or more frequent use (Bryant et al 2016; Wand et al 2016). The use of illicit substances other than cannabis was not common, with use being more prevalent in urban areas; this was attributed to increased ease of access (Bryant et al 2016; Wand et al 2016).

Indigenous Australians have less access to alcohol and other drug treatment programs. The gap in service availability is contributing to the ongoing harms experienced by Indigenous Australians (Brett et al 2016). However, in 2020 17% of those entering alcohol and other drug treatment services were Indigenous Australians (AIHW 2021a).

The Fitzroy Crossing project is an example of courage and resilience among a group of Aboriginal women in the remote Kimberley region of Australia who wanted to address the rising rate of alcohol use among their community (George Institute for Global Health 2023). The group came together, with the support of many men within the First Nation's community, to ban full-strength alcohol in their community. Ultimately, the collaboration of researchers, human rights advocates and the women themselves led to the reduction in rates of domestic violence and alcohol abuse in the community (George Institute for Global Health 2023).

Aotearoa New Zealand Māori

The most recent data available on alcohol consumption and related harm among Māori show that Māori have similar rates of alcohol consumption as the total Aotearoa New Zealand population, but have higher rates of hazardous drinking (this trend remained consistent over 3 years) (Ministry of Health 2018b). This places them at high risk of short-term harm from alcohol use and contributes to statistics that demonstrate more alcohol-related harm occurring among Māori, particularly Māori women, than non-Māori (Ministry of Health 2018b). There is a greater representation of young Māori people drinking hazardously when compared to non-Māori populations, which may be directly contributing to the increased harm experienced by Māori people in Aotearoa New Zealand (Ministry of Health 2018a).

A 2015 survey indicated that Māori men were 2.1 times more likely and Māori women were 2.3 times more likely to use cannabis compared with non-Māori (Ministry of Health 2015). Weekly cannabis use is higher in the most deprived areas of Aotearoa New Zealand (45%) compared with the least deprived areas (20%) (Ministry of Health 2015). For a more detailed discussion of Indigenous Australian and Torres Strait Islander mental health, and Māori health, see chapters 6 and 7.

Pregnancy, Lactation and Parenting

The proportion of women consuming alcohol during pregnancy has been steadily declining since 2007 (AIHW 2017). In 2016, the majority of women abstained from alcohol while they were pregnant (56%), and of those who continued to drink alcohol, 81% reported drinking monthly or less (AIHW 2017). A much smaller proportion of women continued to use illicit substances after finding out that they were pregnant (1.8%) (AIHW 2017). There is a plethora of evidence demonstrating the link between heavy alcohol use in pregnancy and miscarriage, premature birth, stillbirth and the development of gestational hypertension (Cesconetto et al 2016; Dumas et al 2018; The Royal Women's Hospital 2018a). Alcohol passes rapidly through the placenta and into the baby's blood stream, which can lead to a deterioration, or malfunction, in the baby's developing central nervous system (CNS) (Cesconetto et al 2016; The Royal Women's Hospital 2018a).

In order to reduce the risk of harm towards an unborn child, it is now recommended that women who are pregnant or planning pregnancy should not drink alcohol at all (National Health and Medical Research Council (NHMRC) 2020). Further, the NHMRC (2020) has identified that there is a lack of robust and high-quality human studies examining the effects of maternal alcohol consumption on lactation, development and fetal behaviour. As such, it is not possible to establish a "safe" level of alcohol consumption while breastfeeding (NHMRC 2020).

Data collection regarding rates of alcohol use in the prenatal period is essential to identifying neonates at risk of developing fetal alcohol spectrum disorder (FASD) (Cesconetto et al 2016). FASD is a chronic disorder that causes physical and/or neurodevelopment impairment as a result of fetal exposure to alcohol (NOFASD 2018). FASD is characterised by a range of neurodevelopmental problems, as well as facial and other physical abnormalities (although physical anomalies may not always be present; see Table 13.1 for diagnostic criteria and key features of a FASD assessment) (Bower & Elliot 2016).

Smoking during pregnancy has been identified as the single most common preventable risk factor for complications (AIHW 2018). In 2016, one in 10 mothers smoked at some point during their pregnancy and those women were associated with fewer antenatal care visits than those who did not smoke (AIHW 2018). Smoking tobacco during pregnancy is associated with a reduction in the supply of oxygen and blood to the developing baby (The Royal Women's Hospital 2018b). Nicotine causes an increase in heart rate in both the mother and the fetus, which can contribute to the narrowing of blood vessels, thereby reducing the flow of blood through the umbilical cord (The Royal Women's Hospital 2018b). Smoking tobacco during pregnancy is associated with miscarriage, low birth weight and premature birth (The Royal Women's Hospital 2018b).

Although evidence is limited, universal screening for alcohol and other drug use in pregnancy (including tobacco) is recommended (NHMRC 2020; American College of Obstetricians and Gynaecologists 2017). This reduces targeted screening of groups that are marginalised, reduces stigma and reduces the under-identification of alcohol and other drug use in pregnancy. Pregnancy is a critical time to address maternal alcohol and other drug use; however, any changes to substance use during pregnancy must be carefully considered due to the significant stress that a withdrawal syndrome can cause the fetus.

LGBTIQA+ people

Substance use rates among the gender and sexually diverse community are consistently proportionally higher when compared to the general population. It is important to note that the LGBTIQA+ acronym does not necessarily capture the true diversity of identities, sexualities and relationships experienced within the community; however, it is an invaluable term when considering the experience of stigma and discrimination which contributes to the increased rates of substance use (Meridian 2021). Increased rates of alcohol and other drug use among the LGBTIQA+ community has been associated with unique stressors that this population faces with regards to social isolation, marginalisation and discrimination (Hill et al 2022). This is further complicated by peer pressure, high and early exposure to substance use and high concentrations of licensed venues in LGBTIQA+ communities (Demant et al 2018).

TABLE 13.1 Fetal Alcohol Spectrum Disorder

Diagnostic Criteria	DIAGNOSTIC CRITERIA	
	FASD With 3 Sentinel Facial Features	FASD With < 3 Sentinel Facial Features
Prenatal Alcohol Exposure	*Confirmed or Unknown*	*Confirmed*
Neurodevelopmental domains: • brain structure/neurology • motor skills • cognition • language • academic achievement • memory • attention • executive function, including poor impulse control and hyperactivity • affect regulation • adaptive behaviour, social skills or social communication	Severe impairment in at least 3 neurodevelopmental domains	Severe impairment in at least 3 neurodevelopmental domains
Sentinel facial features: • short palpebral fissure • smooth philtrum • thin upper lip	Presence of 3 sentinel facial features	Presence of 0–2 sentinel facial features
Key features of FASD diagnostic assessment: • history: Presenting concerns, obstetric, developmental, medical, mental health, behavioural, social • birth defects: Dysmorphic facial features, other major and minor birth defects • adverse prenatal and postnatal exposures (including alcohol) • known medical conditions including genetic syndromes and other disorders • growth		

Adapted from FASD Hub 2016.

Compared to heterosexual and cis-gender Australians, LGBTIQA+ people are 1.5 times more likely to smoke tobacco, 3.9 times more likely to have used methamphetamine in the last 12 months and overall more likely to have used some form of illicit substance in the past 12 months (LGBTIQ Health 2020). The LGBTIQA+ community is therefore recognised as a priority population as part of the National Drug Strategy due to these persistently high rates of substance use (LGBTIQ Health 2020).

Homelessness

People experiencing homelessness struggle with a range of health and social inequalities. Further exacerbating this is the strong association between homelessness, substance use and mental health changes. From 2021 to 2022, 9% of clients in Australia accessing specialist homelessness services reported concurrent alcohol or other drug use (AIHW 2022a). In Melbourne, Victoria, 43% of the homeless population reported using alcohol and/or other drugs (AIHW 2022a). From 2019 to 2020, 31% of clients with harmful substance use disorders reported current mental health changes and experiencing some form of family or domestic violence, which contributed to episodes of homelessness (AIHW 2022a). Unfortunately, higher levels of substance use have been correlated with prolonging periods of homelessness, which then further contributes to difficulties with accessing health and social support service providers (AIHW 2022a).

PHARMACOLOGY OF PSYCHOACTIVE DRUGS

Pharmacological Aspects of Addiction

When people take drugs, drink alcohol, eat, exercise, gamble or have sex, multiple neurotransmitters are released as part of the pleasure and reward feedback system in the brain. In particular, dopamine is released along the mesolimbic dopamine pathway in the ventral tegmental area (Berridge & Kringelbach 2015; Moore et al 2014). The release of dopamine reinforces the behaviour by producing positive feelings and a sense of wellbeing. It is a central mechanism and communicates to the person that the activity is vital for survival and should be focused upon

(Robertson et al 2015). Importantly, it is the activation of the mesolimbic dopamine pathway by psychoactive substances and other behaviours not associated with the maintenance of life (e.g. gambling) that can lead to addiction. The repeated activation of this pathway contributes to the inability of people with substance use disorders and behavioural addictions to prioritise activities of daily living appropriately. Neurotransmission in the dependent person's brain is fundamentally different from that of the general population, creating a sense that their substance use, or other behaviour, is vital to their survival (Nutt et al 2015).

This psychoactive effect includes changes in mood, arousal, perception, thinking and behaviour. Drugs may be produced in a laboratory (e.g. amphetamines, ecstasy) or extracted from plants (e.g. heroin, cocaine). They can be legal (e.g. alcohol) or illegal (e.g. heroin).

Using categories can greatly assist with identifying similar features of intoxication and withdrawal; for example, alcohol and benzodiazepines are both depressants, so present very similarly during periods of acute intoxication (Australian Government 2021). Some drugs have multiple actions and therefore can be placed in more than one category (Australian Government 2021) (see Table 13.2 for the classification of substances based on their impact on CNS). The common effect of all psychoactive drugs, at least in the early stages of use, is to produce euphoria and a change in conscious state.

Over time, as tolerance develops, many individuals will experience fewer positive effects of substance use (e.g. euphoria). Rather, persistent use simply reduces the onset of withdrawal symptoms, which can be a significant driver of ongoing and longer-term substance use.

Novel Psychoactive Substances

The class of substances known as "novel psychoactive substances" refers to a class of drugs that are essentially similar, but not identical, to other currently available drugs (Burns et al 2014). Novel psychoactive substances are chemically produced to mimic the effects of other drugs (e.g., methamphetamine or cocaine); however, they possess a different chemical structure so may avoid detection by law enforcement agencies (UNODC 2023).

TABLE 13.2 Classification of Substances

Category	Description	Examples
Sedative Hypnotics	Depressants are drugs that slow the activity of the brain and the CNS (it is important to note that this is not associated with mood). When used in small doses they can produce euphoria, relaxation or drowsiness. In larger doses, they can produce a loss of consciousness similar to a deep sleep, impaired coordination, depression, coma and death by respiratory depression.	Alcohol (ethanol) Benzodiazepines (e.g. diazepam, alprazolam) Opioids (e.g. heroin, morphine, codeine) Barbiturates (e.g. phenobarbitone) Volatile substances (e.g. solvents or petrol)
Stimulants	Stimulant drugs increase activity in the CNS and increase the body's level of arousal. Small doses increase awareness and concentration and decrease fatigue. Increasing amounts produce irritability, nervousness and insomnia. At high doses some people experience delusions and hallucinations. Toxic doses lead to convulsions and death via heart attack (myocardial infarction), stroke (cerebrovascular accident) or muscle meltdown (rhabdomyolysis) (Ries et al 2014). Methamphetamine is broken down into three further categories: base, powder and crystal. Ecstasy previously contained only MDMA; however, it is now being cut with a range of different adulterants, in particular, crystal methamphetamine.	Amphetamines (e.g. "speed") Methamphetamine (e.g. crystal methamphetamine or "ice") 3,4-methylenedioxymethamphetamine Cocaine Nicotine Caffeine D-amphetamine (dexamphetamine) Methylphenidate (Ritalin)
Hallucinogens	Hallucinogens (also called "psychedelics") share properties with depressants and stimulants. However, their specific function is to distort perception and consequently induce hallucinations (auditory, tactile and visual). In small doses, some hallucinogens reduce inhibitions and cause the user to become relaxed and feel more sociable. Some amphetamine derivatives such as MDMA (ecstasy) are chemically related to mescaline and have both stimulant and hallucinatory properties. These drugs may be placed in both categories for classification purposes.	Lysergic acid diethylamide (LSD) Psilocybin ("magic mushrooms") Mescaline (part of the Mexican cactus "peyote") Datura ("angel's trumpet")

Continued

Category	Description	Examples
Opioids	While opioids are generally considered sedative hypnotics or depressants, it is important to consider opioids in their own classification due to the rising harm associated with prescription opioids. Opioids are morphine-like substances that work by binding to the opioid receptors which are predominantly located in the CNS, peripheral nervous system and GIT. Opioids as a classification include both endogenous (those created naturally by the body), exogenous (those administered from the external environment), natural (e.g. morphine) and synthetic (e.g. fentanyl). Opioids are used clinically for their potent analgesic effects, anti-diarrhoeal properties and cough-suppressant effects. Short-term adverse effects involve sedation, constipation, nausea and vomiting. When given at high doses, opioids may result in respiratory depression leading to death (Government of South Australia 2023).	Heroin Morphine Oxycodone Codeine Fentanyl Tramadol Tapentadol Methadone Buprenorphine Hydromorphone
Other	Cannabis is often difficult to classify in pharmacological terms because it has a mixture of mood, cognitive, motor and perceptual effects and does not clearly belong with any one drug class (Kleinloog et al 2014). Cannabis taken in low doses produces a mixture of stimulatory and depressant effects; at high doses the effects are mainly depressant. The effects of cannabis include euphoria, relaxation and a feeling of wellbeing, as well as perceptual distortions such as altered time sense. Memory, cognition and skilled task performance are impaired, although many users may feel confident and highly creative. Other physical effects include tachycardia, vasodilation and hypotension (Kleinloog et al 2014; Martin-Santos et al 2012). Cannabis stimulates the appetite and is also an antiemetic; people who have taken cannabis often experience "the munchies", when they feel hungry and crave certain foods. As with all psychoactive drugs, the effects vary between people depending on the amount taken, the manner of administration, the frequency of use, concurrent use with other drugs, past exposure and the environment in which the drug is used (Kleinloog et al 2014).	Cannabis Hashish Marijuana

TABLE 13.2   Classification of Substances—cont'd

Novel psychoactive substances may be known as "legal highs", "bath salts" or "research chemicals" (UNODC 2019). These substances are constantly being developed and modified to stay ahead of legal restrictions. To avoid confusion, UNODC (2019) clearly defines these substances as: "substances of abuse, either in a pure form or a preparation, that are not controlled by the 1961 Single Convention on Narcotic Drugs or the 1971 Convention on Psychotropic Substances, but which may post a public health threat".

Determining the pharmacology and toxicity of novel psychoactive substance is challenging as new variations are being constantly developed and often involve slight alterations to existing formulations (UNODC 2023). See Table 13.3 for further details on different forms of novel psychoactive substances currently in circulation.

Synthetic Cannabinoids

Delta-9-tetrahydrocannabinol (THC) is the active component in natural cannabis and is a partial agonist of the CB1 and CB2 cannabinoid receptors (Akram et al 2019). In contrast, synthetic cannabinoids tend to be full agonists at cannabinoid receptor sites and, as a result, causes them to be more potent than natural cannabis (Akram et al 2019; Sud et al 2018). This creates more intense symptoms during periods of intoxication and withdrawal, as well as placing users at higher risk of longer-term psychological changes. Common street names for synthetic cannabinoids include "Spice", "K2", "Kroc", "Purple Haze" and "Buddha" (Akram et al 2019).

Synthetic cannabinoids are generally distributed as a green, leafy product that is sprayed with a chemical containing synthetic cannabinoids (Clancy et al 2018). One of the major difficulties with the treatment and management of synthetic cannabinoids is that new variations are constantly being developed. Each chemical variation is associated with different risk factors and complications of use. Synthetic cannabinoid users present with a range of behavioural, affective and cognitive changes (Clancy et al 2018). Acute effects may involve CNS depression presenting as lethargy and bradycardia (Sud et al 2018). Synthetic cannabinoids have also been associated with an increased risk of seizures. Synthetic cannabinoids do not show up on conventional urine drug screens, so their use has become more widespread among individuals in workplaces that require regular drug screening.

✸ HISTORICAL ANECDOTE 13.2
Cocaine and Methamphetamine as Medicine?

Cocaine has been used in South America since ancient times (processed from the leaves of the Erythroxylon cocoa plant). Sigmund Freud wrote about the mental health benefits of cocaine as an antidepressant, eventually developing an addiction to the drug. By the early 1900s it became hugely popular in America and was used as an active ingredient in many popular products, including cocoa leaf cigarettes and the soft drink Coca-Cola. Methamphetamine was widely marketed by pharmaceutical companies as a powerful antidepressant. It was used by both the Allies and German armies during World War II to improve soldiers' aggression and endurance. Adolph Hitler became addicted to methamphetamine and opium.

Read More About It
Rasmussen N 2011 Medical science and the military: The Allies' use of amphetamine during World War II. J Interdiscipl History, 42(2): 205–233.

TABLE 13.3 Novel Psychoactive Substances

Drug	Similar to/Effects	Examples
Aminoindanes	Similar to amphetamines and MDMA. Creates similar CNS activity as stimulants. Later versions of these drugs have been able to mimic empathogenic and entactogenic effects of drugs such MDMA.	"M-DAI Gold" (5,6-methylenedioxy-animoindane) "Pink champagne" (2-aminoindane) Commonly found in powder form or crystals for ingestion.
Phencyclidine-type substances	Similar to CNS stimulants such as phencyclidine (PCP). Creates dissociative effects via modulation of NMDA receptors.	Limited information about PCP analogues; known as "research chemicals". Ketamine Ingestion is the most common route of administration for this class of substances. Ketamine is also intravenously and intramuscularly injected.
Phenethylamines	Includes amphetamines (methamphetamine/MDMA), amphetamine variations (2C series and D series drugs) and hallucinogen variations (stimulants with some hallucinogenic effects). These substances act as either CNS stimulants or as hallucinogens. This class includes synthetic analogues of mescaline (potent hallucinogens).	2C agents: 2C1, 2CB, 2CT, 2CE "Europa", NBom, PMMA (para-Methoxy-N-methylamphetamine) "4-MMA" D Series: DOC, DOI Dihydrofuran substances: "FLY", "Dragonfly", "Bromo-Dragonfly" Ingestion is the most common route of administration for this class of substances.
Piperazines	Similar effects to hallucinogens, with some stimulant activity. Termed "failed pharmaceuticals" because some of the substances found in this class have been trialled as potential therapeutic agents.	BZP – trialled as an antidepressant, however, had similar properties to amphetamines. "Pep pills"
Synthetic cannabinoids	Synthetic cannabinoids are added to plant material. Initially, these were synthetic analogues of delta-9-tetrahydroncannabinol; however, different groups of synthetic cannabinoids have since been developed with significant variance in chemical makeup.	"K2", "Kroc", "Black Mamba", "Purple Haze", "Spice", "Genie" Smoking is the most common route of administration for this class of substances.
Synthetic cathinone	Chemically similar structure to amphetamine and methamphetamines. Cathinone is the principal agent in khat plant and is considered the basis on which many synthetic cathinones are developed.	Mephedrone, methadone, methylone, meow, M-Cat, "drone", "bath salts", "plant food" Ingestion is the most common route of administration for this class of substances.
Tryptamines	Primarily derivatives of hallucinogens such as psilocybin and DMT. These substances tend to mimic the effects of existing hallucinogens; however, they may also possess stimulant activity.	"Foxy-methoxy", "alpha-o", "5-MEO" Ingestion is the most common route of administration for this class of substances.

Musselman & Hampton 2014 and United Nations Office on Drugs and Crime 2023.

CONTRIBUTING FACTORS TO SUBSTANCE USE DISORDER

The development of a substance use disorder is complex and multifaceted. Consideration must be given to the interplay between the person's environment, social situation and genetic influences. Adolescents may turn to substance use in response to social isolation, peer pressure, poor academic achievement, family disruption, poor attachment or simple curiosity (SAMHSA 2017). This is further influenced by society and the way various substances are portrayed in the media (e.g. the consequence-free use of drinking and smoking cigarettes in movies and television series) (SAMHSA 2017). Risk factors for developing a substance use disorder will vary significantly according to age, social/psychological development, ethnic/cultural background and environmental surroundings (SAMHSA 2017). SAMHSA (2017) advocates for a greater focus on protective factors against substance use (see Table 13.4).

During adolescence, the brain undergoes significant development; this increases a person's susceptibility to stress and high-risk behaviours. Direct causal mechanisms behind substance use are still relatively unknown; however, twin studies are starting to clearly demonstrate hereditary influences (Boisvert et al 2019; Waaktaar et al 2018). Substance use disorders may also develop later in life in response to a range of stressors, although are often influenced by early life events, such as childhood adverse experiences. Alcohol use disorders are most common among older persons and are frequently associated with retirement, age-related impairments that create difficulties with activities of daily living (ADLs) or the loss of a partner (Lehmann & Fingerhood 2018). Problems with prescription medication may also occur during adulthood and later life in the absence of earlier influencing factors. Chronic pain is more prevalent among older adults, and there is a tendency for adults to more easily access benzodiazepines in response to stressful life events (Lehmann & Fingerhood 2018).

THE EXPERIENCE OF A SUBSTANCE USE DISORDER

The experience of a substance use disorder will vary significantly among individuals, and treatment approaches should be adjusted accordingly. No one treatment pathway will be the same, and nurses should adopt a flexible approach when working with someone with a substance use disorder. The concept of hope and the idea that recovery is possible are important. Health professionals can easily, and inadvertently, become frustrated at the rates of relapse associated with substance use disorders. Further, many people with substance use disorders face significant levels of stigma from

---

TABLE 13.4 Protective Factors for Adolescents

Individual Factors	• Positive temperament
	• Social skills (e.g. problem-solving, ability to stand up for beliefs and core values)
	• Positive social orientation (e.g. engaging in activities that contribute to healthy personal development, accepting rules and community values, identifying with school and choosing friends who don't use harmful substances)
	• Belief in one's ability to control what happens to adapt to change
Family Factors	• Unity, warmth and attachment between parents and children
	• Parental supervision
	• Contact and communication between and among parents and children
Environmental Factors	• Positive emotional support outside of the family such as friends, neighbours and elders
	• Supports and resources available to the family (e.g. crisis lines, programs for individuals with trauma experiences, stress management supports or family counselling)
	• Community and school norms, beliefs and standards regarding substance use
	• Access to education that focuses on commitment and achievement

Adapted from Substance Abuse and Mental Health Services Administration 2017.

healthcare providers, which is often driven by a lack of education and understanding as to how to work with people with substance use disorders. This may present as a fear of being deceived by this patient population and a mistrust of the patient's motives for presentation to healthcare providers (Biancarelli et al 2019). It is therefore imperative that healthcare providers, including nurses, recognise any pre-existing judgements to enable them to continue to work towards instilling hope and fostering self-efficacy as tools in developing rapport with this particularly vulnerable population (Chapman et al 2020).

There is increasing recognition and support for the implementation of lived experience workforce across the hospital, mental health and alcohol and other drug sectors (Chapman et al 2020). Nurses should aim to work closely with the lived, or peer, workforce to assist in breaking down some of these barriers to access care (Chapman et al 2020). See Personal perspectives: Consumer's story 13.1 to 13.3 for a range of addiction experiences.

👤 PERSONAL PERSPECTIVES

Consumer's Story 13.1: Anonymous

Life for me has always been a huge struggle and I could never understand why. From a young age, I stopped being able to process emotions like my friends and family could. I felt immense pain just being me. So, when drugs and alcohol came along at age 14, I thought I'd found my solution. But once I started I couldn't stop, and my life got progressively worse and more unmanageable. After 8 years of a toxic spiral of feeling guilt, shame and remorse and then using again, I landed in a recovery rehab. It was my last option. Something had to change or I would eventually die.

I was introduced to community-based self-help groups. I was introduced to the solution. I now had a program to feel everything I had been so afraid to feel; and I didn't have to go through any of it alone. There was always a woman with more clean time who had been through what I had been through. I worked the recovery program and my self-esteem and self-worth started to grow. For the first time I started to create a relationship with myself by believing in a higher power. I am now nearly 9 months clean from all drugs and alcohol, and I've honestly never been happier.

👤 PERSONAL PERSPECTIVES

Consumer's Story 13.2: Sari

I grew up in a small country town and was very much loved. I can only say that now looking back though, because at the time, despite presenting as a happy child who did well at school and sports, I often felt scared, sad, confused, unlovable and not good enough. My father committed suicide when I was a baby, so I always felt different to everyone else. I do distinctly remember though always hating drugs, wanting to do the right thing, and to be a good person. As a young adult, I left the farm and became a nurse in the city. I loved my job, and helping others seemed to soothe that feeling of unworthiness.

In my early 20s I had a bad car accident and began to develop chronic pain. I was able to manage this mostly with over-the-counter pain relief; however, after my second child was born in my late 20s the pain became unbearable and my doctor put me onto a short course of oxycodone. Before I knew it this short course quickly became 3 years of hell. The first year I must admit was great. I could get everything done! I could function incredibly as a wife, mother, nurse, daughter, sister, friend, human being. I truly believed I had found the one thing that filled the vague hole in my chest. Unfortunately, after that first year things quickly went downhill. I was needing more and more to get me through, and

I was withdrawing from life and everyone in it. All I wanted was to be alone with my drugs; I couldn't answer the phone, the door, or open my mail, and doctor shopping became a full-time job. I was consumed by my need for them and felt like I would die without them in my system. After only 3 short years my drug addiction had completely brought me to my knees, and I knew I could no longer live like this. I felt I was so broken that I had no choice but to finally ask for help and I began to pay attention to my faintly growing hope that there might possibly be a better way for me to live.

I went into rehab with the firm belief that this was just a physical condition that would resolve once I had detoxed and had a break, but I soon found out I was wrong. My addiction had changed me. The day I was to be discharged I was overwhelmed with absolute terror of thinking, how on earth do I function without something in my system? It's hard to describe, but it was like my skin had been ripped off and all my fears and secrets were there to be seen. I relapsed that very day on over-the-counter opiates just to quieten the intense anxiety I was feeling. I was back in that rehab within 2 weeks feeling even more ashamed, afraid and angry than ever before. I was truly broken now and willing to do anything at

Consumer's Story 13.2: Sari

all to fix it. In the weeks prior, during my first stay in rehab, I'd been introduced to a 12-step fellowship and despite my medical background had become open to the idea that perhaps this wasn't just a physical problem, but also a mental and spiritual illness. I knew that I felt deeply depressed, lost and hollow, but still with the slightest glimmer of hope that life could be better. I also came to understand that no one else could fix me and this was a journey that I could only take alone, with a full commitment to being open, honest and completely abstinent from all mood- and mind-altering drugs, including alcohol. This was a hard truth to accept – everyone else drinks! But I wasn't like everyone else anymore. I knew that my brain worked differently now, and I was highly susceptible to relapse.

I was incredibly lucky in the fact that the desire to use a drug left me very quickly, roughly within a week, but I did still have some residual physical withdrawal symptoms almost 3 months later. I should also add that I have never struggled with chronic pain since. I put this down to taking care of my physical health, but also because I took the mental and spiritual aspect of the disease very seriously. I had never seen myself as someone who suffered from mental health issues before, but

since finding recovery it's something I must assess and monitor regularly. And despite my medical background, I firmly believe that learning to care for my spiritual health is what saved my life. I no longer have that hole in my chest and for the most part, feel content and happy within myself. If I hadn't been shown how to nurture all three aspects of my life then I wouldn't have a life worth living today, and if I neglect any one of them for too long then the other two will suffer soon after.

I'm certainly not proud of the places my addiction took me to, and having to swallow my pride, admit defeat and ask for help was possibly the hardest thing I've ever done. But I am forever grateful that I had faith in that little spark of hope and for the people who showed me that recovery was possible and forever within my grasp. I didn't choose to be an addict, but I do choose to recover and live my life to the best of my abilities. If there is one piece of advice I could ever give, it's that pride, fear and shame are powerful motivators to keep an addict sick in the cycle of misery. But willingness, honesty and hope are the keys to recovery and a new life. No one is ever completely hopeless or unworthy and recovery is possible for anyone.

Consumer's Story 13.3: Anonymous

I was trapped in the vicious cycle of addiction for 13 years. Being a young, carefree child was quickly ripped away and in crept relentless feelings of hopelessness and despair. Any hopes and dreams I had as a child seemed to have completely vanished from the horizon. I was resigned to the fact my life was effectively over; I really had thrown it all away and was destined to suffer a miserable existence. It was an incredibly painful and helpless place to be. From being in that place of utter despair, never would I have imagined it possible to be where I am today.

Today I am in recovery, 15 months clean and sober. I went to rehab for four and a half months and to supported accommodation from there. I was truly desperate to get clean and seek a better life for myself and my loved ones. Recovery is freedom like I never thought possible. Today I have a desire to live. I have hope, and I truly believe that if I remain clean and continue to say "yes" to change I will have a future beyond my wildest dreams. Connection is the cornerstone of recovery and I would never have been able to do it without the help and love of others. Abstaining from drugs and alcohol was just the beginning; I had to change everything – my thinking, the way I dealt with my emotions and what I thought I already knew about life. I wouldn't have it any other way. I like the man I am becoming and I'm very proud. Recovery is a lifelong process and a work in progress. It must come first in my life, for all that I have depends on it. It has given me my life back and for that I'm eternally grateful.

Signs and Symptoms

Intoxication

Acute intoxication on alcohol or other drugs can lead to an increased risk of aggression and disruptive behaviours. Intoxicated people can present in the clinical setting as frightened, disruptive and extremely upset at times. It is important to consider how we approach intoxicated clients to ensure the safety of the individual and those around them. Authoritarian approaches can provoke anger and aggression and should be avoided where possible.

When speaking with the client, ensure you use their name and speak in a slow, distinct voice using short, simple sentences. It is important to be genuine in your approach and to avoid using confusing or overly medical terminology. Maintain eye contact, without being intrusive, and do not attempt to engage in complex reasoning. (See Chapter 4 for useful skills in managing aggression and violence.)

It is important to consider the significant medical risks associated with acute intoxication on alcohol and other drugs (e.g. aspiration secondary to vomiting while acutely intoxicated on alcohol). The presence of other organic contributing factors for an acute change in mental state should also be considered (e.g. the presence of an acute delirium). Airway management is the primary concern in those who are unconscious (see Box 13.2). Careful consideration must be given to using sedating medications (e.g. benzodiazepines) in those who are acutely intoxicated on CNS depressants due to the increased risk of respiratory depression.

BOX 13.2 General Principles of Managing Intoxication

- Maintenance of airway is a priority.
- Any patient presenting as confused, disoriented or drowsy should be treated as per head injury until proven otherwise.
- Intoxicated patients must be kept under observation until the level of intoxication diminishes.
- A thorough physical and mental status examination will assist with determining the level of intoxication.
- Patients who appear intoxicated may also be suffering from other concurrent conditions, so if the intoxication does not diminish with falling serum drug levels, the patient must be assessed for other possible causes of their condition.
- If an intoxicated person cannot walk, stand or get up from a chair they must be closely monitored.
- Intoxicated patients should be treated with respect. Speak slowly and simply. Treat them in a low-stimulus environment where possible and provide clear information to reduce the risk of further harm such as falls.
- Patients should be continually assessed for withdrawal. Alcohol withdrawal can occur before a zero-blood alcohol reading is noted.
- Multiple and concurrent substance use is becoming increasingly prevalent. It is important to consider the effect of multiple agents and subsequent interactions.
- Any patient presenting with seizures should be assessed for alcohol withdrawal, benzodiazepine withdrawal or stimulant intoxication, as well as other possible causes. The seizures must be treated according to policy and the patient observed for at least 4 hours after the seizure using the Glasgow Coma Scale score (see Table 13.12).

Withdrawal

The signs and symptoms of withdrawal will vary among the substance classes. The dose and duration of drug use affects the withdrawal process in terms of symptoms experienced and the severity of the withdrawal syndrome (see Box 13.3 for diagnostic criteria for withdrawal) (see Table 13.5 for a summary of key features of withdrawal). Withdrawal can lead to significant and potentially life-threatening complications and, as such, requires close monitoring (Manning et al 2018).

The treatment of withdrawal can occur in a range of different settings and is often driven by client preference. In Australia, there are four different environments in which withdrawal may occur – residential withdrawal units ("detox"), medical detoxification in a hospital-based

---

BOX 13.3   Diagnostic Criteria for Withdrawal

The essential feature of withdrawal is the development of a range of substance-specific behavioural, psychological and cognitive changes to the cessation, or acute reduction in, heavy and long-term substance use. Specifically, the following four criteria must be met:

A – Cessation of, or reduction in use, that has been heavy and prolonged

B – Two (or more) of the following, developing within several hours to a few days after the cessation (or reduction) of the substance:
- autonomic hyperactivity (e.g. sweating or racing heart; pulse greater than 100 bpm)
- insomnia (trouble sleeping)
- increased hand tremors

- nausea or vomiting
- psychomotor agitation
- anxiety
- seizures (usually generalised tonic–clonic type – rhythmic jerking movement, especially of the limbs)
- transient visual, tactile or auditory hallucinations or illusions

C – The signs or symptoms in criterion B cause clinically significant distress or impairment in social, occupational or other important areas of functioning

D – These symptoms are not attributable to another medical condition and are not better explained by another mental disorder including intoxication or withdrawal from another substance.

TABLE 13.5   Key Features of Alcohol and Other Drug Withdrawal Syndromes

Drug	Onset	Duration	Clinical Features
Alcohol	Within 24 hours and up to 48 hours (depending on blood alcohol concentration (BAC), hours after last drink and level of neuroadaptation)	3–7 days (up to 14 in severe withdrawal)	Anxiety, agitation, sweating, tremors, nausea, vomiting, abdominal cramps, diarrhoea, craving, insomnia, elevated blood pressure, heart rate and temperature, headache, seizures, confusion, perceptual distortions, disorientation, hallucinations, seizures, delirium tremens, arrhythmias and Wernicke's encephalopathy
Nicotine	4–12 hours after last use	Peaks days 2–7 and continues in attenuated form for 2–4 weeks	Irritability, anger, anxiety, sadness, restlessness, sleep disturbance, increased hunger, sore throat, headache and difficulty concentrating
Cannabis	1–2 days after last use	Acute phase: 2–6 days, subsiding after 2–3 weeks. May persist for some months	Anger, aggression, irritability, anxiety, nervousness, decreased appetite or weight loss, restlessness, sleep disturbances, chills, depressed mood, shakiness and sweating
Benzodiazepines	1–10 days (depending on half-life of drug) after last use	3–6 weeks (or longer depending on the half-life of the drug)	Anxiety, headache, insomnia, muscle aching, twitching and cramping, nausea, vomiting, diarrhoea, perceptual changes, feelings of unreality, depersonalisation, seizures, agitation and confusion/psychosis
Opioids	Withdrawal from heroin and morphine can begin within 24 hours, while methadone and buprenorphine typically start later (days 3–5)	Heroin withdrawal typically peaks quickly (day 3), with more severe symptoms, subsiding fully within a week. Methadone and buprenorphine withdrawal result in a more protracted withdrawal, with a less abrupt peak and longer duration of symptoms	Runny eyes and nose, sneezing and sweating, agitation, irritability, loss of appetite, craving, abdominal cramps, diarrhoea, anxiety, irritability, disturbed sleep, fatigue, joint and muscle aches, nausea/vomiting and moodiness
Stimulants	Crash phase: Within hours of last use. Withdrawal: 1–4 days after last use	2–4 days. Acute phase: 7–10 days. Subacute phase: A further 2–4 weeks	Cravings, dysphoria, anhedonia, increased appetite, fatigue, agitation, anxiety, increased sleep, vivid, unpleasant dreams and slowing of movement
Ketamine	Within 24 hours of last use	4–6 days	Cravings, decreased appetite or weight loss, fatigue, chills, sweating, restlessness, tremors, disturbed sleep, anxiety, depression and irregular or rapid heartbeat
GHB	Within 12 hours of last use	Up to 15 days	Confusion, agitation, anxiety, depression, paranoia, hallucinations, disturbed sleep, cramps, tremors, sweating and rapid heartbeat

Adapted from Manning et al 2018.

withdrawal unit, medical withdrawal within a general hospital, or non-residential home-based withdrawal as an outpatient.

Alcohol withdrawal. The severity of an alcohol-related withdrawal syndrome is on a continuum from mild to severe (Manning et al 2018). Withdrawal will begin anywhere from 6 to 24 hours after the person's last drink and will peak between 36 and 72 hours. Symptoms will generally resolve after 5–7 days (see Fig. 13.1). The presence of other medical conditions and multiple substance use disorders will vary over the time course and severity of a withdrawal syndrome (Manning et al 2018).

Assessment scales can assist with tracking the severity of a withdrawal syndrome and responses to treatment. Rating scales available include the Alcohol Withdrawal Scale (AWS) and the Clinical Institute Withdrawal Assessment for Alcohol (Revised) (CIWA-Ar). Accurate utilisation of the CIWA-Ar for alcohol withdrawal management within the hospital system may significantly improve quality of care and patient safety (Melkonian et al 2019). However, these scales must be used with caution as concurrent medical, surgical and mental health conditions will complicate interpretation and confound scoring systems.

Medically managing and treating an alcohol withdrawal syndrome generally involves using benzodiazepines (Manning et al 2018). Diazepam is the most commonly used benzodiazepine due to its long half-life, active metabolites and anticonvulsant properties (St Vincent's Hospital Melbourne 2019). Shorter acting benzodiazepines, such as oxazepam, must be considered for those with compromised liver function, brain injuries or in the elderly (Manning et al 2018) (see Table 13.6 for recommended medical and non-medical management options).

There are some factors that predict the likely severity of alcohol withdrawal syndrome. One is whether the client has a long history of regular heavy alcohol use – for example, drinking 4 L of wine every day for the past 20 years. Another is the use of other psychoactive drugs, particularly CNS depressants such as benzodiazepines. Furthermore, if the person has a history of a complicated withdrawal syndrome – for example, delirium tremens or seizures – this places them at greater risk of withdrawal complications again in the future.

Benzodiazepine withdrawal. Benzodiazepine withdrawal will vary significantly depending on the duration of use and half-life of the benzodiazepine being used. Using short-acting benzodiazepines over an extended period can result in a complex withdrawal syndrome similar to that of alcohol, including similar risks of seizures, delirium and death if left untreated (Manning et al 2018). See Table 13.7 for a summary of expected withdrawal symptoms. Due to the variable nature of benzodiazepine withdrawal and potential complexities with concurrent other substance use, specialist consultation should be sought. Nurses should advocate for the continuation of regular benzodiazepines to avoid the onset of withdrawal until a planned taper can be developed in consultation with the client.

Opioid withdrawal. Opioid withdrawal varies significantly based on the substance being used, the route of administration, duration of use and the person's general health (Manning et al 2018). Longer acting opioids (e.g. methadone) are associated with a much slower onset of symptoms and an overall longer withdrawal syndrome when compared with short-acting opioids (e.g. heroin) (Manning et al 2018). Specialist consultation should be sought for individuals with prescription opioid use disorders.

Withdrawal from heroin is not generally life threatening for those clients who have limited co-occurring disorders and who are provided with adequate hydration and electrolyte replacement (Manning et al 2018). However, the risk of post-withdrawal relapse is very high in heroin users and withdrawal provides an opportunity to discuss opioid agonist treatment (e.g. methadone or buprenorphine). Heroin-related withdrawal will start 6–12 hours after the last use, peaks around 24–48 hours and subsides after 5–7 days (Manning et al 2018). Withdrawal symptoms include dilated pupils, runny eyes and nose, yawning, sweating, piloerection, agitation, irritability, fevers, loss of appetite, muscle aches and joint pain, nausea/vomiting and cravings.

Encourage clients to consider opioid agonist treatment because this will rapidly diminish the symptoms of withdrawal and support longer term reductions in illegal or non-prescribed opioid use. Symptomatic treatment can be used, but should be avoided where possible because multiple different agents are required to manage the withdrawal syndrome (e.g. metoclopramide for vomiting, loperamide for diarrhoea, hyoscine butylbromide for stomach and abdominal cramps, ibuprofen for muscle aches and pain, clonidine for excessive sweating and benzodiazepines, such as diazepam for anxiety and agitation) (Manning et al 2018).

In contrast, either a buprenorphine taper or short acting opioids can be used (depending on the clinical setting) and now present the mainstay treatment approaches for those not wanting to go onto

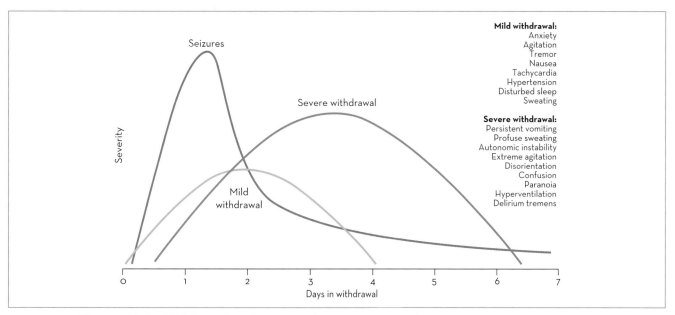

FIG. 13.1 Alcohol Withdrawal Time Course and Symptoms. (Adapted from NSW Department of Health 2008.)

TABLE 13.6   Alcohol Withdrawal Treatment and Management

Non-Medical Management	• Use an alcohol withdrawal scale (1–4-hourly reviews depending on the patient's needs and complexity). • Reduce external stimuli (e.g. visitors, light and noise from the television). • Use dim lighting at night-time to reduce the risk of misinterpreting the physical environment. • Provide regular reassurance and re-orientation to the date, time and place. • Provide written orientation prompts (e.g. writing the current day and date on a board). • Provide ongoing explanations about symptoms and expected time course. • Consider risks (e.g. falls) when the patient is confused or delirious. • Provide regular observation given absconding risk (particularly if there is evidence of delirium).
Medication Management	• Diazepam is the first-line treatment options for adults **without** concurrent severe liver dysfunction or significant medical comorbidities. • Shorter acting benzodiazepines such as oxazepam or lorazepam should be used in the elderly or those with severe liver dysfunction. • A maximum of 120 mg every 24 hours is generally sufficient to manage withdrawal. If doses exceed this, consult with specialist services. • Other underlying conditions should be considered when diazepam doses exceed 120 mg in 24 hours (e.g. delirium, hypoxia, Wernicke's encephalopathy, sepsis or paradoxical responses to medication). • Due to the long half-life and active metabolites of diazepam, prolonged dose tapering is not usually required (unless the patient is concurrently dependent on benzodiazepines). • Diazepam can generally be ceased within 72–96 hours. • Specialist services (e.g. addiction medicine) should be consulted when there is severe liver disease or other co-occurring substance use disorders. • People who are alcohol-dependent are likely to require higher than usual doses of diazepam to achieve clinically significant responses (e.g. 20 mg diazepam every 2–4 hours). • For excessive agitation, aggression or hallucinations, consider the use of low dose antipsychotics (e.g. olanzapine 2.5–5 mg 4/24 prn or haloperidol 1–2 mg PO/IMI 4/24).
Other Medication	• Thiamine deficiency is a potentially serious complication of long-term, heavy alcohol use. • Thiamine should be administered parenterally for the first 3 days, 300 mg, three times per day. After 3 days the dose can be decreased to 100 mg, oral, daily. • High-dose thiamine is required (500 mg TDS), until resolution in symptoms, for those patients with a history of, or who are presenting with, suspected Wernicke's encephalopathy. • Thiamine 100–200 mg, twice per day, can be utilised when access intravenously is not possible. Clotting deficiencies must be excluded before beginning intramuscular thiamine. • Intravenous fluids if there is excessive sweating. • Electrolyte replacement (e.g. calcium, phosphate, magnesium and potassium). Consider the risk of a refeeding syndrome. • Hypomagnesaemia is common in those with alcohol use disorders. People with low magnesium appear to be at greater risk of a severe and complicated withdrawal syndrome. Thiamine absorption appears to be diminished in the presence of magnesium deficiency. • There is some evidence to support the use of beta-blockers to assist with reducing the severity of withdrawal symptoms. However, beta-blockers should be used with caution due to the suppression of symptoms that are monitored via alcohol withdrawal scales. • Current best practice does **not** support the use of alcohol in managing withdrawal for hospital inpatients.

Adapted from St Vincent's Hospital Melbourne 2019.

TABLE 13.7   Benzodiazepine Withdrawal Symptoms

Stage of Withdrawal	Psychological Symptoms	Physiological Symptoms
Intoxication	Drowsiness, relaxation and sleepiness	Sedation and decreases in alertness and concentration
Acute withdrawal	Anxiety, panic attacks, depression, insomnia, poor memory/concentration, anger, irritability and disordered perceptions	Agitation, tremor, headaches, weakness, dizziness, nausea, vomiting, diarrhoea, constipation, palpitations, fatigue and flu-like symptoms
Protracted withdrawal	Anxiety, depression, insomnia, irritability, muscle aches, restlessness, poor concentration and memory problems	Diarrhoea, constipation and bloating
Potential withdrawal complications	Transient hallucinations (visual, tactile, auditory), delirium and psychosis	Withdrawal seizures (1–2% of patients)

Royal Australian College of General Practitioners 2015.

opioid agonist treatment. Buprenorphine should not be administered for at least 6–12 hours after the last use of other shorter acting opioids due to the risk of precipitated withdrawal. Once withdrawal symptoms start to emerge, a flexible approach should be adopted (see Table 13.8 for an example of a dosing regimen). Many individuals may struggle to wait until early withdrawal presents to be able to commence buprenorphine treatment. As such, high doses of short acting opioids should be used if they are receiving treatment within an inpatient setting.

Amphetamine withdrawal. Most people with amphetamine use disorders are able to undertake withdrawal in the community. The severity of the withdrawal syndrome is influenced by the amphetamine being used, the duration of use, the frequency of use, the method of administration and concurrent other substance use. Amphetamine withdrawal generally starts 24 hours after the last use, will peak around 24–72 hours and slowly resolve over the following 7–10 days (Manning et al 2018). Many amphetamine users experience protracted withdrawal symptoms such as poor sleep and mood instability, which can persist for up to 3 months after cessation. Amphetamine-related withdrawal can be broken into three distinct stages: The "crash", acute withdrawal and protracted withdrawal. The crash phase is characterised

TABLE 13.8 Buprenorphine Dosing Regimen

Day	Buprenorphine Dose	Recommended Total Daily Dose
Day 1	4 mg at onset of withdrawal 2–4 mg can be added at night as required	4 mg (max. 8 mg)
Day 2	4 mg in the morning 2–4 mg can be added at night as required	4 mg (max. 8 mg)
Day 3	4 mg in the morning 2 mg can be added at night as required	4 mg (max. 6 mg)
Day 4	2 mg in the morning 2 mg can be added at night as required	0 mg (max. 4 mg)
Day 5	2 mg as required	0 mg (max. 2 mg)

Gowing et al 2014.

by exhaustion, irritability, increased appetite, restlessness and anxiety. Acute withdrawal involves strong cravings, mood fluctuations, disturbed sleep, anhedonia, general aches and pains, headaches, muscle tension, poor concentration and disturbed thoughts, which may include paranoid ideations and hallucinations (Manning et al 2018).

There are no standard guidelines for stimulant withdrawal and no clear replacement pharmacotherapies. The primary focus of treatment is on supportive management and symptom-triggered medication management. Benzodiazepines (e.g. diazepam) and antipsychotics (e.g. olanzapine) are often used to support acute withdrawal from amphetamines (Manning et al 2018).

Cannabinoid withdrawal. Most patients withdrawing from cannabis do not require pharmacological treatment and can be managed at home. However, the severity of the withdrawal syndrome should be assessed carefully, with consideration of the individual's perception of how severe their withdrawal will be. Abrupt cessation of cannabis use after a period of regular, heavy use is associated with a clear withdrawal syndrome characterised by agitation, anxiety, irritability, flat mood, insomnia, vivid nightmares, poor appetite, tremors, sweating, fever and chills (Manning et al 2018). Symptoms of withdrawal generally start 24 hours after the last use of cannabis, peak at 2–3 days and subside after 7 days (Manning et al 2018).

Symptomatic treatment involves using long-acting benzodiazepines (e.g. diazepam), non-steroidal anti-inflammatories (e.g. paracetamol) and anti-emetics (e.g. ondansetron) (Manning et al 2018). Supportive therapies and relaxation techniques have been found to be very useful for some clients undergoing cannabinoid withdrawal.

Nicotine withdrawal. Nicotine withdrawal can impact on healthcare provision and should be carefully assessed. Nurses must consider the impact of cessation of tobacco products (e.g. cigarettes and tobacco pipes) and nicotine vaping products (e.g. e-cigarettes). Withdrawal syndromes will present similarly across these formulations.

Importantly, abrupt cessation of nicotine in the hospital setting is a leading contributor to episodes of agitation, aggression and anxiety and is frequently cited as a contributing cause to code grey utilisation. People with mental health conditions who also smoke tobacco must be treated with particular caution (Qurashi et al 2019). Smoking tobacco may alter the metabolism of many medications used in the treatment of psychotic disorders, in particular clozapine and olanzapine (Qurashi et al 2019). Abrupt cessation of tobacco smoking can then lead to an increase in plasma levels of these medications (Qurashi et al 2019).

Using a rating scale, such as the Fagerstrom nicotine dependence scale (see Table 13.9), can assist with treatment planning and the initiation of appropriate nicotine replacement therapy (NRT). Withdrawal will commence within 24 hours of a cessation, or reduction, in tobacco or nicotine vaping product use. Symptoms include irritability, frustration, anxiety, poor concentration, restlessness, increased appetite,

TABLE 13.9 Fagerstrom Test for Nicotine Dependence

Question	Answer	Score
How soon after you wake up do you smoke your first cigarette?	Within 5 minutes	3
	6–30 minutes	2
	31–60 minutes	1
	After 60 minutes	0
Do you find it difficult to refrain from smoking in places where it is forbidden?	Yes	1
	No	0
Which cigarette would you hate to give up the most?	The first one in the morning	1
	All others	0
How many cigarettes per day do you smoke?	10 or fewer	0
	11–20	1
	21–30	2
	31 or more	3
Do you smoke more frequently during the first hours after waking than during the rest of the day?	Yes	1
	No	0
Do you smoke if you are so ill that you are in bed most of the day?	Yes	1
	No	0

High dependence: 5 >
Moderate dependence: 2–4
Low dependence: 1
Not dependent: 0

Data from: Heatherton T, Kozlowski L, Frecker R & Fagerström K. The Fagerström test for nicotine dependence: A revision of the Fagerström tolerance questionnaire. Br J Addict, 1991. 86(9),1119–1127.

depressed mood, mood instability and insomnia (Manning et al 2018). The mainstay treatment for nicotine withdrawal is NRT, for example, nicotine patches or lozenges (see Table 13.10). Many forms of NRT can be nurse-initiated; however, this will vary depending on individual workplaces and settings. See Perspectives in practice: Nurse's story 13.1 to 13.3 for experiences of working with different types of addiction.

TABLE 13.10 Nicotine Replacement Therapy Dosing Guidelines

NRT Product	Recommended Dose
Patch 24 hour: 21 mg, 14 mg, 7 mg. 16 hour: 25 mg, 15 mg, 10 mg	Begin with full strength if smoking more than 10 cigarettes/day
Mouth spray 1 mg per spray	1–2 sprays every 30–60 mins, max 4 sprays/hour or 64 sprays per day
Lozenges 2 mg, 4 mg	2 mg and 4 mg: 9–15/day (4 mg if time to first cigarette < 30 mins)
Mini lozenges 1.5 mg, 4 mg	1.5 mg: 9–20/day 4 mg: 9–15/day (use 4 mg if time to first cigarette < 30 mins)
Gum 2 mg, 4 mg	2 mg: 8–20/day 4 mg 4–10/day (use 4 mg if time to first cigarette < 30 mins)
Inhalator 15 mg per cartridge	3–6 cartridges/day

NRT is contraindicated as a first-line treatment in those who have significant or active cardiovascular disease or sensitives to nicotine.

Mendelsohn et al 2015.

PERSPECTIVES IN PRACTICE

Nurse's Story 13.1: Maureen

The ultimate challenge and "high" of working in drug and alcohol nursing is the experience of assisting a client and seeing them creating a happier life out of what is sometimes chaos. My part in providing the information and the skills that help that process of recovery gives me a sense of wellbeing and achievement about what I do.

I am only talking about small steps here. Every small step, no matter how hesitant, is cause for celebration and joy. You cannot do the client's work for them, but you can provide assistance to them on the journey they must make. That is where skill is needed. The skill is assessing where the client is on the motivational cycle and being able to provide assistance that helps them towards their recovery, yet recognising that everyone has different recovery goals and that each person's needs are unique. So, the passion for me is in feeling that I am doing something to help people out of this mess. Even if it is only by offering my respect, recognition, skills and time.

The downside is that you cannot do it for them, and the struggle with addiction and dependence is a hard and lonely one. At those times when people give up on their goals, I remind myself that these problems were a long time developing and will be a long time in being resolved, and that a step back is just that, not the end of the game.

PERSPECTIVES IN PRACTICE

Nurse's Story 13.2: Inga

A question I get asked regularly, not only in the workplace but also at dinner parties, is: "Why do you want to work with drug addicts?" To be honest I have never really been able to come up with a clear answer, but I will give it a go.

I have nursed in drug and alcohol for 15 years. I enjoy the job.

A skill learnt early in my career was to engage clients honestly and openly with the expectation that this would be reciprocated. I find it a great privilege to be allowed into the complex layers of drug and alcohol dependency, allowing me the opportunity to offer solutions to health and social needs. There is great scope in working with clients holistically and not merely with their first presenting issue.

I have a very strong belief that as nurses we are not in a position to judge who is worthy of health care. Some of my colleagues treat drug-dependent clients with little respect and understanding. Part of my job is to challenge those beliefs, address fears, educate and assist clients in receiving non-discriminatory health care.

One rare gem that comes with drug and alcohol nursing is that of working with a team of people who know how to look after each other. Having a black sense of humour and being able to share a bottle of wine and many laughs keeps balance in your life and the ability to enjoy a fantastic career.

PERSPECTIVES IN PRACTICE

Nurse's Story 13.3: Sue

I have found, from 25 years' experience working in a mental health unit, that almost every person admitted to a mental health unit has a co-occurring diagnosis or at least a problem with alcohol and/or drugs. My advice is: "Don't be concerned – expect it as the norm." Stop expecting to deal only with your "bit" of the person. You need to be able to deal with the whole person. The mental health nurse has a responsibility to find out more about substance abuse, even if it is only how to recognise symptoms and how and when to refer to other services.

PHYSICAL HEALTH AND SUBSTANCE USE DISORDERS

In Australia, the National Health and Medical Research Council (NHMRC) recommends an intake of no more than 10 drinks in one week and no more than 4 standard drinks on any single day (NHMRC

2020). See Table 13.11 for a summary of acute and chronic physical health consequences of substance use. Unfortunately, people with substance use disorders also struggle with higher rates of physical health complications and yet remain very stigmatised within mainstream healthcare settings.

Assessment Areas

Substance use disorders may occur in all settings of healthcare. Specific assessment tools and criteria are available to assist with obtaining accurate histories of substance use over time. It is important to carefully elicit alcohol and drug use to make a diagnosis, so that an appropriate management strategy can be implemented. Many substance use problems are misdiagnosed or remain undetected, which can lead to significant negative outcomes.

Presentation and Setting

The process of assessment depends on the nature of the presentation and the setting. Careful consideration for the environment must occur; this will assist with assessment processes and rapport development.

Substance Use History

A patient's substance use (prescribed and non-prescribed) must be measured to determine whether the level of use may cause harm or whether withdrawal is imminent. A recent substance use history will determine the type of substance used, the level of use, the frequency of use and whether a withdrawal state could occur, in order to ensure that appropriate treatment planning occurs. This information is also important to identify triggers for initiating use, risk of relapse and to be able to implement an appropriate harm minimisation framework. A developmental and family history should be documented to identify the age at which the client first used a substance, how this use has developed over time, when the client thought the use became problematic, when there were periods of abstinence and when there were any changes to patterns of use (New South Wales Health 2013).

Taking a Substance Use History

When asking about substance use, approach the topic in an open way and speak about substance use as an accepted behaviour. Approach the assessment with a plan and consider the impact of any pre-existing judgements before entering the assessment. Ask questions about legal and more socially acceptable substances first (e.g. alcohol, tobacco and prescription medication) before asking about illicit drug use, which is often heavily stigmatised. This will be less confronting for the patient and help in developing rapport throughout the assessment.

In a substance use assessment, it is essential to cover the domains listed below. Individual health services may use standard substance use assessment forms that cover each of these elements. Systematic assessment of all patients should include a thorough examination of:

- indicators of risk (e.g. history of drink driving, loss of consciousness with multiple head strikes, overdose history)
- medical history (in particular, any history of medical problems associated with substance use such as pancreatitis secondary to chronic alcohol use, hepatitis C, HIV or infective endocarditis associated with injecting drug use)
- psychosocial issues (e.g. housing, social connections, domestic violence)
- physical signs and symptoms (e.g. ascites associated with alcohol use or extensive intravenous injection sites beyond the cubital fossa region)
- mental health status
- pathology results.

No single sign, symptom or pathology test is conclusive evidence of an alcohol or drug-related issue (New South Wales Health 2013).

TABLE 13.11   Physical Health Consequences of Substance Use

Substance	Acute	Chronic
Alcohol	• Dizziness • Poor judgement • Loss of coordination • Memory loss • Vomiting • Headaches • Accidental injury (e.g. road accidents, falls) • Aggression/violence • Alcohol poisoning/overdose (can lead to fatalities)	• Decreased concentration • Short-term and long-term memory impairments • Increased risk of stroke • Alcohol-related brain injury • Alcohol-related dementia • Alcohol-related psychosis • Hypertension • Tachycardia • Cardiomyopathy • Increased risk of acute myocardial infarction • Liver cirrhosis • Liver cancer • Fatty liver • Stomach ulcers • Stomach and oesophageal cancer • Oesophageal varices • Gastro-oesophageal reflux disorder • Gastritis • Pancreatitis (acute and chronic) • Reduction in testosterone, sperm counts and overall fertility in men • Changes to menstruation in women • Fetal alcohol spectrum disorder
Cannabis	• Short-term effects are heavily influenced by the individual's prior experience and setting • Short-term euphoria, poor concentration, psychomotor retardation, amotivation, anxiety • Increased risk of car accidents • Increased risk of relapse in psychotic illness • Increased appetite, hyperemesis • Reddening of eyes, decreased intraocular pressure • Dry mouth	• Impaired learning, impaired concentration, neurocognitive impairments, exacerbation of underlying psychosis, insomnia • Poor appetite • Cardiovascular disease • Respiratory disease (associated with mechanism of administration)
Amphetamines	• Pupil dilation, headache, bruxism • Hyperventilation, dyspnoea, cough, chest pain, wheezing, exacerbation of asthma, pulmonary oedema • Tachycardia, hypertension, palpitations, arrhythmia, acute myocardial infarction/cardiogenic shock • Agitation, psychosis, tremor, hyperreflexia, muscle twitching, seizures, cerebral haemorrhage, cerebral oedema • Nausea, vomiting, bowel infarction/perforation • Diuresis, acute renal failure • Mild fever, increased overall body temperature, malignant hyperthermia • Increased sensory acuity, increased energy, increased motivation, increased concentration, decreased reaction time • Increased risk of sexually transmitted infections (chem-sex) • Amphetamine overdose • Acute psychosis • Rhabdomyolysis	• Anxiety, confusion, insomnia, mood instability, aggression • Chronic psychotic and mood disorders • Impaired decision making, memory loss, poor concentration • Weight loss, severe tooth decay, skin discolouration and sores • Dilated cardiomyopathy • Cardiovascular disease • Chronic obstructive pulmonary disease and exacerbation of asthma (associated with mechanism of administration) • Increased risk of blood-borne viruses (e.g. hepatitis C and HIV) in those who inject
Opioids	• Euphoria, "rush" • Warm flushing, dry mouth, heaviness in extremities • Nausea, vomiting, constipation • Bradycardia, hypotension • Opioid toxicity/overdose	• Increased risk of mortality over time with doses exceeding 100 mg morphine equivalence • Hypothalamic–pituitary–adrenal axis suppression • Sleep apnoea • Opioid-induced hyperalgesia • Constipation • Immune suppression • Prolongation of QT interval (particularly with long-term methadone treatment) • Increased risk of blood borne viruses (e.g. hepatitis C and HIV) in those who inject

TABLE 13.11 Physical Health Consequences of Substance Use—cont'd

Substance	Acute	Chronic
Hallucinogens	• Tachycardia, hypertension • Insomnia, tremor, poor coordination, psychomotor retardation • Sparse or incoherent speech • Respiratory depression • Cardiac arrest • Acute psychosis, anxiety, depression, violence, confusion, loss of control, lethargy, disorientation	• Relatively unknown as there are very few long-term users of hallucinogens • Anxiety, flashbacks and nightmares or "bad trips"
Nicotine/tobacco	• Tachycardia • Hypertension • Dizziness • Increased activity of the gastrointestinal tract • Nausea • Vomiting • Reduction in appetite • Alterations in taste • Cough • Asthma exacerbation • Reduction in muscle tone • Some relaxation effects	• Stroke • Cardiovascular disease • Narrowing of blood vessels • Persistent tachycardia • Stroke • Emboli • Deep vein thrombosis • Chronic obstructive pulmonary disease (emphysema and chronic bronchitis) • Lung cancer • Exacerbation of asthma • Cancer (bladder, blood, cervix, colon and rectum, oesophagus, kidney and ureter, larynx, liver, oropharynx, pancreas, stomach, trachea and bronchus) • Preterm delivery • Stillbirth • Low birth weight • Sudden infant death syndrome • Ectopic pregnancy • Orofacial clefts in infants • Miscarriage • Reduction in male fertility • Reduction in bone density • Gum disease • Increased risk of tooth loss • Increased risk for cataracts • Age-related macular degeneration • Type 2 diabetes mellitus • Rheumatoid arthritis • Poor immune function

The Cancer Council 2018, Centre for Disease Control and Prevention 2018, Government of South Australia 2019, Karila et al 2014, Lawn et al 2016, National Institute on Drug Abuse 2019, Substance Abuse and Mental Health Services Administration 2004, World Health Organization 2018.

Key Elements of Assessment

The following key elements should be clarified and explored as part of the assessment process:

- type of drug (if you are unfamiliar with the substance being used or the colloquial term being used, ask the client to explain it further)
- types of beverage the client usually consumes (it is important with alcohol to distinguish what sort of alcohol is being consumed and what quantity is being purchased, such as drinking one 5 L cask of wine per day or a dozen 375 mL bottles of heavy beer).
- route of administration
- frequency of use
- dose (if you are unsure about the amount due to colloquial terms, ask the patient to explain the quantity they purchase their substance in and how long that lasts for, or ask them to explain their dosing system further)
- duration of use
- time and amount of the last dose (e.g. milligrams of methadone, grams of cannabis)
- any substance-free days
- any previous experiences of withdrawal.

Note: It is important to ask the person if they are using more than one drug at a time and to record each substance separately. Poly-substance use can greatly increase the risk of complicated withdrawal and negative health consequences associated with use. It can be difficult for some people to discuss their substance use with someone they do not know; subsequently, developing rapport is a priority (see Box 13.4 for strategies to assist with the assessment process).

Observations

An assessment of a person's physical and mental state may reveal evidence of recent substance use such as the smell of alcohol or objective signs of withdrawal. A person who has misused substances for some time might have a decline in global functioning, which might be evidenced by a decline in health status and poor hygiene. An assessment should include the following:

- Assess their general appearance. Look for evidence of malnutrition (the person looking gaunt) and for signs of agitation, which might indicate stimulant use or withdrawal from a substance. People who regularly inject drugs will often wear long sleeves and long trousers, even in hot weather, in an attempt to cover up injection marks (see also Box 13.5).

BOX 13.4 Strategies to Assist With Obtaining an Accurate Substance Use History

- Ensure the environment is as quiet and private as possible.
- If it is not possible to be completely private, speak quietly to encourage open discussion.
- When you are interviewing the client, note any inconsistencies in what you are being told.
- If the client becomes upset or distressed, leave the question and rephrase it later. Ensure the client is aware that they are driving the conversation and, if there are any topics they are not comfortable talking about, that these will not be discussed.
- A substance use history can also be elicited from the client's friends or family; however, this should be used with caution because it may not always be an accurate reflection of current substance use patterns and patient privacy needs to be considered.
- How questions are posed is important. Clients may drink well in excess of recommended levels but not see their use as problematic. It is important to remain non-judgemental.
- Overestimate how much someone is using to encourage more accurate accounts of quantities. For example, ask: "how long would it take you to smoke 40 cigarettes?" rather than asking the person to specify how much they are using on their own.
- Illegal substance use may elicit a range of emotions among healthcare providers. It is important to remember that substance use is a health issue, not a moral one. Although illicit substance use may be involved, the primary concern is the individual's health and not the legal aspects to their use.
- Phrase questions to evoke acceptance. For example, ask: "What is your favourite drink?" or "What do you like to drink?", "If you had to pick your drug of choice what would it be?"
- Phrase questions that assume the individual does drink or use substances. For example, "So, how much cannabis would you smoke in a month?" or "When was the last time you drank enough to be merry or even drunk?".
- Use open-ended questions, summaries and validating statements to encourage discussion of topics: "You were talking about how you used heroin in the past and have managed to stay clean for 2 years. That's brilliant. You must be proud of yourself for staying clean for so long. Talk me through what you did during that time."

BOX 13.5 Signs of Intravenous Drug Use

- Puncture marks
- Cellulitis
- Phlebitis
- Skin abscesses
- Erosion or irritation around nostrils/septum
- Irritation around mouth or nose
- Tenderness or liver pain

Reproduced by permission, NSW Health © 2016.

- Look for signs of intoxication such as ataxia (lack of coordination of muscle movements), confused thinking, being argumentative, restricted or dilated pupils, or the smell of alcohol on the person's breath.
- Look for signs of withdrawal such as tremors and sweating, particularly of the hands and face. Consider objective signs of withdrawal rather than self-reported symptoms (e.g. bilateral tremor, diaphoresis and tachycardia versus the patient reporting that they feel sick).

- Look for stigmata such as abscesses at injection sites (see Box 13.6), inflammation of the nasal septum, bruising and scars associated with falls, petechiae, jaundice, or flushed face.
- Investigate pulse rate, blood pressure and evidence of head injury, which may indicate recent substance use (New South Wales Health 2013).

The Glasgow Coma Scale is a neurological scale that aims to give a reliable objective way of recording the conscious state of a person for initial as well as subsequent assessment, and may be required for medical and trauma patients, particularly if they are intoxicated (see Table 13.12).

Tests
Mental Status Examination

A mental status examination is essential (see Chapter 9), paying attention to:
- clouding of consciousness
- perceptual abnormalities, especially visual, auditory and tactile hallucinations (e.g. believing insects are crawling under the skin) – look for evidence of responding to perceptual disturbances (e.g. Do they look distracted? Are they picking at unseen stimulus? Are they muttering to themselves when no one is around?) rather than self-reported experiences only.
- thought abnormalities, especially paranoid ideation and changes to how the patient is expressing themselves (e.g. Are they making sense? Are they struggling to form their thoughts into a meaningful sentence?)
- suicidal ideation
- altered cognition (e.g. are they orientated? Do they know where they are?)

Laboratory Tests

Laboratory tests may provide evidence of substance misuse. Physiological markers of consumption such as mean corpuscular volume and gamma glutamyl transferase are most widely used to verify a diagnosis of substance use; however, these should not be relied upon because progressive liver failure may significantly impact on enzyme production. Other reasons for alterations in these markers should always be considered. Consider blood alcohol levels and urine drug screens (with gas chromatography/mass spectrometry) for patients who are unable to provide a history. Note: There is always a risk of false positives and false negatives with urine drug screening, so presumptive screening tests (e.g. immunoassay) should always be interpreted with caution! Routine pathology should always be considered with clients with a substance use disorder, particularly if acutely substance affected or intoxicated on alcohol. Many features of acute intoxication will mask comorbid physical health changes and this should be considered carefully. Importantly, blood-borne virus screening should be offered to any client with a history of injecting substance use.

Screening Tests

Screening tests may also be used and are not associated with urine drug screening. These instruments usually take the form of self-reported questionnaires and are used for diagnostic purposes. One of the most widely used screening instruments is the Alcohol Use Disorders Identification Test (AUDIT), which is designed to screen for a range of drinking problems, particularly harmful and hazardous use. It is especially suitable for primary healthcare settings and has reliability across cultural groups and a range of specific populations. The AUDIT is a self-report measure comprising 10 items, which are scored by totalling the items (see Box 13.6). The AUDIT is in the public domain and can be used without cost. There is an altered

BOX 13.6   Alcohol Use Disorders Identification Test (AUDIT) Screening Instrument

Please circle the answer that is correct for you.

1. How often do you have a drink containing alcohol?
   Never
   Monthly or less
   2–4 times a month
   2–3 times a week
   4 or more times a week

2. How many drinks containing alcohol do you have on a typical day when you are drinking?
   1 or 2
   3 or 4
   5 or 6
   7 to 9
   10 or more

3. How often do you have six or more drinks on one occasion?
   Never
   Less than monthly
   Monthly
   Weekly
   Daily or almost daily

4. How often have you found that you were not able to stop drinking once you had started?
   Never
   Less than monthly
   Monthly
   Weekly
   Daily or almost daily

5. How often during the last year have you failed to do what was normally expected of you because of drinking?
   Never
   Less than monthly
   Monthly
   Weekly
   Daily or almost daily

6. How often during the last year have you needed a first drink in the morning to get yourself going after a heavy drinking session?
   Never
   Less than monthly
   Monthly
   Weekly
   Daily or almost daily

7. How often during the last year have you had a feeling of guilt or remorse after drinking?
   Never
   Less than monthly
   Monthly
   Weekly
   Daily or almost daily

8. How often during the last year have you been unable to remember what happened the night before because you had been drinking?
   Never
   Less than monthly
   Monthly
   Weekly
   Daily or almost daily

9. Have you or someone else been injured as a result of your drinking?
   No
   Yes, but not in the last year
   Yes, during the last year

10. Has a relative or friend or a doctor or other health worker been concerned about your drinking or suggested you cut down?
   No
   Yes, but not in the last year
   Yes, during the last year

World Health Organization 2001.

TABLE 13.12	Glasgow Coma Scale	
Eye opening	Spontaneous	4
	To speech	3
	To pain	2
	None	1
Verbal response	Oriented	5
	Confused conversation	4
	Words (inappropriate)	3
	Sounds (incomprehensible)	2
	None	1
Best motor response	Obeys commands	6
	Localises pain	5
	Flexion withdrawal from pain	4
	Abnormal flexion to pain	3
	Extension to pain	2
	None	1
Total score	3/15–15/15	

Rosenfeld 2012.

version of AUDIT, called the Drug Use Disorders Identification Test (DUDIT), which is used to screen for a range of other substance use problems. The ASSIT (Alcohol, Smoking and Substance Involvement Screening Test) is a validated questionnaire developed by the World Health Organization. It screens for all levels of problem or risky substance use in adults (WHO 2015). Finally, the ATOP (Australian Treatment Outcomes Profile) has been rolled out in a number of alcohol and other drug treatment services as a means to monitor drug use patterns qualitatively over time (Lintzeris et al 2020).

INTERVENTIONS

Early and Brief Interventions

Studies have shown that early and brief interventions (talking to people at an early stage in their substance use) are effective ways to prevent later possible complications of substance use (Marsh et al 2013; Moyer & Finney 2015; Vasilaki et al 2006; Wild et al 2007). Brief interventions for substance use involve sessions of 5–15 minutes and often include providing self-help materials such as pamphlets or substance use diaries. This may extend to a brief assessment and providing advice (in a one-off session), as well as assessing the client's readiness to change (motivational interview), harm reduction and follow-up.

The components of brief interventions include:

- assessment
- providing feedback to the client on risk or impairments due to drug use
- listening to the client's concerns and advising the client about the consequences of continued drug use
- defining treatment goals such as reducing or ceasing drug use
- discussing and implementing strategies for treatment (e.g. identifying triggers for drug use and strategies to overcome them and offering a follow-up session) (Marsh et al 2013).

Brief interventions are recommended for clients experiencing relatively few problems related to their substance use and who have low levels of dependence, and, in general, can be completed by most healthcare professionals. They are also recommended for clients with a dependence on nicotine, a low-to-moderate dependence on alcohol or a low-to-moderate dependence on cannabis. Brief interventions are not recommended for clients with severe dependence. If a brief intervention consists of only one session, it should include giving advice on how to reduce drug use or drinking to a safer level, providing harm-reduction information and discussing harm-reduction strategies (Marsh et al 2013; Moyer & Finney 2015; Vasilaki et al 2006; Wild et al 2007).

Motivational Interviewing

Motivational interviewing using the Transtheoretical Model of Change is an intervention developed by Prochaska, DiClemente and Miller to work with clients to assess and then enhance the motivation to change their level of substance use (Lundahl et al 2013; Miller & Rollnick 2009; Prochaska & DiClemente 1984). Motivational interviewing is one of the most widely used interventions and has been adopted for a range of challenging behaviours beyond just substance use disorders. Perspectives in practice: Nurse's story 13.3 provides a practical example of motivational interviewing in action (see Box 13.7 for more details about the stages of changes). Motivational interviewing also provides a framework for effectively interviewing clients abbreviated to "OARS":

O – Open-ended questions

A – Affirmation. This involves acknowledging hard work and any difficulties the client may be having.

R – Reflective listening. Active listening is central to motivational interviewing and can demonstrate empathy, compassion and understanding.

S – Summary. Providing summary statements assists with demonstrating understanding and clarifying any areas of confusion. It will assist with ensuring that the client is aware that you are engaged and actively listening.

Cognitive behaviour therapy (CBT)

CBT involves identifying self-destructive thoughts ("Everything has to be perfect", "I always do the wrong thing") and replacing them with more realistic thoughts ("Not everything has to be perfect. Not always", "I don't always do the wrong thing. Sometimes I do good things"). By replacing self-destructive thoughts with more realistic thoughts (cognitions), emotions and behaviour should change for the better as a result. CBT may be effective for substance use and other co-occurring conditions, including post-traumatic stress disorder and depression (McGovern et al 2015; Riper et al 2014). Motivational interviewing and CBT are important counselling approaches in the alcohol and other drugs treatment sector.

BOX 13.7 The Transtheoretical Model of Change Within Motivational Interviewing

Pre-contemplation

The client has no intention of changing. They are in "denial" about the need for change. The therapist works to increase the client's awareness of the problem while consistently remaining non-judgemental and respectful. The therapist provides information and consciousness raising at the same time. It is vitally important that the therapist does not disengage at this stage. The therapist needs to continue to try to connect with the client and raise awareness of the dangers of their alcohol and substance use even if the client does not initially show interest. Rapport is essential during this phase.

Contemplation

The client is aware of their problem, but remains ambivalent about change. The therapist acknowledges the client's ambivalence while working to tip the decisional balance by weighing the pros and cons of change versus the risks and benefits of continuing substance use. Responsibility for change remains with the client.

Preparation

The client intends to change, but might be confused about the best way to do so. The therapist inspires realistic hope, offers a menu of choices to help determine the best course of action and demystifies the change process. Both work to create a plan for change.

Action

Actual behaviour change commences. The client implements a collaborative, realistic plan. Both the therapist and the client monitor the client's progress, highlighting and valuing even small successes, and progressively problem solving.

Maintenance

Behaviour change has been achieved and the client has developed a new lifestyle. The therapist and the client are vigilant to avoid relapse. They have realistic hopes and avoid exaggerated expectations.

Clients may slip back to a previous stage (e.g. from preparation to pre-contemplation) and work their way up again. This is an expected part of the process and relapses should be anticipated. The principle is to ascertain which stage of "readiness to change" the client is at and then to provide information and support to move them on to the next stage. If the client understands what is occurring, they are more likely to change, and it is imperative that the therapist rolls with any resistance presented by the client along their pathway.

Centre for Youth AOD Practice Development n.d.

DETOXIFICATION

Detoxification and withdrawal management are among the first stages of treatment for people with substance use disorders. People enter into supervised treatment, either medical or non-medical, to reduce the severity of the withdrawal syndrome and to manage any potential significant complications. It can take place in an in-patient unit or in the person's own home. The client may require medication, depending on the severity of the withdrawal, substance being used, and the client's wishes. Symptoms of withdrawal range in severity from mildly uncomfortable to life threatening; however, careful assessment and management can alleviate many of the symptoms. Nursing management of withdrawal focuses on five main areas:

- minimising progression to severe withdrawal

- decreasing risk of injury to self/others
- eliminating risk of dehydration, electrolyte and nutritional imbalance
- reducing risk of seizures
- identifying the presence of concurrent illness that masks/mimics withdrawal (New South Wales Health 2013).

RELAPSE PREVENTION

There is a distinct difference between a lapse and a relapse. A lapse is a "slip" in which the person uses a substance again, possibly a couple of times, then returns to their previous reduced level of use or abstinence. At this stage, the person may decide to keep using or learn from their lapse and stop using. A relapse occurs when a person resumes substance use and is not able to maintain abstinence or their reduced level of use (Marsh et al 2013). A lapse does not always result in a relapse, and clients should be encouraged to consider this during any relapse prevention work.

All clients should have a plan, so that if they do lapse, they have support and strategies available to avoid the more dangerous relapse. A lapse should be viewed as a learning experience for both the client and the clinician. For example: What were the triggers that led to the lapse? How did the client manage to contain their substance use to a lapse and not relapse into old behaviours? Within a CBT or motivational interviewing framework, the clinician explores the client's underlying thoughts and feelings that resulted in the lapse. The clinician's role is to assist the client to work through the thoughts that contributed to the lapse and replace them with less damaging thought processes for the future (Marsh et al 2013).

OTHER HEALING APPROACHES

It is always best to offer a wide spectrum of treatment approaches. Residential treatment services may be effective for some people. For others, pharmacotherapy, such as acamprosate (Campral) and naltrexone decreases cravings to drink alcohol. For yet other clients, a 12-step program can be effective; these are peer support programs such as Alcoholics Anonymous (AA) and Narcotics Anonymous (NA) (Alcoholics Anonymous 2001). These groups are based on an abstinence philosophy (Humphreys et al 2014; Kelly et al 2013). Community drug and alcohol services provide a range of interventions, including individual and group counselling, pharmacotherapies (e.g. methadone and buprenorphine maintenance for opiate-dependent clients), CBT and motivational interviewing.

Harm Minimisation and Harm Reduction

Harm reduction is part of a three-pronged international approach to problematic substance use that allows agencies to provide an integrated and collaborative approach to care (National Drug Strategy 2017). The terms "harm reduction" and "harm minimisation" are often used interchangeably. Harm reduction has been particularly successful in its contribution to containing the spread of HIV/AIDS, as well as being the core philosophy for many clinical interventions (e.g. methadone treatment to reduce the number of times someone will inject heroin daily without necessarily abstaining) (National Drug Strategy 2017), and encourages the acceptance that not all individuals are ready for abstinence. The successful use of harm minimisation strategies is one of the most powerful interventions for demonstrating acceptance and a non-judgemental approach. In particular, harm minimisation is robustly supported in the literature as being one of the most effective interventions for engaging with people who use substances and for reducing the harms for both individuals and their broader communities (Harm Reduction Australia 2020; McMillan et al 2021; National

Drug Strategy 2017; Pitakowski et al 2022). Ultimately, harm minimisation strategies aim to reduce the risk of medical and psychological problems associated with substance use for both the individual and the extended community.

Harm minimisation strategies may include the following:

- *Needle and syringe programs* – primary needle and syringe programs extended beyond just providing sterile injecting equipment, to providing primary healthcare and a range of social support programs. Australia and Aotearoa New Zealand have well established needle and syringe programs, which have led to a significant reduction in spread of blood-borne viruses when compared with other western countries.
- *Suggestions for alternative routes of drug administration* – such as inhaling or oral use rather than intravenous use.
- *Alternative injecting sites* – this is particularly useful for long-term injecting drug users who may have significantly damaged or impaired veins; it also assists users with understanding high-risk injecting sites (e.g. the groin or neck), and how to avoid these areas.
- *Take-home naloxone and associated training* – naloxone is a rapid-acting opioid antagonist that has been used for a long time in emergency settings to reverse opioid overdoses (injecting drug users are now trained in administering naloxone, which can be life-saving while awaiting emergency services). Take-home naloxone is now readily available to people who inject drugs, and those dependent on prescribed opioids, as a life-saving intervention to reduce the risk of overdose leading to death.
- *Training in safe injecting practices* such as using sterile equipment, filters, tourniquets and how to access emergency healthcare services.
- *Medically supervised injecting facilities*
- *Provision of methadone and buprenorphine* (opioid agonist treatment; see below)
- *Programs that inform alcohol drinkers* of the dangers of driving while intoxicated, the advantages of having a designated driver and night-time transport schemes from hotels and nightclubs
- *Pill testing* to assess purity of various illicit substances, particularly at festivals.

Another major harm-reduction strategy is opioid agonist treatment (previously known as opioid replacement therapy). The long-acting opioids methadone and buprenorphine are administered as substitution treatment for heroin or other opioid addiction and are considered "essential medicines" for this purpose (WHO 2019). As substitution opioids have the potential to be diverted and intravenously injected, deterrent strategies have been introduced. Naloxone was added to buprenorphine, which created Suboxone (subutex + naloxone). Suboxone was marketed with the information that if the combination drug was injected, it would produce little euphoria but withdrawal symptoms in those already dependent, and this would deter diversion (Larance et al 2014; Yokell et al 2011). In 2011 in Australia, a sublingual film version of buprenorphine with naloxone was introduced to make dosing of buprenorphine easier to supervise and so reduce the risk of further diversion. In 2019, long-acting injectable buprenorphine (LAIB) was approved for use in Australia. LAIB has dramatically altered the provision of opioid agonist treatment through a more accessible formulation of buprenorphine, with less frequency of attendance for administration (with weekly and monthly formulations available) and significantly decreased costs.

CO-OCCURRING SUBSTANCE USE DISORDERS

Several terms are used to describe someone who has more than one disorder concurrently; mental health, alcohol and drug nurses tend to use the terms "comorbid disorders", "comorbidity", "co-existing disorder" and "dual diagnosis" interchangeably (Drake & Wallach 2000; Mills et al 2008). However, more recently co-occurring substance use disorder has become the more accepted way of describing these presentations. Clients with a mental health problem are often drawn to alcohol and drugs with serious and sometimes fatal consequences (e.g. depression and alcohol, psychosis and methamphetamines, bipolar disorder and methamphetamines). There are many theories outlining this relationship, and no one model will definitively predict the relationship between mental health changes and substance use, but can assist with treatment planning:

1. **Direct causal relationship theory** (one disorder produces the other disorder) – for example, a chronic crystal methamphetamine user might start to develop psychosis and the psychosis becomes the predominant problem. Alternatively, a mental illness may cause the drug use. Someone with depression may drink alcohol to relieve their symptoms of depression. The alcohol use then becomes the most debilitating problem.

2. **Indirect causal relationship theory** – for example, depression during childhood might lead to poor school results. This in turn might lead to a less satisfying career, frustration with one's life and subsequent drinking of alcohol to treat the depression. Depression causes the drinking, but in an indirect way and as a result of multiple social influences.

3. **Common causal factors** – for example, traumatic experiences or a family history of mental illness and drug abuse produce both mental health and drug and alcohol problems, but one disorder does not directly initiate the other. Both disorders occur simultaneously as a result of the early trauma.

The client is one person, not two or more separate disorders. Nurses need to consider the impact of the substance use on each person's overall treatment and, as such, be aware of treatment options. Unfortunately, there continues to be a "silo" approach to treatment that can often create difficulties for people when attempting to access services (NSW Ministry of Health 2020).

Tobacco smoking is an important issue when considering co-occurring disorders. Features of schizophrenia include a lack of energy and a lack of interest in activities that would normally bring the individual pleasure (anhedonia). Sedation is also one of the side effects of antipsychotic medication used to treat psychosis. Stimulants like tobacco provide energy (at least in the short term) and people with psychotic disorders may be drawn to the short-term energy enhancing effects of smoking. Furthermore, when considering adolescent mental health, the relationship between tobacco smoking and psychosis becomes even more pertinent (Kanniah & Kumar 2023). There is evidence to suggest that the adolescent brain may be more susceptible to the influence of nicotine in those with early onset psychotic disorders (Kanniah & Kumar 2023).

The relationship between mental health changes and tobacco smoking needs to be considered carefully. Nicotine is well known to interact with and affect the metabolism of a range of medications, in particular, neuroleptic medications such as clozapine, olanzapine and some benzodiazepines (Manning et al 2018). Subsequently, serum levels of these medications can change with abrupt cessation of cigarette smoking.

Clinical significance of a co-occurring diagnosis

There is evidence to suggest that clients with co-occurring disorders have poorer outcomes than those with either a single mental health problem or a distinct substance use disorder. These patients can be more difficult to manage due to their complex health and social needs, and have higher rates of non-adherence with treatment (Hughes et al

2017; Wise et al 2017). Clients with a comorbid diagnosis are more likely to have a chronic disability and consequently require more service utilisation (Hughes et al 2017). These clients have fewer treatment options and increased risks of experiencing difficulties with relationships, poor employment prospects, social isolation, poor health and chronic financial difficulties (Roussy et al 2017). They often have a number of surrounding issues that combine and add to the complexity of their treatment goals and outcomes – for example, children placed in care due to parental substance abuse, legal problems, housing difficulties and psychological problems (Marsh et al 2013).

Managing clients with a co-occurring disorder

People with co-occurring substance use disorders and mental health changes often struggle with mainstream treatment approaches. Nurses need to develop the ability to distinguish between a psychotic disorder that is part of a mental illness and one that is substance-use related (see Box 13.8). Patients with co-occurring disorders often evoke powerful and unpleasant feelings in health professionals that are commonly associated with the frequent attendances at hospital. There is often a lack of a clear pathway for clients attempting to access services. In addition, clients may feel stigmatised by a focus on abstinence within mental health settings that is in direct contrast to the harm-minimisation model supported by the drug and alcohol sector and National Drug Strategy (Roussy et al 2017; National Drug Strategy 2017).

This client group generally struggles to maintain simultaneous wellness with regards to both their mental health and substance use. Developing a collaborative therapeutic alliance is essential, and the nurse needs to adopt an empathetic and non-judgemental approach towards this population. Historically, services have required that a client's mental state be relatively stable before attempting detoxification or modifying use. However, there is growing recognition that this is not always possible, and healthcare providers need to be flexible in their responses. Brief interventions can be used in both outpatient and inpatient settings. For management principles for clients with psychotic disorders and substance abuse, see Box 13.9.

BOX 13.8 Guidelines for Differentiating Between a Primary Psychotic Disorder and a Substance-Induced Disorder

- Substance-induced psychotic symptoms can result from intoxication, chronic use or withdrawal.
- Prolonged heavy use of psychostimulants (e.g. amphetamines) can produce a psychotic picture similar to schizophrenia.
- Hallucinogen-induced psychosis is usually transient but may persist if use is sustained.
- Heavy alcohol use has been associated with alcohol-related hallucinations.
- Psychotic symptoms can also occur during withdrawal (e.g. delirium tremens) and delirious states.
- A non-substance-induced psychotic disorder should be considered when:
  - psychosis preceded the onset of substance use
  - psychosis persists for longer than one month after acute withdrawal or severe intoxication
  - psychotic symptoms are not consistent with the substance used
  - there is a history of psychotic symptoms during periods of abstinence greater than one month
  - there is a personal or family history of a non-substance-induced psychotic disorder.

Lubman & Sundram 2003 © Copyright *The Medical Journal of Australia*. Reproduced with permission.

BOX 13.9 Management Principles for Clients With Psychotic Disorders and Substance Abuse

Assessment

- Screen clients with psychosis for substance misuse.
- Determine the severity of use and associated risk-taking behaviours (e.g. injecting practices, unsafe sex).
- Exclude organic illness or physical complications of substance misuse.
- Seek collateral history – family or close supports should be involved where possible.

Treatment

- First engage the client using a non-judgemental attitude.
- Educate the client.
- Give general advice about the harmful effects of substance misuse.
- Advise about safe and responsible levels of substance use.
- Support the individual to develop links between substance misuse and mental health changes (e.g. methamphetamine use and worsening paranoia).
- Educate the person about safer practices (e.g. safe sexual practices).
- Help the client to establish the advantages and disadvantages of current use and support consideration of change.
- With medical staff, evaluate the need for concurrent pharmacotherapy (e.g. methadone, acamprosate, nicotine replacement therapy).
- Refer the client to appropriate community services.
- Devise relapse-prevention strategies that address both psychosis and substance misuse.
- Identify triggers for relapse (e.g. meeting other drug users, family conflict) and explore alternative coping strategies.

Lubman & Sundram 2003 © Copyright *The Medical Journal of Australia*. Reproduced with permission.

As with all aspects of nursing care, safety is the main concern. If a client has been admitted to a mental health facility in a psychotic state, it is essential that any acute risks are managed as a priority, and this should include consideration of withdrawal risk. If the client is at risk of withdrawal from one or more substances, withdrawal strategies as outlined earlier in this chapter need to be implemented immediately. Careful consideration should be taken regarding the expected severity of the withdrawal syndrome because it may not be appropriate for the withdrawal process to occur within a mental health facility and the client may require more intensive support from medical teams. When the client is more settled, the nurse can begin to explore reasons for the client's substance use, including the relationship of the substance to the client's psychiatric symptoms, treatment for the client's mental illness and feelings of social isolation related to their negative symptoms.

The client's readiness to change for both their mental health and substance use disorder should be explored. If the client is not considering changing their substance use, it is imperative that education is provided regarding harm minimisation strategies. Remember, clients may be at different stages of change regarding their problematic substance use and their mental illness, and interventions need to reflect this. It is important to set small and achievable goals with this client population. Larger goals should be broken down into a series of steps that are manageable rather than focusing on larger and longer-term goals (e.g. rather than obtaining employment focus on establishing a daily routine first). People frequently become isolated from family and friends during the course of their drug use. In

feeling socially isolated they can become vulnerable to relapse if they lack the skills to form new and healthier friendship groups. The re-establishment of new social groups that are not associated with substance use is essential in re-learning how to live without daily use. See Case study 13.1 to read about the experiences of a community health services client.

CASE STUDY 13.1: Helen

Helen has been a client of community health services for approximately 6 months receiving care for a leg ulcer, which is exacerbated by type 2 diabetes. She is 63 years old and lives by herself. Her husband died approximately 12 months ago. She has one married daughter and three grandchildren, who live overseas. On previous visits, Helen was well groomed, her house was clean and she seemed pleased to see the community nurse, offering her cups of tea and cakes that she had cooked. Recently, though, Helen seemed to have lost interest in caring for herself. On the last visit she appeared unkempt; her clothes were wrinkled and had food stains on them. Her hygiene was poor, and the smell of urine and body odour was quite strong. The community nurse noticed two empty flagons of sherry on the table and a half-full sherry bottle. Helen was irritable and her words were slurred. She said that she felt lonely and bored without her daughter and husband, and that "the sherry helps me to forget". Helen denied any previous problems with alcohol or other substances, but she did say that sherry had helped her to cope with the death of her husband, and that the doctor had then given her some pills and gradually they had made her feel better. Helen thinks that she "mostly remembers" to take her diabetes medication, but she does not know what all the fuss is about because there is "nothing wrong" with her.

? CRITICAL THINKING EXERCISE 13.1

1. When assessing a client for possible substance abuse, which of the following would alert the nurse to opioid intoxication?
   a. pupillary constriction
   b. unsteady gait (ataxia)
   c. slurring of words
   d. a strong smell of alcohol on the person's breath
2. Which of the following would alert the nurse to possible alcohol withdrawal?
   a. tremor and sweating
   b. wearing long sleeves and trousers on a very hot day
   c. inability to concentrate
   d. reddened eyes
   e. tachycardia

? CRITICAL THINKING EXERCISE 13.2

With reference to the case study about Helen (Case study 13.1), assume that you are working in a community mental health centre and have arranged to visit Helen. The community nurse has given you Helen's history in her referral letter.

1. How will you prioritise this situation?
2. What types of assessment will you initiate?
3. What questions might you ask?
4. Who will you discuss Helen's situation with?
5. What follow-up plan might you implement?

CHAPTER SUMMARY

Alcohol and other drug use is commonplace in Australia and Aotearoa New Zealand. Many people do not experience problems with their use, but some do and at harmful levels. People who have co-occurring substance use disorders and mental health changes are at greatest risk. There is evidence that these people experience more social problems and have less positive treatment outcomes. As a nurse, it is important to assess every client for alcohol or other drug use and to offer timely and effective treatment. Careful assessment is the key to offering targeted treatment to those presenting with substance use disorders. It is imperative that appropriate withdrawal management is implemented early in a client's treatment program to reduce the risk of adverse events. Treatment might take the form of brief interventions that can be offered in the alcohol and other drug or mental health setting. Alternatively, drug and alcohol and mental health services might need to find ways of working together to offer appropriate services to these clients.

Rates of tobacco use are high among clients with co-occurring disorders, and interventions should be made available to assist clients in reducing or ceasing their tobacco use, as this can dramatically impact on treatment outcomes. Alcohol is still the most used substance and nurses need to undertake an accurate history and follow area health service protocols to minimise the risk of withdrawal and associated complications. Despite the high prevalence of co-occurring disorders, there is little evidence about the nature of best practice for this client group. However, early recommendations from the research literature suggest that a program treating both disorders concurrently, with preference given to an integrated model of treatment, is most beneficial. Clients should be matched with treatments that work for them; there should be an emphasis on the relationship between the healthcare provider and the client. Clients are not separate diagnoses; they are a single person.

REVIEW QUESTIONS

1. Discuss the following questions with your group.
   a. What would you do if you were working on a ward or in a community setting where there were negative attitudes and feelings towards clients with alcohol and drug disorders? Would you challenge your colleagues or refrain from commenting? What would you do if their attitudes impacted on client care? When would you challenge them and what could you do?
   b. How would you feel if you observed another nurse drinking vodka during a lunch break when you were both working together on a ward? What would you do?
   c. Are you aware of your own negative attitudes and feelings that might impede your interactions and therapeutic response to a client with a substance-related disorder? If you have such attitudes, how would you overcome them to establish a therapeutic relationship with the client?
   d. What role does the Australian Health Professional Registration Authority (Ahpra) or the Nursing Council of New Zealand have in responding to a complaint about a nurse using substances when on duty?

2. A 36-year-old man is admitted with the following symptoms: T 38.1, P 106, R 28, BP 189/93, profuse perspiration and tremulousness. He appears highly agitated. A mental status examination reveals confusion, disorientation and visual and tactile hallucinations. His partner advises that he had been a heavy drinker, but he stopped 2 days ago. What substance-induced disorder is the client possibly experiencing?
   a. substance-induced psychosis
   b. alcohol withdrawal syndrome
   c. delirium tremens
   d. substance-induced anxiety disorder

3. When the nurse does an initial admission interview on a client being admitted for detoxification, which of the following areas is it critical to assess?
   a. type(s) of drug used
   b. family history
   c. reason for admission
   d. physical history

USEFUL WEBSITES

Amohia te Waiora: www.alcohol.org.nz

AUDIT – the Alcohol Use Disorders Identification Test: www.who.int/publications/i/item/WHO-MSD-MSB-01.6a

Australian alcohol guidelines revised: www.health.gov.au/news/australian-alcohol-guidelines-revised

Cochrane Library, evidence-based healthcare decision making: www.cochranelibrary.com

Glasgow Structured Approach to Assessment of the Glasgow Coma Scale: www.glasgowcomascale.org

Harm Reduction Australia: www.harmreductionaustralia.org.au

Harm Reduction Victoria: www.hrvic.org.au

ICD-11: www.who.int/classifications/icd/en/

Matua Raki, National Addiction Workforce Development: www.tepou.co.nz/stories/the-matua-raki-name-returns-home

Mental Health Coordinating Council (MHCC): www.mhcc.org.au

National Centre for Education and Training on Addictions (NCETA): nceta.flinders.edu.au

National Drug and Alcohol Research Centre: ndarc.med.unsw.edu.au

National Drug Research Institute: ndri.curtin.edu.au

National Institute on Drug Abuse: Advancing Addiction Science: nida.nih.gov

New South Wales Health – Clinical guidelines for nursing and midwifery practice in NSW: www.health.nsw.gov.au/aod/professionals/Pages/clinical-guidelines-nursing-and-midwifery.aspx

Queensland Alcohol and Drug Research and Education Centre: public-health.uq.edu.au/research/mental-health-tobacco-control-and-substance-abuse

Substance Abuse and Mental Health Services Administration (SAMHSA): www.samhsa.gov

Te Pou o Te Whakaaro Nui, national centre of evidence-based workforce development for the mental health, addiction and disability sectors in New Zealand: www.tepou.co.nz

Thorne Harbour health: thorneharbour.org

Turning Point Alcohol and Drug Centre: www.turningpoint.org.au

United Nations Office on Drugs and Crime: www.unodc.org

Victorian Responsible Gambling Foundation: www.responsiblegambling.vic.gov.au

REFERENCES

Akram, H., Mokrysz, C., Curran, H.V. 2019. What are the psychological effects of using synthetic cannabis? A systematic review. J Psychopharmacol, 33(3), 271–283.

Alcohol and Drug Foundation (ADF) 2022. Understanding dual diagnosis. Online. Available at: https://adf.org.au/insights/understanding-dual-diagnosis/

Alcoholics Anonymous (AA) Australia 2001. Alcoholics Anonymous world service. Online. Available at: https://aa.org.au/

American College of Obstetricians and Gynaecologists (ACOG) 2017. Opioid use and opioid use disorder in pregnancy. ACOG, 711, 1–14.

American Psychiatric Association (APA) 2022. Diagnostic and Statistical Manual of Mental Disorders, 5th Edition Text Revision (DSM-5 TR). APA, New York.

Australasian College for Emergency Medicine 2020. Alcohol and methamphetamine harm in emergency departments: Findings from the 2019 snapshot survey. ACEM, Melbourne. Online. Available at: https://acem.org.au/getmedia/f7bec2c4-6573-471f-8cf4-f9a0bc466506/Alcohol-Snapshot-Report_R6

Australian Bureau of Statistics (ABS) 2017. Causes of death Australia, 2016. ABS cat. no. 33030.0. ABS, Canberra.

Australian Criminal Intelligence Commission 2020. National Wastewater Drug Monitoring Program, Report 17. Online. Available at: www.acic.gov.au/sites/default/files/2022-10/national_wastewater_drug_monitoring_program_report_17.pdf

Australian Government 2021. Types of drugs. Online. Available at: www.health.gov.au/topics/drugs/about-drugs/types-of-drugs

Australian Institute of Health and Welfare (AIHW) 2022a. Alcohol, tobacco & other drugs in Australia. Online. Available at: www.aihw.gov.au/reports/alcohol/alcohol-tobacco-other-drugs-australia/contents/about

Australian Institute of Health and Welfare (AIHW) 2022b. Illicit opioids including heroin. Online. Available at: www.aihw.gov.au/getmedia/96719b23-a2cf-453f-8b21-87a484e213fd/PHE-221-Factsheets-Heroin.pdf.aspx

Australian Institute of Health and Welfare (AIHW) 2022c. Methamphetamine and other stimulants. Online. Available at: www.aihw.gov.au/getmedia/c5f95930-b056-40cb-97f9-30f9e7be0a8b/phe-221-factsheets-meth.pdf.aspx

Australian Institute of Health and Welfare (AIHW) 2022d. Pharmaceuticals. Available www.aihw.gov.au/getmedia/d16d63c0-1686-4f6b-8ddb-ffa51bc32b61/PHE-221-Factsheets-Pharmaceuticals.pdf.aspx

Australian Institute of Health and Welfare (AIHW) 2021a. Aboriginal and Torres Strait Islander health performance. Online. Available at: www.indigenoushpf.gov.au/

Australian Institute of Health and Welfare (AIHW) 2021b. Gambling in Australia. Online. Available at: www.aihw.gov.au/reports/australias-welfare/gambling

Australian Institute of Health and Welfare (AIHW) 2018. Australian mothers and babies 2016: in brief. Online. Available at: www.aihw.gov.au/reports/mothers-babies/australias-mothers-babies-2016-in-brief/contents/summary

Australian Institute of Health and Welfare (AIHW) 2017. National drug household survey 2016: Detailed findings. Drug statistics series no. 31. AIHW, Canberra.

Berridge, K.C., Kringelbach, M.L. 2015. Pleasure systems in the brain. Neuron 86(3), 646–664.

Biancarelli, D.L., Biello, K.B., Childs, E., Drainoni, M., Salhaney, P. et al., 2019. Strategies used by people who inject drugs to avoid stigma in healthcare settings. Drug Alcohol Depend, 198(1), 80–86.

Boisvert, D.L., Connolly, E.J., Vaske, J.C., et al., 2019. Genetic and environmental overlap between substance use and delinquency in adolescence: An analysis by same-sex twins. Youth Violence Juv Justice 17(2), 154–173.

Bower, C., Elliot, E.J. 2016. Report to the Australian Government Department of Health: Australian guide to the diagnosis of fetal alcohol spectrum disorder (FASD). Online. Available at: www.fasdhub.org.au/siteassets/pdfs/australian-guide-to-diagnosis-of-fasd_all-appendices.pdf

Brett, J., Lee, K., Gray, D., et al., 2016. Mind the gap: What is the difference between alcohol treatment need and access for Aboriginal and Torres Strait Islander Australians? Drug Alcohol Rev, 35, 456–460.

Bryant, J., Ward, J., Wand, H., et al., 2016. Illicit and injecting drug use among Indigenous young people in urban, regional and remote Australia. Drug Alcohol Rev. 35, 447–455.

Burns, L., Roxburgh, A., Matthews, A., et al., 2014. The rise of new psychoactive substance use in Australia. Drug Test Anal, 6(7–8), 846–849.

Centre for Disease Control and Prevention 2018. Health effects of cigarette smoking. Online. Available at: www.cdc.gov/tobacco/data_statistics/fact_sheets/health_effects/effects_cig_smoking/index.htm

Centre for Youth AOD Practice Development n.d. Youth AOD Toolbox. Online. Available at: www.youthaodtoolbox.org.au/stages-change

Cesconetto, P.A., Andrade, C.M., Cattani, D., et al., 2016. Maternal exposure to ethanol during pregnancy and lactation affects glutamatergic system and induces oxidative stress in offspring hippocampus. Alcohol Clin Exp Res, 40(1), 52–61.

Chamberlain, S.R., Stochl, J., Redden, S.A., et al., 2017. Latent class analysis of gambling sub-types and impulsive/compulsive associations: Time to rethink diagnostic boundaries for gambling disorder? Addict Behav, 72, 79–85.

Chapman, J., Roche, A.M., Kostadinov, V., Duraisingam, V. & Hodge, S. 2020. Lived experience: Characteristics of workers in alcohol and other drug non-government organizations. Contemp Drug Prob, 47(1), 63–77.

Clancy, R.V., Hodgson, R.C., Kendurkar, A., et al., 2018. Synthetic cannabinoid use in an acute psychiatric inpatient unit. Int J Ment Health Nurs, 27(2), 600–607.

Demant, D., Hides, L., Kavanagh, D.J. & White, K.M. 2018. LGBT communities and substance use in Queensland, Australia: Perceptions of young people and community stakeholders. PLoS One, 13(9), doi.org/10.1371/journal.pone.0204730.

Drake, R.E., Wallach, M.A. 2000. Dual diagnosis: 15 years of progress. Psychiatr Serv, 51(9), 1126–1129.

Dumas, A., Toutain, S., Hill, C., et al., 2018. Warning about drinking during pregnancy: Lessons from the French experience. Reprod Health, 15(20), 1–9.

FASD Hub 2016. FASD diagnosis: Australian guide to the diagnosis of FASD. Online. Available at: www.fasdhub.org.au/fasd-information/assessment-and-diagnosis/guide-to-diagnosis/

George Institute for Global Health 2013. Fighting for a future. The story of the women of Fitzroy Crossing. Online. Available at: www.georgeinstitute.org.au/projects/fighting-for-a-future-the-story-of-the-women-of-fitzroy-crossing

Government of South Australia 2023. Opioids. Online. Available at: www.sahealth.sa.gov.au/wps/wcm/connect/public+content/sa+health+internet/clinical+resources/clinical+programs+and+practice+guidelines/medicines+and+drugs/opioids/opioids

Government of South Australia 2019. Adverse effects due to long-term opioids – medical staff information. Online. Available at: www.sahealth.sa.gov.au/wps/wcm/connect/f190e680499f905480cbde9b6ca12d15/Fact%2Bsheet.adverse%2Beffects%2Bdue%2Bto%2Blongterm%2Bopioids.medical.pdf?MOD=AJPERES&CACHE=NONE&CONTENTCACHE=NONE

Gowing, L., Ali, R., Dunlop, A., et al., 2014. National guidelines for medication-assisted treatment of opioid dependence. Department of Health, Canberra.

Grant, J.E., Odlaug, B.L., Chamberlain, S.R. 2017. Gambling disorder, DSM-5 criteria and symptom severity. Compr Psychiatry 75, 1–5.

Grant, J.E., Odlaug, B.L., Schreiber, L.R.N. 2014. Pharmacological treatment in pathological gambling. Br J Clin Pharmacol, 77(2), 375–381.

Harm Reduction Australia. 2020. What is harm reduction? Online. Available at: www.harmreductionaustralia.org.au/what-is-harm-reduction/

Hill, A.O., Amos, N., Lyons, A., Jones, J., McGowan, I., et al., 2022. Illicit drug use among lesbian, gay, bisexual, pansexual, trans and gender diverse, queer and asexual young people in Australia: Intersections and associated outcomes. Drug Alcohol Rev 42(3), 714–728.

Hughes, J.A., Sheehan, M., Evans, J. 2017. Treatment and outcomes of patients presenting to an adult emergency department involuntarily with substance misuse. Int J Ment Health Nurs, 27(2), 593–599.

Humphreys, K., Blodgett, J.C., Wagner, T.H. 2014. Estimating the efficacy of Alcoholics Anonymous without self-selection bias: An instrumental variables re-analysis of randomized clinical trials. Alcohol Clin Exp Res, 38(11), 2688–2694.

Ishizuka, H. 2010. Carlyle's nervous dyspepsia: Nervousness, indigestion and the experience of modernity in nineteenth-century Britain. In: Salisbury, L., Shail, A. (eds), Neurology and Modernity: A Cultural History of Nervous Systems, 1800–1950. Palgrave Macmillan, London.

Kanniah, G. & Kumar, R. 2023. A selective literature review exploring the role of nicotinic system in schizophrenia. General Psychiatry 36(2), gpsych. bmj.com/content/36/2/e100756.

Karila, L., Roux, P., Rolland, B., et al., 2014. Acute and long-term effects of cannabis use: A review. Curr Pharm Des, 20(25), 4112–4118.

Kelly, J.F., Stout, R.L., Slaymaker, V. 2013. Emerging adults' treatment outcomes in relation to 12-step mutual-help attendance and active involvement. Drug Alcohol Depend, 129(1–2), 151–157.

Kleinloog, D., Roozen, F., De Winter, W. et al., 2014. Profiling subjective effects of delta9-tetrahydrocannabinol using visual analogue scales. Int J Psychiatr Res 23(2), 245–256.

Larance, B., Lintzeris, N., Ali, R., et al., 2014. The diversion and injection of a buprenorphine-naloxone soluble film formulation. Drug Alcohol Depend, 136, 21–27.

Lawn, W., Freeman, T.P., Pope, R.A., et al., 2016. Acute and chronic effects of cannabinoids on effort-related decision making and reward learning: An evaluation of cannabis amotivational hypotheses. Psychopharmacology (Berl), 233, 3537–3552.

Lehmann, S.W., Fingerhood, M. 2018. Substance-use disorders in later life. N Engl J Med, 379(24), 2351–2360.

LGBTIQ Health 2020. Media statement: The national drug strategy household survey key findings. Online. Available at: www.lgbtiqhealth.org.au/the_national_drug_strategy_household_survey_2019_key_findings

Lintzeris, N., Mammen, K., Holmes, J., Deacon, R., Mills, L., et al., 2020. Australian Treatment Outcomes Profile (ATOP) Manual 1: Using the ATOP with individual clients. COQI, Surry Hills, NSW.

Lubman, D., Sundram, S. 2003. Substance misuse in patients with schizophrenia: A primary care guide. MJA 178 (Suppl. May), 71–75.

Lundahl, B., Moleni, T., Burke, B.L., et al., 2013. Motivational interviewing in medical care settings: A systematic review and meta-analysis of randomized controlled trials. Patient Educ Couns, 93(2), 157–168.

Manning, V., Arunogiri, S., Frei, M., et al., 2018. Alcohol and Other Drug Withdrawal: Practice Guidelines, 3rd ed. Turning Point, Richmond.

Marsh, A., Dale, A., O'Toole, S. 2013. Addiction Counselling: Content and Process, 2nd ed. IP Communications, Melbourne.

Martin-Santos, R., Crippa, J.A., Batalla, A., et al., 2012. Acute effects of a single, oral dose of delta9-tetrahydrocannabinol (THC) and cannabidiol (CBD) administration in healthy volunteers. Curr Pharm Des, 18(2), 2966–4979.

McGovern, M.P., Lambert-Harris, C., Xie, H., et al., 2015. A randomized controlled trial of treatments for co-occurring substance use disorders and post-traumatic stress disorder. Addiction, 110(7), 1194–1204.

McMillan, S., Chan, H. & Hattingh, L.H. 2021. Australian community pharmacy harm minimization services: Scope of service expansion to improve healthcare access. Addict Ment Health Pharm, 9(2), 95.

Melkonian, A., Patel, R., Magh, A., Ferm, S & Hwang, C. 2019. Assessment of a hospital-wide CIWA-Ar protocol for management of alcohol withdrawal syndrome. Mayo Clin Proc Innov Qual Outcomes, 3(3), 344–349.

Mendelsohn, C.P., Kirby, D.P., Castle, D.J. 2015. Smoking and mental illness: An update for psychiatrists. Australas Psychiatry 23(1), 37–43.

Meridian 2021. Our communities. Online. Available at: www.meridianact.org.au/our_communities

Miller, W.R., Rollnick, S. 2009. Ten things that motivational interviewing is not. Behav Cogn Psychother, 37(2), 129–140.

Mills, K., Deady, M., Proudfoot, H., et al., 2008. Guidelines on the management of co-occurring alcohol and other drug and mental health conditions in alcohol and other drug treatment settings. National Drug and Alcohol Research Centre, University of New South Wales, Sydney.

Ministry of Health 2018a. Alcohol use in New Zealand: Key results of the 2016/2017 New Zealand Alcohol and Drug Use Survey. Ministry of Health, Wellington.

Ministry of Health 2018b. Alcohol and other drug use in New Zealand: Key results 2017/2018. Ministry of Health, Wellington.

Ministry of Health 2015. Cannabis use 2012/13: New Zealand Health Survey. Ministry of Health, Wellington. Online. Available at: www.health.govt.nz/publication/cannabis-use-2012-13-new-zealand-health-survey

Moore, T.J., Glenmullen, J., Mattison, D.R. 2014. Reports of pathological gambling, hypersexuality, and compulsive shopping associated with dopamine receptor agonist drugs. JAMA Intern Med, 174(12), 1930–1933.

Moyer, A., Finney, J.W. 2015. Brief interventions for alcohol misuse. CMAJ, 187(7), 502–506.

Musselman, M.E., Hampton, J.P. 2014. Not for human consumption: A review of emerging designer drugs. Pharmacother 34(7), 745–757.

National Drug Strategy 2017. Intergovernmental committee on drugs: National Drug Strategy 2017–2026. Online. Available at: www.health.gov.au/resources/collections/national-drug-strategy

National Health and Medical Research Council (NHMRC) 2020. Australian guidelines to reduce health risks from drinking alcohol. Commonwealth of Australia, Canberra. Online. Available at: www.nhmrc.gov.au/about-us/publications/australian-guidelines-reduce-health-risks-drinking-alcohol#block-views-block-file-attachments-content-block-1

National Institute on Drug Abuse 2019. Methamphetamine: What are the long-term effects of methamphetamine misuse? Online. Available at: www.drugabuse.gov/publications/methamphetamine/what-are-long-term-effects-methamphetamine-misuse

New South Wales (NSW) Department of Health 2008. NSW Drug and Alcohol Withdrawal Clinical Practice Guidelines. NSW Department of Health, Sydney.

New South Wales Health 2013. Clinical guidelines for nursing and midwifery practice in NSW. In: Identifying and Responding to Drug and Alcohol Issues. NSW Health, Sydney.

New Zealand Drug Foundation 2018. Nicotine. Online. Available at: www.drugfoundation.org.nz/info/drug-index/tobacco/

NOFASD 2018. FASD Informed. Online. Available at: www.nofasd.org.au/.

North Richmond Community Health (NRCH), 2022. Medically Supervised Injecting Room (MSIR). Online. Available at: Https://nrch.com.au/services/medically-supervised-injecting-room/

NSW Department of Health 2018. Nursing and Midwifery Clinical Guidelines: Identifying and responding to drug and alcohol issues. Online. Available at: www.health.nsw.gov.au/aod/professionals/Pages/clinical-guidelines-nursing-and-midwifery.aspx

NSW Ministry of Health 2020. Effective models of care for comorbid mental illness and illicit substance use: Evidence check review. Online. Available at: www.health.nsw.gov.au/mentalhealth/resources/Publications/comorbid-mental-care-review.pdf

Nutt, D.J., Lingford-Hughes, A., Erritzoe, D., et al., 2015. The dopamine theory of addiction: 40 years of highs and lows. Nat Rev Neurosci, 16(5), 305–312.

Otasowie, J. 2020. Co-occurring mental disorder and substance use disorder in young people: Aetiology, assessment and treatment. Br J Psychiatry, 27(4), 272–281.

Pitakowski, T.M., Hides, L.M., White, K.M., Obst, L.P. & Dunn, M. 2022. Understanding harm reduction perspectives of performance and image enhancing drug consumers and health care providers. Perform Enhanc Health, 10(3), 10.1016/j.peh.2022.100223.

Prochaska, J., DiClemente, C., 1984. The Transtheoretical Approach: Crossing Traditional Boundaries of Therapy. Dow/Jones Irwin, Homewood, Ill.

Qurashi, I., Stephenson, P., Nagaraj, C., Chu, S., Drake, R., et al., 2019. Changes in smoking status, mental state and plasma clozapine concentration: Retrospective cohort evaluation. BJ Psych Bulletin, 43(6), 271–274.

Rasmussen, N. 2011. Medical science and the military: The Allies' use of amphetamine during World War II. J Interdisc Hist, 42(2), 205–233.

Ries, R., Fiellin, D., Miller, S., et al., 2014. American Society of Addiction Medicine: Principles of Addiction Medicine. Wolters Kluwer, Philadelphia.

Riper, H., Andersson, G., Hunter, S.B., et al., 2014. Treatment of comorbid alcohol use disorders and depression with cognitive behavioural therapy and motivational interviewing: A meta-analysis. Addiction 109(3), 394–406.

Robertson, C.L., Ishibashi, K., Mandelkern, M.A., et al., 2015. Striatal D1- and D2-type dopamine receptors are linked to motor response inhibition in human subjects. J Neurosci, 35 (15), 5990–5997.

Rosenfeld, J.V. 2012. Practical Management of Head and Neck Injury. Churchill Livingstone, Sydney.

Roussy, V., Thomaco, N., Rudd, A., et al., 2017. Enhancing health-care workers' understanding and thinking about people living with co-occurring mental health and substance use issues through consumer-led training. Health Expect, 18(5), 1567–1581.

St Vincent's Hospital Melbourne 2019. Alcohol Withdrawal Syndrome: Clinical Practice Guidelines. St Vincent's Hospital, Melbourne.

Substance Abuse and Mental Health Services Administration (SAMHSA) 2023. Co-occurring disorders and other health conditions. Online. Available at: www.samhsa.gov/medications-substance-use-disorders/medications-counseling-related-conditions/co-occurring-disorders

Substance Abuse and Mental Health Services Administration (SAMHSA) 2017. Focus on prevention: Strategies and programs to prevent substance use. Online. Available at: store.samhsa.gov/system/files/sma10-4120.pdf

Sud, P., Gordon, M., Tortora, L., et al., 2018. Retrospective chart review of synthetic cannabinoid intoxication with toxicologic analysis. West J Emerg Med, 19(3), 567–572.

The Cancer Council 2018. Measures of tobacco dependence. Online. Available at: www.tobaccoinaustralia.org.au/chapter-6-addiction/6-12-measures-of-tobacco-dependence

The Royal Women's Hospital 2018a. Women's Alcohol and Drug Service. Alcohol and pregnancy. Online. Available at: www.thewomens.org.au/images/uploads/fact-sheets/YAYB-Alcohol-and-pregnancy-250818.pdf

The Royal Women's Hospital 2018b. Cigarettes and tobacco. Online. Available at: www.thewomens.org.au/images/uploads/fact-sheets/YAYB-Cigarettes-and-tobacco-250818.pdf

United Nations Office on Drugs and Crime (UNODC) 2023. UNODC-Early warning advisory on new psychoactive substances. Online. Available at: www.unodc.org/LSS/Page/NPS

United Nations Office on Drugs and Crime (UNODC) 2022. World Drug Report 2022: Global overview of drug demand and supply. United Nations, Vienna.

United Nations Office on Drugs and Crime (UNODC) 2020. UNODC/WHO International Treatment Standards. Online. Available at: www.unodc.org/documents/drug-prevention-and-treatment/UNODC-WHO_International_Treatment_Standards_March_2020.pdf

Uniting 2022. Medically Supervised Injecting Centre (MSIC) overview. Online. Available at: www.uniting.org/community-impact/uniting-medically-supervised-injecting-centre--msic

Vasilaki, E.I., Hosier, S.G., Cox, W.M. 2006. The efficacy of motivational interviewing as a brief intervention for excessive drinking: A meta-analytic review. Alcohol, 41(3), 328–335.

Victorian Responsible Gambling Foundation 2022. Expenditure on gambling in Victoria. Online. Available at: www.responsiblegambling.vic.gov.au

Victorian Responsible Gambling Foundation. 2020. Lived experience of help-seeking in the presence of gambling related harms and co-existing mental health conditions. Online. Available at: responsiblegambling.vic.gov.au/documents/1012/VRGF_RR-AUG2021_Lived_Experience_Jul20_8TvUDXc.pdf

Waaktaar, T., Kan, K.J., Torgerson, S. 2018. The genetic and environmental architecture of substance use development from early adolescence into young adulthood: A longitudinal twin study of comorbidity of alcohol, tobacco and illicit drug use. Addiction, 113 (4), 740–748.

Wand, H., Ward, J., Bryant, J., et al., 2016. Individual and population level impacts of illicit drug use, sexual risk behaviours on sexually transmitted infections among young Aboriginal and Torres Strait Islander people: Results from the Goanna survey. BMC Public Health 16(1), 1–9.

Wild, T.C., Cunningham, J.A., Roberts, A.B. 2007. Controlled study of brief personalized assessment – feedback for drinkers interested in self-help. Addiction 102(2), 241–250.

Wise, E.A., Streiner, D.L., Gallop, R.J. 2017. Predicting change in an integrated dual diagnosis substance abuse intensive outpatient program. Subst Use Misuse 52(7), 848–857.

World Health Organization (WHO) 2022. Alcohol. Online. Available at: www.who.int/news-room/fact-sheets/detail/alcohol

World Health Organization (WHO) 2019. Methodone use for treatment of opioid dependence. Online. Available at: www.who.int/data/gho/indicator-metadata-registry/imr-details/2545

World Health Organization (WHO) 2018. International Classification of Diseases (ICD-11), 11th revision. Online. Available at: https://icd.who.int/en/

World Health Organization (WHO) 2015. ASSIST (Alcohol Smoking and Substance Involvement Screening Test). Online. Available at: www.who.int/publications/i/item/978924159938-2

World Health Organization (WHO) 2001. AUDIT: The Alcohol Use Disorders Identification Test. Guidelines for use in primary healthcare, 2nd edn. Online. Available at: www.who.int/publications/i/item/WHO-MSD-MSB-01.6a

Yokell, M.A., Zaller, N.D., Green, T.C., et al., 2011. Buprenorphine and buprenorphine/naloxone diversion, misuse, and illicit use: An international review. Curr Drug Abuse Rev, 4(1), 28–41.

14

Psychosis and Schizophrenia

Catherine Daniel and Elizabeth Currie

KEY POINTS

- Most people diagnosed with psychotic disorders such as schizophrenia can recover if they are supported in ways they identify as most valuable.
- Mental health nurses who focus on working in partnership and are compassionate, human-to-human relationships can be invaluable in supporting people labelled as psychotic.

- The aetiology of schizophrenia is poorly understood. Despite this, theories are often promoted as explanations of its origins.
- Experiences of mental ill health, such as experiencing a psychosis, can be understood by many people as meaningful responses to life experiences such as trauma, social stressors and chronic mis-attunement to individual needs.

KEY TERMS

Alternative theories
Dominant models of understanding
Ecological System Framework and psychosis

Language, labels, stigma and discrimination
Positive and negative symptoms
Psychotherapy and psychopharmacology

Recovery
Social determinants
Trauma informed care

LEARNING OUTCOMES

The material in this chapter will assist you to:
- understand the prevalence and social determinants of people diagnosed with schizophrenia
- develop awareness of the influence of language, culture, ideology and power embedded within current dominant approaches to psychosis

- build familiarity with commonly used descriptions of signs and symptoms associated with psychosis and schizophrenia
- outline modern alternative approaches to working with psychosis, including the Power Threat Meaning Framework, Open Dialogue and Intervoice: The International Hearing Voices Network.

INTRODUCTION

The human mind controls an amazing, relational and embodied process that regulates the flow of energy and information, processing millions of pieces of information from myriad micro and macro experiences every day (Siegel & Drulis 2023). Given its remarkable complexity, there should be little surprise that the mind is sensitive to anomalies. This chapter is concerned with how to provide nursing care to people whose minds experience distortions in perception and thoughts, broadly referred to as psychosis and schizophrenia-related phenomena. Additionally, this chapter offers information on the clinical evaluation and treatment of people who are experiencing psychosis, across multiple theoretical orientations and diverse populations.

The word "psychosis" stems from the ancient Greek term meaning "illness of the mind", and records show that people have had such experiences ever since the beginning of recorded history. In the modern era, psychosis has become a term used to describe a disease of the brain, a phenomenon in which people experience a move away from regular perception into an inner world, in which patterns of thinking,

feeling and behaving become distorted. Many people experience psychosis as confusing, bizarre and frightening. For others, however, psychosis can be more bearable than their "real world".

Like other mental illnesses, experiences currently labelled as psychosis and schizophrenia-type disorders do not have any laboratory tests or other diagnostic procedures that can either confirm or refute diagnoses. Often, psychosis is not only strange for the person who experiences it, but becomes confusing for the people around them. Unfortunately, fear created by this confusion then leads people who receive diagnoses to be treated in discriminatory ways. People diagnosed with conditions such as schizophrenia are often considered unpredictable and dangerous. While there is a small increased risk of violence associated with psychosis, portrayal of violence is often exaggerated; in fact, the reverse is true in that people who experience psychosis have far higher chance of being victims of crime and violence (Ross et al 2020). Despite modern education campaigns, research reveals that people who have experienced psychosis feel that the effects of stigma are as bad as or indeed worse than the effects of the psychosis itself.

Many people fear that experiencing a psychotic episode means they will inevitably be burdened with a lifetime diagnosis of schizophrenia; this may be based on the initial findings by Emil Kraepelin (1856–1926), a German psychiatrist who was influential in defining the illness as a "progressive deterioration". It is now known that this is not entirely accurate. Long-term studies have shown that early effective interventions may lead to social and functional recovery (Onitsuka et al 2022). Given such evidence, this chapter takes a recovery-oriented approach to understanding psychosis and schizophrenia-related phenomena. It is assumed that the focus of mental health nursing is working with the issues experienced by consumers whatever their diagnosis, as well as supporting their families and carers. This chapter addresses how people who receive a diagnosis such as "psychosis" and "schizophrenia" are understood, cared for and treated. Descriptions of common symptoms, such as disorganisation, delusions and hallucinations, are provided, along with alternative modern approaches to working with people who experience psychosis.

PREVALENCE AND SOCIAL DETERMINANTS

Schizophrenia affects approximately 24 million people or 1 in 300 (0.32%) worldwide. The lifetime prevalence of schizophrenia and related psychotic disorders range between 0.33% and 0.75% (Howell et al 2019; Onitsuka et al 2022). There is some variability in the reported rates in individual studies due to the research design, study setting, sample size and differing definitions of psychosis and schizophrenia-spectrum disorders across cultural groups.

Modern psychiatric literature, such as the *Diagnostic and Statistical Manual for Mental Disorders*, 5th Edition (DSM-5) (American Psychiatric Association (APA) 2013), estimates prevalence at similar figures and that the schizophrenia rarely occurs before adolescence, with onset most common in the early to mid-20s. There are also statistics to indicate the median male/female ratio, which indicates that more men are diagnosed with schizophrenia than women (Onitsuka et al 2022). Unfortunately, due to stigma and historically poor care and approaches, people who experience psychosis and schizophrenia-type conditions are far more likely to experience disadvantage through poverty, incarceration and homelessness. These factors are potentially modifiable, but require societal change and governmental resources, commitment, and investment.

Prison populations in Australia and Aotearoa New Zealand and similar populations overseas continue to have a disproportionately high number of people diagnosed with psychosis and schizophrenia-type conditions (Chowdhury et al 2019). There could be mitigating circumstances for this over-representation; for example, a shoplifter might offend because of lapses of memory and concentration, or because of confusion due to a psychotic episode, comorbid drug or alcohol use. Nonetheless, the existence of an association between mental illness and crime contributes to the stigma that mentally ill people experience.

Cultural meaning and understanding are also often overlooked when a person is labelled as being psychotic. This is despite the rich knowledge and understanding among many First Nations peoples of the experiences of what we in the western world call psychosis. The work of Taitimu and colleagues (2018), *Ngā Whakāwhitinga (standing at the crossroads): How Māori understand what Western psychiatry calls "schizophrenia"*, describes how First Nations peoples understand the experience that modern approaches refer to as schizophrenia, with strong cultural and spiritual overlays.

In the Organisation for Economic Co-operation and Development (OECD) nations, psychotic disorders such as schizophrenia also tend to be more prevalent among the socially disadvantaged. The homeless population is one example where there are higher rates of the condition, and people of different cultural backgrounds, including Aboriginal and Torres Strait Islander people, also have a higher prevalence (Grech & Raeburn 2019).

The main societal costs related to psychosis are due to lost productivity caused by high unemployment and under-employment of people with mental illness, along with health service costs, which commonly include in-patient hospital, criminal justice system and community-based psychiatry costs. Schizophrenia has the highest median societal costs for mental illnesses, with those costs being highest in relation to people with negative symptoms (Kotzeva et al 2023). It is important to note that studies show young people who experience psychosis want to work; however, they are less likely to be employed compared to their peers (Aguey-Zinsou et al 2022).

THE POWERFUL ROLE OF LANGUAGE AND LABELS

In many parts of society language is a tool that has been used to control, threaten and coerce people who experience mental ill health into line or to modify behaviours. Nurses need to be aware of the power of language and communication, both verbal and non-verbal. Language needs to be well considered, respectful, honest and genuine in ways that enhance the process of therapeutic engagement and alliance. Language also needs to be both inclusive, and not used to perpetuate stigma and discrimination.

The modern label "schizophrenia" was coined in 1911 by Swiss psychiatrist Eugen Bleuler (1857–1939) as an amalgam of two Greek words: S*chizo*, meaning "split", and *phrenia*, meaning "mind". Bleuler intended the term to symbolise the schism between the external world of the individual and the internal conflict of the individual's mind. (His emphasis was on the split or lost connections between thoughts and the split connections between thought, emotion and will.) Despite this, a dominant societal myth equating schizophrenia with a "split personality" developed. This belief equated schizophrenia with a sort of "Jekyll and Hyde" manifestation, wherein an apparently "normal" person may turn unpredictably into a person who is irrational and dangerous. Unfortunately, popular film and media characterisations of people who experience psychosis often fail to accurately depict the manifestations of the experience and often perpetuate such common myths, stereotypes and stigma.

Descriptions of signs and symptoms of psychosis are therefore heavily reliant on cultural and linguistic terms. Such terms have been invented due to the neurotypical human desire to group experiences into clusters that appear to be similar. Despite the ever-changing language and lack of objectivity that surrounds how mental disorders such as psychosis are described, it is nonetheless important for nurses to familiarise themselves with the current dominant ways of thinking and talking about mental ill health.

Inclusive language in mental health is another contemporary area that is now being addressed. Diverse communities, such as lesbian, gay, bisexual, transgender, intersex, queer, asexual+ (LGBTIQA+), have been identified as having increase risks, due to gender minority stress which can lead to higher degrees of psychological distress and mental ill-health (Ventriglio et al 2022). A study that explored data obtained from an online psychosis screening and support program identified that individuals who identified as LGBTQ reported psychosis-like experiences but were reluctant to seek support, mainly due to fear of discrimination (Savill et al 2022). Research from Barr and colleagues (2021) concurs with this data in that they found higher rates of psychotic disorders in transgendered people. Greater consideration and inclusive language towards gender diversity in psychosis research will support clinical care. Thus, mental health nurses need to familiarise themselves with nationally and locally developed language guides to support their understanding of the use of universal and inclusive language to promote therapeutic engagement. The Victorian Department of Health has developed such a guide, considering the nuances across different generations and cultures (see Useful websites at the end of the chapter).

The signs and symptoms described in the section below are abridged descriptions from the 2013 DSM-5, which is the most used source for descriptors for symptoms of mental ill health in modern healthcare systems. These next two sections should be read with the concerns previously outlined regarding language, culture, ideology and power in mind.

SIGNS AND SYMPTOMS

Psychotic disorders such as schizophrenia are characterised by one or more of the following five types of symptoms: delusions; hallucinations; disorganised thinking (speech); grossly disorganised or abnormal motor behaviour (including catatonia); or negative symptoms. Each of these states are outlined below.

Delusions are fixed beliefs that are not amenable to change in light of conflicting evidence. Their content may include a variety of themes (e.g. persecutory, referential, somatic, religious, grandiose). Examples include:

- paranoid delusions, such as a belief that the person is being followed or monitored (e.g. "My neighbour is plotting to kill me")
- grandiose delusions, where a person may believe they have special abilities or "powers" (e.g. "I can fly" or "I'm on a mission from God")
- thought broadcasting, which is the belief that the person's thoughts are being broadcast to or heard by others
- thought withdrawal, which is the belief that others are taking their thoughts
- thought insertion, which is the belief that thoughts are being placed in their mind against their will.

Hallucinations refer to distortions in perception. People with psychosis may experience hallucinations in any of the five senses, hearing, seeing, feeling, smelling or tasting sensations that do not appear to be real. Common hallucinations include:

- auditory hallucinations, which commonly include hearing voices talking to them or about them, or hearing music and other noises when there is no sound (e.g. hearing someone call their name when they are at home alone)
- visual hallucinations, such as seeing things that are not there, or seeing things in a strange way (e.g. seeing unusual shapes, colours or lights, or seeing an image of someone standing before them)
- tactile hallucinations involving feeling something touch or something happening in their body when there is nothing there (e.g. feeling as though ants are crawling on their skin)
- olfactory hallucinations, which involve smelling things when there are no smells around (e.g. smelling rotting fish in the house, even though there are no fish there)
- gustatory hallucinations, which refer to tasting things in a strange way (e.g. tasting metal in their mouth).

Disorganised thinking is inferred from a person's speech. It is commonly characterised as including speech that switches rapidly from one topic to another; this may be described as "derailment" or "loose associations". A person may reply to questions with answers that are tangential, which means they are oblique or unrelated. Sometimes speech may be incomprehensible, and it may be described as incoherent or "word salad". Nurses conducting a mental health assessment need to remember that mildly disorganised speech is common and

non-specific, so symptoms must be severe enough to substantially impair effective communication. Severity of the impairment may be difficult to evaluate if the person making the diagnosis comes from a different linguistic background than that of the person being examined. Less severe disorganised thinking or speech may occur during the prodromal and residual periods of schizophrenia. Speech may include:

- "neologisms", which involves using words that don't exist
- "echolalia", which is repeating words/phrases used by other people in conversation
- "perseveration", whereby the person uses excessive continuation/ repetition of a single response or idea.

Disorganised behaviour may be exhibited in a variety of ways, ranging from childlike "silliness" to unpredictable agitation. Problems may be noted in any form of goal-directed behaviour, leading to difficulties in performing activities of daily living (ADLs). Catatonic behaviour is a marked decrease in reactivity to the environment. This can include:

- resistance to instructions (negativism)
- maintaining a rigid, inappropriate or bizarre posture
- a complete lack of verbal and motor responses (mutism and stupor)
- purposeless and excessive motor activity without obvious cause (catatonic excitement).

Other features include repeated stereotyped movements, staring, grimacing, mutism and the echoing of speech. Although catatonia has historically been associated with schizophrenia, catatonic symptoms are non-specific and may occur in other mental disorders (e.g. bipolar or depressive disorders with catatonia) and in medical conditions (catatonic disorder due to another medical condition).

Negative symptoms are absences or reductions of thought processes, emotions and behaviours that were present before the onset of the illness, but have since diminished or are absent following the onset of the illness. These symptoms are substantial in schizophrenia, but less common in other psychotic disorders.

Diminished emotional expression includes reductions in the expression of emotions in the face, eye contact, intonation of speech and movements of the hand, head and face that normally give an emotional emphasis to speech.

Avolition refers to a decrease in motivated self-initiated purposeful activities. The person may sit for long periods of time and show little interest in participating in work or social activities. Other negative symptoms include alogia, anhedonia and asociality:

- Alogia manifests in diminished speech output.
- Anhedonia is the decreased ability to experience pleasure from positive stimuli or a degradation in recalling pleasure previously experienced.
- Asociality refers to the apparent lack of interest in social interactions and may be associated with avolition, but it can also be a manifestation of limited opportunities for social interactions.

Symptoms of psychosis often contribute to deterioration in interpersonal relationships. Heightened levels of anxiety are experienced as the person identifies a perceived conflict between what is and what should be. Anger may occur when others appear to disregard what the person acknowledges as their reality, and attempts are made to refocus and reorient. The person may feel their need for safety and security are threatened by their attempt to cope with an "alien world".

It is important to remember that the signs and symptoms described above are the opinion and view of the APA – the organisation that constructed the DSM-5. Such descriptions are therefore layered with cultural understandings from an American/western point of view and, as previously stated, lack objective scientific evidence. When a person seeks to dispute the construct of schizophrenia, nurses can play a pivotal role in supporting and advocating for the legitimate views and experiences of the person in distress towards forming a collaborative understanding.

In Personal perspectives: Consumer's story 14.1, James talks about how he found validation for his experiences in the "hearing voices"

movement, which is an example of the emerging influence of consumer-led understandings and involvement. International Hearing Voices Network groups operate at a wide variety of locations in Australia, Aotearoa New Zealand and overseas. Relevant weblinks can be found in the Useful websites list at the end of this chapter.

PERSONAL PERSPECTIVES

Consumer's Story 14.1: James

I had used illicit drugs since my early teens. I had lived overseas and experienced homelessness, and I could see little future in my life when at the age of 21 I went with my mother to see a general practitioner (GP). The GP was concerned about my focus on suicide, sense of hopelessness and reported drug use, so following liaison with the mental health team, he arranged for a direct admission to a psychiatric hospital. Although I had many friends growing up, I had few functional relationships in my life at this time and my family was very concerned about my wellbeing. They had little knowledge about mental health problems at this stage.

Although I was assessed by a consultant psychiatrist and a nurse, I felt that the nurse heard me most clearly and appeared to be less concerned by my diagnosis and more concerned with who I might be and the experiences that might have contributed to my condition. I was started on antipsychotic and antidepressant medication and discharged 6 weeks later to my mother's home, with planned GP follow-up. One of the friends I made in hospital killed himself shortly after I left hospital, and not long after this I made an attempt on my own life. I told people I was hearing voices saying that I was worthless and should kill myself. I also heard the voice of a man saying that he was watching me through video cameras at all times, and I became very frightened. I did not try to end my life because the voices were telling me to. I was suicidal in the context of despair and homelessness that was exacerbated by the system's responses.

Several admissions followed during which I had stopped using illicit drugs, yet I still heard derogatory voices and felt a sense that the world and myself were being controlled by an external "force". I was suicidal and I tried to kill myself, following through on a plan I had made. Other frightening psychotic experiences included seeing a cat who I believed attempted to kill me, which led to my imprisoning myself for 3 days until I knew that the cat had gone. I experienced a sense of being an incompetent human being and searched for potential explanations for my experiences, exploring my sexuality and seeking religious justifications. I was admitted to hospital five times, but I felt that the nursing and medical teams never discovered what caused my experiences of psychosis. My unusual realities were considered part of a biomedically informed rationale for a psychotic disorder, and the possibility of my suffering from schizophrenia was not excluded. Nurses spent

a lot of time with me in the unit, but they were task-oriented. I believe that they could have used basic mental health nursing skills, such as building a therapeutic relationship, to develop a more meaningful understanding of the events that contributed to my experiencing psychosis. Treatment focused on medications and electroconvulsive therapy. I was prescribed a concoction of antipsychotic, antidepressant and mood-stabilising medications. I feel now that, as my primary healthcare workers, nurses could have been more assertive in identifying for me the side effects of my medication and their negative impact. A proactive approach on their part might have prevented or addressed a number of the difficulties and problems that arose. I gained 50 kg in 18 months, probably due to medication, a poor diet and reduced exercise, and I became increasingly socially isolated: All of which were perceived by nursing staff as the usual negative symptoms of a psychotic illness. No one talked about recovery, and the concept of a positive personal and clinical journey was not easy to imagine.

During my fifth admission I commenced 2 years of psychotherapy because medication and hospitalisation had not led to an improvement in my symptoms. I went to live in a nurse-led housing community of eight residents with mental health problems, where the person-centred emphasis was less on diagnosis and disease and more on the acceptance of my own experiences and reality, and support for my journey towards my future. I made a number of friends in the mental health system, and that mutual acceptance between peers proved to be a significant factor in making sense of the whole experience, and finally, in accepting myself.

Over time the voices and other psychotic phenomena impacted my life less, and I worked with a psychiatrist to reduce, then stop, all medications. I worked as a volunteer, then found paid employment before moving into my own accommodation. Since the 4-year period when I was "treated" by the mental health system for a psychotic disorder, I have spent 15 years following my life journey, being part of a beautiful family as a husband and a father to three children and developing a successful career in mental health nursing and therapy. Especially valuable in helping me to interpret the cause of the voices that I experienced has been the "hearing voices" approach towards making sense of and understanding psychosis.

TYPES OF PSYCHOSIS AND SCHIZOPHRENIA-RELATED PHENOMENA

There are no laboratory tests or other diagnostic procedures that can either confirm or refute a diagnosis. Making psychiatric diagnoses therefore relies heavily on detailed history-taking, behavioural observation and opinion. Data gained from a comprehensive assessment are then measured against diagnostic criteria published by groups such as the APA (DSM-5) and the World Health Organization (WHO) and the *International Classification of Diseases* 11th Revision, or ICD-11.

Grouping similar signs and symptoms into diagnostic categories is an attempt to increase effectiveness of assessment and treatment of mental ill health and allow clinicians to be consistent in language used to describe psychotic experiences. This is not an evidence-based approach, but remains the dominant model. Common diagnostic terms currently used to describe psychotic disorders and fit within the

umbrella term of schizophrenia spectrum and other psychotic disorders in modern health care include:

- substance-induced psychotic disorder
- brief intermittent psychosis
- delusional disorder
- schizophreniform disorder
- schizophrenia
- schizoaffective disorder.

In clinical settings, you may come across other people with psychotic symptoms that do not meet the criteria under these categories, such as psychosis due to other medical conditions (e.g. traumatic brain injury or temporal lobe epilepsy), as well as the symptoms that may describe prodromal psychosis which can be classified as attenuated psychosis, within conditions for further studies. Disorders such as postpartum psychosis are serious and can result in maternal and infant mortality and morbidity. First episode psychosis (FEP) will be mentioned in brief, just to provide some context to other presentations you may encounter.

Brief summaries below provide abridged versions of descriptions found in *Schizophrenia Spectrum and Other Psychotic Disorders: DSM-5 Selections* (APA 2015).

Substance-Induced Psychotic Disorder

To be diagnosed with substance-induced psychotic disorder, a person needs to have experienced delusions or hallucinations and their health history, physical examination or laboratory findings need to indicate that psychosis developed during or soon after substance intoxication or withdrawal, or after exposure to a medication capable of producing psychotic symptoms. The substance-induced psychosis needs to have caused substantial distress or impairment in social, occupational or other important areas of functioning. Other medical causes, such as delirium, need to be excluded, and it needs to be clear that the psychosis is not better explained by a pre-existing psychotic disorder that preceded the substance/medication use or that persists for a substantial period (at least a month) after the cessation of acute withdrawal or severe intoxication.

Brief Intermittent Psychosis

Brief intermittent psychosis is distinctive because it involves the sudden onset of psychosis and is strictly time-limited, lasting for more than a day but less than a month, with eventual full return to psychosocial functioning. To receive a diagnosis of brief intermittent psychosis, a person needs to exhibit the presence of one (or more) of the following symptoms: delusions, hallucinations, disorganised speech (e.g. incoherence or frequent derailment), grossly disorganised behaviour or catatonic behaviour. Other experiences include mental disorders such as depression or bipolar disorder. The possibility that a person may be affected by drugs or other general medical conditions needs to be excluded. Specific description of a brief intermittent psychosis may also be added if it occurs in response to stressful events, during pregnancy or within 4 weeks' postpartum.

Delusional Disorder

To be diagnosed with delusional disorder, a person needs to have experienced the presence of one (or more) delusions for a month or longer. Second, on assessment it needs to be clarified that the person does not meet diagnostic criteria for schizophrenia, and if hallucinations are present, they must not be prominent or related to the delusional theme. Third, the person's behaviour needs to be interpreted as not being obviously odd or bizarre; social and occupational functioning needs not to have been markedly impaired. Fourth, if manic or major depressive episodes have occurred, these need to have been brief relative to the duration of the delusional periods. Fifth, other illnesses, including mental disorders such as body dysmorphic disorder or obsessive-compulsive disorder or the possibility that the person may be affected by drugs or other general medical conditions, needs to be excluded. On diagnosis, the specific type of delusional psychosis should be described – for example, grandiose, jealous, persecutory, mixed or erotomanic.

Schizophreniform Disorder

For a diagnosis of schizophreniform disorder, a person needs to have exhibited at least two of the following list of symptoms, including at least one from a, b or c:
a. delusions
b. hallucinations
c. disorganised speech (e.g. frequent derailment or incoherence)
d. grossly disorganised behaviour

e. catatonic behaviour
f. negative symptoms (diminished emotional expression or avolition).

Symptoms must last for at least 1 month but less than 6 months. Other disorders, such as schizoaffective disorder and depressive or bipolar disorder with psychotic features, need to be excluded.

Schizophrenia

A diagnosis of schizophrenia requires a person to have experienced at least 6 months of a mixture of negative and positive symptoms. Negative symptoms are characterised by a marked disturbance level of functioning in one or more major areas, such as work, interpersonal relations or self-care, and is markedly below the level achieved before the onset (or when the onset is in childhood or adolescence, there is failure to achieve the expected level of interpersonal, academic or occupational functioning). Within the 6-month period, the person also needs to have experienced at least 1 month of positive symptoms for a substantial period, with at least one of a, b or c being present.
a. delusions
b. hallucinations
c. disorganised speech (e.g. frequent derailment or incoherence)
d. grossly disorganised or catatonic behaviour
e. negative symptoms (i.e. diminished emotional expression or avolition).

Other conditions, such as schizoaffective disorder and depressive or bipolar disorder, need to be excluded and the symptoms must not be attributable to any other physiological cause or substance use.

Schizoaffective Disorder

Schizoaffective disorder describes a long-term condition in which a person experiences a mood episode (major depression or mania), along with symptoms fulfilling the primary criteria for schizophrenia. Diagnoses must exclude the effects of a substance (a drug of abuse, a medication) and other medical conditions as causative. If a manic episode is part of the presentation, the schizoaffective disorder may be specified as "bipolar type". If major depressive episodes occur, it may be classified as "depressive type".

First Episode Psychosis

It is important to mention first episode psychosis (FEP) within this section for your nursing considerations. There is evidence to suggest that many people (not all) prior to first episode of psychosis have symptoms of impairment in social and occupational functioning (prodromal). There can be noticeable indicators, such as trouble thinking clearly, spending more time alone, increasing worry about school or work performance and/or suspiciousness. Some people have retrospectively stated inappropriate emotional responses and or no emotion/feeling at all. First episode psychosis is usually evident in adolescence and early adulthood and manifests as acute psychotic symptoms of the illness. It can be classified on the onset of symptoms, either within the month, or gradual (symptoms within 6 months), or insidious (symptoms that can occur after 6 months or longer) (Brasso et al 2021). The clinical outcome for FEP is multifactorial (background, risk factors and treatment choices) and will not be explored in detail here. Psychosocial impairment can occur for individuals who experience a chronic course of the illness or have full symptom remission. There needs to be further evidence and robust studies on outcomes of FEP; however, this is limited by the scarcity of long-term follow-up of greater than 20 years (Peralta et al 2021).

Postpartum Psychosis

The rarity of a mental health condition still warrants discussion, such is the case for postpartum psychosis. This condition is known to only effect 1–2:1000 women who give birth, yet the severity of the condition can result in high risks for both the mother and child if left untreated (Spinelli 2021; Ungvarsky 2023).

Symptoms can include:

- delusions or strange beliefs (e.g. thinking their newborn is possessed or someone is trying to harm the child).
- hallucinations (more commonly visual and olfactory in nature)
- thoughts of harm to self and baby
- increased irritation
- hyperactivity
- severe depression or flat affect
- lability of mood
- decreased need for or inability to sleep.

These symptoms can alter rapidly and there may be noticeable changes in the person behaving uncharacteristically, such as signs of paranoia or suspiciousness of those around her (Ungvarsky 2023). The condition is frequently associated with infanticide (murder of the baby); and statistics have indicated increased maternal death by suicide of up to 20% in the first postpartum year (Spinelli 2021).

ALTERNATIVE APPROACHES TO PSYCHOSIS AND SCHIZOPHRENIA-RELATED PHENOMENA

While the definitions listed above tend to be the dominant descriptions used in modern health services, it is important for nurses to know that there is a growing disquiet regarding the lack of effectiveness, overly biomedical and concrete nature of such diagnostic terms. Frustration with systems such as the DSM-5 have led people working with allied health professionals and people with lived experience of mental ill health to develop a range of emerging, alternative approaches to understanding experiences currently labelled as psychosis and schizophrenia.

Brief summaries of four promising modern alternative approaches are outlined as follows.

The Power Threat Meaning Framework

The Power Threat Meaning Framework (PTMF) provides a conceptual and intellectual alternative to diagnostic and medicalised thinking and practice in the treatment of mental ill-health. This framework considers aspects of human experience, such as the operation of power, the links between threats and fear responses, and the autonomy of people within personal, social, economic and material environments (Boyle 2022).

Individual personal stories offer rich and meaningful alternatives to psychiatric diagnosis. The discussion of power is one of interest and the suggestion that where this operation is not central to the person the emotional distress and troubling behaviour can be more evident. This PTMF sits well along the notion of adverse childhood experiences (ACE) (Boyle 2022). Often there is failure to find a biological cause, yet this framework suggests evidence for psychosocial causes for people who present with schizophrenia and psychosis is evident. Read the quote below to understand the shift in one psychiatrist's thinking.

In the last two decades, it has become obvious that child abuse, urbanization, migration, and adverse life events contribute to the aetiology of schizophrenia and other psychoses. This has been a big shift for me! My preconceptions had made me blind to the influence of the social environment.

British psychiatrist Robin Murray (2016, p. 255).

Considering the highly debatable nature of psychosis and schizophrenia-related phenomena, the PTMF provides a more pragmatic way to develop a collaborative formulation of people's experiences, empowering individuals to formulate their own meaning and sense of whether they have a disorder or not. Language associated with schizophrenia diagnosis has become something of a chimera of the psychiatric paradigm, heavily embedded in the power imbalance of psychiatric relationships. Nurses may therefore find the PTM framework useful to understand the negative experience of power in people's lives and the potential for the positive use of power when a person is supported to find meaning in the context of threat.

Dissociachotic Theory

Developed by mental health nurse practitioner Matthew Ball, dissociachotic theory provides an alternative way of understanding experiences traditionally referred to as psychosis (Ball & Picot 2021). Dissociachotic theory contends that experiences currently mistakenly labelled as psychotic disorders are in fact meaningful forms of dissociation that serve to create experiential separation from perceived threats. Building on the seminal work of Corstens and colleagues (2008) on working with voices, and the polyvagal theory developed by Porges (2011), dissociachotic theory contends that extraordinary experiential realities are often mislabelled as abhorrent symptoms like hallucinations and delusions. The theory suggests such phenomena should be viewed as meaningful human coping strategies, designed to satisfy the innate human need for social, emotional and physical safety.

Traditionally, psychological theories have suggested that threat responses generally emerge from one of three instinctual coping strategies, known as fight, flight or freeze responses. Dissociachotic theory proposes that as the human brain has evolved and the prefrontal cortex has become increasingly linked to executive function, a fourth instinctual threat response, known as "dissociachotic phenomena", has developed. The theory contends that experiences currently labelled as psychotic symptoms are in fact dissociachotic phenomena, which provide animated meaningful responses to threatening experiences.

Early work indicates that when dissociachotic theory is put into practice, the role of nurses and other supporters becomes focused on uncovering the meaning that dissociachotic phenomena holds for people and using therapeutic communication to explore and remedy the sense of threat and need for safety experienced by the individual concerned. As a reduction in sense of threat and increase in safety is achieved, the theory suggests that dissociachotic phenomena subside, thereby explaining the episodic nature of such phenomena. Dissociachotic theory is consistent with nursing approaches that emphasise the importance of interpersonal relationships and is supported by social constructionist philosophy that legitimises the differences in reality experienced by every individual.

THEORIES OF CAUSATION/AETIOLOGY

To date, research has failed to demonstrate the aetiology or cause of psychotic disorders. Despite this, many theories have attempted to explain them. The causes of schizophrenia remain unknown (Zwicker et al 2018). There are several theoretical perspectives that support the possible causation of the illness, which include biological, psychological and social theories.

Three commonly posited biological theories are brain anatomy, genetics and brain biochemistry. It would be erroneous to consider these three factors as mutually exclusive, and it may be more likely that there is a relationship between the three and with the person's environment. Schizophrenia has often been referred to as a "neuropsychological disorder", which implies that the origins of the psychological disturbance lie in the neurological structure and function of the brain. This biological perspective supports the neurodevelopment hypotheses that the disorder emerges from brain dysfunction and consideration to structural abnormalities in the cerebral cortex have all been well researched

(Zwicker et al 2018). Modern imaging techniques have been used to suggest lower brain tissue volume and higher cerebrospinal volumes in people with schizophrenia, but these findings are not conclusive, and these factors are now being demonstrated as being a side effect of anti-psychotic medication. There is, however, a growing body of modern evidence related to the influence of traumatic life experiences in developing psychotic disorders. Recognising the dose response between adverse childhood experiences and reduced health and social outcomes is important (Chase et al 2018). Research of 41 robust studies examining adverse childhood experiences in people who had developed psychosis indicated that they were 2.8 times more likely to have experienced one or more childhood traumas (such as sexual and/or physical abuse, emotional abuse, neglect, bullying or parental death) (see Morrison & Waddingham 2020). The "trauma-genic neurodevelopmental model of psychosis" that demonstrates, through functional magnetic resonance imaging (MRI), five primary changes in brain chemistry and structure that are used to justify similar states to schizophrenia are also found in people who have experienced cumulative childhood trauma (Read et al 2020).

Evidence from an epidemiological study found that health professionals do not routinely inquire about trauma, knowing the evidence that adverse experiences are common among people with psychosis (Turner et al 2020). The stress-vulnerability-protective factors model has been used to explain psychotic symptoms and symptomatic relapses. The model attempts to integrate environmental, biological and traumagenic theories, suggesting that people are exposed to stressful events in the course of their lives and that these events may precipitate symptoms in some people who have a biological (genetic) predisposition to mental ill-health (Lecomte et al 2019). Essential to this theory is the notion that some people are more vulnerable to mental ill-health than others. For example, people with psychosis and/or schizophrenia may have additional stressors related to childhood adversity and trauma; however, where they have strong protective factors, such as family, social skills and adherence to treatment, this may in fact serve as a buffer against the effects of stress health (Lecomte et al 2019).

The family is part of the person's environment and culture and has the potential to affect the course of psychosis. More specifically, people with lived experience of psychosis from families that showed high levels of expressed emotion typified by excessive criticism, hostility or emotional over-involvement appeared to struggle more than people with lived experience who were from families with patterns of relating that were not high in expressed emotion.

What is well known is that the disorder may have groupings of similar symptoms, as noted earlier; however, the consideration to the uniqueness of the individual and how they relate to their mental ill-health, the environment and others fits well within a biopsychosocial approach to the illness, and partners well with a recovery approach.

Assessment

Because mental health has no objective scientific instruments or tests to rely upon (such as blood tests or x-rays), the assessment process is heavily influenced by the knowledge and understanding of the person conducting the assessment. Any assessor's knowledge is limited, meaning that the safest way to conduct mental health assessment is to collaborate with the person being assessed to identify strengths and challenges and to assist them and the people they live with towards a more satisfying life. Nurses need to be as interested in people's abilities and activities as they are in indicators that suggest mental ill health. It is crucial for nurses to remember that:

- a mental health assessment should never be a mental illness assessment,
- assessment can be helpful or unhelpful,
- assessment is a process, not a single event,

- assessment can be an intervention in itself,
- misinformation can misinform future actions, and
- incomplete or ill-informed assessment may be considered worse than no assessment.

Fusar-Poli and colleagues (2020) indicate the presence of low-grade (subthreshold) psychotic symptoms, poor functioning, depression and disorganisation as predictors of an overt psychotic episode. In addition, comorbid features, such as substance abuse and depression, should not be overlooked. Because the onset of schizophrenia may occur during adolescence or in early adulthood, this constellation of negative symptoms tends to interfere with education, employment and the development of meaningful connections with others in a social setting. Negative symptoms may sometimes cause conversations to be limited and responses to be short, often monosyllabic. Symptoms such as alogia and avolition (described previously) leave the person feeling numb and unable to respond to the demands of daily living. There is often a significant loss of drive, and the person has difficulty initiating and completing activities. Both the illness and the treatment can introduce impairments, such as difficulty learning new concepts and disturbances in attention, which further impact on treatment and rehabilitation efforts since they undermine the acquisition of new skills. It is important to remember that assessment focuses on the hypothesis distilled into the DSM-5 symptomology and is not a scientific approach.

The early phase of a psychotic disorder may sometimes be confused by parents as a "normal" one because parents are aware that adolescent children are known to need increased privacy and to seek separation from parental surveillance. Limited social engagement means the person finds it difficult to develop and sustain stimulating and rewarding social relationships and partnerships at a time when most people are socialising, seeking life partners and training for their future careers. Instead of beginning to earn an income and seek personal independence, a person who is developing schizophrenia might find themselves hospitalised or dependent on their parents for help with personal hygiene, nutrition and motivation to undertake physical activity.

Course and outcome cannot be reliably predicted for every person, but a variable course with sometimes lengthy periods of remission and intermittent relapses is common, although the illness can become chronic in a proportion of people. Early onset is associated with poorer outcomes and later onset results in better outcomes; for most people, negative symptoms predominate later in the course of the illness (APA 2013). Factors associated with a better prognosis include:

- a good level of premorbid adjustment
- sudden and later onset
- self-awareness and resilience
- having identifiable triggers for episodes
- concurrent mood disturbance
- short periods of acute illness
- higher levels of functioning between episodes
- fewer residual symptoms
- good neurological function.

With reference to schizophrenia, the DSM-5 (APA 2013) specifies whether the symptoms are "continuous" or in "full" or "partial" remission. Continuous symptoms "fulfil the diagnostic symptom criteria of the disorder for the majority of the illness course" (APA 2013, p. 100). A long-term course appears to be favourable in about 20% of people with schizophrenia, and a small number of these recover completely. Of the other 80%, most will require assistance with daily living activities; exacerbations and remissions of active symptoms; while others may experience a course of progressive deterioration. Psychotic symptoms usually diminish over time, but negative symptoms and cognitive deficits, which are closely related to prognosis, tend to persist (APA

2013, p. 102). It is important to note that there is a bias in the DSM-5 to support its own argument, with most commentators or professional associations recognising that the recovery rate is significantly higher.

Although nurses are taught to use the mental state examination, this is especially problematic in the context of psychotic disorders. The key aspects of assessing "insight" and "judgement" of an individual can de-legitimise the experience of the person, dismissing the possibility they may experience alternative realities. Such an approach rarely facilitates meaningful outcomes. Instead, nursing assessment should focus on principles of mutual learning and sharing the experience of being human, as described by mental health nursing theorists Joyce Travelbee developed in 1971 (Shelton 2016) and Gertrud Schwing (1954). Schwing skillfully demonstrated the value of human connection and creating an environment that the person could be in human relationship.

✳ HISTORICAL ANECDOTE 14.1
Pseudo-Patients

Lack of objectivity in diagnoses related to psychosis was exposed by an experiment conducted by a group of psychologists in 1968. Led by University of Stanford psychology professor David Rosenhan and published by the journal *Science* in 1973, the experiment involved three women and five men (including Rosenhan himself), who briefly acted as pseudo-patients feigning auditory hallucinations in an attempt to gain admission to psychiatric hospitals in five different states in North America. Despite none of them really being ill, all of the pseudo-patients were admitted and diagnosed with psychiatric disorders. After admission, each pseudo-patient began to act normally and informed staff that they felt fine and were no longer experiencing any further psychosis. Despite this, to be released all pseudo-patients were forced to agree they had a mental illness and to take antipsychotic drugs as a condition of discharge. The average time that the pseudo-patients were kept in hospital for treatment was 19 days. Following the experiment, one of the hospitals involved challenged Rosenhan to send pseudo-patients to its facility, whom it guaranteed its staff would then detect. Rosenhan agreed and, in the following weeks, out of 193 new patients, hospital staff identified 41 people as pseudo-patients, with 19 of them receiving suspicion from at least one psychiatrist and one other staff member. In fact, Rosenhan had sent no further pseudo-patients to the hospital.

Read More About It:
Rosenhan DL 1973 On being sane in insane places. Science 179(4070): 250–258.

NURSING INTERVENTIONS

Any mental health nursing intervention should focus on the holistic understanding of the person seeking support. This is often overlooked, and disorder-specific approaches are then developed. As outlined previously, using psychiatric approaches to psychosis and schizophrenia-related phenomena are generally thought to share the common characteristics of severe disturbances in perception, cognition and thinking. While the term "psychosis" is most strongly associated with schizophrenia, it may also be a feature of other disorders such as bipolar disorder, depression, dementia and delirium. When conducting health assessments, nurses need to be aware that the current approaches that seek to assess mental health disorders, such as psychosis and schizophrenia, are questionable and contentious. Common interventions delivered by nurses in the process of caring for people who experience psychosis and schizophrenia-related phenomena include assessment, therapeutic communication, trauma-informed care, psychopharmacology, physical health promotion, social advocacy, relapse prevention and recovery and wellness care planning. Each of these interventions is briefly discussed as follows.

Therapeutic Communication

Overcoming mental ill-health can be intense. Like a rollercoaster ride, movement towards personal and clinical recovery can bring with it lots of highs and lows. As part of this process, nurses may adopt a range of modes of communication in delivering individual assistance, including approaches such as acceptance, mutuality, giving gentle reality feedback, teaching new thinking and strengthening existing or developing new coping skills. How nurses communicate with people who experience psychosis and schizophrenia-type conditions plays a vitally important role in their recovery. People with positive relationships with their nurses and other carers are more likely to experience recovery outcomes.

There are a number of nursing behaviours that might assist in building a therapeutic alliance, such as building trust, active listening, providing empathy and validating the client's experience, as well as engaging in a collaborative approach with the person in need of care. Working together as a team and using statements like "we" and "us" will help inspire collaboration.

Nurses have the most frequent and regular contact with people who experience psychosis and schizophrenia, their family and other support people, so nurses are in the best position to assist them with stressors, provide education and establish a therapeutic relationship. Nurses can learn effective communication strategies that will better enable them to "be with" the person with schizophrenia or psychotic disorders. For example, the advice offered by the New Zealand Early Intervention in Psychosis Society (see Useful websites) could be useful if the person is distracted by their symptoms, experiencing difficulties with attention and concentration, and/or distressed and isolated. This advice includes the following:

- Respect the person's privacy and autonomy.
- Keep communication and choices clear.
- Check that the person and nurse have a shared understanding about what has been said.
- Do not dismiss them, even if what they are saying sounds unusual or doesn't make sense to you.
- Recognise that what the person says seems very real to them.
- Listen respectfully to what they are saying.
- Avoid arguing or getting into a debate unless safety is an issue.

At times, much of a nurse's use of therapeutic communication may need to focus on the so-called negative symptoms (lack of motivation, blunted emotions, loss of drive, social withdrawal and inattention), which are major determinants of social disability. A person having experiences described as "psychotic" usually struggles to function at a level that they might previously have achieved. Early manifestations might include poor or deteriorating school performance, poor social relations, decreased self-care and a failure to achieve expected developmental milestones. In addition to the decline in social and occupational performance, common to the prodromal phase of the illness, the person may present with all or some of the symptoms listed in Table 14.1.

Trauma-Informed Care (TIC)

Using the principles of trauma-informed care (TIC) to support people experiencing psychosis has begun to be explored in more depth. The theory of developmental trauma is that the impact of repeated adverse childhood events has correlations with potential risks of development of psychosis (Bloomfield et al 2020). As mental health nurses, we can employ the five principles of TIC – Safety, Choice, Collaboration, Trustworthiness and Empowerment – to assist and support people who are assessed as having trauma and experience losing touch with reality as a result.

People who are managing their mental ill-health may benefit from safety planning in collaboration with the multidisciplinary team, their

TABLE 14.1 Adverse Effects of Antipsychotic Medications and Nursing Interventions

Adverse Effect	Nursing Intervention
Weight gain, especially with clozapine, olanzapine and chlorpromazine	Stress the importance of activity and exercise and accompany the person, if possible, to overcome lethargy. Assess current dietary intake and suggest modifications if required. Be aware not to blame the person for the challenges in managing the effects of medication.
Parkinsonian effects: Blank, mask-like expression, drooling, tremor, muscle rigidity, stiffness and shuffling gait	Reassure the person that these adverse reactions subside with time. Monitor for Parkinsonian effects and administer anticholinergics as prescribed and prn. Be open with the person about the limited value of additional medication in managing some side effects.
Akathisia, which may disturb both sleep and rest with the incessant urge to move the limb and to change position	Report this to the medicine prescriber, who might need to review the antipsychotic if adverse reactions cannot be tolerated. Anticholinergics might ameliorate adverse reactions.
Neuroleptic malignant syndrome, which is serious and life-threatening; usually develops quickly, but could occur any time the person is taking a higher potency typical antipsychotic (e.g. haloperidol)	This is a medical emergency, which literature suggests has a mortality rate between 3% and 27%, with a lowering trend since the advent of atypical antipsychotic medications (Guinart et al 2021). Symptoms are hyperthermia, severe motor rigidity, disturbances in levels of consciousness, cardiovascular functioning, blood pressure, sweating, pyrexia, hypotension, tachycardia, stupor and muscular rigidity. Cease antipsychotic immediately and refer to a medical practitioner. Nursing care consists of vigilance for the syndrome in those who are taking high-potency drugs such as haloperidol; hydration; monitoring; and reduction of body temperature.
Tardive dyskinesia (TD; "late-occurring movement disorder"), a devastating, irreversible adverse reaction to long-term conventional antipsychotic medication (e.g. haloperidol), but less frequently atypical antipsychotics	Effects range in severity from mild to incapacitating and include: Uncontrollable coarse tremor; spasm-like movements of the body, arms and legs; rolling of the tongue; and smacking of the lips. TD continues after cessation of antipsychotics and is often made worse by administering antiparkinsonian drugs such as benztropine. Refer involuntary movements to the medical practitioner to cease, lower or taper off the dose and assess.
Acute dystonic reaction (spasm) – muscle spasms in the trunk and neck (opisthotonos and torticollis); eyes can roll up uncontrollably (oculogyric crisis); life-threatening when muscles of the larynx spasm and occlude the airway	This is a medical emergency demanding swift nursing intervention. Acute dystonic reactions respond swiftly to intravenous, intramuscular or oral (route depends on the level of acuity) administration of antiparkinsonian drugs, such as benztropine, followed by careful observation. In the case of laryngeal spasm, the person may require airway support and oxygen therapy until it resolves.

families, carers and/or supporters. Providing opportunities for choice in helping to control the person's trauma disclosure is aimed to empower them and support therapeutic engagement. Importantly, mental health staff need to have training and education in TIC principles. This will help in providing safe childhood trauma assessments; however, staff supervision is vital in employing any TIC principles to reduce the risks of re-traumatisation of the consumer, and vicarious trauma and associated burnout for staff (Mitchell et al 2021). Many people accessing mental health services who experience psychosis are often not asked about their developmental trauma histories. Evidence now supports mental health clinicians to ask about a person's trauma if they are educated on how to implement TIC and participate in regular supervision (Bloomfield et al 2020).

Read the three-phase Delphi method study to further your understanding of the principles of TIC in early intervention of psychosis (see Mitchell et al 2021).

Cognitive Behavioural Therapy (CBT)

Cognitive behavioural interventions may be suited to some people in later stages of recovery or as maintenance therapy when they are well. The underlying assumption behind cognitive behaviour therapy (CBT) is that people can positively influence their symptoms by changing their thinking and behaviour. Moreover, the symptoms currently experienced are the result of habits in thinking and behaviour learnt in the past and have a detrimental effect in the present. The approach to therapy is therefore to unlearn the destructive ways of the past and to replace them with more constructive approaches for the future. Unlike antipsychotic medication, CBT has no adverse effects, but has the potential to improve a person's quality of life long after treatment ceases.

For example, a person who hears frightening hallucinations while travelling on public transport may discover that listening to music through headphones and a portable device can drown out the voices, and no one can detect that they are talking to "voices" if they speak into a mobile phone. In addition, the person can be encouraged to view hallucinations as part of an illness that can be managed, and that these voices are harmless. People experiencing delusional thinking can be encouraged to explore the content of these delusions through CBT approaches.

Open Dialogue

Open dialogue therapy (ODT) is a therapeutic approach developed in the 1980s in Scandinavia for treating psychosis. The primary goal of ODT is increased engagement of a person's social network/family in therapy, with a view to creating a more open dialogue about experiences related to psychosis in the home environment. There have been some parallels between open dialogue and hearing voices, although the two have been developed independently. Seven core principles are embedded in ODT. The first is a requirement for providing immediate help, meaning that access to health services must occur within 24 hours of the first contact between the health team and the consumer, their family or carer or referral service, and thereafter the person must receive immediate support from health professionals during any crisis.

The second principle involves the ongoing inclusion of a social network within the therapeutic sessions. This social network is selected by the person and may consist of relatives, friends, neighbours, employers, co-workers or other care agencies, and, as such, is fundamental to the therapy sessions through sharing stories of the consumer. As well as listening to one another, the consumer and the health team providing treatment, this social network also provides support to the consumer.

The third principle of ODT is flexibility and mobility, which refers to the need for services to be flexible and thus adapt to the changing requirements of the patient and the support network. In practice, this allows a range of psychotherapeutic approaches to be adapted to the needs of the client, such as psychodynamic theory, systemic family therapy and dialogical theory, as well as pharmacological and social constructionism. Meetings are preferably conducted within the patient's home with the consent of the client and their family.

The fourth and fifth principles of ODT are responsibility and psychological continuity. These refer to the importance of the initial team that assesses the consumer coordinating treatment throughout the entire process so that psychological continuity of therapy is maintained.

The final two principles of ODT are tolerance of uncertainty and dialogism. Tolerance of uncertainty refers to the fact that the recovery journey is full of ups and downs and that all involved need to be willing to accept risks that are included in recovery. Dialogism refers to the openness that is needed between the consumer, their social network and clinicians as they move along their recovery journey. Family connectedness is improved as they discuss the client's "difficulties and problems". Rather than a formal interview approach, the team adapts to the language and way of speaking the family is used to (Buus & McCloughen 2022).

Intervoice: The International Hearing Voices Network

Developments in understanding the impact of trauma on the brain has led to the creation of the International Hearing Voices Network (see Useful websites). Founded by Professor Marius Romme and a group of people with lived experience, Intervoice reasons that psychotic experiences such as voices (also known as auditory hallucinations) need to be understood from the perspective of their meaning for the person who experiences them. The network also supports theories that traumatic experiences can often be the origin of voice hearing rather than interpreting voices as being an aberrant symptom of schizophrenia (Longden 2013).

Psychopharmacology

Psychotropic medications are used in the treatment for psychosis and schizophrenia (Stroup et al 2019). These medications can affect the mind, emotions and behaviour. Some main drug classes of psychotropics include antidepressants, mood stabilisers, anxiolytics (also known as hypnotics) and antipsychotics. Antipsychotics are considered to be the first-line treatment for people experiencing schizophrenia and are known to be effective for some consumers in reducing psychotic symptoms such as hallucinations and delusions. Although their effectiveness is supported by evidence, antipsychotics on their own are often inadequate to address all symptoms and many produce unwanted side effects, including producing sedative effects (Stroup et al 2019).

As mental health nurses, our role is to respectfully engage with the consumer, their families and carers about their physical health goals, medication management, including self-management (when possible). Medication therapy can positively impact a person's capacity to achieve their personal recovery goals. The nurse can assist them to optimise the use of psychotropic medications. Some examples of this include the following:

- Taking a medication history – explore what the person found helpful or unhelpful.
- Asking about the reasons for ceasing medication. Was it due to intolerable side effects, stigma, little or no perceived benefits or financial costs? Talk to them about the potential withdrawal effects.
- Exploring concurrent or adjunct treatment options. Some medications can take up to 2–4 weeks to be effective.
  - Discuss the "stay-low and go slow" approach, where medications are used in low doses while other treatment approaches are provided, such as psychotherapy, sensory modulation.
  - Additionally, medication can be slowly titrated, taking a cautious, gradual approach to increasing the dose of medication

as needed, assessing the effects of the medication at each dose increase.
- Reducing risks of polypharmacy. There may be a need to introduce other adjunct medications to manage some symptoms and levels of distress. Be transparent in your discussions with the consumer and review the evidence on reduced risks. Although you are not the prescriber, your role is administering medications. Your medication knowledge is vital in these conversations and will help the consumer with their supported decision-making processes.
- Understanding the indications for use for all psychotropics and other medications used for physical health needs.
- Being aware of the balance between the risks and benefits (e.g. reduced positive symptoms but increased weight gain).
- Advocating for the consumer and their families and carers about medication choices and decisions.
- Understanding the interactions of these medications with alcohol and other drugs.

The Victorian Equally Well Framework was developed in 2019 to support the physical health of people with serious mental illness (e.g. schizophrenia). This framework acknowledges the complex interplay with mental ill health and the individual's life. Understanding the person's values and beliefs about psychotropic medication will help build a safe therapeutic environment where medications, such as antipsychotics, can be discussed; for example, the strength, dose, effects and potential side effects. The mental health nurse's role is to provide medication information to consumers, their families and carers, so that they can take responsibility for treatment decisions affecting their physical health and weigh up the risks and benefits of the chosen medication.

Joanna Moncrieff (2021), a psychiatrist, refers to a drug-based, not diagnosis-based approach that invites the person to describe the way they would like to feel if they were to take medication and avoid suggesting that the medication specifically targets "disease", explaining that this idea cannot be objectively proven. Such an approach reflects interpersonal and ethical nursing values.

Side Effects

Many psychotropics, particularly antipsychotics, have serious side effects that can reduce life expectancy, such as metabolic syndrome and cardiovascular disease. People experience a wide range of negative side effects caused by antipsychotics. It is common for these medications to have peripheral nervous system side effects, such as dry mouth, headaches, constipation, urinary hesitancy, photophobia, decreased lacrimation (tear production) and sexual dysfunction. Central nervous system side effects may include sedation, Parkinsonian effects, akathisia and lowered seizure threshold. Other unwanted side effects include photosensitivity, retinal deterioration and hormonal interference. The most commonly experienced symptoms in schizophrenia are negative symptoms. Unfortunately, antipsychotic medications are largely ineffective against negative symptoms and can make them worse, giving rise to the so-called neuroleptic-induced deficit syndrome, which includes apathy, lack of initiative, indifference, blunted affect and reduced insight into their experiences.

Other severe adverse reactions are acute dystonic reaction, agranulocytosis, neuroleptic malignancy syndrome and tardive dyskinesia.
- *Acute dystonic reactions* are painful muscle spasms in the face, neck, trunk, pelvis or extremities that may last for either short or long periods. Although treatable with anticholinergics and rarely life-threatening, the spasms cause substantial distress.
- *Agranulocytosis* is a potentially fatal blood disorder with prodromal signs similar to those observed in influenza. Symptoms include sudden fever, chills, sore throat, muscle weakness and sore mouth.

Early recognition is essential and is facilitated through monitoring of laboratory findings. Stopping antipsychotic medication immediately is mandatory if agranulocytosis develops.

- Common symptoms of *neuroleptic malignancy syndrome* include high body temperature (fever), excessive sweating and mouth saliva, muscle stiffness, altered mental status and big swings in blood pressure. Early recognition is essential, and stopping antipsychotic medication immediately is mandatory if neuroleptic malignancy syndrome is identified.
- *Tardive dyskinesia* is a syndrome involving gross motor movements of the entire muscular system. Characteristically, the client displays hyperkinetic activity of the mouth, such as sucking/smacking of the lips and protrusion of the tongue, along with side-to-side movements of the chin. Facial grimaces, tics and spastic distortions are also evidenced. This condition usually appears in patients after long-term therapy and is irreversible.

Anticholinergic medications (or antiparkinsonian agents) are a group of drugs found to be helpful at counteracting the negative side effects of antipsychotics. As outlined above, these can include muscle rigidity, akinesia, tremor, akathisia and a range of other effects. Anticholinergics work by blocking acetylcholine in neural synapses. Three common anticholinergic agents are benztropine mesylate, trihexyphenidyl and biperiden. The objective of treatment is to provide maximum relief of uncomfortable symptoms and to promote normal physical function. Unfortunately, when anticholinergics are started, many people experience dry mouth, dizziness, blurred vision, nausea and increased nervousness. Other problems can include constipation, tachycardia, urinary hesitancy or retention, drowsiness, weakness, vomiting and headache. In addition, these medications can increase CNS stimulation, which is usually manifested by increased restlessness and agitation, disorientation, memory loss, confusion, delirium or visual hallucinations.

Iatrogenesis

The term "iatrogenesis" refers to harm or unintended adverse outcome caused by a healthcare intervention that is not normally considered part of the natural course of the illness being treated. Modern-day health services tend to maintain biomedical approaches to mental health treatment that emphasise the use of long-term antipsychotic medication, which places nurses in a challenging position regarding administration of antipsychotic drugs.

Table 14.2 lists what the nurse can do to help a person who is experiencing some of the more common side effects caused by antipsychotics. A useful resource is a systematic review of the impact of antipsychotics on symptoms, sense of self and agency, which can guide collaborative approaches to drug treatments in schizophrenia and psychosis (Thompson et al 2020).

TABLE 14.2 Nursing Approaches to Psychotic Disorders

Issue	Nursing Response
Delusional thinking	• Attempt to understand the content of the delusional thinking. Delusional ideas can often provide a clue to themes occurring in the person's thinking. Consider alternative language (preferably adopting the language of the person) and acknowledge that you believe the delusions are real to the person concerned. This conveys a concerned understanding and helps develop trust. • Be authentic in acknowledging that you and the person may have different experiences and views of a situation or reality – this is not collusion but a demonstration that you accept the person's experience of reality. • Collaborate with the person to identify different aspects of the environment that may be valuable to adjust to create a safer experience for the individual.
Auditory hallucinations	• Engage with the person to understand their realities. • If the voices are suggesting certain actions, explore the resources the person has to make choices over their own actions. Voices may suggest a person takes actions that impact on personal safety – work with the person to understand that the voices may have important metaphorical meaning related to past distress and that they are distinct from the individual in terms of choice in acting on the voices. • Discuss and explore the potential value of increased support from the nurse, a peer worker or other person to manage any distress being caused by the voices. • Work with the person to identify activities that appear to stimulate hallucinations and devise ways of coping with such situations. • In partnership with the person, identify actions that reduce the impact of hallucinations such as listening to music through headphones, rituals, play or creativity. • When in acute distress, a person may value prn medication; this should be considered in collaboration with the individual.
Fear/anxiety/paranoia	• Reflect on any fear, anxiety or paranoia the person may be experiencing. • Discuss fears and experiences and consider any supports that might be of value. • Be aware of your own behaviour and how it could be misinterpreted. Ensure your approach is quietly confident and mindful of the person's need for generous personal space. • Physical contact should always be by consent and should only be considered as an approach to reassurance and support in collaboration with the person. Considering the likely presentation as a stress/trauma response will support such consideration. • Always seek to work in partnership with the person as a mutual human being.
Disordered thinking	• Spend time exploring experiences with the person. • Reflect on the impact of disordered thinking in the person's life. • In collaboration with the person, consider if medication may be useful, but be mindful not to suppress the individual's personal expression. • Consider physical activity as a mechanism for assisting the person to regain a sense of ownership over their body and personal sense of safety. • Working with the person, reflect on any factors that may be increasing the feelings of unsafety.
Stress/trauma response	• Consider a stress/trauma-related response as a common reason for a person being in distress experiencing a "psychotic" state. • Understanding what has happened, not what is wrong, is vital in collaborating on the most supportive approach from a nurse. • Consider the impact of distress of any psychotic experiences, especially on daily living and broader acute and chronic wellbeing.

Promotion of Health and Wellbeing, Including Physical Health Promotion

People with serious mental illness (SMI) have higher rates of mortality and morbidity than the general population (Morgan et al 2021). Individuals with schizophrenia die on average 20 years earlier, with "natural causes" accounting for 80% of premature deaths (Seeman 2019). Australian evidence indicates the seriousness in the reduced life expectancy for this population group (up to 30%) (Roberts 2019). People with SMI are:

- six times more likely to die from cardiovascular disease
- five times more likely to smoke
- four times more likely to die from respiratory disease
- likely to die between 14 years and 23 years earlier than the general population and account for approximately one-third of all avoidable deaths (National Mental Health Commission 2016).

> *The high rate of physical comorbidity, which often has poor clinical management, drastically reduces life expectancy for people with mental illness, and also increases the personal, social and economic burden of mental illness across the lifespan.*
>
> **(Firth et al 2019, p. 676).**

The evidence presented in Fig. 14.1 highlights the risk of premature deaths to the ratio of risk for people with a mental illness, with a notable increase in risk of death for a person experiencing psychosis.

Lower rates of screening for cardiovascular risk, such as blood pressure and cholesterol, and the increased risk of developing metabolic syndrome, given the high use of psychotropic treatments, in particular, newer antipsychotics such as Clozapine, contribute to the worsening of the metabolic profile in this population (Howell et al 2019). Although the data is not new, the 2010 Australian National Psychosis Survey indicated that one-quarter of users were at risk for a cardiovascular event (Harris et al 2018). Over the years, these statistics have improved minimally, if at all.

Consumers also have lower rates in participation of national screening programs and prevention programs, such as bowel cancer screening, mammograms and flu shots (Seeman 2019). Additionally, dental hygiene is poor in this group (Morgan et al 2021). These are all modifiable risks, and as mental health nurses, we can work in collaboration with the consumer, their family and carers to address and improve their physical health needs.

For many people who have experienced a harsh outcome to their battle with experiences labelled as schizophrenia or psychotic illness, especially the homeless and the destitute, access to much-needed healthcare remains a major issue. For many, the additional stress of the illness, the risk of poverty and the increased stigma, all have high impacts on the individual's personal and clinical recovery, as do the detrimental side effects of many antipsychotic medications (e.g. weight gain, sexual dysfunction) (Seeman 2019).

Understandably, adherence to treatment is often problematic, and many choose to cease taking medication, which often results in a return to clinician perceptions of mental illness and repeated admissions. The pattern of a consumer returning to health services for treatment is often referred to in mental health contexts as the "revolving-door syndrome". It is important to be aware of the contexts of revolving-door syndrome, which can include nurses (in collaboration with psychiatrists) limiting the potential for alternatives to medication and hospital. It is also important to understand non-adherence as a legitimate right of any person contrary to the opinion of a prescriber. In people who experience psychosis, this legitimate right is often overlooked and limited by professionals who take a single-minded, risk-focused perspective that has limited evidence. The evidence for positive risk-taking in the context of mental health and recovery is a new discovery that is now a more considered approach.

Physical and mental wellbeing for an individual needs to shift from a deficit and difficulties base to a positive way where we promote abilities and strengths. Social supports, having meaningful activity in one's life and making healthy behaviour choices can improve the health outcomes for people experiencing schizophrenia and psychotic disorders.

Mental health nurses are in a good position to promote the health of the whole person. Implementation of physical health priorities, such as metabolic screening, are ways to ensure the person experiencing mental ill-health has rights to access care that is equitable and in their best interest. Encouraging the consumer and their families and carers to have choice and control about their health needs promotes the principles of recovery and engages the person in the care and treatment which is likely to lead to improved health outcomes.

The impacts of medication on weight and physical health have begun to be addressed, with consideration of alternative treatment options, although not common, being the focus for contemporary mental health reform. Increasing access to GP care, private healthcare and financial assistance, to fresh food, good nutrition and exercise, needs to be a priority for government and health services to provide. Coordination between acute and primary healthcare is needed to support the reduction in re-admission rates. It is recommended that regular health checks be implemented for people who commence antipsychotic medication, gathering information and data from the consumer and their families and carers on:

- history/family history
- lifestyle risk factors (such as diet, physical activity, smoking, alcohol and other drugs)
- weight (including Body Mass Index (BMI))
- HbA_{1c} or fasting glucose

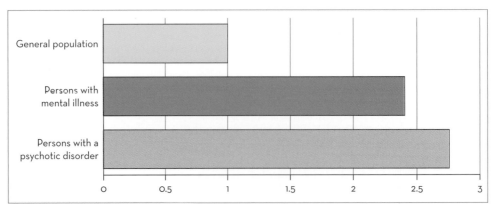

FIG. 14.1 Risks of Premature Deaths.

- lipids
- blood pressure
- prolactin
- ECG (electrocardiograph)
- use of statins and antihypertensives where increased risk of cardiovascular disease is known
- metformin use, where metabolic risks cannot be managed by diet and exercise
- shared care arrangement (GP and mental health professionals).

Advocacy

People who have experiences being labelled as having psychosis or schizophrenia often confront social challenges. These impact on issues of everyday life, which the unaffected person seems to carry out with relative ease. Impacts may include misinterpreting one's external social environment accurately, resulting in feelings of threat or peril, social isolation, poor self-esteem and challenges with expressing emotions and understanding how others accept these expressions. The role of social advocacy in supporting a person to manage impacts arising from their experience is just as important as treating symptoms and is central to any treatment. A nurse's ability to provide useful social advocacy relies on establishing a therapeutic relationship that addresses individual needs. Perspectives in practice 14.1: Nurse's story: Jane recounts the experiences of a nurse whose role was to advocate for a consumer with schizophrenia.

 PERSPECTIVES IN PRACTICE

Nurse's Story 14.1: Julie

A person (pronouns he/him) with schizophrenia was scheduled to come to hospital for a colonoscopy. He was being cared for in a community care unit (CCU) and there were concerns that he would not cope well with a medical admission. The focus of pre-hospital discussions focused on the risk to others and the potential for him to not want to stay for the procedure. There was discussion about the need for an additional nurse to watch this person the whole time he was in hospital. He was engaged in his treatment and there were no acute concerns for his mental health. Given the high rates of medical comorbidity, facilitating medical investigations should be prioritised. I as the specialist mental health nurse was notified of these discussions. I spoke with the consumer and contacted his carers, with consumer consent, to develop a plan. My role was to advocate for the consumer and to understand what fears or concerns they had in relation to this procedure. The consumer's concerns were identified and included not having his own bathroom while having bowel preparation for the colonoscopy, and he is usually a smoker. Although he would usually have this as a day procedure, he had a shared bathroom in the community care unit and didn't feel comfortable with this.

The need for one-to-one nursing was discussed because he had schizophrenia; however, this was not commenced as there was no indication for this. An alternative plan was developed where his regular staff would spend time with him in hospital and help him settle in. The need for one-to-one nursing was raised based on his diagnosis and stigma rather than his need to feel comfortable in hospital. This person had capacity to make decisions and the staff were reminded that he had rights – the right to refuse treatment, consent to treatment, and to smoke outside the hospital if he wanted to.

Despite extensive pre-hospital concerns, this procedure went ahead with no concerns raised by the staff and/or the consumer. Hospitals can be confronting places for anyone and even more so when there is stigma and fear of a person with a mental illness. These reasons can impact the person's care.

The key message as a mental health nurse is the importance of our role as an advocate for the consumers, their families, carers and supporters.

Work, education and socioeconomic status are key aspects of most people's lives, and those who have experiences with psychosis and or schizophrenia often suffer significant disruption and disadvantage. Lack of employment opportunities represent a form of social exclusion facing those experiencing the effects of schizophrenia. Unemployment rates are very high in people who experience psychoses, and of those who are engaged in employment, a significantly large period of time is lost to sick leave. There is a great need for research into the area of the beneficial effects of work on those who experience schizophrenia, as well as the factors that either facilitate or inhibit finding work or returning to work. Often the transition back into work is easier if voluntary work is undertaken initially. Each Australian state has disability discrimination legislation that may have a bearing on the type of assistance the workplace is required to undertake. In most cases, the employer is responsible for providing a workplace that is both safe and free from adverse responses from the employer and other employees. This is often difficult given the societal stigma that a disorder such as schizophrenia carries.

Having a safe home that is conducive to a sense of security and wellbeing is an essential human need, yet this need goes unmet for a great number of people who are diagnosed with schizophrenia, a common mental illness among people who are homeless. Studies have shown that psychosis and homelessness are interrelated in several ways and are intersected with trauma and adversity, gender, race and other social determinants (Grech & Raeburn 2019). Unusual realities can result in the disruption of home life and the destruction of relationships. So-called positive symptoms may affect the relationship between a person with schizophrenia who is a tenant and the owner of a property, in some cases resulting in eviction of the individual with the disorder. This is, of course, a form of discrimination and perpetuates stigma and lack of knowledge and awareness by the public. Negative symptoms often affect the person's ability to form and maintain attachments with others. Coupled with negative symptoms are the everyday challenges of work, which may result in failure to meet commitments associated with tenancy and housing repayments.

However, this is not the only way in which mental illness and homelessness are related. For some, mental illness develops after the person becomes homeless and is probably associated with the immense stress associated with the conditions of homelessness: frequent assaults, rapes, robberies, malnourishment, lack of support and lack of access to health services. Clearly, suffering from schizophrenia and being homeless is destructive. According to the literature, the death rate for those who find themselves in both situations is four times that of the general population and twice that of those experiencing schizophrenia but who have a home (Ayano et al 2019). The great challenge for mental health policymakers and clinicians is to provide comprehensive healthcare to the homeless mentally ill and to promote access to housing and health agencies for people who are diagnosed with schizophrenia (see Table 14.3).

Recovery and Wellness Planning

Recovery and wellness planning is encouraged to support all people to actively participate in their own mental health care and decision-making by recording consumers' goals and care preferences (Gieselmann et al 2018). It may take the form of an advance directive or advance statement, which documents the consumer's wishes and treatment preferences in the event of a mental health emergency or crisis (Gaillard et al 2023). Additionally, it aims to empower people who may be experiencing psychosis to be supported in their decisions when they may have lost decision-making capacity. Once a mental health crisis has developed, options for negotiated care become more challenging to the nursing professional, with a greater likelihood that people will be hospitalised and treated under mental health legislation. For young people

TABLE 14.3	Resources to Support the Consumer, Family and Carer Advocacy	
Advocacy Service	**What Can They Provide?**	**Website**
Independent Mental Health Advocacy (IMAR)	This advocacy service supports Victorians who are accessing public mental health services inpatient and community. The service is guided by the principles of the *Mental Health Act 2014*, and has a focus on the individual's recovery and a holistic approach to mental health care. The service has information about the mental health rights of consumers and support with the National Disability Insurance Scheme (NDIS).	www.imha.vic.gov.au
Victorian Mental Illness and Awareness Council (VMIAC)	This service provides advocacy at all levels individual and systemic advocacy. It provides support and resources for people with a mental illness and advocates for a "life full of choices", rights and embedding principles of advocacy within the broader society. They also like IMAR and provide NDIS advocate support.	www.vmiac.org.au/
Tandem	This service is a Victorian peak body representing families, carers and supporters who support people living with mental health issues. Tandem advocate for family and carer involvement in planning and care and service participation and is a member of Mental Health Carers, a national advocacy group.	https://tandemcarers.org.au/

IMAR – Independent Mental Health Advocacy
NDIS – National Disability Insurance Scheme

who are experiencing first episode psychosis (FEP) and their families and carers, they are often faced with a range of complex decisions, including risk–benefit considerations in times of crisis where they are most vulnerable. Having an advance statement in place would support their involvement in their decisions and may strengthen positive therapeutic relationships with the health professionals (Valentine et al 2021).

Advance statements are negotiated with consumers when their distress has reduced, and they are able to communicate their preferences more intentionally and skillfully.

An advance directive or statement is a legal document and might be used to specify medication the consumer does or does not wish to receive, who should be contacted for support (e.g. nominated person) and what strategies have been found helpful in past crises (Gieselmann et al 2018).

Consumers need to be supported in developing their directives and statements, usually by a friend or family member. They may also wish to involve a lawyer. The plan should be discussed with the consumer's treatment team and a copy kept in the consumer's file. Nurses can assist consumers to initiate advance care directives and can advocate for advance care plans to be incorporated into the consumer's treatment plan. Nurses also need to be aware of the content of the advanced statements, who the consumer's nominated person is and of their ethical responsibility to respect the choices recorded (James et al 2023). Advance directives and statements are not binding on clinicians, but every attempt should be made to provide care that is in keeping with the consumer's expressed wishes.

Relapse Prevention

Longer-lasting forms of psychotic disorders such as schizophrenia are usually episodic, relapsing and remitting, with periods of acute psychosis alternating with periods of relative stability.

Relapse for people experiencing schizophrenia may be frequent, particularly within the first year of a diagnosis, and may contribute to psychological and social distress, not just for the consumer, but for their families, carers and supporters (Takeuchi et al 2019). People can experience a relapse of an acute episode within a year of being hospitalised, so it is essential to be able to detect the early signs and triggers of a potential relapse and to support a person to finding meaningful ways to support themselves in different environments and relationships to reduce the likely re-experience of threat and distress.

Relapse is a major obstacle to recovery in schizophrenia. Eighty per cent of those diagnosed with first episode schizophrenia will relapse within 5 years. The discontinuation of antipsychotic treatment is the most critical factor in relapse.

Rodolico and colleagues (2022) found that the key to relapse prevention was working closely with families and other supporters, who are often more likely than consumers to detect the onset of relapse. This approach, of course, needs to be collaboratively agreed with the individual.

Relapse prevention involves several steps: establishing a therapeutic relationship that is positive, engaging and honest, and ongoing education; identifying the early signs of relapse; monitoring for signs of relapse; and intervening early when or if these signs are observed. Unfortunately, family and carers are often overlooked as allies in consumer care. Relatives and carers expect to be included in care planning as a good source of information about the consumer, but can feel actively distanced or underprepared and undereducated to make confident and correct decisions (Lal et al 2019).

Some studies have identified that antipsychotic treatment responses in the context of a relapse may be delayed following on from first-episode psychosis. Therefore, consideration of adjunct therapies during this time may be an appropriate treatment intervention. For some consumers, continuous antipsychotic medications to prevent relapse is encouraged, yet there are many reasons for consumers (e.g. side effects, financial costs) to not adhere to the recommended treatment. Additionally, some research indicates a diminished antipsychotic treatment response can occur in second and subsequent psychotic episodes (Takeuchi et al 2019). The term "treatment resistant" is often used in clinical settings to describe the poor treatment responses to the medication therapies; however, this term is not well accepted across the recovery principles and frameworks.

A FINAL WORD REGARDING STIGMA

Many people who receive a diagnosis of schizophrenia labour under the stigma associated with the mental illness, which can be highly damaging to the person, their families and carers at various levels, such as public stigma, structural stigma and self-stigma (Valery & Prouteau 2020). The effects of stigma are many, and may include poor self-esteem, internalised negative beliefs and feelings associated with stigmatised conditions – social and psychological reactions. Society's institutions, including health services, health professionals and the media can often legitimatise and, in fact, perpetuate stigma for people experiencing mental ill-health (Valery & Prouteau 2020).

Research conducted on public stigma showed that among the mental illnesses, schizophrenia was associated with the worst representation (e.g. incompetency, violence and dangerousness) in the general population (Valery & Prouteau 2020).

The news media has an enormous influence on the way people view mental illness, and even when no harm is intended, the words "schizophrenic", "crazy" or "insane" are inappropriately used as terms of description. These terms are often used by the layperson as a way of conceptualising aberrant behaviours that they may not fully understand. These repetitive references add to the general public's confusion and lack of clarity about mental illness.

In the depths of their illness, the person can rarely concentrate on societal norms, such as appropriate dress, social etiquette and personal hygiene because of the intensity of their symptoms. In addition, some of the medications used to treat schizophrenia have unsightly adverse effects, which serve to further identify and alienate the person experiencing the illness.

Mental health nurses need to increase their knowledge in the area of stigma and its associated causes in order to advocate and support the fight against discrimination and the promotion of diversity.

The media can also play a crucial role in challenging public stigma by providing more balanced and accurate framing of information, including the use of images, video footage and social media, which can reduce stigmatising attitudes about people with severe mental ill-health (Ross et al 2019; Ross et al 2020).

SANE Australia maintains the Stigma Watch website (see Useful websites). This program promotes responsible reporting of mental ill-health and suicide in the Australian media. The program highlights instances of mockery or vilification, such as occasions on which people who have committed violent or horrible crimes, and how they are reported by news media. SANE Australia and the Australian Press Council have implemented reporting Mindframe's guidelines to ensure that media professionals report responsibly. These guides help the media to make use of appropriate language and not reinforce stereotypes when discussing people with serious mental illness, such as schizophrenia. Other social media environments seek to provide alternative understandings to reduce stigma and increase public knowledge of the disorder. One example is ISPS Australia, the Australian branch of ISPS International, which campaigns for psychological and social approaches to schizophrenia. The website provides information, resources, ideas and a connection for people who have an interest in this area (see Useful websites).

CHAPTER SUMMARY

Psychosis and schizophrenia-related phenomena refer to experiences that are often debilitating and affect around 1% of the population. These experiences often occur early in a person's adult life and can affect perception, behaviour, mood, thinking ability and social and occupational functioning. Despite their prevalence and impact, psychosis and schizophrenia-related phenomena have yet to be fully understood. They continue to be erroneously associated with "split personality" or "multiple personality", and people who are diagnosed with schizophrenia or psychotic disorders are often mistrusted, feared and discriminated against. Aetiology is probably due to several causes, including social, environmental, psychological and biological factors; all are current focuses of research and theory development. The consumer movement has greatly influenced the ways in which the aetiology, terminology, prognosis and recovery from schizophrenia and psychotic disorders are viewed. Strong advocacy of capable consumers is necessary when the stigma of violence and dangerousness is over-emphasised by a great many in society, compounding the difficulties faced by people experiencing the clinical manifestations of these illnesses.

Nurses play an important role in assisting people who experience psychosis and schizophrenia-related phenomena to recover from illness, maintain their health and achieve their optimal level of wellness. Nurses use the information gained from mental health assessment, including both subjective and objective data, to plan and implement care designed to assist people to predict and prevent relapse and to take responsibility for their own style of recovery. The great challenge to improve the lives of those who experience these illnesses is far from over. Understanding schizophrenia and psychotic disorders, the symptoms and some ways in which the people who experience such conditions can be assisted enables nurses to contribute to meeting this challenge.

ACKNOWLEDGEMENT

We would like to acknowledge Toby Raeburn and Matthew Ball for their contribution to the previous edition.

USEFUL WEBSITES AND OTHER RESOURCES

The Humane Clinic is a psychotherapy centre that values the autonomy and empowerment of individuals in navigating the experiences of being human and provides an alternative to diagnosis-led approaches. www.humaneclinic.com.au/

International Hearing Voices Network: www.hearing-voices.org/ Hearing Voices Network Aotearoa New Zealand: hearingvoicesnet workanz.wordpress.com; hearingvoicesnetworkanz.wordpress.com/ support-groups

Intervoice online: www.intervoiceonline.org

ISPS Australia: ispsaustralia.com

LGBTIQA+ Inclusive language guide. Victorian Department of Health: www. vic.gov.au/inclusive-language-guide

New Zealand Early Intervention in Psychosis Society: www.earlypsychosis.org. nz/index.php/about-psychosis/support-from-family-friends

One Door Mental Health: www.onedoor.org.au/

Orygen Youth Health: www.orygen.org.au/

Safehaven model of care: www.seslhd.health.nsw.gov.au/sites/default/files/ groups/Mental_Health/Consumer_Representation/SafeHaven_Program_ Framework_February_2021_v1.3.pdf

Safer Care Victoria: www.safercare.vic.gov.au/improvement/projects/mh/ safe-haven-cafe

SANE Australia: www.sane.org/ StigmaWatch: www.sane.org/get-involved/advocacy/stigmawatch Discussion regarding schizophrenia: www.sane.org/spotlight-on/ schizophrenia

Second Life virtual world was utilised in a study by Australian Professor Peter Yellowlees designed as an educational tool to simulate the frightening experiences of hallucinations associated with mental illness in order to develop greater understanding among non-sufferers: www.youtube.com/ watch?v=P4-PUF3ScL0

Voice hearer and psychologist Eleanor Longden talks about her journey back to mental health and makes the case that it was through learning to listen to her voices that she was able to survive: www.ted.com/talks/eleanor_ longden_the_voices_in_my_head

World Health Organization: Fact sheet: Schizophrenia: www.who.int/news-room/fact-sheets/detail/schizophrenia

REFERENCES

Aguey-Zinsou, M., Scanlan, J.N., & Cusick, A. 2022. A scoping and systematic review of employment processes and outcomes for young adults experiencing psychosis. Comm Ment Health J, 1–28.

American Psychiatric Association (APA), 2015. Schizophrenia Spectrum and Other Psychotic Disorders: DSM-5 Selections. American Psychiatric Publishing, Washington DC.

American Psychiatric Association (APA), 2013. Diagnostic and Statistical Manual of Mental Disorders, 5th Edition. APA, Washington DC.

Ayano, G., Tesfaw, G., Shumet, S. 2019. The prevalence of schizophrenia and other psychotic disorders among homeless people: A systematic review and meta-analysis. BMC Psychiatry, 19(1), 370.

Ball, M., & Picot, S. 2021. Dissociachotic: Seeing the non-psychosis that we share. J Humanist Psychol, 63(2), 002216782199366.

Barr, S.M., Roberts, D., & Thakkar, K.N. 2021. Psychosis in transgender and gender non-conforming individuals: A review of the literature and a call for more research. Psychiatry Res, 306, 114272.

Bloomfield, M.A., Yusuf, F.N., Srinivasan, R., Kelleher, I., Bell, V., et al., 2020. Trauma-informed care for adult survivors of developmental trauma with psychotic and dissociative symptoms: A systematic review of intervention studies. The Lancet Psychiatry, 7(5), 449–462.

Boyle, M. 2022. Power in the power threat meaning framework. J Constructiv Psychol, 35(1), 27-40.

Brasso, C., Giordano, B., Badino, C., Bellino, S., Bozzatello, P., et al., 2021. Primary psychosis: Risk and protective factors and early detection of the onset. Diagnostics, 11(11), 2146.

Buus, N. & McCloughen, A. 2022. Client and family responses to an open dialogue approach in early intervention in psychosis: A prospective qualitative case study. Iss Ment Health Nurs, 43(4), 308–316.

Chase K.A., Melbourne, J.K., Rosen C., McCarthy-Jones S., Jones N., et al., 2018. Traumagenics: At the intersect of childhood trauma, immunity and psychosis. Psychiatry Res, 273, 369–77.

Chowdhury, N.Z., Albalawi, O., Wand, H., Adily, A., Kariminia, A., et al., 2019. First diagnosis of psychosis in the prison: Results from a data-linkage study. BJ Psych Open, 5(6), e89.

Corstens, D., Escher, S., & Romme, M. 2008. Accepting and working with voices: The Maastricht Approach. In: Moskowitz, A., Schafer, I. & Dorahy, M.J. (eds), Psychosis, trauma and dissociation: Emerging perspectives on severe psychopathology. Wiley-Blackwell, Oxford.

Firth, J., Siddiqi, N., Koyanagi, A.I., Siskind, D., Rosenbaum, S., et al., 2019. The Lancet Psychiatry Commission: A blueprint for protecting physical health in people with mental illness. Lancet Psychiatry, 6(8), 675–712.

Fusar-Poli, P., de Pablo, G.S., Correll, C.U., Meyer-Lindenberg, A., Millan, M.J., et al., 2020. Prevention of psychosis: Advances in detection, prognosis, and intervention. JAMA Psychiatry, 77(7), 755–765.

Gaillard, A.S., Braun, E., Vollmann, J., Gather, J., & Scholten, M. 2023. The content of psychiatric advance directives: A systematic review. Psychiatric Serv, 74(1), 44–55.

Gieselmann, A., Simon, A., Vollmann, J., & Schöne-Seifert, B. 2018. Psychiatrists' views on different types of advance statements in mental health care in Germany. Int J Soc Psychiatry, 64(8), 737–744.

Grech, E., Raeburn, T. 2019. Experiences of hospitalised homeless adults and their health care providers in OECD nations: A literature review. Collegian 26, 204–211.

Guinart, D., Misawa, F., Rubio, J.M., Pereira, J., de Filippis, R., et al., 2021. A systematic review and pooled, patient-level analysis of predictors of mortality in neuroleptic malignant syndrome. Acta Psychiatrica Scandinavica, 144(4), 329–341.

Harris, B., Duggan, M., Batterham, P., Bartlem, K., Clinton-McHarg, T. et al., 2018. Australia's mental health and physical health tracker: Background Paper. Australian Health Policy Collaboration. Technical paper No. 2018–06, AHPC, Melbourne.

Howell, S., Yarovova, E., Khwanda, A., & Rosen, S.D. 2019. Cardiovascular effects of psychotic illnesses and antipsychotic therapy. Heart, 105(24), 1852–1859.

James, R., Maude, P., & Searby, A. 2023. Promoting and hindering factors in the use of advance statements by Australian mental health clinicians. J Psychiatric Ment Health Nurs, 30(4), 743–760.

Kotzeva, A., Mittal, D., Desai, S., Judge, D., & Samanta, K. 2023. Socioeconomic burden of schizophrenia: A targeted literature review of types of costs and associated drivers across 10 countries. J Med Econom, 26(1), 70–83.

Lal, S., Malla, A., Marandola, G., Thériault, J., Tibbo, P., et al., 2019. "Worried about relapse": Family members' experiences and perspectives of relapse in first-episode psychosis. Early Intervent Psychiatry, 13(1), 24–29.

Lecomte, T., Potvin, S., Samson, C., Francoeur, A., Hache-Labelle, C., et al., 2019. Predicting and preventing symptom onset and relapse in schizophrenia – a metareview of current empirical evidence. J Abnorm Psychol, 128(8), 840–854.

Longden, E. 2013. The voices in my head. Ted Talk. Available: www.ted.com/talks/eleanor_longden_the_voices_in_my_head/transcript?language=en

Mitchell, S., Shannon, C., Mulholland, C., & Hanna, D. 2021. Reaching consensus on the principles of trauma-informed care in early intervention psychosis services: A Delphi study. Early Intervent Psychiatry, 15(5), 1369–1375.

Moncrieff, J. 2021. A Straight Talking Introduction to Psychiatric Drugs: The Truth About How They Work and How to Come Off Them. Blackwell, Oxford.

Morgan, M., Peters, D., Hopwood, M., Castle, D., Moy, C., et al., 2021. Being equally well – a national policy roadmap to better physical health care and longer lives for people with serious mental illness. Mitchell Institute, Victoria University, Melbourne, August 2021.

Murray. R.M., 2017. Mistakes I have made in my research career. Schizophr Bull, 43(2), 253–256.

National Mental Health Commission, 2017. The 2016 Report on Mental Health and Suicide Prevention. National Mental Health Commission, Sydney.

Onitsuka, T., Hirano, Y., Nakazawa, T., Ichihashi, K., Miura, K. et al., 2022. Toward recovery in schizophrenia: Current concepts, findings, and future research directions. Psychiatry Clin Neurosci, 76(7), 282–291.

Peralta, V., Moreno-Izco, L., Garcia de Jalon, E., Sánchez-Torres, A.M., Janda, L., et al. & SEGPEPs Group 2021. Prospective long-term cohort study of subjects with first-episode psychosis examining eight major outcome domains and their predictors: Study protocol. Front Psychiatry, 12, 643112.

Porges, S.W. 2011. The polyvagal theory: Neurophysiological foundations of emotions, attachment, communication, and self-regulation. W.W. Norton, New York.

Read, J., Morrison, T., & Waddingham, R. 2020. Traumas, adversities, and psychosis: Investigating practical implications. Psychiatric Times, 37(7), 48–51.

Roberts, R. 2019. The physical health of people living with mental illness: A narrative literature review. Charles Sturt University, NSW.

Rodolico, A., Bighelli, I., Avanzato, C., Concerto, C., Cutrufelli, P., et al., 2022. Family interventions for relapse prevention in schizophrenia: A systematic review and network meta-analysis. Lancet Psychiatry, 9(3), 211–221.

Rosenhan, D.L. 1973. On being sane in insane places. Science, 179 (4070), 250–258.

Ross, A.M., Morgan, A.J., Jorm, A.F., & Reavley, N.J. 2019. A systematic review of the impact of media reports of severe mental illness on stigma and discrimination, and interventions that aim to mitigate any adverse impact. Soc Psychiatry Psychiatric Epidemiol, 54, 11–31.

Ross, A.M., Morgan, A.J., Wake, A., Jorm, A.F., & Reavley, N.J. 2020. Guidelines for news media reporting on mental illness in the context of violence and crime: A Delphi consensus study. Aust Journalism Rev, 42(2), 293–311.

Savill, M., Nguyen, T., Shim, R.S., & Loewy, R.L. 2022. Online psychosis screening: Characterizing an underexamined population to improve access and equity. Psychiatric Serv, 73(9), 1005–1012.

Schwing, G., 1954. A Way to the Soul of the Mentally Ill. International Universities Press, New York.

Seeman, M.V. 2019. Schizophrenia mortality: Barriers to progress. Psychiatric Quart, 90(3), 553–563.

Shelton, G., 2016. Appraising Travelbee's Human-to-Human Relationship Model. J Adv Practice Oncol, 7(6), 657–661.

Siegel, D.J. & Drulis, C. 2023. An interpersonal neurobiology perspective on the mind and mental health: Personal, public, and planetary well-being. Ann Gen Psychiatry, 22, 5. doi.org/10.1186/s12991-023-00434-5

Spinelli, M. 2021. Postpartum psychosis: A diagnosis for the DSMV. Archives of Women's Mental Health, 1–6.

Stroup, T.S., Gerhard, T., Crystal, S., Huang, C., Tan, Z., et al., 2019. Comparative effectiveness of adjunctive psychotropic medications in patients with schizophrenia. JAMA Psychiatry, 76(5), 508–515.

Taitimu, M., Read, J., McIntosh, T. 2018. Ngā Whakāwhitinga (standing at the crossroads): How Māori understand what Western psychiatry calls "schizophrenia". Transcult Psychiatry 55(2), 153–177.

Takeuchi, H., Siu, C., Remington, G., Fervaha, G., Zipursky, R.B. et al., 2019. Does relapse contribute to treatment resistance? Antipsychotic response in first vs. second-episode schizophrenia. Neuropsychopharmacology, 44(6), 1036–1042.

Thompson, J., Stansfeld, J.L., Cooper, R.E., Morant, N., Crellin, N.E. et al., 2020. Experiences of taking neuroleptic medication and impacts on symptoms, sense of self and agency: A systematic review and thematic synthesis of qualitative data. Soc Psychiatry Psychiatric Epidemiol, 55(2), 151–164.

Turner, S., Harvey, C., Hayes, L., Castle, D., Galletly, C., et al., 2020. Childhood adversity and clinical and psychosocial outcomes in psychosis. Epidemiol Psychiatric Sci, 29, e78.

Ungvarsky, J. 2023. Postpartum psychosis. Salem Press Encyclopedia of Health: Research Starters.

Valentine, L., Grace, D., Pryor, I., Buccilli, K., Sellars, M., et al., 2021. "When I'm thinking straight, I can put things in place for when I'm not." Exploring the use of advance statements in first-episode psychosis treatment: Young people, clinician, and carer perspectives. Comm Ment Health J, 57, 18–28.

Valery, K.M., & Prouteau, A. 2020. Schizophrenia stigma in mental health professionals and associated factors: A systematic review. Psychiatry Res, 290, 113068.

Ventriglio, A., Castaldelli-Maia, J.M., Torales, J., Chumakov, E., De Berardis, D., et al., 2022. New approaches for mental health of social minorities. Int Rev Psychiatry, 1–10.

Zwicker, A., Denovan-Wright, E.M., Uher, R. 2018. Gene-environment interplay in the etiology of psychosis. Psychology Med, 48, 1925–1936.

15

Eating Disorders

Peta Marks and Bridget Mulvey

KEY POINTS

- Eating disorders are mental illnesses associated with significant morbidity and mortality; anorexia nervosa has the highest mortality rate of any mental illness.
- Recovery is always possible, and outcomes improve with early identification, intervention and appropriate treatment.
- Many myths and stereotypes are associated with eating disorders. Nurses need to be aware of their own values, attitudes and biases that may impact on their capacity to work effectively with the person.

- Psychological distress associated with eating disorders is high; ambivalence and resistance to treatment are part of the illness and are to be expected.
- Nurses working across all clinical settings need an understanding of eating disorders because patients will present to varied clinical settings (primary care, emergency department, general medical, and inpatient or outpatient mental health services) often experiencing complex medical and mental health consequences and complications.

KEY TERMS

Anorexia nervosa
Binge eating disorder
Body image disturbance
Bulimia nervosa
Cognitive behaviour therapy

Family-based therapy
Motivational intervention
Nutritional rehabilitation
Other specified feeding or eating disorder (OSFED)

Psychoeducation
Refeeding syndrome
Specialist supportive clinical management
Therapeutic meal support

LEARNING OUTCOMES

The material in this chapter will assist you to:
- develop an understanding of eating disorders and disordered eating behaviours, within individual, family and social contexts
- identify areas of health and wellbeing – including physical health, mental health, nutritional status, social and behavioural patterns – affected by eating disorders, and to understand the genuine struggle with ambivalence to treatment typically experienced by a person with an eating disorder

- understand the importance of a collaborative and compassionate nursing approach to positive clinical outcomes across all treatment settings and describe important aspects of nursing care for hospitalised patients with anorexia nervosa
- identify various approaches to treatment including specialist supportive clinical management, cognitive behaviour therapy, interpersonal therapy, motivational interventions, family-based therapy, psychoeducation and pharmacotherapy.

INTRODUCTION

This chapter discusses the eating disorders including anorexia nervosa, bulimia nervosa, binge eating disorder, other specified feeding or eating disorder (OSFED) and avoidant/restrictive food intake disorder (ARFID). Eating disorder symptoms are known to exist on a continuum from risk-taking behaviours such as disordered eating and dietary restriction, to moderately serious, higher prevalence illnesses (e.g. bulimia nervosa and binge eating disorder) to very serious relatively low prevalence disorders (e.g. anorexia nervosa).

While a person cannot be simultaneously diagnosed with anorexia nervosa, bulimia nervosa and OSFED, disordered eating behaviours can fluctuate between these illnesses over time. OSFED is a more recently defined category of eating disorder (American Psychiatric Association (APA) 2013) that has not been as well described in the research literature. It encompasses those who meet most, but not all, of

the diagnostic criteria for anorexia nervosa or bulimia nervosa, but who still have significant illness – often as severe and complex as the other eating disorders. OSFED's predecessor, "eating disorder not otherwise specified", differed from OSFED in that it included binge eating disorder (which has now been categorised separately) and was well researched, demonstrating that subclinical disorders can also have a significant impact on health, wellbeing, quality of life, morbidity and mortality (Miskovic-Wheatley et al 2023).

Eating disorders are characterised by one or more seriously disturbed eating behaviours, such as food restriction or recurrent episodes of uncontrolled eating, and weight-control behaviours including self-induced vomiting, excessive exercising or the misuse of laxatives or diuretics. A person with an eating disorder is preoccupied with their weight, and their self-worth is dependent largely, or even exclusively, on their perceived ability to control their shape and weight. Because of stigma and because eating disorders are often hidden, most people in the community who experience them do not seek treatment. As such, there is substantial unmet need regarding awareness and identification, diagnosis and treatment (Fitzsimmons-Craft et al 2019).

Nurses across all clinical settings need to develop an evidence-based understanding of how eating disorders are developed and maintained, identifying those at risk and gaining the skills required to intervene early and to work with people towards their recovery. Educating the community, providing effective person-centred treatment and supporting better outcomes for people and their families are the focus. As with all other physical and mental health disorders, "early recognition and timely intervention based on a developmentally appropriate, evidence-based, multidisciplinary team approach (medical, psychological and nutritional) is the ideal standard of care" (Koreshe et al 2023).

Eating disorders are among the most serious and misunderstood of all mental illnesses, with myths and stereotypes impacting significantly on those who experience them (Bryant et al 2023). Eating disorders are not lifestyle choices driven by vanity or a desire for attention. They are complex and potentially lethal illnesses associated with significant emotional distress, that generally require medium- to long-term treatment. People with eating disorders do not bring the illness on themselves and cannot simply choose to stop dieting or easily change the negative self-destructive behaviours that form part of the illness. As well as having significant negative health effects, eating disorders are associated with significant quality of life impairment and impact on a person's personal, work/education and social/emotional life.

TYPES OF EATING DISORDERS

Anorexia Nervosa

Anorexia nervosa is a complex and serious mental illness that has impairment outcomes comparable to schizophrenia and high rates of psychiatric comorbidity, medical morbidity and mortality. It is characterised by intense fear (and avoidance of) weight gain or of being "fat", which motivates persistent and severe dietary restriction and other weight loss behaviours. Low body weight or low body mass index (BMI) is the central diagnostic feature for anorexia nervosa; however, for atypical anorexia nervosa (which is covered by an OSFED diagnosis), the person is not usually underweight. Anorexia nervosa usually starts in early to middle adolescence (but it can emerge at any age) and begins with dieting or restricting food that is perceived to be fattening or "unhealthy" (e.g. "clean eating"). This dietary restriction becomes more rigid and extreme as the illness progresses and is generally accompanied by worsening depressed mood, increasing anxiety and obsessive-compulsive features, as well as cognitive impairment. Common weight-loss behaviours include excluding entire food groups (e.g. carbohydrates), excessive exercise, self-induced vomiting or purging and, less commonly, using appetite suppressants or diuretics. Young people who develop anorexia nervosa may fail to make expected weight gains or maintain normal developmental trajectories (as opposed to losing weight). If the onset of anorexia nervosa is pre-pubertal, the sequence of pubertal events will be delayed or even arrested (e.g. in girls the breasts do not develop and there is primary amenorrhoea, and in boys the genitals remain juvenile) and menstruation in women may or may not occur.

Body mass index (BMI) can be used to stage severity of illness (APA 2013) – that is, BMI < 15 kg/m^2 = extreme; BMI 15–15.99 kg/m^2 = severe; BMI 16–16.99 kg/m^2 = moderate; and BMI > 17 kg/m^2 = mild. However, it is important to remember that if someone is presenting with atypical anorexia nervosa (which is more common), they may experience all the symptoms and complications of anorexia nervosa but not meet the weight/BMI criterion.

Personal perspectives: Consumer's story 15.1 describes the early development of an eating disorder.

PERSONAL PERSPECTIVES

Consumer's Story 15.1: Rebecca

Rebecca is a 16-year-old in Year 11, living with her parents and older sister, and doing her Higher School Certificate. Rebecca has lost a significant amount of weight over the past few months by engaging in very restrictive eating and excessive exercise behaviours, but she remains at the lower healthy weight range. She was previously sporty, sociable and a high academic achiever, but this year has struggled with changes to her peer group at school, as well as bullying by exclusion and having shame-inducing comments posted to her Facebook page, which has caused her to feel anxious, embarrassed, sad and very distressed at times. Her mother, a dietitian, has tried to help Rebecca to eat healthily, but this has been ineffective, and she is worried her daughter has an eating disorder. When Rebecca fainted at school, her mum took her to a GP. The GP found that Rebecca had lost 8–10 kg over the preceding 2 months and was medically unstable (low body temperature, low pulse, blood pressure changes on standing and an irregular ECG). She referred Rebecca immediately to the local hospital emergency department for further assessment.

At the hospital, the triage nurse was overheard telling the doctor: *I've got a 16-year-old in bed 5 who is medically unstable for you to see. She doesn't look skinny, but apparently the GP and mother are worried she's got an eating disorder. I really don't get people who starve themselves to be beauty queens.*

Learning Point

Stereotyping, stigma and discrimination can affect a practitioner's attitude and approach, which in turn impacts on a consumer's help-seeking behaviour and potentially their health outcome. It is important to share your knowledge with other health practitioners, in an effort to dispel some of the myths and stereotypes that surround eating disorders.

People experiencing anorexia nervosa often feel that their identity becomes synonymous with the eating disorder and through the disorder they experience a sense of control over their environment or satisfaction at achieving weight-loss goals. This is despite the significant nutritional compromise and life-threatening medical complications the person experiences as a result of dietary restriction, weight loss and malnutrition, and the often-debilitating psychological distress, difficulties with emotion regulation and poor cognitive flexibility that accompany the illness (Dann et al 2023). There are real feelings of body weight and shape distortion, where the person feels globally overweight or focuses on particular body parts (typically buttocks, thighs or abdomen) as being "too fat". The idea of weight gain is seen as an unacceptable failure of self-control, so regardless of how underweight a person with anorexia nervosa may become (or how unwell they may be feeling), there remains an overwhelming fear of becoming fat, a desire to lose more weight and an increasing preoccupation with strategising for continued restriction and weight loss.

Bulimia Nervosa

Bulimia nervosa is characterised by regular, overwhelming urges to overeat large amounts of food (binge), followed by compensatory behaviours to avoid weight gain, such as self-induced vomiting, excessive exercise, food avoidance or laxative misuse. Like people with anorexia nervosa, people with bulimia nervosa overvalue weight and shape and fear weight gain. They often experience symptoms of anxiety and depression. The word "binge" is often used inaccurately – a "binge" is defined as eating an excessive amount of food that is definitely larger than most individuals would eat, over a similar period of time, under similar circumstances. There is always a sense of lack of control associated with binge eating (Citrome 2019).

One of the main triggers for binge eating is hunger; a cycle is often established where food is restricted during the day and binge eating behaviour occurs in the afternoon/evening. Other triggers can be interpersonal stressors, intense emotions, boredom or negative feelings related to self-worth, body weight and shape. Binge eating continues until the person is uncomfortably or painfully full and leads to feelings of guilt, self-recrimination and self-disgust. Fear of weight gain triggers vomiting or other compensatory behaviours, further reinforcing the person's poor sense of self-worth and, as they resolve to do better with "dieting" the next day, helps maintain the bulimic cycle.

The key feature distinguishing bulimia nervosa from anorexia nervosa is weight: people with bulimia nervosa are likely to have normal or near-normal body weight. They are less likely to require renourishment in in-patient hospitalisation; however, that is not to say that bulimia nervosa is a harmless illness. In fact, the fluid and electrolyte disturbances created by purging can create serious and potentially fatal medical problems (e.g. cardiac arrhythmias, oesophageal tears, gastric rupture) that may require treatment in hospital.

Personal perspectives: Consumer's story 15.2 describes a consumer presenting to her general practitioner (GP) with a request for laxatives; however, the issue is disordered eating and elimination patterns.

👤 PERSONAL PERSPECTIVES

Consumer's Story 15.2: Mandy

Mandy is a 25-year-old who presented to a new GP for a laxative prescription because her usual doctor was unavailable. She was booked in to see the nurse first because it had been some time since she had visited a doctor. Mandy reported that she had been having problems with abdominal pain, said she was constipated and wanted to see the doctor for a stronger laxative. She had tried most over-the-counter laxatives, but they were not effective. Mandy admitted she had problems with stress, controlling her weight and managing her diet. She thought she had been suffering from food allergies – probably lactose and gluten intolerance (she avoided both in her diet). She had just started a new job, was not eating regularly and was skipping meals. She also experienced tiredness, moodiness and erratic menstrual periods. She was thin and pale, but was not clinically constipated on examination.

The primary care nurse said: *Mandy, I don't see any clinical signs of constipation when I feel your tummy, so let's have a think about what else might be going on. Some people who worry about constipation say they have difficulties with their eating. Would you say that this is an issue for you?*

Learning Point

Asking about disordered eating behaviours in a matter-of-fact, non-judgemental way is important for early identification and intervention. Using a simple evidence-based screening tool such as the IOI-S (Bryant et al 2021) can help to start the discussion. It is available online at https://insideoutinstitute.org.au/screener.

Binge Eating Disorder

Binge eating disorder is the most common eating disorder and has demonstrated impacts on a person's health and quality of life. Someone with binge eating disorder experiences recurrent episodes of binge eating but without the use of compensatory behaviours. Similar to people with other eating disorders, binge eating is accompanied by a sense of lack of self-control while eating and, after a binge, marked distress (guilt, disgust) and feelings of anxiety and depression. Binge eating disorder can occur in people who are normal weight, overweight or obese. Not all people who are obese engage in binge eating, but those who do experience greater functional impairment, poorer quality of

life, greater subjective distress and psychiatric comorbidity than those who do not. Nearly three-quarters of people who experience binge eating disorder have a co-occurring mental disorder – this significant psychiatric comorbidity is comparable with anorexia and bulimia nervosa (Giel et al 2022).

Other specified feeding or eating disorder

At times, people experience eating disorders that cause clinically significant distress or impairment in important areas of functioning (e.g. social, occupational), but that do not meet the full criteria for diagnosis as an eating disorder. Examples include those with atypical anorexia nervosa, as described above, or someone who meets all the criteria for bulimia nervosa or binge eating disorder, except the criteria around frequency of binge eating or other compensatory behaviours. OSFED also includes purging disorder, where a person purges without binge eating, and night eating syndrome. The UK's National Institute for Health and Care Excellence published a guideline recommending that treatment should be the same as the eating disorder the person is most closely experiencing (Riesco et al 2018).

Avoidant/restrictive food intake disorder (ARFID)

ARFID is a more recently defined illness (APA 2013), where the person restricts their eating due to a lack of interest in eating or food, avoidance of foods because of textural issues, or due to fear of an adverse consequence of eating (e.g. nausea, pain, reflux, vomiting), often as a response to a previously upsetting food-related experience. While there is limited research into ARFID, it is estimated to be common in clinical settings and in the general population, and those with ARFID commonly experience other co-morbidities (such as anxiety disorder and autism spectrum disorder) (Sanchez-Cerezo et al 2022). A multidisciplinary approach that provides psychological interventions (such as behavioural therapy, cognitive behavioural therapy (CBT) and family-based therapy), along with nutritional interventions and support of physical health, is recommended, but as yet, no evidence-based treatments exist (Willmott et al 2023).

In addition to ARFID, there are a number of eating or feeding disorders that are identified, but will not be discussed in this chapter because they are not focused on body weight and shape concerns: pica, where the person craves and eats non-food substances such as dirt; and rumination disorder, where the person regurgitates, re-chews and swallows food.

INCIDENCE AND PREVALENCE

There is a common misperception that eating disorders are very rare. While we know that incidence and prevalence rates for eating disorders are difficult to determine as the result of a range of factors (such as individual, illness-related factors like denial and shame; stigma and discrimination impacting on detection rates in primary care and other settings; low investment in eating disorder research and inconsistent application of study design and measures (Hay et al 2023)), a recent rapid review (Hay et al 2023) identified that eating disorders are a global phenomenon present in all ages and gender groups, that prevalence rates are increasing, and age of onset is getting younger (Morris et al 2022). At least one in 20 adults has an eating disorder and they are known to emerge in adolescence and early adulthood – the highest prevalence rates are seen in children and adolescents. Various cohort studies of adolescents have estimated prevalence at roughly 15–22% (Mitchison et al 2020). These are not rare disorders in young people.

The early stages of the COVID-19 pandemic made matters worse for people with eating disorders with changes in daily routine, social media, restricted access to support people and changes to treatment causing eating disorder symptoms to worsen for those with existing illness, and presentations for eating disorder to increase in Australia and overseas (Miskovic-Wheatley et al 2022) – a trend that has not abated.

Eating disorders are common in Aboriginal and Torres Strait Islander peoples. There is limited research but the evidence identifies an increase in some eating disorders (over-eating type disorders – such as night eating syndrome in adolescents (Burt et al 2020b) and unspecified feeding and eating Disorders (UFED) with binge eating in adults than for the general population (Burt et al 2020a). Food security issues, food trauma and other issues may contribute (The Australian Eating Disorders Research and Translation Centre 2022). Eating disorders appear more prevalent in young people from sexually/gender diverse groups and there is emerging research from a range of sources that there is also intersectionality between eating disorders and neurodiversity (Cobbaert & Rose 2023), particularly ADHD. However, we also know that males, particularly people from diverse sexual, gender, cultural and neurodiverse backgrounds, are under-researched, and most people with eating disorders do not access treatment, so we are likely to be underestimating the impact of eating disorders across all population groups (Hay et al 2023; InsideOut Institute 2021).

In adolescents, the presentation is likely to be sub-clinical, with disordered eating behaviours highly prevalent (Hay 2023). We also know that adolescents whose body weight is over the most healthy weight, in the obese category, are twice as likely to have an eating disorder, but that this might not just be a binge eating type disorder, it could also be an atypical restricting or purging disorder. In the older age groups – late teens, early 20s – eating disorders are also very common (Tavolacci et al 2021).

Australian research has identified that in primary care most people with eating disorders are not identified (Ivancic et al 2021), most people with eating disorders don't seek treatment (less than 30%) and of those who do access treatment, it is unlikely to be evidence-based (Kazdin et al 2017).

Eating Disorders and Gender

Most people who experience eating disorders are assigned female at birth; however, eating disorders also occur in those assigned male at birth (especially in children). Eating disorders occur in pregnant women, in older adults, in the LGBTIQA+ population, in people across all age and cultural groups and across the socioeconomic spectrum, in people with other mental health problems, in people with other physical health problems, and in people who are over their most healthy weight or living in a larger body.

Eating disorders and disordered eating behaviours are increasingly identified in those who have been historically underdiagnosed and under-represented in eating disorder research and clinical practice (see Personal perspectives: Consumer's story 15.3).

Some researchers state that eating disorders tend to be diagnosed earlier for males than females (Zerwas et al 2015); other research has found onset of eating disorders is later for males (Mitchison & Mond 2015). Binge eating disorder is the most common eating disorder experienced in adult males (at almost equal prevalence as females), followed by bulimia nervosa and anorexia nervosa.

Significant differences may exist between males and females in terms of predisposing, precipitating and perpetuating factors for an eating disorder. For example, males who have an eating disorder are more likely to have been pre-morbidly mild to moderate obesity, whereas women tend to have a normal weight history, but feel fat before losing weight; males with bulimia nervosa, binge eating or binge eating disorder are less likely to engage in vomiting or laxative abuse and more likely to use excessive exercise as a compensatory behaviour than women. Men report that anger can trigger a binge, whereas suppressing anger is a more likely trigger for women (Strother et al 2012).

PERSONAL PERSPECTIVES
Consumer's Story 15.3: Vahid

Vahid grew up in a bigger body and always felt self-conscious and ashamed because he was fat. Teased at school, he turned to food as a coping mechanism, for comfort. By the time he was 25 he decided that he would diet and exercise, losing a significant amount of weight through extreme dietary restriction and trying to bulk up his muscles at the gym. Despite having what his friends thought of as an "ideal" body, 28-year-old Vahid was miserable. The rigid dieting became too much and Vahid began to binge eat, in secret, especially if he'd had a few drinks at a party and his guard was down. He felt so guilty and distressed about what he'd eaten that he would sometimes vomit and sometimes just double down at the gym and not eat for a few days at a time, to avoid putting on weight. Although he thought that he probably needed help to stop the binge–purge–starve cycle that he found himself in, Vahid also felt ashamed that he had a "girl's" problem and feared that nobody would believe him.

Internalisation of the thin ideal, weight-based self-worth, food restriction and body dissatisfaction have been reported in lesbian women, gay men, transgender and non-conforming adults (Bell et al 2018; Cervantes-Luna et al 2019). And transgender youth are reported to experience increased internalisation, body surveillance, disordered eating and body shame (Chaphekar et al 2022).

Body dysmorphic disorder (listed within the "Obsessive compulsive and related disorders" section of the *Diagnostic and Statistical Manual of Mental Disorders* (DSM-5) (American Psychiatric Association (APA) 2013) rather than in the "Eating disorders" section) and anorexia nervosa, share a number of significant overlaps – "sociodemographic characteristics, severity of body image concerns, level of body dissatisfaction and preoccupation, degree of perfectionism, altered experience of emotion, degree of obsessive-compulsive disorder comorbidity and deficits in body size estimation" (Phillipou et al 2019, p. 136). And muscle dysmorphia, a subtype of body dysmorphic disorder, is widely thought to be more prevalent in males than females. It is characterised by a preoccupation with muscularity and achieving a low degree of body fat and is associated with eating disorder symptoms (like body checking, body avoidance), as well as greater psychopathology, psychosocial impairment and suicide risk than other body dysmorphic disorders.

HISTORICAL ANECDOTE 15.1
Eating disorders affect all genders

Descriptions of disordered eating practices can be found in ancient religious texts. Puritanical Christian groups in the 1600s promoted fasting methods for spiritual enlightenment, suggesting starvation could be used to assert control over bodily desires for purification and a more spiritual life. Interestingly, early descriptions of eating disorders rarely viewed them as conditions experienced by males. Dr William Gull, who coined the term "anorexia nervosa" as early as 1873, described it as a condition in "females between the ages of fifteen and twenty-three characterised by extreme emaciation". Early treatment approaches focused on separating women who experienced anorexia nervosa from their family because they were viewed as "thin-blooded and emotional", causing distress within the family unit. It wasn't until the aftermath of the First World War and the increasing emergence of several war-related mental health conditions, such as "shell-shock" (post-traumatic stress disorder), that mental health clinicians began to accept that "male anorexia" was also a condition that needed attention.

Read More About It:
Zhang C 2014 What can we learn from the history of male anorexia nervosa? J Eat Disord, 2(1), 138.

Eating Disorders in Children and Adolescents

Children with eating disorders can get sicker more quickly than adults. Emaciation and medical complications can occur more rapidly because young people have lower energy stores and dehydrate sooner. As a result, rapid weight loss in children is more likely to result in life-threatening complications (DerMarderosian et al 2018).

Children under 12 years of age who present with an eating disorder may present with similar psychological symptoms as adolescents and adults. However, they are less likely to report fear of fatness or weight gain, less likely to appreciate just how severe the illness is, more likely to present with non-specific symptoms, more likely to be boys and more likely to have lost weight rapidly (Hay et al 2014). They are also less likely to vomit or abuse laxatives and more likely to be diagnosed with an unspecified feeding or eating disorder (Hay et al 2014).

Early and more aggressive nutritional rehabilitation is needed for children and adolescents with eating disorders to prevent potentially irreversible complications affecting development, such as growth retardation, delayed pubertal maturation and irreversible and long-term effects on bone development, as well as structural and morphological changes in different organ systems (including the brain), pubertal delay/arrest and chronicity of illness (Campbell & Peebles 2014; DerMarderosian et al 2018).

CRITICAL THINKING EXERCISE 15.1

1. How would you describe a "normal" interest in body image, eating and dieting versus an "obsessive" interest?
2. Is your answer different for males and females?
3. Does age affect what you consider to be "normal"?
4. Severe dieting is the single biggest risk factor for the onset of an eating disorder. There is also a focus on preventing obesity and a high incidence of dieting behaviour in the community. How might it be possible to balance these messages of risk and prevention?

CONTRIBUTING FACTORS

There are several factors that increase a person's vulnerability to developing an eating disorder. Some of these are modifiable risk factors, others are not. For example, being female, 10–25 years old and living in an industrialised society are the top three unmodifiable risk factors; genetic predisposition, early puberty, a perfectionistic temperament and a history of traumatic life experiences are also unmodifiable. Dieting, disordered eating behaviours and excessive exercise, as well as body dissatisfaction, are modifiable risk factors – variables that are potentially a focus for targeted prevention activities. In terms of risk, high-frequency (or severe) dieting is the strongest predictor for developing any eating disorder and early onset of dieting is associated with poorer physical and mental health, more disordered eating, extreme body dissatisfaction and more frequent general health problems, such as reduced bone mineral density, as well as family conflict and depressed mood in adolescents (Barakat et al 2023; Koreshe et al 2023).

A number of risk factors are described below. Remember, though, that most people are exposed to many of these factors and do not develop an eating disorder, so it is likely that an intricate interplay exists between the risk and protective factors, and that for each individual, the illness develops in a unique way.

Biological and Genetic Factors

Anorexia nervosa, bulimia nervosa and binge eating disorder are all heritable conditions influenced by genetic and environmental factors and evidence for genetic risk factors for other eating disorders is growing. Anorexia nervosa is a complex heritable phenotype (i.e. it has characteristics that result from interaction of genes with environment) that has significant genetic correlations with other eating disorders (e.g. bulimia nervosa), other psychiatric disorders (e.g. obsessive-compulsive disorder), with educational attainment and with multiple metabolic traits (Barakat et al 2023). First-degree relatives of people who have had anorexia nervosa are up to 11 times more likely to develop the disorder than someone from the general population, and are significantly more likely to develop an eating disorder in general. Maternal eating disorders have also been linked with negative pregnancy effects (e.g. diabetes, pre-eclampsia and gestational hypertension), complications during delivery (e.g. prolonged labour, induced delivery), impacts on prenatal and neonatal growth (Watson et al 2018) and poor respiratory outcomes (Popovic et al 2018).

Biological sequalae that occur as a result of dietary restriction and disordered eating, or of excessive exercise, as well as weight loss associated with physical illness or the presence of an illness such as diabetes mellitus (which requires dietary restriction), also increase the risk of developing an eating disorder.

Individual Psychological Factors

Personality traits seem to differ across the eating disorders; however, some features, such as lack of emotional awareness, are common to all eating disorders. Perfectionism is common in people with anorexia nervosa and those with bulimia nervosa, obsessiveness is strongly associated with people who have anorexia nervosa and people with binge-purge type illnesses experience higher levels of impulsivity and emotional dysregulation (Barakat et al 2023).

A range of emotion regulation difficulties are also common, including feelings of guilt, disgust and shame, avoidance and negative problem-solving, comparing themselves with others and submissive behaviours, worry and rumination, and using emotional suppression to avoid conflict (Oldershaw et al 2015).

Childhood adversity, family disruption and childhood trauma (e.g. neglect, emotional abuse, sexual abuse) and other traumatic experiences (e.g. criticism, teasing, bullying around weight and shape, loss and grief) are known to be risk factors for binge/purge type disorders in particular (i.e. those with anorexia nervosa binge purge type, bulimia nervosa, binge eating disorder, purging disorder) (Barakat et al 2023).

Social theories about eating disorders are explored in Box 15.1.

BOX 15.1   Social Theories About Eating Disorders

Cognitive behaviour theory suggests the restriction of food and other characteristic behaviours are related to the person's beliefs about weight and eating and that these beliefs reinforce the overvaluation of restrained eating, as well as the underlying body shape and weight concerns. *Sociocultural theories* of eating disorders relate to the environmental factors that impact on how people view themselves and compare themselves with others, and how prevailing social norms (e.g. the thin ideal) are internalised. *Feminist theories* see eating disorders in relation to the messages women receive from society about their bodies and the relationship with success, admiration and control — and that the thin ideal is society's attempt to fight against increasing independence and power of women. From a *psychodynamic theoretical perspective*, issues of separation and autonomy, involving enmeshed relationships, as well as difficulties with the expression of anger and psychosexual development, are described (Smolak & Levine 2015).

Sociocultural and Environmental Influences

Sociocultural influences include unrealistically thin media (and social media) images, the stigmatisation of people who are overweight – stereotyping them as lazy and unintelligent – as well as the increasing use of injectables and cosmetic surgery by people seeking a "perfect" face and body, with the cultural acceptance of thinness as being more highly valued than almost any other strength or quality. Body image dissatisfaction is exacerbated for many people by this social and cultural pressure to conform to a particular "thin" ideal of beauty. Comparing one's body with others (e.g. peers, family, famous people or "influencers") and appearance-related bullying/teasing and "fat shaming" are recognised as factors that contribute to body dissatisfaction, dieting and symptoms of disordered eating. There is a strong and consistent association between the use of social media and body image and eating concerns in adolescents and young women, with the use of social networking sites that utilise photo-posting and "liking" activities contributing to body comparison and dissatisfaction; driving a desire for thinness, dietary restraint and disordered eating; and, reinforcing the internalisation of thinness ideals (de Vries et al 2016; Hummel & Smith 2015; McLean et al 2015; Sidani et al 2016; Tiggemann & Slater 2016). For middle-aged women, menopausal status and anxiety around ageing are also associated with body image dissatisfaction and for developing or exacerbating eating disorder symptoms (Thompson & Bardone-Cone 2019). Body image dissatisfaction is a predictor for the development of eating disorders (Rhode et al 2015).

In recent years, pressure has been applied to the fashion, media, marketing and advertising industries to encourage the employment of models with a greater diversity of more realistic weight and body shapes. As a result, "real body" campaigns have been launched and promoted. However, unhealthy images (including "pro-anorexia", "thinspiration/thinspo/thinfluencer" and "fitspo", as well as those posing as "recovery") and nutritional advice can be promulgated by anyone, and algorithms support promotion of these types of accounts (CCDH 2022). Given the continuing rise, influence and impact of social media, targeted social media literacy and focus on social media platform's role in amplifying unhealthy content may make a greater impact.

Sports, hobbies or careers where body weight, shape and appearance are emphasised (e.g. modelling, gymnastics, body building and ballet dancing) are high-risk activities, particularly for those in the at-risk population (Voelker & Galli 2019).

✳ HISTORICAL ANECDOTE 15.2

Jane Fonda

French doctor Pierre Janet first described people exhibiting bulimic behaviours in 1903, but it was not until 1979 that Gerald Russell published the first formal paper on bulimia nervosa. He described it as a distinct variant of anorexia. In 1987, the DSM-III-R listed bulimia as a separate disorder for the first time. Jane Fonda, a pioneer of the women's fitness and fashion industry, struggled with body image and bulimia from her early teenage years in the 1960s. Although she grew up in a physically safe home, Fonda has described emotional pressure from her father and the society she grew up in to "look perfect". Such pressure had a major impact on her self-concept. She battled low self-esteem and poor self-image during adolescence and her struggles soon morphed into bulimia, which she failed to finally overcome until middle age.

Read More About It

Bosworth P 2011 Jane Fonda: The Private Life of a Public Woman. Houghton Mifflin Harcourt, Boston.

Interpersonal Relationships

Family Relationships

Some family factors can play a role in the genesis or maintenance of eating disorders; however, this does not mean that families are to blame for the eating disorder, There is no research that proves a causative link between family functioning and the onset of eating disorders (Giles et al 2022). Some of the family issues that will be explored in treatment may include any significant changes in parental structure, parenting and communication styles, conflict around mealtimes, modelling eating-disordered behaviours (e.g. dieting, compulsive exercise) and eating disorder attitudes (e.g. body dissatisfaction). Any issues identified during assessment will be addressed as part of treatment. Eating disorders place incredible stress on families – including impacting on health. Families need reassurance and assistance to develop the knowledge and skills they will need to support their loved one to recover. In most instances, the person's family are the primary resource – the support and understanding they can provide are very often vital to the recovery process. Evidence shows that family involvement is useful in reducing psychological and medical morbidity, especially for children and younger adolescents but also with older adolescents and emerging adults – particularly those with a short duration of illness (less than 3 years) (Brown et al 2016).

Peer and Other Important Relationships

Adolescence is a time when the relationships that develop within peer groups begin to overshadow the importance of family for many young people. It is important to consider the impact of all peers, including friends and connections that young people have in their online community – the ubiquitous use of social media by young people means they are particularly vulnerable to overuse, which may have a range of negative effects on wellbeing and mental health depending on the "unique dispositional, social-context, and situational factors that guide their SMU and moderate its effects" (Valkenburg et al 2022, p. 66). Access to, and the impact of, relationships developed in the context of the "pro-Ana" movement, which exist across all social media platforms, are also particularly influential and potentially dangerous, where "thinspiration tips and tricks" of weight loss are shared and the "community" support each other to maintain focus and motivation on extreme thinness – claiming anorexia nervosa as a lifestyle choice, not an illness (Bert et al 2016).

Peer groups that have a high level of body-related competitiveness, or where there is pressure to diet or to be thin, people of influence (e.g. a weight-focused coach or personal trainer) can reinforce the overvaluation of appearance that some young people experience and are vulnerable to. Bullying or teasing around appearance is related to shame and body dissatisfaction – this can be online or in person. Peer groups that diet together and compare body weight and shape (whether overtly or covertly) are extremely influential for young people. Body comparison is a common behaviour among young people and in social media, but it contributes to peer competition and comparison and is associated with negative outcomes (McLean & Paxton 2019). For example, we know that posting selfies, particularly where there is significant investment in taking and editing the selfie, is associated with body dissatisfaction, overvaluation of shape and weight (the internalisation of the thin ideal) and dietary restraint (Lonergan et al 2019; McLean et al 2015). In the more recent "fitspiration" and "clean eating" movement on Instagram and other social media platforms, images of a thin, muscular body ideal have been promoted, often including "inspirational" quotes (of which 11.3% are dysfunctional) (Tiggemann & Zaccardo 2018). Research has demonstrated that fitspo inspires people to improve fitness and eat more healthily, but is also associated with significant increases in body dissatisfaction (Tiggemann & Zaccardo 2015). Almost one-fifth (17.5%) of women who post on fitspiration are thought to be at risk for a clinical eating disorder (Holland & Tiggemann 2017).

Prevention and Protective Factors

Given the significant life impact, illness severity and treatment complexity of eating disorders, prevention is an important public health goal. Individual protective factors include good social and emotional skill development (emotional wellbeing), assertiveness, being self-directed and having a positive coping style – developing resilience. Media literacy and the ability to critically process media images are also important. Protective family factors may include family connectedness, being part of a family where the emphasis is on recognising strengths and skills unrelated to weight and appearance (rather than being weight and physical appearance focused), and a harmonious, consistent, parenting approach. One of the simplest and best protective behaviours for families, across eating disorders and a range of other mental health concerns, is to have shared family meals (Utter et al 2017). From an environmental and sociocultural perspective, a climate where a range of body shapes and sizes are accepted, where performance is valued over physical attractiveness and where relationships (e.g. peers, teachers, community members) are supportive and caring, rather than competitive and critical, may be protective (Breithaupt et al 2017). Prevention programs that incorporate novel interventions associated with, for example, social media literacy, mindfulness, self-compassion are promising, but more research is needed (McLean & Paxton 2019).

💡 CRITICAL THINKING EXERCISE 15.2

1. Think about your personal body image, weight and shape perception. What do you notice about these aspects of how you view yourself?
2. What do you believe have been the major influences on your own body image, or weight and shape perception?
3. To what extent have images in the media, including social media, affected your body image?
4. How might your own body image, weight and shape beliefs impact on how you provide nursing care and a therapeutic relationship with a person who has an eating disorder?

SIGNS AND SYMPTOMS

Physical Health

Measures of weight or BMI are not necessarily good indicators of the degree of potential medical compromise. People who lose weight rapidly can become medically compromised at higher weights than those who lose weight slowly over time, even if they are still at high BMIs. It is important to note that many potentially life-threatening medical sequelae are difficult to detect or are nondetectable with medical testing, and patients who die from medical complications of their illness often have normal laboratory test values (DerMarderosian et al 2018).

Malnutrition affects every organ in the body, and the related medical complications can be life-threatening. Acute complications of anorexia nervosa include bradycardia and cardiac compromise, hypotension, hypothermia, electrolyte disturbance (generally associated with purging, dehydration, starvation), gastrointestinal motility disturbances, renal problems, infertility and perinatal complications. Most of the medical complications of anorexia nervosa (except osteoporosis and necrotic bowel) can be reversed with nutritional rehabilitation and maintenance of a healthy weight range. However, the long-term effect of malnutrition on cognition and brain structure and functioning requires further research.

The abnormalities seen in a person with bulimia nervosa, particularly electrolyte disturbances, are usually related to frequent vomiting or laxative and diuretic misuse. Binge eating disorder carries similar medical risks and long-term consequences to those seen in obesity, such as hypertension, high blood cholesterol, heart disease and increased risk of diabetes and stroke (Table 15.1). Again, these medical complications are usually treated effectively with nutritional management, normalisation of weight and cessation of purging behaviours where these exist (Voderholzer et al 2020).

Mental Health

The psychological and emotional aspects of eating disorders are significant and can be devastating for the person and their family.

The underlying psychological and emotional issues that are related to the onset and maintenance of the eating disorder will be the issues that will need to be addressed over longer-term treatment. Most people with eating disorders experience co-occurring mental health issues – particularly with anxiety disorders (generalised anxiety disorder and social anxiety), obsessive-compulsive disorder, mood disorders (particularly major depression), substance use disorders, post-traumatic stress disorder and personality disorder. Anxiety disorders frequently predate the onset of an eating disorder and anxiety may also develop or worsen as treatment progresses and weight is restored. There is emerging evidence from a range of sources that eating disorders also co-occur with those who have neurodevelopmental disorders, particularly ADHD and autism spectrum disorder (Hambleton et al 2022). It is important to remember that the cognitive and psychological effects of starvation and the symptoms of the illnesses themselves can complicate the mental health picture. For example, symptoms of depression, such as low mood, irritability and social withdrawal, are common in people with eating disorders and are associated with malnutrition. These symptoms do not necessarily warrant a separate diagnosis of major depression because they often reverse with nutritional rehabilitation. Caution is always required, however, particularly as suicide is one of the leading causes of death of people with eating disorders (Hambleton et al 2022).

The increased anxiety and emotional distress that accompany treatment (requiring weight gain, normalising eating and addressing underlying psychological issues) can be harrowing for the person and their family. Supportive nursing interventions, including validation, empathy, externalising the illness and working collaboratively with the person and their family, are therefore very important.

ASSESSMENT

A comprehensive multidisciplinary assessment will determine whether the criteria for diagnosis of a specific eating disorder are met and identifies symptoms and behaviours that require intervention in the person's treatment program. This is also the opportunity for clinicians to establish rapport with the person and to get to know them as an individual. A collaborative approach to assessment and treatment planning is an important part of engaging the person with recovery.

Physical Assessment

The physical assessment, including blood chemistry, urinalysis and ECG, helps detect any significant medical complications. It is also important to exclude other causes of weight loss. A medical examination includes weight and height measures, vital signs, cardiovascular and peripheral vascular function, metabolic status, dermatological manifestations and evidence of self-harm.

TABLE 15.1 Effects of Malnutrition

Body System/ Organ	Effects
Cardiovascular effects	Bradycardia, hypotension and cardiac arrhythmias
	ECG abnormalities – prolonged QTc interval and non-specific ST segment depression or T wave changes – are associated with electrolyte disturbances and malnutrition
	Cardiac arrest can result from arrhythmias
	Hospitalisation and cardiac monitoring are recommended for people presenting with bradycardia or a prolonged QTc interval on ECG (see Fig. 15.1)
Electrolyte abnormalities	Electrolyte abnormalities – including low potassium, chloride and sodium levels – in bulimia nervosa and people with anorexia nervosa who purge
	Frequent vomiting can result in metabolic alkalosis and hypokalaemia, whereas laxative misuse can lead to metabolic acidosis, hyponatraemia and hypokalaemia
	Refeeding syndrome can be fatal
Renal dysfunction	Reduced glomerular filtration rate, elevated serum urea nitrogen and hypovolaemia can occur in both anorexia and bulimia nervosa
	Reduced urine production can indicate severe dehydration or progressive renal insufficiency
	Associated renal failure is sometimes seen in adult patients, especially in those whose illness has become chronic
Gastrointestinal effects	Feeling bloated or full even after eating small amounts of food can indicate shrinking of the stomach or delayed gastric emptying
	Binge eating can lead to gastric dilation and, in rare cases, stomach rupture or death
	Diarrhoea can be a sign of laxative abuse; constipation can result from inadequate food (and fibre) intake, dehydration or decrease in gastric motility
	Common household food supplies such as artificial sweeteners, chewing gum and diet drinks can have laxative effects
	Recurrent vomiting can lead to enlarged parotid and salivary glands, oesophagitis or oesophageal or gastric tears
	Abdominal pain or involuntary regurgitation of food can be associated with both the trauma and the frequency of vomiting
Endocrine effects	Irregular menstrual periods or amenorrhoea due to chaotic eating and/or the effect of malnutrition on central regulatory structures such as the pituitary gland and the hypothalamus, in combination with decreased secretion of leptin, a hormone secreted by fat cells
	Decreased serum testosterone levels and accompanying loss of libido are commonly found in underweight males
	Thyroid function (in particular, T3 levels) may be depressed in people with anorexia nervosa and is consistent with clinical findings such as dry skin and brittle hair, fatigue and cold intolerance
Musculoskeletal effects	Osteopenia, osteoporosis and associated risk of fractures are common in long-term/severe anorexia nervosa
	Irreversibly decreased bone mineral density is associated with prolonged malnutrition, low oestrogen levels and amenorrhoea for longer than 6 months, and decreased muscle mass
	A dual-energy x-ray absorptiometry (DEXA) scan is generally ordered to assess bone mineral density when a woman with an eating disorder has experienced amenorrhoea for longer than 6 consecutive months
	Linear growth retardation can occur in children when the onset of an eating disorder occurs before closure of the epiphyses
Dental and oral effects	Dental erosion and subsequent cavities can occur with recurrent self-induced vomiting
	Riboflavin deficiency may cause fissures of the lips, especially in the corners of the mouth, and iron and zinc deficiencies cause glossitis and loss of taste sensation
Skin/integumentary effects	Malnutrition leads to loss of subcutaneous fat
	Lanugo – a fine, downy hair that grows on the face and body – is often seen and is believed to be an adaptation to loss of body fat and it functions to help preserve body temperature
	Cool hands and feet with bluish discolouration (peripheral cyanosis), calluses on the dorsum of the dominant hand due to repeated self-induced vomiting, brittle nails and dry skin are commonly seen
Neurological effects	Structural and functional changes have been reported in anorexia nervosa; some reverse with refeeding and maintenance of normal weight, while others persist beyond recovery
	Structural changes in the brain including loss of brain volume, cerebral atrophy and ventricular dilation have been reported in anorexia nervosa
	Reduced total white matter volume and global grey matter volume are consistently reported; grey matter volume atrophy has been reported in a range of areas of the brain including the frontal lobe (responsible for executive functions) and temporal lobe (involved in memory, language, emotion and integration of sensory information), which are both critical for flexible eating, reward and motivation
Cognitive effects	Impaired concentration and memory
	Cognitive inflexibility, characterised by perseverative, rigid, circular and inflexible thinking with significant deficits in the ability to use "bigger picture thinking" or holistic thinking strategies
	A pervasive preoccupation with food, body shape and weight-related issues, one of the core diagnostic criteria of anorexia nervosa
	In children and adolescents, poor concentration can lead to difficulties keeping up with schoolwork, and special consideration should be requested from education departments for exams and assessments and amounts of classroom time may need to be tailored to the individual's stage of recovery
	The profound effects on cognitive function, and in particular executive functioning, impair the person's ability to engage in psychological interventions; this impairment underscores the need for nutritional rehabilitation beyond a minimum healthy weight such that the person is able to engage in, and make effective use of, psychological interventions and, ultimately, reach physical, emotional and psychological recovery

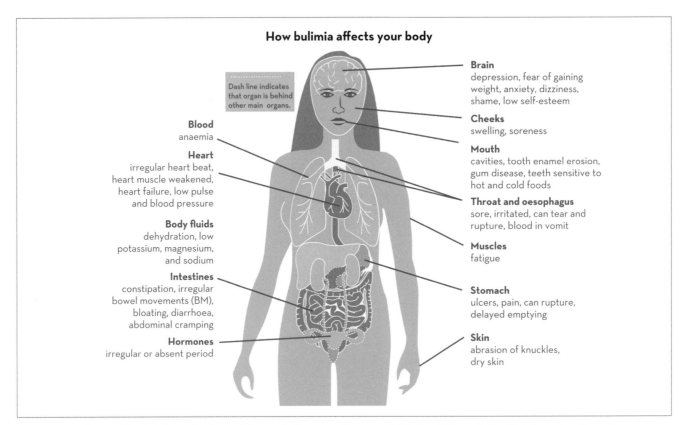

FIG. 15.1 Medical Complications of Anorexia Nervosa. (Courtesy Of National Women's Health Information Center.)

BOX 15.2   Calculation of Body Mass Index

To calculate body mass index (BMI), divide the person's weight (in kilograms) by their height (in metres squared). For example, an adult who is 163 cm (1.63 m) tall and weighs 55 kg would have a body mass index of 20.70, which is within the normal range. To calculate:

$$1.63 \times 1.63 = 2.656$$
$$55 \div 2.656 = \text{a BMI of } 20.70$$

An online calculator can be accessed at: www.heartfoundation.org.au/BMI-calculator

BMI percentile (rather than just BMI) is used to determine expected height, weight and growth trajectories in children and teenagers (see www.cdc.gov/healthyweight/assessing/bmi/).

Medical complications develop at higher weights in those who lose weight rapidly, and recording the history of highest and lowest weights helps to assess the rapidity and course of weight loss and estimate the healthy weight range for an individual. It is also useful to note any significant relationships between life events and weight loss because this gives insight into potential contributing factors that can be addressed in treatment. In adults, height and weight are used to calculate BMI (see Box 15.2), which helps determine the degree of starvation. Children and adolescents younger than 16 years of age are assessed on percentage of ideal body weight or gender-specific standardised growth charts.

Mental Health Assessment

A mental health assessment will confirm the specific diagnosis, identify co-occurring mental illness and exclude possible differential diagnoses such as major depression, which can present as loss of appetite and weight loss, without the body image disturbance and fear of weight gain seen in eating disorders. Other aspects of the person's mental health status that influence the clinical course and outcome will be assessed, including mood and anxiety, substance use, motivation to engage with treatment, personality traits and family support (Hay et al 2014).

A mental state assessment should be conducted and cognitive changes that may have occurred due to starvation should be identified – in particular, slowed thought processes, short-term memory impairments, changes in cognitive flexibility, difficulty with attention and poor concentration. Psychosocial factors that should be reviewed in the mental health assessment include the person's family history (including eating disorders and other mental illness in family members), attachment and developmental issues, any interpersonal problems or relationship issues that are particularly impacting on the person, as well as trauma or significant life events (Hay et al 2014).

Denial of illness and minimisation of symptoms are common in people with anorexia nervosa and can complicate the assessment process. Parents or carers of children and adolescents are generally interviewed as part of the assessment to help validate findings and provide a family history that is helpful in identifying risk and protective factors.

Body Image Assessment

It is useful to understand the person's perception of their weight and body shape, and to identify any significant events that might have triggered negative responses to body image, such as teasing, bullying or criticism about weight or body shape. Assessing the degree and nature of body image disturbance and fear of weight gain assists in diagnosis, in understanding the severity of the disorder and in guiding treatment. Assessment of body image has several components:

1. **Body image distortion:** a multidimensional phenomenon consisting of perceptual disturbance, cognitive-affective and behavioural

components in which people describe their body or parts of it as large or fat despite concrete evidence to the contrary (Smolak & Levine 2015).

2. **Body image dissatisfaction:** a disturbance of cognition and affect that leads to a negative evaluation of physical appearance. Body image dissatisfaction may be considered "normative" because it is highly prevalent in the general community, not just in people with eating disorders. However, this is not to say that it is harmless. Even in those without eating disorders, body image dissatisfaction is associated with significant quality of life impairment and impacts on mental health, psychosocial functioning and physical health (McLean & Paxton 2019).

3. **Body-related avoidance:** avoidance behaviours can be personal or situational and are driven by the fear and anxiety processes associated with eating disorders (Butler & Heimberg 2020). Avoiding confrontation with one's own body (e.g. by not looking in mirrors or avoiding taking baths where the body is clearly visible) is thought to be related to body image distortion. Body-related avoidance behaviour significantly contributes to body size overestimation. Situational avoidance involves avoiding environments or social situations that provoke anxiety about the body, like going to the beach.

4. **Body checking behaviours** should also be assessed over time: such as feeling bones (e.g. collar bones, ribs); checking weight many times a day; checking the body's silhouette in the mirror or other reflective surfaces; for example, lifting up the shirt to check the tummy after eating and at other times in the day; checking one specific body part regularly; for example, thigh gap or spread of thighs when sitting; pinching or grabbing at the body parts to measure "fat"; measuring wrists and thighs (for example) with fingers or hand; taking photos of the body or body parts or in specific clothes.

Simple questions that can provide insight into the person's experience of their body include:

- "People often *feel* fat, even when they are not. How do you feel about your body?"
- "Some people weigh themselves many times a day. Do you do this?"
- "When you look in the mirror, do you focus on one particular part of your body or look at your body as a whole?"
- "What weight do you think is the right weight for you? What weight would you like to be?"

Suicide Assessment

People with eating disorders are at risk of suicide and self-harm, with some disorders conferring more risk than others. In particular, anorexia nervosa is associated with high rates of death by suicide (Smith et al 2018), and about 20% of people with anorexia nervosa engage in non-suicidal self-harm (Bodell et al 2019; Davico et al 2019). Self-harm is also common in people with other eating disorders: they are more frequent in adolescents, those with comorbid mental health problems and those whose eating disorder includes binge and purge symptoms (Smith et al 2017). Asking the person about suicidal ideation and active self-harm is important. Questions such as, "Have things been so bad with the eating that you have wanted to harm yourself in any way?" will not trigger the person towards suicidal or self-harm behaviours. More likely, the person will be relieved to know that someone understands how severe the disorder has become and how bad they are feeling. Nurses need to respond to all expressions of suicidality in this very high-risk group. See Chapter 9 for further information on suicide assessment.

Nutritional and Exercise Assessment

A dietary history is used to identify specific deficiencies and should include information about the person's nutritional (food and fluid) intake, as well as any behaviours designed to reduce or control appetite (e.g. caffeine, smoking, vaping), alcohol use, use of supplements (e.g. vitamins, herbal preparations) and frequency of self-measurement of weight. Energy input and output are assessed, including the amount and types of food eaten and avoided, and the degree of any compensatory behaviours, including over-exercising, bingeing and purging used to control weight gain. Many people with eating disorders avoid whole food groups (typically meat protein, dairy products and/or carbohydrates). Because of the person's beliefs about uncontrollable weight gain, some foods can be considered "fear foods".

Excessive exercise is estimated to occur in 30–80% of people with eating disorders (Renz et al 2017), more commonly in those with anorexia than bulimia nervosa (Dittmer et al 2018). It can be used as a compensatory behaviour to avoid weight gain, or as a weight loss mechanism. Excessive exercise can be identified where a person experiences negative emotionality (e.g. intense guilt) when exercise is missed or postponed, or where hard exercise is focused primarily on influencing weight or shape (instead of on enjoyment). Asking people what the goal of their exercise is will help determine if it is excessive and associated with the eating disorder and help develop a graded approach to return to exercise during nutritional and psychological recovery (Dobinson et al 2019).

Assessing Disordered Eating Behaviours and Rituals

Disordered eating behaviours are driven by fear of weight gain. In inpatient settings, nurses can assess the extent of the person's struggle with food when observing mealtime behaviours. Box 15.3 provides examples of some frequently observed eating disorder behaviours.

People with eating disorders sometimes utilise excessive amounts of some condiments or foods that they perceive may be of benefit in terms of weight loss. Large quantities of fluid can help suppress hunger, and it is not unusual for a person with an eating disorder to drink copious amounts of fluid if they perceive this as helpful in avoiding weight

---

BOX 15.3 Examples of Eating Disorder Behaviours

- Refusing to eat
- Cutting out particular foods (e.g. cake, cheese, chocolate) or whole food groups (e.g. carbohydrates, fats, proteins)
- Cutting up food into tiny pieces and then eating the pieces individually, or by colour, or in groups of numbers (e.g. two peas followed by two pieces of carrot)
- Attempting to remove any oil and fats from food (e.g. pressing food into absorbent serviettes and scraping butter from sandwiches)
- Restricting foods, so as to eat the same thing every day
- Fear of touching food or having different food groups touch on the plate
- Eating painfully slowly and without enjoyment
- Constantly fidgeting at the table – this could be related to anxiety or to the physical hyperactivity that can be activated by starvation
- Obsessive kilojoule counting and/or measuring of all food quantities
- Leaving the table during or immediately after the meal to purge or throw away food hidden during the meal
- Excessive use of diet foods or diet products
- Excessive preoccupation with the preparation and serving of food to others, but not eating it
- Avoiding eating with others in a social context
- Binge eating (eating more than someone else would eat within a specific period of time)
- Using compensatory behaviours such as vomiting, laxatives or excessive exercise to "earn" food

gain. Drinking just prior to being weighed (water loading) may occur in an attempt to give the impression of weight gain.

People with bulimia nervosa commonly skip or restrict intake during breakfast and lunch, and then binge eat at night in response to the body's hunger signals. Bingeing can be spontaneous or planned, and it can occur in a ritualistic manner; for example, the binge may occur at the same time and place every day, or it may only happen on certain nights of the week when there is no one else around, or the binge may progress with foods in a particular order. It can cause great anxiety to a person if their planned binge episode is prevented or interrupted, or events outside their control impact on them carrying out the ritual. Some people with bulimia will, over time, choose food that is easily regurgitated or food that is economical if they cannot finance their binges (which can be very expensive). A binge episode is usually terminated in response to abdominal fullness, distension and pain, running out of food and/or social interruptions.

Self-induced vomiting usually follows a binge episode, and techniques used to induce vomiting include putting the fingers or another implement like a toothbrush down the throat, or regurgitation after eating may be spontaneous.

Signs that vomiting may be occurring in people with anorexia nervosa include weight loss or no weight gain despite apparent adherence to a prescribed nutritional program, leaving the dining table immediately after a meal to go to the shower or toilet, or the smell or presence of vomit in the toilet, sink or shower. Low potassium or raised amylase can indicate purging.

Diuretics cause fluid loss and laxatives work on the large bowel – after most of the nutrients from food have already been absorbed in the small intestine (Kiela et al 2016).

It is important for nurses to approach discussing disordered eating behaviours and rituals sensitively and in a curious and non-judgemental way. The person may be deeply embarrassed by some of their behaviours, which they may perceive as disgusting and shameful; they may also be protective of the behaviours as part of the disorder or worried that they will be forced to change what they are doing immediately, causing "massive" weight gain. Asking questions about disordered eating behaviours can be made less threatening by using statements that indicate that other people also experience similar issues; for example, "Many people who experience an eating disorder do things that they feel help them to control their eating or weight, like vomiting or using other ways of getting rid of food. Has this ever been something that you have tried?"

Family Assessment

When undertaking a family assessment, it is important to assess the quality of family relationships, the level of support available within the family, the way family members communicate with each other, family attitudes towards eating and appearance, and the effect the eating disorder has on family and social relationships. A family history of eating disorder, mental illness or substance use may have implications for treatment. During the assessment, be mindful that many families and carers are emotionally exhausted by their own struggle to help their family member to manage the eating disorder, and that feelings of guilt, failure, anger, blame and fear are common. Feeling blamed is harmful and could impair the desire, willingness and capacity to participate actively and constructively in the process of treatment and recovery, so it is important to convey a warm, encouraging, non-judgemental and collaborative approach (Dalle Grave et al 2019).

While family involvement is strongly encouraged, confidentiality issues must be considered for both adolescents and adults, and these should be clearly discussed during the assessment period. The decision to involve families, spouses and/or partners of adult patients should be made in consultation with the patient.

The importance of the nurse's role in supporting families through the treatment process cannot be overstated. At the family assessment stage, providing information around the eating disorder and helping family members to understand the challenges and opportunities that are associated with the disorder can be useful.

INTERVENTIONS

Recovery from an eating disorder is always possible and should be the goal. The illness duration can range from less than a year in children and adolescents who are identified and treated early, to a long-term illness, with remission and relapse of symptoms occurring.

Treating people with eating disorders occurs in primary care, outpatient and day-patient programs and inpatient care in medical, paediatric or mental health settings. Determining the most appropriate treatment service will depend on the person's age and their physical and mental health, as well as the availability of expert local healthcare providers. A multidisciplinary team approach is needed as medical and nursing care, nutritional rehabilitation, psychological therapy and, particularly in children and adolescents, family-based therapy are all integral parts of treatment. The priorities for treating someone with an eating disorder, regardless of the practice setting, include:

- engaging with the person using a non-judgemental, inclusive, empathic and curious approach
- engaging with the person's family and enlisting their support in appealing to the "healthy" part of their loved one
- conducting a thorough assessment, as outlined above
- providing information about normal eating (including healthy nutrition and eating patterns) and supporting the person to establish regular eating, which reverses the cognitive effects of starvation
- monitoring medical stability and responding to medical complications
- providing structured psychological treatment, including support and psychoeducation, building the therapeutic relationship in the first instance, and later, when the person is sufficiently stabilised from a medical/nutritional/cognitive perspective in terms of the effects of starvation, individualised therapy (Hay et al 2014).

People with binge eating disorder are generally treated in a community setting through primary care. The aims of treatment include normalising eating patterns, reducing or eliminating binge episodes, stabilising weight within a healthy weight range, effectively treating any underlying psychopathology and preventing relapse.

Hospitalisation

People with an eating disorder are generally admitted to hospital when they require nursing care. They may be at imminent risk of serious medical sequelae or complications of the illness, they may be experiencing significant mental health symptoms associated with the illness, or outpatient treatment may not be working (Hay et al 2014).

People with anorexia nervosa or OSFED are more likely to become medically compromised and require hospitalisation than those with bulimia nervosa. Indicators for admission include medical instability, significant risk of self-harm or suicide, psychiatric symptoms (severe low mood, suicidality, psychosis) and severe family dysfunction or abusive relationships. Compulsory treatment may be used where necessary. All nurses should be aware of the local policies related to admission for people with eating disorders.

Treating someone in a hospital setting includes:

- safely refeeding the person – avoiding refeeding syndrome (see p. 238) and underfeeding

- reducing and eliminating (where possible) binge eating and purging behaviours
- medical stabilisation and treating physical complications
- supporting and enhancing the person's ability to restore healthy eating patterns and engage fully with treatment
- helping the person to assess and address the psychological aspects of the illness (including their thoughts, feelings, attitudes, beliefs, motives, conflicts)
- treating a co-occurring mental health issue, including anxiety or mood disorder, and addressing issues such as impulse control, emotion regulation and other self-esteem and behavioural issues that contribute to maintaining the illness
- discharge treatment planning that involves psychological therapy, regular monitoring by a GP and dietetic support
- engaging with the person's family or significant others to enlist their support
- providing psychoeducation, family therapy or individual counselling where possible and appropriate.

In public hospitals in Australia and New Zealand, in-patient admission generally consists of either a short-term admission for medical stabilisation or a longer admission for weight restoration and normalisation of eating. Restoration of weight to a minimum healthy BMI is recommended because this facilitates the person's ability to cognitively engage in ongoing outpatient psychotherapy. A brief admission for 24–48 hours for medical stabilisation only is not conducive to recovery and may be likely to result in rapid readmission with the person in a worse physical or psychological condition. A longer admission to a medical or paediatric unit in a general hospital for medical stabilisation and initiation of nutritional rehabilitation does occur, in both Australia and Aotearoa New Zealand. Ideally, this should include meal support and psychological support from consultation–liaison mental health nurses, as well as dietetic and psychiatric support.

Specialist in-patient programs aim to provide a structured yet nurturing environment that includes behavioural modification strategies targeted towards weight gain and challenging and addressing abnormal eating behaviours. Behavioural programs are usually based on an "activity level system", through which the patient progresses as they are nutritionally rehabilitated. These programs usually incorporate strict bed rest while the person is physically compromised, ambulation on then off the ward, and then increasing the time out of hospital to practise normal eating behaviours in the home and community environment. When the person is medically stable, increasing levels of supervised activity/physiotherapy, including stretching and strengthening exercises, help the person to regain muscle and bone health. For children and adolescents, ongoing school education during hospitalisation is incorporated into the inpatient program whenever possible.

It is essential to have realistic expectations and clear goals for the admission. It is important for everyone to understand that hospitalisation is just one part of the recovery process: no one leaves hospital "cured" from an eating disorder – recovery can be a long process involving ongoing weight restoration, normalisation of eating patterns and talking therapy. Ideally, when someone leaves hospital, they will be medically stable, on the way towards weight restoration and, as a result, have a greater cognitive capacity to engage effectively with a psychotherapeutic intervention, be that individual or family-based (or both).

Like any mental illness, recovery from an eating disorder is a challenging personal journey that takes time and courage. It requires self-knowledge, self-compassion and the support of friends, family and health professionals. Return of symptoms and multiple admissions to hospital are not uncommon (see Personal perspectives: Consumer's story 15.4: Lizzie). To avoid the person feeling defeated and like a failure, or becoming helpless and institutionalised after

several admissions, it is particularly important that every hospitalisation involves collaboratively developing a plan for the admission that includes clearly defined goals. Nurses also need to be mindful of their approach and how important this is to how a person feels about the admission and what they can achieve. Nurses need to be aware of any attitudes, beliefs or values that they hold that may impact on (or impair) their clinical efficacy.

👤 PERSONAL PERSPECTIVES

Consumer's Story 15.4: Lizzie

Lizzie is a 24-year-old woman who has been admitted to the acute mental health unit for the third time in 18 months. She has a 10-year history of anorexia nervosa and, although she has spent most of the last 10 years out of hospital and has completed her university studies, she has not been able to achieve a healthy weight since she was first diagnosed. Lizzie has been having individual psychotherapy on and off for the past five years and is estranged from her family. Two years ago Lizzie was sexually assaulted one night on the way home from the library. She has been extremely unwell since that time.

Lizzie is admitted, having lost all the weight she put on at the last hospital admission. She is very medically compromised, tearful, defeated and psychologically unwell, requiring one-to-one nursing care. She struggles desperately with the eating disorder and, by her own admission, hides food, tampers with the nasogastric tube (even though she has agreed to have it inserted) and exercises in secret when she gets an opportunity. Lizzie says that she wants to recover and feels like nobody can help her.

Nursing Response Option 1
The staff roll their eyes when they hear that Lizzie is back. "What a surprise…She's never going to get better. I don't know why we bother! I don't know why she bothers! She's such a difficult patient. What a waste of a bed. Don't give her to me – I just don't get it."

Nursing Response Option 2
The nursing staff in the handover empathise with Lizzie's struggle. They know how difficult Lizzie is finding recovery; they are cognisant of the trauma she has experienced and the toll the illness is taking on her physical and mental health. They understand that recovery from anorexia nervosa can be a long-term process. They are keen to know why the discharge plan didn't adequately support Lizzie to maintain her weight after discharge. They are determined to support Lizzie to pick up the pieces and they hold hope for her recovery. "Lizzie must be feeling so defeated being back here so soon. I wonder what happened when she left here last time?"

❓ CRITICAL THINKING EXERCISE 15.3

Read Consumer's story 15.4: Lizzie.
1. What do you envisage might be the impact on Lizzie of the two different nursing responses outlined above?
2. How would you respond to staff who were expressing the type of response seen in option 1?

Nursing Care of People Who are Medically Unstable

Nurses working with people who have severe and complex eating disorders and who are medically unstable require both medical and mental health knowledge and skills. Medical resuscitation and stabilisation of any medical instability always take priority if the patient has been admitted to hospital with life-threatening complications. If the patient is bradycardic on admission, continuous cardiac monitoring and daily 12-lead ECGs are recommended. Four-hourly vital sign measures, including heart rate, temperature and blood pressure are recorded until normal readings are sustained for at least a minimum of 72 hours. Overnight vital sign measurements and blood sugar levels, taken when the body is most at rest, provide invaluable insight into the body's ability to maintain homeostasis. Nasogastric feeds, administered either continuously or overnight, are vital in reversing medical instability when patients are unable to consume enough kilojoules orally.

Examples of nursing responsibilities in this situation include:

- monitoring the patient's physical safety
- documenting vital signs and acting as per local protocols when vital signs indicate medical instability – every service treating people with eating disorders needs to have clear guidelines for managing medical instability
- empathising with any distress the person expresses and validating their experience and efforts
- initiating and encouraging the prescribed refeeding process
- inserting and ensuring the patency of any nasogastric tubes and acting to prevent the patient from tampering with feeds (remember, they will likely be very fearful of rapid weight gain)
- documenting nutritional intake
- monitoring for clinical signs of refeeding syndrome
- observing for and managing challenging behaviours such as covert exercise, weight manipulation, vomiting, hiding food in an empathic and supportive way (using externalisation can help, e.g. "I notice that the eating disorder is trying to get you to hide food. That must be very stressful for you when you know that you need to eat to recover.")
- talking with the person about their emotional response to admission and providing therapeutic support and psychoeducation to help contain the anxiety and distress of both the patient and their family
- administering prescribed medication.

Psychological and emotional care of the person requires that nurses:

- understand that eating disorder behaviours are driven by fear of weight gain and overwhelming anxiety
- work with the person and their family to develop skills to contain anxiety and distress
- facilitate and encourage motivation to change, rather than imposing or enforcing behavioural change – getting to know the person, their plans for the future, hopes, dreams and desires will help them (and you) to see the bigger picture
- provide supportive meal supervision designed to achieve nutritional rehabilitation, normalised eating behaviours and reduction in compensatory behaviours
- consistently adhere to the plan of care
- ensuring all limits set have a clear and transparent purpose and are discussed with the person at the outset
- attend multidisciplinary case reviews to contribute to treatment planning
- engage in clinical supervision or other professional support to help with managing the interpersonal conflicts and intense emotions that may arise in the nurse.

Refeeding Syndrome

Refeeding syndrome is a rare but potentially fatal complication that can occur in the first 1–2 weeks of commencing refeeding for people who are severely malnourished. It is important for nurses in all clinical settings to be vigilant for the signs and symptoms of refeeding syndrome, which is a medical emergency that can be variable, unpredictable and may occur without warning.

Refeeding syndrome involves disturbances in insulin and serum electrolytes, specifically changes in phosphate, potassium and magnesium, vitamin deficiencies and sodium and fluid retention. If serum phosphate levels drop significantly, especially during the first week of refeeding, this can cause cardiac, neurological and haematological complications and sudden death. Electrolyte abnormalities should be monitored daily until they have stabilised within normal ranges.

People with eating disorders who are particularly at risk of refeeding syndrome include those who have:

- severe malnutrition, particularly where it has been prolonged
- rapid weight loss greater than 1 kg per week over several weeks
- a very low BMI (less than 14, although the syndrome has been reported in patients with a normal BMI)
- abnormal electrolytes prior to refeeding
- a history of severe dietary restraint or not eating for a week or more
- vomiting, laxative misuse or bingeing
- concurrent medical conditions such as diabetes, infection or major organ failure (Friedli et al 2018).

During the first 1–2 weeks of refeeding, nurses monitor for clinical signs of refeeding syndrome (confusion, delirium or other mental status changes, seizures, cardiac arrhythmias, fluid retention and oedema) and ensure prophylactic phosphate and vitamin and mineral supplements are administered. If signs of refeeding syndrome become evident, urgent medical consultation should be sought to normalise electrolyte levels and prevent cardiovascular and other organ system failure and death. Prophylactic phosphate supplements, carefully prescribed rates of refeeding and daily monitoring of electrolyte levels during the first 1–2 weeks of starting refeeding minimise the risk of a patient developing refeeding syndrome. Ideally, the patient will ultimately obtain all their vitamin and mineral requirements through food, but initially vitamin and mineral supplements are routinely prescribed.

Therapeutic Relationships

Effective nursing management requires developing a therapeutic alliance *with* the person and *against* the eating disorder. Without this, it is likely that the person will see the eating disorder as their ally or their only friend and feel that their parents, friends and health practitioners are all against them. The therapeutic alliance is enhanced by validating the person's experience ("recovery is really hard"), empathetic discussion, consistent positive regard, reassurance, motivational enhancement and supporting the person to develop new insights and accept change. Perspectives in practice: Nurse's story 15.1 describes the experience of providing nursing care for adolescents with anorexia nervosa.

Positive regard for the person can be displayed by "externalising" the eating-disordered thoughts and behaviours as separate from the person; for example, "Is *the anorexia* making it really difficult for you to eat today?", "I know it's hard for you to eat when the anorexia is telling you not to. How can I best help you to fight *those eating disorder* thoughts?" Putting this distance between the illness and the person is a very important first step towards helping the person see that the things they value (e.g. health, friendships, doing well at school, having a great career) are incompatible with the long-term maintenance of an eating disorder. It is also very useful for families to learn to identify and externalise the person's disordered eating thoughts and behaviours as part of their illness rather than as wilful behaviour on the part of their child or family member.

Unless a particular situation is life-threatening, confrontation and invasion of privacy (e.g. observing a patient in the bathroom) are generally unnecessary and are destructive for both developing therapeutic

PERSPECTIVES IN PRACTICE

Nurse's story 15.1: Gail

When I first started working with adolescents who have anorexia nervosa, I was scared that I would say or do the wrong thing. As a paediatric nurse, I didn't understand the complexity of the illness or why it was so difficult for them to eat normally and maintain a healthy weight.

Previously, I had always tried to meet my patients' needs and advocate for them, but I could see that if I supported the disordered eating behaviours, I would collude with the illness and the person would only lose more weight. When I first tried to talk to them about the behaviours, they would lie to me or get angry, and I initially found this hard to understand and quite frustrating.

Luckily, I work with a great team and was able to learn "on the job". My senior nursing colleagues spent a lot of time teaching me about the illness and about how the behaviours I was seeing were not directed at me personally, but rather reflected the strength of the anorexic thoughts and the person's overwhelming fear of change.

I realised that I wasn't responsible for making the person gain weight. Rather, I tried to understand what it was like for them to experience the illness, work collaboratively with them to see the illness for what it is, and help them to increase their motivation and capacity to recover. I soon found that by taking a different approach, I could encourage patients to better manage their fears and start taking responsibility for making small but positive changes in their behaviours.

Now that I understand just how difficult it is for people who experience eating disorders to change, I am better able to support them in managing their anxiety, I am better at working collaboratively and I am able to gain the person's trust so they communicate honestly with me.

Along with a greater understanding of people who experience eating disorders came a sense of confidence in my role as a nurse and a feeling of satisfaction with my job, rather than frustration. I enjoy my work with these young people now and feel that I am making a positive difference in their lives.

relationships and for promoting the person's self-responsibility and motivation for change. Even if these behaviours are necessary, it is possible to address them in a collaborative (rather than demoralising) way and to provide choice wherever possible. For example, "I know that you find it difficult to resist the eating disorder when it demands you exercise in the shower. I'd like to help you regain control of that. Let's look at the options …"

Food avoidance and the use of compensatory behaviours will be reflected to a great extent in the person's pattern of weight gain (and in their blood and urine test results). Generally, if they fail to gain the expected amount of weight each week in hospital, they have either restricted their oral intake or participated in compensatory behaviours. Invading privacy or engaging in confrontation will result in an angry, defensive response rather than encouraging positive growth and motivation for change. The following statement is an example of a comment that would lead to an angry eating disordered response: "It's pretty clear by your weight loss that you've been cheating on the program. You're never going to get out of here if that's your approach." Taking control of eating and ceasing compensatory behaviours are ultimately the responsibility of the patient. The goal for nurses is therefore not to enforce change, but to encourage the person's motivation to change by exploring and challenging their individual perspective on, and experience of, their disordered eating behaviours. For example: "I see that your weight has gone down

today and I'm wondering if we can talk about that? Usually, weight loss is either from not eating enough, or from exercising or vomiting. I'm wondering if you have felt so bad in the last few days, or so pushed around by the eating disorder, that you've been doing any of those things?"

Younger children, however, may need a more directive approach than adolescents and adults, especially when they have not yet developed abstract thought processes. For example: "We noticed that your weight has gone down and it is important for us to sort that out … because to get better, you need to get back to eating normally and into a healthy weight range. I've noticed you haven't been finishing all your meals, even though we've talked about you needing to do that to get better. How can we help you to make sure that you finish all your meals?"

Nutritional Rehabilitation, Normalising Eating Patterns and Meal Support

The cornerstones of nutritional treatment are education, meal planning, establishing regular eating patterns and discouraging dieting. Everyone with an eating disorder will be fearful of weight gain, particularly in the early stages of treatment, where regular eating is initiated, and often there is heightened distress as a person approaches weight milestones. Psychoeducation about the effects of extreme dietary restriction/starvation, bingeing, purging, disordered eating and the need to reverse these is important.

Depending on the treatment setting and the type of eating disorder, a meal plan designed to achieve a prescribed weekly weight gain or to normalise eating behaviours should be developed. The meal plan will be individualised and takes into consideration the person's tastes, their cultural background, their physical needs and their clinical picture. It will also identify portion sizes and gradually introduce foods that have been avoided. The aim is that the diet will include all the food groups and that fear foods (i.e. foods that have been withdrawn or avoided as part of the illness) have been habituated, with nursing staff providing reassurance and encouragement and validating how difficult the recovery process can feel.

For those who are struggling with their intake, nutritional supplementation may be required. These are given either as a drink or via a nasogastric tube, which is usually considered when the person is medically compromised and is not able to eat enough food to reverse the medical complications and achieve adequate nutritional rehabilitation. When initiated, nasogastric feeds should initially be given slowly enough so as not to cause refeeding syndrome, but not so slowly as to underfeed the person (Mosuka et al 2023). Continuous feeding over a 24-hour period helps to avoid low blood sugar levels from the effects of delayed insulin phase and metabolic changes and the supplemental feed should restrict the percentage of daily energy provided by carbohydrate to help mitigate against the risk of refeeding syndrome (Haas et al 2020).

People's reactions to nasogastric feeds are varied. Some express relief that they do not have to eat what they perceive to be enormous amounts of food required for weight gain and view positively the fact that the initial responsibility for weight gain has been taken away from them. Others struggle with the invasive nature of the tube and the lack of control they feel they have over their nutritional intake. "Nasogastric feeding is less likely to be perceived negatively if the procedure has been fully explained, demystified and medicalised" (Robinson & Nicholls 2015, p. 22). Regardless of how they are delivered, nutritional supplements are given for the shortest possible time – ultimately, the person needs to relearn how to eat food normally – and so the goal is always transition to an oral meal plan as soon as possible. Transition to a full oral diet including three meals and three snacks needs to occur before discharge.

Supporting the person to cope with the distressing thoughts that accompany nutritional rehabilitation is an important role for nurses. This will include helping the person to develop a range of strategies that help – for example, distraction, cognitive challenging and mindfulness. In inpatient settings, nurses can help by providing therapeutic meal support, having clear boundaries around expected mealtime behaviours and acting as a role model for healthy eating behaviour. The goals of meal support are to help the person to normalise their eating behaviours, begin the process of weight gain or at least ensure weight maintenance, reintroduce the concept of eating as a pleasant social experience, assist the person to address and decrease food rituals, and increase their ability and confidence in making healthy food choices and eating a "normal" amount.

The 3-Hour Rule

People who have eating disorders need to understand that if they undereat or restrict their food intake, have lost an understanding of hunger and satiety, or engage in non-hungry eating, then working to establish a regular eating pattern and introducing the 3-hour rule will be important. The 3-hour rule simply means eating something every 3 hours and eliminating dieting. Since hunger is the primary trigger for binge eating, maintaining consistent intake is the first step in ceasing binge/purge behaviours. Establishing a pattern of eating something every 3 hours often creates anxiety and fear of rapid, uncontrolled weight gain in many patients. Nurses need to reassure the person that research and clinical experience demonstrate that this does not occur and that, in fact, the body's metabolism increases with regular eating.

Monitoring Intake and Weight Gain

Monitoring dietary intake is an important tool that helps identify food/eating patterns and gives the person and the team an overview of what and how much the person is really eating. In hospital, monitoring will generally be done by the nursing staff, but the person may also do this themselves, provided the record is accurate.

Monitoring the person's thoughts and feelings in response to their dietary intake can also be a helpful tool for nurses and other health professionals to review with them. These forms (or online tools) ask the person to identify their thoughts and feelings in association with their eating or restricting behaviours, exposing how the person responds to emotions like guilt, anger and sadness through their intake, and identifying how the eating disorder bullies them into behaving in a certain way. The Recovery Record App (for example) enables the primary therapist to prescribe evidence-based strategies to help the person manage these responses, and to observe intake in real time.

As weight restoration (or partial weight restoration) is the primary goal of treatment for someone who has anorexia nervosa or who is underweight, and demonstrating that regular eating does not necessarily lead to weight gain as a person with bulimia nervosa or binge eating disorder may fear, weight needs to be regularly and accurately monitored. Patients are often highly anxious about being weighed and so weighing should be done in a sensitive and straightforward manner. Describing a person's weight as "the number on the scale" rather than "your weight" is a CBT technique designed to help the person separate that number from how they feel about themselves – particularly because every scale is different and certain behaviours, such as drinking water, can change the number within a matter of minutes. Because symptoms of starvation include perseveration and rigid thinking, it is not helpful to have an emphasis on a "goal weight" that a patient will likely become fixated on. Instead, advise the person that reviewing medical parameters, such as improved cardiovascular status and blood results and ultimately the return of ovulation and a normal menstrual cycle, as well as psychological recovery in terms of the person's mood and thinking, will inform ongoing nutritional rehabilitation.

Most treatment facilities aim for an average weekly weight gain of 1–2 kg in inpatient settings and 0.5 kg in outpatient settings. The frequency of weighing, or monitoring of expected weight gain, varies between treatment settings, but twice a week is enough to monitor and reward progress. In an outpatient setting, any team member can undertake monitoring of weight gain, but in the hospital environment it is generally a nurse's responsibility. Patients are usually weighed early in the morning wearing only a hospital gown and before consuming any food or drink. At times, patients who are struggling use techniques to falsely increase their weight, including drinking large amounts of water just prior to weighing and hiding weights on their body. Therefore, patients are usually asked to empty their bladder just before weighing and urinalysis will identify if water loading (if the specific gravity is low (< 1.01)) or purging (if a high pH (8–9) is recorded) has occurred. A sudden increase in weight, or an increase that is inconsistent with the observed eating behaviour, will alert you that weight manipulation may be occurring, and discussion should ensue about possible behaviours that may account for this. A random (unexpected/spot) weight measurement can be undertaken outside the normal weighing time if there is concern that the person is manipulating their real weight.

It is important to remember that if someone is attempting to manipulate their weight, they are doing so out of fear and distress and because they are really struggling with the ambivalence that the eating disorder generates. They will probably be feeling very anxious that their behaviours will be detected, but at the same time will be relieved when the secret is out. Nurses need to respond in a sensitive, respectful and empathic way when discussing these issues with the person, to avoid them feeling humiliated, judged and hopeless. For example: "I can see by this spot weigh that your weight is actually quite a lot lower than what it was yesterday. I'm guessing that you have felt really worried about weigh days because you've been struggling so much with the eating … Is that right? Can you tell me what you've been doing to keep your weight measurements from going up?"

Psychotherapeutic Techniques and Treatments

General principles of treatment for people with eating disorders, regardless of the type include (Hay et al 2014):

- person-centred, informed decision-making
- involving a person's family and significant others
- recovery-oriented and trauma-informed practice
- least restrictive treatment context
- multidisciplinary approach
- stepped and seamless care
- a dimensional and culturally informed approach to diagnosis and treatment.

Examples of some of the psychotherapeutic techniques and treatments currently used for people with an eating disorder are discussed below. In clinical practice, a combination of these therapies, or other psychotherapies not described below (e.g. psychodynamic psychotherapy, dialectical behaviour therapy and narrative therapy), may be used. When considering therapy for an eating disorder, the person's medical status, age, family supports, cognitive capacity, duration of illness and the accessibility of services are all considered. Perspectives in practice: Nurses story 15.2 describes the role of a primary care mental health nurse.

PERSPECTIVES IN PRACTICE

Nurse's Story 15.2: Peta

I am a credentialled mental health nurse and family therapist who specialises in working with people who have eating disorders – mostly anorexia nervosa, but also those with OSFED or people with severe bulimia nervosa complicated by another physical or mental health condition. I have undertaken relevant postgraduate training in family therapy and have done a lot of professional development (cognitive behaviour for eating disorders, acceptance and commitment therapy, dialectical behaviour therapy, family-based therapy for eating disorders) and studied some manualised eating disorder treatments – there is always more to learn. This is definitely an area of practice that really challenges the mental health nurse to use the breadth of mental health nursing knowledge and skills. Our background in biological science means we also have the knowledge and skills to assess and respond to a person's physical health status and monitor the impact of medications.

Cognitive Behaviour Therapy

Enhanced CBT for eating disorders (CBT-E) is structured to focus on the processes associated with maintenance of the eating disorder. CBT-E uses a variety of cognitive and behavioural interventions, but uses strategic behaviour change to modify thinking, rather than the direct cognitive restructuring usual in other forms of CBT. CBT-E is delivered in three stages, typically over 40 sessions. The first stage involves engaging the person in treatment and change, jointly creating the formulation, establishing self-monitoring practices, weekly weighing, establishing regular patterns of eating and providing education to the person and significant others. Stage 2 is brief and incorporates a review of stage 1 and planning for stage 3. The final stage is the main body of treatment, where the over-evaluation of shape and weight, dieting rules, interpersonal problems, perfectionism and self-esteem issues are addressed. The focus here is on eliminating dieting, problem-solving and modifying thoughts that link body and weight with self-esteem, as well as relapse prevention and developing skills to manage stressors. CBT-E is an effective treatment for many outpatients with eating disorder (Fairburn et al 2015) and can be delivered through supported self-help eTherapy, with good outcomes for people with bulimia nervosa (Barakat et al 2021) and binge eating disorder (Rom et al 2022).

There is only tentative evidence that usual CBT is effective for relapse reduction after weight restoration in anorexia nervosa, and it is not an appropriate treatment for those with anorexia nervosa who are not weight restored. However, evidence for using CBT with people who have bulimia nervosa is strong (when used to address the cycle of dieting, binge eating and purging or other extreme weight-control behaviours). CBT has also been developmentally adapted for adolescents with binge eating disorder and bulimia nervosa.

Preliminary studies on treatment for people with ARFID indicate that CBT for ARFID (CBT-AR) may be promising for adults (Thomas et al 2020a) and for children and adolescents (Thomas 2020b).

Family-Based Treatment

There is moderate research to support family therapy as an effective treatment for younger children and adolescents who live with their families and who have experienced anorexia nervosa for less than 3 years. The focus of family therapy approaches varies, but the general theme is that the family are involved in treatment and support weight restoration and recovery. Models of family intervention have been developed for adults and couples, but these have not been evaluated.

Family therapy is the treatment of choice for most children and adolescents with anorexia nervosa, but is not demonstrably effective for those over 18 years of age (Hay et al 2014).

Families play an important role in the assessment and treatment of young people with eating disorders. Unless contraindicated, families are best placed to support their loved one to manage the burden of the illness. Families need to understand the illness and be involved and engaged as an important resource by the treating team. To facilitate change, families need to develop effective coping strategies for managing the behaviours that support and maintain the illness and adopt interactional patterns that accommodate the young person's normal growth and development.

Sometimes families can inadvertently reinforce the eating disorder (particularly when the person's distress around eating is so intense) by giving into, accommodating or colluding with the eating disordered behaviours (e.g. making family meals consisting only of "safe" foods). If families of children and adolescents are not engaged with, and committed to, the treatment program, or are unable to work together to provide clear, firm boundaries regarding food and disordered eating behaviours, relapse is more likely.

One particular model of family therapy designed for children and adolescents with anorexia nervosa, Maudsley family-based therapy, has proven to be effective for some families (Lock & Le Grange 2012). This therapy is delivered in three phrases. The first phase involves the parents taking control of their child's eating until 90% of ideal body weight is achieved; the second phase involves the family gradually giving control over eating back to the young person while continuing to supervise them until they reach their healthy weight range; and the final phase involves supporting the young person to address any unresolved individual concerns, as well as assisting the family to return to the normal family life cycle by addressing any unresolved family or marital interactional problems.

Family-based therapy has also been adapted for use with families who have a young person with bulimia nervosa, prodromal presentations of anorexia nervosa, paediatric obesity and ARFID. The emphasis shifts from weight restoration to normalisation of eating, eating new/fear foods, regular family meals and supporting parents to model healthy eating (Rienecke 2017).

MANTRA (Maudsley Model of Anorexia Nervosa Treatment for Adults)

MANTRA is a cognitive-interpersonal manual-based outpatient treatment for adults with anorexia nervosa developed by the Maudsley Hospital team in London designed to address the underlying worries the person experiences, including interpersonal difficulties, fear of rejection, negative perception of self and the experience of negative emotions (Schmidt et al 2014). It uses a motivational interviewing approach that is highly strategic in looking out for and creating "teachable moments" that will support the person to shift the balance towards change and recovery.

Interpersonal Therapy

Interpersonal therapy for people with eating disorders is based on the premise that interpersonal difficulties result in the development of disturbances in self-esteem and mood, which then give rise to eating disorder symptoms. Interpersonal therapy is a structured, time-limited psychotherapy that focuses on resolving interpersonal difficulties and encouraging the development of affirming relationships, thereby providing a viable alternative to the eating disorder in attaining positive self-esteem, affect and problem-solving skills. The symptoms of the eating disorder are not themselves the focus of therapy. Interpersonal therapy appears to have long-term efficacy for those with bulimia nervosa and people with binge eating disorder (Reas & Grilo 2014).

Motivational interventions

Motivation is a key issue for people with eating disorders. In particular, a person's motivation to change at the outset of treatment is thought to be helpful in predicting outcome (Sansfacon et al 2020). Motivational interventions typically target denial, ambivalence and resistance to change. They are commonly used with people who have eating disorders – either before they participate in other psychological interventions or as a key element of other therapies such as MANTRA. Understanding motivation and where a person is at in terms of their motivation is important because delivering interventions or elements of treatment that are targeted towards a person in the action stage are likely to be ineffective if the person is pre-contemplative and denying that there is a problem. This can create difficulties where action is required to ensure a person's medical safety, but the person does not believe there is a problem. For this reason, collaboration with the person and targeting issues that they see as important is essential, as is taking a respectful approach. Acknowledge that changing, when you're not that convinced there is a problem, is very challenging, and support the person using motivational interviewing techniques to begin to develop an understanding of the impact of the illness.

Psychoeducation

Psychoeducation involves providing information about the eating disorder to enable the person with an eating disorder (and their families/carers) to better understand the illness and its effects and to develop more effective coping strategies to overcome difficulties they are experiencing. Psychoeducation is an essential part of treatment for all types of eating disorder. It is much easier for people with eating disorders to change the eating disorder behaviours when they understand the interplay between the behaviours and the illness and their dual role in keeping them trapped.

Some examples of psychoeducation topics are:

- the short- and long-term medical and psychological effects of starvation
- the biological factors that regulate weight – this includes discussion of how dieting largely works against the body's weight regulators, causing stress to both physical and psychological functioning
- regular eating and myths about dieting
- the physical side effects of vomiting and laxative and diuretic abuse
- the binge–purge cycle and how it affects self-esteem – nurses can help the person to identify and manage cues for bingeing and purging behaviours, learn distraction or relaxation techniques to decrease the urge to vomit immediately after meals and understand the benefits of eating regularly throughout the day, thereby reducing the physical and psychological drive to binge in the evenings
- the importance of establishing a healthy pattern of exercise based on enjoyment and focusing on muscle strengthening and bone health, rather than focusing on burning up kilojoules for weight control or controlling body shape
- the effects of anxiety on the body and techniques for coping (e.g. mindfulness practices, cognitive challenging).
- The Western Australian Centre for Clinical Interventions (see Useful websites at the end of the chapter) provides a range of psychoeducation materials specific to eating disorders for use in clinical practice.

Psychoeducation on an individual or a group basis can also be extremely useful for engaging parents and family members in the treatment program, increasing their understanding of the complexity of the illness, developing realistic expectations and facilitating useful strategies to better manage the person's disordered eating behaviours. The more informed families are, the less anxious or blaming they become and the more open they will be to making positive changes that can support and improve the person's health outcome.

There are many web-based resources available for families, as well as state-based eating disorders associations, that provide parent and carer support programs throughout Australia and New Zealand (see Useful websites).

Specialist Supportive Clinical Management

Specialist supportive clinical management (McIntosh et al 2005) combines features of supportive psychotherapy and clinical management to establish a "supportive therapeutic context". The person is encouraged to explore issues that impact on and promote change, and they are encouraged to actively make changes to core symptoms by increasing their weight, eating less restrictively and decreasing the use of inappropriate compensatory behaviours. The process focuses on facilitating normal eating, weight restoration and psychoeducation about anorexia nervosa, as well as addressing other life issues that may be identified by the person as relevant to the eating disorder. Supportive psychotherapy is a generalised therapy that has been used to treat people with eating disorders and can be implemented in primary care and general mental health settings. Techniques such as active listening, verbal and nonverbal attending, using open-ended questioning, encouraging reflection, providing reassurance and praise are key. Advice-giving and therapist self-disclosure are also used. Specific components of supportive therapy include reassurance, explanation, guidance, suggestion, encouragement and permission for catharsis or sharing of pent-up feelings, such as fear, grief, sorrow, concern and frustration.

Self-help programs

Evidence-based self-help programs are now recommended as a possible first-stage intervention for bulimia nervosa and binge eating disorder in people aged 18 years or older (National Institute for Health and Care Excellence 2017). Self-help programs that include direct support from health professionals are termed "guided" or "supported" self-help. They have been found to have better adherence and treatment outcomes than "pure" self-help (Beinther et al 2014); however, Australian evidence has demonstrated that eTherapy for people with bulimia nervosa contributes to significant post-treatment reductions in eating disorder symptoms for supported and purely self-help (Barakat et al 2021). There is less evidence available on the effectiveness of self-help and supported self-help for underweight people with anorexia nervosa, and for adolescents and younger people.

Pharmacotherapy

Pharmacotherapy is not used as a first-line treatment for people with anorexia nervosa. Evidence for pharmacological treatment is weak, but low-dose antipsychotics (e.g. olanzapine) may be helpful for some people to reduce anxiety, rumination and obsessive thinking (Hay et al 2014), and have shown promise in diminishing thought intrusions and distorted body image. Selective serotonin reuptake inhibitors are not indicated in the acute or maintenance stages of anorexia nervosa for young people (Hay et al 2014). The potential role of anxiolytics and antidepressants is best assessed after nutritional rehabilitation in low-weight patients with anorexia nervosa, as food and nutritional rehabilitation can be the best "medicine" for improving mood.

Pharmacotherapy has been shown to be a helpful adjunctive treatment (along with CBT-E) for people with bulimia nervosa and binge eating disorder (Hay et al 2014). If psychological therapy is not readily available, pharmacological treatment for people with bulimia/binge eating disorder is supported by evidence. However, the first-line treatment for both disorders is therapist-led CBT or CBT-E (Hay et al 2014).

A FINAL WORD ON THE NURSE'S ROLE

Nurses in all clinical settings are ideally placed to make a significant impact on the health and mental health of the many children from Australia and Aotearoa New Zealand, young people, women and men who experience eating disorders. Nurses have the skills required to work holistically and collaboratively, to empathise, to validate and to support people with eating disorders through this complex and challenging life experience. Recovery is always possible, at any stage of the illness. What is required is that, as nurses, we are kind and hold hope for the person when they are not able to hold hope for themselves; we understand the difficulties the person is experiencing in their struggle to recover; we do not buy into the stereotypes about eating disorders which result in stigmatising and discriminatory attitudes towards people who experience them; we support families who are frightened and bewildered and questioning themselves; and, we critically reflect on our own practice to ensure we are offering high-quality evidence-informed practice that supports the person's recovery and optimises their outcome.

Working with people who have eating disorders is a rewarding professional experience. These are complex illnesses that stretch our knowledge and skills and require us to reflect on the impact of our values and attitudes on our nursing practice. Nurses who choose to specialise in working with people who have eating disorders undertake additional training and professional development and engage in regular clinical supervision (e.g. credentialled mental health nurses, mental health nurse practitioners working in primary care or private practice may provide psychological therapy, family-based therapy, CBT-E or other specialised treatment).

The following is an extract from a letter written by a recovering young adult:

It's now been six years since I was first diagnosed with anorexia nervosa. I know I still have many years ahead to learn about life and to learn from my mistakes and experiences, but this recovery process has taught me so much about confronting myself, challenging myself and training my mind to think positively and it does work. Thank you for firmly confronting my disorder when I couldn't and for hanging in with me, keeping me alive and supporting me long enough for me to finally get to the point where I feel strong enough as a person to not need or want this illness any more.

(Private communication)

Professional aspects of working with a person who has an eating disorder in an inpatient setting include:
- maintaining clear professional boundaries, which includes not being over-involved, or dismissive and under-involved
- developing and regularly reviewing an evidence-based local behavioural program for patients that is achievable for nurses within their specific work environment
- having realistic expectations regarding what can be achieved during a hospital admission given the complexity and chronicity of the illness; this includes the awareness that relapse and re-admission are common and are not a sign of failure, but an opportunity to review the relapse plan
- being aware of one's own personal emotional wellbeing and participating in adequate clinical supervision and support
- enjoying the challenge of caring for individuals with an eating disorder and assisting them to understand and care for themselves in more healthy ways
- validating the person's experience and maintaining positive regard for the person in the face of their ambivalence and resistance to treatment.

CHAPTER SUMMARY

This chapter has provided an introduction to the eating disorders encountered in nursing practice and has included a focus on psychological factors, medical complications, assessment and treatment. Eating disorders are complex, multidimensional illnesses that encompass a range of psychological and physical health issues. The severity of impact of these disorders in terms of quality of life, morbidity and mortality is high and these are common illnesses in children, adolescents and young people. Many sufferers encounter difficulties in accessing appropriate services and this difficulty, coupled with the shame, denial and ambivalence to treatment commonly associated with these disorders, on top of stereotyping, stigma and discrimination associated with eating disorders in particular and mental illness in general, can result in delayed treatment. This is of particular concern because of the known effectiveness of early treatment in preventing or reducing progression to severe, complex and enduring illness.

So, what of the future? In modern western societies there seems to be an ever-increasing concern with body image, weight, shape and appearance for both women and men. For some, this leads to severe distress, disruption and diagnosis with one of a growing list of disorders including the eating disorders. A greater emphasis on establishing evidence-based prevention strategies is required – with targets including the very young, all genders and people from all cultural groups.

A multidisciplinary approach to treatment of eating disorders is crucial and nurses committed to caring for people with an eating disorder have much to contribute in inpatient, outpatient, community and primary care treatment settings. Patients are admitted to hospital when they require 24-hour nursing care – this might be in mental health, paediatric, cardiac care, emergency department or general medical settings. In order that optimal care is provided, it is essential that all nurses understand and develop skills to manage the biopsychosocial complexity of these very challenging illnesses, relative to their scope of practice and clinical setting.

More research is needed to better understand the relative importance of biological and psychosocial risk and protective factors, and to continue developing more effective, individualised treatments, both for early intervention and for those with more complex needs. One needs only to look at the outcome data to see that new therapeutic treatments need to be developed to enhance outcomes and decrease the high levels of associated morbidity and mortality. Furthermore, more emphasis needs to be placed on early and more aggressive nutritional rehabilitation to enable those with an eating disorder to cognitively engage in therapeutic psychological interventions. Nurses are in a key position to undertake research designed to better understand eating disorders and promote evidence-based effective nursing strategies that will enhance care and outcomes for people experiencing an eating disorder.

REVIEW QUESTIONS

1. In a group, discuss the influence of the media, marketing, the advertising industry and popular role models on the development of eating disorders among young women and men.
2. Discuss the reasons why body image dissatisfaction tends to increase during adolescence.
3. Do a search on the internet for Ancel Keys' 1950s Starvation Study. Identify the physical, psychological, social and emotional aspects that relate to starvation, which people with eating disorders commonly experience. Some people think that eating disorders are self-inflicted and purposeful, or that they are a type of personality disorder. Having reviewed this study, what aspects of it challenge these kinds of assumptions?
4. Working with the person to find their strengths is an important part of recovery from an eating disorder. Make a table with two columns. In one column, list the self-defeating thoughts that a person with an eating disorder may experience. In the other column, suggest alternatives that are self-supporting behaviours and thoughts.
5. "Fat talk" has been said to be a common motif of female culture, particularly with young women in developed countries. Girls and women are encouraged to aspire to the thin "ideal" body type and often say self-disparaging things or communicate with others around this theme. Consider the following commonly heard statement: "I feel so fat today". This expression is made more commonly by young women than men and is repeated over and over. But, in fact, the person is actually feeling another emotion, such as worry, guilt, anger or frustration. The expression of emotion is covered up by referring instead to an outward physical presence (being fat). So "fat talk" is actually a metaphor for a feeling. When this notion is identified as a metaphor, it is possible for it to be challenged and replaced. What are some more productive metaphors or statements that you could suggest young women could make to help them to express their emotions more accurately?
6. Some health practitioners say that people with eating disorders engage in manipulative and "splitting" behaviours. We know that "splitting" is actually a process whereby a team of practitioners fails to be consistent or to work collaboratively towards shared goals. We also know that words like "manipulative" can be very damaging and labelling. How will you protect yourself against taking up judgemental and non-therapeutic language and ideas when you are working as a clinical nurse?

USEFUL WEBSITES

Australian Eating Disorders Research and Translation Centre: www.eatingdisordersresearch.org.au/
Australian and New Zealand Academy for Eating Disorders: www.anzaed.org.au/
Butterfly Foundation for Eating Disorders: www.thebutterflyfoundation.org.au/
Eating Disorders Association of New Zealand: www.ed.org.nz/
Eating Disorders Queensland: eatingdisordersqueensland.org.au/
Eating Disorders Victoria: www.eatingdisorders.org.au/
InsideOut Institute for Eating Disorder Research: insideoutinstitute.org.au/
Journal of Eating Disorders – peer-reviewed journal publishing leading research in the science and practice of eating disorders: jeatdisord.biomedcentral.com/
National Eating Disorders Collaboration (NEDC): nedc.com.au/
South Australia Statewide Eating Disorder Service (SEDS): www.sahealth.sa.gov.au/
The Victorian Centre for Excellence in Eating Disorders (CEED): ceed.org.au
The Western Australian Centre for Clinical Interventions: www.cci.health.wa.gov.au

Other resources
National ED Helpline: 1800 ED HOPE/1800 33 4673
Email: support@thebutterflyfoundation.org.au or phone the helpline to speak to a counsellor 8 am to midnight 7 days a week.

REFERENCES

American Psychiatric Association (APA), 2013. Diagnostic and Statistical Manual of Mental Disorders, 5th Edition (DSM-5). APA, Washington DC.
Barakat, S., McLean, S.A., Bryant, E., Le, A., Marks, P., et al., 2023. Risk factors for eating disorders: Findings from a rapid review. J Eat Disord, 11(1), 8.
Barakat, S., Touyz, S., Maloney, D. et al., 2021. Supported online cognitive behavioural therapy for bulimia nervosa: A study protocol of a randomised controlled trial. J Eat Disord, 9, 126.
Beinther, I., Jacobi, C., Schidt, U.H., 2014. Participation and outcome in manualized self-help for bulimia nervosa and binge eating disorder – a systematic review and metaregression analysis. Clin Psychol Rev, 34(2), 158–176.
Bell, K., Rieger, E., Hirsch, J.K., 2018. Eating disorder symptoms and proneness in gay men, lesbian women and transgender and non-conforming adults: Comparative levels and a proposed mediational model. Front Psychol, 9, 2692.
Bert, F., Gualano, M.R., Camussi, E., et al., 2016. Risks and threats of social media websites: Twitter and the Proana movement. Cyberpsychol Behav Soc Netw, 19(4), 233–238.
Bodell, L.P., Cheng, Y., Wildes, J.E., 2019. Psychological impairment as a predictor of suicide ideation in individuals with anorexia nervosa. Suicide Life Threat Behav, 49(2), 520–528.
Bosworth, P., 2011. Jane Fonda: The Private Life of a Public Woman. Houghton Mifflin Harcourt, Boston.
Breithaupt, L., Eickman, L., Byrne, C.E., et al., 2017. Enhancing empowerment in eating disorder prevention: Another examination of the REbeL peer education model. Eat Behav, 25, 38–41.
Brown, A., McClelland, J., Boysen, E. et al., 2016. The FREED Project (first episode and rapid early intervention in eating disorders): Service model, feasibility and acceptability. Early Interv Psychiatry, 12, 250–257.
Bryant, E., Miskovic-Wheatley, J., Touyz, S.W., Crosby, R.D., Koreshe, E., et al., 2021. Identification of high risk and early stage eating disorders: First validation of a digital screening tool. J Eat Disord, 6;9(1), 109.
Bryant, E., Touyz, S. & Maguire, S. 2023. Public perceptions of people with eating disorders: Commentary on results from the 2022 Australian national survey of mental health-related stigma and discrimination. J Eat Disord, 11, 62 doi.org/10.1186/s40337-023-00786-z
Burt, A., Mannan, H., Touyz, S., Hay, P. 2020a. Prevalence of DSM-5 diagnostic threshold eating disorders and features amongst Aboriginal and Torres Strait Islander peoples (First Australians). BMC Psychiatry, Sep 11; 20(1), 449.
Burt, A., Mitchison, D., Dale, E., Bussey, K., Trompeter, N., et al., 2020b. Prevalence, features and health impacts of eating disorders amongst First-Australian Yiramarang (adolescents) and in comparison with other Australian adolescents. J Eat Disord Mar, 12;8(1), 10.
Butler, R.M. & Heimberg, R.G., 2020. Exposure therapy for eating disorders: A systematic review. Clin Psychol Rev, 78, 101851.
Campbell, K., Peebles, R., 2014. Eating disorders in children and adolescents: State of the art review. Pediatrics, 134 (3), 582–593.
CCDH (Center for Countering Digital Hate) 2022. Deadly by design. TikTok pushes harmful content promoting eating disorders and self-hate in users'

feeds. Online. Available at: Counterhate.com/wp-content/uploads/2022/12/CCDH-Deadly-by-Design_120922.pdf

Cervantes-Luna, B.S., Ponce de Leon, C.S., Ruiz, E.J.C., et al., 2019. Aesthetic ideals, body image, eating attitudes and behaviors in men with different sexual orientation. Rev Mex Trastor Aliment (Mex J Eat Disord), 10 (1), 66–74.

Chaphekar, A.V., Vance, S.R., Garber, A.K. et al., 2022. Transgender and other gender diverse adolescents with eating disorders requiring medical stabilization. J Eat Disord, 10, 199, doi.org/10.1186/s40337-022-00722-7.

Citrome, L. (2019). Binge eating disorder revisited: What's new, what's different, what's next. CNS Spectrums, 24(S1), 4–13.

Cobbaert, L. & Rose, A. 2023. Eating disorders and neurodivergence: A stepped care approach. Online. Available at: nedc.com.au/assets/NEDC-Publications/Eating-Disorders-and-Neurodivergence-A-Stepped-Care-Approach.pdf

Dalle Grave, R., Eckhardt, S., Calugi, S. et al., 2019. A conceptual comparison of family-based treatment and enhanced cognitive behavior therapy in the treatment of adolescents with eating disorders. J Eat Disord, 7, 42.

Dann, K.M., Hay, P., & Touyz, S., 2023. Interactions between emotion regulation and everyday flexibility in anorexia nervosa: Preliminary evidence of associations with clinical outcomes. Eating Disorders, 31(2), 139–150.

Davico, C., Amianto, F., Gaiotti, F. et al., 2019. Clinical and personality characteristics of adolescents with anorexia nervosa with or without non-suicidal self-injurious behavior. Compr Psychiatry 94, 152115.

DerMarderosian, D., Chapman, H.A., Tortolani, C. et al., 2018. Medical considerations in children and adolescents with eating disorders. Child Adolesc Psychiatr Clin N Am, 27, 1–14.

de Vries, D.A., Peter, J., de Graaf, H. et al., 2016. Adolescents' social network site use, peer appearance-related feedback, and body dissatisfaction: Testing a mediation model. J Youth Adolesc, 45, 211–224.

Dittmer, N., Jacobi, C., Voderholzer, U., 2018. Compulsive exercise in eating disorders: Proposal for a definition and clinical assessment. J Eat Disord, 6(42), doi.org/10.1186/s40337-018-0219-x

Dobinson, A., Cooper, M., Quesnel, D., 2019. The Safe Exercise at Every Stage (SEES) guideline: A clinical tool for treating and managing dysfunctional exercise in eating disorders. Online. Available at: www.safeexerciseateverystage.com

Fairburn, C.G., Bailey-Straebler, S., Basden, S. et al., 2015. A transdiagnostic comparison of enhanced cognitive behaviour therapy (CBT-E) and interpersonal therapy in the treatment of eating disorders. Behav Res Ther, 70, 64–71.

Fitzsimmons-Craft, E.E., Balantekin, K.N., Graham, A.K., Smolar, L., Park, D., et al., 2019. Results of disseminating an online screen for eating disorders across the U.S.: Reach, respondent characteristics and unmet treatment need. Int J Eat Disord, 52, 721–729.

Friedli N, Stanga Z, Culkin A, et al., 2018. Management and prevention of refeeding syndrome in medical inpatients: An evidence-based and consensus-supported algorithm. Nutrition, 47, 13–20.

Giel, K.E., Bulik, C.M., Fernandez-Aranda, F. et al., 2022. Binge eating disorder. Nat Rev Dis Primers, 8, 16.

Giles, E.M., Cross, A.S., Matthews, R.V. et al., 2022. Disturbed families or families disturbed: A reconsideration. Eat Weight Disord, 27, 11–19.

Haas, V., Kohn, M., Korner, T., Cuntz, U., Garber, A.K., et al., 2020. Practice-based evidence and clinical guidance to support accelerated re-nutrition of patients with AN. J Am Acad Child Adolesc Pyschiatry, 60(5), 555–561.

Hay, P., Aouad, P., Le, A. et al., 2023. Epidemiology of eating disorders: Population, prevalence, disease burden and quality of life informing public policy in Australia – a rapid review. J Eat Disord, 11(1), 23.

Hay, P., Chinn, D., Forbes, D., et al., 2014. Royal Australian and New Zealand College of Psychiatrists clinical practice guidelines for the treatment of eating disorders. Aust N Z J Psychiatry, 48(11), 977–1008.

Hambleton, A., Pepin, G., Le, A., Maloney, D., NEDRC, Touyz, S., et al., 2022. Psychiatric and medical comorbidities of eating disorders: Findings from a rapid review of the literature. J Eat Disord, 10, 132.

Holland, G., Tiggemann, M., 2017. "Strong beats skinny every time": Disordered eating and compulsive exercise in women who post fitspiration on Instagram. Int J Eat Disord, 50 (1), 76–79.

Hummel, A.C., Smith, A.R., 2015. Ask and you shall receive: Desire and receipt of feedback via Facebook predicts disordered eating concerns. Int J Eat Disord, 48, 436–442.

InsideOut Institute 2021. Australian Eating Disorders Research and Translation Strategy 2021–2031. A national project funded by the Australian Government, Department of Health. Online. Available at: www.eatingdisordersresearch.org.au/static/3c9b6cd8ecea7f09dc9b8853aa913435/australian_eating_disorders_research_translation_strategy_2021-2031.pdf

Ivancic L, Maguire S, Miskovic-Wheatley J, Harrison C, Nassar N. 2021. Prevalence and management of people with eating disorders presenting to primary care: A national study. Aust N Z J Psychiatry, 55(11), 1089–1100.

Kazdin, A.E., Fitzsimmons-Craft, E.E. & Wilfley, D.E. 2017. Addressing critical gaps in the treatment of eating disorders. Int J Eat Disord, 50(3), 170–189.

Kiela, P.R., Gishan, F.K. 2016. Physiology of intestinal absorption and secretion. Best Pract Res Clin Gastroentorol, 30(2), 145–159.

Koreshe, E., Paxton, S., Miskovic-Wheatley, J. et al., 2023. Prevention and early intervention in eating disorders: Findings from a rapid review. J Eat Disord, 11, 38.

Lock J, Le Grange D. 2012. Treatment Manual for Anorexia Nervosa: A Family-Based Approach, 2nd ed. Guilford Press, New York, NY.

Lonergan, A.R., Bussey, K., Mond, M., et al., 2019. Me, my selfie, and I: The relationship between editing and posting selfies and body dissatisfaction in men and women. Body Image, 28, 39–43.

McIntosh VVW, Jordan J, Carter FA, Luty SE, McKenzie JM, et al., 2005. Three psychotherapies for anorexia nervosa: A randomized, controlled trial. Am J Psychiatry, 162(4), 741–747.

McLean, S.A., Paxton, S.J., 2019. Body image in the context of eating disorders. Psychiatr Clin North Am, 42, 145–156.

McLean, S.A., Paxton, S.J., Wertheim, E.H., et al., 2015. Photoshopping the selfie: Self photo editing and photo investment are associated with body dissatisfaction in adolescent girls. Int J Eat Disord, 48, 1132–1140.

Miskovic-Wheatley, J., Bryant, E., Ong, S.H. et al., 2023. Eating disorder outcomes: Findings from a rapid review of over a decade of research. J Eat Disord, 11, 85.

Miskovic-Wheatley, J., Koreshe, E., Kim, M. et al., 2022. The impact of the COVID-19 pandemic and associated public health response on people with eating disorder symptomatology: An Australian study. J Eat Disord, 10, 9.

Mitchison, D. & Mond, J. 2015. Epidemiology of eating disorders, eating disordered behaviour, and body image disturbance in males: A narrative review. J Eat Disord, 3(1), 1–9.

Mitchison D, Mond J, Bussey K, Griffiths S, Trompeter N, et al., 2020. DSM-5 full syndrome, other specified, and unspecified eating disorders in Australian adolescents: Prevalence and clinical significance. Psychol Med, 50(6), 981–990.

Morris, A., Elliott, E., Madden, S., 2022. Early-onset eating disorders in Australian children: A national surveillance study showing increased incidence. IJED, 55(12), 1838–1842.

Mosuka E.M., Murugan A., Thakral A., et al., 2023. Clinical outcomes of refeeding syndrome: A systematic review of high vs. low-calorie diets for the treatment of anorexia nervosa and related eating disorders in children and adolescents. Cureus, 15(5), e39313.

National Institute for Health and Care Excellence (NICE), 2017. Eating disorders: Recognition and treatment. In: NICE Guideline NG69. NICE, London.

Oldershaw, A., Lavender, T., Sallis, H., et al., 2015. Emotion generation and regulation in anorexia nervosa: A systematic review and meta-analysis of self-report data. Clin Psychol Rev, 39, 83–95.

Phillipou, A., Castle, D.J., Rossell, S.L., 2019. Direct comparisons of anorexia nervosa and body dysmorphic disorder: A systematic review. Psychiatry Res, 274, 129–137

Popovic, M., Pizzi, C., Rusconi, F., et al., 2018. The role of maternal anorexia nervosa and bulimia nervosa before and during pregnancy in early childhood wheezing: Findings from the NINEFA birth cohort study. Int J Eat Disord, 51(8), 842–851.

Reas, D.L., Grilo, C.M., 2014. Current and emerging drug treatments for binge eating disorder. Expert Opin Emerg Drugs, 19(1), 99142.

Renz, J.A., Fisher, M., Vidair, H.B., et al., 2017. Excessive exercise among adolescents with eating disorders: Examination of psychological and demographic variables. Int J Adolesc Med Health, 31(4), doi.org/10.1515/ijamh-2017-0032.

Rienecke, R., 2017. Family-based treatment of eating disorders in adolescents: Current insights. Adolesc Health Med Ther, 8, 69–79.

Riesco, N., Aguera, Z., Granero, R., et al., 2018. Other specified feeding or eating disorders (OSFED): Clinical heterogeneity and cognitive-behavioural therapy outcome. Eur Psychiatry, 54, 109–116.

Robinson, P.H., Nicholls, D., 2015. Critical Care for Anorexia Nervosa: The MARSIPAN Guidelines in Practice. Springer, London.

Rohde P., Stice E., Marti C.N., 2015. Development and predictive effects of eating disorder risk factors during adolescence: Implications for prevention efforts. Int J Eat Disord, 48(2), 187–198.

Rom, S., Miskovic-Wheatley, J., Barakat, S., Aouad, P., Fuller-Tyszkiewicz, M., et al., 2022. Evaluating the feasibility and potential efficacy of a brief eTherapy for binge-eating disorder: A pilot study. IJED, 55(11), 1614–1620.

Sanchez-Cerezo, J., Nagularaj, L., Gledhill, J. & Nicholls, D., 2022. What do we know about the epidemiology of avoidant/restrictive food intake disorder in children and adolescents? A systematic review of the literature. Europ Eat Disord Rev, 31(2), 226–246.

Sansfacon J., Booij, L., Gauvin, L., Fletcher, E., et al., 2020. Pretreatment motivation and therapy outcomes in eating disorders: A systematic review and meta analysis. IJED, 53(12), 1879–1900.

Schmidt, U., Wade, T.D., Treasure, J., 2014. The Maudsley model of anorexia Nervosa treatment for adults (MANTRA): Development, key features, and preliminary evidence. J Cogn Psychother, 28 (1), 48–71.

Sidani, J.E., Shensa, A., Hoffman, B., et al., 2016. The association between social media use and eating concerns among US young adults. J Acad Nutr Diet, 116(9), 1465–1472.

Smith, A.R., Zuromski, K.L., Dodd, D.R., 2018. Eating disorders and suicidality: What we know, what we don't know, and suggestions for future research. Curr Opin Psychol, 22, 63–67.

Smith, KE., Hayes, NA., Steer, DM., Washburn, JJ. 2017. Emotional reactivity in a clinical sample of patients with eating disorders and nonsuicidal self-injury. Psychiatry Res, 257, 519–525.

Smolak, L., Levine, M.P., 2015. The Wiley Handbook of Eating Disorders, Assessment, Prevention, Treatment, Policy, and Future Directions. John Wiley & Sons, Chichester.

Strother, E., Lemberg, R., Stanford, S.C., et al., 2012. Eating disorders in men: Underdiagnosed, untreated and misunderstood. Eat Disord, 20 (5), 346–355.

Tavolacci, M.P., Ladner, J., Déchelotte, P., 2021. Sharp increase in eating disorders among university students since the COVID-19 pandemic. Nutrients. Sep 28;13(10), 3415.

The Australian Eating Disorders Research and Translation Centre, 2022. Key Thinkers Forum: Eating disorder, wellbeing and a need for research. Online. Available at: www.eatingdisordersresearch.org.au/events/2022-01-22-research-centre/

Thomas, J.J., Becker, K.R., Breithaupt, L., et al., 2020a. Cognitive-behavioural therapy for adults with avoidant/restrictive food intake disorder. J Behav Cognit Ther, 31(1), 47–55.

Thomas JJ, Becker KR, Kuhnle MC, Jo JH, Harshman SG, et al., 2020b. Cognitive-behavioral therapy for avoidant/restrictive food intake disorder: Feasibility, acceptability, and proof-of-concept for children and adolescents. Int J Eat Disord, 53(10), 1636–1646.

Thompson, K.A., Bardone-Cone, A.M., 2019. Disordered eating behaviours and attitudes and their correlates among a community sample of older women. Eat Behav, 34, 101301.

Tiggemann, M., Slater, A., 2016. Facebook and body image concern in adolescent girls: A prospective study. Int J Eat Disord, 50(1), 80–83.

Tiggemann, M., Zaccardo, M., 2018. "Strong is the new skinny": A content analysis of #fitspiration images on Instagram. J Health Psychol, 23(8), 1003–1011.

Tiggemann, M., Zaccardo, M., 2015. "Exercise to be fit, not skinny": The effect of fitspiration imagery on women's body image. Body Image, 15, 61–67.

Utter, J., Denny, S., Peiris-John, R., et al., 2017. Family meals and adolescent emotional well-being: Findings from a national study. J Nutr Edu Behav, 49(1), 67–72.

Valkenburg, P.M., Meier, A., Beyens, I., 2022. Social media use and its impact on adolescent mental health: An umbrella review of the evidence. Curr Opin Psychol, 44, 58–68.

Voderholzer, U., Haas, V., Correll, C.U., Körner, T. 2020. Medical management of eating disorders: An update. Curr Opin Psychiatry, 33(6), 542–553.

Voelker, D.K., & Galli, N. 2019. Eating disorders in competitive sport and dance. In: Anshel, M.H, Petrie, T.A. & Steinfeldt, J.A. (eds), APA Handbook of Sport and Exercise Psychology, Vol. 1. Sport Psychology. American Psychological Association, New York.

Watson, H.J., Zerwas, S., Torgersen, L., et al., 2018. Maternal eating disorders and perinatal outcomes: a three-generational study in the Norwegian mother and child cohort study. J Abnorm Psychol, 126 (5), 552–564.

Willmott, E., Dickinson, R., Hall, C., Sadikovic, K., Micali, N., et al., 2023. A scoping review of psychological interventions and outcomes for avoidant and restrictive food intake disorder (ARFID). Int J Eat Disord, 57(1), 27–61.

Zerwas, S., Larsen, J.T., Petersen, L., et al., 2015. The incidence of eating disorders in a Danish nationwide register study: Associations with suicide risk and mortality. J Psychiatr Res, 65, 16–22.

16

Personality Disorders

Katrina Campbell and Marika Van Ooyen

KEY POINTS

- Personality disorders are common conditions, with borderline personality disorder being the most likely of these disorders that nurses will encounter in their practice.
- A wide range of terms are used to describe personality disorders. Section 2 of the *Diagnostic and Statistical Manual of Mental Disorders, 5th Edition, Text Revision* (DSM-5-TR) groups personality disorders into three broad clusters: (A) odd or eccentric; (B) dramatic, emotional or erratic; and (C) anxious or fearful. Although diagnosis is useful to enable access to treatment, in some cases diagnosis can be harmful and fails to acknowledge the uniqueness of the individual's experience.

- Effective nursing care of people with a personality disorder involves practising in a trauma-informed way to foster a safe environment to develop a therapeutic relationship and empower the person to regain the life they so desire.
- Self-care, self-awareness and clinical supervision help nurses to reflect on their practice, to gain insight and understanding into a person's behaviours, help to improve practice and also help to process our emotions, to ensure we are looking after our own mental health.

KEY TERMS

Borderline	Family	Recovery
Diagnosis	Hospital	Trauma
Dialectical	Mood	
Disorder	Personality	

LEARNING OUTCOMES

The material in this chapter will assist you to:
- discuss the development of personality
- identify the main characteristics of each of the three clusters of personality disorders
- develop an understanding of responses that nurses and other health professionals may experience when working with people who have a personality disorder

- identify effective nursing approaches to work with people who have a personality disorder, in particular borderline personality disorder.

INTRODUCTION

Personality disorders are described as a group of disorders whereby patterns of a person's thought processes and behaviours differ significantly from social norms and cultural expectations, leading to distress and functional impairment (American Psychiatric Association (APA) 2022). The three groups of personality disorders (referred to as clusters) will be discussed later in this chapter. It is not uncommon for people with a personality disorder to present to health services seeking help for a co-occurring condition, such as a substance use disorder, depression and anxiety. In fact, people with a personality disorder are frequent service users (Kavanagh et al 2021) and often present with self-harm, thoughts of self-harm and/or suicidal ideation. Nurses will encounter these presentations in a variety of health environments, so it is important for all nurses to understand how best to provide care and effectively work with people experiencing a personality disorder to facilitate positive health outcomes.

A comprehensive understanding of psychological trauma and the ongoing implications this can have on a person's functioning is essential when working with people with a personality disorder. Many people diagnosed with a personality disorder have experienced trauma throughout their life (Campbell et al 2020; Grenyer 2019), and in some cases, they may have experienced prolonged exposure to a trauma. Trauma can be acute (i.e. exposure to a catastrophic event or accident) or chronic in nature (i.e. domestic violence, abuse, repeated exposure to multiple traumas). The exact rates of psychological trauma in people with a personality disorder is unknown; however, there is clear evidence of a link between people with borderline personality disorder and childhood trauma (Bozzatello et al 2021). Acknowledging and empathising with the effect that trauma may have had in the lives of people with personality disorders is therefore essential. There are national practice recommendations for providing trauma-informed care for mental health services, and the incorporation of trauma-informed principles in the care of people with a personality disorder will be explored later in this chapter.

This chapter describes how personality disorders are currently categorised and identifies the defining characteristics of different types of personality disorders according to the *Diagnostic and Statistical Manual of Mental Disorders, 5th Edition, Text Revision* (DSM-5-TR) (APA 2022). Considerations surrounding diagnosis are provided; however, the chapter focuses on the assessment and interventions for working with people with personality disorders. Borderline personality disorder (BPD), a cluster B disorder, will be the primary focus for discussions surrounding assessment and treatment because it is the most common of the personality disorders with high rates of service use (Papathanasiou & Stylianidis 2022).

WHAT IS PERSONALITY?

Each of us has a personality and a commonsense understanding of what that means. We may describe others as "outgoing", "assertive", "withdrawn" or "shy", for example. Some individuals have personalities that seem to draw people to them – they may be described as charismatic, outgoing, friendly, good team players, helpful or kind. Others seem to have difficulty attracting others or maintaining relationships – they may appear to be unreceptive, cold, aloof, isolative, eccentric or perhaps moody, aggressive or reckless. Our personality may be thought of as the expression of our feelings, thoughts and patterns of behaviour that evolves over time. Genetics, family, life events, culture and the society we live in all contribute to shaping our personality. Personality manifests via our general disposition, behavioural patterns and approach to the world, and is especially evident during interactions with others.

Enduring aspects or features of our personality are referred to as "personality traits" and these traits are what differentiate us from one another. Social mores provide unwritten boundaries for what constitutes a "normal" personality trait. For example, if a student expresses concern at having to present their work to the class because they are shy and public speaking makes them nervous, most people would understand their difficulties. With perseverance and support, most students will incrementally gain confidence and participate in tutorials regardless of some level of continuing discomfort. However, some people are so averse to public speaking that they will eventually avoid social situations where this might be required of them, to the extent of dropping out of an interesting course or a good job or from contact with friendship groups. Such extreme behaviour is beyond what is socially regarded as shyness. The personality trait has moved beyond normal boundaries to a point where it may be understood in terms of psychopathology. Some people display personality traits that seem to be beyond the scope of what is considered reasonable, as observed by their behaviour and attitudes to others. These traits may be inflexible and maladaptive, resulting in distress, significant relational difficulties, and functional impairment to the individual, and it is only then are they considered personality disorders (APA 2022).

Before a diagnosis of a personality disorder is made there are a number of factors which must be considered. A person's culture can directly influence certain aspects of one's personality (APA 2022). For example, different historical periods, societies and cultures describe personalities differently and encourage or discourage certain personality types. We may associate different temperaments with different cultures (Crocq 2013). Additionally, certain behaviours may be acceptable in one culture and not another (APA 2022). For example, people raised in regimes such as the former East Germany, where the secret police network was widespread and intruded into families, would more likely be secretive, suspicious of others and unforthcoming. Similarly, contemporary indigenous cultures that are group-oriented may endorse mutual friendliness, sharing and fitting in at the expense of competitiveness and individualism.

TYPES OF PERSONALITY DISORDER

When personality manifestations interfere significantly with a person's general functioning, the person may then meet the criteria for a personality disorder. As with personality types, traits associated with personality disorders are often apparent in childhood and persist through adolescence to adulthood. The difference is largely of degree: the characteristics associated with a personality disorder are more inflexible and are often considered maladaptive. The characteristics of people with a personality disorder manifest in problems across their emotional regulation, interpersonal function, cognitive processes and impulse control, which impacts their day to day functioning both socially and occupationally (APA 2022). What a personality disorder is not is an acute emotional or behavioural reaction in response to a distressing situation (i.e. the experience of a traumatic loss). Given that norms relating to behaviour are socially and culturally constructed, when is the expression of someone's personality to be considered disordered? Herein lies the challenge for nurses to consider the context in which the person's symptomology is present and the extent in which that response would be considered socially appropriate.

Signs and Symptoms

If one considers that people with personality disorders demonstrate maladaptive and inflexible patterns of thinking and ways of behaving, the nature of the symptoms experienced are often associated with the individual's intrapersonal and interpersonal functioning (Kavanagh et al 2021). As a way of categorising and explaining personality disorders, the DSM-5-TR has grouped personality disorders into three clusters based on their descriptive similarities: Cluster A (odd–eccentric), B (dramatic–erratic) and C (fearful–anxious). Table 16.1 lists each of the personality disorders and their associated diagnostic criteria.

Prevalence

There is limited contemporary data available in Australia regarding the prevalence of personality disorders. However, it has been reported that 6.5% of the Australian population has a diagnosed personality disorder (Grenyer et al 2017). Globally, estimates of the prevalence of personality disorders range from 7.8% (Winsper et al 2020) to 12.16% (Kavanagh et al 2021). Certain personality disorders are diagnosed more in men (antisocial personality disorder) than women (borderline personality disorder); however, limited data exists which confirms personality disorders are more prevalent in one gender over the other (APA 2022). For those using mental health services, the prevalence of personality disorders is much higher, at approximately 45.5% (Quirk et al 2017). Increased rates of substance use, co-occurring mental health conditions, self-injurious behaviours and suicide are commonly associated with people with a personality disorder (Kavanagh et al 2021; Papathanasiou & Stylianidis 2022). Personality disorders are associated with higher service use, increased comorbidities and higher mortality rates, resulting in an increased economic burden on society (Kavanagh et al 2021; Papathanasiou & Stylianidis 2022). Possible reasons for the increased economic burden are believed to be associated with the impairments in interpersonal functioning which can impact the treatment received and chronicity of the disorder and have implications on the individual's social supports and ability to work (Kavanagh et al 2021).

TABLE 16.1 Criteria for Classifying Personality Disorders

Cluster A (odd or eccentric)	Criteria
Paranoid personality disorder APA 2022, p. 737	A. A pervasive distrust and suspiciousness of others such that their motives are interpreted as malevolent, beginning by early adulthood and present in a variety of contexts, as indicated by four (or more) of the following: 1. Suspects, without sufficient basis, that others are exploiting, harming or deceiving him or her. 2. Is preoccupied with unjustified doubts about the loyalty or trustworthiness of friends or associates. 3. Is reluctant to confide in others because of unwarranted fear that the information will be used maliciously against him or her. 4. Reads hidden demeaning or threatening meanings into benign remarks or events. 5. Persistently bears grudges (i.e., is unforgiving of insults, injuries, or slights). 6. Perceives attacks on his or her character or reputation that are not apparent to others and is quick to react angrily or to counterattack. 7. Has recurrent suspicions, without justification, regarding fidelity of spouse or sexual partner. B. Does not occur exclusively during the course of schizophrenia, a bipolar disorder or depressive disorder with psychotic features, or another psychotic disorder and is not attributable to the physiological effects of another medical condition. **Note:** If criteria are met prior to the onset of schizophrenia, add "premorbid", i.e. "paranoid personality disorder (premorbid)".
Schizoid personality disorder APA 2022, p.741	A. A pervasive pattern of detachment from social relationships and a restricted range of expression of emotions in interpersonal settings, beginning by early adulthood and present in a variety of contexts, as indicated by four (or more) of the following: 1. Neither desires nor enjoys close relationships, including being part of a family. 2. Almost always chooses solitary activities. 3. Has little, if any, interest in having sexual experiences with another person. 4. Takes pleasure in few, if any, activities. 5. Lacks close friends or confidants other than first-degree relatives. 6. Appears indifferent to the praise or criticism of others. 7. Shows emotional coldness, detachment, or flattened affectivity. B. Does not occur exclusively during the course of schizophrenia, a bipolar disorder or depressive disorder with psychotic features, another psychotic disorder or autism spectrum disorder, and is not attributable to the physiological effects of another medical condition. **Note:** If criteria are met prior to the onset of schizophrenia, add "premorbid", i.e. "schizoid personality disorder (premorbid)".
Schizotypal personality disorder APA 2022, p.744	A. A pervasive pattern of social and interpersonal deficits marked by acute discomfort with, and reduced capacity for, close relationships, as well as by cognitive or perceptual distortions and eccentricities of behaviour, beginning by early adulthood and present in a variety of contexts, as indicated by five (or more) of the following: 1. Ideas of reference (excluding delusions of reference). 2. Odd beliefs or magical thinking that influences behaviour and is inconsistent with subcultural norms (e.g. superstitiousness, belief in clairvoyance, telepathy, or "sixth sense"; in children and adolescents, bizarre fantasies or preoccupations). 3. Unusual perceptual experiences, including bodily illusions. 4. Odd thinking and speech (e.g. vague, circumstantial, metaphorical, over-elaborate, or stereotyped). 5. Suspiciousness or paranoid ideation. 6. Inappropriate or constricted affect. 7. Behaviour or appearance that is odd, eccentric, or peculiar. 8. Lack of close friends or confidants other than first-degree relatives. 9. Excessive social anxiety that does not diminish with familiarity and tends to be associated with paranoid fears rather than negative judgements about self. B. Does not occur exclusively during the course of schizophrenia, a bipolar disorder or depressive disorder with psychotic features, another psychotic disorder or autism spectrum disorder. **Note:** If criteria are met prior to the onset of schizophrenia, add "premorbid", e.g. "schizotypal personality disorder (premorbid)".
Cluster B (Dramatic, erratic and emotional)	**Criteria**
Antisocial personality disorder APA 2022, p.748	A. A pervasive pattern of disregard for and violation of the rights of others, occurring since age 15 years, as indicated by three (or more) of the following: 1. Failure to conform to social norms with respect to lawful behaviours, as indicated by repeatedly performing acts that are grounds for arrest. 2. Deceitfulness, as indicated by repeated lying, use of aliases, or conning others for personal profit or pleasure. 3. Impulsivity or failure to plan ahead. 4. Irritability and aggressiveness, as indicated by repeated physical fights or assaults. 5. Reckless disregard for safety of self or others. 6. Consistent irresponsibility, as indicated by repeated failure to sustain consistent work behaviour or honour financial obligations. 7. Lack of remorse, as indicated by being indifferent to or rationalising having hurt, mistreated, or stolen from another. B. The individual is at least age 18 years. C. There is evidence of conduct disorder with onset before age 15 years. D. The occurrence of antisocial behaviour is not exclusively during the course of schizophrenia or bipolar disorder.

Continued

TABLE 16.1 Criteria for Classifying Personality Disorders—cont'd

Cluster B (Dramatic, erratic and emotional)	Criteria
Borderline personality disorder APA 2022, p.752	A pervasive pattern of instability of interpersonal relationships, self-image, and affects, and marked impulsivity, beginning by early adulthood and present in a variety of contexts, as indicated by five (or more) of the following: 1. Frantic efforts to avoid real or imagined abandonment. (**Note:** Do not include suicidal or self-mutilating behaviour covered in Criterion 5.) 2. A pattern of unstable and intense interpersonal relationships characterised by alternating between extremes of idealisation and devaluation. 3. Identity disturbance: markedly and persistently unstable self-image or sense of self. 4. Impulsivity in at least two areas that are potentially self-damaging (e.g. spending, sex, substance abuse, reckless driving, binge eating). (**Note:** Do not include suicidal or self-mutilating behaviour covered in Criterion 5.) 5. Recurrent suicidal behaviour, gestures, or threats, or self-mutilating behaviour. 6. Affective instability due to a marked reactivity of mood (e.g. intense episodic dysphoria, irritability or anxiety usually lasting a few hours and only rarely more than a few days). 7. Chronic feelings of emptiness. 8. Inappropriate, intense anger or difficulty controlling anger (e.g. frequent displays of temper, constant anger, recurrent physical fights). 9. Transient, stress-related paranoid ideation or severe dissociative symptoms.
Histrionic personality disorder APA 2022, p. 757	A pervasive pattern of excessive emotionality and attention seeking, beginning by early adulthood and present in a variety of contexts, as indicated by five (or more) of the following: 1. Is uncomfortable in situations in which he or she is not the centre of attention. 2. Interaction with others is often characterised by inappropriate sexually seductive or provocative behaviour. 3. Displays rapidly shifting and shallow expression of emotions. 4. Consistently uses physical appearance to draw attention to self. 5. Has a style of speech that is excessively impressionistic and lacking in detail. 6. Shows self-dramatisation, theatricality and exaggerated expression of emotion. 7. Is suggestible (i.e. easily influenced by others or circumstances). 8. Considers relationships to be more intimate than they actually are.
Narcissistic personality disorder APA 2022, p.760	A pervasive pattern of grandiosity (in fantasy or behaviour), need for admiration, and lack of empathy, beginning by early adulthood and present in a variety of contexts, as indicated by five (or more) of the following: 1. Has a grandiose sense of self-importance (e.g. exaggerates achievements and talents, expects to be recognised as superior without commensurate achievements). 2. Is preoccupied with fantasies of unlimited success, power, brilliance, beauty or ideal love. 3. Believes that he or she is "special" and unique and can only be understood by, or should associated with, other special or high-status people (or institutions). 4. Requires excessive admiration. 5. Has a sense of entitlement (i.e. unreasonable expectations of especially favourable treatment or automatic compliance with his or her expectations). 6. Is interpersonally exploitative (i.e. takes advantage of others to achieve his or her own ends). 7. Lacks empathy: is unwilling to recognise or identify with the feelings and needs of others. 8. Is often envious of others or believes that others are envious of him or her. 9. Shows arrogant, haughty behaviours or attitudes.

Cluster C (Anxious and fearful)	Criteria
Avoidant personality disorder APA 2022, p.764	A pervasive pattern of social inhibition, feelings of inadequacy, and hypersensitivity to negative evaluation, beginning by early adulthood and present in a variety of contexts, as indicated by four (or more) of the following: 1. Avoids occupational activities that involve significant interpersonal contact because of fears of criticism, disapproval, or rejection. 2. Is unwilling to get involved with people unless certain of being liked. 3. Shows restraint within intimate relationships because of the fear of being shamed or ridiculed. 4. Is preoccupied with being criticised or rejected in social situations. 5. Is inhibited in new interpersonal situations because of feelings of inadequacy. 6. Views self as socially inept, personally unappealing, or inferior to others. 7. Is unusually reluctant to take personal risks or to engage in any new activities because they may prove embarrassing.

TABLE 16.1 Criteria for Classifying Personality Disorders—cont'd

Cluster C (Anxious and fearful)	Criteria
Dependent personality disorder APA 2022, p.768	A pervasive and excessive need to be taken care of that leads to submissive and clinging behaviour and fears of separation, beginning by early adulthood and present in a variety of contexts, as indicated by five (or more) of the following: 1. Has difficulty making everyday decisions without an excessive amount of advice and reassurance from others. 2. Needs others to assume responsibility for most major areas of his or her life. 3. Has difficulty expressing disagreement with others because of fear of loss of support or approval. (**Note:** Do not include realistic fears of retribution.) 4. Has difficulty initiating projects or doing things on his or her own (because of a lack of self-confidence in judgement or abilities rather than a lack of motivation or energy). 5. Goes to excessive lengths to obtain nurturance and support from others, to the point of volunteering to do things that are unpleasant. 6. Feels uncomfortable or helpless when alone because of exaggerated fears of being unable to care for himself or herself. 7. Urgently seeks another relationship as a source of care and support when a close relationship ends. 8. Is unrealistically preoccupied with fears of being left to take care of himself or herself.
Obsessive-compulsive personality disorder APA 2022, p.771	A pervasive pattern of preoccupation with orderliness, perfectionism, and mental and interpersonal control, at the expense of flexibility, openness and efficiency, beginning by early adulthood and present in a variety of contexts, as indicated by four (or more) of the following: 1. Is preoccupied with details, rules, lists, order, organisation, or schedules to the extent that the major point of the activity is lost. 2. Shows perfectionism that interferes with task completion (e.g. is unable to complete a project because his or her own overly strict standards are not met). 3. Is excessively devoted to work and productivity to the exclusion of leisure activities and friendships (not accounted for by obvious economic necessity). 4. Is overconscientious, scrupulous, and inflexible about matters of morality, ethics, or values (not accounted for by cultural or religious identification). 5. Is unable to discard worn-out or worthless objects, even when they have no sentimental value. 6. Is reluctant to delegate tasks or to work with others unless they submit to exactly his or her way of doing things. 7. Adopts a miserly spending style towards both self and others; money is viewed as something to be hoarded for future catastrophes. 8. Shows rigidity and stubbornness.
Personality disorder not otherwise specified	**Criteria**
APA 2022, p.778	This category applies to presentations in which symptoms characteristic of a personality disorder that cause clinically significant distress or impairment in social, occupational, or other areas of important functioning predominate but do not meet the full criteria for any of the disorders in the personality disorders diagnostic class. The other specified personality disorder category is used in situations in which the clinician chooses to communicate the specific reason that the presentation does not meet the criteria for any specific personality disorder. This is done by recording "other specified personality disorder" followed by the specific reason (e.g. "mixed personality features").

From the MSD Manual Professional Version, edited by Sandy Falk. Copyright © 2024 Merck & Co., Inc., Rahway, NJ, USA and its affiliates. All rights reserved. Available at: www.msdmanuals.com/professional.

Cluster A

Cluster A describes personalities of an odd or eccentric nature. The three disorders within this group are paranoid, schizoid and schizotypal personality disorders. Although difficult to ascertain the exact prevalence of cluster A personality disorders in Australia, it has been reported that 4.2% of the global population has a cluster A personality disorder. This group of personality disorders has a higher incidence in higher income earning countries despite being associated with a lower prevalence of clinical presentations (Winsper et al 2020).

Cluster B

Cluster B refers to the dramatic, erratic and emotional disorders, and includes histrionic, borderline, narcissistic and antisocial personality disorders. The cluster B personality disorders are generally considered to be the most prevalent of all three clusters. However, the prevalence varies between countries due to differences in social and cultural expectations. For example, borderline personality disorder (BPD) is not acknowledged

in the Chinese diagnostic classification system; similarly, antisocial personality disorder is seldom seen in Taiwan due to stronger social control mechanisms which inhibit the development of such behaviours (Winsper et al 2020). As a result of these differences, the global prevalence of cluster B personality disorders is estimated at 2.8% (Winsper et al 2020).

The most common and most complex personality disorder encountered in the clinical setting is BPD. The prevalence of BPD in other countries among the general population is estimated at approximately 1–4% (Campbell et al 2020), and prevalence rates of BPD among people who use psychiatric services is estimated at up to 67% (Papathanasiou & Stylianidis 2022).

Cluster C

Cluster C comprises the anxious and fearful group of personality disorders. Avoidant, dependent and obsessive-compulsive personality disorders belong in the cluster C group. It is estimated that approximately 5% of the population globally have a cluster C personality disorder (Winsper et al 2020). Cluster C personality disorders are more commonly seen in higher income earning countries.

DIAGNOSTIC CONSIDERATIONS

It is difficult to determine the exact prevalence of personality disorders for a multitude of reasons, which stem beyond cultural and social differences. The categorical nature of the DSM-5-TR presents personality disorders and their symptoms as distinct syndromes. Within Australia, categorical diagnosis is by and large used within the health system to determine funding (Campbell et al 2020). By contrast, the ICD-11, used in Europe, favours a dimensional approach in which people are assessed to either meet the criteria of a general personality disorder or not. Then the severity of dysfunction is determined (mild–moderate or severe), followed by evaluating the five main personality domains (negative affectivity, dissociality, disinhibition, anankastia and detachment) (Campbell et al 2020). This approach acknowledges each disorder on a continuum, with a specific focus on the impact that symptoms have on the individual's functioning. For us as nurses, it is important that we understand how a person is impacted by their symptoms, more so than which condition the person meets the diagnostic criteria for. Understanding what the person is experiencing and how a person is impacted will allow us to tailor our care to the individual and support them through their recovery journey.

Assessment and diagnosis of personality disorders can be challenging because a person who exhibits symptoms of one type of personality disorder invariably also exhibits symptoms of other disorders. A person may exhibit symptoms from multiple categories of personality disorders, as well as other mental health conditions. This can be problematic if we are defining people's problems as one personality disorder or another instead of focusing our care on the symptoms or distress the person presents with. In the past, the most common clinically documented personality disorder diagnosis was that of the residual category, "Not otherwise specified", which means that the clinician cannot decide between two or more possibilities. This may not reflect a limitation in the clinician's diagnostic ability, but rather a realistic acknowledgement that a person may experience a number of symptoms from different personality disorders, but may not strictly meet the criteria for one specific personality disorder.

While the layperson might be excused for believing that diagnoses are clear-cut, nurses need to be aware that all psychiatric diagnoses lack clarity in some situations and overlap at times. This means that debates about whether a given person has a specified disorder are often legitimate. Psychiatry is an inexact science, and even when a definitive personality disorder diagnosis can be made, the optimal approach to treatment is not always clear (Campbell & Lakeman 2021). As in previous editions, the DSM-5-TR (APA 2022) issues a cautionary statement to clinicians about interpreting its diagnostic categories; indeed, they are advised that specific diagnostic criteria serve only to inform professional judgement, not to override it. This is especially the case with personality disorder, where the diagnosis is often debated.

Historically, psychiatric diagnoses have often become pejorative labels, where those bearing the descriptors have been prejudged and stereotyped, especially by health professionals (Campbell et al 2020; Papathanasiou & Stylianidis 2022). In the case of BPD, this is arguably the most stigmatised condition of all mental health conditions (Papathanasiou & Stylianidis 2022), and therefore labelling should be done with caution. The current taxonomy of personality disorders, alongside the use of checklists and abstract diagnostic criteria, is generally considered inadequate because it leads to narrow, subjective assessments that ignore life events, the person's history and their social circumstances (Campbell et al 2020).

CAUSAL AND CONTRIBUTING FACTORS

The precise causes of a personality disorder are largely unknown; however, there are a number of factors which have been found to be linked to the development of a personality disorder. The presence of trauma in a person's presentation is arguably the most common factor associated with a personality disorder. Research consistently reveals that people who have experienced childhood physical, emotional or sexual abuse or emotional neglect, as well as those raised in families characterised by withdrawal or violence, are much more likely to display behaviours consistent with a personality disorder diagnosis than those who have not been abused or neglected (NHMRC 2012). An important consideration of note here though, is that not all people who experience trauma will develop a personality disorder (Grenyer 2019). One of the possible explanations for this is the heredity (or genetic) factors, which have been found to influence the likelihood of developing personality traits consistent with a personality disorder. For example, there is evidence that people with BPD inherit vulnerabilities for hypersensitivity and emotional dysregulation, meaning they are more likely to perceive interpersonal interactions as traumatic (Grenyer 2019). Regardless, a combination of biological, psychological and social risk factors, including heredity, life experiences and environmental factors, influence the development of a person's personality traits, which may become rigid and result in ongoing distress and functional impairment. Herein lies the importance of adopting a trauma-informed approach when working with people with personality disorders, particularly given the high prevalence of traumatic experiences in this population.

THE EXPERIENCE OF PEOPLE WITH A PERSONALITY DISORDER: STIGMA

People are rarely admitted to in-patient mental health settings simply because of their personality disorder. Rather, they are admitted because of conditions that coexist with their disorder, such as anxiety, depression, substance misuse, or for assessment due to difficulties managing distress or regulating their emotions. People with a diagnosis from cluster A, odd and eccentric personality disorders, are the least likely to seek treatment. Those with cluster C, anxious and fearful disorders, more frequently require treatment. However, it is those with cluster B, dramatic and emotional personality disorders, who most frequently find themselves the recipients of care from mental health clinicians (Papathanasiou & Stylianidis 2022).

When one reviews the characteristics of people who have these disorders, it is easy to appreciate why this may be so. As previously mentioned, people with BPD have high rates of health service use and have a high prevalence in both in-patient and out-patient services alike (Campbell et al 2020). Quite often, people with this disorder present in crisis following an interpersonal conflict (i.e. relationship breakdown) or increased life stressors (Campbell et al 2020). Impulsivity, self-harm, suicidal gestures and engaging in high-risk behaviours (substance use) tend to bring people with BPD into contact with healthcare services. These behaviours can be confronting for health professionals to witness, particularly when someone is actively trying to harm themselves, which contributes towards the development of stigma towards this condition (Campbell et al 2020).

People with a personality disorder experience high rates of stigma and discrimination from within the health system in comparison to people diagnosed with other mental illnesses (Grenyer 2019; Klein et al 2021). This is particularly true for BPD. Stigma can lead to the misdiagnosis of a personality disorder as another mental health condition, reluctance to diagnose or treat someone with a personality disorder, and delayed access to appropriate and timely treatment and support for consumers and carers alike, resulting in poor health outcomes (Grenyer 2019).

Help-seeking behaviours and attendance to healthcare services is generally viewed as a strength and mitigates risk when providing mental health care. It is unfortunate that in the case of BPD, what would ordinarily be viewed as a strength is viewed as a pitfall; the very nature of BPD that provides an avenue for support and treatment conversely drives stigmatisation of this group by health professionals. People with BPD experience overwhelming distress leading to recurrent suicidality and thoughts of self-harm and often seek help to manage their overwhelming distress (Klein et al 2021). However, help-seeking through contact with acute care and emergency services, presentations to emergency departments (EDs) and seeking in-patient admissions is often met by stigmatising responses, leading to exacerbation of distress and re-traumatisation (Klein et al 2021). It is therefore important that we provide care that is free from bias and does not discriminate.

When considering the socioecological approach outlined in Chapter 2 of this text, and the importance of interactions between a person and their environment, this is inclusive of the person's experience with health systems. When the person with borderline personality disorder faces stigmatisation when seeking help this impedes the recovery process and causes further negative impacts on their mental health.

INITIAL ASSESSMENT

Nursing assessment of people with personality disorder can take place in a variety of settings; this may include general and mental health settings, as well as in-patient and community settings. The assessment may occur in the context of a crisis such as in the ED or with a crisis team. The assessment may take place at the initial point of access, such as a GP clinic or other community health clinic. Alternatively, the assessment might be undertaken as part of general nursing duties when the person is admitted as an in-patient or out-patient.

HISTORICAL ANECDOTE 16.1

On the "Border"

Use of the term "borderline" to describe people's mental state began in the early 20th century. Professor Carl Pelman (1838–1916) at Bonn University in Germany wrote a paper using the term "borderline" to describe a range of mental health problems that did not fit a description of "psychosis", which was the dominant diagnostic category back then. By 1938 the term "borderline" had begun to be associated with personality, when psychoanalysts began describing people who failed to fit into either the psychotic or psychoneurotic groups, which were the two main diagnostic categories of the time. The phrase "borderline" was therefore used to describe dominant symptoms, such as narcissism and insecurity. The diagnostic term we associate with borderline personality disorder today has changed and modernised in various editions of the DSM.

Read More About It
Howell, E. 2018. From hysteria to chronic relational trauma disorder: the history of borderline personality disorder and its connection to trauma, dissociation, and psychosis. In: Moskowitz A, Dorahy MJ, Schäfer I (eds). Psychosis, Trauma and Dissociation: Evolving Perspectives on Severe Psychopathology. John Wiley & Sons, Hoboken, pp. 83–95.

Assessment is a continuous process drawing on high-level communication and listening skills, and keen observation. Assessing someone with a personality disorder is not dissimilar to assessing people with other mental health complaints; It needs to be holistic, considering the person's present relationships, as well as childhood experiences and traumatic events. It is important to remember that the findings of your assessment may be considered provisional, at least until further corroborating material is gathered. Although the assessment process doesn't necessarily differ for someone with a personality disorder, there are considerations when communicating, and a trauma-informed approach is essential.

An empathetic approach during assessment is required in order to build a therapeutic relationship with a person who has a personality disorder and who may struggle with establishing and maintaining both professional and personal relationships due to past relational difficulties. Project Air (2015, p. 6) provides some key principles for working with people with personality disorders:

- Be compassionate and demonstrate empathy.
- Listen to the person's current experience and maintain a non-judgemental approach. Take their experience seriously – remember, one of the characteristics of BPD is chronic suicidal gestures.
- Validate the person's current emotional state, particularly when emotional dysregulation is present. There are some cases where the person may have experienced ongoing invalidation which has contributed to the development of their condition. Dismissing or further invalidation can result in increased distress.
- Be aware of your own emotions and body language. Remain caring, but recognise the person's level of distress and project a sense of calm.
- Remain respectful.
- Engage in open communication and foster trust to allow strong emotions to be freely expressed.
- Be human and be prepared to acknowledge both the serious and the funny side of life where appropriate.
- Be clear, consistent, and reliable.
- Remember aspects of challenging behaviours have survival value given past experiences.
- Convey encouragement and hope about their capacity for change while validating their current emotional experience.

These principles can help to anchor the clinician in the assessment and minimise negative reactions to expressions of distress, such as resistance, rejection, suicidality and thoughts of self-harm. They also adopt a trauma-informed approach. See Personal perspectives: Consumer's Story 16.1, which recounts the experiences of Charlie.

PERSONAL PERSPECTIVES

Consumer's Story 16.1: Charlie

Charlie is a 21-year-old who lives in a unit by themselves and has a pet cat called Mali. Charlie grew up in a single-parent household and rarely had contact with their father, due to domestic violence, and has no siblings. Charlie's mother describes them as an irritable baby and found Charlie difficult to soothe. Charlie was diagnosed as having ADHD as a young child. During primary school, Charlie struggled with the other kids at school, and often got into fights with their peers. From the onset of puberty, Charlie experienced a rapid rise in emotional instability, impulsive behaviour and aggression. Charlie was in and out of home care, because their mother couldn't cope with the emotional instability, aggression and impulsive behaviours Charlie displayed. Charlie experienced a sexual assault when they were 14 years old. Charlie tried to report this to their home care case manager; however, no formal police report was made and Charlie states, "No one believed me". At age 17 Charlie ran away from their foster home and lived with an older male. Charlie dropped out of school and did not complete Year 12.

Historically, when Charlie has met someone, they tend to form intense friendships, with high hopes that this would help Charlie feel better about themselves, but these relationships are short-lived and usually end on bad terms. Charlie has an extensive history of tumultuous relationships, being the victim of domestic violence (DV), most recently having taken out a DVO on their latest partner.

Charlie works at a local cafe full-time, but has recently missed a few shifts. Charlie has also recently broken up with their boyfriend of 4 months. Charlie describes the relationship as "good until a few weeks ago". Charlie has a limited social support and struggles to identify people they can trust in their inner circle. Charlie is well known to the mental health service and was last in the emergency department one week ago following an episode of impulsive self-poisoning with Citalopram tablets. This presentation was in response to a fight with their boyfriend. Charlie often presents to the ED in the context of life or relationship stressors, usually accompanied by self-harm (cutting to their thighs, arms or stomach) and thoughts of suicide.

Charlie is not currently engaged with mental health services and they do not have a regular GP. Charlie tells you that they have been referred to psychologists in the past, but "none of them understand, they think I am just attention seeking. The last lady I saw told me I needed to accept responsibility for my actions and so I didn't go back."

? CRITICAL THINKING EXERCISE 16.1

After reading Charlie's story, discuss the following questions with your group:
1. Based on the information provided, what factors do you think could influence the development of Charlie's personality?
2. What questions would you ask Charlie to develop a therapeutic alliance and obtain further information in your assessment to develop a plan of care?
3. What potential barriers might a person like Charlie experience when presenting to the emergency department seeking help and why?

A TRAUMA-INFORMED ASSESSMENT

A trauma-informed approach shifts the tone of the assessment from blame/problem focus – "What is wrong with you?" – to inquire and attempt to understand the person by exploring "What happened to you?" (Kezelman & Stavropoulos 2020). (See Chapter 9 for more about assessment.) At any assessment stage, the principles of trauma-informed care provide a clear basis for establishing and maintaining the therapeutic relationship. The principles of trauma-informed care are: safety, trustworthiness, choice, collaboration, empowerment and respect for diversity (Kezelman & Stavropoulos 2020). When working with people with personality disorders, the principles of trauma-informed care are even more pertinent due to the high prevalence of experiences of trauma for people accessing mental health services (Grenyer 2019; Isobel & Edwards 2017). Each of the six principles of trauma-informed care are discussed in relation to working with people with BPD below.

Safety and Trustworthiness

People who have experienced trauma have often had unsafe relationships in both childhood and adulthood; therefore, a sense of safety can feel alien to them (Kezelman & Stavropoulos 2020). For people with BPD, safety can feel fractured and unattainable, often due to past experiences of unstable relationship patterns. This can mean it is difficult for these people to trust others, including healthcare professionals. Consistency is essential to building a sense of safety and establishing trust, and is often illusive in health settings due to difficulties with staffing consistencies and differences in communication styles. For example, some health professionals may set boundaries that are too

firm and come across as authoritarian and punitive, while others may have looser boundaries that cross the professional relationship and lead to inconsistencies across teams. Inconsistent approaches create an unsafe relationship for the person with a personality disorder because they negatively influence the therapeutic relationship, derail trust in individual health professionals and services, and negatively affect treatment, access to services and recovery. As stated in the Project Air principles (2015) for working with people with personality disorders, it is important to be clear, consistent and reliable. Trust is essential to any person's sense of safety and to build trust we need to provide clear messages that are reflected in our actions. Well-documented treatment plans across services such as EDs, mental health acute care services, general wards and mental health in-patient wards are an excellent tool to ensure safety and consistency.

When we relate the principles of safety and trustworthiness to Charlie's story we can see that they lacked safety in their home from a young age with a father who was violent towards their mother and largely absent. Charlie's mother then struggled to care for Charlie and they were in and out of home care, leading to a lack of solid foundation through adolescence and people they could put their trust in. They experienced a sexual assault, leading to a further diminution in a sense of safety and felt they weren't believed by professionals involved in their care at the time. Charlie has then gone on to have unstable personal and professional relationships, stating that they felt a psychologist saw them as attention-seeking. Charlie brings their own experiences to their interaction with us as nurses; while part of them wishes to reach out for help and support, another part of them is likely to be wary and defensive. The best way we can approach Charlie is to be consistent in our interactions and to share this consistency across our teams. A practical way to do this is if we say we will come and see Charlie in an hour but find ourselves busy at that time, we can take a moment to explain this to Charlie, give a specific time for when we will return and stick to this time. Small actions like this can help to build trust that you will follow through with what you say.

Choice, collaboration and empowerment

Recovery from borderline personality disorder involves developing and strengthening one's sense of self (Ng et al 2019). Treating teams can foster this developing sense of self by providing choice in treatment strategies, collaborating "with" the person in all aspects of care rather than doing "to" or "for" them and therefore empowering them to be the driver in their own recovery process (Kezelman & Stavropoulos 2020). This approach can be built upon during each interaction with health services from initial assessment, and will aid in developing safety and trust. We can see from Charlie's story that they may feel a low sense of control over their own life, particularly during childhood and adulthood when they experienced traumatic events that were beyond their control. Charlie has likely felt things were done to them: they were in and out of home care, they were sexually assaulted and this was not reported to authorities. Charlie has not been given many opportunities to feel empowered in their own life. As nurses, we can work collaboratively with Charlie by asking them what they would like to happen when they present to the ED in distress, asking them how self-harm helps them to manage difficult emotions in a non-judgemental way and how they manage suicidal ideation in those times when they don't present to health services, while encouraging their help-seeking in instances when they do present. There are evident strengths in Charlie's story; they have managed to hold down a full-time job and have continued to seek help despite feeling let down by professional care providers in the past. As nurses, we can support Charlie to draw on those strengths and feel empowered in their own care.

Respect for diversity

Inclusive services that respect all forms of diversity are essential to a trauma-informed approach (Kezelman & Stavropoulos 2020). People from culturally and linguistically diverse (CALD) communities, those who experience disability, First Nations people, and people who are perceived to be abnormal by society experience ongoing marginalisation within institutions and health services (Kezelman & Stavropoulos 2020). Additionally, two-thirds of sexual and gender diverse people have experienced a mental health condition, and also have experienced difficulty in accessing services due to a lack of specific or safe options (NSW Ministry of Health 2022). The high incidence of mental health concerns and low incidence of access to support services is driven by stigma, discrimination and a lack of understanding of diverse experiences of identity (NSW Ministry of Health 2022). A key example is misgendering of people accessing health services, a person may identify as a different gender and/or name than is reflected on their medical record. It is important to take this into account when working with people with borderline personality disorder; when nurses refer to the person by the wrong name or gender, this negates any safety or trust in the service or individual and means the person is unlikely to continue to access support.

RISK ASSESSMENT

Often assessment and management of risk form a large component of the treatment plan for people with a personality disorder, particularly people with cluster B personality disorders, such as BPD. The experience of emotional dysregulation is so powerful and consuming it can lead to thoughts of harm to self and, more rarely, thoughts of harm to others. The nature of this disorder results in interpersonal dysfunction, which impacts on the person's ability to form and maintain stable supportive relationships, often resulting in behaviours which leave the person quite vulnerable to exploitation and abuse from others. Chapter 9 provides detailed information on risk assessment processes. Below are some considerations when conducting a risk assessment for people with BPD.

Risk of self-harm and suicide

People with BPD experience high rates of self-harm and suicidal ideation/attempts in comparison to other mental health conditions. Although risk of self-harm and risk of suicide are often assessed and documented independently, they are often intrinsically linked. It is estimated that 60–90% of people with BPD have self-harmed, experience suicidal ideation or have attempted suicide (Broadbear et al 2020). One of the common characteristics of BPD includes recurrent self-harm or suicidal gestures (APA 2022). It is important that the nurse assesses both the person's risk of self-harm and the person's suicidal ideation. Nurses may be reluctant to ask about thoughts of suicide or self-harm, worrying that they may increase the person's level of distress and suicidal or self-harm thoughts (Townsend et al 2021). This is not the case; by asking directly about suicidal ideation or thoughts of self-harm, nurses can build safety and trust with the person, give them a chance to discuss a topic that is difficult for them to talk about with friends or family, and encourage help-seeking (Townsend et al 2021). It is important that the nurse does not dismiss the seriousness of the suicidal thoughts held by the person with BPD. Suicidal ideation/gestures is often a chronic experience for those with BPD and this, coupled with their impulsivity, can place them at a high risk of suicide or misadventure.

Risk of Suicide

The mortality rate of suicide in people with BPD is 10%, which makes the risk of suicide one of the highest in this population of all mental health conditions (Papathanasiou & Stylianidis 2022). While a risk assessment can help to identify the level of suicide risk the person may be experiencing, we cannot always eliminate the risk in its entirety. Rather, the risk assessment provides opportunities for the treating team to mitigate and reduce risk where possible. It is essential that nurses use a socioecological approach to their clinical assessments, which adopts a holistic view of the context in which the person is experiencing suicidal ideation. A collaborative meaningful risk assessment considers the person's current healthy coping strategies, including how they have managed their suicidal thoughts in the past, the supports they have in their lives, what may increase or decrease their suicidal ideation, and how they can bolster their current personal and professional supports. Safety planning is a useful tool to use in conjunction with risk assessments, and to provide a basis for discussions around supports and protective factors.

Safety planning. Safety planning is an evidence-based, collaborative process that results in a detailed, individualised plan that defines steps that a consumer, their supports and health services can take to recognise and respond when in crisis and thoughts of self-harm or suicidal ideations are present. Individuals who completed a safety plan were half as likely to exhibit suicidal behaviour and twice as likely to present for outpatient mental health appointments (Labouliere et al 2020). High-quality, detailed and personalised plans are associated with fewer subsequent hospitalisations (Ferguson et al 2022). Safety planning is a collaborative process between the person and the nurse that can be shared across teams and services to ensure a consistent approach to working with the person experiencing suicidal thoughts. They draw on the person's own supports, coping strategies and knowledge of their warning signs. Safety plans are a standard document that can be in paper format, written into the medical record and are also available on the Beyond Blue app.

Safety plans include:
- My warning signs that I may be heading into a crisis …
- Things I can do to make my space safe …
- My reasons to live and to continue my recovery are …
- My personal coping strategies …
- People and places I can connect with that distract me or take my mind off things …
- People I know who I would feel comfortable reaching out to for help when I am distressed …
- Professional supports I can call on are …
- Contact details for supports that are available after hours such as Lifeline and the Suicide Call Back Service.

Risk of Self-Harm

Self-harm is an example of a maladaptive coping strategy, often seen in the presentations of those with BPD. Self-harming behaviours include, but are not limited to, cutting, head-banging, deep scratching with or without an implement, and self-burning with cigarettes or lighters.

Self-harming behaviours are also a significant risk factor for suicide. However, just because someone engages in self-harm does not mean they are attempting to take their own life. It is important that the difference between suicide and self-harm be clearly established as, although they are linked, they are not the same. Self-harm occurs without the intent to end one's life. There are a number of reasons someone might engage in self-harm. However, in the case of BPD, people often engage in self-harm as a means to regulate their emotions or communicate distress. Indeed, self-harm is a coping strategy, although it is not the most ideal coping strategy, which is why we refer to it as a maladaptive coping strategy. A suicide attempt/gesture, on the other hand, differs from self-harm because it is with the intent to end one's life. It is important when conducting a risk assessment to distinguish between the two, which can be tricky, particularly when the person struggles to articulate their emotions and verbalises their wish to not "be here" any longer. When assessing a person's risk of self-harm, there are key considerations the nurse should explore. Some key considerations include:

- the means of self-harm
- the reasons behind why the person is self-harming (this helps us also determine if the person has intent to end their life or not)
- how often the person self-harms
- how helpful they find self-harming to be.

Self-harming behaviours are confronting and distressing and undoubtedly contribute to negative attitudes towards people with BPD and feed into stigmatisation (Campbell et al 2020; Papathanasiou & Stylianidis 2022). Moreover, nurses often find it especially confronting and describe working with people who self-harm as difficult. As Feigenbaum (2010, p. 115) succinctly states, from a person's perspective, self-harm is "the solution not the problem". Needless to say, many clinicians continue to see self-harm as the problem, not a part of the solution, and, with good treatment, a temporary or interim solution. The reality is that expecting people to simply give up self-harming actions can precipitate intense panic and anxiety because they are effectively being asked to give up a tried and true way of managing rage, shame and alienation from self and others that works for them. Understanding the reasons for self-harm may help nurses and other mental health clinicians to face their own reactions and increase their self-awareness, enabling them to provide high-quality and stigma-free care.

Sensory interventions. Sensory modulation can be described as the process of regulation and organisation of the nature and intensity of responses to sensory input, which occurs in a graded manner (Matson et al 2021). The mediums by which sensory modulation might be delivered include the use of physical items, activities or environmental changes (Matson et al 2021). The idea behind sensory modulation is that arousal levels of the person are regulated. Given that people with BPD experience significant emotional dysregulation, it is not surprising that sensory interventions would be beneficial for this population.

Sensory interventions are often used in in-patient settings as a way of adapting healthier coping strategies that help to regulate distress and intense emotions. Sensory approaches aim to stimulate the senses as a method of self-soothing; strategies include using weighted blankets, massage chairs, calming lights and pictures, kinetic sand and fidget toys, and aromatherapy (Matson et al 2021). Sensory modulation has also been found to be beneficial in reducing urges to self-harm. Examples of sensory strategies which reduce self-harm include fidget toys and bracelets or items a person can bite or throw without causing harm to themselves or other people (Matson et al 2021). Sensory modulation is also considered to be trauma-informed because it facilitates empowerment by providing the person with a more active means of coping, meaning they can engage in this independently, reducing reliance on their existing supports (Matson et al 2021). Personal perspectives: Consumer's story 16.2, continues Charlie's experiences.

PERSONAL PERSPECTIVES

Consumer's Story 16.2: Charlie

Today, Charlie has self-presented to the mental health crisis team in the ED at the local hospital with suicidal ideation and self-harm following a recent break-up with their partner. Upon assessment, Charlie is of thin build and is dressed casually in a shirt and jeans and has brightly coloured short hair. Charlie has obvious scarring down their left forearm and has a small bandage over their wrist from cutting with a razor earlier in the day. When you initially see Charlie, they are obviously distressed and tearful, and they avoid eye contact with you. Charlie repeatedly tells you, "I don't want to be here anymore". Charlie tells you they have voices that are derogatory in nature, telling them to "kill myself". Charlie tells you that "everyone hates me and I'm not worth living for", "everyone just leaves me anyway!"

CRITICAL THINKING EXERCISE 16.2

In your groups, discuss the following questions:
1. What risks do you think you would be likely to explore with Charlie?
2. What questions will you ask to assess Charlie's risk?
3. What strategies could you consider using to help reduce Charlie's level of distress?

CRISIS INTERVENTION

Crisis intervention and stabilisation are often the first priorities in responding to acute distress in people with BPD (NHMRC 2012). Nurse interactions with people with BPD will often occur when they present in crisis to EDs, mental health acute care teams and mental health in-patient units. When the person with borderline personality disorder is presenting in crisis they are likely to exhibit high levels of emotional distress, which may be accompanied by urges to self-harm, self-harm injury, suicidal attempts or ideation, drug and alcohol misuse, risk-taking behaviours and a reduced capacity to problem-solve (Pierce & Critchlow 2019; Project Air Strategy for Personality Disorders 2015). Working with people when they are in crisis can be challenging and confronting for nurses due to the high level of emotional distress the person is experiencing (Campbell et al 2020). They may present to EDs and mental health services frequently and with similar symptoms, leading to frustration for nurses, and it may also be difficult for the person to articulate how they are feeling and the reasons behind their distress (Pierce & Critchlow 2019; Project Air Strategy for Personality Disorders 2015). It is important to keep in mind that when people are presenting in crisis, we are seeing them at their worst and that they are accessing services to seek help to manage their overwhelming distress (Pierce & Critchlow 2019; Project Air Strategy for Personality Disorders 2015).

On initial interaction with the person in crisis, the level of imminent risk needs to be assessed collaboratively with the person presenting, and safety provided. If the risk is high and changeable, this would involve being admitted to an ED or a mental health in-patient unit for observation while distress remains high, and the risk of self-harm or suicide is acute. If the risk is manageable in the community, the person may go home with professional and personal supports. It is important when assessing risk that the person experiencing the crisis feels their concerns regarding risk are also acknowledged and taken into account in the plan (Proctor et al 2021). Hospital admissions are generally not considered appropriate for treatment of BPD; however, in the event that imminent risks are present to the person, a brief hospital admission may be beneficial (Proctor et al 2021). The goal of care during crisis is to help the person manage their distress, assist the person to stabilise and provide a safe, consistent approach that does not further exacerbate the feelings of judgement or rejection that people with BPD are highly attuned to (Pierce & Critchlow 2019; Project Air Strategy for Personality Disorders 2015). This can feel difficult to navigate for the nurse caring for the person in crisis; however, using the six principles of trauma-informed care as a framework can aid in this safe, consistent approach.

People with BPD have often developed methods they use for managing high levels of distress, some of which may be considered unhealthy or risky in themselves, such as self-harm, while others may be non-harmful and useful to draw on in a hospital setting; for example, distraction techniques, including listening to music, journalling, art, and contact with friends or family. A safety plan made in collaboration with the person in crisis can help to identify coping strategies. A point worth highlighting here is that it is essential that

BOX 16.1 The TIPP Technique

TIPP is a common approach used in Dialectical Behaviour Therapy that is found to be helpful for managing overwhelming emotions and is often used for those experiencing the urge to self-harm. The TIPP acronym stand for: Temperature, Intense exercise, Paced breathing and Progressive muscle relaxation. Nurses can talk the person experiencing distress through these techniques to help the person manage their distressing thoughts.

Temperature:
- Put cold water on the face or run hands under cold water
- Hold an ice cube or cold pack (make sure it is wrapped in fabric so burns do not occur and that the person does not hold it for too long)

Intense exercise:
- Expend the body's stored up energy by short bursts of running, walking fast, jumping, playing a physical game or doing a video workout

Paced breathing:
- Breathe deeply, counting breaths in and out, breathe out for more counts than you breathe in (for example, 5 seconds in and 7 seconds out)

Progressive muscle relation:
- While breathing in, deeply tense your body muscles
- Notice the tension in your body
- While breathing out say the word "relax" in your mind
- Let go of the tension and notice the difference in your body. (You can find guided muscle relation audio and videos online.)

Linehan 2015.

if a safety or management plan is being developed that the person is genuinely involved and consulted throughout its development. Failure to develop such a plan in a collaborative manner can be detrimental to the person's recovery and future engagement with the health service (Proctor et al 2021). Having honest discussions with the person about what helps and doesn't help during crisis can assist the nurse to develop a plan of care that can be shared with the treating team and used to provide a consistent approach. Box 16.1 explains the TIPP technique.

COLLABORATIVE TEAM APPROACHES

The nature of the symptoms characteristic of BPD sees that people with this condition experience marked emotional dysregulation, unhelpful cognitions and misattributed empathy, all of which directly impact interpersonal relationships (Noor et al 2022). Health professionals also experience the impacts of these symptoms when attempting to develop a therapeutic alliance with people with BPD, which presents unique challenges during therapeutic interactions (Noor et al 2022). Often, the way in which someone with BPD will interact with health professionals can be chaotic in nature, which can be confronting and elicit feelings of confusion from nurses and other health professionals. Attitudes towards people with BPD differ greatly between individual clinicians and disciplines; however, a pervasive negative attitude is reported across all health professionals, with terms such as "manipulative", "attention-seeking" and "difficult" often used to describe people with this diagnosis (Day et al 2018).

These negative attitudes towards people with BPD generate emotional responses in healthcare professionals, including frustration and helplessness, and can lead to approaches to care that include avoidance, dismissiveness and intolerance. Within a team, some staff may experience negative attitudes towards people with BPD, while others may not, causing inconsistencies in the way care is provided and discord among a treating team. This discord creates a "split" in the team approach (Green 2018).

When working in mental health services, you are likely to hear the term "staff splitting" in relation to people with personality disorders.

While it is important that differing approaches are recognised, this term places the blame and onus for change on the person with BPD rather than prompting the team to look at how they can provide consistent care that enhances safety and trust in service provision for the consumer (Green 2018). It is therefore important that the treating team are consistent with their approaches when providing care. Nurses are in a unique position to be able to provide consistent and collaborative care as they often spend the most time with these people, particularly when they are acutely distressed.

Care plans are one way in which the treating team can provide consistent care, limiting disparities between different staff approaches (Project Air Strategy for Personality Disorders 2015). Care plans or treatment plans need to be created in collaboration with the person with BPD to empower them to have choice in their treatment. There are a number of factors which contribute to a successful care plan:

- Care plans need to involve ALL staff members in the treating team to ensure consistency.
- The family members or carers who the person wants involved in their care should be included.
- If multiple service providers are involved in care provision, the care plan should also be shared to these.
- The care plan should be clearly documented in the person's medical record so that it is easily located.

The overarching goal of the care plan is to provide a clear overview of care provision for the person with BPD. Challenging expressions of emotional distress need firm, consistent limits so they don't devolve into further harmful behaviours and damage to interpersonal relationships, both personal and professional (Project Air Strategy for Personality Disorders 2015). Information included in the care plan might include the person's goals, early warning signs to reduce possible crisis, crisis survival strategies (i.e. tips or coping strategies the person may use to diffuse their crisis), and both personal and professional support contact details (Project Air Strategy for Personality Disorders 2015). In addition to the above, care plans can also be used to outline clear boundaries or limits of care. For example, the care plan may articulate the parameters for hospital admissions. Historically, the terms "boundaries" and "limit setting" have resulted in negative connotations for the person with BPD because they can accompany punitive and paternalistic approaches (Project Air Strategy for Personality Disorders 2015). However, when the boundaries and limits are clear and transparent for the person, and consistent across the treating team(s), punitive responses are limited and stability is provided, which helps to build **trust** in service providers.

TREATMENT

There is an array of interventions and evidence-based treatments available for the spectrum of symptoms people with personality disorders may experience. For this discussion, focus will be placed on the interventions and treatments for those with a borderline personality disorder, as this consumer group has a high prevalence of healthcare service use in comparison to the other personality disorders. Treatments for BPD focus on strengthening the person's sense of self, improving emotional resilience and management of distress and building healthy interpersonal relationships (Grenyer 2019). It is important to approach treatment in a collaborative manner and work with the person to achieve recovery. Additional considerations include the nature of the person's presentation and the symptoms they are experiencing; for example, not everyone with BPD has experienced trauma, so providing a therapy that targets trauma may not necessarily be appropriate. However, in order to determine the most appropriate treatment, we need to provide support to work through the current crisis.

Psychotherapy

Psychotherapy is considered the most effective treatment for BPD (Stoffers-Winterling et al 2022a). There are a number of psychotherapies which have been proven to be beneficial in the treatment of personality disorders. Some of these therapies target specific types of distorted cognitions, thus having a specific focus in the conditions they will help. In the case of BPD, despite there being a number of psychotherapies which are beneficial to this condition, dialectical behaviour therapy is considered the gold standard for treatment because it targets emotional dysregulation and interpersonal skills (Campbell & Lakeman 2021). However, evidence exists that one of the reasons psychotherapy is so effective is because individual clinicians use a combination of elements of the different psychotherapies to tailor their treatment to the individual's symptoms and needs (Campbell & Lakeman 2021). Another consideration as to why psychotherapy is beneficial for this particular population is that unstable relationships so often accompany their presentations, and the stability and consistency which arises from the relationship between an empathetic therapist and person with BPD is therapeutic in itself (Campbell & Lakeman 2021). Nonetheless, the basis for effective treatment requires a skilled therapist and a person who is willing and ready to engage in the therapy process.

The most well-known, and often the foundation of other psychotherapies, is cognitive behaviour therapy (CBT). CBT uses aspects of both cognitive therapy (which targets unhelpful beliefs) and behavioural therapy (which aims to change non-constructive or damaging behaviours). CBT aims to help people to develop more effective coping mechanisms by equipping them with strategies that promote more adaptive ways of thinking about and responding to everyday situations (Stoffers-Winterling et al 2022a). Research generally supports the conclusion that CBT is an effective treatment modality for people with a range of personality disorders.

Dialectical behaviour therapy (DBT) is based on CBT, and research shows it is useful for people with BPD (Stoffers-Winterling et al 2022a). DBT is what is known as a multimodal therapy, in that it combines a combination of individual therapy, group skills training, and crisis phone coaching (if warranted) (Lakeman et al 2022a). The focus of this therapy is: (1) the attenuation of parasuicidal and life-threatening behaviours; (2) the attenuation of behaviours that hinder therapy; and (3) the attenuation of behaviours that frustrate the person's ability to improve their quality of life. Essentially, this therapy, developed by Marsha Linehan (1998; 2000), conceptualises people with personality disorders as having significant problems in regulating their emotions and behaving in accordance with social norms, often as a result of unsupportive, socially chaotic or traumatic life histories (Lakeman et al 2022a). DBT involves an intensive, highly structured approach to treatment, including both individual and group sessions that focus on identifying strengths and overcoming negative coping habits. Therapy teaches new skills and facilitates practice of replacement behaviours in a range of social contexts. Common components of a DBT program include:

- *individual therapy* – focused on strengths identification, reflecting on recent challenges and using the therapist–person relationship as a template for practising new coping skills
- *group therapy and teaching sessions* – focused on four core themes of interpersonal effectiveness, distress tolerance, emotion regulation and mindfulness
- *role-playing* – behaviour rehearsals, practised in either individual or group therapy sessions
- *homework* – often involving practising social skills in real-life contexts
- *telephone coaching* – unlike many other approaches, telephone contact between therapist and person is encouraged in between individual sessions (Lakeman et al 2022b).

DBT has a growing body of evidence, including randomised controlled trials and systematic literature reviews, that suggests it can be useful for a range of personality disorders (Lakeman et al 2022a; Lakeman et al 2022b; Stoffers-Winterling et al 2022a). Nurses can complete short courses in DBT skills to use both with people currently undergoing DBT and to help people manage acute distress. The TIPP technique is an example of one of these skills.

Other psychotherapies with an evidence base in the treatment of BPD include mentalisation-based therapy (MBT), interpersonal psychotherapy–BPD (ITP–BPD) and dynamic deconstructive psychotherapy (DDP). Mentalisation-based therapy is similar to DBT, in that it comprises both individual and group sessions, but it focuses on helping people to identify and understand their experiences of the self and others (Stoffers-Winterling et al 2022a). MBT is grounded in psychoanalysis and draws from both attachment and cognitive theory. Interpersonal psychotherapy–BPD is an adaptation of the "interpersonal therapy", which was originally developed as a treatment for mood disorders. IPT-BPD adopts the standpoint that BPD is a chronic mood disorder and focuses on the interpersonal context in which one is experiencing their distress and uses the therapeutic relationship to help the person process these experiences (Stoffers-Winterling et al 2022a). Dynamic deconstructive therapy is also specifically developed for the treatment of BPD, but has also been found to be particularly useful for people with a co-occurring substance use disorder or antisocial personality disorder (Stoffers-Winterling et al 2022a). DDP aims to repair the distorted cognitions surrounding one's experiences through guiding the person to identify their emotions surrounding a particular interaction and find other ways to interpret and understand this situation, therefore altering the polarised thinking so commonly seen in people with BPD.

Pharmacological Interventions

Reviewers of pharmacological treatments conclude that there is limited evidence to justify using medication in people with a personality disorder (Stoffers-Winterling et al 2022b). Yet, people who have BPD are often prescribed multiple psychotropic drugs for use over a prolonged period of time, despite the limited evidence supporting their benefit (Stoffers-Winterling et al 2022b). Doctors often prescribe psychotropic medications for off-label use (meaning they are not used for the condition they were designed for) to ameliorate symptoms and enable people to undertake the therapies discussed earlier in this chapter. Particular symptoms targeted include mood dysregulation (selective serotonin reuptake inhibitors), impulsivity (mood stabilisers, anticonvulsants, carbamazepine), limited sociability (atypical neuroleptics) and cognitive distortions (atypical neuroleptics) (NHMRC 2012). Chapter 21 provides more information about these medications. Personal perspectives: Consumer's Story 16.3 discusses a comprehensive assessment of Charlie's situation.

👤 PERSONAL PERSPECTIVES

Consumer's Story 16.3: Charlie

After a period of time in the emergency department, Charlie's level of distress reduces greatly, enabling you to undertake a more comprehensive assessment. Throughout your discussion, Charlie mentions they had never had a sense of who they are as a person and struggles to articulate their likes, dislikes, values or aspirations when asked. Charlie indicates they have very few friends or social supports. When questioning Charlie about suicidal ideation, they tell you "I'm permanently like this and have been since I was 10". When attempting to brainstorm ideas with Charlie surrounding treatment, Charlie says "I don't know what the point of talking to you is, you never do anything to help anyway". Charlie becomes increasingly irritable, stating "I'm not going to kill myself, so can I just go home?".

Although Charlie presents to the ED frequently, they have not had an admission into the mental health unit for 2 years.

CRITICAL THINKING EXERCISE 16.3

In your group, discuss the following questions:
1. What could you say to Charlie in this situation to encourage engagement in a plan?
2. What approach do you think might be appropriate for Charlie's presentation?

SELF-CARE OF THE NURSE

From the discussion in this chapter so far, it is clear that nurses and other members of the healthcare team face a range of personal, interpersonal and professional challenges when working with people with personality disorders. Nurses working with people in acute distress face difficult, emotionally charged situations that can have immediate and long-term effects on their own wellbeing and performance in their role (Delgado et al 2020). Reflection and developing self-awareness can help nurses to manage these challenges and develop resilience that will be protective throughout their careers (Delgado et al 2020). Delgado and colleagues (2022) explored how nurses build and maintain their emotional resilience and found three themes:

- "Being attuned to self and others" (p. 1263): through developing self-awareness and maintaining empathy for others.
- "Having a positive mindset grounded in purpose" (p. 1263): staying connected to the positive aspects of their work and why they do the work they do.
- "Maintaining psychological equilibrium through proactive self-care": both personal self-care strategies, such as hobbies and exercise, that allows the nurse to focus on non-work-related activities and keep their body and mind healthy, and professional self-care; for example, advancing professional development through education or changing a task during the day to have a break from one that is emotionally intensive.

Working with people with personality disorders often evokes strong emotions in health professionals. These emotions may be positive or negative in nature. It is important to remember that we are human, and experiencing emotions is part of being human. What this means is that it is not necessary to eliminate all emotional responses you may experience throughout your role as a nurse; rather, it is about being aware of those emotions you experience and managing those emotions accordingly. There are times when you will experience an emotion towards someone in your care which may trigger an emotive reaction from you which can impact the care you are delivering. For example, you may be providing care to someone who is experiencing emotional dysregulation and has a diagnosis of BPD that evokes feelings of anxiety and incompetence, which can result in you avoiding the person or providing substandard care, which in turn can impact health outcomes negatively. This experience is called counter-transference and can occur in a therapeutic relationship where you as the health professional project emotions onto the person you are providing care to, in turn negatively impacting care provision. Moreover, counter-transference is something many health professionals experience when providing care to people with personality disorders (Prasko et al 2022). One of the ways

we can recognise and respond to these types of experiences is through clinical supervision.

Clinical supervision provides an avenue for reflection and learning through feedback that can help nurses manage the challenges in working in emotionally intense situations (Delgado et al 2020). Clinical supervision provides a safe place for nurses to discuss and explore their own feelings and reactions to working with people with personality disorders. Through our work with people with personality disorders, we can use education and clinical supervision to enrich our own self-growth and better understand ourselves and the people we work with. The key to working with people with personality disorders is a trusting and optimistic relationship that benefits the consumer, their families and significant others, and our own nursing practice. Perspectives in practice: Nurse's Story 16.1 relates how nurse Vanessa was able to engage Charlie in therapy and some of the issues that arose.

 PERSPECTIVES IN PRACTICE

Nurse's Story 16.1: Vanessa

Vanessa, the credentialled mental health nurse leading the DBT program at a community health centre, felt an immediate empathy for Charlie because they reminded her of one of her younger siblings. Vanessa engaged Charlie in regular one-to-one therapy and psychotherapy using a DBT approach and provided oversight for group sessions run by a psychologist at the centre. Vanessa also monitored Charlie's continuation on the antidepressant medication (Citalopram) prescribed by the referring psychiatrist.

Early in therapy, Vanessa was very encouraging of Charlie, telling them they could ring her at any time. Charlie agreed and immediately warmed to Vanessa's empathetic approach, telling her that she was "The best counsellor I've ever met … way better than the psychiatrist who is only interested in what pills I am taking". While Vanessa appreciated Charlie's enthusiasm, she was aware of the way that people with personality disorders can exhibit dependent traits and so made a mental note to reflect on and discuss Charlie's case during her monthly clinical supervision session.

Despite Charlie's enthusiasm and assurances, within a couple of months they began calling multiple times a day, just "to have someone to talk to". This created further stress because Vanessa was not always able to take the calls and Charlie would leave messages indicating "if I die, it's your fault", "You are the reason I am cutting myself". Vanessa found this extremely difficult because she couldn't stop thinking about the relationship problems she had experienced with her sibling, who had behaved in a similar way before taking their own life. Vanessa often found herself drinking extra wine and struggling to sleep following workdays when she received these calls from Charlie.

 CRITICAL THINKING EXERCISE 16.4

Group discussion:
1. What is Vanessa likely to be experiencing in this situation?
2. What strategies could Vanessa be aware of and implement to ensure she maintains professional boundaries but also looks after herself?

CHAPTER SUMMARY

Working with people with personality disorders can be a challenging experience for nurses, but it can also be very rewarding and provide an avenue for personal and professional growth as we learn the skills to support people through distress and navigate interpersonal

relationships within our practice. This chapter has focused on borderline personality disorder (BPD), as nurses are most likely to work with people with this personality disorder due to high rates of service use (Papathanasiou & Stylianidis 2022). Emerging treatments and improved understandings of BPD have shown that full recovery is possible, with the majority of people diagnosed with BPD experiencing symptomatic remission within 15 years if diagnosed at a young age (Balaratnasingam & Janca 2020; Campbell et al 2020). Awareness and management of the stigmatised views within health services is one of the challenges nurses face when providing care to these people. An additional consideration is that nurses should ensure their own practice comes from the trauma-informed perspective of "What happened to you?" rather than "What's wrong with you?", and uses the principles of trauma-informed care: safety, trustworthiness, choice, collaboration, empowerment and respect for diversity to frame their work with people with BPD (Kezelman & Stavropoulos 2020). Consistency across individuals and teams, improving your own knowledge of personality disorders and self-awareness and reflection can make working with this cohort an extremely rewarding experience.

The six principles of trauma-informed care – safety, trustworthiness, choice, collaboration, empowerment and respect for diversity – assist nurses and others to work in collaboration with this group of people (Kezelman & Stavropoulos 2020).

USEFUL WEBSITES

National Health and Medical Research Council: www.nhmrc.gov.au/guidelines-publications/mh25

National Institute for Health and Care Excellence – borderline personality disorder treatment and management: www.nice.org.uk/guidance/cg78

National Institute of Mental Health: www.nimh.nih.gov/health/publications/borderline-personality-disorder/index.shtml

Project Air: www.projectairstrategy.org/index.html

Royal College of Psychiatrists: www.rcpsych.ac.uk/healthadvice/problemsdisorders/personalitydisorder.aspx

REFERENCES

American Psychiatric Association (APA) 2022. Diagnostic and Statistical Manual of Mental Disorders: 5th Edition, Text Revision (DSM-5-TR). APA Publishing, New York.

Balaratnasingam, S., & Janca, A. 2020. Recovery in borderline personality disorder: Time for optimism and focused treatment strategies. Curr Opin Psychiatry, 33(1), 57–61.

Bozzatello, P., Rocca, P., Baldassarri, L., Bosia, M., & Bellino, S. 2021. The role of trauma in early onset borderline personality disorder: A biopsychosocial perspective. Front Psychiatry, 12, 721361.

Broadbear, J.H., Dwyer, J., Bugeja, L., & Rao, S. 2020. Coroners' investigations of suicide in Australia: The hidden toll of borderline personality disorder. J Psychiatric Res, 129, 241–249.

Campbell, K., & Lakeman, R. 2021. Borderline personality disorder: A case for the right treatment, at the right dose, at the right time. Iss Ment Health Nurs, 42(6), 608–613.

Campbell, K., Clarke, K.A., Massey, D., & Lakeman, R. 2020. Borderline Personality Disorder: To diagnose or not to diagnose? That is the question. Int J Ment Health Nurs, 29(5), 972–981.

Crocq, M.-A. 2013. Milestones in the history of personality disorders. Dialogues Clin Neurosci, 15(2), 147–153.

Day, N.J.S., Hunt, A., Cortis-Jones, L., & Grenyer, B.F.S. 2018. Clinician attitudes towards borderline personality disorder: A 15-year comparison. Personal Ment Health, 12(4), 309–320.

Delgado, C., Roche, M., Fethney, J., & Foster, K. 2020. Workplace resilience and emotional labour of Australian mental health nurses: Results of a national survey. Int J Ment Health Nurs, 29(1), 35–46.

Feigenbaum, J. 2010. Self-harm–the solution not the problem: The dialectical behaviour therapy model. Psychoanalytic Psychother, 24(2), 115–134.

Ferguson, M., Rhodes, K., Loughhead, M., McIntyre, H., & Procter, N. 2022. The effectiveness of the safety planning intervention for adults experiencing suicide-related distress: A systematic review. Arch Suicide Res, 26(3), 1022–1045.

Green, H. 2018. Team splitting and the "borderline personality": A relational reframe. Psychoanalytic Psychother, 32(3), 249–266.

Grenyer, B.F.S. 2019. Integrating trauma-informed care for Personality Disorders – The Project Air Strategy. In: Benjamin, R., Haliburn, J., King, S. (eds). Humanising Mental Health Care in Australia (1st ed.). Routledge, New York.

Grenyer, B.F.S, Jenner, B.A., Jarman, H.L., Carter, P., Bailey, R.C. et al., 2015. Treatment guidelines for personality disorders. Illawarra Health and Medical Research Institute.

Grenyer, B.F.S., Ng, F.Y.Y., Townsend, M.L., & Rao, S. 2017. Personality disorder: A mental health priority area. ANZ J Psychiatry, 51(9), 872–875.

Isobel, S., & Edwards, C. 2017. Using trauma informed care as a nursing model of care in an acute inpatient mental health unit: A practice development process. Int J Ment Health Nurs, 26(1), 88–94.

Kavanagh, B.E., Gwini, S.M., Pasco, J.A., Stuart, A.L., Quirk, S.E., et al., 2021. the added burden of personality disorder on subsidized Australian health service utilization among women with mental state disorder. Frontiers Global Women's Health, 2, 615057.

Kezelman, C.A., & Stavropoulos, P. 2020. Organisational Guidelines for Trauma Informed Service Delivery. Blue Knot Foundation, Milsons Point.

Klein, P., Fairweather, A.K., Lawn, S., Stallman, H.M., & Cammell, P. 2021. Structural stigma and its impact on healthcare for consumers with borderline personality disorder: Protocol for a scoping review. Systematic Reviews, 10(1), 23.

Labouliere, C.D., Stanley, B., Lake, A.M., & Gould, M.S. 2020. Safety planning on crisis lines: Feasibility, acceptability, and perceived helpfulness of a brief intervention to mitigate future suicide risk. Suicide Life-Threaten Behav, 50(1), 29–41.

Lakeman, R., Hurley, J., Campbell, K., Hererra, C., Leggett, A., et al., 2022a. High fidelity dialectical behaviour therapy online: Learning from experienced practitioners. Int J Ment Health Nurs, 31(6), 1405–1416.

Lakeman, R., King, P., Hurley, J., Tranter, R., Leggett, A., et al., 2022b. Towards online delivery of Dialectical Behaviour Therapy: A scoping review. Int J Ment Health Nurs, 31(4), 843–856.

Linehan, M.M. 2015. DBT® Skills Training Handouts and Worksheets, 2nd ed. Guilford Press, New York.

Linehan, M.M. 2000. Commentary on innovations in dialectical behavior therapy. Cogn Behav Pract, 7(4), 478–481.

Linehan, M.M., 1998. An illustration of dialectical behavior therapy. In Session: Psychother Pract 4(2), 21–44.

Matson, R., Kriakous, S., & Stinson, M. 2021. The experiences of women with a diagnosis of borderline personality disorder (BPD) using sensory modulation approaches in an inpatient mental health rehabilitation setting. Occupat Ther Ment Health, 37(4), 311–331.

National Health and Medical Research Council (NHMRC) 2012. Clinical Practice Guideline for the Management of Borderline Personality Disorder. National Health and Medical Research Council, Melbourne.

Ng, F.Y.Y., Townsend, M.L., Miller, C.E., Jewell, M., & Grenyer, B.F.S. 2019. The lived experience of recovery in borderline personality disorder: A qualitative study. Bord Personal Disord Emot Dysreg, 6(1), 10.

Noor, N., Rufino, K.A., Patriquin, M.A., Oldham, J.M., & Rohr, J. C. 2022. Impact of personality dysfunction on interdisciplinary treatment team working alliance in an inpatient psychiatric population. Personality disorders: Theory, Res Treat, 14(2), 216–222.

NSW Ministry of Health. 2022. NSW LGBTIQ+ Health Strategy 2022–2027. Online. Available at: www.health.nsw.gov.au/lgbtiq-health/Publications/lgbtiq-health-strategy.pdf

Papathanasiou, C. & Stylianidis, S. 2022. Mental health professionals' attitudes towards patients with borderline personality disorder: The role of disgust. Int J Psychiatr Res, 5(1), 1–13.

Pearce, S. & Critchlow, G. 2019. People with personality disorders and developmental conditions on an inpatient ward. In: Barrera, A., Attard, C., Chaplin, R. (eds). Oxford Textbook of Inpatient Psychiatry. Oxford University Press, Oxford.

Prasko, J., Ociskova, M., Vanek, J., Burkauskas, J., Slepecky, M., et al., 2022. managing transference and countertransference in cognitive behavioral supervision: Theoretical framework and clinical application. Psychol Res Behavior Manage, 15, 2129–2155.

Proctor, J. M., Lawn, S., & McMahon, J. 2021. Consumer perspective from people with a diagnosis of borderline personality disorder (BPD) on BPD management—How are the Australian NHMRC BPD guidelines faring in practice? J Psychiatric Ment Health Nurs, 28(4), 670–681.

Project Air Strategy for Personality Disorders 2015. Treatment Guidelines for Personality Disorders, 2nd ed. University of Wollongong. Online. Available at: www.projectairstrategy.org/content/groups/public/@web/@ihmri/documents/doc/uow189005.pdf

Quirk, S.E., Berk, M., Pasco, J.A., Brennan-Olsen, S.L., Chanen, A.M. et al., 2017. The prevalence, age distribution and comorbidity of personality disorders in Australian women. ANZ J Psychiatry, 51(2), 141–150.

Stoffers-Winterling, J.M., Storebø, O.J., Kongerslev, M.T., Faltinsen, E., Todorovac, A., et al., 2022a. Psychotherapies for borderline personality disorder: A focused systematic review and meta-analysis. Br J Psychiatry, 221(3), 538–552.

Stoffers-Winterling, J.M., Storebø, O.J., Pereira Ribeiro, J., Kongerslev, M.T., Völlm, B.A. et al., 2022b. Pharmacological interventions for people with borderline personality disorder. Cochrane Database of Systematic Reviews, 11(11), CD012956.pub2.

Townsend, M.L., Barr, K.R., & Grenyer, B.F.S. 2021. Early identification of personality disorder: Helping to understand youth suicide risk. Aust J Gen Pract, 50(5), 332–334.

Winsper, C., Bilgin, A., Thompson, A., Marwaha, S., Chanen, A.M., et al., 2020. The prevalence of personality disorders in the community: A global systematic review and meta-analysis. Br J Psychiatry, 216(2), 69–78.

Zimmerman, M. 2023. Paranoid Personality Disorder (PPD). MSD Manual. Merck & Co. Online. Available at: www.msdmanuals.com/en-au/professional/psychiatric-disorders/personality-disorders/paranoid-personality-disorder-ppd

17

Mental Health in Childhood and Adolescence

Lucie Ramjan and Greg Clark

KEY POINTS

- The term "childhood" spans the period from birth to adolescence. According to the World Health Organization (WHO), adolescents are aged 10–19 years; however, some health services cater to young people up to the age of 25 years. As such, in this chapter people aged 0–25 years will at times be referred to collectively as children and young people; however, the terms child, adolescent, youth and young person/people will be used as appropriate to the context.
- The prevalence of mental health conditions in the early years of life can range from 10% to 20% internationally, including in Australia and Aotearoa New Zealand.
- Anxiety and depression are among the most common mental health problems experienced by adolescents.
- Half of all mental disorders arise before the age of 14, but often go undetected. Although the highest prevalence of mental health problems occurs in 18–24-year-olds, precursors to serious mental illness that are identified and managed during childhood and adolescence (i.e. early intervention) can serve to reduce this statistic.

- Mental health problems do not occur in isolation from other aspects of children and young people's lives.
- Evidence of a child or adolescent experiencing behavioural or emotional problems may be indicative of difficulties with family, peers or school.
- It is essential to clarify the person's perception of their experiences and their goals for "treatment", as well as their parents' perceptions and desired outcomes, while working safely to protect the young person's right to confidentiality.
- "Engagement" is the establishment of a therapeutic alliance, or rapport, in collaboration with the young person and their family to achieve desired outcomes and goals. This occurs from the initial interview. Understanding young people's language and their style of communicating is integral to effectively engaging with them.
- Nurses involved in the care of children and adolescents may have to deal with legal issues relating to duty of care, child protection and mental health legislation.

KEY TERMS

Assessment
Depression
Engagement
Family

Gillick competence
Internalising and externalising problems
Psychoeducation
Psychosis

Resocialisation
Suicide

LEARNING OUTCOMES

The material in this chapter will assist you to:
- develop an introductory understanding of childhood and adolescent mental health and the mental health problems they may experience
- gain awareness of the extent of childhood and adolescent mental health problems in Australia and Aotearoa New Zealand and internationally

- appreciate the range of mental health services available to children and young people
- explore the role of nurses working with children and adolescents with mental health needs and supporting their families.

INTRODUCTION

Children and adolescents cannot simply be considered as "little adults". Within the field of mental health there are distinct differences between early life and adulthood. In recognition of the specific needs of children and young people, youth services (including mental health services) often extend their age range to include young adults up to 25 years of age.

This chapter introduces the field of child and adolescent mental health nursing. It explores the role of nurses and, using case studies from clinical practice, provides examples of disorders experienced by

children and adolescents. Furthermore, it describes interventions that nurses can implement to assist young people and their families.

Although some disorders are intergenerational (i.e. experienced by people across age groups), they may differ in their form of presentation during different developmental stages. For example, children with depression may present as agitated or with a variety of somatic symptoms, whereas adolescents with depression might appear antisocial, aggressive or withdrawn, or become involved in substance use (Rey et al 2020). Mental health concerns in adults may start in childhood or be influenced by events that occurred early in life. Some problems may resolve with neurological development, emotional maturity or a stable, supportive environment. Likewise, with effective intervention and treatment, there will be problems from which the young person can achieve a complete recovery.

Anxiety, depression and self-harm are among the most common mental health problems experienced during adolescence (World Health Organization (WHO) 2019). The onset of the first mental disorder generally occurs before 14 years in one-third of individuals (34.6%), before 18 years in nearly half (48.4%) and before 25 years in over half (62.5%) of individuals who experience mental disorders as adults (Solmi et al 2022). The highest prevalence of all mental health problems, including substance disorders, occurs in the 16–24 age group, with suicide being the third highest cause of death worldwide (Gore et al 2011; Naghavi 2019). In Australia, the COVID-19 pandemic has impacted on the psychological wellbeing of young people, and suicide and self-inflicted injury remain high in young men and anxiety disorders in young women aged 15–24 years (Australian Institute of Health and Welfare (AIHW) 2021). With statistics such as these, it is crucial that the mental health of children and young people is a priority for society as a whole.

An important factor in considering the effect of any kind of illness on young people is the disruption it may bring to their development and education. In adulthood, our lives can be dramatically impacted by illness, yet we have usually completed the basic developmental tasks of life and have finished the foundations of education. For a child or adolescent, however, various problems may develop simply due to the life interruption caused by an illness. Similarly, a child's experiences during early development and onwards can influence subsequent developmental progress, mental health and wellbeing, giving rise to problems in adolescence and later life.

Despite the prevalence of child and adolescent mental health disorders, mental health issues continue to go unrecognised and untreated in children and young people, leading to poorer outcomes in areas such as health and wellbeing, education and occupation. In addition to the human cost to the individual, their family or supports and the community, this can result in a vast economic cost to society. Specialised child and adolescent mental health services are frequently unavailable or difficult to access from regional and remote areas of Australasia; many young people are therefore unable to access appropriate early recognition and support (Oostermeijer et al 2021). It is with this in mind that health service policy, planning and models of care for children and young people should be targeted towards strategies such as mental health promotion, prevention and early intervention, to support tomorrow's adults and reduce the associated burdens to the community (Oostermeijer et al 2021; WHO 2014; 2019).

DIAGNOSIS IN CHILD AND ADOLESCENT MENTAL HEALTHCARE

Unlike previous editions of the American Psychiatric Association's *Diagnostic and Statistical Manual of Mental Disorders*, 5th edition – DSM-5 TR (2022) places emphasis on non-stigmatising language and a developmental and lifespan perspective, accepting that a significant proportion of mental health problems begin in childhood and adolescence. Symptoms exhibited by young people may be transient, dynamic and change over time, and may not always fall easily into a diagnostic category. While acknowledging that these problems are not limited to a specific age group, there is a higher frequency of occurrence during periods such as early childhood, middle childhood and adolescence. There are a range of mental health issues typically experienced in childhood and adolescence and described in the DSM-5 TR (APA 2022), including:

- neurodevelopmental disorders (e.g. attention deficit hyperactivity disorder (ADHD); autism spectrum disorder; communication disorders; specific learning disorders; tic disorders)

BOX 17.1 Child Behaviour Checklist

General Areas
- **Internalising problems:** Inhibited or over-controlled behaviours such as anxiety or depression
- **Externalising problems:** Antisocial or under-controlled behaviours such as delinquency or aggression

Specific Areas
- **Somatic complaints:** Recurring physical problems that have no known cause or cannot be medically verified; these may include headaches or a tendency to develop signs and symptoms of a medical disorder
- **Delinquent behaviour:** Behaviour where rules set by parents or communities are broken, such as property damage, theft of cars and other items
- **Attention problems:** Concentration difficulties and an inability to sit still, including school performance problems
- **Aggressive behaviour:** Bullying, teasing, fighting and temper tantrums
- **Social problems:** Where individuals have impairment of their relationships with peers
- **Withdrawal:** Where the individual is specifically inhibited by shyness and being socially isolated
- **Anxious/depressed behaviour:** A range of feelings of loneliness, sadness, feeling unloved, a sense of worthlessness, anxiety and generalised fears
- **Thought disorders:** What might be seen as bizarre behaviour or thinking

Adapted from Sawyer et al 2007.

- elimination disorders (e.g. enuresis, encopresis)
- disorders related to impulse control and conduct (e.g. conduct disorder; intermittent explosive disorder; oppositional defiant disorder)
- disorders related to trauma or other stressors (e.g. acute stress disorder; adjustment disorder; post-traumatic stress disorder; reactive attachment disorder)
- disorders related to mood (e.g. major depressive disorder, bipolar disorder) or anxiety (e.g. generalised anxiety disorder, social anxiety, separation anxiety, panic disorder)
- disorders related to feeding and eating (e.g. anorexia nervosa, avoidant/restrictive food intake disorder, binge-eating disorder, bulimia nervosa)
- disorders related to psychosis (e.g. brief psychotic disorder, delusional disorder, schizoaffective disorder, schizophrenia).

The child behaviour checklist (see Box 17.1) places stronger emphasis on behaviour and problems rather than diagnostic categories. Viewing problems within such a framework helps us understand young people as having issues related to predominant personality traits, developmental factors or incidents and influences within their family and wider social environment. By contrast, static diagnostic systems can mask the fluid, changing and reorganising nature of young people's experience as they progress towards adulthood, and may also run the risk of encouraging a focus on one "problem" in isolation, rather than exploring a child's functioning in different settings and from different sources of information (Achenbach & Ndetei 2020; Laver-Bradbury et al 2021). For this reason, this chapter describes mental health problems in the context in which symptoms are observed, rather than in relation to categorical diagnostic criteria.

INCIDENCE AND EXPRESSION OF MENTAL ILLNESS IN YOUNG PEOPLE

Writers in various western countries have often expressed concern about the prevalence of emotional problems in the earlier years of life. Within countries surveyed, the incidence ranges from 10% to 20%

(WHO 2018). This pattern is reflected in Australasia, with the Second Australian Child and Adolescent Survey of Mental Health and Wellbeing noting that 13.9% of 4- to 17-year-olds have had a mental health disorder in the past 12 months. Of this number, 59.8% had a mild mental disorder, 25.4% had a moderate disorder and 14.7% had a severe disorder (Lawrence et al 2015).

Psychosis usually emerges in late adolescence or early adulthood, with 80% of people experiencing their first episode of psychosis between the ages of 18 and 30 years (Orygen 2016). There is a small number of adolescents who experience psychosis at a younger age, but this is fortunately a rare phenomenon; fortunate, because psychosis is very disruptive to a younger adolescent's developmental trajectory and life in general. Adolescents and young people experience the same symptoms as anyone with a psychotic illness. These symptoms include thought disorder, hallucinations, delusional thinking, poor concentration, lack of energy/motivation and emotional blunting. However, not all these symptoms will be present in every young person, and it is not uncommon for younger adolescents to present with a limited range of symptoms. In many cases, there is a period of deterioration leading up to the emergence of a fully developed psychotic illness. This is known as the "prodromal" stage and intervention at this early stage is known to have long-term benefits. It is therefore important for problems to be identified as early as possible to offset the impacts that may occur with untreated psychosis. General practitioners (GPs) are often the first port of call when these subtle changes are first recognised, and efforts have been made to educate GPs to recognise these early changes (Orygen 2016).

Depression and risk of suicide are major concerns in the community, and, while the number of completed suicides of young people appeared to have decreased over the past 20 years, recent data suggests figures are again rising in western countries, with social media being a cause for concern (Jans et al 2020). In Australia, considering all causes of death in 2017, suicide accounted for 2% of deaths among males and 1.2% of deaths among females aged 0–14 years. This increased to 36.4% of deaths among males and 32.9% of deaths among females aged 15–19 years, and 38.5% of deaths among males and 30.6% of deaths among females aged 20–24 years (Australian Bureau of Statistics (ABS) 2018). Particularly vulnerable groups at risk include LGBTIQA+ youth (Rivers et al 2018) and Indigenous Australian youth (Campbell et al 2016), with a study in the Kimberley region identifying a correlation between death by suicide with the "wet season", being Indigenous, male and under the age of 25 years (Campbell et al 2016). In contrast, rates of suicide in pre-pubertal children remain very low. This is possibly due to their lack of understanding of the concept of suicide and that they are less likely to be faced with the risk factors associated with puberty.

Self-harm is reasonably common in young people, with a prevalence rate of 371.4 per 100,000 of the population among females aged 15–19 years. The highest rate for males, at 163.4 per 100,000, occurs in the 30- to 34-year age group (Hungerford et al 2018). Overall lifetime prevalence is 16.9%, with a mean starting age of 13. The most frequent reason for self-harm is to achieve relief from thoughts or feelings, and the most frequent self-harm behaviour is cutting (Gillies et al 2018), although a wide variety of self-harm behaviours are seen in practice. Young people who self-harm commonly present to GP or hospital emergency departments (EDs) to have their injuries attended to. Frequently, they are brought in or sent to hospital by parents, teachers or concerned friends.

The response of the WHO to the need for better adolescent health promotion and prevention strategies, including mental health, has been *Global Accelerated Action for the Health of Adolescents (AA-HA!): Guidance to Support Country Implementation* (2017), which provides guidance to policymakers and program managers and highlights the importance of co-production of programs *with* adolescents (WHO 2017).

✳ HISTORICAL ANECDOTE 17.1

Young People Who Experience Mental Ill Health Can Become Leaders

Clifford Beers (1876–1943) was a young person with lived experience who became a pioneer of modern community-based mental health services. When he was 18 years old and studying at Yale University in the United States, Beers' brother was diagnosed with epilepsy. Beers subsequently developed obsessional ideas and anxiety, fearing that he would develop epilepsy himself. He wrote that, "The more I considered it and him, the more nervous I became and the more nervous, the more convinced that my own breakdown was only a matter of time" (Beers 1908, pp. 7–8). Beers became so unwell that he was admitted several times to mental hospitals. His experiences within mental hospitals of the early 20th century led him to publish a memoir of his experiences titled *A Mind that Found Itself*. He went on to establish America's National Committee for Mental Hygiene, which was later renamed the National Association for Mental Health.

Read More About It
Beers CW 1908 A mind that found itself: An autobiography. Longmans, Green.

DEVELOPMENTAL ISSUES

There is a range of theories and models addressing physical, psychological and cognitive development pertaining to children and young people. Knowledge of these various models can be helpful when working with children and adolescents because they provide us with guidance about what to look for when assessing children and adolescents, as well as guide our interactions with them, based on their cognitive or emotional stage of development. For example, knowing that the capacity for abstract thinking does not develop until approximately 12 years of age can help us with the language and concepts we use with younger children. In practice, this means using terms like being "unhappy" or "sad" rather than being "depressed". Younger children can usually understand "unhappy" or "sad", whereas "depressed" is an abstract concept that they may not understand or relate to.

Physical milestones usually occur within an age range, and knowledge of these normal ranges can alert us to the need to consider potential problems. For example, most babies learn to walk between 12 and 18 months of age, and a delay in acquiring this skill may indicate a physical or cognitive problem.

Jean Piaget, a Swiss psychologist, identified a number of important milestones in a child's emotional and cognitive development. The first milestone is acquiring a sense of object permanence, which occurs around 9 months of age. The baby comes to realise that things continue to exist even when they are out of sight. This can lead to the baby becoming distressed when their primary caregiver is absent or leaves the room and helps explain why this behaviour begins around the age of 9 months. Between 18 months and 24 months, children develop the capacity for symbolic play and use their imagination in play. This is frequently the time when young children begin to develop their language skills and they can therefore describe what is happening in their play. Language involves using symbols to represent something else, so it is not surprising that these developments occur at around the same time.

Around the age of 7 years, children develop an understanding of the conservation of volume. This is a further development of symbolic thinking. For example, if you show a younger child a tall, skinny container and a low, wide container, they will invariably tell you that the tall skinny container contains more liquid. Once they develop understanding of conservation of volume, they realise this is not always the case and the child may experiment with the containers to determine which has the largest volume.

The final stage in Piaget's framework is developing the capacity for abstract thinking at around 12 years of age. Piaget described this as being capable of reasoning, not only based on objects but also on the basis of hypotheses or of propositions (Piaget 1962). The capacity for abstract thinking is a sign of sound cognitive development and informs us that the child is developing as expected.

There are other developmental models including the social ecological model (Bronfenbrenner 1979; 1992) where complex relationships within the child's social environment, such as family, school, health services, social and cultural norms, all influence development. Piaget's model and the social ecological model are probably the more useful approaches in mental health work, but it is not the only way to think about developmental issues. Those who have an interest in this area can investigate other possibilities, such as Freud's psychosexual developmental theory, Erikson's psychosocial developmental theory, Bowlby's attachment theory and Bandura's social learning theory.

Knowledge of developmental processes and normal ranges can help us identify any delays in development. Delays can be due to a range of factors, including difficulties during the birthing process, such as restricted oxygen intake resulting from compression of the umbilical cord, or from exposure to domestic violence or poor caregiving. The importance of responsive caregiving, early learning, optimal nutrition and supporting maternal mental health in promoting child development cannot be underestimated (WHO 2020). Nurses can play a key role in early identification and resolution of problems in these areas. It is important for all nurses in all clinical settings to identify and delineate the nature of any developmental concerns and make referrals to the most appropriate service.

 CRITICAL THINKING EXERCISE 17.1

1. Why do nurses (general and specialist) have such a vital role to play in early detection of mental health problems in children and young people?
2. What interventions might nurses (general and specialist) provide?

MENTAL ILLNESS IN CONTEXT

Because mental health issues can affect many aspects of young people's lives, their experiences must be seen in context. It is often the case that the more significant the mental health concern, the greater the possibility of complications and impacts in other areas of life. Furthermore, parents and other family members' wellbeing, lifestyle and activities (such as employment) may be affected. While more needs to be understood about the long-term outlook for these young people, it is important for professionals to see the problems in the context of the child's everyday experiences. For example, help may be needed across a broad range of life issues, including with family functioning, social skills or school. While the mental health problem may have caused the difficulties, it is equally important to consider that a life issue may have been the trigger *or* a contributing factor in the development of the disorder. We need to understand the context to inform prevention strategies (Gunnell et al 2018). We must take a balanced view so that causal factors are not attributed to one area without adequately observing what is happening in other aspects of the young person's life. It may be that the issues the child or adolescent is presenting with are acting as a "barometer" for broader concerns; for example, the young person may be presenting with symptoms that reflect problems in the family or between parents. This may not be recognised initially and may be revealed only after exploration over time, which is why exploring the family's functioning and coping skills is an important aspect of assessment.

 HISTORICAL ANECDOTE 17.2

Historical Labels

In 1856 French psychiatrist Benedict Morel began describing young people exhibiting signs of mental ill health as experiencing "dementia praecox" (meaning precocious or early dementia). In 1902, German psychiatrist Emil Kraepelin (1956–1926) used the term "dementia praecox" to differentiate psychosis from what he referred to as manic depression (bipolar disorder). Morel and Kraepelin linked "dementia" with psychotic features because they theorised that the illness was neurologically based, like forms of dementia, and that the clinical pathway led to deterioration and chronicity, similar to dementia. This view was far from optimistic, and the prognosis left minimal hope for the individual's recovery. It is more widely accepted today that it is possible for young people who experience episodes of mental ill health to recover.

Read More About It

Kendler KS 2018 The development of Kraepelin's mature diagnostic concepts of paranoia and paranoid dementia praecox: A close reading of his textbooks from 1887 to 1899. JAMA Psychiatry 75(12), 1280–1288.

ASSESSMENT AND CARE PLANNING

A myriad of factors contribute to and affect the mental health of young people, which can make assessing the mental health of children and young people very complex. Familial or genetic predisposition to mental illness, the presence of a coexisting medical or neurological problem, developmental problems or growing up in a chaotic or deprived environment, are just a few of the considerations nurses should be mindful of during assessments of young people and their families. These factors will also affect the direction taken with goal planning and nursing interventions.

It may not be the young person who identifies a specific problem or seeks assistance. Rather, referrals are often received from an adult (parent, teacher, health worker) presenting their view of the problem, thus providing an interpretation of what they perceive is occurring for the child. It is the responsibility of the nurse to then establish a therapeutic alliance with all parties involved, ensuring each person feels heard, valued and respected.

Assessment of a young person will follow a similar structure to that undertaken in an adult mental health context. In the process of gathering information, an assessment should include not only talking with the child or young person on their own, but also asking their consent to talk to others (and explaining the rationale for this), such as their parents, carers, friends and teachers, to gain alternative perspectives. It is helpful to obtain relevant information from several people, given that problems may be interpreted and represented in a variety of ways by others involved in a child's life. Using a biopsychosocial assessment approach can be time-consuming and is often best managed over several short sessions, rather than in one go.

A sound knowledge of expected developmental milestones enables the nurse to differentiate between the responses and developmental challenges of life and the significant psychological problems that may be occurring. Many mental health problems in children and young people may go undetected because signs of the problem are exhibited through their behaviour, physical manifestations or school performance. Exploring the prevalence, persistence, pervasiveness and negative impact of the problem helps appraise and conceptualise its nature and severity so that appropriate interventions can be implemented.

Similarly, gaining an appreciation of the hopes, fears and expectations of each person present – while exploring strengths and protective factors, parenting styles and relationships between family members – can assist in placing the identified problems in context. For example, issues such as poverty, unemployment, parental substance misuse and cultural isolation can all have a detrimental impact on a child's mental health. Therefore, it is important to collect information that enables the nurse to see the problem through a wider lens, so they can work effectively with the child and family (Mitchell 2022).

Discrete observation plays a critical role when assessing mood and behaviour, and children and adolescents' interactions with peers, family, friends and others. Behaviour and the information provided may not always be congruent, so observing interactions, non-verbal communication and each person's responses can highlight family dynamics and lead to further understanding of what may be happening for the young person within their family or their other social contexts. Observation of these factors, considered in the broader psychosocial context, will enable the nurse to achieve a more comprehensive understanding of the factors contributing to the current difficulties experienced by the young person and their family. Ongoing discussion with parents (carers) should clarify which specific factors may be contributing to the person's current experience.

Finally, assessing risk is an essential part of any child and adolescent mental health assessment (Mares & Woodgate 2020). In Australia and Aotearoa New Zealand, health professionals are required by law to report any children who they believe are at risk. Mental health nurses therefore have a statutory obligation to report any suspicion of risk to a child or young person with whom they are working. Significant harm or the likelihood of experiencing significant harm from abuse (physical, sexual, emotional, neglect or a combination) must be reported. To ensure a unified response, multi-agency collaboration and cohesion is essential in cases where abuse is suspected or disclosed. Risk assessment cannot be achieved through a "tick box" exercise, since risks concerning children and adolescents are often multifactorial and complex. Risk must be assessed not only from a mental health perspective, but also within the caregiving context. Risk factors can include an immediate threat to the child's safety, as in cases of child abuse, or be cumulative, such as a child who is exposed to multiple risk factors such as adversity, neglect, parental illness or family violence.

Being sensitive to the presence of child abuse and the impact of abuse on a child's health and psychological wellbeing is essential in any assessment. The long-term effect of abuse and associated trauma can have profound consequences on brain development, leading to mental health problems, drug and alcohol dependence and associated risk-taking (Child Welfare Information Gateway 2019).

It can be helpful to have a framework from which all aspects of the assessment are completed (see example in Box 17.2). Ultimately, undertaking a comprehensive mental health assessment will enable the mental health nurse to gather the facts and ensure that any decisions made are in the best interests of the child and family.

With a more specific diagnosis and an understanding of all the issues that the young person is experiencing, the nurse and family may

begin the process of exploring solutions (planning), and referral to mental health services may be warranted. Any solutions agreed with the family are best implemented with the family's support and commitment, maximising the probability of positive change.

SERVICES AVAILABLE TO CHILDREN AND YOUNG PEOPLE

In many western countries, specialised input is most often provided by child and adolescent mental health services (CAMHS) or child and youth mental health services (CYMHS), or mental health services targeted specifically towards young people (such as Headspace in Australia). These services have expanded their scope considerably, offering a range of specialist assessment and treatment options. A limitation remains that these services are often found only in metropolitan areas. However, regional and remote areas throughout Australia and Aotearoa New Zealand may have the benefit of eCYMHS and other services, with access to online psychiatry, nursing and allied health input.

To offer a comprehensive stepped care service that meets the mental health needs of children and adolescents, universal services (such as primary health care, education and social and community workers) need to identify those at risk of, and those who are experiencing early symptoms, and effectively implement mental health promotion, prevention and early intervention strategies. These professionals, by the nature of their roles, work daily with children and adolescents and are in a prime position to recognise and manage mental health issues early in their development. A range of broad psychosocial strategies, education and general advice can be offered, and those experiencing more complex mental health issues can be identified and referred to specialist services as required.

This stepped care approach is consistent with the pyramid framework, as advocated by the World Health Organization (2009) (see Fig. 17.1). When planning and organising service delivery, involving people such as nurses working in general practice, rural and remote nurses, teachers, social workers, GPs and youth workers would reflect the largest tier of the multilayer pyramid (universal informal community

---

BOX 17.2 Example of a Framework to Guide the Assessment Process

- Presenting concerns
- Family history
- Social history
- Developmental assessment
- Cultural issues
- Psychometric tools
- Mental state assessment
- Observation of interactions
- Risk assessment

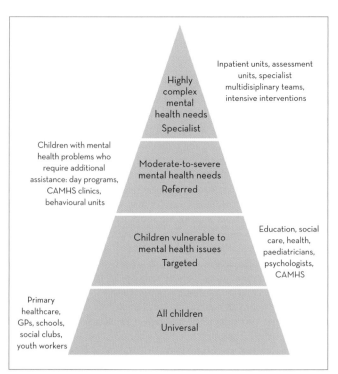

FIG. 17.1 A Stepped Approach to Care Based on a Pyramid Framework of Healthcare Delivery. (Adapted from WHO 2009.)

care). This tier represents services that are frequently needed and includes interventions that can be provided at a moderately low cost. Nurses working in EDs and generalist clinical settings, and child and family nurses, can provide primary care mental health services (universal and targeted support), which may include digital self-help and supported self-help interventions. The top tier of the pyramid reflects specialist services, which are often expensive and required for only a small percentage of children and young people; for example, those with moderate to severe and highly complex mental health disorders, who require input from specialist health professionals such as mental health nurses (Pretorius et al 2019; Servili 2020). Nationally in Australia and Aotearoa New Zealand, there is active collaboration among the various government and community-based agencies providing care to young people and their families, resulting in considerably less overlap or duplication of services. This has led to various inter-agency education and training opportunities for workers in the field.

For adolescents, in particular, simply providing a traditional outpatient or in-patient service may not be enough. Many teenagers worry about what others would think if they asked for help, while others say they prefer to take care of their own problems, as they struggle with their sense of identity and relationships with adults. A variety of unhealthy or "at-risk" behaviours may be present. Despite the National Drug Strategy Household Survey (AIHW 2020) reporting a decline in the use of tobacco, alcohol and illicit substances in young people, prevalence rates remain fairly high and show a rise in cannabis use. This highlights the need for more collaboration and more funding for generalised adolescent health services and outreach programs that can support young people with mild-to-moderate mental health issues.

In some centres in Australia and Aotearoa New Zealand, there are adolescent health centres where no appointment is needed, and teenagers can attend unaccompanied. These centres provide a wide range of services and programs for all health and lifestyle matters. They are often based on a model of primary care promoting early intervention for several health needs and are delivered by a range of multidisciplinary professionals. Such a place in Australia is Headspace, a national youth mental health foundation (see Useful websites), which offers a youth-friendly environment where young people with mental health issues can attend for a range of issues, such as general health, mental health, drug and alcohol issues and education or vocational support (Perera et al 2019; Rickwood et al 2019). Headspace has been so effective in working with young people that a number of primary and tertiary health services have adopted its assessment interview, known as HEEADSSS (Home, Education and Employment, Activities, Drugs, Sexuality, Suicide/Depression, Safety) to assist in identifying psychosocial and mental health issues (Hirani et al 2018).

There is variation between regional services in the types of intervention and treatments available. As with adult services, there is usually a range of walk-in clinics and mobile crisis and support teams, backed up by separate residential units for adolescents and for children; some with programs for families to be admitted in specific circumstances. However, there are significant barriers to access primary mental health providers, especially in regional and remote areas where there are often limited mental health professionals, with long waiting lists and frequently gap fees that are prohibitive.

Treatment provided also varies from centre to centre, depending on what has led the young people to present, their age, the treatment philosophy, theoretical models, expertise available and the living circumstances of the young person and their family. Interventions may include cognitive behaviour therapy (CBT), play therapy, psycho-dynamic individual or group work, socialisation and social skills programs, systems-based family therapy, couples therapy, parenting programs or individual therapy for a parent. Sometimes approaches are combined to achieve better outcomes. For example, a child may benefit from CBT to help

them, while their parents and siblings may benefit from learning positive ways of functioning together. As with adult services, nurses have a range of roles, often developing expertise in various modes of therapy.

THE NURSING ROLE

Children and adolescents are still developing as individuals, so an intervention while they are young can often have a dramatic positive impact for the rest of their life. Early intervention is often more effective than managing difficulties that have extended into adulthood. With adequate care and a supportive environment, young people can develop resilience – emotionally, psychologically and physically. All nurses have a key role in implementing stepped care arrangements, including services for young people with, or at risk of, mental illness.

Working within a child and adolescent mental health team provides the opportunity to use a wide range of dynamic clinical treatment strategies and therapies. A multidisciplinary team approach is most frequently used. Nurses often play a significant role in various aspects of care, including that of therapist for children, adolescents and families. It is usually expected that a nurse wishing to enter this field will have some years of experience as a mental health nurse and further education, therefore possessing a solid grounding in theory and clinical practice.

Apart from graduate nursing programs, child and adolescent mental health nurses have options available for advanced studies in specialist areas of mental health through postgraduate and Master's programs. In addition, nurses can take further training in counselling programs, such as family therapy, solution-focused therapy and psychotherapy. Australian child and adolescent mental health services require workers with a high level of knowledge and skills. While Australia does not currently have a set of national competencies relating specifically to nursing in child and young people mental health settings, services have adopted guidelines for practice based on the standards of practice developed by the Australian College of Mental Health Nurses (2010). Likewise, some states have developed a competency framework based on those already developed in Aotearoa New Zealand (NSW Ministry of Health 2011; Wharaurau 2021). These frameworks acknowledge the unique knowledge and skills regarded as fundamental for all professionals and focus on a number of universal key areas, each with further identified core knowledge and skills to work effectively with children and young people experiencing mental health problems. See Perspectives in practice: Nurse's story 17.1 for a nurse's experience of working with young people.

Identifying Vulnerable Children and Young People

Parental illness, and specifically mental illness, may have a significant impact on a child's life and mental health. For example, the child may have to take on extra responsibilities, may experience inconsistent parenting or may observe behaviour that is difficult to comprehend, depending on their age. As a result, children of parents who have a mental illness often have social, emotional and psychological support needs that are different from those of children with healthy parents, or those with parents who have chronic physical health conditions. Research has shown that some adult children of parents with mental illness recalled childhood experiences of fear and mistrust, loneliness and isolation that continued into adulthood (Murphy et al 2018). Over many years the Australian Infant, Child, Adolescent and Family Mental Health Association has campaigned for support for these young people. Since 2001 the Australian Government has provided funds for an initiative known as Children of Parents with a Mental Illness (COPMI) to enable the provision and sharing of resources and support for various groups around Australia working with these families (see Useful websites).

PERSPECTIVES IN PRACTICE

Nurse's Story 17.1: Kristin Henderson

As an experienced mental health nurse, I'd regarded myself as a spontaneous, reflective clinician, confident that my interactions with patients were at all times respectful, helpful and kind. I was taken by surprise, then, when I began working with young people in an inpatient mental health setting – surprised that I now felt hesitant and doubtful about how to respond. What was appropriate? What would be a better response? My confidence and spontaneity had given way to feeling stilted and unsure … until a defining moment when I realised that I should open my senses to cues within myself and from others, taking time to reflect upon what I was seeing in myself. This could deepen my understanding of how others see themselves. This is my story…

With his bath finished and his pyjamas on, 8-year-old Cobey and I stand in front of the full-length mirror looking straight at ourselves, occasionally glancing across at each other's reflection, then back to our own. As we look at our reflections, I wonder what we are really seeing. I see myself: Casually dressed, complete and unchanging … oh, and looking a wee bit tired! I suspect that Cobey, like me, sees an image of himself, but I can only speculate what self-image that might be…

I kneel down beside Cobey to try to observe his reflection as he might be seeing it. I note a small crack in the glass near where Cobey is standing. The mirror has been damaged, but because of the safety component of the glass, it has not shattered but simply absorbed the knock, leaving three fractures darting out from the one stress point. As I had anticipated, his image is disjointed, and the symbolic implications momentarily tug at me.

"What do you see?" I ask quietly.

No answer. He continues looking into the broken mirror. He is observing fragmented self – lots of small pieces, together, but not quite. He moves bodily up and down and sideways, all the time trying to piece together his reflection in a harmonious union. But it is not to be – whichever position he views himself from, he is in several pieces, a fragmented whole.

"I'm in pieces … nothing fits together properly," he eventually says, giggling. Then for a few more minutes he moves about, trying to find where he might place himself so that the pieces of him do come together, as they should. In a short while, in frustration, he curses the mirror and leaves the room. I stand stunned. Cobey's complex and distressing childhood history symbolically laid bare before the mirror. So much about us both, reflected in this brief encounter.

Other groups of children who may be deemed vulnerable, or at increased risk of developing mental health problems, include: children in care, such as those in foster care or residential care homes, or who are adopted; young offenders; young people with a physical or intellectual disability; young people from culturally diverse backgrounds; homeless children; refugees and asylum seekers; and young people with diverse sexual orientation or gender identity experiences (Australian Health Ministers' Advisory Council 2013). In responding to children and young people who present with complex needs, nurses may need to work with several agencies, each with a different agenda. Under these circumstances, it is important that the nurse remains flexible and has clear guidelines for what is expected in their role.

Perinatal Mental Health Nursing

Historically, perinatal mental health included only the postpartum stage of childbirth with a focus on the mother's mental health and wellbeing. As more evidence arises, there is a better understanding that both mother and baby require sensitive assessment and the earliest possible intervention to maximise mental wellness for them both. Perinatal mental health encompasses not only the mental health of the mother and the child but also the child–mother relationship, the emotional and psychological wellbeing of other family members and social factors that may impact on

the overall health of individuals within the family. Starting from preconception, perinatal mental health includes the antenatal and the postnatal periods, usually until the child is 24 months old. However, an Australian study shows that women experience mental health symptoms in pregnancy and well beyond the 24-month period, with the highest symptoms after the child has reached 4–5 years of age (Bryson et al 2021).

Nevertheless, whether a mother has a pre-existing mental health condition or develops one in the antenatal or postnatal stage, it can have direct and indirect consequences for the child. Research indicates that mothers experiencing mental distress may not be as sensitive or responsive to their infant's needs and can struggle to complete several activities associated with caring for an infant (Sliwerski et al 2020). With a strong evidence base demonstrating the importance of secure attachments between a child and their primary caregiver, interactions between a mother experiencing mental illness and her infant can have a detrimental impact on the bonding relationship. Evidence also suggests that the children of mothers who experience longer term illness, such as postnatal depression, may be prone to experiencing developmental delays in areas such as social functioning, language, cognition and behaviour (Goodman 2019).

Recent advances in screening for perinatal mental health issues and a multitude of training courses designed to identify and manage perinatal issues in primary care are now available throughout Australia. Midwives and nurses in all clinical settings need to be aware of mental health during the perinatal period and use these opportunities to identify, assess and refer as necessary. The role of a mental health nurse working in child and adolescent mental health services is to assess and take account of any perinatal mental health issues when undertaking a psychosocial assessment. Part of planning care for a child or young person may involve referring the mother or carer to a more appropriate service to manage their own mental health.

ENGAGING WITH CHILDREN AND ADOLESCENTS

Mental health nurses can become a significant resource for their clients. To be able to intervene effectively, the nurse needs to master the art of engaging with children and young people as individuals and with their parents or carers, in the context of *their* families. *Engagement* is the process of forming a relationship based on person-centred interactions where there is an ongoing conversation or acknowledgement of a partnership (Doherty et al 2020). Engagement between the nurse, the young person and their family is fundamental to developing a relationship based on trust. A relationship founded on trust will foster a willingness to work together towards change. This involves communicating in a way that is appropriate within the context of the child's development (Wharaurau 2021). For example, the communication skills and language used when working with a 5-year-old would differ significantly from those used when working with a 16-year-old. Essentially the nurse is required to master a diverse range of communication skills that not only encourages children and teenagers to listen, but also foster effective active listening so that the young person is more likely to communicate in response.

An important element of engagement is rapport building, which encompasses not only the formal aspects of mental health care, such as completing a diagnostic interview, but also the social interactions and non-verbal communications that occur. Geldard and colleagues (2018) state that non-verbal forms of communication may be more significant than verbal interactions when interviewing and engaging young people with mental health problems.

The full participation of young people and their family in their mental health care is more likely in environments where young people feel welcomed and valued. Organisations have a lot to learn from consumers about planning environments that are sensitive to the needs of young people. "Family-friendly" environments also need to include processes that respond to the specific needs of younger people, in particular those who are experiencing significant emotional or mental health difficulties.

Engaging young people and families across cultural contexts is key to relationship building, accurate diagnoses and comprehensive treatment planning. There are implications for the way in which mental health professionals approach assessing clients and families in both Australia and Aotearoa New Zealand. The nurse's understanding of (and attempts to understand) specific cultural practices and beliefs held by clients is imperative to developing trust and will promote confidence in the care provided. This requires the nurse to ask for information in such a way that recognises cultural norms, practice in a culturally safe way, and acknowledge that the person's perspectives and understanding may be different to their own. Clients are more likely to provide accurate information if they believe the nurse has an understanding of their cultural needs and a genuine respect and commitment to a recovery plan that is culturally sound.

Engagement Issues Specific to Adolescents

When adolescents and their family (carers) present to a healthcare facility, there is an expectation on their part that treatment will achieve the desired outcomes, in terms of the physical, emotional and mental state of the young person. However, it is possible that these outcomes may not be achieved because of many situational factors. One such factor may be the young person's lack of willingness to be part of the referral, assessment and treatment process due to shame, guilt or embarrassment, or to not recognising or acknowledging that a significant problem exists. Nurses working with adolescents need to acknowledge that possible influencing factors such as poor insight, resistance to treatment or challenging of authority may be part of normal adolescent behaviour. Mental health nurses should attempt to form a relationship with the young person through engagement and foster a sense of purpose with the treatment plan.

Language and Engagement

Language is the key to open communication and creating an environment that can augment engagement. Keep in mind that young people may still be determining who they are and their identity; be it sexual or gender identity. So communicating in a respectful and inclusive way by using gender-neutral language and asking the young person what pronoun/s they prefer (she, her, hers/they, them, theirs) is important in building trust. Young people may use language and jargon that differs according to their age group or subculture, especially when it comes to "street lingo". They may have a culture that at times seems alien to their parents, caregivers and health professionals. Young people, particularly adolescents, may use words and phrases that have a significantly different meaning from that to which adults may be accustomed – for example, "sick", "deadly", "bad" or "gross" may mean "good". Health professionals may need to clarify with the young person what they actually mean by their phrases or words, if the professional does not understand them. This may be particularly relevant when discussing illicit drugs and the street names used for marijuana, amphetamines or hallucinogens. Understanding language and communicating effectively is integral to engaging with young people and vital to the success of their ongoing treatment.

Nurses should also be aware that language that is used in mental health services and about mental illness can be confronting for young people and their families. For example, psychosis (rather than schizophrenia) is the preferred term for use in child and adolescent mental health services and in early intervention services for young people with first-episode presentations. This is due to the negative associations and stigma attached to the term "schizophrenia" (as well as the fact that some people experience an acute and transitory episode of psychosis that does not meet the criteria for a schizophrenia diagnosis and which resolves completely). It is important to provide information in a sensitive way that aims to reduce the negative impacts and experiences that may occur at what is, for most, a very difficult time.

WORKING WITH FAMILIES

Nurses working with children and adolescents experiencing mental health issues should be aware that it is best that this client group should, if possible and appropriate, not be seen, assessed or treated in isolation. Ideally, nurses and all members of the family who have a significant role within the household should be included. This ensures the "identified consumer" is not treated as the family scapegoat. A family scapegoat is used to divert attention away from other problems that may exist in a family, such as difficulties in the parental relationships. It is also the case that children and adolescents live within and depend on their families for sustenance and emotional support, and families need to be involved in helping their young person manage whatever difficulties they face. At times, this may involve changes in the way the family operates in terms of support and discipline. Therefore, a major component of the nursing role is involving the family in treatment through family work.

Families are often unaware of what they can do or need to do to support their young person. Ultimately, families provide the lion's share of support for their family members, and supporting them to do this in an effective and helpful way can have significant benefits for both the young person and the family. In addition, it is important to be aware of the effects that a diagnosis of mental illness in their young family member can have on families. They may respond to this with feelings of grief that their child's future potential may be lost or fear about what will happen over time. Family members may also feel helpless in knowing what to do to help their family member achieve their dreams and aspirations and to manage the day-to-day impacts of the illness. It is important for us to understand how the family reacts to the diagnosis, so we can support them through this process.

It should be remembered that the nursing care plan is in fact a recovery plan for the young person and family; therefore, the goals must be achievable, the plan must be collaboratively developed and the strategies must be practical and able to be implemented by the child and parents (with nursing support). If the plan is based on what the nurse can achieve rather than what the young person and their family want and can realistically accomplish, then the medium- to long-term success for recovery may be severely impaired and continuity of care lost.

In recent times there has been a shift in focus towards family-centred mental health nursing, which includes family-based assessments and treatments, spreading the attention across the whole family rather than focusing on the identified client. Family work is based on the principles of family therapy, which requires a specific way of working and requires specialist training.

Case studies 17.1 to 7.3, and the exploration of the issues discussed, illustrate some key concepts.

CASE STUDY 17.1: Adam

A mother takes her four-year-old daughter for an immunisation and mentions to the general practice nurse that she's worried about her 9-year-old son, Adam, who she describes as "becoming increasingly anxious" and who has developed "a fixation with tidiness", so much so that it is causing disruption in the family. The family consists of two female siblings, aged 11 and 4, and a father who is an accomplished musician and frequently travels for extended periods performing

Continued

CASE STUDY 17.1:   Adam—cont'd

nationally and internationally. The nurse empathises with the mother and validates her concerns, referring her to the GP and recommending she contacts the community CYMHS. The mother decides to contact CYMHS. The mental health nurse receiving the call assures the mother that her concerns warrant a further assessment by a member of the mental health team, as her child appears to be highly anxious. He is unable to relax and appears to be developing maladaptive behaviours (excessive tidying). Furthermore, his anxiety is having an adverse effect on his relationship with his siblings. The nurse gathers more specific information by phone and explains to the mother that this referral will be discussed at the next team meeting and that she will receive a call within a week regarding an appointment for her, her husband and their son, for further assessment.

Discussion of Case Study: Adam

Within the first minutes of a mother's description of her son's problem, the mental health nurse was able to predict a role for the mental health team in assisting this family. The mother was assured that her concerns were well founded. The nurse spent a little more time gathering only the information necessary to discuss the case (assessment) with the clinical team so a plan for a further face-to-face interview could be made. The mother was reassured by the prospect of another appointment (implementation) and felt her initial concerns had been validated. A therapeutic alliance has been initiated between the family and the mental health service.

This early process reflects the beginning of the nurse's role in engaging the family in the therapeutic alliance and emphasises how important each team member's role is in promoting a positive impression on the family (even before meeting them personally). The impression the family gains from an initial phone call can colour their perception of further interactions with the mental health team. Furthermore, the parents' feelings of confidence in the mental health nurse and other team members will most likely have an impact on the confidence that the child and siblings experience. This is important because all family members will be involved in the child's recovery.

The foundation and building of a therapeutic relationship with the young person and the family will usually begin at the time of the initial phone call or face-to-face interview. This interview can be difficult for the young person, who may not perceive that there is a problem and therefore may not fully understand why they are attending an assessment at a mental health service. A skilled mental health nurse will use this opportunity to establish the young person's understanding of their need for an appointment. If the young person seems unsure (or unwilling to concede), they can often be encouraged to describe some difficulties that are occurring at home that they think may have led to their needing this appointment.

It is essential to clarify the child or young person's perception of the problem and their goals for treatment, as well as those of the parents. The nurse's role is to facilitate expression of the difficulties and to make explicit the goal(s) that the client and family have regarding recovery. This is necessary so that all parties (child, family and mental health team) agree on the treatment plan.

Case study 17.2 illustrates these key issues. While a diagnosis such as attention deficit hyperactivity disorder might possibly be indicated in this situation, the case illustrates that it is important to concentrate on the presenting problems and any associated difficulties, rather than giving priority to diagnostic classification. Involving diagnostic controversies can potentially misdirect the focus of care from the individual needs of the child and family.

CASE STUDY 17.2:   Tim

Tim is a 6-year-old boy who is attending his first appointment at a community CYMHS, accompanied by his parents. He is the oldest of three children and has a young brother and baby sister. His parents report an escalation in Tim's behaviour just before he turned three: "It's like he never grew out of the 'terrible twos'. He just kept on going at a hundred miles an hour," reported his mother. Tim's father concurred: "The more limits I set, the worse he gets." Tim's reply when asked if he knew why he was here was simply: "I've been naughty."

Discussion of Case Study: Tim

A skilled mental health nurse will attempt to clarify these comments using objective language and will eventually identify specific behaviours that the parents regard as priorities for change. The nurse will attempt to match the parents' goals with those of their son.

The nurse's response to Tim's perception that he has been "naughty" might be: "Naughty? What do you mean?" The aim for the nurse is to guide Tim to use specific words to tag specific behaviours, and if these match those identified by his parents, a simple goal may be developed to achieve an outcome that is satisfying to both parties. Tim's descriptions of how he sees what's going on may also help the nurse to establish more accurately what the relevant issues might be. Consider this further exchange between Tim and the nurse:

Nurse: Naughty? What does that mean?

Tim: When I run away or squeal.

Nurse: So, you run away?

Tim: My brother … he's three. He runs away too. When he runs away from Mummy, she chases him.

Nurse: And does your brother squeal?

Tim: No, but when my baby sister squeals, Daddy helps Mummy play with her.

This exchange demonstrates how, through active listening, the nurse has gathered some very specific information about the family dynamics that provides a possible explanation for some of Tim's behaviour. It could be that he is mimicking the behaviours of his younger siblings to receive the same attention from his parents that he perceives his brother and sister receive when they run away or squeal.

Encounters with children and adolescents and their families, as illustrated in these case studies, demonstrate how the nurse and other team members can engage young people in ongoing treatment, and how treatment will be influenced by further findings. Initiating a sound therapeutic alliance with the child and family is an achievement, although the alliance also requires nurturing.

Generally, a therapeutic alliance is accomplished when respect is paramount in the nurse–client relationship. Like adults, young people respond most positively to being treated with genuine respect. Young people feel respected when they are listened to and given opportunities to make choices and contribute to solving problems. As Roberts and colleagues (2015) identify, making choices gives the child valuable practice in making decisions, and opportunities for problem solving give them courage to follow things through independently. A commitment by the mental health nurse to facilitating choice and promoting problem-solving opportunities for young people will be further enhanced by a belief in the humanistic idea that all behaviour has meaning. If mental health nurses explore the meaning behind the behaviours we observe, we can plan appropriate strategies to modify behaviour and promote positive change.

Within Australia and Aotearoa New Zealand, CYMHS work with many young people who present in acute emotional distress. Some will internalise their distress and may become withdrawn and depressed. Others may externalise their emotional pain. When this occurs, the child will demonstrate altered behaviours, which may include rigid thinking, compulsive patterns of behaviour, agitation, impulsivity and, in severe cases, aggression. If the nurse has established a therapeutic alliance with the child, the shared trust and respect will provide a foundation for choice-giving and problem solving. An example from practice (Case study 17.3) will best illustrate this concept.

CASE STUDY 17.3: Fiona

Fiona is 12 years old and is attending the CYMHS for the first time, accompanied by her mother, with whom she lives. Her younger brother has lived with their father since their parents separated 3 years ago. Fiona's mother is extremely concerned about a gradual change in Fiona's mood over the past 2 years. She has reportedly become angry and unpredictable, a dramatic change from the quiet but confident child she used to be. Her mother describes instances where Fiona will impulsively run from home and engage in risky behaviours such as riding her bike recklessly on their busy street. When met by members of the mental health team, Fiona is at first passive, refusing eye contact, seeming to ignore the conversation between her mother and the nurse and refusing to respond when spoken to directly. Several times during the conversation, however, Fiona interrupts with a hostile comment, countering information provided by her mother.

Discussion of Case Study: Fiona
Skills Required
Even though Fiona is refusing to be involved in the initial assessment, her behaviour and her brief interjections are a valuable source of assessment information. The nurse will document Fiona's behaviour and her comments. In context, this will reflect some family dynamics and give some indication of how Fiona currently feels about life. The challenge for the nurse will be to initially engage Fiona in a shared interest of hers that is non-emotional and therefore less threatening.

Rather than attempting to engage Fiona too early, the nurse wisely chooses to wait for an opportunity. This does not arise until the very end of the initial interview, when the nurse announces that the assessment is almost complete.

"About time", Fiona grumbles, "I just want to get in the car and listen to my new CD." The nurse grasps this opportunity:

Nurse: Ah, a new CD … which group?
Fiona: No one you'd know.
Nurse: Maybe not … but try me.

To Fiona's surprise, the nurse has recently bought the same CD and although Fiona feigns horror that an adult would even know the band, she cannot completely disguise her admiration.

Nurse: See you in a fortnight then?
Fiona: If I'm not too busy with my music.

Fiona's choice of words ("If I'm not too busy …") indicates that she is trying to sound uninterested while still leaving her options open.

Approach Taken and Outcome Achieved
Children and adolescents are not always easily engaged. Often the factors contributing to their need for mental health support have affected their ability to trust others; in many cases they have felt let down by adults. The nurse who recognises this will allow time for the young person to engage, initially on their own terms, so the fragile therapeutic alliance can gradually strengthen. Fiona's hostility was ignored; the nurse chose instead to preserve Fiona's fragile sense of dignity. Respecting Fiona's ability to make sound decisions, the nurse did not assume that she would be returning in a fortnight, but rather posed it as a question; this approach was aimed at reassuring Fiona that she had a choice. Her choice to return in a fortnight would demonstrate her courage in recognising that a problem exists and her willingness to explore some supports.

🅠 CRITICAL THINKING EXERCISE 17.2

1. What might the outcomes have been if the nurse had persisted in asking Fiona questions early in the interview?
2. What assumptions could be made regarding Fiona's need to interrupt while her mother and the nurse were speaking?

In some cases, family work is contraindicated. This applies where there is violence or physical abuse in a family or where there is a suspicion of sexual abuse. Engaging all members of the family in therapeutic work can have negative consequences for the young person because they may be held responsible for exposing the family to outside scrutiny.

Family therapy has been constantly evolving since its inception in the middle of the 20th century. Traditionally, it has focused on the identified problems with the child or adolescent and how the family has dealt with these issues from a particular theoretical perspective. There is a wide variety of theoretical frameworks operating in the family therapy space, and family therapists usually adhere to the framework in which they are trained. Family therapy works within the following principles:

- Problems in families are best understood and treated from a circular rather than a linear perspective. A linear perspective uses a straightforward cause-and-effect relationship, whereas a circular approach considers all contributing factors, some of which may not seem, on the surface, to be directly related to the issues at hand. For example, difficulties in the parental relationship may be played out through relationships with the children, particularly where one child is favoured above others by one of the parents.
- Families experiencing problems need to be supported to develop their own problem-solving abilities.
- The ability of family members to change depends on their ability to alter their perception of the problem.
- A family's understanding of problems does not itself lead to changes in behaviour.

- A therapeutic context for change must be created for families.
- Problems or symptoms may serve a positive family function.
- Outcomes are more positive if problems are treated from an eco-systemic perspective (Dallos & Draper 2015).

From these key aspects of family involvement, nurses can formulate their own methods of working with families that best suit their clinical environment. Undertaking family work can be both challenging and rewarding. It is recommended that nurses involved in such work or working in child and adolescent teams undertake specialist training and engage in ongoing clinical supervision to ensure that optimal patient/family–nurse relationships are maintained and that the family achieves their desired outcomes.

Working with families is discussed in more detail in Chapter 5.

EDUCATION AND PSYCHOSOCIAL INTERVENTION

Adolescence is a period of rapid development encompassing a range of important tasks such as achieving a sense of individuality and independence, which can be derailed by a mental illness. It is also the time when adolescents are engaged in education, and any disruption to this process can have long-term consequences. Maintaining the young person's connections with their peer group and education has short- and long-term benefits. Some special education facilities for young people with mental health problems are available, and these should be sought out and accessed whenever possible. These facilities provide a more personalised approach and usually have smaller classes with specially trained teachers who have expertise in educating young people with special needs. Where these specialist schools are not available, the mental health nurse might work with the school counsellor and classroom teachers to help ensure the young person remains connected to their education.

Another option is distance education, which requires considerable support from parents. Mental health nurses may need to provide support to the parents to facilitate this process. Nurses need to know what relevant support services are available in the local area, the referral criteria and how to access these services. Schools often work collaboratively with mental health services, and establishing a positive working relationship with the school has benefits for all concerned.

Given the potential impacts of mental illness on the developmental trajectory of adolescents, psychosocial interventions are also important. Supporting young people to stay connected with their peer group can require creativity and innovation. Having some knowledge of the young person's interests and activities prior to development of the mental health concern provides insight as to what might be effective.

 CRITICAL THINKING EXERCISE 17.3

As a small group exercise, discuss some strategies that nurses can use to foster engagement with an adolescent who is sullen and guarded.

MEDICATION AND PSYCHOEDUCATION

For some mental health conditions, treatment routinely involves medication. Providing psychoeducation about medication customised to the person's age and developmental stage is a key nursing role. This includes information about the effects of the medication (what it is intended to do) and information about side effects and how to manage them. For example, in psychosis, medication options usually focus on newer atypical antipsychotics such as risperidone and paliperidone. Benzodiazepines such as diazepam or lorazepam may be used in the initial period of treatment while waiting for the antipsychotic medications to take effect. Benzodiazepines can help with agitation and sleep problems and provide a calming effect as an interim measure. Benzodiazepines should not be used long term due to their high potential for dependence. The golden rule when using medication in young people is to start low and go slow. The aim is to find the lowest possible effective dose to help manage the symptoms of psychosis (Orygen 2016). Using the lowest possible effective doses of medication helps to limit the negative impacts of side effects. Young people experience the same side effects as anyone else taking these medications. However, atypical medications, such as risperidone and paliperidone, have fewer adverse effects than other medications and are less sedating so have fewer negative impacts on the person's ability to function. These medications are less prone to increase appetite, a leading cause of weight gain and subsequent risk of metabolic syndrome – a group of physical health problems related to weight gain that increase the risk of cardiac problems. They are also prone to elevate prolactin levels in some people, and this can lead to sexual dysfunction (Stahl 2019). Young people may be embarrassed to discuss this last side effect, so it is important to establish a good therapeutic relationship that supports and encourages open discussion about sensitive topics, and to ask directly about sensitive issues, using a matter-of-fact tone that reduces the potential for embarrassment.

In some cases, where side effects are more troubling, it may be necessary to try a different medication, and it is important to educate patients about the need for these changes. It is especially important to highlight that a change of medication is not a failure of treatment; rather, it is done to find the most effective medication with the least side effects. This approach is driven by the need to maintain hope in the young person, an important aspect of mental health nursing work.

Having to take regular medication can be a major issue for adolescents, regardless of the condition. Many young people do not want to be different from their peer group. This may include not wanting to be seen as being different by needing to take tablets. Through psychoeducation, the rationale for taking medication should be explained and adverse effects discussed, together with how to reduce any potential complications of medication therapy. Problem solving with the young person about ways to discreetly include taking the prescribed medication in their daily lifestyle will be of benefit. The risk of taking non-prescribed medications

and taking medications in addition to illegal substances and alcohol should also be highlighted. This can be achieved by maximising therapeutic interventions. In adolescent mental health, engagement through developing rapport and trust are key elements to achieving change. Without these elements, minimal change might be achieved.

Behavioural Issues

Behavioural issues in childhood and adolescence can be complex and difficult to resolve. Generally, early intervention is the most effective approach and naturally this requires early identification of behaviours of concern. This might occur in preschools or the early stages of formal education. GPs, paediatricians, child and family nurses, school nurses and nurses working in other primary care settings can also be involved in identifying behavioural problems early.

The causes of behavioural issues in children and adolescents are multifaceted. In some cases, difficult behaviour is a response to exposure to neglect or abuse such as domestic violence or physical, emotional or sexual abuse. Trauma has a significant impact on a young person's capacity to manage their behaviour. Children flourish in consistent, reliable, safe and predictable environments. Some parents, perhaps due to their own experience of poor parenting or other life challenges, have a limited understanding of how best to support children to develop in healthy and adaptive ways. The bonding process between a mother or other primary caregiver and a baby is referred to as "attachment", and ruptures in this attachment relationship (e.g. where a mother is experiencing postnatal depression) can create difficulties that manifest as disturbed behaviour as the child develops. The primary task of the attachment relationship is to provide a secure base for the infant from which they can venture out into the world, knowing that they can always return to their safe base.

Parents who teach their children emotional regulation provide a language for emotions and help them manage the ups and downs of life. Where parents are not able to support the child to develop these skills, for whatever reason, children can experience greater difficulty regulating their behaviour.

The most effective intervention for problematic behaviours in children and adolescents involves working with the parents or caregivers to support them to develop skills and provide them with strategies to manage difficult behaviours and foster the development of more appropriate behaviours. Constant monitoring (evaluation) of behavioural interventions and responses by family members is essential to ensure the mental health team, the young person and their family continue to share a common understanding about managing the problem and a commitment to recovery.

This is specialised work that is undertaken by a multidisciplinary team, including mental health nurses, who have training in various approaches and techniques. Some interventions can be counterintuitive, which is why training is essential. Success in these therapeutic endeavours takes time and persistence, so developing a positive and supportive relationship with all members of a family is required over the longer term.

Supporting a child or young person to more effectively manage their behaviour increases the likelihood that they will succeed in all areas of life, especially their education, family relationships and other social relationships (American Academy of Child and Adolescent Psychiatrists 2007). The American Academy of Child and Adolescent Psychiatrists (2007, p. 136) provides a brief list of useful interventions that focus on parent management training:

1. Reduce positive reinforcement of disruptive behaviours.
2. Increase reinforcement of prosocial and acceptable behaviour. Positive reinforcement varies widely, but parental attention is predominant. A consequence usually consists of a form of time out or loss of privileges.
3. Apply consequences and/or punishment for disruptive behaviour.
4. Make the parental response predictable, contingent and immediate.

Case study 17.4 looks at a young man experiencing his first episode of psychosis.

CASE STUDY 17.4: David

A 15-year-old boy, David, has been admitted to hospital. He is experiencing a psychotic episode as a result of smoking marijuana for several months. He has been hearing auditory hallucinations (voices telling him he is useless and a nuisance to be around). In the past 6 months there has been a decline in David's academic performance, and he has been isolating himself from his friends and family. Within the past 2 months he has been verbally and physically abusive towards his parents and siblings.

Discussion of Case Study: David

The presentation of a young person like David experiencing a first episode of psychosis is not uncommon. In considering David's care, the nurse's first priority is to ensure David is physically safe and that those around him also feel safe. When a person's thinking is altered by psychotic phenomena, they may act irrationally as a consequence of feeling fearful and insecure. This may include aggressive behaviour, which is often a response to feeling frightened, threatened or overwhelmed. It is important that the nurse appears calm but confident and offers reassurance and guidance with statements such as, "David, what you are experiencing must be frightening. You are safe here. We will help you." Short, clear statements made firmly but quietly and with genuine empathy will be reassuring for David and his family. It is important that it is made clear that, whatever David says or does, he has been heard. At this stage, the nurse should avoid disputing any irrational thoughts David may verbalise. Rather, he should be encouraged to verbalise his confusion and distress. This may assist in diffusing his agitation and may lead to his feeling calmer, thereby reducing the risk of him becoming aggressive.

Another important priority is involving David's family as early as possible, providing them with much-needed support so that they can, in turn, support David. The family will usually be most helpful in providing an accurate history of family health. This will assist in identifying any familial predispositions to mental illness and the nature of onset. This information may help the mental health team to establish the likely severity and prognosis for the illness and organise an individualised treatment plan that will have a higher probability of a positive outcome. Recovery from mental illness demands a high level of support from family, friends and agency staff. The best prognosis and quality of life are achieved when all work collaboratively.

Working with adolescents experiencing psychosis can be extremely challenging. However, where the mental health nurse engages effectively with the young person and can support the client and family through the difficult times towards recovery, it can also be very rewarding work. Once safety has been established and the young person and their family have adjusted to the shock of the initial experience and begun to engage with staff, the medium- to long-term relief of symptoms and psychoeducation towards recovery can begin.

Recovering from psychosis may require a range of interventions including resocialisation through group therapy and individual goal setting that focuses on peer support and re-establishing a social network. Individual goal planning, peer support and group therapy can each promote socially adaptive and acceptable behaviour. Adolescence is a period of personal development involving challenging authority and pushing against the norms of society. The "normal" adolescent behaviours should not be stifled through treatment but recognised and supported so the young person can return to his or her peer group and family with minimal residual effects of the psychotic episode. One aspect of hospitalisation that can have negative longer term effects is labelling David's condition.

Depression and Suicide

The psychological and physical trauma experienced by young people who have attempted suicide may be difficult for everyone to come to terms with, including the resulting fear and grief expressed by their parents/carers. The young person should be reassured that their safety is the treatment team's priority while at the same time providing support to the family. Youth suicide and attempts at self-harm may challenge health professionals and family members to consider their own mortality and the question of why people attempt and complete suicide. It is important that nurses develop skills that enable them to feel comfortable addressing these issues directly with the young person and their family – this is particularly essential for nurses working in clinical areas where contact with young people who have attempted suicide is more common (nurses working in EDs, nurses working in rural and remote medicine, mental health nurses working in acute care teams or CYMHS).

Engaging with young people who are depressed or suicidal can be extremely difficult due to their tendency towards socially withdrawn and isolative behaviour, or due to cognitive impairment. Nurses can engage through routine nursing care, social interactions, groups and individual therapy. In an in-patient setting, it is often a nurse who spends long hours with the young person and is present with them as their mood shifts throughout the day and who may be alerted to a subtle increase in risk to the young person's emotional or physical safety. A nurse's ability to reassure young people of their availability as needed helps young people feel free to discuss issues with the nurse when the time seems most appropriate for them.

An issue that can be confusing for nurses is that at times adolescents who are clinically depressed may present with aggressive traits or behaviours. Some adolescents are not able to communicate their emotions verbally. As a result, their only means of expressing distress may be through verbal or physical aggression, towards themselves or others. Getting involved in physical activity, sport, music or art may help engagement. Sharing the young person's physical space and activities may help in forging a therapeutic alliance. Using diversional activities can enable mental health nurses to further engage the young person and progress the therapeutic relationship. Establishing a confidante may be the turning point in the young person's treatment.

Self-Harm and Young People

Self-harm refers to a specific set of behaviours, but the term is used somewhat loosely to cover a wider range of issues including suicidal behaviour and thinking. In this section, self-harm refers specifically to intentional self-injury or poisoning that does not have suicidal intent. This does not mean that self-harm is never associated with suicidal thinking or behaviour, but it is important to make a clear distinction between self-harm without suicidal intent and self-harm in the context of suicidal thinking (Hungerford et al 2018). The reasons for this distinction are concerned with the different causes and interventions that are needed to manage non-suicidal self-harm compared with suicidal behaviour and thinking. It is important to bear in mind that self-harm is an expression of personal distress, not an illness, and there are many varied reasons for a young person to engage in self harm (NICE 2022).

Self-harm is used as a coping mechanism to manage feelings of distress arising from a variety of sources, including abuse and trauma. In some cases, an adolescent might engage in self harm in an effort to fit in with a peer group or to engender care or concern from friends. It is therefore important when assessing young people who are engaging in self-harm to understand the motivations for the behaviour. Where a history of abuse or trauma is revealed as a potential underlying cause, it is important to gain an understanding of the nature and extent of this issue. This can be difficult due to the high levels of shame and embarrassment that accompany the experience of abuse and trauma which may be particularly difficult for a young person to talk about. An underlying mental illness such as anxiety, depression or psychosis may also contribute to self-harm behaviour, and it is helpful for this to be identified as part of any assessment of a young person who engages in self-harm (Hungerford et al 2018).

It is important for all members of the healthcare team to treat young people who engage in self-harm with respect and courtesy, using a non-judgemental, non-critical approach. This includes nurses working in triage, assessment and treatment, as well as nurses conducting mental health assessments. People who self-harm are frequently ashamed of their behaviour and fear judgement and discrimination from others due to a lack of understanding about self-harming behaviour. Adopting a stance of genuine curiosity and acceptance can have powerful therapeutic effects.

Immediate interventions for self-harm need to focus on managing any injuries that have occurred. This may involve stitches, dressings or managing intentional poisoning. Once the person's physical healthcare needs have been addressed it is usual for mental health staff to conduct an assessment. This should be conducted as soon as possible and can be done before physical health care has been completed, if it is safe to do so. All staff who have contact with people who self-harm need to adopt an accepting, respectful, non-critical approach. Remembering that people who self-harm are managing their distress in the only way they know how can help with this process. Those who self-harm, particularly those who have been subject to abuse or trauma, are usually hypersensitive to the reactions of the people around them so it is important to maintain a positive therapeutic stance. This is a particularly important strategy because people who self-harm can be seen in a negative light by some staff, possibly due to lack of understanding about the levels of distress these people experience and the apparently ineffective methods used to manage this distress.

The aim of assessment with people who self-harm is to gain an understanding of the extent and frequency of their behaviours. It is also important to gain an understanding of the motivations for self-harming behaviour. This can help us work with the person to develop interventions that will address the underlying problems.

Some people who self-harm find it extremely difficult to stop their behaviours for a range of reasons including ongoing exposure to trauma and abuse. In such situations, identifying harm-reduction strategies, accepting that self-harm will most likely continue into the foreseeable future, should be the focus. Harm reduction involves working with the person to find less harmful ways to manage their distress and thereby minimise the damage that may result from self-harming behaviour. This can be something as simple as getting the person to attach a rubber band to their wrist and to flick the rubber band when they feel the need to self-harm. The pain from the rubber band mimics the pain from cutting and can serve the same purpose as cutting. In the longer term, various psychological and talking therapies can be helpful for people who self-harm. This includes cognitive behaviour therapy and dialectical behaviour therapy. These therapies are delivered by suitably trained and qualified practitioners including mental health nurses (NICE 2022).

As with all areas of work with children and adolescents, working with family or carers (wherever possible and appropriate) is an important part of interventions for young people who self-harm, and most parents want to be involved with the treatment process. Helping parents and caregivers gain an understanding of self-harm behaviour can reduce interpersonal conflicts within the family. Working to help family members develop strategies to support their young family member can also be beneficial. Knowing about self-harming behaviours and developing ways to provide support and care to their young family member and being open to talking about the issues can help ameliorate the distress and difficulties resulting from self-harm. Parents may also benefit from accessing mental health support for themselves to manage their own overwhelming emotions. Those who are reluctant may benefit from being provided access to psychoeducational self-help resources (Zhao et al 2022).

Case study 17.5 looks at a 14-year-old girl who is engaging in self-harm.

CASE STUDY 17.5: Julia

Julia is a 14-year-old who, over the past year, has become increasingly withdrawn from her peer group. She was previously an A-grade student in a select school, but over the past 4 months her school grades have dropped noticeably and she is not completing her homework. She no longer has an interest in playing netball or attending her athletics club. Julia's mother says that Julia has been aggressive towards her and has been harming herself by cutting her wrists with any sharp object available. Julia's GP prescribed antidepressant medication 6 weeks before admission, but there has been minimal change in her mental state.

Discussion of Case Study: Julia
Julia requires intensive therapy, which may include cognitive behaviour therapy, family therapy, individual psychotherapy and a review of her medication. Psychosocial issues also need to be considered during Julia's treatment. This may include exploring school issues, as well as whether there is any risk of Julia having been physically, emotionally or sexually abused. Also, there may have been significant losses that have contributed to her depression.

In assisting young people like Julia, the mental health nurse will need to establish rapport and maintain engagement. It will be important to gain the client's confidence from the initial meeting because there will be many sensitive issues to address. Adolescents seeking help from adults will not always commit time for a therapeutic relationship to grow if they doubt in any way the sincerity of the person in whom they are confiding.

In some instances, the action of inflicting harm upon oneself can provide a sense of relief from severe emotional distress and psychic pain. It is therefore essential that the nurse recognises this possibility and, while working with the young person, makes every effort for them to feel respected and not judged on the behaviour that has led to them seeking help. Medical care, such as attention to a wound, should be addressed discreetly and professionally. The key aspect of providing care for the young person is establishing their current level of safety and working with them on how this can best be achieved. It will be helpful to ensure the young person has adequate support networks so they can strengthen these connections with a view to obtaining help in more adaptive ways in the future.

❓ CRITICAL THINKING EXERCISE 17.4

List the potential barriers to establishing a therapeutic alliance with Julia.

Risk-Taking and Young People

Some problematic or risk-taking behaviours among adolescents and young people are often seen to be part of "normal" development and the transition from adolescence to adulthood. Problematic or risk-taking behaviours can take a number of forms including tobacco use, binge drinking, cannabis or other drug use, reckless driving (e.g. texting while behind

the wheel) and risky sexual activity. The adolescent brain is still maturing during adolescence, and young people are strongly influenced by peers in their decision making, which leads to increased impulsivity and risk-taking behaviours – often in an attempt to avoid peer exclusion. There also appears to be a neurobiological link and correlations between certain personality factors and risk-taking in youth, and these include greater levels of risk tolerance, sensation, thrill seeking and impulsivity (Nagel 2019). For some young people, engaging in risk-taking is experimental and forms part of their search for identity and values, social and financial independence, and peer networks (Sanci et al 2018). However, in Australia, Grigg (2020) identified some concerning trends at outdoor music festivals,

BOX 17.3 HEEADSSS Assessment

- **H**ome environment
- **E**ducation and employment
- **E**ating and exercise
- Peer-related **A**ctivities
- **D**rugs, tobacco and alcohol
- **S**ex and sexuality
- **S**uicide, depression and other mental health issues
- **S**afety from injury, violence, abuse, and safety precautions to reduce sun damage and vaccine preventable infections

Klein et al 2024.

with normalisation of ecstasy/MDMA, an increase in the use of cannabis, and the use of nitrous oxide ("nangs") among festival-goers, with 90% combining the illicit drugs with alcohol (polydrug use). For around one in four adolescents, risk-taking can affect their mental and physical wellbeing (Sanci et al 2018), and may be a maladaptive coping strategy for young people who are already experiencing poor mental health.

Education and role-modelling within the home, school and community is crucial in teaching young people how to act in a socially responsible way. As a clinician, early detection is important. Take any opportunity that presents to talk with young people about risk-taking behaviours. Young people may be reluctant to disclose and access healthcare services, but value the advice of clinicians (Sanci et al 2018). Some of the barriers for young people in accessing healthcare services include cost and issues of convenience (e.g. transport), worries about confidentiality, clinicians who aren't sensitive to the young person's developmental stage or who lack the clinical skills (such as communication) required to work with young people, and developmental issues (Tylee et al 2007).

Building resilience is key and using the HEEADSSS health assessment (Box 17.3) supports a clinician to explore protective factors that the young person already has in their lives and ways to strengthen these, while respecting choices and decisions. Bear in mind, that while peers may be a risk factor, in some cases they may also be the people who take steps or intervene to prevent harm, so greater knowledge of peers about the potential risks of behaviours can be empowering.

 CRITICAL THINKING EXERCISE 17.5

Either individually or in a group, have a brainstorming session and list all the skills that a child and youth mental health nurse would require. Subdivide these into skills that you think may be specific to either a community mental health nurse or a mental health nurse working in an inpatient setting.

Technology and Young People

Children and young people are spending more and more time online or connected to devices. Nine out of 10 Australian teenagers aged 14–17 years have a mobile phone, and nearly all have a smartphone (Roy Morgan 2016). There are benefits to the social connectedness that technology and social media affords, and there are also risks. Cyberbullying is when technology is used in a negative and unhealthy way and can include sending or sharing hurtful, embarrassing or abusive emails/messages, humiliating others online through videos or posting of images, spreading rumours online, excluding others or threatening others, making people feel afraid (Kids Helpline 2019). Cyberbullying is a real risk and can be the source of emotional disturbances and substance use; it can lead to self-harm and thoughts of suicide in children and young people (Kwan et al 2020; Li et al 2022). Four in ten (44%) of Australian children aged 12–17 years have reported at least one negative online

experience over a 6-month period (AIHW 2021). The potential danger of cyberbullying is that the reach is much greater because of the internet, technology and mobile phones, which provide access to worldwide communication options such as text, email and private messaging, as well as through social media platforms such as Snapchat, Instagram and Tik-Tok. There is also greater anonymity for the perpetrator and difficulty in removing statements or images once shared publicly because we leave our "digital footprints" (Ophir et al 2019).

Family members may notice if their child or young person is affected by cyberbullying. Signs can include greater isolation from peers or social activities, trouble sleeping, complaints of somatic symptoms, poor school performance, seeming unhappy or stressed after being on their mobile phone or computer, or receiving more messages than usual by text or on social media. Health professionals should be aware of the potential mental health risks associated with cyberbullying and how social support from school and family can be a protective mechanism (Giumetti & Kowalski 2022). Family can be instrumental in encouraging the young person to talk openly about what is happening and their feelings or, alternatively, helping them find someone safe to talk to such as a health professional or accessing counselling supports such as the Kids Helpline, eheadspace or Lifeline. Family members, school staff and health professionals can also help the young person to develop a plan or steps to respond and cope with the bullying. Steps can include not responding and blocking the bully in privacy settings, collecting evidence and reporting the abuse to the service or social media outlet for removal of material and, depending on the severity of the offence, reporting it to an e-safety agency such as the Office of the eSafety Commissioner in Australia or law enforcement (eSafety Commissioner 2019).

With the rise in the need to be "connected", there has also been a rise in young people's use of social media with the emergence of platforms such as Facebook (2004), Twitter (X) (2006), Instagram (2010) and Snapchat (2011). Gunnell and colleagues (2018, p. 1) explain that "social media use may result in less face to face communication, overdependency on being 'liked' for social validation (particularly for girls), and pressure to keep up with discussions 24 hours a day, leading to poor sleep". "Fear of missing out" has come to the fore among young people who feel the need to be continually connected with what others may be doing to avoid missing out, having significant effects on their mental wellbeing (Stephen & Edmonds 2018). Similarly, problem gaming, particularly for boys, may be a symptom of factors such as being lonely or feeling anxious or depressed. And while there is debate about whether it should be classified as a disorder, the amount of time a young person spends gaming can have significant negative effects on daily life (relationships, school or work, health and wellbeing) (Orlando 2019).

Greater access to the online environment and technology also means young people are exposed to pornography and sexting behaviours (e.g. sending sexually explicit text messages, images or videos). Research shows that nearly half of children 9–16 years of age experience regular exposure to sexual images, and young males are more likely to seek out pornography and do so frequently. The impact of this exposure can increase sexual behaviour and risk-taking in teenagers, with pornography associated with unsafe sexual health practices, such as multiple partners and not using condoms because they don't see this as "normal", increasing risk for unplanned pregnancies and sexually transmitted infections (Quadara et al 2017).

Taking this all into account, nurses should support recommendations for appropriate screen time, encouraging 8–12 hours of sleep and 1 hour of exercise each day as a priority over screen time. Nurses can also support families with setting screen time guidelines and family media agreements to help young people "stay safe", "think first" (before posting), "stay balanced" and "communicate openly". An example of an agreement can be found on the Common Sense Media website (see Useful websites).

CRITICAL THINKING EXERCISE 17.6

Imagine you are contacting a health service about worries and concerns you have for a family member. What nursing attributes and skills would you find reassuring during the first phone contact?

CONFIDENTIALITY

An important issue for young people is being able to understand how the information shared during interactions with team members is documented and knowing who has access to these records. It is important to them that their need for confidentiality be maintained; however, there are constraints on the confidentiality available to children and adolescents. One such constraint is the presence of risk factors. The young person must know that nurses and their colleagues are bound to share information that has a direct effect on their safety or the safety of others. The age of the young person is another issue we need to consider. There is no statute law covering confidentiality or consent and, as such, case law (see Chapter 10) and health service policy should guide action in this area. When working with families in the child and adolescent sphere it is unwise to promise complete confidentiality when working with young people. For young people aged 14 years or older, it is generally wise to let them know that information may be shared with others and that this will be discussed and negotiated with the young person before this is done. Exceptions to this process should also be discussed in the early stages of the therapeutic relationship. The exceptions are generally related to issues of safety such as the emergence of suicidal thinking, the young person engaging in dangerous behaviours like drug taking or revelations about abuse. It is not necessary to list every possible exception. A general statement about issues of concern or safety is usually enough. If the young person is forewarned that there are exceptions to confidentiality, this can lead to a more open and productive relationship.

Interviews with adolescents should not be restricted to the formality of interview rooms. So long as safety can be assured, some adolescents may prefer to be interviewed in a more public place such as a courtyard. Flexibility (and not a small dose of ingenuity!) is the key to providing a quality service that will encourage young people to return when needed.

LEGAL ISSUES

Nurses caring for young people admitted to mental health services often have to deal with legal issues relating to duty of care, child protection and mental health legislation. In the developed world, children and younger adolescents (usually aged 13 years or under) must have a parent's or guardian's consent to seek treatment for any form of medical intervention, including mental health assessments and treatment. Young people in Australia aged 14 years or older can give their own consent to receive medical or nursing treatment, as long as their parents are aware and the health professionals believe that the young person is competent to give consent.

The ability for young people to consent to medical treatment or seek medical consultations is referred to as "Gillick competence" (*Gillick v. West Norfolk and Wisbech Area Health Authority 1986*). Medical and nursing staff may question whether the young person is "Gillick competent" or has the cognitive ability to make an informed judgement to give their own consent for treatment. The legal precedent is the case where a parent took a local health authority to court after one of her children received treatment from a GP without her consent. This case has had a major impact on the provision of paediatric healthcare and, consequently, health workers must consider each child's competence on a case-by-case basis, assessing both the competence and the maturity of the child (Daly 2020).

In mental health, as with general health care, consent could be challenged by parents and doctors; however, to ensure the safety and wellbeing of young people, mental health legislation provides strong guidelines and rights of appeal. Mental health nurses working with young people aged under 16 years should be aware that it is unethical and legally unsafe to engage a young person in treatment without informing their parent(s). Healthcare agencies and inpatient units tend to have specific protocols and policies to address this issue.

The legal process by which young people can be admitted involuntarily to mental health agencies is similar to that for adults. This ensures legal processes and due process are followed regarding human rights, issues of liberty and protecting the rights of others. It is always preferable that young people are admitted voluntarily. However, if their safety (or the safety of another) is at risk and they are unable to consent to voluntary treatment, the relevant mental health Act can be invoked. Younger people, aged 13 or under, are usually regarded as voluntary if their parents have provided consent. If a young person is aged 14 or 15 it is beneficial, if possible, to gain their consent to treatment, as well as a parent's consent.

The other main legal issues that need to be observed in child and adolescent mental health are child protection and statutory orders regarding custody. As stated above, nurses are mandatory reporters under child protection legislation, and all nurses need to be familiar with the legislation in their jurisdiction. Aotearoa New Zealand and the states and territories of Australia have their own legislation governing child protection and guardianship. However, the overriding principles are those of the WHO and the United Nations Convention on the Rights of the Child (Parliament of the Commonwealth of Australia Joint Standing Committee on Treaties 1998). In theory, all children and adolescents have legal rights to education, health and wellbeing.

CHAPTER SUMMARY

This chapter has highlighted knowledge and skills that a beginning nurse requires when working for the first time with children and adolescents in the mental health field. It has focused primarily on engagement – establishing a therapeutic relationship and forging a therapeutic alliance. Nurses must first master strategies for engaging young people and their families before more advanced skills in mental health nursing can be consolidated effectively. Engaging young people and families early and developing a therapeutic relationship will enhance the quality of assessment information clients provide. Furthermore, a sense of trust will promote commitment to a shared treatment plan created in partnership between the young person, their parents and the mental health team.

The case studies in this chapter have sought to reinforce the importance of engagement and working in partnerships. Demonstrating empathy and performing with absolute sincerity are important factors in caring for children and young people. It is important that young people feel that they are the priority for the nurse at this particular time.

REVIEW QUESTIONS

1. Contact your nearest CYMHS and ask for information on the services available to children and young people. Share this information with your group.
   - Are these services proactive and responsive?
   - Does the service actively promote early intervention?
2. Contact a nurse working in a community setting and another from an inpatient unit and ask them to speak to your group about their roles. Note any differences between the mental health nursing of young people in the community and that of young people in an inpatient setting.
3. In small groups, nominate one person to act as a mental health nurse and another to play the role of a sullen, guarded adolescent.

Remaining group members are to observe and document the difficulties presented in establishing rapport.

4. Contact a child and youth mental health agency or community youth shelter and arrange to speak with a person who has experience with depressed or suicidal youth. Then clarify your responses to Critical thinking exercise 17.5.
5. Seek out the mental health and child protection Acts applicable in your state, territory or region. Summarise key points in applying these to establishing safety for young people. Share your findings.

USEFUL WEBSITES

Children of Parents with a Mental Illness (COPMI): www.copmi.net.au/
Common Sense Media: www.commonsensemedia.org/family-media-agreement
headspace: headspace.org.au/
Kidshelpline: www.kidshelpline.com.au/

REFERENCES

Achenbach, T.M., Ndetei, D.M., 2020. Clinical models for child and adolescent behavioral, emotional, and social problems. In: Rey, J.M. & Martin, A. (eds), IACAPAP E-Textbook of Child and Adolescent Mental Health. International Association for Child and Adolescent Psychiatry and Allied Professions, Geneva.

American Academy of Child and Adolescent Psychiatrists, 2007. Practice parameter for the assessment and treatment of children and adolescents with oppositional defiant disorder. J Am Acad Child Adolesc Psychiatry, 46(1), 126–141.

American Psychiatric Association (APA), 2022. Diagnostic and Statistical Manual of Mental Disorders: 5th Edition Text Revision. (DSM-5-TR). APA Publishing, Washington, DC.

Australian Bureau of Statistics (ABS), 2018. Causes of death, Australia, 2017. Catalogue 3303.0. Commonwealth of Australia, Canberra.

Australian College of Mental Health Nurses, 2010. Standards of practice for Australian mental health nurses: 2010. Online. Available at: acmhn.org/Web/Resources/Best-practice-resources.aspx .

Australian Health Ministers' Advisory Council, 2013. A national framework for recovery-oriented mental health services: Guide for practitioners and providers. Commonwealth of Australia, Canberra.

Australian Institute of Health and Welfare (AIHW) 2021. Bullying and negative online experiences, AIHW, Australian Government. Online. Available at: www.aihw.gov.au/reports/children-youth/negative-online-experiences

Australian Institute of Health and Welfare (AIHW), 2020. National Drug Strategy Household Survey 2019: Detailed findings 2019. Drug Statistics Series No. 32. Cat. no. PHE 270. AIHW, Canberra.

Beers, C.W., 1908. A Mind That Found Itself: An Autobiography. Longmans, Green, New York.

Bronfenbrenner, U 1979, The Ecology of Human Development. Harvard University Press, Cambridge, MA.

Bryson, H., Perlen, S., Price, A., et al., 2021. Patterns of maternal depression, anxiety and stress symptoms from pregnancy to 5 years postpartum in an Australian cohort experiencing adversity. Arch Women's Ment Health, 24, 987–997.

Campbell, A., Chapman, M., McHugh, C., et al., 2016. Rising Indigenous suicide rates in Kimberley and implications for suicide prevention. Australas Psychiatry 24(6), 561–564.

Child Welfare Information Gateway, 2019. Long-term consequences of childhood abuse and neglect. Online. Available at: www.childwelfare.gov/pubs/factsheets/long-term-consequences/

Dallos, R., Draper, R., 2015. An Introduction to Family Therapy: Systemic Theory and Practice, 4th ed. McGraw-Hill Education, Maidenhead.

Daly, A. 2020. Assessing children's capacity. Int J Children's Rights, 28(3), 471–499.

Doherty, M., Bond, L., Jessell, L., et al., 2020. Transitioning to person-centered care: A qualitative study of provider perspectives. J Behav Health Serv Res, 47 (3), 399–408.

eSafety Commissioner, 2019. Cyberbullying. Online. Available at: www.esafety.gov.au/esafety-information/esafety-issues/cyberbullying

Geldard, K., Geldard, D., Foo, R.Y., 2018. Counselling Children: A Practical Introduction, 5th ed. Sage, London.

Gillies, D., Christou, A, Dixon, A.C., Featherston, O.J. Rapti, I. et al., 2018. Prevalence and characteristics of self-harm in adolescents: Meta-analyses of community based studies 1990–2015. J Am Acad Child Adolesc Psychiatry, 57(10), 733–741.

Giumetti, G.W., Kowalski, R.M., 2022. Cyberbullying via social media and well-being. Curr Opin Psychol, 45, 101314.

Goodman, J.H., 2019. Perinatal depression and infant mental health. Arch Psychiatr Nurs, 33 (3), 217–224.

Gore, F.M., Bloem, P.J.N., Patton, G.C., et al., 2011. Global burden of disease in young people aged 10–24 years: A systematic analysis. Lancet 377, 2093–2102.

Grigg, J. 2020. A Mixed Methods Study of Drug Use at Outdoor Music Festivals in Western Australia and Victoria. PhD thesis. Curtin University.

Gunnell, D., Kidger, J., Elvidge, H., 2018. Adolescent mental health in crisis. BMJ 361, k2608.

Hirani, K., Cherian, S., Mutch, R., et al., 2018. Identification of health risk behaviours among adolescent refugees resettling in Western Australia. Arch Dis Child, 103, 240–246.

Hungerford, C., Hodgson, D., Bostwick, R., et al., 2018. Mental Health Care, 3rd ed. John Wiley, Milton.

Jans, T., Vloet, T.D., Taneli, Y., Warnke, A., 2020. Suicide and self-harming behaviour (update 2018). In: Rey, J.M. & Martin, A. (eds), IACAPAP E-Textbook of Child and Adolescent Mental Health. International Association for Child and Adolescent Psychiatry and Allied Professions, Geneva.

Kendler, K.S., 2018. The development of Kraepelin's mature diagnostic concepts of paranoia and paranoid dementia praecox: A close reading of his textbooks from 1887 to 1899. JAMA Psychiatry 75(12), 1280–1288.

Kids Helpline, 2019. Cyberbullying. Online. Available at: kidshelpline.com.au/teens/issues/cyberbullying

Klein, D.A., Goldenring, J.M., Adelman, W.P. 2014. Probing for scars: How to ask the essential questions. Contemp Pediatr, 31(1), 16–28.

Kwan, I., Dickson, K., Richardson, M., MacDowall, W., Burchett, H., et al., 2020. Cyberbullying and children and young people's mental health: A systematic map of systematic reviews. Cyberpsychol, Behavior, Soc Network, 23(2), 72–82.

Laver-Bradbury, C., Thompson, M.J.J., Gale, C., Hooper, C.M., 2021. Child and Adolescent Mental Health: Theory and Practice, 3rd ed. CRC Press, Boca Raton.

Lawrence, D., Johnson, S., Hafekost, J., et al., 2015. The mental health of children and adolescents. Report on the second Australian Child and Adolescent Survey of Mental Health and Wellbeing. Department of Health. Canberra.

Li, C., Wang, P., Martin-Moratinos, M. et al 2022. Traditional bullying and cyberbullying in the digital age and its associated mental health problems in children and adolescents: A meta-analysis. Eur Child Adolesc Psychiatry. https://doi.org/10.1007/s00787-022-02128-x

Mares, S., Woodgate, S., 2020. The clinical assessment of infants, preschoolers and their families. In: Rey, J.M. & Martin, A. (eds), IACAPAP E-Textbook of Child and Adolescent Mental Health. International Association for Child and Adolescent Psychiatry and Allied Professions, Geneva.

Mitchell, A.E. 2022. Supporting families to manage child behaviour and sleep patterns, and promote optimal child development. In: Fraser, J., Waters, D., Forster, E., Brown, N. Paediatric nursing in Australia and New Zealand, 3rd ed. Cambridge University Press, UK.

Murphy, G., Peters, K., Wilkes, L., et al., 2018. Adult children of parents with mental illness: Parenting journeys. BMC Psychology, 6, 37.

Nagel, M.C., 2019. The neurobiology of risk taking and impulsivity. Encycl Child Adolesc Dev, doi:10.1002/9781119171492

Naghavi, M., 2019. Global, regional, and national burden of suicide mortality 1990 to 2016: Systematic analysis for the Global Burden of Disease Study 2016. BMJ 316, 194.

NICE, 2022. Self-harm: Assessment, management and preventing recurrence. National Institute for Health and Care Excellence. Online. Available at: www.nice.org.uk/guidance/ng225

NSW Ministry of Health, 2011. NSW Child and Adolescent Mental Health Services (CAMHS) Competency framework. NSW Government, Sydney.

Oostermeijer, S., Bassilios, B., Nicholas, A. et al., 2021. Implementing child and youth mental health services: Early lessons from the Australian Primary Health Network Lead Site Project. Int J Ment Health Syst 15, 16, doi.org/10.1186/s13033-021-00440-8.

Ophir, Y., Asterhan, C.S.C., Schwarz, B.B., 2019. The digital footprints of adolescent depression, social rejection and victimization of bullying on Facebook. Computers Human Behav, 91, 62–71.

Orlando, J., 2019. How to know if your child is addicted to video games and what to do about it. The Conversation. Online. Available at: http://theconversation.com/how-to-know-if-your-child-is-addicted-to-video-games-and-what-to-do-about-it-118038

Orygen. The National Centre for Excellence in Youth Mental Health, 2016. Australian Clinical Guidelines for Early Psychosis, 2nd ed. Orygen Youth Health, Melbourne.

Parliament of the Commonwealth of Australia Joint Standing Committee on Treaties, 1998. United Nations Convention on the Rights of the Child, 17th report. Commonwealth of Australia, Canberra.

Perera, S., Hetrick, S., Cotton, S., et al., 2019. Awareness of headspace youth mental health service centres across Australian communities between 2008 and 2015. J Ment Health, 29(4), 410–417.

Piaget, J., 1962. The stages of the intellectual development of the child. Bull Menninger Clin, 26 (3), 120–128.

Pretorius, C., Chambers, D., Coyle, D., 2019. Young people's online help-seeking and mental health difficulties: Systematic narrative review. J Med Internet Res. 21(11), e13873. doi: 10.2196/13873.

Quadara, A., El-Murr, A., Latham, J., 2017. The Effects of Pornography on Children and Young People: An Evidence Scan. Australian Institute of Family Studies, Melbourne.

Rey, J.M., Bella-Awusah, T.T., Jing, L., 2020. Depression in children and adolescents. In: Rey, J.M. & Martin, A (eds), IACAPAP E-Textbook of Child and Adolescent Mental Health. International Association for Child and Adolescent Psychiatry and Allied Professions, Geneva.

Rickwood, D., Paraskakis, M., Quin, D et al 2019. Australia's innovation in youth mental health care: The headspace centre model. Early Interv Psychiatry, 13(1), 159–166.

Rivers, I., Gonzalez, C., Nodin, N., et al., 2018. LGBT people and suicidality in youth: A qualitative study of perceptions of risk and protective circumstances. Soc Sci Med, 212, 1–8.

Roberts, J., Fenton, G., Barnard, M., 2015. Developing effective therapeutic relationships with children, young people and their families. Nurs Child Young People, 27(4), 30–35.

Roy Morgan, 2016. 9 in 10 Aussie teens now have a mobile (and most are already on to their second or subsequent handset). Press Release Finding No. 6929. Australia. Online. Available at: www.roymorgan.com/findings/6929-australian-teenagers-and-their-mobile-phones-june-2016-201608220922

Sanci, L., Webb, M., Hocking, J., 2018. Risk-taking behaviour in adolescents. Aust J Gen Pract, 47, 829–834.

Sawyer, M.G., Miller-Lewis, L.R., Clark, J.J., 2007. The mental health of 13–17-year-olds in Australia: Findings from the National Survey of Mental Health and Wellbeing. J Youth Adolesc, 36, 185–194.

Servili, C., 2020. Organizing and delivering services for child and adolescent mental health. In: Rey, J.M. & Martin, A (eds), IACAPAP E-Textbook of Child and Adolescent Mental Health. International Association for Child and Adolescent Psychiatry and Allied Professions, Geneva.

Sliwerski, A., Kossakowska, K., Jarecka, K., et al., 2020. The effect of maternal depression on infant attachment: A systematic review. Int J Environ Res Public Health, 17(8), 2675.

Solmi, M., Radua, J., Olivola, M. et al., 2022. Age at onset of mental disorders worldwide: Large-scale meta-analysis of 192 epidemiological studies. Mol Psychiatry 27, 281–295.

Stahl, S.M., 2019. Stahl's Prescriber's Guide: Children and Adolescents. Cambridge University Press, Cambridge.

Stephen, R., Edmonds, R., 2018. Briefing 53: Social Media, Young People and Mental Health. Centre for Mental Health, London.

Vasta, R. (ed.) 1992, Six Theories of Child Development. Revised Formulations and Current Issues. Jessica Kingsley, London.

Wharaurau, 2021. Real Skills Plus ICAMH/AOD Competency Framework. Wharaurau, Auckland.

World Health Organization (WHO) 2020, Improving early childhood development: WHO guideline, WHO, Geneva.

World Health Organization (WHO), 2019. Coming of age: Adolescent health. Online. Available at: www.who.int/news-room/spotlight/coming-of-age-adolescent-health

World Health Organization (WHO), 2018. Adolescent mental health. Online. Available at: www.who.int/news-room/fact-sheets/detail/adolescent-mental-health

World Health Organization (WHO), 2017. Global accelerated action for the health of adolescents (AA-HA!): guidance to support country Implementation. Online. Available at: www.who.int/publications/i/item/9789241512343

World Health Organization (WHO), 2014. Health for the World's Adolescents: A Second Chance in the Second Decade. WHO, Geneva.

World Health Organization (WHO), 2009. Improving health systems and services for mental health. Available: www.who.int/publications/i/item/9789241598774

Zhao, Y., Liu, Z., Li, Y., Liu, D., Yi, J., 2022. The lived experiences of parents providing care to young people who self-harm: A meta-aggregative synthesis of qualitative studies. Int J Ment Health Nurs, 32(2), 402–419.

18

Mental Health in Older Age

Jim Xu and Kerry Capelin

KEY POINTS

- People are living longer and, as populations age, understanding the mental disorders and needs of older people, and considering the factors that impede care, such as ageism, stereotyping and stigma, is important.
- Throughout life's trajectory, changes that influence and impact on a person as they age should be considered.
- Functional deterioration is a normal part of ageing, and, although mental illness may increase with age, not all older age people will require health and social support.
- Nursing management of mental illness in older people should be person-centred, including listening to the person, encouraging an active and healthy lifestyle, and cultivating an interactive, therapeutic nurse–patient relationship.
- Nurses' attitudes are important in influencing the delivery of care to older people. In assessing an older person, avoid making ageist assumptions, such as assuming that dementia is the cause of changes in behaviour and activity.
- Common mental health disorders in old age include depression, anxiety, delirium, dementia and schizophrenia. Substance misuse is also an issue.

KEY TERMS

Aboriginal and Torres Strait Islander Australians/New Zealand Māori
Ageing
Ageism
Alzheimer's disease
Anxiety

Cognitive assessment tools
Delirium
Dementia
Depression
LGBTIQA+ (lesbian, gay, bisexual, transgender, intersex, queer/questioning or asexual)

Mental disorders
Schizophrenia
Stepped care
Substance misuse
Suicide

LEARNING OUTCOMES

The material in this chapter will assist you to:
- understand the difference in ageing for young–old to old–old people
- develop knowledge to help identify risks and respond in context to older aged people
- identify life trajectory changes that can contribute to new or established mental disorders
- apply new knowledge and support strategies in caring for older aged people experiencing depression, anxiety, substance misuse, delirium, dementia, schizophrenia and suicide risk
- support consumers to improve mental health in older age.

INTRODUCTION

Ageing brings with it many life-changing events. Older aged people (65+ years) have lifelong experiences and some have pre-existing health disorders. With this in mind, it is important to have an understanding of the changes that occur in ageing, including physical changes and mental disorders that can coincide with, and impact on, health care. Mental health problems are common among older people, and mental disorders can have a big impact on older people's ability with activities of daily living (ADLs), independence and quality of life. Unfortunately, mental disorders are often undiagnosed and untreated, and the needs of older people with mental disorders are often unmet.

This chapter presents an insight into the mental disorders and mental health challenges that are common in older people. The principles underlying nursing diagnosis, assessment and management are explored.

Strategies to promote mental health and reduce negative attitudes to enhance the quality of care for older aged people as consumers of mental health care are discussed.

DEMOGRAPHY OF AGEING

Older age is categorised into three broad groups: young–old (65–74 years), middle–old (75–84 years) and old(est)–old (85+ years).

The Australian Institute of Health and Welfare (AIHW) reports that in 2020 one in six Australians was aged 65 years or older (AIHW 2020), with more than half of older people (56% or 2.4 million) aged 65–74, around one-third aged 75–84 (31% or 1.3 million), and 13% aged 85 or older (528,000). It was estimated that the population aged 65+ in Australia would be 4.2 million by mid-2021 (Australian Bureau of Statistics (ABS) 2020), and it is projected to be 6.66 million by 2041 (Wilson & Temple 2022). By 2066 it is projected there will be over 4.5 million people aged 65–74 in Australia, people aged 75–84 will account for 34% (3.5 million) of the population and one in five older people will be aged 85 or older (21% or 2.2 million) (ABS 2018). The proportion of older adults in New Zealand is similar, with one in six of the population aged over 65 years (Statistics New Zealand 2022), and projections that one in five of the population will be aged over 65 years in 2028, and one in four by 2050. With average life expectancy increasing, the number of New Zealanders aged 65 years or older is expected to grow by nearly 40% over the next decade (Te Pou 2019) and the number of people in these older ages could reach 1.3 million in 2040 and 1.5 million in 2050 (Statistics New Zealand 2022). Older populations are increasingly diverse across cultural backgrounds and ethnicity, religious and spiritual beliefs, gender identity, relationships and sexuality (older adults who identify as lesbian, gay, bisexual, transgender, intersex, queer/questioning, asexual (LGBTIQA+)).

In 2022, only 5.6% of Indigenous Australians were aged 65+ compared to 17% of non-Indigenous Australians (ABS 2021), reflecting the life expectancy gap between Indigenous and non-Indigenous Australians and the lower proportion of Indigenous people aged 65 years or older. Aboriginal and Torres Strait Islanders Health Performance Framework Summary report recognises the generally poorer health of Aboriginal and Torres Strait Islanders compared with other Australians (AIHW 2023). In New Zealand, Māori account for 15% of the total population; however, only 5.8% of older people aged 65 and over are Māori (Statistics New Zealand 2019). Both New Zealand Māori and Aboriginal and Torres Strait Islanders have poor health as they age as a result of the compounded negative effects of the legacy of colonisation resulting in intergenerational disadvantage and a lower life expectancy than the non-Māori and non-Indigenous populations (Te Pou 2019).

Mental disorders are thought to be more common in the older population (Petrova & Khvostikova 2021). The World Health Organization (WHO) world mental health report (WHO 2022) reported in 2019 that around 13% of older people aged 70 and over had a mental disorder, and depression and anxiety were the most prevalent mental disorders in this age group with estimated rates of 5.4% and 4.4% respectively, although dementia was not included in the report. Dementia has become a key public health concern and is estimated to have a prevalence of 6.9% in people aged 65 and over (WHO 2021).

"Ageism" was a broad term introduced in the late 1960s by Dr Robert Butler in response to the dismissive attitude towards older people in the United States (Butler 1969). Age does not always reflect a person's abilities or capabilities, and some older aged people may not identify with being old or with their living age. Older aged people may feel discriminated against because of their chronological age, which to them may be simply a number. This in itself leads to anxiety and stress and missed opportunities for seeking support and a positive mental health outcome (Lyons et al 2018). Ageism is negatively associated with older people's mental health (Kang & Kim 2022) and it is a risk factor for increased stress, depression, anxiety and lowered life satisfaction (Ayalin et al 2019). In older people, ageism and stigma are often compounded (Banerjee et al 2021) and are deemed a consequence of losing or gradually losing independence, whether it be physical or functional, and results in tactless stereotyping. Although ageism is experienced almost universally by older people, younger people have also reported having ageist views reciprocated against them (Wilson 2019). Ageist views may affect the recorded prevalence rates of mental illness in the older population through misdiagnosis or unwillingness to diagnose individuals because their experiences are stereotyped as being related to their age. Ageism can also influence assessment and treatment – for example, where conclusions are drawn too quickly about what the person is experiencing and why, or where treatment is withheld due to perceived

value and the person's age. Self-stigma around ageing may also influence health literacy, help-seeking and health outcome.

The concept of health literacy has three themes including a) knowledge of health, health care and health system, b) ability to process and use information in relation to health and health care, and c) ability to maintain health through self-management and by working partnership with health care providers (Liu et al 2020). Health literacy is considered as a modifiable factor of socioeconomic inequalities in health, and it has the potential to improve health outcomes and to enhance the resilience and empowerment of older people (Smith et al 2021).

SCREENING AND ASSESSMENT OF OLDER PEOPLE

The world is full of active and healthy older people, and most older people do not require additional health and social support. How each person ages is individual and unique. Some of these characteristic changes are noticeable, such as the extrinsic effects on the skin, thinning of hair and stature, but many are not.

There are several theories about ageing:
- It occurs as the result of pre-programmed switching on and off of certain genes.
- It is the result of normal "wear and tear" or a biological deteriorative process.
- It is an environmental process due to the links between chronic inflammation, DNA damage and metabolic factors influenced by diet (Bektas et al 2018).

Whatever theory you support, the life changes that can occur in older people – including physical illness and chronic disease, as well as emotional, financial and social factors – may contribute to developing new mental health issues or exacerbate pre-existing mental illness.

BIOPSYCHOSOCIAL FACTORS AND LIFE-STAGE TRANSITION

Biopsychosocial factors and life-stage transition points (e.g. retirement, death of a spouse, outliving friends or children (Fig. 18.1)) can

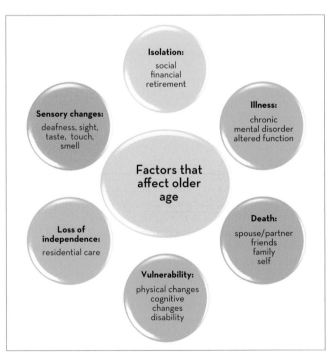

FIG. 18.1 Experiential Impacts in Ageing.

interact and lead to changes in a person's physical and mental health. For example, a person's physical activity level may alter, given changes in motivation as the result of a change in relationship or social circumstance, a chronic disease, pain, injury or increasing frailty (or a combination of these). As a consequence of a more sedentary lifestyle, a person may be more predisposed to obesity, although diet and poor oral health can also contribute, particularly if nutrition becomes poorer as the result of selecting convenience meals or making food choices based on cost. Social isolation and loneliness have a significant impact on older people's health and are particularly associated with depression, anxiety and dementia (Berg-Weger & Morley 2020).

Ageing and becoming older can also affect a person's independence. Living arrangements can change from being a homeowner, transitioning to retirement lifestyle accommodation, to requiring supportive care in a residential aged care facility. The move from home into residential aged care is one of most stressful life experiences for older people and is associated with the onset of depression and anxiety (Polacsek & Woolford 2022). Panthi (2022) conducted qualitative research on loneliness and boredom in residential care settings in New Zealand and findings indicated that older people experience loneliness and boredom despite there being a person-centred care policy in place. Moreover, older adults often struggle to adjust to live in an environment where there are a lot of people, noises and unfamiliar routines. All these factors would increase an older person's vulnerability to mental illness.

When assessing an older adult, it is important to identify what is meaningful for them, what gives them purpose and what offers connectedness. Meaning is crucial, but to continue finding or having meaning in one's life can be challenging. Meaning can be as simple as what gets you up every morning to start the day. Having "purpose" is similar, but describes a deeper sense of meaning and relates more to existential issues, such as the meaning of life. While meaning and purpose impact on how we are connected, the idea of "connectedness" also includes spirituality and closeness to others (Drageset et al 2017). In Critical thinking exercise 18.1, consider some of the uncertainty that may develop in older age.

? CRITICAL THINKING EXERCISE 18.1

Paul is 88 years old and his wife died 2 years ago, yet he could tell you exactly to the day/hour/minute how long it has been. He uses words like "nothingness", "hatred", "anger" and "emptiness" when he is talking about life and feels he is now a nuisance to all. He also feels worn out and disappointed that he too has not yet died.

From this short scenario, consider where meaning, purpose and connectedness is evident (or not). What more would you want to know about Paul?

When communicating with an older age person, allow extra time, use simple sentences (but don't speak down to the person) and do not rush. It is important for nurses to remember the person may be experiencing sensory or cognitive impairment, or both. Sight, hearing and memory may be affected. Avoid speaking in an environment filled with distractions or background noise, and sit opposite them to enable eye contact. Always listen and give the person time to respond or to ask you questions. To know if you have been understood, you can summarise the discussion. Help the person to focus on activities that may enable meaning, purpose and connectedness.

CHRONIC DISEASE AND MENTAL HEALTH

Ageing is a risk factor for developing chronic disease. The association between chronic diseases and mental health disorders have been well

established (Daré et al 2019). It is important for nurses to be aware that chronic diseases can negatively impact on mental health, and vice versa. A person's health outcomes are better when their mental health is addressed, and worse when it is not. The following list outlines some of the mental health impacts of chronic disease:

- Chronic heart failure shares some pathological pathways, physical and cognitive symptoms with depression (Sbolli et al 2020). More than 50% of patients with chronic heart failure had symptoms of depression and anxiety (Tsabedze et al 2021). Neurotransmitters or neurohormonal dysfunction contribute to the onset and worsening of the symptoms related to depression. The implication of cortisol, which is a steroid hormone, is released at times of stress, and this can exacerbate cardiac conditions and subsequently bring out depressive symptoms.

- Chronic respiratory diseases, such as chronic obstructive pulmonary disease and asthma, are commonly comorbid with mental health conditions such as depression and anxiety (Hunter et al 2021), and can affect longevity. Respiratory dysfunction can lead to, or exist with, other comorbidities and loss of physical function. Cognitive impairment is common in people with chronic obstructive pulmonary disease due to poorer physical fitness and the ability to manage own care (Yohannes et al 2017).

- Neurological injury can lead to depression and a significantly increased risk of mortality, given the functional disability incurred. Depression is a common post-stroke complication (Wijeratne & Sales 2021). It impacts recovery and quality of life, and also contributes to higher risks of stroke recurrence and mortality. The functional decline resulting from this life-threatening event can also bring about anxiety.

- Late-onset type 2 diabetes also has implications for depression as well as functional impairment and increased mortality. People who are well and manage their diabetes are at lesser risk. Studies indicate that diabetic patients with hypoglycaemic episodes are at increased risk of dementia (Huang et al 2022), and hypoglycaemia is known to effect microvascular changes which can lead to cardiac events. As a preventative strategy, guidelines suggest that an older person's glycaemic level should be slightly higher than in people with younger onset diabetes (The Royal Australian College of General Practitioners 2020).

- Chronic kidney disease and resultant end-stage renal disease are associated with an increased mortality rate and are linked to psychological distress, depression and anxiety that negatively impact the wellbeing and quality of life of patients (Guerra et al 2021). Mental health disorders are commonly comorbid with chronic kidney disease (Dalal et al 2022). Severe mental disorders reportedly increase the risk of chronic kidney disease and psychotropic medications also increase the risk of renal impairment (Taylor et al 2021). Careful monitoring of kidney function is important during psychotropic treatment.

- Arthritis, osteoarthritis, osteoporosis and pain are common and debilitating in older aged people. Onset can occur in early to midlife and becomes more severe in later years. Commonly, joints, hips, knee(s) and hands are most affected. Chronic pain has a bidirectional relationship with depression, particularly in the older population, which has the highest prevalence of comorbid chronic pain and depression (Roughan et al 2021).

- Cancer is well evidenced to affect cognition, mental and physical health. In older aged people, this can be a subjective experience and there are many physical and psychological factors that can lead to mental disorders. Cancer is often considered a chronic disease and can be emotionally disabling. Cancer-related cognitive impairment is evident in the cancer survivors, and various mechanisms are probably responsible, including chronic neuroinflammation and neurotoxic injury associated with cancer treatment (Országhová et al 2021).

SCREENING AND OBSERVATION

The main reasons for assessing older people are:
- to obtain a baseline assessment of function – this can assist in avoiding unrealistic goals
- to demonstrate positive changes to clients and to gather evidence for relatives, nurses and other health professionals
- for selection purposes (e.g. in research) to ensure that groups of people are of similar levels
- to evaluate a new approach, treatment program or service
- for legal purposes (e.g. complications following a head injury)
- to assist with diagnosis, treatment planning and expectations about prognosis.

Most of the time, nurses are involved in obtaining a baseline assessment of function and assisting with diagnosis and determining the factors relevant to prognosis. Cognitive assessment should be included in any evaluation of older adults. When a client is experiencing psychological distress, there may be limited time to conduct a full assessment. The use of observation skills and a brief assessment of the client's cognitive functioning provides valuable baseline data on which to base subsequent observations and care. Cognitive changes can affect memory and retention, orientation to place and time, and the ability to complete simple and complex tasks through executive functioning.

When making a diagnosis of mental illness, cultural concepts related to physical and mental wellbeing must be considered. The Mini-Mental State Examination (MMSE) (Folstein et al 1975), which must be purchased to use, is available in a number of different language versions that take into consideration an individual's educational attainment and culture (see Useful websites at the end of the chapter). The consequence of using the standard MMSE in groups that differ on cultural and linguistic grounds is the potential to attribute low scores to pathological processes rather than to other factors such as education level, literacy and cultural differences in cognitive and perceptual information processing. The Mini-Addenbrooke's Cognitive Examination (Mini-ACE), developed by Hsieh and colleagues (2015), is the recommended cognitive impairment screening tool in New Zealand (New Zealand Dementia Foundation 2020). The Mini-ACE has a high sensitivity for the diagnosis of dementia and mild cognitive impairment with a low specificity, and it is an acceptable testing tool for the cognitive screening in the community (Williamson & Larner 2018). The Mini-ACE is free and easy to use (see Useful websites). The Rowland Universal Dementia Assessment Scale (RUDAS) is a short cognitive screening instrument designed to minimise the effects of cultural learning and language diversity (Storey et al 2004). The RUDAS instrument and guide is freely available (see Useful websites).

When screening older people, use instruments that consider the attributes of older people, as well as reporting other conditions. For example, the Cornell Scale for Depression in Dementia is useful for identifying depression in older people with dementia (Snowdon 2010). In addition, the Mini-Cog is a short screening tool that combines the clock drawing test and three-word recall. While some studies report the superior screening properties of the Mini-Cog compared with the MMSE (Borson et al 2005; Milian et al 2012), others report similar screening results (Borson et al 2003; Dougherty et al 2010). The Mini-Cog assessment and instructions are freely available (see Useful websites).

Comprehensive geriatric assessment is a multi-dimensional assessment that includes medical, psychological and functional assessments aiming to evaluate older people's impairments, functional capacity and needs and to develop a holistic care plan (Parker et al 2018). Comprehensive geriatric assessment needs to be performed for older people with complex comorbidities, multimorbidity, frailty or polypharmacy (Kok & Reynolds 2017).

Obtaining a health history and nursing assessment

The determinants of health are grouped into four categories:
- physical environment – housing
- social environment – education, employment, relationships
- economic environment – income
- individual environment – sex, physical or mental determinants (WHO 2016).

Pay attention to each of these determinants when obtaining a health history in older aged people, particularly where the person has comorbidities and a mental disorder, to ensure you identify all the issues that may inform nursing care and management (Talley & Jones 2018). A methodical approach to history-taking is necessary because older aged people tend to under-report symptoms and problems. Building a rapport will foster trust. Remember not to use terms of endearment, which can feel patronising. Use the person's name. Wherever possible, have a carer or relative present to assist in gathering collateral information.

Establish what is the presenting issue and obtain an in-depth history. Asking about a person's social history and the physical environment where they live can help to flag any difficulties or habits that may be influencing their symptoms or impacting on their activities of daily living. Follow through with a review of body systems. This can be modified to reduce the burden of answering questions, which may have already been asked on many occasions, to specific areas such as mobility and falls, elimination, diet, vision and hearing. Ask about current medications, why the person is taking them and whether they adhere to what has been prescribed. You may also have access to previous health records and you can check medications with the person's general practitioner or prescriber if you are unsure.

A dementia assessment is only appropriate if suspected. Complete Critical thinking exercise 18.2 before moving onto the next section, where specific assessment tools are discussed.

 CRITICAL THINKING EXERCISE 18.2

List the specific areas you have observed a medical or nursing colleague perform in a health history assessment for an older age person. What did you notice is different from a younger person's assessment?

Cognitive Assessment Tools

Assessment tools are often used to assist in care strategies and are well validated globally to the general population. However, in a recent Australian study involving Aboriginal and Torres Strait Islander peoples, the findings suggested considering the efficacy of alternative assessment tools for visual and motor impairment, and people with lower education levels (Lavrencic et al 2018). Culturally specific adaptions, such as "logical memory" support the use of stories for memory assessment in this cohort (Lavrencic et al 2018). Logical memory involves being told a story and asking the person to recall it 30 minutes later.

The most commonly used validated cognitive assessment tools are:
- The Standardised Mini Mental-State Examination (Molloy & Standish 1997)
- The Abbreviated Mental Test Score (Hodkinson 1972)
- The Clock Drawing Test (Rakusa et al 2018)
- Montreal Cognitive Assessment (Nasreddine et al 2005)

- The Mini-Addenbrooke's Cognitive Examination (Hsieh et al 2015)
- The Addenbrooke's Cognitive Examination – Revised (Beishon et al 2019).

Tools developed for use with people from culturally diverse backgrounds are:
- Mini-Cog (Seitz et al 2018)
- Rowland Universal Dementia Assessment Scale (Komalasari et al 2019)
- Kimberley Indigenous Cognitive Assessment short form (LoGiudice et al 2010).

Capacity and Competence

Older adults are certainly at increased risk for impaired decisional capacity. However, psychiatric illness and dementia do not invariably impair decisional capacity. Dementia is often the most prominent illness in clinicians' minds when considering impaired decisional capacity. Psychosis and depression may also impair decisional capacity in older adults via emotional factors, such as paranoid delusions or severe hopelessness.

Given the variety of validated tools available, complete the Critical thinking exercise 18.3.

 CRITICAL THINKING EXERCISE 18.3

Choose a tool and try it on yourself and then a friend. How was the experience for you? Discuss the experience with your friend and comment on how useful the tool was.

MENTAL HEALTH DISORDERS IN OLDER AGE

Although a number of conditions, including anxiety disorders, depression, suicide, substance misuse, delirium, dementia and schizophrenia, fall within the context of mental illness in old age, they do not occur *because* of ageing. Approximately 15% of people aged 60 or older experience a mental disorder (Kenbubpha et al 2019).

Older people often present with and focus on physical symptoms, such as pain or difficulty sleeping, cognitive concerns and associated stress, rather than reporting psychiatric symptoms, such as depression and anxiety (Herman 2022). All psychological symptoms should be assessed in the context of medical or cognitive impairments to ensure the most appropriate treatment is provided (Crocco et al 2017). Often differential symptom presentation can be difficult because survey criteria specifically for older aged people (e.g. "fear of burden on family") is not included (Balsamo et al 2018). Older people may fear situations or objects, experience memory impairment or confusion, and their symptoms may coexist with another mental illness, such as depression and dementia (Balsamo et al 2018).

Common mental health disorders are explored in the following sections with relation to older people and also in separate chapters devoted to the relevant disorder.

Anxiety Disorders

Anxiety disorders are highly prevalent in later life (Byrne & Pachana 2021) and are one of the most common mental disorders experienced by older adults. However, anxiety disorders are largely underdiagnosed and undertreated in older people (Grenier et al 2019). Anxiety disorders are highly comorbid with depression, substance use disorder and sleep disorder (Hellwig & Domschke 2019). They can continue through life from an early onset, or can manifest later in life, but are often under-recognised, perhaps in part because older adults have lower mental health literacy around anxiety than younger people (Beaunoyer

et al 2019). A presentation of anxiety in older people is similar to that in younger people. However, as with depression, diagnosis is complicated by the tendency of older adults to focus on physical rather than psychological illness and by sensory deficits, medical comorbidities and cognitive impairment (Creighton et al 2018). The most common anxiety disorders in older adults are generalised anxiety disorder and phobias. Anxiety disorder is negatively associated with cognition, especially executive functions related to working memory (Nyberg et al 2021).

There is insufficient research examining the aetiology of anxiety disorders in older adults. However, evidence suggests that while risk factors are similar to those for depression, social factors such as low affective support during childhood, negative parenting and experiencing negative life events are uniquely associated with anxiety (Zhang et al 2015). Women experience higher prevalence of anxiety disorders (Grenier et al 2019), and residents of residential aged care facilities are at high risk for developing an anxiety disorder (Creighton et al 2018). Discrimination experienced by older people in the LGBTIQA+ community has been considered a factor for anxiety related to disclosing sexual orientation and gender identity, with 34% hiding their sexuality when seeking healthcare (Australian Human Rights Commission 2015).

Co-occurring anxiety and depression are common and affect treatment and outcome. Anxiety worsens the severity of depression in later life, but doesn't change psychopathology (An et al 2019). Co-occurring anxiety disorder in people with major depression lowers the rate of recovery and is also associated with a higher rate of cognitive decline and suicide (Santini et al 2015). The presence of anxiety symptoms decreases the efficacy of depression treatment, and, although treatment for depression may reduce anxiety, this is not always the case, with anxiety symptoms persisting despite the resolution of other depressive symptoms (van der Veen et al 2015). Those experiencing a cognitive disorder and behaviour problems often have a more rapid functional loss when they also present with anxiety symptoms (Crocco et al 2017).

Given that anxiety is so frequently under-diagnosed, awareness of how anxiety presents and routine screening in older adults is an important nursing role – regardless of the clinical setting. Talking and building a rapport that is therapeutic can help to identify anxiety and enables early intervention, treatment and referral as appropriate. Treatment strategies involve individual planning with the person and may require modifications in lifestyle and addressing psychosocial stressors. Depending on the severity of the illness, the comorbidities and the clinical setting, nurses can assess the capacity of the older age person to engage with different types of therapy and support skill development (e.g. mindfulness and breathing techniques, online self-help). The Royal Australian and New Zealand College of Psychiatrists' clinical practice guidelines recommend cognitive behaviour therapy (CBT), either face-to-face or digital, as first-line management (Andrews et al 2018). Digital CBT, whether via a computer, hand-held device or mobile phone, has been shown to be effective even in people with mild cognitive impairment (Andrews et al 2018). CBT is one modality of talking therapy, providing psychoeducation working on cognition and behaviour by addressing maladaptive thought patterns, and gradual exposure to anxiety-provoking situations (Munir & Takov 2022).

In terms of pharmacological options, selective serotonin reuptake inhibitors (SSRIs) and serotonin norepinephrine reuptake inhibitors (SNRIs) are the first-line choices for older adults with anxiety disorders as they are proved to be efficacious and well tolerated. Treatment duration varies from 3–6 months to years (Garakani et al 2021).

The Three Ds: Depression, Delirium and Dementia

Depression is not unique to older age. It can manifest at different times in a person's life and may be untreated for many years. Delirium and dementia are also not necessarily age-related and can occur in younger people. However, because depression, delirium and dementia are common in older adults and are frequently confused, it is important to understand the differences and similarities. Keep in mind that an older age person may present with more than one of these disorders and the symptoms may overlap as shown in Table 18.1.

Depression

There is a common perception that older people become depressed as a part of the normal ageing process. This is not so, but older people are vulnerable to developing a depressive illness because of age-related biochemical changes and psychological factors.

Depression is one of the most prevalent disorders of older age and it is associated with increased risks of disability and mortality in older people. The cause of depression remains unclear; however, depression in late life is thought to be related to the complex psychological, biological and social factors a person might experience (Zenebe et al 2021). There is also a lack of clarity around the interrelationship between depression, cognitive decline and dementia, with some reporting depression as a dementia risk factor and others naming depression as a consequence of cognitive decline. There was a suggestion that depression may be associated with lower frontal lobe blood perfusion (Brandao et al 2019). Furthermore, diagnosis may be hindered if the person also has a physical illness, which leads health professionals to believe that the person's depressive symptoms are understandable given their physical status – depression is frequently associated with many common medical conditions found in later life such as stroke, cancer, myocardial infarction, diabetes, rheumatoid arthritis and Parkinson's disease (Julien et al 2016).

As described above, significant life changes that are associated with growing older can also place older people at risk of depression. It is suggested that lower social support and even hospitalisation can be factors in developing distress that can lead to depression (Liguori et al 2018). Prevalence increases for people aged 85 years or older, those who are hospitalised and those living in residential aged care facilities. Factors associated with depression include female gender, poor education, early trauma, chronic somatic illness, cognitive impairment, stressful life events (e.g. bereavement), medications, a decrease in activity and losses related to physical illness, financial security, accommodation and independence (Kok & Reynolds 2017).

Presentation. Although older people may exhibit the cardinal features of depression, such as low mood and loss of interest, they often attribute these feelings to their physical condition; this will then be the focus of the presentation rather than an acknowledgement of feeling depressed. Complaints might include fatigue, weight loss, pain, problems with self-care, memory concerns or unexplained medical symptoms (Hegeman et al 2015; Kok & Reynolds 2017).

Depression and dementia share common features, such as poor concentration, low mood and social isolation and may both present with psychomotor slowing, apathy, impaired memory, fatigue, sleep disturbance and poor concentration. Distinguishing between grief and depression can also be difficult, since they also share many symptoms. Grief, however, tends to fluctuate, with the person experiencing good and bad days, whereas feelings of emptiness and despair are constant in a person with depression.

Screening and assessment. Initiating a conversation with an older age person about their mood is a good starting point to identifying depression and ensuring appropriate care and treatment are implemented. In evaluating symptoms of depression, the person's context is important; remember that concurrent diagnoses contribute to (and complicate) the clinical picture. Interviewing the person's family or carer can both corroborate the person's history and substantiate a professional assessment, as well as gather additional information to assist in the assessment. Family or a carer will commonly report changes that the person has not recognised such as social withdrawal, irritability, avoiding family and friends, poor hygiene and memory change. Losses such as status, income and bereavement can contribute to feelings of dejection.

Undiagnosed and untreated depression places the person at risk of mental suffering, poor physical health, social isolation and suicide. Screening for depression should be undertaken for people who are recently bereaved and, in particular, when they have unusual symptoms, such as marked functional impairment, mood-congruent delusions and psychomotor retardation. It is important to note that older people may use different language to describe their depressed mood. For example, rather than describing sadness they may talk about "their nerves".

The Geriatric Depression Scale (short form) (Box 18.1) is an age-specific screening tool for use in those who are cognitively intact (Sheikh & Yesavage 1986; Yesavage et al 1983). There is also a longer version of 30 items, although it does not measure physical symptoms. The GDS is available in many languages (see Useful websites).

The Patient Health Questionnaire or PHQ9 (Spitzer et al 1994) is another simple screening tool that may help identify depression. In particular, there are three questions that ask directly if there is a loss of mood or sense of hopelessness, a lack of interest and thoughts of death.

The possibility of a depressive illness should also be considered in older people if they develop anxiety or cognitive impairment. Depression has a high degree of overlap with dementia, and can have further impairment on cognition and function (Kverno & Velez 2018). The best practice is early diagnosis and early treatment.

To assist with the diagnosis of depression:

- check for the presence of depressive symptoms using a screening instrument for this age group, such as the GDS, but note that the reliability of the GDS is reduced when clients have cognitive impairment. Remember that people can experience depression, a physical disorder and/or dementia all at the same time. Do not assume that symptoms can be easily related to the person's life circumstances or their age.

BOX 18.1   Geriatric Depression Scale (Short Form)

A series of yes and no questions, with the answer in bold equalling one point.

1.	Are you basically satisfied with your life?	**No**
2.	Have you dropped many of your activities or interests?	**Yes**
3.	Do you feel that your life is empty?	**Yes**
4.	Do you often get bored?	**Yes**
5.	Are you in good spirits most of the time?	**No**
6.	Are you afraid that something bad is going to happen to you?	**Yes**
7.	Do you feel happy most of the time?	**No**
8.	Do you feel helpless?	**Yes**
9.	Do you prefer to stay at home, rather than go out and do things?	**Yes**
10.	Do you feel that you have more problems with memory than most?	**Yes**
11.	Do you think it is wonderful to be alive now?	**No**
12.	Do you feel pretty worthless the way you are now?	**Yes**
13.	Do you feel full of energy?	**No**
14.	Do you feel that your situation is hopeless?	**Yes**
15.	Do you think that most people are better off than you are?	**Yes**

When a score of more than five is indicated, a more thorough clinical investigation should be undertaken.

This short version has been adapted by many organisations.

Yesavage 1988.

Where clients have significant cognitive impairment the Cornell Scale for Depression in Dementia (CSDD) should be used. The CSDD was developed to assess the severity of depressive symptoms of people with dementia (Alexopoulos et al 1988) and it is a screening tool and is not diagnostic. The nurse will interview the client's caregiver on the 19 items of the scale. The caregiver then reports their observations based on the previous week.

Treating depression in older people. The most effective treatment for depression is early intervention. Nurses are often in the unique position of being able to identify behaviour changes and specific symptoms early or at onset because they have more contact with clients in hospital and community settings. Documenting what you have observed clearly in the person's medical record and escalating a referral for further assessment and treatment by health professionals who are skilled and educated in the care and management of older people with mental illness is essential (Haugan et al 2013).

Nurses can support people to engage in regular exercise, which has been identified as effective for improving physical and mental health in older adults with mental illness, particularly for those who are experiencing depression (Chen et al 2018). Mental health nurses provide psychotherapeutic support and interpersonal psychotherapy to enable clients to problem-solve and to talk about their feelings. Psychotherapy is recommended for older adults experiencing mild to moderately severe depression and is as effective as antidepressants (Kok & Reynolds 2017). Acceptance and commitment therapy, cognitive therapy, CBT, mindfulness-based cognitive therapy, compassion-focused therapy, group therapy and counselling are useful, especially when the depressive illness is loss-related. CBT needs to be adapted to older people's special needs in order to be effective (Dafsari et al 2019). Mindfulness-based cognitive therapy is a meditation-based intervention that has been reported as a promising and cost-effective treatment for older adults with depression and anxiety (Foulk et al 2014). Mindfulness-based cognitive therapy is also potentially effective for people with depression in dementia (Douglas et al 2022).

Although pharmacological treatment is often effective in treating depression, adverse events due to medical comorbidities and medication interactions can be problematic in older people. Selective serotonin reuptake inhibitors (SSRIs) and serotonin norepinephrine reuptake inhibitors (SNRIs) are the first-line pharmacological intervention for late life depression as they are generally safe and well tolerated (Kverno & Velez 2018). However, it is crucial that the introduction (and discontinuation) of antidepressants is titrated (tapered) gradually to ensure the drug is tolerated (and to ensure relapse or recurrence does not occur). Problems with polypharmacy can be minimised through a tool such as the Screening Tool of Older Persons Prescriptions and Screening Tool to Alert doctors to Right Treatment (STOPP/START), which supports prescribing doctors to make appropriate medication prescriptions and avoid undertreatment (Kok & Reynolds 2017). Electroconvulsive therapy is strongly recommended in all patients (including older people) with severe and treatment-resistant major depressive disorder (Zilles 2018) and it was shown to be safe with no increased risk of dementia (Osler et al 2018).

Delirium. Delirium (or acute confusion) is the most prevalent neurocognitive disorder and is a serious acute reversible medical condition whereby a person's mental ability is affected (an acute decline in consciousness and cognition). It develops over a short period of time (usually within hours or days) and symptoms tend to fluctuate throughout the day. Delirium mostly affects patients who are older and hospitalised for medical treatment; delirium is often underdiagnosed by clinicians, so careful history review and physical examination are important to detect delirium associated with underlying medical conditions (Keenan & Jain 2022).

Older aged people are at risk of developing delirium if they:
- are acutely unwell or have a chronic illness
- have a pre-existing diagnosis of dementia or depression
- are 70 years of age or older
- have sensory impairment such as poor eyesight
- are taking multiple medications
- are in drug withdrawal, including from alcohol
- are undergoing a surgical procedure requiring general anaesthetic (e.g. hip fracture) (Lee et al 2017).

The causes of delirium can include physical illness, urinary tract infection, constipation, dehydration, pain, polypharmacy, excessive alcohol consumption and abruptly withdrawing from alcohol or medications. Presenting symptoms can vary and are often masked by comorbid symptoms of other diseases. Symptoms include confusion and forgetfulness, inattention, unusual behaviour, agitation or withdrawn behaviour, night wakening and day sleeping, exhibiting fear or upset, mood change, hallucinations and incontinence (Lee et al 2017). It is imperative to determine the causal factors and treat the underlying problem if possible. Taking a comprehensive history in consultation with the family and including medical, physical, cognitive, social and behavioural function will help identify the underlying condition and inform interventions to reverse delirium.

The approach to delirium. The Confusion Assessment Method is a tool developed for non-psychiatrically trained clinicians and researchers (Inouye et al 1990). This tool is available in a short form, which has four items commonly used for screening and a long form, which has 10 items for diagnostic confirmation, subtyping and research (Inouye 2018). To support a diagnosis of delirium, there must be evidence of an acute onset and fluctuating changes in the person's condition. The presence of inattention, with either disorganised thought processes or an altered level of consciousness, is required.

Although there is no specific pathology test for diagnosing delirium, there are studies that suggest an association with raised inflammatory markers C-reactive protein and inteleukin-6 (Inouye 2018).

Prior to an older person undergoing surgery, it is important that the nurse assesses the person to ensure any changes in behaviour following surgery can be detected and early intervention given. There are two established risk factors for older people undergoing surgery: previous alcohol/drug abuse and prolonged operating time under a general anaesthetic. Evidence supports a preventive approach including all staff being aware of delirium risk factors, reductions in the use of medications that increase risk and delirium-friendly post-surgery medication orders, addressing constipation and other known risk factors, and attending to sensory impairment and individual complications (Freter et al 2016). Managing delirium includes supportive therapy and pharmacological management. Supportive therapy that nurses can offer includes ensuring patient safety, attention to fluid and nutrition and reorientation (e.g. memory cues, including calendars, clocks and photographs of family and pets).

Dementia

Prevalence. There are more than 100 diseases, including brain injury or trauma, that can cause dementia, but it is not a normal part of ageing. However, as the prevalence of dementia increases exponentially with age, the number of people living with dementia is increasing in Australia and New Zealand because more people are living longer. In 2021 it was estimated that between 386,200 and 472,000 Australians were living with dementia (AIHW 2021). The number of people diagnosed with young-onset dementia (before the age of 65) is also increasing, with approximately 27,800 people affected, including people as young as 30 years of age (AIHW 2021). Dementia is the second leading cause of death in Australia and the leading cause of death in women

(Australian Bureau of Statistics 2018). In Aboriginal and Torres Strait Islander people aged over 65 years, dementia is three times higher than for the wider Australian older age population (AIHW 2018a; Radford et al 2015). New Zealand estimates are similar – in 2016, the prevalence estimate of dementia in New Zealand was 62,287 people (Deloitte Economics 2017) – a 29% increase since the estimate of 48,182 in 2011. This number is also predicted to increase to 170,212 (2.9% of the population) by 2050 (Deloitte Economics 2017). Māori and Pacific Islanders in New Zealand have higher prevalence of dementia (Cheung et al 2022).

In the early stages of dementia, people usually live in the community, while people with higher levels of cognitive impairment are often accommodated in residential aged care facilities.

"Dementia" is the common umbrella term used for Alzheimer's disease, vascular dementia and Lewy body dementia, and is the single greatest cause of disability in older Australians (AIHW 2018a). Other types of dementia are frontotemporal lobe, substance/medication use, traumatic brain injury, HIV infection and many more. Another term for dementia is "major neurocognitive disorder"; for the purpose of this section, dementia will be referred to in this context.

Clinical features. Older aged people with dementia experience cognitive decline/impairment and behavioural and/or psychological symptoms. Cognitive impairment can also result in the person displaying problems that may be identified by care staff as being challenging to manage. "Sundowning" is a term to describe unsettled presentation and worsening neuropsychiatric symptoms of people with dementia in the afternoon and early evening (Valletta et al 2021). The clinical features of sundowning include worsening disorientation and anxiety, and associated wandering, agitation and aggression. This increase in disorientation has variously been attributed to diurnal variations in hormones and light, as well as to fatigue and a search for familiar surroundings in which to rest. However, in some people this pattern is reversed – they are more disoriented in the morning. Apathy and depression are often misinterpreted and underdiagnosed. Excluding other causes for the fluctuations in behaviour, such as pain or infection, should be considered.

Assessing the following cognitive domains helps to establish the presence of dementia and determine severity:

- Complex attention – includes sustained attention, divided attention, selective attention and information processing speed
- Executive function – includes planning, decision-making, working memory, responding to feedback, inhibition and mental flexibility
- Learning and memory – includes free recall, cued recall, recognition memory, semantic and autobiographical long-term memory and implicit learning
- Language – includes object naming, word finding, fluency, grammar and syntax and receptive language
- Perceptual-motor function – includes visual perception, visio-constructional reasoning and perceptual-motor coordination
- Social cognition – includes recognition of emotions, theory of mind and insight.

Nursing management of people with dementia. Nurses can support the person with dementia to manage their feelings and thoughts, to deal with their stresses, to link them to their community (including a safe environment) and to support the individual and family to build resilience. A person-centred approach to care aims to understand the person and seeks to engage with and respond appropriately to their individual situation.

Distraction, redirection, reassurance and reorientation form the core behavioural interventions. Observe for triggers that pre-empt behavioural symptoms – an individualised care plan should identify and address the person's triggers and behaviours (Macfarlane &

O'Connor 2016). People with dementia are often highly responsive to the environment they find themselves in. Therefore, wherever possible, the environment needs to be made safe and familiar, with objects that have meaning for the person (e.g. family photographs). Avoid unnecessary changes to routines.

However, not all people with dementia have behavioural problems, as Stephen's story presents.

PERSPECTIVES IN PRACTICE
Nurse's Story 18.1: Stephen

As a newly qualified registered nurse commencing in aged care, I had not considered that LGBTIQA+ issues would have to be considered. It came to my attention with the admission of Alex (61 years), who was brought to the facility by his partner, James. James reported that Alex had been displaying strange behaviours for the past two years. He had been an architect in a small local company, and one of the senior partners had contacted James with concerns about his quality of work, which was deteriorating. James had also noted that Alex was becoming increasingly dependent on him in decision-making. At this point James took Alex to see his general practitioner and he was diagnosed with early dementia and referred to an aged care assessment team (ACAT). Alex then moved into an aged care facility; however, he experienced loneliness, new surroundings and the absence of his lifelong partner. The ACAT occupational therapist introduced Alex to art therapy. Initially this was enjoyed, but Alex thought the people who were there were odd, and this was getting him down. He thought of them as unfamiliar and "old". Alex's niece mentioned to James that she had met some of his old acquaintances at a community centre, which prompted connecting with their old network of friends and the social life they both had led. Some of his friends attended social functions at the aged care facility. Alex's friends helped staff to understand Alex's personality and values, as well as gaining a better understanding of things that would help him to feel more accepted and comfortable in his new environment. These social events also helped Alex to adjust to the changes in his environment and staff noticed that he was more accepting and engaged with other residents.

Treating People with Dementia

There currently is no cure for dementia, with the main focus of care being to maintain quality of life and ensure that a person's functional abilities and independence are maximised for as long as possible. Focus of care from nurses should be to promote a healthy lifestyle, including regular exercise, good diet and socialisation, which can also help to improve quality of life. Medications that can help somewhat are acetyl-cholinesterase inhibitors (donepezil, memantine and galantamine), which can prolong the action of the deficient neurotransmitter in the brain and might improve the cognition of people with dementia and delay the progression of the dementia (Marucci et al 2021). It is important that people with dementia and their families understand the limited effects that these medications can have, and that disease progression will continue despite them being prescribed.

Behavioural and psychological symptoms are common in people with dementia. Non-pharmacological interventions are recommended as the first treatment choice for the behavioural and psychological symptoms of dementia (BPSD) (Masopust et al 2018). Non-pharmacological principles for dementia care include safe environments that are familiar, using cues to assist the individual, such as routines, and using familiar repetitive activities. This may be in the form of music, art, household chores or having personal belongings that connect to their past, activity engagement with pets or sensory stimulation (Scales et al 2018). Pharmacological interventions should only be used for BPSD if non-pharmacological interventions are ineffective, and associated

TABLE 18.1 Comparison of Dementia, Delirium and Depression

Features	Dementia	Delirium	Depression
Onset and duration	Slow deterioration over time – months to years	Sudden onset – hours or days	Mood change over 2 weeks and may coincide with a life event or change such as the death of a loved one
Course	Slow and progressive cognitive decline; non-reversible	Sudden, short and fluctuating; reversible underlying cause	Diurnal fluctuations – can be worse of a morning or evening; reversible with treatment
Signs and symptoms	Wandering, agitation, sleep disturbance, fluctuations in behaviour during the day, generally alert, depression may be present, difficulty with word recall	Restless and uneasy, with fluctuations in agitation, restlessness and hallucinations, impaired attention, mood changes from anger, tearful outbursts and fear, disorganised thinking	Withdrawn, apathetic, feelings of hopelessness and alert, though attention fluctuates with mood; appetite may be increased or diminished

risks are high and acute (Masopust et al 2018). Demonstrated efficacy of pharmacological interventions in BPSD management is limited, and the medications used (i.e. antidepressants, antipsychotics, acetylcholinesterase inhibitors, mood stabilisers and benzodiazepines) are associated with potentially severe side effects (Masopust et al 2018). Therefore, pharmacological interventions in BPSD management should constantly consider risk verse benefit, and treatment should be discontinued once symptoms are improved or risk outweighs benefit.

To recap, depression, delirium and dementia may present with similar features. Table 18.1 provides an overview of the onset and duration, course, activity, alertness, attention mood and thinking pattern.

Substance Use

Substance use is a growing problem within the older age population (Rao et al 2019). In 2018 the AIHW reported that older people aged 70 years or older were more likely to exceed lifetime risks and alcohol-related harm, with alcohol consumption more than 5 days per week (AIHW 2018b). The 2016 National Drug Strategy House Survey reported an increase in the proportion of older Australians using illicit drugs, indicating that there is now an ageing cohort of drug users (AIHW 2017). In 2016–17 the principal drugs of concern for those aged over 50 years old were alcohol (66%), followed by 9% for cannabis, 7% for amphetamines and 5% for heroin (AIHW 2018b). Problematic use is clearly under-reported, with drug use prevalence occurring in baby boomers and post-baby boomers (Carew & Comiskey 2018). In New Zealand, alcohol is the most commonly used substance in the older population, and other substance use among older people is also increasing with time (Te Pou 2019). Older people are reported to have the highest increases in morbidity and mortality associated with substance use conditions (Thompsell et al 2019).

Triggers for increased substance use in older age may be associated with tolerance to previously used substances, although life-changing events, as well as planned and unplanned stressors, have a significant influence – for example, retirement, unforeseen financial strain, death of a spouse, chronic illness (both physical and mental), family disputes/estrangement, sleep disturbances or change of living arrangements.

Cannabis use in older Australians is also increasing, particularly given the contemporary influence of medicinal cannabinoids (Kostadinov & Roche 2017). Opioid use for chronic pain is also not without risk. Pain is diverse, with long term co-occurring conditions and concerns. Benzodiazepines prescribed for sleep deprivation are among the most frequently prescribed drugs for older people (Musich et al 2019). This in itself is problematic because benzodiazepines are highly addictive and increase the risk of falls. Symptoms of substance use can also be masked by symptoms of chronic illness, such as diabetes, or even depression and dementia. Review the possible symptoms in Critical thinking exercise 18.4.

CRITICAL THINKING EXERCISE 18.4

Signs and symptoms of substance use can be both behavioural and physical. Substance use may manifest with many overlapping symptoms with chronic illness. Access the following NARCONON web link and review the listed signs and symptoms. Which do you believe may be misinterpreted as a chronic illness?

NARCONON web link: www.narconon.org/drug-abuse/signs-symptoms-of-drug-abuse.html

Substance use should always be explored during the nursing assessment. Ascertaining the substances used, when and how much, is the primary goal. And ask for specifics. Rather than asking someone whether they drink alcohol, ask: "How much alcohol do you drink per day?" If they say "not much" or "I only drink socially", ask them to tell you exactly how much alcohol this involves. Many people may relate that they do not drink "much", but may be unaware of the guidelines and consider their intake to be less harmful than it is (see also Chapter 13 for more information). Given the complexity of older age care, targeted age-appropriate interventions should be implemented (Kostadinov & Roche 2017; Musich et al 2019). Meeting the individual needs of an older age person can be complex because withdrawal symptoms may be delayed, so ongoing nursing observation and assessment is required. Providing social and emotional support requires an interdisciplinary team approach. Escalation of care should be considered during detoxification.

Schizophrenia

Psychosis usually onsets in the early 20s; however, in 15–20% of those with a diagnosis of schizophrenia, symptoms appear in middle to later life (Cohen 2018). Precise age of onset is difficult to determine given it may be based on the person's age when clinically assessed, but it is estimated 17% of the general older age have mild cognitive impairment (Cohen 2018). Older-onset schizophrenia is more likely in women given physiological changes, such as oestrogen depletion after menopause, which is thought to affect neuron function and decrease cognition (Cai & Huang 2018). In older aged people, paranoia is common and not necessarily due to cognitive changes.

As with other mental health disorders in old age, assessment is complicated by co-occurring conditions, and stigma is also an issue. There is also a relationship between schizophrenia and risk of dementia, specifically in women, which is associated with loneliness and women being more prone to mood swings, insomnia, irritability, anxiety and depression (Cai & Huang 2018). If we consider the symptoms of schizophrenia in the older aged (65 years or older), there are common features with dementia, though dementia is characterised by a progressive loss of cognition and function.

In older people, psychosis in schizophrenia is often associated with brain abnormalities such as stroke, tumours and trauma, with marked neuropsychological impairment (Cai & Huang 2018). Behaviours can be challenging to manage, and determining the underlying factors is crucial. In people with Alzheimer's and psychosis related to schizophrenia (rather than to dementia), remission is common. Management should be collaborative, with clinical symptom management and involving the older age person in addressing any concerns affecting their daily life. CBT and social skills training are useful strategies. Social contact and education of caregivers can reduce associated anxiety and normalise the person's environment.

The use of second-generation antipsychotics has increased in older people even though the side effects may cause serious harm in older age (Kjosavik et al 2017). Antipsychotics should always be used cautiously and critically (Gebauer & Lukas 2022). Clinicians should constantly evaluate the treatment effects and monitor potential side effects while antipsychotics are being prescribed.

✳ HISTORICAL ANECDOTE 18.1

Basket Cases and Bedlam!

After St Marys of Bethlehem was established in 1247, the monks there became known as "basket men" for their habit of carrying baskets to collect and distribute food and alms for the sick – this led to our modern stigmatising term "basket case". By 1377, St Marys had become known as "Bethlem", which local townspeople vulgarised to "Bedlam". The modern-day term "bedlam", meaning uproar and confusion, is derived from the asylum's name. Like many asylums of the Middle Ages, Bedlam was overcrowded and maladministered. A dehumanising practice developed in the mid-1700s when, for the price of a penny, a visitor could spend what was advertised as a "very amusing" afternoon touring the facility observing the "old loonies". During visits, people were provided with a glimpse of the horrific, yet socially acceptable, treatment of people in grisly living conditions receiving bizarre, painful, dehumanising treatments.

Read More About It
Clarke BFL 1975. Mental disorder in earlier Britain: exploratory studies. University of Wales Press, Cardiff.

✳ HISTORICAL ANECDOTE 18.2

Treatment or Neglect?

History teaches that treatment of mental illness has been used to justify healthcare and nursing negligence. During the 1960s and '70s, a program referred to as "deep sleep therapy" was practised (in combination with electroconvulsive therapy) by Dr Harry Bailey at Chelmsford Private Hospital in Sydney. Deep sleep therapy involved long periods of barbiturate-induced unconsciousness. It was prescribed for conditions ranging from schizophrenia and depression to addiction. Twenty-six patients died due to the therapy during that time. After the failure of medical agencies to investigate or address complaints, a series of newspaper articles in the early 1980s in the *Sydney Morning Herald* and television coverage exposed the abuses at the hospital.

Read More About It
Walton M 2013 Deep sleep therapy and Chelmsford Private Hospital: Have we learnt anything? Australasian Psychiatry, 21(3): 206–212.

Suicide

Older aged people have a significantly higher rate of death by suicide in Australia than the younger population. In 2021, there were 3144 suicide deaths in Australia, with 18.1% of people over the age of 65 years; males aged over 85 years had the highest age-specific suicide rate of any age group (ABS 2021). In New Zealand, the rate of suicide in people aged over 65 years is significantly lower. However, across all age groups, men and Māori were highly represented in the figures, with 401 men dying by suicide in 2021–22, a rate of 14.9 per 100,000. The rates of Māori who died by suicide, not age specific, in 2020–21, was 23.9 per 100,000 in males and 9.2 per 100,000 in females; that was about 1.4 and 2 times higher than non-Māori males and females respectively (Te Whatu Ora 2022).

Risk Factors for Suicide in Older People

Older aged people may be vulnerable to suicide, particularly where there is an increase in the complexity of lifelong stressors. Significant issues may enhance feelings of loss: losing or having lost a life partner; bereavement and becoming socially isolated; feeling a lack of social support; or being lonely or alone. Other risks include cognitive impairment or decline, whether from a physical or neurodegenerative cause. Chronic illness, physical/psychological pain, substance use and mental health disorders are also key risk considerations, as are previous suicide attempts. Depression and dementia, stroke and a new or existing diagnosis of a life-limiting disease such as cancer may contribute to suicidal ideation due to loss of (or fear of loss of) physical and cognitive function (Ahmedani et al 2017). Unmistakably, suicide risk is linked to poor physical health. In an American study, 17 physical health conditions were associated with increased suicide in older people (Ahmedani et al 2017).

Building an awareness of these risks places nurses in a position to be more involved in mental health promotion and early intervention focused on preventing suicidal behaviours in older aged people. Like anyone who says they are experiencing suicidal thoughts, an older age person who talks about suicide must be taken very seriously – never assume that because someone is an older person and hospitalised, or accessing aged care services or living in a residential aged care facility, that they are not capable of a suicide attempt. The person offering information about their intended suicide, identifying how, when and by what means, will enable the level of risk to be assessed (see Chapter 9 for risk assessment).

A suicide intent may not always be obvious, as Peter's story shows.

🕮 PERSPECTIVES IN PRACTICE

Nurse's Story 18.2: Peter

I had been allocated an older male client, Bill, who had been bounced around to different organisations before securing funding with the non-government organisation I was working at. Because of Bill's circumstances (socioeconomic, health and age), he qualified for several care packages. So, two community support workers were allocated to work with him across the week for nominal hours. I visited Bill in the first week and began to establish a relationship with him. My co-worker was on sick leave, so my 1-hour visit was the only support Bill had received for the first week. In the second week, Bill received support from both packages (total of 3 hours). During this visit, I noted Bill to be comfortable to verbalise that he was feeling unsure about his future, though we spoke of his long-term goals. In his younger years he had been interested in studying computing at TAFE, so he agreed that in our next visit we would focus on short-term achievable goals. Two days after this visit, he died by suicide.

I had mixed emotions about this. I had a duty of care to Bill. Did I miss something? Were there signs that I should have picked up? Am I qualified enough to be dealing with these types of people? I became angry – the system had let Bill down. Why had he been bounced around? Would the outcome have changed with a more consistent approach to his care? I even questioned if this reflected on my capacity to manage people with mental health disorders as a community support worker. To rationalise this, I tried to weigh up how much I could really achieve in such a short time with him. We had a total of 2 hours together.

Suicide prevention in old age should greatly expand its intervention and pay more attention to socio-environmental conditions that particularly affect old people, such as decreased physical health, social isolation and loneliness, and financial difficulties (De Leo 2022). Health and stress factors increase the complexity of the explanatory model for suicide in older age (Conejero et al 2018). Psychological pain and somatic distress have been implicated in people who have had lifelong suicide ideation (Concjero et al 2018). It was suggested that suicide risk assessment should be part of the older age assessment (van Orden & Deming 2018).

One approach to restoring recovery is through a chronic care model. The chronic care model, developed by Dr Edward Wagner (2014), is based on organisational and patient–provider relationships, which aims to address the management of long-term conditions that may result in depression and potentially lead to suicide ideation (Conejero et al 2018).

In Jill's story, she shares her experience with the suicide of her friend.

PERSONAL PERSPECTIVES

Consumer's Story 18.1: Jill

I had what I thought was an honest and strong relationship with Margaret. I was introduced to her at a stroke support group meeting, and she was a lot older than me. We had consistently communicated for around 9 months. She shared with me on different occasions when she was feeling anxious about being alone with her thoughts for too long. She would say things like: "Make sure you are coming on Thursday – I know I'll need to see someone by then".

Coming from a rural community originally, we had long-term plans to visit her family home because her much older brother, Jim, I think he was 82 years old, was still living there. The chosen weekend was approaching and despite me noticing a decline in her mood, Margaret insisted that she would be alright and that this would be good for her. She called it her "out". I contacted her brother and, without breaking Margaret's confidence, I indicated that she was not well and hoped Jim could keep an eye on her. The drive was uneventful, and she seemed happy to see her home and her brother. After her first night with Jim, she died by suicide on the property.

Working with older people and responding appropriately to early cues is a proactive approach. Assessment for depression, if not already an underlying mental disorder, can be an effective strategy, and providing timely therapeutic management may help. Interventions to prevent experiences of loneliness, hopelessness and isolation can be explored by nurses working in primary care and community settings with older people, as well as by those working in aged care and residential aged care services. Monitoring and reviewing current care strategies for effectiveness and escalating care to the appropriate mental health or crisis intervention service when it is required is vital.

Be mindful that it is important to engage in self-care when working with people who are expressing suicidal thoughts, attempting suicide or dying by a catastrophic event like suicide (see Chapter 8).

NURSING MANAGEMENT OF OLDER PEOPLE

Health professionals, as well as the public, often have negative attitudes towards ageing and poor attitudes to and tolerance of mental illness. Stereotypical images of older people and ageist beliefs can affect the quality of nursing care and therefore on a person's health outcomes (Rush et al 2017). For nurses, an important aspect of managing older people is reflecting on your own attitudes and biases, and how these might affect care.

Several nursing interventions are known to assist older people:
- Listen to the person in an active way; in particular, try to notice the feelings and emotions behind the words.
- Encourage older people to participate in physical and social activities that invite them to focus on aspects of their life apart from illness.
- Assist older people to understand disease processes, how to take medications and to maintain a physically and mentally active lifestyle.
- Help older people to find coping strategies to assist them with any losses such as a decline in health or financial status or bereavement.
- Support the person to work through the pain of grief and to adjust to an environment where the deceased is no longer available.
- Identify informal supports such as social networks and support services.

Use a person-centred care approach – develop a collaborative and respectful partnership with the person and respect the contribution that the older person can bring. This approach requires the nurse to get to know the person – their needs, preferences and life history – and to empower them by encouraging them to be involved in the decisions that affect their health and wellbeing as much as possible. Providing flexible and accessible services that respond to the individual's needs is vital.

Nurses can assist older people in maintaining function by ensuring they have small, frequent meals, are well hydrated and maintain bowel function through a high-fibre diet, hydration and exercise. Clients should be encouraged to mobilise and be independent, and nurses should ensure they have undisturbed rest and relaxation. Other therapies that older people may find therapeutic include listening to music they enjoy, hand and back massage and pet therapy (Moyle 2014). Massage, for example, can induce a calming sensation that may reduce anxiety (Moyle et al 2013a). In addition, companion robots such as animal robots have also been reported to reduce agitation and improve quality of life, in particular for older people with non-communicable disease, such as Alzheimer's, cancer, stroke and many more (Moyle et al 2013b).

These interventions are generalised and so it is important to evaluate care processes regularly to ensure the interventions are appropriate for the situation. As previously highlighted, it is also imperative that health professionals consider the person's culture, as decisions about care may be affected by cultural differences. For example, institutional care for family members is not an accepted way of providing care in some cultures. People from non-English-speaking populations often present at later stages of mental illness due to low levels of English proficiency or unfamiliarity with mental health services. People who come to Australia and New Zealand as refugees or asylum seekers have frequently experienced extreme hardship and trauma in their country of origin and/or in their migration journey. The effects of displacement and trauma place them at high risk of developing post-traumatic stress disorders and depression, but the stigma associated with mental-health-related conditions can affect a person's desire to seek help (Procter 2016). (See Chapter 3 for more information about trauma, crisis, loss and grief.)

When mental health nurses are providing psychological therapy, they will need to consider the needs of the individual and the underlying conditions or circumstance. For example, cognitive behavioural therapy (CBT) has demonstrated social wellbeing along with lower levels of depression; fewer physical symptoms and sleep complaints have also been evidenced (Friedman et al 2017). CBT could be used to help address fears of falling and lead to adaptive behaviours such as exercising regularly (Liu et al 2018). Not all older aged people will be able to participate in psychological therapy given the level of their cognitive or sensory impairment, but given the complexities associated with the use of medicines in older people, wherever possible, non-pharmacological treatments should be used.

POLYPHARMACY FOR OLDER AGE AND MEDICATION SAFETY

Polypharmacy in older aged people can be complex and is not without risks (Wallis et al 2018). Risks such as inappropriate prescribing, medication omission and adverse reactions due to interactions of drug groups are of concern. Adjunct to this is a possible acute illness and admission to hospital, multiple prescribers, and inaccurate/incomplete medical records. There is also the issue of older aged people memory recall on which medications they are taking, how much and when. Confusion over generic names versus trade names and over-the-counter medications may contribute to pharmacy errors at point of care. Non-adherence to prescribed regimens is another problem and may be related to memory or an issue such as being unable to pay for the number of scripts that have been issued. The provision of verbal and written drug information may allay some of these issues.

Prescribing in this context requires sound knowledge of ageing physiology, geriatric medicine and pharmacotherapy to reduce potential error (Lennox et al 2019). Physiological changes, chronic illness and nutrition affect drug pharmacokinetics and pharmacodynamics (Lavan et al 2016) – in particular, absorption, distribution, metabolism and excretion (Australian Medicines Handbook 2019; Lavan et al 2016). As previously discussed, physical ageing, especially renal function and chronic co-morbidities, can impact on sensitivity to specific drugs and may contribute to the person's presenting symptoms. Take the time to ponder Critical thinking exercise 18.5.

？ CRITICAL THINKING EXERCISE 18.5

It is important to consider polypharmacy, as up to 40% of people over the age of 60 may take five or more different medications. How should prescribing in older age be approached to prevent adverse effects?

The role of antipsychotics and antidepressants to manage symptoms in older aged people requires special consideration. Using antipsychotics can increase the risk of stroke and death when beginning treatment. It is recommended to use lower starting doses of any medication and gradually titrate to reduce side effects and to limit the period of use (Australian Medicines Handbook 2019). Although in Australia there has been a reduction in prescribing frequency, there has been an increase in "prn" prescribing (Westbury et al 2018). In an Australian study, off-label prescribing of antipsychotics occurred in 63% of people over 75 years of age with dementia for behavioural and psychological symptoms (Kjosavik et al 2017). Yet, antipsychotic use can worsen behavioural and psychological symptoms of dementia (Westaway et al 2018).

Note the following precautions for antipsychotics that are used in acute and chronic psychoses:
- respiratory failure or respiratory depression – exacerbated by alcohol use
- hyperthyroidism – check thyroid function routinely
- hypo/hyperthermia – may lead to shock
- gastrointestinal obstruction, urinary retention, myasthenia gravis – may be exacerbated by anticholinergic effects
- diabetes – may have raised glycaemic levels
- neurological effects – can aggravate Parkinson's or tremors, cognitive deterioration in Lewy body dementia, risk of seizures
- cardiovascular effects – risk of arrhythmias and prolonged Q-T intervals
- use of antipsychotics in older people – associated with increased risk of stroke (Australian Medicines Handbook 2019).

Given the ongoing dialogue within the literature, antidepressants, SSRIs and SNRIs are most suited to managing specific mental health disorders in older age (Andrews et al 2018). Side effects should be monitored and observed for any metabolic effects (Australian Medicines Handbook 2019). Both SSRIs and SNRIs have a risk of serotonin toxicity and require tapering of the dose over at least 4 weeks to prevent withdrawal effects. Common adverse effects include gastrointestinal upset, nausea, diarrhoea, agitation, insomnia/drowsiness, decreased libido, myalgia and rash (Australian Medicines Handbook 2019). Blood pressure and sodium levels (risk of hyponatraemia) should be monitored, with a baseline measurement taken before treatment.

To recap, providing older aged people with information about their medications and associated effects is crucial. Any new medication should be started at a low dose to monitor effect. It is also preferable to only begin one new treatment at a time to enable any side effects to be identified. Critical thinking exercise 18.6 provides an opportunity for you to review pharmacology.

？ CRITICAL THINKING EXERCISE 18.6

Complete the following table to consolidate your learning about pharmacology in the following mental health disorders. Complete the missing information and provide the precautions, adverse effects and any practice point pertaining to older aged people.

Mental Health Disorder	Drug Group	Precaution	Adverse Effects	Practice Point for Older People
Depression	Antidepressant			
Dementia	Benzodiazepine			
Anxiety	SSRI			
Schizophrenia	Antipsychotic			

CHAPTER SUMMARY

Healthy ageing involves more than promoting good mental and physical health; it includes social and emotional wellbeing. Nurses can support older people to maintain social connections and regular engagement with supports and community. As people age, they experience psychosocial factors such as bereavement and may experience loss of physical and/or mental functioning, placing them at risk of mental disorders and, in particular, depression or anxiety, which are both common and treatable. However, mental disorders are not a normal part of ageing, and clients require adequate assessment and diagnosis

to ensure their symptoms are not related to other issues such as adverse effects of medications or underlying physical disease. The diagnosis and treatment of mental disorders in older adults can be complex and are complicated by the presence of co-occurring conditions. Negative stereotypical ageist assumptions are also problematic.

Nurses have an important role to play with older people experiencing mental disorders. Establishing a therapeutic relationship provides the opportunity for nurses to recognise the symptoms of mental illness and to suggest/provide/refer for further assessment and treatment as required. The knowledge that older people have a high risk of suicide means it is imperative that they are assessed and treated appropriately and effectively. Skills in establishing a therapeutic relationship, and in using psychotherapeutic support such as CBT, can assist older people

to address the impacts of grief and bereavement, role disputes and transitions, or interpersonal issues, and can, along with pharmaco-therapy and at times electroconvulsive therapy, improve older people's quality of life.

USEFUL WEBSITES

Alzheimers New Zealand: alzheimers.org.nz/
Australasian Delirium Association: www.delirium.org.au/
Australian and New Zealand Society for Geriatric Medicine: www.anzsgm.org/
Beyond Blue: www.beyondblue.org.au/
Black Dog Institute: www.blackdoginstitute.org.au/clinical-resources/depression
Capital Health Network: www.chnact.org.au/mental-health-programs-hp
Dementia Australia: www.dementia.org.au/
Dementia New Zealand: dementia.nz/
Dementia Training Australia: www.dta.com.au/
Geriatric Depression Scale: web.stanford.edu/~yesavage/GDS.html
Head to Health – Australian Government: headtohealth.gov.au/supporting-someone-else/supporting/aged-and-elderly
Health Direct: www.healthdirect.gov.au/older-people-and-mental-health
HELP: www.hospitalelderlifeprogram.org/about/
Khan Academy: www.khanacademy.org/science/health-and-medicine/mental-health/dementia-delirium-alzheimers/v/what-is-delirium
Mental Health Commission of NSW: nswmentalhealthcommission.com.au/mental-health-and/older-people
Mental Health Foundation suicide prevention: www.mentalhealth.org.nz/suicideprevention
Mental Health Foundation. mentalhealth.org.nz/
Mind and Body: mindandbody.co.nz/
Mini-ACE is available: www.nzdementia.org/mini-ace
Mini-Cog assessment and instructions: mini-cog.com/
Mini-Mental State Examination (MMSE): www.parinc.com/Products/Pkey/237
Narconon Drug Rehab and Drug Education Centre: www.narconon.org/drug-rehab/centers/narconon-melbourne-australia.html
National Depression Initiative: www.depression.org.nz
RUDAS is available: www.health.qld.gov.au/tpch/html/rudas.asp
SANE Australia: www.sane.org/images/PDFs/GrowingOlderStayingWell.pdf
Te Pou New Zealand: www.tepou.co.nz/
World Health Organization: www.who.int/mental_health/en/

REFERENCES

Ahmedani, B.K., Peterson, E.L., Hu, Y., Rossom, R.C., Lynch, F., et al., 2017. Major physical health conditions and risk of suicide. Am J Prev Med, 53(3), 308–315.
Alexopoulos, G.A, Abrams, R.C., Young, R.C., Shamoian, C.A., 1988. Cornell scale for depression in dementia. Biol Psychiatry, 23(3), 271–84.
An, M.H., Park, S.S., You, S.C., Park, R.W, et al., 2019. depressive symptom network associated with comorbid anxiety in late-life depression. Front Psychiatry, 10, 856.
Andrews, G., Bell, C., Boyce, P., et al., 2018. Royal Australian and New Zealand College of Psychiatrists clinical practice guidelines for the treatment of panic disorder, social anxiety disorder and generalised anxiety disorder. Aust N Z J Psychiatry, 52(12), 1109–1172.
Australian Bureau of Statistics (ABS), 2021. Causes of Death, Australia. ABS, Canberra. www.abs.gov.au/statistics/health/causes-death/causes-death-australia/latest-release.
Australian Bureau of Statistics (ABS), 2020. National, state and territory population. ABS cat. no. 3101.0. ABS, Canberra.
Australian Bureau of Statistics (ABS), 2018. Population projections, Australia. ABS cat. no. 3222.0. ABS, Canberra.

Australian Human Rights Commission (AHRC), 2015. Resilient individuals: Sexual orientation, gender identity & intersex rights 2015. AHRC, Sydney.
Australian Institute of Health and Welfare (AIHW), 2023. Aboriginal and Torres Strait Islander Health Performance Framework Summary report 2023. AIHW, Canberra.
Australian Institute of Health and Welfare (AIHW), 2021. Dementia in Australia 2021: Summary Report. AIHW, Canberra.
Australian Institute of Health and Welfare (AIHW), 2020. National, state and territory population. ABS cat. No. 3101.0. ABS, Canberra.
Australian Institute of Health and Welfare (AIHW), 2018a. Older Australia at a glance. AIHW, Canberra.
Australian Institute of Health and Welfare (AIHW), 2018b. Alcohol and other drug treatment services in Australia 2016–17. Drug treatment services series no. 31. Cat. no. HSE 207. AIHW, Canberra.
Australian Institute of Health and Welfare (AIHW), 2017. National Drug Strategy Household Survey 2016: Detailed findings. Drug statistics series no. 31. Cat. no. PHE 214. AIHW, Canberra.
Australian Medicines Handbook, 2019. Australian Medicines Handbook. Online.
Balsamo, M., Cataldi, F., Carlucci, L., et al., 2018. Assessment of anxiety in older adults: A review of self-report measures. Clin Interv Aging 13, 573.
Banerjee, D., Rabheru, K., Ivbijaro, G., et al., 2021. Dignity of older persons with mental health conditions: Why should clinicians care? Front Psychiatry 12, 774533.
Beaunoyer, E., Landreville, P., Carmichael, P.H. 2019. Older adults' knowledge of anxiety disorders. J Gerontol B Psychol Sci Soc Sci, 74(5), 806–814.
Beishon, L.C., Batterham, A.P., Quinn, T.J., et al., 2019. Addenbrooke's Cognitive Examination III (ACE-III) and mini-ACE for the detection of dementia and mild cognitive impairment. Cochrane Database Syst Rev, (12), CD013282.
Bektas, A., Schurman, S.H., Sen, R., et al., 2018. Aging, inflammation and the environment. Exp Gerontol, 105, 10–18.
Berg-Weger, M., Morley, J.E., 2020. Loneliness in old age: An unaddressed health problem. J Nutr Health Ageing, 24, 243–245.
Borson, S., Scanlan, J.M., Chen, P., et al., 2003. The Mini-Cog as a screen for dementia: Validation in a population-based sample. J Am Geriatr Soc, 51, 1451–1454.
Borson, S., Scanlan, J.M., Watanabe, J., et al., 2005. Simplifying detection of cognitive impairment: Comparison of the Mini-Cog and Mini-Mental State Examination in a multiethnic sample. J Am Geriatr Soc, 53, 871–874.
Brandao, D.J., Fontenelle, L.F., da Silva, S.A., Menezes, P.R., Pastor-Valero, M. 2019. Depression and excess mortality in the elderly living in low- and middle-income countries: Systematic review and meta-analysis. Int J Geriatr Psychiatry, 34, 22–30.
Butler, R.N., 1969. Age-ism: Another form of bigotry. Gerontologist 9(4 Pt 1), 243–246.
Byrne, G.J., Pachana, N.A., 2021. Epidemiology, risk and protective factors. In: Byrne, G., & Pachana, N. (eds), Anxiety in older people: Clinical and research perspectives. Cambridge University Press, Cambridge.
Cai, L., Huang, J., 2018. Schizophrenia and risk of dementia: A meta-analysis study. Neuropsychiatr Dis Treat, 14, 2047.
Carew, A.M., Comiskey, C., 2018. Treatment for opioid use and outcomes in older adults: A systematic literature review. Drug Alcohol Depend, 182, 48–57.
Chen, L.J., Ku, P.W., & Fox, K.R., 2018. Exercise for older people with mental illness. In: Stubbs, B., Rosenbaum, S. (eds), Exercise-Based Interventions for Mental Illness: Physical Activity as Part of Clinical Treatment. Academic Press, Cambridge.
Cheung, G., To, E., Rivera-Rodriguez, C., et al., 2022. Dementia prevalence estimation among the main ethnic groups in New Zealand:

A population-based descriptive study of routinely collected health data. BMJ Open, 12:e062304.

Clarke, B.F.L., 1975. Mental Disorder in Earlier Britain: Exploratory Studies. University of Wales Press, Cardiff.

Cohen, C.I., 2018. Very late-onset schizophrenia-like psychosis: Positive findings but questions remain unanswered. Lancet Psychiatry, 5(7), 528–529.

Conejero, I., Olié, E., Courtet, P., et al., 2018. Suicide in older adults: Current perspectives. Clin Interv Aging, 13, 691.

Creighton, A., Davidson, T., Kissane, D., 2018. The assessment of anxiety in aged care residents: A systematic review of the psychometric properties of commonly used measures. Int Psychogeriatr, 30(7), 967–979.

Crocco, E.A., Loewenstein, D.A., Curiel, R.E., Alperin, N., Czaja, S.J., et al., 2018. A novel cognitive assessment paradigm to detect Pre-mild cognitive impairment (PreMCI) and the relationship to biological markers of Alzheimer's disease. J Psychiatr Res, 96, 33–38.

Dafsari, F.S., Bewernick, B., Biewer, M., Christ, H., et al., 2019. Cognitive behavioural therapy for the treatment of late life depression: Study protocol of a multicentre, randomized, observer-blinded, controlled trial (CBTlate) BMC Psychiatr, 19(1):423.

Dalal, P.K., Kar, S.K., Agarwal, S.K. 2022 . Management of psychiatric disorders in patients with chronic kidney diseases. Indian J Psychiatry, 64(Suppl 2), S394–S401.

Daré, L.O., Bruand, P.E., Gérard, D., et al., 2019. Co-morbidities of mental disorders and chronic physical diseases in developing and emerging countries: A meta-analysis. BMC Public Health, 19, 304.

De Leo, D., 2022. Late-life suicide in an aging world. Nature Aging, 2, 7–12.

Deloitte Economics, 2017. Dementia Economic Impact Report 2016. Alzheimers New Zealand. Online. Available at: cdn.alzheimers.org.nz/wp-content/uploads/2021/05/Economic-Impacts-of-Dementia-2017.pdf

Dougherty, J.H., Cannon, R., Nicholas, C.R.N., et al., 2010. The computerized self-test (CST): An interactive, internet accessible cognitive screening test for dementia. J Alzheimers Dis, 20, 185–195.

Douglas, S., Stott, J., Spector, A., Brede, J., Hanratty, É., et al., 2022. Mindfulness-based cognitive therapy for depression in people with dementia: A qualitative study on participant, carer and facilitator experiences. Dementia (London), 21(2), 457–476.

Drageset, J., Haugan, G., Tranvåg, O., 2017. Crucial aspects promoting meaning and purpose in life: Perceptions of nursing home residents. BMC Geriatr 17 (1), 254.

Folstein, M.F., Folstein, S.E., McHugh, P.R., 1975. Mini-Mental State: A practical method for grading the state of patients for the clinician. J Psychiatr Res, 12, 189–198.

Foulk, M.A., Ingersoll-Dayton, B., Kavangh, J., et al., 2014. Mindfulness-based cognitive therapy with older adults: An exploratory study. J Gerontol Soc Work, 57, 498–520.

Freter, S., Dunbar, M., Koller, K., et al., 2016. Prevalence and characteristics of pre-operative delirium in hip fracture patients. Gerontology 62, 396–400.

Friedman, E.M., Ruini, C., Foy, R., et al., 2017. Lighten UP! A community-based group intervention to promote psychological well-being in older adults. Aging Ment. Health 21 (2), 199–205.

Garakani, A., Freire, R.C., & Murrough, J.W., 2021. Pharmacotherapy of anxiety disorders: Promises and pitfalls. Front Psychiatry, 12, 662963.

Gebauer, E.M., Lukas, A., 2022. Prescriptions of antipsychotics in younger and older geriatric patients with polypharmacy, their safety, and the impact of a pharmaceutical-medical dialogue on antipsychotic use. Biomed, 10(12), 3127.

Grenier, S., Payette, M., Gunther, B., Askari, S., Desjardins, F., et al., 2019. Association of age and gender with anxiety disorders in older adults: A systematic review and meta analysis. Int J Geriatr Psychiatry, 34(3), 397–407.

Guerra, F., Di Giacomo, D., Ranieri, J., Tunno, M., Piscitani, L., et al., 2021. Chronic Kidney Disease and Its Relationship with Mental Health: Allostatic Load Perspective for Integrated Care. J Pers Med, 1;11(12), 1367.

Haugan, G., Innstrand, S.T., Moksnes, U.K., 2013. The effect of nurse–patient interaction on anxiety and depression in cognitively intact nursing home patients. J Clin Nurs, 22, (15–16), 2192–2205.

Hegeman, J.M., de Waal, M.W., Comijis, H.C., et al., 2015. Depression in later life: A more somatic presentation? J Affect Disord, 170, 196–202.

Hellwig, S., Domschke, K., 2019. Anxiety in late life: An update on pathomechanisms. Gerontology, 65(5), 465–473.

Herman, B., 2022. PTSD Assessment and treatment in older adults. PTSD: National Center for PTSD. Online. Available at: www.ptsd.va.gov/professional/treat/specific/assess_tx_older_adults.asp

Hodkinson, H.M., 1972. Evaluation of a mental test score for assessment of mental impairment in the elderly. Age Ageing, 1(4), 233–238.

Hsieh, S., McGrory, S., Leslie, F., Dawson, K., Ahmed, S., et al., 2015. The Mini-Addenbrooke's Cognitive Examination: A new assessment tool for dementia. Dement Geriatr Cogn Disord, 39, 1–11.

Huang, L., Zhu, M. & Ji, J., 2022. Association between hypoglycemia and dementia in patients with diabetes: A systematic review and meta-analysis of 1.4 million patients. Diabetol Metab Syndr 14, 31.

Hunter, R., Barson, E., Willis, K. and Smallwood, N., 2021. Mental health illness in chronic respiratory disease is associated with worse respiratory health and low engagement with non-pharmacological psychological interventions. Intern Med J, 51, 414–418.

Inouye, S.K., 2018. Delirium – a framework to improve acute care for older persons. J Am Geriatr Soc, 66(3), 446–451.

Inouye, S.K., van Dyck, C.H., Alessi, C.A., et al., 1990. Clarifying confusion: The confusion assessment method: A new method for detection of delirium. Ann Intern Med, 113(12), 941–948.

Julien, C.L., Rimes, K.A., Brown, R.G., 2016. Rumination and behavioural factors in Parkinson's disease depression. J Psychosom Res, 82, 48–53.

Kang, H., Kim, H., 2022. Ageism and psychological well-being among older adults: A systematic review. Gerontol Geriatric Med, 8. doi: 10.1177/23337214221087023.

Keenan, C.R., Jain, S., 2022. Delirium. Med Clin N Am, 106(3), 459–469.

Kenbubpha, K., Higgins, I., Wilson, A., et al., 2019. Psychogeriatrics, testing psychometric properties of a new instrument "Promoting Active Ageing in Older People with Mental Disorders Scale" from a cross-sectional study. Psychogeriatrics, 19(4), 370–383.

Kjosavik, S.R., Gillam, M.H., Roughead, E.E., 2017. Average duration of treatment with antipsychotics among concession card holders in Australia. Aust N Z J Psychiatry, 51(7), 719–726.

Kok, R.M., Reynolds, C.F., 2017. Management of depression in older adults: A review. JAMA, 317(20), 2114–2122.

Komalasari, R., Chang, H.C., Traynor, V., 2019. A review of the Rowland Universal Dementia Assessment Scale. Dementia, 18(7–8), 3143–3158.

Kostadinov, V., Roche, A., 2017. Bongs and baby boomers: Trends in cannabis use among older Australians. Australas J Ageing, 36 (1), 56–59.

Kverno, K., & Velez, R. 2018. Comorbid depression and dementia: The case for integrated care. J Nurse Practition, 14(3), 196–201.

Lavan, A.H., Gallagher, P.F., O'Mahony, D., 2016. Methods to reduce prescribing errors in elderly patients with multimorbidity. Clin Interv Aging, 11, 857.

Lavrencic, L.M., Richardson, C., Harrison, S.L., et al., 2018. Is there a link between cognitive reserve and cognitive function in the oldest-old? J Gerontol A Biol Sci Med Sci, 73(4), 499–505.

Lee, M., Kim, T., Ahn, S., et al., 2017. Effectiveness of antipsychotics on delirium in elderly patients. J Psychiatry, 20, 4.

Lennox, A., Braaf, S., Smit, D.V., et al., 2019. Caring for older patients in the emergency department: Health professionals' perspectives from Australia – the Safe Elderly Emergency Discharge project. Emerg Med Australas, 31(1), 83–89.

Liguori, I., Russo, G., Curcio, F., et al., 2018. Depression and chronic heart failure in the elderly: An intriguing relationship. J Geriatr Cardiol, 15(6), 451.

Liu, C., Wang, D., Liu, C., et al., 2020. What is the meaning of health literacy? A systematic review and qualitative synthesis. Fam Med Comm Health, 8, e000351.

Liu, T.W., Ng, G.Y., Chung, R.C., et al., 2018. Cognitive behavioural therapy for fear of falling and balance among older people: A systematic review and meta-analysis. Age Ageing, 47(4), 520–527.

LoGiudice, D., Strivens, E., Smith, K., et al., 2010. The KICA screen: The psychometric properties of a shortened version of the KICA (Kimberley Indigenous Cognitive Assessment). Australas J Ageing, 30, 215–219.

Lyons, A., Alba, B., Heywood, W., et al., 2018. Experiences of ageism and the mental health of older adults. Aging Ment Health, 22(11), 1456–1464.

Macfarlane, S., O'Connor, D., 2016. Managing behavioural and psychological symptoms in dementia. Aust Prescr, 39(4), 123–125.

Marucci, G., Buccioni, M., Dal Ben, D., Lambertucci, C., Volpini, R., Amenta, F., 2021. Efficacy of acetylcholinesterase inhibitors in Alzheimer's disease, Neuropharmacol, 190, 108352.

Masopust, J., Protopopova, D., Valis, M., Pavelek, Z., Klimova, B., 2018. Treatment of behavioural and psychological symptoms of dementias with psychopharmaceuticals: A review. Neuropsychiatric Dis Treat, 14, 1211–1220.

Milian, M., Leiherr, A.M., Straten, G., et al., 2012. The Mini-Cog versus the Mini-Mental State Examination and the Clock Drawing Test in daily clinical practice: Screening and value in a German memory clinical. Int Psychogeriatr, 24(5), 766–774.

Molloy, D.W., Standish, T.I., 1997. A guide to the standardized Mini-Mental State Examination. Int Psychogeriatr, 9(S1), 87–94.

Moyle, W., 2014. Evidence-based nursing interventions: Fostering quality of life. In: Moyle, W., Parker, D., Bramble, M. (eds), Care of Older Adults: A Strengths-Based Approach. Cambridge University Press, Sydney.

Moyle, W., Cooke, M., Beattie, E., et al., 2013a. Foot massage versus quiet presence on agitation and mood in people with dementia: A randomized controlled trial. Int J Nurs Stud, 51, 856–864.

Moyle, W., Cooke, M., Beattie, E., et al., 2013b. Exploring the effect of companion robots on emotional expression in older people with dementia: A pilot RCT. J Gerontol Nurs, 39, 46–53.

Munir S, Takov V 2023. Generalized anxiety disorder. In: StatPearls [Internet]. Treasure Island (FL): StatPearls Publishing; 2023 Jan–, Available at: www.ncbi.nlm.nih.gov/books/NBK441870/.

Musich, S., Wang, S.S., Slindee, L., et al., 2019. Prevalence and characteristics associated with high dose opioid users among older adults. Geriatr Nurs (Minneap), 40(1), 31–36.

Nasreddine, Z.S., Phillips, N.A., Bédirian, V., Charbonneau, S., Whitehead, V., 2005. The Montreal Cognitive Assessment, MoCA: A brief screening tool for mild cognitive impairment. J Am Geriatr Soc, 53, 695–699.

New Zealand Dementia Foundation, 2020. Introducing the Mini-ACE. Auckland. www.nzdementia.org/mini-ace

Nyberg, J., Henriksson, M., Wall, A. et al., 2021. Anxiety severity and cognitive function in primary care patients with anxiety disorder: A cross-sectional study. BMC Psychiatry, 21, 617.

Országhová, Z., Mego, M., Chovanec, M., 2021. long-term cognitive dysfunction in cancer survivors. Front Mol Biosci, 8, 770413.

Osler, M., Rozing, M.P., Christensen, G.T., Andersen, P.K., Jorgensen, M.B., 2018. Electroconvulsive therapy and risk of dementia in patients with affective disorders: A cohort study. Lancet Psychiatry, 5(4), 348–356.

Panthi, M., 2022. Loneliness and boredom in residential care: Voices of older adults. Aust NZ Soc Work Rev, 34(1), 88–99.

Parker, S.G., McCue, P., Phelps, K., McCleod, A., Arora, S., et al., 2018. What is comprehensive geriatric assessment (CGA)? An umbrella review. Age Ageing. 47, 149–155.

Petrova, N.N., & Khvostikova, D.A. 2021. Prevalence, structure, and risk factors for mental disorders in older people. ADV Gerontol, 11(4), 409–415.

Polacsek, M., Woolford, M., 2022. Strategies to support older adults' mental health during the transition into residential aged care: A qualitative study of multiple stakeholder perspectives. BMC Geriatr, 22(1), 151.

Procter, N.G., 2016. Person-centred care for people of refugee background. J Pharm Pract Res, doi.org/10.1002/jppr.1222.

Radford, K., Mack, H.A., Draper, B., et al., 2015. Prevalence of dementia in urban and regional Aboriginal Australians. Alzheimers Dement, 11, 271–279.

Rakusa, M., Jensterle, J., Mlakar, J., 2018. Clock drawing test: A simple scoring system for the accurate screening of cognitive impairment in patients with mild cognitive impairment and dementia. Dement Geriatr Cogn Disord, 45(5–6), 326–334.

Rao, R., Crome, I., Crome, P., & Iliffe, S., 2019. Substance misuse in later life: Challenges for primary care: A review of policy and evidence. Prim Health Care Res Dev, 20, e117.

Roughan, W.H., Campos, A.I., García-Marín, L.M., Cuéllar-Partida, G., Lupton, M.K., et al., 2021. Comorbid chronic pain and depression: Shared risk factors and differential antidepressant effectiveness. Front Psychiatry, 12, 643609.

Rush, K.L., Hickey, S., Epp, S., et al., 2017. Nurses' attitudes towards older people care: An integrative review. J Clin Nurs, 26(23–24), 4105–4116.

Santini, Z.I., Koyanagi, A., Tyrovolas, S., et al., 2015. The association of relationship quality and social networks with depression, anxiety, and suicidal ideation among older married adults: Findings from a cross-sectional analysis of the Irish Longitudinal Study on Ageing (TILDA). J Affect Disord, 179, 134–141.

Sbolli, M., Fiuzat, M., Cani, D., O'Connor, C. M., 2020. Depression and heart failure: The lonely comorbidity. Eur J Heart Fail, 22, 2007–2017.

Scales, K., Zimmerman, S., Miller, S.J., 2018. Evidence-based nonpharmacological practices to address behavioral and psychological symptoms of dementia. Gerontologist, 58 (Suppl. 1), S88–S102.

Seitz, D.P., Chan, C.C., Newton, H.T., et al., 2018. Mini-Cog for the diagnosis of Alzheimer's disease dementia and other dementias within a primary care setting. Cochrane Database Syst Rev, (2), CD011415.

Sheikh, J.I., & Yesavage, J.A. 1986. Geriatric Depression Scale (GDS): Recent evidence and development of a shorter version. Clin Gerontol, 5(1–2), 165–173.

Smith, G.D., Ho, K.H.M., Poon, S., Chan, S.W.-C., 2022. Beyond the tip of the iceberg: Health literacy in older people. J Clin Nurs, 31, E3–E5.

Snowdon, J., 2010. Depression in nursing homes. Int Psychogeriatr, 22(7), 1143–1148.

Spitzer, R.L., Williams, J.B.W., Kroenke, K., et al., 1994. Utility of a new procedure for diagnosing mental disorders in primary care: The PRIME-MD 1000 study. JAMA, 272, 1749–1756.

Statistics New Zealand, 2019. Population projection tables. Wellington.

Statistics New Zealand, 2022. National population projections: 2022(base)– 2073. Wellington.

Storey, J., Rowland, J., Basic, D., et al., 2004. The Rowland Universal Dementia Assessment Scale (RUDAS): A multicultural cognitive assessment scale. Int Psychogeriatr, 16(1), 13–31.

Talley, N.J., Jones, S., 2018. Clinical Examination: A Guide to Specialty Examinations, vol. 2, 8th ed. Elsevier, Sydney.

Taylor, D.M., Barnes, T.R., Young, A.H., 2021. The Maudsley Prescribing Guidelines in Psychiatry. Wiley-Blackwell, UK.

Te Pou, 2019. Working with older people: Mental health and addiction workforce development priorities. Te Pou, Auckland.

Te Whatu Ora, 2022. Suicide web tool. Online. Available at: www.tewhatuora. govt.nz/our-health-system/data-and-statistics/suicide-web-tool/

The Royal Australian College of General Practitioners, 2020. Management of type 2 diabetes: A handbook for general practice. RACGP, East Melbourne.

Thompsell, A., Sachdev, K., Das-munshi, Rao, T., 2019. Substance misuse in older adults with frailty. BMJ, 364, 1958.

Tsabedze, N., Kinsey, J.H, Mpanya, D., Mogashoa, V., Klug, E., Manga, P., 2021. The prevalence of depression, stress and anxiety symptoms in patients with chronic heart failure. Int J Ment Health Syst, 15, 44.

Valletta, M., Canevelli, M., Blasi, M.T., Bruno, G., 2021. Sundowning in patients with dementia: Prevalence and clinical features. J Neurol Sci, 429, 118056.

van der Veen, D.C., van Zelst, W.H., Schoevers, R.A., et al., 2015. Comorbid anxiety disorders in late-life depression: Results of a cohort study. Int Psychogeriatr, 27, 1157–1165.

van Orden, K., Deming, C., 2018. Late-life suicide prevention strategies: Current status and future directions. Curr Opin Psychol, 22, 79–83.

Wagner, E., 2014. The chronic care model and integrated care. [Video file]. Available at: www.youtube.com/watch?v=K-z6HjRkKSc

Wallis, K.A., Elley, C.R., Lee, A., et al., 2018. Safer Prescribing and Care for the Elderly (SPACE): Protocol of a cluster randomized controlled trial in primary care. JMIR Res Protoc, 7(4), www.researchprotocols.org/2018/4/e109

Walton, M., 2013. Deep sleep therapy and Chelmsford Private Hospital: Have we learnt anything? Australas Psychiatry, 21(3), 206–212.

Westaway, K., Sluggett, J., Alderman, C., et al., 2018. The extent of antipsychotic use in Australian residential aged care facilities and interventions shown to be effective in reducing antipsychotic use: A literature review. Dementia, doi: 10.1177/1471301218795792

Westbury, J., Gee, P., Ling, T., et al., 2018. More action needed: Psychotropic prescribing in Australian residential aged care. Aust N Z J Psychiatry, 53(2), 136–147.

Wijeratne T, Sales C., 2021. Understanding why post-stroke depression may be the norm rather than the exception: The anatomical and neuroinflammatory correlates of post-stroke depression. J Clin Med, 10(8), 1674.

Williamson J, C, Larner A, J., 2018. MACE for the diagnosis of dementia and MCI: 3-year pragmatic diagnostic test accuracy study. Dement Geriatr Cogn Disord, 300–307.

Wilson, D.M., 2019. Where are we now in relation to determining the prevalence of ageism in this era of escalating population ageing? Ageing Res Rev, 51, 78–84.

Wilson, T. & Temple, J. 2022. New populations projections for Australia and the states and territories with a particular focus on population ageing. CEPAR Working Papers 2022/11. Available from: www.researchgate.net/publication/362666686_New_population_projections_for_Australia_and_the_States_and_Territories_with_a_particular_focus_on_population_ageing

World Health Organization (WHO), 2022. World mental health report: Transforming mental health for all. WHO, Geneva.

World Health Organization (WHO), 2021. Global status report on the public health response to dementia. WHO, Geneva.

World Health Organization (WHO), 2016. Health Impact Assessment (HIA) – The Determinants of Health. WHO, Geneva.

Yesavage, J.A., Brink, T.L., Rose, T.L., 1983. Development and validation of a geriatric depression rating scale: A preliminary report. J Psychiatr Res, 17, 27.

Yohannes, A.M., Chen, W., Moga, A.M., et al., 2017. Cognitive impairment in chronic obstructive pulmonary disease and chronic heart failure: A systematic review and meta-analysis of observational studies. J Am Med Dir Assoc, 18(5), 451–e1.

Zenebe, Y., Akele, B., Selassie, M., Necho, M., 2021. Prevalence and determinants of depression among old age: A systematic review and meta-analysis. Ann Gen Psychiatry, 20(1), 55.

Zhang, X., Norton, J., Carriere, I., et al., 2015. Generalized anxiety in community-dwelling elderly: Prevalence and clinical characteristics. J Affect Disord, 172, 24–29.

Zilles, D., 2018. Beneficial effects of electroconvulsive therapy in elderly people. Lancet Psychiatry, 5(9), 697–698.

19

Autism Spectrum Disorder and Intellectual Disability

Andrew Cashin

KEY POINTS

- Person-centred care necessitates a conscious effort to understand how the person at the centre of care thinks and processes information.
- Autism encompasses a different style of thinking and information processing to that experienced by neurotypical thinkers.

- Intellectual disability relates to the volume of information that can be handled at any one time, the speed of processing this information and the associated functional impairment.
- Assessment and intervention needs to be adjusted to be meaningful for people with autism spectrum disorder and/or intellectual disability.

KEY TERMS

Ability versus disability
Autism and intellectual disability

Diagnosis and difference
Information processing

Neurotypical thinking
Nursing and difference

LEARNING OUTCOMES

The material in this chapter will assist you to:

- understand the thinking and information-processing styles that characterise autism spectrum disorder and intellectual disability
- distinguish between neurotypical thinking and the differences experienced by those with autism spectrum disorder and/or intellectual disability

- identify what is meant by diagnostic overshadowing and appreciate the impact of this phenomenon on health outcomes for people with disability
- design adjustments to mental health nursing interventions to be used with people with autism spectrum disorder and/or intellectual disability to promote better and more equitable health outcomes.

INTRODUCTION

Understanding how people think and process information is essential for mental health nurses. This understanding includes denoting what are transitory changes in thinking related to the symptoms of a mental illness, such as that experienced in psychosis, and what are permanent traits that result from a developmental process. This chapter contains essential knowledge to progress the development of this understanding.

Person-first language will be used in this chapter in full acknowledgement that it is understood that people are not defined by an illness or disability. This approach is consistent with person-centred nursing, a concept embedded in nursing standards in Australia and Aotearoa New Zealand (Cashin et al 2017; Nursing Council of New Zealand 2022). However, it is acknowledged that, in the context of autism, this use of language is contested by proponents of identity-based language. In the case of identity-based language, it is conceptualised that a trait may define who a person is. If we were to adopt identity-based language, as an example, in place of referring to a person with autism, we would refer to the person as autistic. In practice, it is important as part of person-centred care to identify how the person you are working with understands what is going on for them and to identify if they have a preference of identifying language and what it is (Shakes & Cashin 2018).

Autism and intellectual disability are conceptualised as spectrums. For autism this is represented in the diagnostic nomenclature of autism spectrum disorder (ASD). For intellectual disability, the spectrum is signified in the diagnostic nomenclature of the level of disability that ranges from mild to severe. The diagnostic classifications in both the *Diagnostic and Statistical Manual of Mental Disorders, 5th Edition* (DSM-5) (American Psychiatric Association (APA) 2013) and the *International Classifications of Disease*, 11th edition (ICD-11) (World Health Organization (WHO) 2019) will be explored in the discussion of the types of disorder.

Autism represents a fundamental difference in thinking and information processing that results from a developmental process. In the world there are two recognised styles of thinking and information processing. One is autism, and the second, far more common style, is typical thinking (Cashin & Barker 2009). The term used to describe those with a typical thinking style is commonly accepted to be "neurotypical". Thinking differences that underpin behaviours recognised as difference in people with ASD include impaired abstraction (the ability to recognise like and similar as opposed to concrete black and white), impaired linguistic processing with a relative strength in visual processing and impaired theory of mind (the awareness that people all have minds and these minds are particular to individuals, with the ability to put oneself figuratively in another person's shoes and guess what they are thinking and feeling) (Cashin 2020). The impact of these differences is significant and tends to compound, resulting in a lack of formation of a unified base of knowledge about the world, a central characteristic of neurotypical thinking. While thinking changes are a frequent symptom of mental illness, they are often transitory in the form of psychotic phenomena. At times, people become stuck in such thinking patterns for long periods and people refer to such things as fixed thinking or chronicity; however, these changes became superimposed on what was originally a typical thinking style.

At this point, an astute reader may wonder about the negative or deficit symptoms of schizophrenia. Negative symptoms commonly include decreased emotional expression and decreased abstraction. Similar to that experienced in ASD, there is often impaired theory of mind and executive functioning (Nylander et al 2008). Such an example brings to our attention that boundaries between disorders are artificial constructions as we attempt to linguistically construct our world and demarcate understanding (Cashin 2016). Boundaries are fluid and will change as our understanding of the brain and genetics improve.

In contrast to ASD, intellectual disability does not represent a different thinking style, but rather a difference in the speed of processing within a person's thinking style and a difference in the volume of information that can be handled at any point in time. While intellectual disability is comorbidly experienced in a larger proportion of people who also have ASD, as compared to neurotypical thinkers, overall it is still experienced by the minority in that population (Cashin & Yorke 2016).

With the incidence of approximately 1% of the population having ASD and approximately 1% overall having an intellectual disability (APA 2013), all nurses will at some time care for someone with these disabilities, even in generalist services. Working with people with ASD and with people with intellectual disability is a specialty area of practice. An emerging and even more specialised area of practice is work in specialty services that support care for people with ASD and/or intellectual disability and comorbid mental illness. These services do not yet exist in a way to meet the required demand and are not evenly geographically spread.

THE SOCIAL MODEL OF DISABILITY

The social model of disability has a focus on the disabling structures in society that prevent people with identified impairments from full inclusion (Barnes 2019). The aim is to promote inclusion and quality of life. While individual impairment in physical, cognitive or mental health is acknowledged, the model is primarily concerned with the disabling structures in society. The model uses the medical model as the contrast, in which it posits that the primary focus is the individual impairment and the intention, it is posited, is curative (Pracilio et al 2022). The model underpins contemporary disability policy in Australia and Aotearoa New Zealand. While the model has many strengths, a consequence of the model in many cases is that nursing is seen as aligned with the medical model and the scope of nursing that is discussed is constrained. This limitation has flowed through to funding arrangements for services, which have seen the exclusion of mental health nurses as eligible providers (Pracilio et al 2022).

TYPES OF DISORDER

Autism Spectrum Disorder

Autism spectrum disorder (ASD) is the current diagnostic entity for autism and encompasses the diagnoses previously used colloquially,

and in the DSM and ICD. The diagnostic entities used in versions of the DSM up to DSM-5 of autistic disorder, Asperger's disorder and pervasive developmental disorder not otherwise specified, have now been encompassed by the term "autism spectrum disorder". In the ICD, atypical autism was used as an equivalent descriptor to pervasive development disorder not otherwise specified, which appeared in the DSM. Both terms were frequently employed to denote a sub-threshold diagnosis and less frequently to diagnose someone where symptoms were not recognised until later in life.

High-functioning autism was never a DSM diagnosis, but a colloquial term at times employed by people to signify ASD without a comorbid intellectual disability. At an earlier phase of understanding autism, some people used it to denote ASD without impairment of speech (note this is the function of speech, not a judgement on communication). While some people still use this term, it is incorrect. To correctly describe the comorbid presence of intellectual disability or language impairment, it should be stated as a comorbidity and the level and type of disability described.

The multitude of terms that have now been collapsed into recognising the spectrum nature of ASD evolved based on the neurotypical thinking trait of needing to name things, followed by the need to define the level or to answer the question of how much of the thing is present. In terms of disability, this often takes the form of a quest to determine if the disability is mild, moderate or severe. In ASD, severity levels have been incorporated into the DSM-5 to accommodate this need. However, there are caveats around the levels based on full acknowledgement that the frequency and intensity of the characteristic behaviours of ASD will fluctuate based on mediating factors, such as anxiety; that is, severity levels are not consistent for a person and will go up and down depending on context. A person with ASD in a very social and unfamiliar environment, as an example, would potentially meet the criteria for a higher severity rating than when in a more familiar and less socially demanding space. Hence transition periods often see a sustained, albeit not permanent, increase in severity ratings.

The ICD-11 and DSM-5 classifications have converged and are more closely aligned than ever before. Both classifications conceptualise autism as based on a dyad of impairment. The two underpinning domains are impaired social communication and the presence of restrictive and repetitive interests, activities and behaviours. This dyad replaces the earlier triad of impairment that underpinned classification symptoms. Previously, autism was conceptualised as being underpinned by impairment in the domains of communication, social skills and behavioural flexibility. It became clear that the separation of communication and social skills was redundant and so the two areas were collapsed into "impaired social communication". The DSM-5 diagnostic criteria is presented in Box 19.1.

ASD is a behavioural diagnosis, as can be seen from the criteria used to diagnose it. There are no physical tests that can be used to diagnose or confirm the diagnosis of ASD. The behaviours, it has come to be recognised, are the outward expression of difference in thinking and information processing. Just like the previously conceptualised triad of behavioural impairment, there is a triad of thinking impairments or difference represented by the diagnosis of ASD. These impairments are impaired abstraction, impaired theory of mind and impaired linguistic processing (having a relative strength in visual processing). Understanding these differences are key to successfully working with a person with autism. This includes work at the assessment phase and the intervention/support phase. The thinking differences will be discussed further under the heading signs and symptoms.

BOX 19.1 Autism Spectrum Disorder Diagnostic Criteria 299.00 (F84.0)

Persistent deficits in social communication and social interaction across multiple contexts, as manifested by all the following, currently or by history (examples are illustrative, not exhaustive):

- deficits in social–emotional reciprocity, ranging, for example, from abnormal social approach and failure of normal back-and-forth conversation, to reduced sharing of interests, emotions or affect, to failure to initiate or respond to social interactions
- deficits in non-verbal communicative behaviours used for social interaction, ranging, for example, from poorly integrated verbal and non-verbal communication, to abnormalities in eye contact and body language or deficits in understanding and use of gestures, to a total lack of facial expressions and non-verbal communication
- deficits in developing, maintaining, and understanding relationships, ranging, for example, from difficulties adjusting behaviour to suit various social contexts; to difficulties in sharing imaginative play or in making friends; to absence of interest in peers.

Specify current severity:

Severity is based on social communication impairments and restricted, repetitive patterns of behaviour.

- Restricted, repetitive patterns of behaviour, interests or activities, as manifested by at least two of the following, currently or by history (examples are illustrative, not exhaustive):
  - stereotyped or repetitive motor movements, use of objects or speech (e.g. simple motor stereotypies, lining up toys or flipping objects, echolalia, idiosyncratic phrases)
  - insistence on sameness, inflexible adherence to routines, or ritualised patterns of verbal or non-verbal behaviour (e.g. extreme distress at small changes, difficulties with transitions, rigid thinking patterns, greeting rituals, need to take the same route or eat the same food every day)
  - highly restricted, fixated interests that are abnormal in intensity or focus (e.g. strong attachment to or preoccupation with unusual objects, excessively circumscribed or perseverative interests)

- hyper- or hypo-reactivity to sensory input or unusual interest in sensory aspects of the environment (e.g. apparent indifference to pain/temperature, adverse response to specific sounds or textures, excessive smelling or touching of objects, visual fascination with lights or movement).

Specify current severity:

Severity is based on social communication impairments and restricted, repetitive patterns of behaviour.

- Symptoms must be present in the early developmental period (but may not become fully manifest until social demands exceed limited capacities or may be masked by learned strategies in later life).
- Symptoms cause clinically significant impairment in social, occupational or other important areas of current functioning.
- These disturbances are not better explained by intellectual disability (intellectual developmental disorder) or global developmental delay. Intellectual disability and ASD frequently co-occur; to make comorbid diagnoses of ASD and intellectual disability, social communication should be below that expected for general developmental level.

Note: Individuals with a well-established DSM-IV diagnosis of autistic disorder, Asperger's disorder or pervasive developmental disorder not otherwise specified, should be given the diagnosis of ASD. Individuals who have marked deficits in social communication, but whose symptoms do not otherwise meet criteria for ASD, should be evaluated for social (pragmatic) communication disorder.

Specify if:

- with or without accompanying intellectual impairment
- with or without accompanying language impairment
- associated with a known medical or genetic condition or environmental factor
- associated with another neurodevelopmental, mental or behavioural disorder
- with catatonia (refer to the criteria for catatonia associated with another mental disorder, pp. 119–120 of DSM-5, for the definition).

APA 2013.

Intellectual Disability

Intellectual disability (intellectual developmental disorder) is the diagnostic nomenclature used in the DSM-5 (APA 2013). The ICD-11 uses the term "disorders of intellectual development", a shift from mental retardation, the terminology used in earlier editions (Girimaji & Pradeep 2018). The shifting terminology again reflects evolution in understanding difference and in this case the developmental aspect of intellectual development.

In Australia and Aotearoa New Zealand, the terminology "intellectual disability" is commonly used. In the United States "developmental disability" is most commonly used, and in the United Kingdom "learning disability" is the preferred nomenclature (Vidyadharan & Tharayil 2019). Just as "mental retardation" is now exiting as a term from the diagnostic vernacular, earlier nomenclature used terms such as "idiocy", "mental deficiency", "moron" and "imbecile", which are now out of use. When reflecting on community attitudes to intellectual disability, it is important to note that these terms have been incorporated as slurs in everyday language use. One point of accessible self-reflection is to consider whether and when you use these terms, and whether it

reflects a position on individual value of people with intellectual disability?

In both the DSM-5 and the ICD-11, intelligence or intellect is now represented as more than that which can be represented by an intelligence quotient (IQ) test alone. Intelligence includes the capability to demonstrate functioning through adaptive behaviour (Girimaji & Pradeep 2018). This situates clinical assessment as an important element of the diagnostic practice alongside the use of standardised tests. Intellectual disability is a disorder, therefore, in which deficits are assessed to occur through IQ testing and assessment of adaptive functioning across the domains of conceptual, social and practical application (DSM-5).

Intellectual disability is the opposite to ASD in our evolution of understanding. In intellectual disability. the original focus was thinking alone, and this has now extended to the acceptance of the need to look at behaviours in the form of adaptive functioning. In ASD, the understanding first evolved in understanding the triad of impaired behaviours and then moved to the underlying thinking and information processing differences. For the DSM-5 diagnostic criteria of intellectual disability see Box 19.2.

BOX 19.2   Intellectual Disability Diagnostic Criteria

Intellectual disability (intellectual developmental disorder) is a disorder with onset during the developmental period that includes both intellectual and adaptive functioning deficits in conceptual, social and practical domains. The following three criteria must be met:

A. Deficits in intellectual functions, such as reasoning, problem-solving, planning, abstract thinking, judgement, academic learning and learning from experience, confirmed by both clinical assessment and individualised, standardised intelligence testing

B. Deficits in adaptive functioning that result in failure to meet developmental and sociocultural standards for personal independence and social responsibility (without ongoing support, the adaptive deficits limit functioning in one or more activities of daily life, such as communication, social participation or independent living, across multiple environments such as home, school, work and community)

C. Onset of intellectual and adaptive deficits during the developmental period.

   Note: The diagnostic term intellectual disability is the equivalent term for the ICD-11 diagnosis of intellectual developmental disorders. Although the term

intellectual disability is used throughout this manual, both terms are used in the title to clarify relationships with other classification systems. Moreover, a federal statute in the United States (Public Law 111-256, Rosa's Law) replaces the term mental retardation with intellectual disability, and research journals use the term intellectual disability. Thus, intellectual disability is the term in common use by medical, educational and other professions and by the lay public and advocacy groups.

   Specify current severity:
- 317 (F70) Mild
- 318.0 (F71) Moderate
- 318.1 (F72) Severe
- 318.2 (F73) Profound.

The various levels of severity are defined based on adaptive functioning and not IQ scores because it is adaptive functioning that determines the level of supports required. Moreover, IQ measures are less valid in the lower end of the IQ range.

APA 2013.

✳ HISTORICAL ANECDOTE 19.1

Autism

The term autism can be traced back to the work of Eugene Bleuler, who as early as 1910 described autism as a symptom of schizophrenia involving an inability to distinguish internal fantasy from reality. Later in 1943 American child psychiatrist Leo Kanner described autism in children as being distinguished by an inability to relate self towards other people and the world from the beginning of life. He described an "extreme autistic aloneness that whenever possible disregards, ignores, shuts out anything that comes to the child from the outside" (Kanner 1943). In 1944, and with no knowledge from Kanner's work, paediatrician Hans Asperger published a paper describing similar types of children in Vienna. He observed children who had high intelligence and creativity but often experienced learning difficulties. They would habitually avoid eye contact and did not speak in a way that was attuned to their listener, but aimed into the distance. Initially

unacclaimed, Asperger's work later become well known and led to the naming of the condition known as Asperger's syndrome. The name of this disorder has been challenged in recent times due to the unearthing of historical documents that revealed Hans Asperger was heavily involved in Nazi eugenics. Further to this, and with greater understanding, it has become clear that the main distinguishing factor between what came to be seen as autistic disorder and Asperger's disorder was the presence of comorbid intellectual disability and both disorders referred to the same thing, so the terms have been collapsed into ASD.

Read More About It
Feinstein A 2011 A history of autism: Conversations with the pioneers. John Wiley & Sons, West Sussex.

🐾 PERSPECTIVES IN PRACTICE

Nurse's Story 19.1: Toby

Michael, aged 25 years, had his first mental health admission when he was 15 years old. The admission was linked to concerns about anxiety and that he had been physically harassing girls at his high school. In addition to having an anxiety disorder diagnosed, a psychometric evaluation revealed that Michael had an intellectual disability. Due to a long history of pre-admission difficulties at school, he was subsequently transferred to a special needs high school. Despite the best efforts of his teachers, whenever he became excited during his senior years at high school Michael had a tendency to get into trouble because he would stand very close to females and sometimes touch them inappropriately, becoming demanding and irritable when told to provide space. Female teachers and students were warned that he was potentially dangerous and that they should not get too close to him. A common term used to describe Michael's behaviour was "predatory". Because of this he experienced very little physical human contact and did not get to attend school excursions or co-ed events unless there were male staff members present. After finishing high school aged 18, Michael started on a Disability Support Pension and became increasingly socially isolated. He spent all his time with his mother at home, who also had an intellectual disability, where they engaged in hoarding behaviour, collecting rubbish from their local neighbourhood and storing it at home.

My work with Michael began following complaints to the local council about his family's hoarding behaviour. After a general practitioner review, I began providing regular consultations with Michael, which were often also attended by his mother as a support person. Following a full case review of his history of care, what came to light was that although he was constantly told his behaviour was inappropriate during high school, the school had made little headway in helping Michael to understand what "appropriate behaviour" was. They told him what not to do, but there was no teaching of what to do (the replacement behaviour). The focus of my treatment from that point on was exploring Michael's interpretation of his world, understanding it from a developmental perspective in that Michael had not really advanced past junior "adolescent type" behaviour in the way he related to females and how he interpreted personal space.

When alone with his mother and engaged in his familiar routine, his anxiety remained low and his behaviour was relatively predictable. But if he visited a shopping centre or used public transport – less predictable situations – his mood could quickly become elevated and he then tended to start invading the personal space of nearby females. My work with him had a strong educational flavour, using graded exposure to teach about personal space and about what was acceptable and non-acceptable social behaviour in public spaces (e.g.

Nurse's Story 19.1: Toby

shaking hands, not hugging or touching others unless they gave him permission). This was combined with work to promote recognition of contexts in which his anxiety was high and symptoms that suggest anxiety levels are rising. Although it took a couple of years of regular consultations, with repetition, which was helpfully supported and reinforced by his mother, Michael eventually learnt the concept of personal boundaries. He became very proud of himself,

enjoying the positive responses he got from people. He became better at regulating his behaviour in unpredictable and anxiety-provoking environments. Michael's mother has since passed away and he now lives in a group home where he receives daily support and works on a production line at a local factory. I have seen him a couple of times since our meetings ended and on each occasion he proudly shook my hand.

PREVALENCE

The prevalence of ASD globally in the general population is reported to be 1% in children and adult populations (APA 2013). Reported prevalence rates in studies vary greatly, depending on whether the study is retrospective or prospective in design.

Prevalence of intellectual disability in the general population is approximately 1%, with the percentage varying by age and severity rating (American Psychiatric Association 2013).

The prevalence of people with ASD having comorbid intellectual disability is estimated to range from 20% to 40%, with most recent data suggesting the co-morbid rate being 27% (Cashin 2021). The variance is based, as in the studies determining prevalence, on the design of the studies.

Contributing Factors

Autism Spectrum Disorder

Causation of ASD has been discussed from a variety of viewpoints across time. We have come to know more clearly what does not cause ASD through the process than to understand the cause.

Parenting as a causative factor was an early point of consideration, progressing from Leo Kanner's observation of a cold and uncaring parenting style in the sample he reported on, to the coining of the term "refrigerator mother" by psychologist Bruno Bettleheim (Bettleheim 1990; Kanner 1943). Bettleheim based his theory on the observation that children with autism shared many characteristics with prisoners he had observed in World War II concentration camps. These factors he attributed to the guards' cold and uncaring behaviours in the camps and he projected this onto parental behaviours in the context of parenting children with autism. This psychogenic theory eventually dissipated, as research demonstrated no relationship between parenting style and causation of ASD.

There was a long debate on the link with the measles, mumps and rubella vaccination and the role of the preservative thimerosal in the vaccine; however, this has not been supported by any evidence despite several large-scale commissions to examine it. The early work of the scientist who proposed this link has now been discredited and withdrawn from the journal in which it was published.

The notion of neurodiversity has been put forward to challenge the logic of the idea of searching for causation. The neurodiversity movement promotes the concept that ASD is not a pathology with a cause but part of the diversity of humanity (Shakes & Cashin 2018). This discourse, while making some strong points, does suffer from an internal inconsistency, in that an entitlement for support is championed, yet parallels are drawn with previous social movements related to race, colour and sexual preference, areas of obvious diversity that are not conceptualised as including the need for support to promote adaptive functioning and comprehension.

The emergence of the strong suspicion of genetic difference, represented by partial dislocation identified on many genes in people with ASD, and the heritability of ASD in that prevalence is higher among biological siblings than the general population, supported suspicions that ASD as a developmental disorder developed in utero and was present at birth as part of the different way of thinking and processing information. As early as 2001, changes had been identified in people with ASD on all chromosomes excepting 14 and 20 (Committee on Children with Disabilities 2001). There is increased prevalence of ASD in groups of people with other genetic conditions, suggesting some shared liability. At this point we are left without known causation of ASD. There is a strong suspicion that ASD as a spectrum disorder is heterogeneous by nature and, as technology develops, what we now cluster under the umbrella of ASD may have different causative trajectories.

Intellectual Disability

Prenatal, perinatal and postnatal factors have been associated with developing intellectual disability (APA 2013). Examples of prenatal factors that affect development include genetic syndromes, environmental factors (e.g. toxins and maternal alcohol consumption), maternal illness (e.g. blood-borne viruses and placental disorders) and structural differences/abnormality in the physical development of the brain. Examples of perinatal factors include delivery-related incidents and development of acute inflammation of the brain. Postnatal factors may include a wide variety of traumas originating from physical injury, infections, syndromes and situations that impair oxygen supply in the brain (APA 2013).

In addition to the examples described above, extreme social deprivation has been associated with developing intellectual disability. While the potential causes are many, it must be emphasised that in many cases no cause can be identified.

THE EXPERIENCE OF INCLUSION AND EXCLUSION

One unifying element in the discourse related to the experience of both ASD and intellectual disability is that of inclusion and a sense of community belonging. Society could be described as "a large group of people who live together in an organized way, making decisions about how to do things and sharing the work that needs to be done" (Cambridge English Dictionary 2020). Around the world, societies are mediated by a complex mix of implicit and explicit rules as elements of governance. The rules determine what is acceptable both in behavioural performance of societal tasks and routines, and also in the process of social mediation.

Belonging in society is determined through participation in activities designed to promote thriving. Participation is predicated on the ability to comprehend both the explicit and the implicit rules and to participate in the social mediation. While often taken for granted, the underpinning abilities required to meet these demands are many and complex.

In ASD the core features of impaired social communication and impaired behavioural flexibility, manifested as restrictive and repetitive behaviour, represent challenges. The abilities of those with ASD in many cases do not align with those complex abilities identified and needed for active participation, and so the deficit in the required abilities, by definition, becomes a disability.

The challenge in intellectual disability is that of being able to handle the volumes of information needed to navigate participation and to have the necessary processing speed to manage the information in a timely manner. The social mediation occurs in real time and requires a multitude of on-the-spot decisions.

SIGNS AND SYMPTOMS

It is useful to discuss the signs and symptoms of ASD and intellectual disability to understand how they shape the requirements needed for adjustments in the mental health assessment and in intervention strategies. Developing capability in assessing the mental health of people with ASD and intellectual disability is essential for mental health nurses, as not only do people with ASD and intellectual disability each represent approximately 1% of the population (APA 2013) but, as population groups, they both have a disproportionate prevalence of mental ill health and mental illness.

Autism Spectrum Disorder

Earlier in the chapter the behavioural dyad of impairment and the underpinning thinking and information-processing triad of impairment was discussed. In this section, the signs and symptoms as manifested in thinking and information processing, and the subsequent behaviour, will be unpacked further. These differences are the characteristic signs and symptoms of ASD.

The thinking and information-processing impairments of ASD are inherent traits. As we discovered in the historical evolution of our understanding of ASD, and our passage through psychogenic theory in which parenting was the focus, we have come to know that the traits are not learnt, and that a new way of thinking cannot be taught. They are gifts, as in the great gift of abstraction, first identified by Aristotle. The differences are most likely linked to genetically mediated differences that affect brain structure and function, although these differences have not yet been conclusively identified. The differences in thinking and information processing are impaired abstraction, impaired theory of mind and impaired linguistic processing of information (with a relative strength in visual processing).

Abstraction is the gift that allows us to recognise like and similar and gradients of things. An impairment in abstraction manifests as the black-and-white thinking characteristic of people with ASD. Impaired abstraction makes understanding homonyms extremely difficult, such as understanding the difference between a tear in your eye and a tear in your pants. As an interesting exercise, think about a fluffy white cat and a small fluffy white dog. Then, without relying on the abstract notion of "catness" and "dogness", describe each on a piece of paper and see if you can identify the difference. While subtle, abstraction is the core unifying element in neurotypical thinking. It provides the glue, or central coherence. The gift of abstraction is the basis of generalisation.

Theory of mind is the gift that allows neurotypical thinkers to know that every person has a mind, that each mind is unique and hence different from each other. The ability to make a guess of what other people are thinking, using context and a self-referential process, is central to neurotypical thought. This is the process of imagining oneself in the other person's shoes and projecting an understanding that, if in that context I would feel *x*, there is a good chance for other person may be experiencing this, and this is the gift of theory of mind.

Theory of mind is impaired in people with ASD. The impairment is on a spectrum from the assumption that if I think it that all people think it, to knowing that other people have a mind separate from one's own, but being mystified by what others are thinking and feeling and what motivates their behaviour. Theory of mind is a central capability in social competence, and impaired theory of mind is manifested in the impaired social communication characteristic of ASD. This manifests in the symptoms of a deficit in the ability to engage in reciprocal conversation. In mental health, reciprocal conversation, in which you put your thoughts out there and then modify your thinking based on the feedback of others, is the essence of reality testing (Cashin 2020).

Neurotypical thinkers are linguistic processors of information. Heidegger famously wrote "to know the world is to name it" (Heidegger, 1962). In typical thought, information is stored based on the stories one tells oneself about the world. The coding would perhaps be most accurately written as a type of mentalese, as opposed to what we understand to be language, but fundamentally it is a linguistically mediated process (Pinker 1997). This form of processing allows typical thinkers to build conceptual knowledge about abstract or nonconcrete entities, such as emotions. This is opposed to visual coding where the thing coded needs to be something concrete that can be seen to allow it to be coded.

Neurotypical thinkers can label emotions in themselves and others. The ability to recognise symptoms of the presence of emotions, and the emotions themselves, are purely a linguistic construct. You can easily describe symptoms of being happy, but you cannot produce and show someone "a happy" as an example. This is because it is an abstract entity. The knowledge of emotions allows typical thinkers to self-monitor for the presence of these abstract entities and to regulate their behaviour based on this monitoring. People with ASD have a relative strength in visual coding of information and a relative deficit in linguistic processing. Even before we consider the compounding effect of the combination of the three impairments, the impact of the deficit in linguistic processing becomes clear. Impaired linguistic processing is linked to impaired self-regulation of behaviour, based on the self-monitoring enabled through identifying emotions.

These impairments in thinking and information processing each by themselves have clearly associated disability. However, the greatest impact comes from the combination of all three impairments globally in the process of thinking and information processing.

The world is unpredictable in many ways and presents each person with a succession of novel circumstances. The novelty may be a truly new situation or a variant of something experienced before. Adaptation, by definition, is the process of adapting in the context of novelty or changed circumstances (Cashin & Yorke 2017). As discussed earlier, society is socially mediated, and adaptation relies on a high degree of social competence.

When an individual is placed in a novel situation, they experience a surge in anxiety. This anxiety is the motivating factor to adapt. A neurotypical thinker is able, often without even being aware of the process, to gather clues to establish context and then reach into their unified in-head filing cabinet and pull forward directions from the closest situation they have been in before. This means they have a clue of how to begin to adapt and their anxiety subsides a little. The person can apply the directions and look for clues as to whether it has been effective. If it is not effective, anxiety will again surge and prompt modification of their coping response. The person will then attempt to change their response in what appears to be the most efficient manner. Anxiety will again drop, and they will look for evidence of success. If not successful, the process will continue until adaptation has occurred. The person has then succeeded in adapting, and, what is more, they then add the new context and directions to their in-head filing cabinet of life information for future use (Cashin 2020).

In these situations, you will notice that, while perhaps initially a long way off the mark, the person had some clue. First the person needed to recognise context. This includes a mixture of concrete and abstract elements. The person then had to reach in their unified base of knowledge of the world to find a like or similar context to have a clue of where to begin and what behavioural direction or strategies to apply. Both the recognition of like and similar, and the presence of a unified base of knowledge about the world, are dependent on abstraction. To judge success of the behaviour and whether adaptation has occurred relies at least in part on the feedback of others through the social mechanism of communication. To recognise anxiety and respond in a targeted manner of focused adaption, as opposed to being pushed into non-adaptive behaviour and thought, such as ritual and obsession, requires a recognition and labelling of the feeling (Cashin 2018). The final step of saving the information for future use and expanding the unified knowledge of the world requires again recognition of like and similar to store the information in a coherent and accessible manner.

When in novel situations people with ASD can in effect not have a clue where to begin. The anxiety, while not monitored for and hence recognised and labelled, still exists. Anxiety is designed to push, as in

the flight and fight mechanism, and will push the person even if not acknowledged. While anxiety is not recognised, the flight or fight system biologically remains unimpaired. There is a link between increased anxiety and increased restrictive and repetitive behaviours, with the behaviours increasing in intensity and frequency as anxiety goes up (Cashin & Yorke 2018). The restrictive and repetitive behaviours have a filtering function where the focus shifts to managing the communicated demand to adapt as opposed to adapting (Cashin & Yorke 2016).

In terms of symptoms of mental illness, people with ASD experience a disproportionately high prevalence of comorbid mental illness. This includes high rates of anxiety disorders, which makes sense given the above description. It also appears that there is a high rate of depression, although much less studied. People with ASD also experience high rates of psychosis, with up to 30% of people with ASD experiencing psychotic phenomena (Cashin 2016). The comorbidity in some cases may be reactive and related to adaption. There is also a strong chance of shared, as yet undefined, biological mechanisms. See Personal perspectives: Consumer's story 19.1 about the experiences of Martin.

PERSONAL PERSPECTIVES

Consumer's Story 19.1: Martin

Martin was a 16-year-old male with a diagnosis of ASD in Year 10 at a public school in Victoria. Martin received his diagnosis when he was 7 years old. Martin had an IQ of 74 when last tested in Year 7 and was attending mainstream classes with homeroom support from a special education teacher and teacher aides. He was taking no medication and had no history of illicit drug use.

Martin had few friends at school and spent most breaks in his homeroom.

Martin became increasingly focused on the idea that males at the school were taking steroids. The intensity of Martin's beliefs increased in the context of acute stress when his parents separated. All of Martin's routines changed as he and his siblings lived between the family home and his father's new apartment. Martin had become panicked when out with his family when he saw males from the schools and explained it as a fear of being near steroid-takers. While able to describe his idea as a fear, Martin was not able to clarify it further and was not ameliorable to any other points of view when his parents tried to discuss it with him. Without warning, first thing on a Wednesday morning Martin walked into the playground and physically attacked a boy. When asked why he attacked the boy, Martin claimed the boy was a steroid-taker.

The attack resulted in a suspension from school and full health assessment. Martin felt no empathy with the boy who he attacked and could not identify if the boy would have been scared or worried. Martin stated that he had been told one year earlier by an older boy that the boy he attacked was "on steroids". Martin ruminated over this idea, even though the boy described was small and

of slight build. Martin had become preoccupied with this thought over the year, but it had increased in intensity since his social situation changed. He was having difficulty falling asleep because he could not get the thought out of his head.

Martin's thoughts were not sequential, and he had difficulty focusing on the discussion, often going onto tangents. Martin said that he infrequently heard voices calling his name when no one was in the room. Martin had no suicidal or homicidal ideation plan or intent and no recent history of physical ill health or injury.

Martin was prescribed risperidone 0.5 mg nocte and was able to return to school in one week after making a written agreement to not attack fellow students. The medication was up-titrated to 1 mg nocte 2 months later in the context of increased stress-related behaviour at school.

Healthcare staff worked with the family to develop firm routines that were made explicit, and if the routine was to change to show Martin with as much warning as possible what the change was and where it fitted. Through discussion, behavioural warning signs of increased stress (Martin does not label his feelings, so cannot rate his own anxiety) were identified and management strategies formed and rehearsed.

Martin, although agreeing to not attack anyone, and able to give a historical account of the evolution of the idea, remained suspicious that it may be true that the boy was on steroids and resented the fact the boy was given a citizenship award at school for not fighting back.

Adapted from Cashin 2016.

Intellectual Disability

A concrete exercise to elucidate the vast number of choices we are continually confronted with, and the information we need to extract to optimise outcomes, is to write down each choice that was made and the action followed from the time you woke this morning up until the time you left the house for work or study. Of course, it is best to choose a morning when you left early because the information you will record will be voluminous.

The exercise may begin with choices such as to hit snooze or not on the alarm, what side of the bed to get out of, what leg to put weight on first as you stand, and so on. Our lives are full of choices, and we are constantly bombarded by stimuli (Gergen 2000). Many of the choices

go underground as they become subconscious, and this is a way of managing the volume. Prejudice or pre-judgement is a typical way of also managing the volume of choice (Gadamer 1960/1985). It may come as a surprise that prejudice is a natural part of typical thought processes and that it has a function in making the volume of choice we are confronted with manageable. A good example is favourite foods, which make choices presented on a menu manageable. An even better example may be coffee choices, in what is often a time-limited rush into the coffee shop to grab a takeaway while often simultaneously engaged in other activities such as a phone call or checking social media updates. Of course when pre-judgements extend to races or groups of people, including those with intellectual disability, it is incumbent on us to make our prejudices as known to ourselves as is possible, to allow us to become aware of what we can modify, as needed, to be consistent with our overall worldview.

Even with prejudices, and many choices moving below the conscious level, it is clear that people are confronted with huge volumes of information that need to be managed and often simultaneously and quickly. Any impairment of the volume of information that can be handled at any one time and the speed at which information can be processed and acted on, will result in serious functional impairments. Even self-care tasks consist of chains of behaviours each preceded by choices. Think of the simple activity of brushing your teeth. An exercise of writing out the chain of steps in brushing your teeth will show how a simple task, taken for granted by typical thinkers, is in fact quite complex.

People with intellectual disability also have a disproportionate prevalence of mental illness (Department of Developmental Disability Neuropsychiatry 2018). This burden may arise from the challenge and stress of adaptation, but also plausibly be related to shared causative biological mechanisms.

✳ HISTORICAL ANECDOTE 19.2

A Dark Chapter in the History of Nursing

Autism, intellectual disability and mental ill health have been used by nurses and other health professionals as justification for taking part in mass sterilisation and extermination. At the start of the 20th century, the philosophy of "eugenics" was developed by social policy experts and scientists in the United States. This philosophy suggested that people with disabilities or mental illness should be eradicated from society. From the 1920s to the 1960s, the influence of this ideology led to government policies that facilitated the involuntary sterilisation of more than 60,000 people with mental and physical disabilities in North America. The philosophy of eugenics was then used by Hitler and the Nazi regime in Germany to justify the extermination of more than 200,000 disabled people during World War II. Much of the extermination was carried out by nurses and doctors in hospitals like Hadamar in Germany.

Read More About It
Iredale R 2000 Eugenics and its relevance to contemporary health care. Nursing Ethics 7(3), 205–214.

PHYSICAL HEALTH AND ASD AND INTELLECTUAL DISABILITY

People with ASD and intellectual disability experience a higher burden of chronic ill health than the general population of people without either disability (Cashin et al 2018; Trollor et al 2018). It would appear that obesogenic factors are prevalent, particularly in the domains of diet and physical activity. The risk for ill health is particularly challenging related to inequitable access to health care and accessible information on self-care.

Autism Spectrum Disorder

There is a marked lack of research focused on the physical health of adults with ASD (Cashin et al 2018). The research with children has highlighted the need to focus intervention on the commonly experienced obesogenic factors and to be aware of ASD-related factors that exacerbate these, including restricted diet and reduced physical activity, such as when engaged in some obsessional behaviours (e.g. gaming) or avoidance of physical activity based on the social demands of participation (Cashin 2020). People with ASD have a higher risk of mortality than those without ASD; in a sample of people with ASD in New South Wales, mortality is 2.06 times more for those with ASD than the population without ASD (Hwang et al 2019). This information is important to guide intervention and particularly from a mental health nursing perspective when prescribing or administering medications associated with an increased risk of chronic illness such as type 2 diabetes, which may further compound the risk of ill health.

Intellectual Disability

People with intellectual disability experience a higher burden of ill health, both physically and mentally, compared to the population without intellectual disability (McCarthy & Duff 2019; Trollor et al 2018). The impact is made even more significant by inequitable access to services. In Aotearoa New Zealand, within the context of limited statistical information, the life expectancy is 22.9 years less for people with intellectual disability than those without (McCarthy & Duff 2019).

Challenges exist both in the Aotearoa New Zealand and Australian contexts related to the identification of intellectual disability in mental health policy, ranging from exclusion to inadequate acknowledgement of the unique needs of the group (Dew et al 2018; McCarthy & Duff 2019). The policy context, as it exists, perpetuates both issues with access to services and an inadequate focus on teaching the required adjustments to provide adequate services to this group, and practitioners need this policy change for services to improve. In Australia, a national roundtable was convened by Parliament to address the inequities in health service provision for people with intellectual disability in 2019. See Personal perspectives: Consumer's story 19.2 about the experiences of Margaret.

👤 PERSONAL PERSPECTIVES

Consumer's Story 19.2: Margaret

Margaret is a 35-year-old woman who normally lives with her mother and has limited support needs. She has a small vocabulary, but can understand much of what is said to her. She can perform self-help tasks and has developed competencies in occupational, leisure and social skills. Diagnostic overshadowing played a large part in the delay between the onset of severe symptoms and diagnosis for this client.

The police brought Margaret into the emergency department late one Sunday after local residents reported that she had been lying on the road outside a shopping centre. Margaret was very distressed and crying, and when asked why she was on the road replied: "You will get run over lying on the road and go to heaven, sorry Mr Policeman". She was able to give her name, phone number and address to the attending mental health nurse and a subsequent phone call found

that Margaret lived at home with her mother and had gone to the local shops for bread. The mental health nurse and the duty psychiatrist decided that Margaret could go home to the care of her mother because there was no history of mental illness and she was able to say where she lived. Lying on the road was dismissed as "behaviour" due to her intellectual disability. This proved to be diagnostic overshadowing.

Two days later, Margaret's mother Jean telephoned the mental health service staff to say that a local shopkeeper had brought Margaret home after he had found her lying on the road. Jean was told that someone from the mental health team would visit in the next couple of days, but this was not regarded as high priority because the behaviour was seen as part of Margaret's intellectual disability. The following afternoon, community mental health nurses visited and

Consumer's Story 19.2: Margaret

questioned Margaret, who became tearful and repeated: "I'll get run over and go to heaven". Jean told the staff that she had heard Margaret crying at night and that she had been awake early in the morning and needed to be told to shower. This was unlike Margaret, but Jean said that she had been sad since her grandmother died 3 months ago and seemed to lack motivation.

On their way back to the community mental health centre the nurses called in to the local shops and discovered that Margaret had been lying on the road intermittently for the past 4 weeks. At first, she would get up as soon as someone called out to her, but over the past 2 weeks she would cry: "No, I'll get run over and go to heaven". The staff, recognising her behaviour as suicidal, arranged for Margaret to be admitted to the mental health unit as an involuntary patient (i.e. she was deprived of her right to discharge herself from hospital on the grounds that there was a reasonable risk that she would harm herself).

In Margaret's case, nursing and medical staff found that she was uncommunicative upon admission to the mental health unit and that she sat gently rocking and averting her gaze from staff. Fortunately, the staff were able to engage Jean in the process of taking a history and for some of the assessment process. After medical staff had performed a physical examination of Margaret, it was decided to take her to her bedroom and continue the assessment process once she had familiarised herself with her new environment. In the interim, a nurse was able to start brief conversations with Margaret using gentle open-ended questions. Margaret was subsequently asked to unpack her suitcase and engage in self-care activities independently.

Margaret lived at home and, in such cases, it is important to work with the family to gain their trust, to ensure the optimal outcome for the client and to obtain a reliable history of the client's mental and physical status. Over the course of the next hour, the nurse was able to ascertain from Jean that Margaret was uncharacteristically withdrawn and that her movements were much slower than usual. Jean also revealed that Margaret's concentration had deteriorated in recent weeks, and Margaret was able to add that she felt terrible and that she didn't "want to live anymore". Apart from these typical signs of clinical depression, staff noted that Margaret's rocking had continued and that she made low, barely audible noises. Jean confirmed that rocking and moaning were atypical signs of Margaret's depression because they were not normally part of her behavioural repertoire.

Having gained the confidence of the new patient, the nurse was able to interview Margaret alone and, after some encouragement, found that she had retained her plan to kill herself by lying down in the middle of a road and being run over by a car. She did not have any other plans for her own death, but repeated that what she really wanted was to die and go to heaven to see her grandmother. Eventually the nurse was able to complete the initial assessments for Margaret, including a physical assessment, mental status assessment, risk assessment, assessment of strengths and assessment of Margaret's risk of vulnerability to exploitation and abuse, and was able to write admission notes that described her signs and symptoms, including the atypical signs of depression.

Margaret was subsequently placed on half-hourly general observations with 4-hourly observations. Although primary nursing was not a part of the unit's policy on patient care, Margaret was allocated a single nurse for each subsequent morning and afternoon "shift" on the first two days of her admission to facilitate communications and to assist in the process of ongoing assessment. Despite these arrangements, Margaret remained largely uncommunicative and chose to speak only with a few of the staff.

Apart from the interventions outlined above, the management of Margaret's depression was much like that afforded to other patients. While she was being stabilised on an antidepressant (in this case, fluoxetine), Margaret was offered grief counselling to help her to cope with the loss of her grandmother. Although Margaret was quick to understand that she needed to take her medication with her morning meals until her doctor said to stop, she was unable to grasp education given to her by staff about the physiology of her depressive illness and the need to be vigilant regarding the symptoms of relapse. She also had a very limited understanding of the way in which her medication was helping her.

At the suggestion of Margaret's mother, and with Margaret's permission, it was decided to devise a mental health support plan to disseminate information about Margaret's management strategies to the people in her circle of support when she was discharged. The plan featured possible relapse signs (such as social withdrawal and "rocking") and management strategies should Margaret again decide to harm herself (such as removing Margaret from harmful circumstances, clarifying Margaret's intentions and contacting the community mental health team if Jean required assistance).

KEY POINTS RELATED TO ASSESSMENT

The good news related to the required adjustments to be discussed in this section of key points related to assessment, and in the following section on interventions, is that incorporating these adjustments into general practice will strengthen the delivery of truly person-centred care (Wilson et al 2022).

Before discussing specific adjustments it is important to acknowledge that an assessment is not an interrogation designed to extract information to allow the formulaic construction of a diagnostic picture. An assessment is an opportunity for the assessor and assessee to build an understanding of the context, in the form of recent and more extensive history, and the personal experience of living within that context. How that understanding is co-constructed needs careful attention. The interview, as discussed earlier, includes coming to consensus on not only what the experience is, but also how it is labelled.

In regards to working with a person with ASD, it is imperative to take into consideration their thinking and information-processing style. Without being mindful of this, it can be like speaking different languages, and while the words may appear common, it can impair the ability to develop shared understanding.

Regarding impaired abstraction, it is important to check if the person makes sense of emotions and self-monitors for these. It may make more sense to explore symptoms of anxiety such as increased engagement in restrictive and repetitive behaviours than ask the person if they feel anxious. Don't assume that rating scales such as 1–10 when discussing the experience of emotions make any sense to the person. Check this out thoroughly with them. If someone presents as sad, again, rather than discussing being depressed, it may make more sense to explore changes in usual behaviours such as sleeping, eating and activity. When discussing the experience of assessment, discuss what will happen in a linear fashion in the order that it will occur. If the person appears distracted, re-ground the interview by discussing where you are at in the order things, and what will occur next, with reference to what happened immediately before, what will happen now and what will follow. Don't expect the person to generalise from past experiences, particularly if these occurred in a different visual context, such as a different emergency department. Even with a history of past assessments for the person, this may be a novel situation. Be concrete in what is being asked. Be careful that your questions will result in discussion of the target information. A good example is the question: "Do you hear voices?" Unless experiencing a hearing deficit, the answer would be yes; that is, if they heard the question. If exploring auditory hallucinations, a rephrased question such as, "Do you hear voices when no one is around and there are no devices capable of delivering sound on?" can help.

In terms of theory of mind, at the outset it needs to be established that the interview is a social process. On top of whatever challenge to health it was that brought the person to the interview, the interview itself can generate significant anxiety. Affect is an important element of a mental health assessment. People with ASD may have a limited range of affect and reduced prosody (variance in pitch and tone) in the voice. Both affect and prosody are learnt behaviours, and the learning is mediated in the social process, beginning with the child–parent relationship and expanding from there, by theory of mind. What the person with ASD is feeling on the inside (e.g. scared) may not be expressed externally through changes in affect or prosody. Ask the person clearly what they are feeling in the concrete context of inquiry. Don't rely on eye contact as a sign of attention. Lack of eye contact may be related to the social aspect of this, or equally that looking and listening is overwhelming and not looking allows full concentration on what is said. When exploring empathy, don't rely on the ability of the person with ASD to guess what others are thinking and feeling and to consider this perspective.

As the person with ASD is not primarily a linguistic processor of information, it is easy to become overwhelmed by words. If the person is appearing confused, reduce the volume of words. If giving instructions, make sure the person with ASD understands what is required and what order it is to be done in. Don't be afraid of doodling and drawing to augment understanding. The art does not have to be high quality; it just needs to promote understanding. Write down any key instructions and what is to happen next because, unlike spoken words, writing and drawing are not transitory.

In regards to intellectual disability, all of the ASD adjustments will be important. In addition, become familiar with characteristic patterns of speech (particularly in people with a higher degree of intellectual impairment) such as echolalia. Be clear that the person is not just repeating the question rather than taking it as a form of confirmation. Be very mindful of changes to usual activity and behaviours, and explore plausible causes thoroughly. For non-verbal individuals, find out how they usually communicate and how this can be incorporated in the assessment. Work closely with family and carers to establish meaning making.

For people with ASD and people with intellectual disability, ensure a thorough physical examination is conducted. Be mindful that they may not describe discomfort or pain in the typical manner or, unless asked, may not disclose it at all.

One common issue that warrants discussion is diagnostic overshadowing. This is the situation where everything is attributed to the primary diagnosis (such as ASD or intellectual disability), and this diagnosis overshadows other important understandings of what is happening. This leads to missing treatable comorbidities and is largely contributing to the increased morbidity and mortality in these groups. This overshadowing can lead to lack of exploration of provisional diagnosis. An example would be the failure to diagnose delusions in people with ASD due to an assumption that because people with ASD think differently, delusional beliefs must be normal for this group. Or that a rise in self-harming behaviour in someone with intellectual disability may just be an increase in self-stimulatory behaviour and have no relationship with self-harming, even though this is a new behaviour for this person.

INTERVENTIONS

Interventions designed to work on thinking need to be modified to be accessible by the participants. Psychotherapies used in typical populations all need adjustments to work with people with ASD and intellectual disability. As an example, modified narrative therapy has been effective in a trial with a small sample of young people with ASD (Cashin et al 2013). The therapy was adjusted based on the principles discussed above to work on the problems of daily living (Cashin 2020). Similar modifications have occurred with cognitive behaviour therapy (CBT).

If we accept that talking therapies are needed by the neurotypical population, there is no logical reason why such therapy is not needed by people with ASD and intellectual disability. Mental health nurses are ideally situated to deliver the therapy, but need to be mindful of the adjustments required to make them accessible and functional for people with ASD and intellectual disability. The health disparity between people with ASD and intellectual disability and the neurotypical population in general is large. Nurses have a role in reducing this and understanding the thinking and information-processing styles is all that is needed to make creative adjustments that can be trialled and evaluated.

DEINSTITUTIONALISATION

In the mid- to late 20th century nurses performed a central role in the care of people with ASD and intellectual disabilities in both Australia and Aotearoa New Zealand. Deinstitutionalisation with the move to community care progressively saw a decline in the involvement of nurses in the care of these groups (Trollor et al 2018). Institutional living was, in many ways, undesirable (Burghardt 2018) and with the evolution of the diagnostic construct of ASD in particular, even if the return of institutional living was seen as an answer, it would not service a large proportion of those diagnosed. However, the return of nursing as a central component of care would undoubtedly lead to better health outcomes.

▌ CHAPTER SUMMARY

Every nurse can make a difference in the lives of people with ASD and intellectual disability. It is every nurse's business (Cashin 2021). This can be in each clinical encounter and through advocacy to make adjustments to practice, so that services can be more accessible. Participation in policy and practice related to inclusion criteria for services, at a local and national level, is also an area where nurses can make an impact. Such adjustments are predicated on understanding the thinking and information processing style inherent in ASD, and the thinking and processing challenges experienced in intellectual disability. The link between thinking and behaviour, once understood, leads to both accessible and hence more effective assessment and intervention.

USEFUL WEBSITES

Autism Science Foundation: autismsciencefoundation.org/
Autism Spectrum Australia: www.autismspectrum.org.au
Carer Gateway (Australian Government): www.carergateway.gov.au/
National Autistic Society (UK): www.autism.org.uk/
Raising Children.net: raisingchildren.net.au/
University of New South Wales – Department of Developmental Disability Neuropsychiatry (3DN): 3dn.unsw.edu.au/content/disability-professionals-elearning

REFERENCES

American Psychiatric Association (APA) 2013. Diagnostic and Statistical Manual of Mental Disorders, 5th Edition. (DSM-5). APA, Washington DC.

Barnes, C. 2019. Understanding the social model of disability: Past, present and future. In: Watson, S., Roulstone, A., Thomas, C (eds). Routledge Handbook of Disability Studies. Routledge, New York.

Bettleheim, B., 1990. Recollections and Reflections. Thames and Hudson, London.

Burghardt, M. 2018. Broken: Institutions, Families and the Construction of Intellectual Disability. McGill-Queen's University Press, Montreal.

Cambridge English Dictionary 2020. Society, Cambridge University Press. Online. https://dictionary.cambridge.org/help/

Cashin, A. 2021. Understanding how to care for and support people with intellectual disability and/or autism is every nurse's business. Aust Crit Care, 34(5), 401–402.

Cashin, A. 2020. Young People, Adults and Autism Spectrum Disorder. Nova Science Publishers, New York.

Cashin, A. 2018. Why do some people with autism have restricted interests and repetitive movements? The Conversation. Online. Available at: theconversation.com/why-do-some-people-with-autism-have-restricted-interests-and-repetitive-movements-94401

Cashin, A. 2016. Autism spectrum disorder and psychosis: A case study. J Child Adolesc Psychiatr Nurs, 29, 72–78.

Cashin, A., Barker, P. 2009. The triad of impairment in autism revisited. J Child Adolesc Psychiatr Nurs, 22, 189–193.

Cashin, A., Browne, G., Bradbury, J., et al., 2013. The effectiveness of Narrative Therapy with young people with autism. J Child Adolesc Psychiatr Nurs, 26, 32–41.

Cashin, A., Buckley, T., Trollor, J.N., et al., 2018. A scoping review of what is known of the physical health of adults with autism spectrum disorder. J Intellect Disabil, 22, 96–108.

Cashin, A., Heartfield, M., Bryce, J., et al., 2017. Standards for practice for registered nurses in Australia. Collegian, 24, 255–266.

Cashin, A., Yorke, J. 2018. The relationship between anxiety, external structure, behavioral history and becoming locked into restricted and repetitive behaviors in Autism Spectrum Disorder. Issues Ment Health Nurs, 39, 533–537.

Cashin, A., Yorke, J. 2017. Conceptualization of a heuristic to predict increase in restricted and repetitive behaviour in ASD across the short to medium term. Autism Open Access, 7(1), doi: 10.4172/2165-7890.1000200.

Cashin, A., Yorke, J. 2016. Overly regulated thinking and autism revisited. J Child Adolesc Psychiatr Nurs, 29, 148–153.

Committee on Children with Disabilities 2001. Technical report: The pediatrician's role in the diagnosis and management of autistic spectrum disorder in children. Pediatrics, 107, e85.

Department of Developmental Disability Neuropsychiatry 2018. Recommendations from the National Roundtable on the Mental Health of People with Intellectual Disability 2018. University of NSW, Sydney.

Dew, A., Dowse, L., Athanassiou, U., et al., 2018. Current representation of people with Intellectual Disability in Australian mental health policy: The need for inclusive policy development. J Policy Pract Intellect Disabil, 15, 136–144.

Feinstein, A., 2011. A History of Autism: Conversations With the Pioneers. John Wiley & Sons, West Sussex.

Gadamer, H., 1960/1985. The discrediting of prejudice by the enlightenment. In: Mueller-Vollmer, K. (ed.), The Hermeneutics Reader. Basil Blackwell, Oxford.

Gergen, K. 2000. The Saturated Self. Basic Books, New York.

Girimaji, S., Pradeep, A. 2018. Intellectual Disability in international classification of Diseases-11: A developmental perspective. Indian J Soc Psychiatry (Suppl. S1), 68–74.

Heidegger, M., 1962. Being and Time. Blackwell, Malden.

Hwang, Y.I., Srasuebkul, P., Foley, K.R., et al., 2019. Mortality and cause of death of Australians on the autism spectrum. Autism Res, 12(5), 806–815.

Iredale, R. 2000. Eugenics and its relevance to contemporary health care. Nurs Ethics, 7(3), 205–214.

Kanner, L., 1943. Autistic disturbances of affective contact. Nerv Child 2, 217–250.

McCarthy, J., Duff, M. 2019. Services for adults with intellectual disability in Aotearoa New Zealand. B J Psych Int 16(3), 71–73.

Nursing Council of New Zealand 2022. Competencies for registered nurses. Nursing Council of New Zealand, Wellington.

Nylander, L., Lugnegard, T., Hallerback, M. 2008. Autism spectrum disorders and schizophrenia spectrum disorders in adults – is there a connection? A literature review and some suggestions for future clinical research. Clin Neuropsychiatry 5, 43–54.

Pinker, S., 1997. How the Mind Works. W.W. Norton and Company, New York.

Pracilio, A., Wilson, N.J., Kersten, M., Trollor, J.N., & Cashin, A. 2022. A discourse analysis of the representation of nursing in the National Disability Insurance Scheme pricing guide and eligibility criteria. Collegian, 30(4), doi: 10.1016/j.colegn.2022.08.007

Shakes, P., Cashin, A. 2018. Identifying language for people on the autism spectrum: A scoping review. Issues Ment Health Nurs, 40(4), 317–325.

Trollor, J., Eagleson, C., Turner, B., et al., 2018. Intellectual disability content within pre-registration nursing curriculum: How is it taught? Nurse Educ Today, 69, 48–52.

Vidyadharan, V., & Tharayil, H.M. 2019. Learning disorder or learning disability: Time to rethink. Ind J Psycholog Med, 41(3), 276–278.

Wilson, N.J., Pracilio, A., Kersten, M., Morphet, J., Buckely, T., et al., 2022. Registered nurses' awareness and implementation of reasonable adjustments for people with intellectual disability and/or autism. J Adv Nurs, 78(8), 2426–2435.

World Health Organization (WHO), 2019. International statistical classification of diseases and related health problems, 11th ed. ICD-11. Available: https://icd.who.int/

20

Physical Health in the Context of Mental Health

Andrew Watkins and Patrick Gould

KEY POINTS

- The prevalence and causes of preventable physical health issues among people with mental illness are a concern for nurses in every practice setting.
- Mental health nurses have an important role in preventing and addressing physical health issues among people with mental illness.

- Nurses need to understand the impact of physical health on mental wellbeing.
- Nurses need to appreciate the challenges and benefits of partnerships and collaboration for improving physical and mental health.

KEY TERMS

Cardiometabolic health
Cardiovascular disease
Metabolic screening
Metabolic syndrome
Nutrition

Obesity
Obstructive sleep apnoea
Oral health
Physical activity
Premature mortality

Sexual health
Type 2 diabetes
Vaccine preventable diseases

LEARNING OUTCOMES

The material in this chapter will assist you to:
- recognise the relationship and common issues between mental health and physical health
- develop an understanding of the experience and needs of people with both physical and mental health issues

- explain and implement the nurse's role in assessing and improving physical health
- describe evidence-based interventions for physical health issues
- apply nursing interventions relevant to physical health issues identified.

INTRODUCTION

People living with mental illness experience much poorer physical health outcomes compared with the general population (Rodrigues et al 2021) . There is a life expectancy gap of 15–20 years between consumers with severe mental illness (SMI), such as schizophrenia and bipolar disorder, and the general population (Nielsen et al 2021). There is also clear evidence that individuals across the range of mental disorders have a significantly reduced life expectancy compared with the general population (Firth et al 2019). In contrast to the commonly held misconception, nearly four in every five of these premature deaths are associated with preventable physical health conditions and not suicide (Correll et al 2022).

The World Health Organization (WHO) describes mental health as "a state of well-being in which every individual realises his or her own potential, can cope with the normal stresses of life, can work productively and fruitfully, and is able to make a contribution to her or his community" (Freeman 2022). WHO also acknowledges a universal right to health that includes the right to control one's health and body, to be free from interference, also including the right to a system of health protection that gives everyone an equal opportunity to enjoy the highest attainable level of health. Historically, the physical health care

of people with mental illness has been neglected (Thornicroft et al 2022). In both Australia and Aotearoa New Zealand, Equally Well has been established with the primary purpose of taking initiatives and creating change to achieve physical health equity for people experiencing mental health issues. Nurses are well placed to take the lead in ensuring that people with mental illness have their physical health needs considered and adequately addressed from the initial assessment, right through the person's mental health journey. It is therefore vital that nurses practise in a holistic way, incorporating physical health care by "keeping the body in mind".

It is beyond the scope of this chapter to address all the physical illnesses experienced by people with mental illness. The authors have therefore chosen to focus on physical health issues that negatively impact on life expectancy, are most prevalent and that most markedly affect wellbeing and quality of life. Factors contributing to physical health risks are shown in Fig. 20.1.

This chapter will discuss metabolic syndrome, diabetes, cardiovascular disease, respiratory diseases, immunisation, oral health, sleep and sexual health. These physical health issues require action, and we believe nurses are well positioned to make a difference to the current trends.

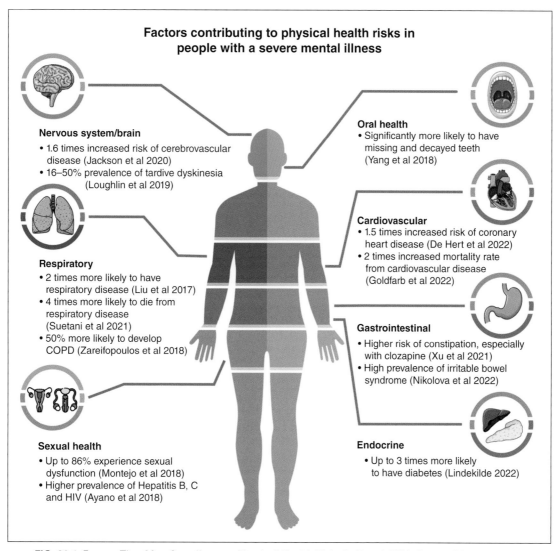

Factors contributing to physical health risks in people with a severe mental illness

Nervous system/brain
- 1.6 times increased risk of cerebrovascular disease (Jackson et al 2020)
- 16–50% prevalence of tardive dyskinesia (Loughlin et al 2019)

Respiratory
- 2 times more likely to have respiratory disease (Liu et al 2017)
- 4 times more likely to die from respiratory disease (Suetani et al 2021)
- 50% more likely to develop COPD (Zareifopoulos et al 2018)

Sexual health
- Up to 86% experience sexual dysfunction (Montejo et al 2018)
- Higher prevalence of Hepatitis B, C and HIV (Ayano et al 2018)

Oral health
- Significantly more likely to have missing and decayed teeth (Yang et al 2018)

Cardiovascular
- 1.5 times increased risk of coronary heart disease (De Hert et al 2022)
- 2 times increased mortality rate from cardiovascular disease (Goldfarb et al 2022)

Gastrointestinal
- Higher risk of constipation, especially with clozapine (Xu et al 2021)
- High prevalence of irritable bowel syndrome (Nikolova et al 2022)

Endocrine
- Up to 3 times more likely to have diabetes (Lindekilde 2022)

FIG. 20.1 Factors That May Contribute to Physical Health Risks in People With Severe Mental Illness.

SOCIO-ECOLOGICAL INFLUENCES IMPACTING PHYSICAL HEALTH

There are multiple reasons for the high levels of physical morbidity that exist among people with mental illness, with many due to socio-ecological influences. Many psychotropic medications prescribed to people with SMI are associated with adverse effects on physical health, including weight gain and endocrine changes. In addition, the symptoms of many mental illnesses, like the negative symptoms of schizophrenia, can contribute to withdrawal, isolation and an increased likelihood of living a sedentary lifestyle. The Australian National Psychosis survey identified that one in three people with SMI were sedentary and the large majority of the remaining two-thirds engaged in low levels of physical activity (Morgan et al 2012). People with SMI also have greater susceptibility to other risk factors for chronic illness, including poverty, smoking, alcohol and drug use, homelessness, unemployment, dental disease, sexually transmitted infections, sleep disorders and a poor-quality diet (Luciano et al 2021; Tanskanen et al 2018).

People with comorbid serious mental and physical illness frequently fall through the gaps between physical and mental healthcare systems (Lawn et al 2021). The healthcare systems in Australia and Aotearoa New Zealand are often divided between services for physical and mental health care, with a lack of integration. In mental healthcare systems, clinicians may focus on symptoms of mental illness, often to the detriment of other health issues, a phenomenon referred to as "diagnostic overshadowing" (Molloy et al 2021). Physical health symptoms regularly go unnoticed or are not addressed, even when people with mental illness report them to health professionals (Morgan et al 2021). Often nurses and others working in mental health do not consider addressing physical health issues as fundamental to their duty of care or they lack the confidence to undertake a physical assessment (Tyerman et al 2021). In the wider health system, there is often a lack of confidence in working with people who have mental illness. Many services, such as medical specialists and allied health services, are commonly financially unavailable to this population. Any of these issues can form an extremely challenging obstacle to care for people with complex chronic comorbid conditions, such as schizophrenia and diabetes. Therefore, this very vulnerable population can be marginalised from health services that are a human right and essential to attaining wellbeing.

Access and availability are not the only barriers to good health faced by people with SMI. The higher rate of physical illness among people with SMI not only leads to a much shorter life expectancy, but also causes a secondary effect of ongoing physical illness on top of a mental illness such as schizophrenia and diabetes. These comorbidities increase the challenge of people being able to actively participate in the workforce and create an increased risk of poverty and welfare dependency. Despite having much higher rates of morbidity than most others in the community, people with SMI are less likely to have their physical health needs met (Morgan et al 2021). A comorbid physical health issue can put extra demands on family, friends and carers of people with mental illness by expanding this role to include physical health care. The economic cost of comorbidities associated with premature death in people living with severe mental illness was estimated in 2016 to be AUD$45.4 billion in Australia and NZD$6.2 billion in Aotearoa New Zealand (Sweeney et al 2016).

METABOLIC SYNDROME

Obesity is associated with metabolic syndrome, which is a clustering of abnormalities that result in an increased risk of developing type 2 diabetes mellitus and cardiovascular disease (CVD). Metabolic syndrome includes a cluster of abnormal clinical and metabolic findings that are predictive of CVD (Fahed et al 2022). These abnormal findings include visceral adiposity, insulin resistance, increased blood pressure, elevated triglyceride levels and low levels of high-density lipoprotein (HDL) (Fahed et al 2022). The complications of metabolic syndrome involve multiple body systems, including the cardiovascular, hepatic, endocrine and central nervous systems. Meeting the criteria for metabolic syndrome causes a fivefold increase in the risk of developing type 2 diabetes and a twofold increase in the risk of developing CVD over the next 5–10 years (Guembe et al 2020). Assertive screening, intervention and follow-up are therefore required when metabolic syndrome risk factors are present.

According to the Australian national survey, *People Living with Psychotic Illness 2010*, of more than 1800 people aged 18–65, three-quarters were overweight or obese, with around half having hypertension, 50% had an abnormal lipid profile with low HDL-cholesterol and/or elevated triglycerides, and one in three had an elevated fasting glucose level (Galletly et al 2012; Morgan et al 2011). More than half of the people surveyed met criteria for metabolic syndrome (see Table 20.1), a rate two to three times higher than the general population (Morgan et al 2011). In Aotearoa New Zealand, mental health service users also have a higher prevalence of severe chronic physical conditions and an age-adjusted mortality rate twice the rate of the general population, but evidence gaps around Māori and Pacific Islander groups remain (Cunningham et al 2020; Lockett et al 2017; Richmond-Rakerd et al 2021).

People with SMI have much higher rates of obesity and abdominal obesity compared to the general population. Similar to the general population, obesity in people with SMI is associated with lifestyle factors, such as a poor diet and lack of physical activity (Firth et al 2019). There are a number of mental illness-related features, such as sedation, amotivation and disorganisation, that exacerbate the likelihood of negative lifestyle factors that promote weight gain (Cimo & Dewa

2018). There is also evidence of medication-induced effects on appetite and food intake (Grajales et al 2019).

Weight gain is a well-established side effect of antipsychotic medications. It is most pronounced at the beginning of treatment and generally continues with long periods of treatment (Bazo-Alvarez et al 2020). Weight gain is usually greatest with clozapine and olanzapine, while quetiapine, risperidone and paliperidone cause a significant but more moderate gain (Burschinski et al 2023). Aripiprazole, lurasidone and ziprasidone are likely to cause less weight gain (Burschinski et al 2023). Without interventions, all antipsychotic medications have been found to result in significant weight gain when they are first initiated (Barton et al 2020). The Healthy Active Lives declaration (see Box 20.1) sets out standards of physical health expectations for people who are newly diagnosed with a psychotic illness. This important declaration and the algorithm will help nurses to integrate the mind and body in nursing care.

Screening for Metabolic Health

In order to identify metabolic syndrome and allow for early treatment it is vital to screen for the presence of factors that increase the risk of CVD and type 2 diabetes. Screening for metabolic syndrome is well within the scope of nurses and should be viewed as an essential activity. Metabolic screening involves taking a person's blood pressure, height and weight, and calculating body mass index (DeJongh 2021). The best indicator of metabolic health is waist circumference, and this is the most important measure to screen (Nilsson et al 2019). In addition to these measures, lipids and glucose complete the metabolic screening process (DeJongh 2021). Screening should occur every 6 months, with the exception of when someone is starting a new medication or if there are concerns about a person's health where monitoring should be more frequent (see Fig. 20.2). More details about how to undertake a metabolic screen are provided in Box 20.2.

DIABETES

Type 2 diabetes is a progressive condition in which the body becomes resistant to the normal effects of insulin and/or gradually loses the

TABLE 20.1 International Diabetes Federation Metabolic Syndrome Criteria

Central Obesity (Waist Circumference in Centimetres)			Plus Any Two of:	
Ethnicity	Male	Female	Triglycerides (mmol/L)	≥ 1.7 mmol/L
Europid	≥ 94	≥ 80	HDL (mmol/L)	< 1.03 (males) < 1.29 (females)
South Asian and Japanese	≥ 90	≥ 80	Blood pressure (mmHg)	Systolic ≥ 130 or diastolic ≥ 85
Central and South America	≥ 90	≥ 80	Fasting blood sugar (mmol/L)	≥ 5.6

Adapted from Alberti et al 2005.

BOX 20.1   Healthy Active Lives Declaration

A group of clinicians, service users, family members and researchers from more than 10 countries joined forces to develop an international consensus statement on improving the physical health of young people with psychosis. The statement, called *Healthy Active Lives* (HeAL), aims to reverse the trend of people with SMI dying early by tackling risks for future physical illnesses proactively. Compared with their peers who have not experienced psychosis, young people with psychosis face a number of preventable health inequalities, including:

- a lifespan shortened by about 15–20 years
- two to three times the likelihood of developing CVD, making it the single-most common cause of premature death (more so than suicide)
- two to three times the likelihood of developing type 2 diabetes
- three to four times the likelihood of being a smoker.

The HeAL statement reflects international consensus on a set of key principles, processes and standards. It aims to combat the stigma, discrimination and prejudice that prevent young people experiencing psychosis from leading healthy active lives and to confront the perception that poor physical health is inevitable. It does this by:

- being tailored to each person
- having a longer duration, with more frequent face-to-face contact
- using multidisciplinary teams (including allied health practitioners).

The HeAL declaration sets out 5-year targets aimed to reduce future cardiovascular risk in youth with psychosis.

HeAL can be downloaded free of charge at www.iphys.org.au/

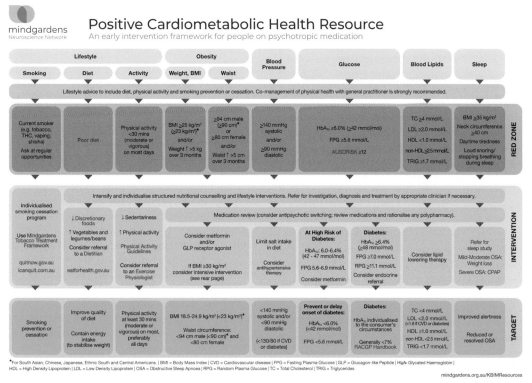

FIG. 20.2 Mindgardens Positive Cardiometabolic Health Framework, p. 1. Watkins et al. 2023a.

BOX 20.2 Screening for Metabolic Health

Weight
First ask the person to remove their shoes, any items from their pockets and bulky clothing.

Height
With their shoes removed, make sure the person's feet are flat on the floor and the person is looking straight ahead.

Body Mass Index
Calculate by dividing the person's weight by their height squared (normal range 18.5–25):

$$\frac{weight}{height\ (m)^2}$$

- A useful online calculator is available at: www.heartfoundation.org.au/BMI-calculator

Waist Circumference
Waist measurements should be taken after exhaling. Consumers should be encouraged to relax and to not contract any abdominal muscles. Align the tape measure at the level of the belly button and circle, the whole way around the body and back to the starting point.

- Make sure the tape is parallel to the ground and not twisted.
- The tape should be snug, without compressing the skin.
- Ask the person to breathe in and out twice and measure on the second out-breath.

Blood Pressure
- Ensure the correct cuff size.
- Measure the person when they are relaxed.
- Measure with their arm resting at the height of their heart.

Pathology
- Ensure the person has fasted. Test for:
  - lipid profile (including HDL/LDL)
  - glucose
  - liver function.

capacity to produce enough insulin in the pancreas (Taylor 2021). Type 2 diabetes greatly increases the risk of CVD, renal failure, amputation and blindness, lowering life expectancy by 10 or more years (Caussy et al 2021). The prevalence of type 2 diabetes in people with schizophrenia, as well as in people with bipolar disorder, is two to three times higher than in the general population (Firth et al 2019). The risk of type 2 diabetes in people with anxiety, depression or depressive symptoms is also elevated compared with those without depression (Firth et al 2019).

There are a multitude of reasons for the elevated risk of type 2 diabetes among people with SMI, including lifestyle factors, genetic predisposition and disease- and treatment-specific effects (Lister et al 2021). Antipsychotic medications carry an increased risk of developing type 2 diabetes, with olanzapine and clozapine particularly associated with carrying an increased risk (Wium-Andersen et al 2022).

Despite a high prevalence of type 2 diabetes among people with SMI, screening rates remain low. This leads to prolonged periods of raised blood glucose levels, hastening the onset of negative consequences associated with type 2 diabetes (Caussy et al 2021). Once diagnosed, people with SMI are more likely to be suboptimally treated and have poor glycaemic control (Scheuer et al 2022). Even when young, after being diagnosed with type 2 diabetes people with SMI experience a rapid decline in health and premature death (Scheuer et al 2022).

PERSONAL PERSPECTIVES

Consumer Story 20.1: Judy

I started taking olanzapine in mid-2008 when I was 20 years old, and within 4 months I had gained over 20 kilograms! I was shocked. I was starting to recover from a serious episode of psychosis, but I became fat so quickly. I didn't feel at all comfortable with my new body shape and started to avoid people because I was ashamed. I found myself being very hungry nearly all of the time and craving food that was fatty and sugary. No one mentioned to me anything about the fact that I'd feel this hungry or put on this much weight.

Over the next few years I tried to lose the weight I had put on, but I couldn't seem to shift it. In fact, I continued to gain weight, although at a slower rate. In 3 years I put on another 15 kg. This was something that was very strange for me, I'd always been a fit and healthy person, and at that point I'd hit 105 kg, a far cry from the 68 kg I was prior to starting medication. I became resigned to the fact that I was going to be fat and there was nothing I could do about it.

I then met a mental health nurse who spoke to me about what my goals in life were. I had already got back into the workforce full-time, so I told her that it was my physical health I wanted to work on. She told me that she'd be very happy to help and measured my weight, took my waist measurement and blood pressure and organised for a blood test. Together we looked at areas that could be improved and she assisted me to find out information on what were the best exercises to do and how I could improve my diet.

My blood test came back and showed a higher than normal cholesterol level. This really had me concerned and I expressed this to my nurse – I was worried that this was going to kill me. She told me that sometimes medications could cause these problems in addition to weight gain. She reassured me that it was possible to make changes to my health, even though things I'd tried in the past had not worked. She came with me to my next doctor's appointment and helped advocate for a change in medication. The doctor agreed and switched me to aripiprazole.

My nurse then suggested we work on some goals that were short term. We started with trying to stop my weight gain and then developed more goals that increased my fitness levels and improved my nutritional intake. I started to find that I could lose weight. I found this support and encouragement gave me a lot of motivation where I had previously given up.

Two and a half years later I have managed to take off all of that weight and am now about the same as I was before I started seeing mental health services. I feel so much happier and have lots more energy now. My cholesterol has returned to normal and I am not feeling burdened by physical health issues like I was.

CRITICAL THINKING EXERCISE 20.1

Imagine you have just gained 20 kg in the past 2 months. Most of the weight gain is around your abdomen.
- How would you feel?
- Consider your current lifestyle. What changes to your life would occur?

Imagine now that you have also been diagnosed with a psychotic disorder.
- What changes to your life would occur?
- How might your psychosis and weight gain affect your self-esteem?
- What might that do to your ability to recover?
- Would you continue to take medication if you thought that it caused you significant weight gain? Why or why not?

CARDIOVASCULAR DISEASE

The term "cardiovascular disease" refers to any disease that affects the heart and blood vessels (Australian Institute of Health and Welfare (AIHW) 2021). Coronary heart disease and cerebrovascular disease are the primary components of CVD. The major risk factors for CVD are smoking, obesity, hypertension, raised blood cholesterol and type 2 diabetes (AIHW 2021). Other factors that increase the risk include genetic factors, an unhealthy diet, physical inactivity and low socioeconomic status (Goldfarb et al 2022).

CVD is the most common cause of death in people with SMI, with prevalence rates approximately twice that of the general population (Lambert et al 2022). In younger people with SMI, CVD rates are three times higher when compared with matched controls (Lambert et al 2022). People with SMI have significantly higher rates of several of the modifiable risk factors when compared with controls; they are more likely to be overweight or obese, to have type 2 diabetes, hypertension or dyslipidaemia and to smoke (Goldfarb et al 2022).

Despite the high CVD mortality among people with SMI, they receive fewer of many specialised interventions or circulatory medications (Galderisi et al 2021). Evidence suggests that people with schizophrenia are not being adequately screened and treated for dyslipidaemia and hypertension (Galderisi et al 2021). Depression is also noted as being an independent risk factor for worsening morbidity and mortality in coronary heart disease (Ogunmoroti et al 2022).

People with SMI have considerably lower rates of surgical interventions, such as stenting and coronary artery bypass grafting (Nielsen et al 2021). This poorer quality of medical care contributes to excess mortality for people with SMI after heart failure (Nielsen et al 2021). An additional significant barrier is the high level of undiagnosed cardiovascular disease among people with SMI, even when engaged in primary care (Heiberg et al 2019).

In addition to weight gain and obesity-related mechanisms, there appears to be a direct effect of antipsychotic medication that contributes to the worsening of CVD risk (Nielsen et al 2021). Type 2 diabetes antagonism can be caused by antipsychotics having a direct effect on developing insulin resistance (Grajales et al 2019). Higher antipsychotic doses predict greater risk of mortality from coronary heart disease and cerebrovascular incidents (Lin et al 2023). Most antipsychotics and some antidepressants are also associated with a change in the heart's electrical cycle, known as QTc prolongation (Edinoff et al 2022). A prolonged QTc puts a patient at significant risk of torsade de pointes, ventricular fibrillation and sudden cardiac death (Howell et al 2019).

CRITICAL THINKING EXERCISE 20.2

Who should be responsible for screening and intervention of physical health problems in people with SMI? Consider the registered nurses' scope of practice, competencies and code of professional conduct. How do these standards influence your thoughts and actions on responsibility?

MANAGEMENT OF CARDIOMETABOLIC HEALTH

While screening for metabolic health is important, it serves little benefit if no action is taken after problems are identified. It is vital that nurses "don't just screen but intervene" for metabolic health. At the centre of managing cardiometabolic health are lifestyle interventions. Nurses are well positioned to advise, encourage and implement lifestyle interventions around tobacco cessation (see Perspectives in practice: Nurse's story 20.1 on p. 315), physical activity and healthy nutrition. People with SMI can benefit enormously from even small lifestyle changes. A positive cardiometabolic health algorithm has been developed to help guide clinicians in managing the leading causes of mortality in people with SMI (see Fig. 20.3).

CRITICAL THINKING EXERCISE 20.3

Consider the HeAL declaration (Box 20.1), then use the cardiometabolic algorithm in Fig. 20.2 and the screening for metabolic health information in Box 20.2 to develop a nursing care plan for a young person who has just started taking antipsychotic medications.
- What information do you need to tailor the plan to the individual?
- How will you get this information?
- What do you consider most important? Why?

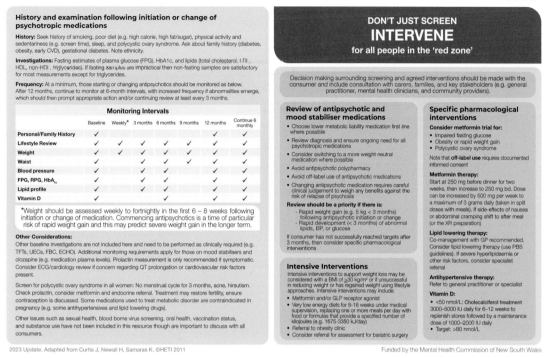

FIG. 20.3 Mindgardens Positive Cardiometabolic Health Framework, p. 2. Watkins et al 2023a.

Core Nursing Interventions

Tobacco-Related Illness and Respiratory Disease

Respiratory diseases were the leading cause of death in psychiatric institutions up until the 1970s (Brown 1997). Today, respiratory diseases are still more prevalent in people with SMI, with approximately one in three people with SMI having either restrictive or obstructive lung disease, a rate double that of the general population (Jaén-Moreno et al 2023). The likelihood of developing pneumonia or COVID-19 complications is also considerably raised (De Hert et al 2021). Not only are these conditions far more common in people experiencing SMI, but they are also more likely to lead to mortality (Jaén-Moreno et al 2023). Tobacco smoking is closely associated with an increased risk of respiratory diseases and, in particular, influences chronic obstructive pulmonary disorder in its development and progression, as well as mixed forms of asthma (Krieger et al 2019).

Respiratory assessment is an essential component of a physical health assessment and nurses should be vigilant and maintain regular and timely screening for respiratory conditions. Additional support and referral may be required, with consideration given to modifiable risk factors such as tobacco smoking, which is closely linked to increased cardiometabolic health risk factors. Physical activity should be promoted, as it might delay decline in lung function (Wu et al 2020).

Very high smoking rates are observed among people with SMI. Two in three people with severe mental illness are tobacco smokers compared to less than 12% of the general Australian population (Greenhalgh et al 2022). People with mental illness also smoke more cigarettes per day and inhale more deeply than other smokers, achieving higher blood levels of nicotine than smokers without SMI (Pettey & Aubry 2018).

Tobacco-related diseases made up approximately half of total deaths seen in people with SMI, and tobacco use represents the highest single factor that contributes to premature death (Krieger et al 2019). The high smoking rate among people with SMI increases their risk of developing cancer and respiratory diseases. Tobacco smoking may be particularly problematic because it amplifies the increased risk of CVD alongside the centralised weight gain associated with using atypical antipsychotic medications (Krieger et al 2019).

The high rate of smoking among people with SMI can be attributed to a high smoking take-up rate that occurs early in life, often before a mental health diagnosis, combined with fewer and less successful quit attempts (Gogos et al 2019). Despite some evidence showing short-term neurocognitive improvements with nicotine use, this does not last and overall nicotine use is associated with more intense clinical symptoms in SMI (Dondé et al 2020). Addressing tobacco use in people with SMI is a major clinical and public health issue, and there is limited clinical attention devoted to tobacco use in these groups (Caponnetto et al 2020).

There is a common misconception that people with SMI do not wish to quit smoking (Lum et al 2018). Despite this misconception, there is a strong interest in smoking cessation in people with SMI, who are motivated for the same reasons as other smokers – to improve their health (Caponnetto et al 2020). An additional motivation to quit is the substantial financial cost of cigarette smoking for people who often have very low incomes, largely derived from social welfare.

Smoking cessation can be successfully delivered within mental health programs for both adult and youth populations (Curtis et al 2018; Gilbody et al 2015). Substantial mental health benefits can be gained from quitting smoking, including reduced symptoms of depression and anxiety (Taylor et al 2021).

Nurses can play a vital role in smoking cessation, influencing tobacco-related mortality. People with SMI are likely to experience more severe withdrawal symptoms compared to the general population and require extra support during cessation attempts (Hawes et al 2021). It is important to realise that people with SMI respond to smoking cessation treatment as well as the general population in the short term, although they generally have worse long-term outcomes (Gilbody et al 2019). The Mindgardens Tobacco Treatment Framework, designed for use with people on psychotropic medications, can be used as a tool to assist nurses in supporting people to quit or reduce their use of tobacco (see Figs 20.4 and 20.5).

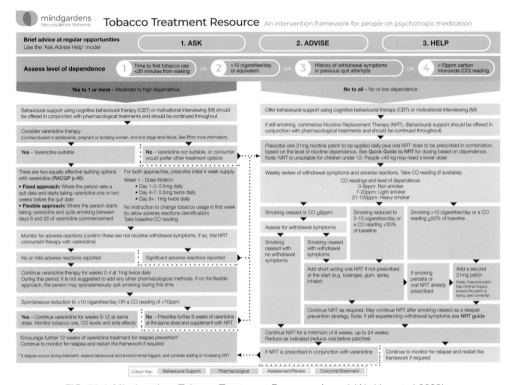

FIG. 20.4 Mindgardens Tobacco Treatment Framework, p. 1. Watkins et al 2023b.

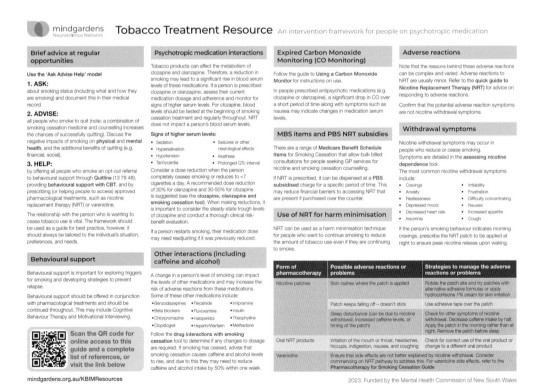

FIG. 20.5 Mindgardens Tobacco Treatment Framework, p. 2. Watkins et al 2023b.

PERSPECTIVES IN PRACTICE

Nurse's Story 20.1: Malcolm

Malcolm has been a nurse for 27 years and now works on an acute inpatient mental health unit. He has been leading a project to help people admitted to the mental health unit in dealing with smoking withdrawal and encouraging them to quit.

"When I first started working as a nurse in mental health, I was a smoker. The senior nurses I was working with at the time told me that a great way to build a relationship with the patients on the unit was to chat to them while we were all having a smoke."

Malcolm ceased smoking 15 years ago after witnessing his aunt dying from lung cancer.

"I saw what my aunty was going through and it was horrible. She was in so much pain and distress. I decided at that time I needed to quit for my health. So, I quit. It wasn't easy at all, especially being around people smoking while I was at work. I persisted though and my health has improved out of sight."

Malcolm decided he wanted to support the patients he was working with to experience the same benefits that he gained after quitting smoking. When he heard about the smoking ban in mental health units, he thought it was an ideal opportunity.

"I thought to myself: If they are not allowed to smoke while they are on the unit, they may as well use it as a launching pad to quit smoking. The worst part of nicotine withdrawal is the first couple of days, so it would make sense if they could make it through that, why couldn't they quit altogether? So, I got myself skilled up on withdrawal symptoms from nicotine and learnt how to adequately prescribe nicotine replacement therapy."

As Malcolm built up the intervention, other nurses took an interest and became involved with the program. This led to a much more comprehensive approach to addressing smoking and not just when Malcolm was on shift.

"The key to the intervention was giving patients who were in nicotine withdrawal support. Nicotine replacement therapy doesn't completely stop the cravings, and talking to patients about how they are going with the withdrawal was really helpful."

The program has become quite a success, with many people successfully quitting and not taking up the habit again. Malcolm and the program have also been recognised with awards.

"Just banning smoking is cruel, but giving people 'smoking leave' from the unit would just restart the withdrawal process again. What's the point in making people withdraw if there is no benefit for the person in the end? What we found was that many people actually wanted to quit and had found it really hard in the past. No one likes withdrawal symptoms, but in hindsight they were often very thankful that we supported them to actually start the quitting process properly."

 ## CRITICAL THINKING EXERCISE 20.4

Discuss the following question: "People with mental illness don't have much enjoyment in life, so why would you want to take another enjoyment away and encourage them to quit cigarettes?"

Nutrition

People experiencing SMI have poorer diets when compared with the general population (Firth et al 2018). Dietary consumption in this population is lower in fruit and fibre and higher in saturated fat compared to the general population (Teasdale et al 2019). Studies that assessed caloric intake found higher intakes in those with SMI (Firth et al 2018), while evidence also demonstrated that the diets of those with SMI are lower in vegetables, legumes and dairy (Teasdale et al 2019). This is a significant and, importantly, modifiable factor that

contributes to severe weight gain, subsequent poor cardiometabolic health and a mortality gap in this population.

People receiving antipsychotic therapy commonly complain of significantly increased hunger and an inability to sense satiety (feeling full), particularly on clozapine and olanzapine (Mutwalli et al 2023). These medications can affect ghrelin and leptin hormones, which regulate hunger and satiety (Mukherjee et al 2022). The highest increases in leptin levels are seen in patients using antipsychotics that produce the most weight gain (Singh et al 2019).

Combining these factors with constant cravings for sugary or processed oily foods, low food preparation skills, low levels of motivation and often-restricted budgets, creates an environmental mix that can lead to weight gain and poor metabolic health. Furthermore, people with SMI have a lower basal metabolic rate than the general population, contributing to rapid weight gain (Singh et al 2019). Additional dietary considerations for this population include fast-eating syndrome, disordered eating habits, such as only eating one main meal per day, constipation and higher levels of dental and coeliac disease (Teasdale et al 2017).

Given these dietary patterns and nutritional side effects, interventions that aim to reduce caloric intake and improve diet quality by increasing core foods and reducing discretionary foods can be seen as key factors in improving the physical health of those with SMI. Core foods in Australia reflect the five food groups: (1) vegetables, (2) fruit, (3) milk, cheese, yoghurt and alternatives, (4) lean meat, fish, poultry, eggs, seeds and nuts, and (5) grains, with some healthy oils such as olive oil. Discretionary foods reflect those that are high in energy (kilojoules/calories) and low in nutrients, and are generally highly processed and refined foods (National Health and Medical Research Council (NHMRC) 2013). Evidence has emerged demonstrating that people following a higher quality diet have better mental health, while those whose diet quality is lower have poorer psychological functioning (Begdache et al 2019).

An alternative dietary pattern shown to be beneficial for mental health by preventing and/or reducing depressive symptoms is the Mediterranean diet (Parletta et al 2019). The Mediterranean diet focuses on fruits and vegetables, fish, nuts/seeds, wholegrains, legumes, olive oil, fetta cheese and moderate intakes of red wine, particularly with meals. In addition to improvements in mental health, this pattern of eating is protective for both type 2 diabetes and CVD (Becerra-Tomás et al 2020).

Key nutrients of concern in SMI include caffeine, omega-3 fatty-acids, folate and magnesium. Caffeine overconsumption is common in patients experiencing schizophrenia – they are twice as likely to consume more than 200 mg (2 cups of coffee) per day (Teasdale et al 2019). There is currently no acceptable daily intake value for caffeine in Australia; however, a review performed by Food Standards Australia New Zealand (FSANZ) suggests an increased risk of anxiety at 95 mg (one cup of coffee or two cans of cola) per day for children and 210 mg for adults (Smith et al 2000). Low levels of omega-3 fatty acids, folate and magnesium have been linked with depression, with increased intake (oral or supplemented) proving to be an effective part of treatment (Lassale et al 2019).

Nutrition interventions in people with SMI to date have generally been scarce; however, studies have demonstrated reduced health risks when these interventions are used in both early and longer term illnesses (Burrows et al 2022). Although future studies need to assess the long-term impacts on anthropometric, biochemical and lifestyle (nutrition and exercise) measures, as well as quality of life, mental health symptomatology and re-admission rates, there is enough evidence to support the use of nutrition interventions in combination with exercise as core components of mental health services.

Nutritional advice and support should be integrated into routine nursing care. When providing nutrition interventions, it is crucial to provide both educational and practical components to ensure adequate knowledge, but also to improve shopping, label reading, food safety and culinary (food preparation) skills. With patients particularly vulnerable to increased hunger, reduced satiety and cravings for high caloric convenience foods and drinks with little nutritional value, mindfulness-based activities may also prove to be an adjunctive intervention.

Physical Activity

Physical activity can be defined as any bodily movement produced by skeletal muscle resulting in increased energy expenditure. The term "physical activity" encompasses both structured forms of activity, such as exercise, and unstructured forms, such as incidental activity. People experiencing mental illness are known to be less physically active than the general population and engage in prolonged periods of sedentary behaviour (Firth et al 2019). Low levels of physical activity are an established risk factor for cardiometabolic dysfunction, including diabetes and obesity. In addition to low levels of physical activity, people with mental illness have poorer cardiorespiratory fitness in comparison with the general population, which is an established risk factor for all-cause mortality and morbidity (Bort-Roig et al 2020). Given the high rates of premature mortality linked to preventable CVD within this population, evidence-based physical activity interventions aimed at reducing sedentary time, increasing overall activity and increasing moderate–vigorous physical activity participation should be considered part of routine care for people living with mental illness (Stubbs et al 2018).

Physical activity and exercise have been shown to have beneficial effects on psychiatric symptomatology, regardless of diagnosis, while a growing body of research has reported on the benefits of exercise for improving cognition (Firth et al 2019). Longitudinal studies have also highlighted the bidirectional relationship between activity and depressive symptoms, with evidence of a protective effect of being physically active (Zhang et al 2021).

Evidence-based strategies to increase physical activity among people with mental illness include behavioural techniques, such as motivational interviewing, face-to-face and group-based exercise sessions (Teychenne et al 2020). In addition, structured exercise prescriptions and individualised interventions reflect individual variations in mood, motivation and access to facilities and resources (Teychenne et al 2020). Exercise is not a one-size-fits-all intervention, and a range of individual factors should be considered when developing individualised exercise interventions. Aside from physical limitations, factors to be considered are severity of psychiatric symptomatology, previous exercise history, motivation and access to services or facilities that may affect the modality and intensity of exercise that individuals are able to undertake (Teychenne et al 2020).

Exercise is a structured subset of physical activity, and exercise prescriptions are typically described according to the "FITT" principle (frequency, intensity, time and type) while incorporating appropriate goal-setting strategies. The World Health Organization (WHO) recommends that adults aim for 150 to 300 minutes per week of moderate intensity physical activity or 75 to 150 minutes of moderate–vigorous activity, in addition to muscle strengthening activities on at least 2 days per week (Bull et al 2020). Further, the WHO advocates that patients should avoid physical inactivity, noting that some level of physical activity regardless of intensity is better than none (Bull et al 2020).

People with SMI should be supported and encouraged to adhere to physical activity recommendations; however, there is growing consensus that such recommendations may be aspirational and unrealistic for many people living with SMI. Positive messaging around pragmatic goals, such as breaking up sitting time throughout the day and aiming to increase short-duration walking should be routinely promoted (Deenik et al 2020). Mental health nurses are well positioned to provide exercise advice and physical activity counselling to mental health consumers (Lundström et al 2020). Examples of pragmatic interventions include using objective monitoring devices such as pedometers (or commercially available accelerometers), individualised advice on ways to accumulate greater light physical activity, such as rising from a chair and moving during television commercial breaks or adding 5-minute walks at structured and specified points throughout the day. This may include, for example, taking less direct routes while walking to dining rooms within in-patient facilities (Czosnek et al 2019). Although such limited interventions may appear trivial, encouraging small and incremental changes may better position sedentary people with SMI to transition to brief bouts of moderate intensity activity that will help them to achieve guideline-specified targets.

VACCINE-PREVENTABLE DISEASES

The Equally Well Australia (2021) *Global Call to Action for fair and equitable access to vaccination for people living with mental illness and substance use disorders* highlights that people living with mental illness have almost five times the rate of being hospitalised, four times the rate of premature death from vaccine-preventable conditions, over seven times the rate of vaccine preventable hospital bed days, and that proactively offering vaccination to people with serious mental illness would save $84 million in hospital costs each year in Australia.

In a study conducted by Sara and colleagues (2021) on potentially preventable hospitalisations due to a vaccine-preventable illness for people with SMI in New South Wales, Australia, it was found that the length of stay for hospitalisation for people with severe mental illness was 11.2 days vs 6 days for the general public, with an age and disadvantage adjusted incidence ratio of 8.7. Sara and colleagues (2021) also found that vaccine-preventable diseases made a significant contribution to 24.5% of excess bed days for the population sampled. Unpublished data from NSW Health agency InforMH shows that people who have recently received mental health care have over three times the rate of vaccine-preventable hospitalisations and bed days compared to other residents of NSW and have an increased risk for all types of vaccine-preventable hospitalisations. There is some evidence that people living with mental illness are under-vaccinated. Burke and colleagues (2018) conducted a study on respiratory disease within mental health in-patients and found that only 14% of consumers in the study had received an influenza vaccine in the past 12 months, while only 4% had ever received a pneumococcal vaccination.

The literature also suggests that people living with mental illness may be more at risk of catching a vaccine-preventable disease. Seminog and Goldacre (2013) identified that having SMI was a risk factor for pneumococcal disease. Lluch and Miller (2019), in a meta-analysis on hepatitis infection in patients with schizophrenia, found that people with schizophrenia had threefold increased odds of contracting a hepatitis disease. Lawrence and Jablensky (2001), in a study in Western Australia, found that there was significant excess mortality for influenza within the SMI population, with influenza having the highest hospitalisation rate for any disease included in the study.

In relation to the recent COVID-19 pandemic, people living with SMI have excess mortality from COVID-19 (De Hert et al 2021; Vai et al 2021). There is some evidence that people who become infected with COVID-19 also have an increase in the incidence of poor mental health outcomes (Xie et al 2022), meaning that if a person with mental illness becomes infected with COVID-19, there is a potential significant impact on both their physical and their mental health.

For mental health nurses the implications of the poor vaccine-related health statistics of people with mental illness are significant. Mental health nurses play a crucial role in advocating for consumers' health needs, including the need for equitable access to vaccinations. Mental health nurses can educate consumers on the benefits of vaccination and the increased risks of being unvaccinated. They can also provide support for consumers who may have concerns about being vaccinated, or who may have difficulty accessing vaccination services. In addition to advocating for vaccination access, mental health nurses can also play a critical role in identifying patients who may be at higher risk for vaccine preventable diseases. Through routine assessments and screenings, mental health nurses can identify patients who may be due for vaccinations and provide education and support to encourage them to get vaccinated. Mental health nurses can also train to become an Accredited Nurse Immuniser to increase their scope of practice to prescribe and administer vaccines within mental health services.

Vaccination is a critical component of healthcare for people living with mental illness and substance use disorders. Mental health nurses

have an important role to play in promoting vaccination access and ensuring that consumers receive the care they need to stay healthy. By staying informed, advocating for consumers and providing education and support, mental health nurses can help improve vaccination rates and ultimately improve the health outcomes of consumers.

? CRITICAL THINKING EXERCISE 20.5

You are a nurse working on a busy acute mental health unit, who is aware of the importance of influenza vaccination.
- What strategies could you develop to improve the vaccination rates of the staff and patients on the unit?
- How can you effectively educate consumers around vaccination, particularly those who may be hesitant or resistant to getting vaccinated?
- How can you collaborate with other healthcare providers, such as general practitioners or public health units, to ensure that their patients receive appropriate vaccinations and other preventive care?

CASE STUDY 20.1: "Keeping the Body in Mind"

The Early Psychosis Program is located at the Bondi Centre in Sydney. It works with young people between the ages of 15 and 25 in the early stages of psychotic illness. The team works with an interdisciplinary model within a community mental health service.

Nurses working with young people experiencing their first episode of psychosis at the Bondi Centre were extremely concerned that, while atypical antipsychotic medications were successful in alleviating people of many of the troubling symptoms of mental illness, they also appeared to be correlated with rapid weight gain and subsequent longer-term risks of diabetes and heart disease.

"We responded to these alarms by developing an assessment tool to measure changes in weight and other metabolic abnormalities. What we found was that young people were all too commonly putting on 10–20 kg, and sometimes more, within their first year with the service and that alterations in a person's metabolic health deteriorated rapidly with this weight gain. These issues included elevated cholesterol and hypertension. Blood glucose levels may become raised, putting these young people at much higher risk of developing diabetes."

Nursing staff also noticed that the young people were experiencing increased rates of stigma and poor self-esteem. This was like a "double whammy" because a young person who was dealing with a new mental health diagnosis, and the fact that they have to take psychiatric medication, was also trying to deal with transformations to their body image. This affected their personal lives, impacting on their work, study and socialisation.

"We realised that just assessing people's health was inadequate. We actually needed to make a difference and so we adopted a mantra of 'Don't just screen, intervene'."

Working in conjunction with a multidisciplinary team, nursing staff established a number of lifestyle interventions and a program called Keeping the Body in Mind (KBIM). This program aimed to prevent weight gain and the accompanying deterioration in metabolic health that might in future lead to heart disease and diabetes. The program is coordinated by a clinical nurse consultant and utilises an exercise physiologist, a dietitian and a peer support worker. The lifestyle intervention program encompasses three elements, including health coaching, dietetic support and a supervised exercise program, which are delivered with an interconnected approach. Each participant's intervention program is tailored to suit the individual.

The program was recently evaluated in a controlled study comparing it against another early psychosis service. The KBIM program was compared against a similar early psychosis program in Sydney, with the exception of the metabolic intervention. Participants in the KBIM group were provided 12-week individualised lifestyle program, while the comparison group ($n = 12$) received standard care. The evaluation study established that the KBIM group had considerably less weight gain at 12 weeks (an average of 1.8 kg over 12 weeks) compared with standard care (an average of 7.8 kg). Only 13% per cent of the intervention group experienced clinically significant weight gain (greater than 7% of baseline weight) compared with 75% in the non-intervention group.

Source: Curtis 2015.

ORAL HEALTH

Oral health is integral to general health and essential for wellbeing. It influences eating, physical appearance, speech and other social and psychological factors (Cai et al 2022). Oral health issues include hygiene, dental caries (cavities), periodontal disease, dental trauma and oral cancers (Sanz et al 2020). Oral health also plays a vital role in cardiometabolic health, with periodontal disease increasing the risk of type 2 diabetes, coronary heart disease and stroke (Sanz et al 2020). People with SMI experience markedly higher rates of oral health problems compared with the general population (Yang et al 2018). The reasons that this population have poorer oral health outcomes in comparison with the general population are multifaceted (Cai et al 2022). Many psychotropic medications can reduce the amount of saliva the mouth produces, leading to a dry mouth or xerostomia (Yang et al

2018). Xerostomia is associated with an increase in periodontal disease (Sanz et al 2020). Symptoms of mental illness, such as depression, amotivation and cognitive impairment can lead to an apathy around dental hygiene, and considerably lower rates of regular teeth brushing and flossing is observed in people with SMI (Yang et al 2018). People with SMI are also more likely to be smokers and consume sugary carbonated drinks, both of which increase the likelihood of dental disease (Cai et al 2022).

Nursing Management of Oral Health

People with SMI are less likely to seek dental treatment than the general population, especially for preventative dental work (Yang et al 2018). Given the higher risk of dental disease in this population, it is essential that people with SMI attend to dental care more frequently than general public recommendations (Cai et al 2022). Mental health nurses have a clear role in encouraging and facilitating access to dental services. This is particularly important in Australia and Aotearoa New Zealand, where most dental services are private and financially out of reach for many people with SMI; people will often require assistance in accessing public dental schemes. It is also important that nurses use clinical interactions as an opportunity to promote oral health as a vital part of general health. Health promotion that focuses on smoking, diet, alcohol use and dental hygiene should be routinely incorporated into mental health nursing care (Cai et al 2022).

 CRITICAL THINKING EXERCISE 20.6

Consider and discuss the social and economic factors that influence an individual's oral health. Consider what nursing actions/strategies you could develop to change these factors.

SLEEP

Good sleep is essential to good physical and mental health. Sleep disturbance is a symptom of almost every mental disorder, from anxiety disorders through to mood disorders and psychosis (Firth et al 2020). Although its significance is often under-recognised (Tobin & Tobin 2017), sleep disturbance can be one of the more distressing and persistent symptoms of mental disorder. Sleep disturbance can also present as one of the first signs of mental illness exacerbation (Freeman 2022). Poor sleep can also independently contribute to causing a mental illness and impede recovery from mental illness (Freeman 2022). Recognising and treating sleep disturbances can therefore be critical to the primary or secondary prevention of mental disorders and their treatment.

Sleep Disturbance

What is normal sleep? Each person has a different sleep requirement and this changes over the life span. On average, most adults need 7–8 hours; children and adolescents 9–10 hours per night and children 11–13 hours or more, depending on their age (Institute of Medicine Committee on Sleep and Research 2006). **Insomnia** is the most common sleep disturbance and is a core feature of mood disorders; it frequently complicates anxiety disorders and psychosis. Anxiety and severe depression are commonly associated with sleep disturbance (Freeman 2022). In schizophrenia, the sleep cycle is often disturbed, with fragmented sleep throughout the cycle or even reversal of the sleep–wake cycle, so that most sleep occurs during the day (Kaskie & Ferrarelli 2020). **Hypersomnia** (excessive sleep) is less common, but can occur in depression and in some cases of bipolar disorder (Bušková et al 2022). Hypersomnia can also occur secondary to some treatments of mental illness, which have sedative side effects.

Given the high rates of obesity in people with mental disorders, the risk of obstructive sleep apnoea in this population is high, so it is important to screen for and treat this disorder (Zhang et al 2022). Obstructive sleep apnoea is the most common form of sleep disorder breathing. Untreated, it is associated with high morbidity and mortality due to increased risks of cardio- and cerebrovascular disease, and worsening of diabetes and hypertension (Yeghiazarians et al 2021).

 CRITICAL THINKING EXERCISE 20.7

In what ways might poor sleep impede a person's mental health recovery? What nursing strategies can you implement to improve sleep for someone who is experiencing insomnia?

- Go to sleep and wake up at roughly the same time each day.
- Maintain regular meal times.
- Avoid daytime naps.
- Don't eat a big meal or exercise within 2 hours of going to bed.
- Avoid caffeinated drinks after midday.
- Minimise alcohol and cease smoking.
- Ensure the bedroom is cool, comfortable, dark, quiet and safe and used for only sleep and sex.
- Engage in exercise (avoid this at night) and exposure to bright outside light each day, preferably in the morning.
- Do not share the bed with children or pets.
- If sleep is not achieved within 20–30 minutes of going to bed, get up and do something relaxing for a few minutes and then try again when feeling sleepy.
- Ensure medications are taken as directed because some can cause sedation or arousal.
- Avoid stimulating activities before bedtime and exposure to the blue light emitted by computer or tablet screens.

Adapted from American Association of Sleep Medicine 2020.

Nursing Assessment and Intervention of Sleep Disorders

The most important primary action for nurses is to ask about a person's sleep. Depending on the clinical setting, there may be an option for nurses to take an active role in diagnosing and managing sleep problems. There are a number of useful screening and diagnostic tools, the most simple of which is a sleep diary (see Useful websites), in which the person documents times spent sleeping and other influential activities such as caffeine and alcohol intake, exercise and sedentary activities such as electronic screen time.

In established sleep disorders, nurses may play an important role in encouraging patients to manage any lifestyle issues that could be contributing to their sleep problems (see Box 20.3). Sedative/hypnotic medications have a place, but should not necessarily be the first form of treatment offered. Benzodiazepines have a propensity for addiction and are associated with an increased risk of falls among other serious potential side effects (see Chapter 21 for more information about medications and their sedative effects).

SEXUAL HEALTH

Sexuality and sexual health are important aspects of every person's health and wellbeing. Sexuality is a complex issue that encompasses not only the physical activity of sex but also gender identity, values and beliefs (Urry et al 2019). Contrary to common belief, most people with SMI show an interest in sex that differs little from the general population (Evans et al 2021; McCann et al 2019). High-risk sexual behaviours are more likely to be observed in people with SMI, including unprotected intercourse, multiple partners, involvement in sex work and illicit drug use (Cloutier et al 2021). The rates of blood-borne viruses, such as HIV and hepatitis C, have been found to be higher among people with SMI (Liang et al 2020).

Social and interpersonal impairments commonly occur in people with SMI and limit the development of stable sexual relationships. Men with SMI, in particular, have poorer social outcomes, less frequent (sexual) relationships and fewer offspring than the general population (Cloutier et al 2021). Women with SMI are more likely to have relatively chaotic patterns of sexual behaviours and a higher rate of unprotected and non-consensual sex than their counterparts without SMI (Lawley et al 2022).

An Australian report found that mental health nurses are reluctant to bring up the topic of sexual health or discuss sex related topics (Urry et al 2019). To enable you to feel comfortable and confident to discuss sexual health you will need to identify any personal issues that affect your ability to openly discuss sexual health and increase your knowledge of sexual issues. Common issues that affect a person's sexuality and sexual health include sexually transmitted infections, body image, gender identity, physiological changes, medications and stigma (Cloutier et al 2021).

? CRITICAL THINKING EXERCISE 20.8

1. Consider and discuss social, cultural and religious beliefs that influence a person's sexuality.
2. Consider your own personal beliefs about sexuality. Do you have any preconceived ideas about mental illness and sexuality? Do you have any concerns about conducting a sexual health assessment?

Medication and Sex

Medication-induced sexual dysfunction is a common but largely ignored side effect of most psychotropic medications (Urry et al 2019). Psychotropic medications are linked with sexual dysfunction, including low libido, delayed ejaculation, orgasm problems like anorgasmia, and impaired erection (Montejo et al 2021). Medication-induced sexual dysfunctions can lead to issues with relationships, medication adherence and quality of life (Hendry et al 2018). Despite people with SMI considering sexual health issues to be highly relevant, it is important to remember that issues like sexual dysfunction are unlikely to be discussed, often due to the reluctance of health professionals and mental health nurses to talk about sex (Hendry et al 2018). This often leads to an underestimation of their prevalence and contribution to decreased adherence to treatment (Cloutier et al 2021). Chapter 21 discusses psychotropic medication and its side effects.

Sexual Health Screening

Health screening includes preventative testing or investigation to prevent or ameliorate future problems. Sexual health screening includes breast, prostate, cervical and sexually transmitted infection screening. Mental health nurses can play an important role in health screening, particularly when access to services is challenging for the person with mental illness. Mental health nurses can refer people directly to a health screening service or they can provide the health assessment. Nurses can offer advice about preventing the contraction and spread of sexually transmitted infections by providing education on safe sex such as the correct use of condoms (Berger-Merom et al 2022).

Breast, prostate and cervical screening services are generally offered by public health services. Given the vulnerability of clients with SMI around their sexual health, it is essential that nurses include sexual health screening as part of holistic care. Nurses should reflect on any personal attitudes or beliefs that might be creating barriers that impede a thorough sexual health assessment.

WHEN PSYCHIATRIC SYMPTOMS ARE NOT A MENTAL ILLNESS

Confusion, vision problems and behaviour changes can be common symptoms for many mental illnesses, but they are also common symptoms of brain tumours, infectious diseases and dehydration. Correct assessment that includes history-taking and checking with relatives will lead to correct diagnoses and avoid missing a physical health issue (see Chapter 9 for more details of accurate assessment). Misdiagnosis or delayed diagnosis of physical health issues presenting with psychiatric symptoms can lead to further damage and complications. For example, brain tumours can grow and cause more harm, and infectious diseases can spread and become more severe if not identified and treated promptly. Therefore, it is crucial for healthcare providers to thoroughly assess a patient's history and consult with their relatives to make an accurate diagnosis. Other medical conditions that may present with psychiatric symptoms include Wilson's disease (a hereditary metabolic disorder), Graves' disease and HIV (McKee & Brahm 2016). Chapter 18 discusses the symptom similarities that can occur with depression, delirium and dementia.

CHAPTER SUMMARY

People who experience SMI have far higher rates of morbidity and mortality across nearly all chronic health conditions. This chapter has highlighted the importance of promoting, assessing and maintaining optimum physical health for people with SMI. Specific health assessments have been highlighted – sexual health, oral health, sleep, metabolic syndrome, CVD, diabetes and respiratory disease; however, it is important to remember that a full physical assessment, including routine health screening, is an essential element of holistic mental health care.

The vital role that nurses can play in improving preventable illness and disease is clear. People with SMI have physical health outcomes that are far worse than the general population. If we are to improve the unacceptable life expectancy gap that is currently experienced by those with an SMI, mental health nurses will need to address this important issue with primary health messages and interventions. Smoking cessation, diet and exercise advice are core interventions crucially required for preventing premature CVD. Awareness and advocating for the screening and intervention of other areas of physical health, especially respiratory, sexual, oral and sleep health, are extremely important to improve overall quality of life. Early intervention and prevention of physical health conditions are key to improving the outcomes of people with mental illness. Mental health nurses need to prioritise physical health care as one of their primary responsibilities, and this involves taking the time to listen and support people's needs in a holistic way.

REVIEW QUESTIONS

1. Maintaining optimum physical health is multifaceted and essential to wellbeing, and nurses play an important role in assessing, treating and preventing physical health issues. Working in groups discuss the following statements:
   a. Sexual health is a human right.
   b. Metabolic syndrome is preventable.
   c. Oral health is an important part of overall health.

   d. People with schizophrenia are likely to die 20–25 years earlier than the general population.
   e. SMI is as much a risk factor of cardiovascular risk as a diagnosis of diabetes.

2. Working with your group, develop nursing interventions and strategies to ensure the issues listed in the statements are assessed, treated and not overlooked. Consider what resources you will need

to implement the strategies you have identified. Are there any barriers? How can these barriers be overcome?

3. Develop a checklist of routine health screenings and assessments that should be conducted for people with SMI. Discuss the importance of each assessment and potential barriers to conducting them in clinical settings.

4. Consider the potential impact of social determinants of health (e.g. poverty, discrimination, lack of access to healthcare) on physical health outcomes for people with SMI. Discuss potential nursing interventions and strategies to address social determinants of health and promote health equity in this population.

5. Discuss the importance of interdisciplinary collaboration in providing holistic physical health care for people with SMI. How can nurses work with other healthcare professionals (e.g. doctors, social workers, dietitians) to ensure that patients receive comprehensive, coordinated care?

USEFUL WEBSITES

Australian Dental Association: www.ada.org.au/
Equally Well Australia: www.equallywell.org.au
Equally Well New Zealand: www.tepou.co.nz/initiatives/equally-well-physical-health/37
International Diabetes Federation: www.idf.org/
Keeping the Body in Mind in Youth with Psychosis: www.iphys.org.au/
Mental Health Foundation of Australia: www.mhfa.org.au/
Mental Health Foundation of New Zealand: www.mentalhealth.org.nz/
New Zealand Dental Association: www.healthysmiles.org.nz/
Sexual Health & Family Planning Australia: familyplanningallianceaustralia.org.au/
Sleep diary: http://sleepeducation.org/docs/default-document-library/sleep-diary.pdf
The New Zealand Sexual Health Society Incorporated: www.nzshs.org/
World Health Organization: www.who.int/en/

REFERENCES

Alberti K.G., Zimmet, P., Shaw, J. & Group, IDFETFC 2005. The metabolic syndrome – a new worldwide definition. Lancet, 366, 1059–1062.

American Association of Sleep Medicine. 2020. Healthy sleep habits. Online. Available at: https://sleepeducation.org/healthy-sleep/healthy-sleep-habits/

Australian Institute of Health And Welfare (AIHW) 2021. Heart, stroke and vascular disease—Australian facts. Online. Available at: www.aihw.gov.au/reports/heart-stroke-vascular-diseases/hsvd-facts/contents/about

Barton, B.B., Segger, F., Fischer, K., Obermeier, M. & Musil, R. 2020. Update on weight-gain caused by antipsychotics: A systematic review and meta-analysis. Expert Opin Drug Safety, 19, 295–314.

Bazo-Alvarez, J.C., Morris, T.P., Carpenter, J.R., Hayes, J.F. & Petersen, I. 2020. Effects of long-term antipsychotics treatment on body weight: A population-based cohort study. J Psychopharmacol, 34, 79–85.

Becerra-Tomás, N., Blanco Mejía, S., Viguiliouk, E., Khan, T., Kendall, C.W., et al., 2020. Mediterranean diet, cardiovascular disease and mortality in diabetes: A systematic review and meta-analysis of prospective cohort studies and randomized clinical trials. Crit Rev Food Sci Nutrit, 60, 1207–1227.

Begdache, L., Chaar, M., Sabounchi, N. & Kianmehr, H. 2019. Assessment of dietary factors, dietary practices and exercise on mental distress in young adults versus matured adults: A cross-sectional study. Nutr Neurosci, 22, 488–498.

Berger-Merom, R., Zisman-Ilani, Y., Jones, N. & Roe, D. 2022. Addressing sexuality and intimate relations in community mental health services for people with serious mental illness: A qualitative study of mental health practitioners' experiences. Psychiatric Rehab J, 45, 170.

Bort-Roig, J., Briones-Buixassa, L., Felez-Nobrega, M., Guardia-Sancho, A., Sitja-Rabert, M. et al., 2020. Sedentary behaviour associations with health outcomes in people with severe mental illness: A systematic review. Eur J Public Health, 30, 150–157.

Brown, S. 1997. Excess mortality of schizophrenia. A meta-analysis. Br J Psychiatry, 171, 502–508.

Bull, F.C., AL-Ansari, S.S., Biddle, S., Borodulin, K., Buman, M.P., et al., 2020. World Health Organization 2020 guidelines on physical activity and sedentary behaviour. Br J Sports Med, 54, 1451–1462.

Burke, A.J., Hay, K., Chadwick, A., Siskind, D. & Sheridan, J. 2018. High rates of respiratory symptoms and airway disease in mental health inpatients in a tertiary centre. Intern Med J, 48, 433–438.

Burrows, T., Teasdale, S., Rocks, T., Whatnall, M., Schindlmayr, J., et al., 2022. Effectiveness of dietary interventions in mental health treatment: A rapid review of reviews. Nutrition & Dietetics, 79, 279–290.

Burschinski, A., Schneider-Thoma, J., Chiocchia, V., Schestag, K., Wang, D., et al., 2023. Metabolic side effects in persons with schizophrenia during mid-to long-term treatment with antipsychotics: A network meta-analysis of randomized controlled trials. World Psychiatry, 22, 116–128.

Bušková, J., Novák, T., Miletínová, E., Králová, R., Košt' Álová, J., et al., 2022. Self-reported symptoms and objective measures in idiopathic hypersomnia and hypersomnia associated with psychiatric disorders: A prospective cross-sectional study. J Clin Sleep Med, 18, 713–720.

Cai, V., Ng, C.P., Zhao, J., Siskind, D. & Kisely, S. 2022. A systematic review and meta-analysis of the association between periodontal disease and severe mental illness. Psychosomat Med, 84, 836–847.

Caponnetto, P., Polosa, R., Robson, D. & Bauld, L. 2020. Tobacco smoking, related harm and motivation to quit smoking in people with schizophrenia spectrum disorders. Health Psychol Res, 8, doi: 10.4081/hpr.2020.9042.

Caussy, C., Aubin, A. & Loomba, R. 2021. The relationship between type 2 diabetes, NAFLD, and cardiovascular risk. Curr Diabetes Rep, 21, 1–13.

Cimo, A. & Dewa, C. S. 2018. Symptoms of mental illness and their impact on managing type 2 diabetes in adults. Can J Diabetes, 42, 372–381.

Cloutier, B., Francoeur, A., Samson, C., Ghostine, A. & Lecomte, T. 2021. Romantic relationships, sexuality, and psychotic disorders: A systematic review of recent findings. Psychiatric Rehab J, 44, 22.

Correll, C.U., Solmi, M., Croatto, G., Schneider, L.K., Rohani-Montez, S.C., et al., 2022. Mortality in people with schizophrenia: A systematic review and meta-analysis of relative risk and aggravating or attenuating factors. World Psychiatry, 21, 248–271.

Cunningham, R., Stanley, J., Haitana, T., Pitama, S., Crowe, M., et al., 2020. The physical health of Māori with bipolar disorder. ANZ J Psychiatry, 54, 1107–1114.

Curtis, J., Zhang, C., Mcguigan, B., Pavel-Wood, E., Morell, R., et al., 2018. y-QUIT: Smoking prevalence, engagement, and effectiveness of an individualized smoking cessation intervention in youth with severe mental illness. Front Psychiatry, 9, 683.

Czosnek, L., Lederman, O., Cormie, P., Zopf, E., Stubbs, B. et al., 2019. Health benefits, safety and cost of physical activity interventions for mental health conditions: A meta-review to inform translation efforts. Ment Health Phys Activity, 16, 140–151.

De Hert, M., Detraux, J. & Vancampfort, D. 2022. The intriguing relationship between coronary heart disease and mental disorders. Dialogues Clin Neurosci, 20(1), 31–40.

De Hert, M., Mazereel, V., Stroobants, M., De Picker, L., Van Assche, K. et al., 2021. COVID-19-related mortality risk in people with severe mental illness: A systematic and critical review. Front Psychiatry, 12, doi: 10.3389/fpsyt.2021.798554.

Deenik, J., Czosnek, L., Teasdale, S.B., Stubbs, B., Firth, J., et al., 2020. From impact factors to real impact: Translating evidence on lifestyle interventions into routine mental health care. Translation Behav Med, 10, 1070–1073.

Dejongh, B.M. 2021. Clinical pearls for the monitoring and treatment of antipsychotic induced metabolic syndrome. Ment Health Clinician, 11, 311–319.

Dondé, C., Brunelin, J., Mondino, M., Cellard, C., Rolland, B. et al., 2020. The effects of acute nicotine administration on cognitive and early sensory processes in schizophrenia: A systematic review. Neurosci Biobehav Rev, 118, 121–133.

Edinoff, A.N., Ellis, E.D., Nussdorf, L.M., Hill, T.W., Cornett, E.M., et al., 2022. Antipsychotic Polypharmacy-related cardiovascular morbidity and mortality: A comprehensive review. Neurol Int, 14, 294–309.

Equally Well Australia 2021. A Global Call to Action – Fair and equitable access to vaccination for people living with mental illness and substance use disorders. Online. Available at: www.equallywell.org.au/declaration/

Evans, A.M., Quinn, C., Mckenna, B. & Willis, K. 2021. Consumers living with psychosis: Perspectives on sexuality. Int J Ment Health Nurs, 30, 382–389.

Fahed, G., Aoun, L., Bou Zerdan, M., Allam, S., Bou Zerdan, M., et al., 2022. Metabolic syndrome: Updates on pathophysiology and management in 2021. Int J Molecul Sci, 23, 786.

Firth, J., Siddiqi, N., Koyanagi, A., Siskind, D., Rosenbaum, S., et al., 2019. The Lancet Psychiatry Commission: A blueprint for protecting physical health in people with mental illness. Lancet Psychiatry, 6, 675–712.

Firth, J., Solmi, M., Wootton, R.E., Vancampfort, D., Schuch, F.B. et al., 2020. A meta-review of "lifestyle psychiatry": The role of exercise, smoking, diet and sleep in the prevention and treatment of mental disorders. World Psychiatry, 19, 360–380.

Firth, J., Stubbs, B., Teasdale, S.B., Ward, P.B., Veronese, N., et al., 2018. Diet as a hot topic in psychiatry: A population-scale study of nutritional intake and inflammatory potential in severe mental illness. World Psychiatry, 17, 365–367.

Freeman, M. 2022. The World Mental Health Report: Transforming mental health for all. World Psychiatry, 21, 391.

Galderisi, S., De Hert, M., Del Prato, S., Fagiolini, A., Gorwood, P., et al., 2021. Identification and management of cardiometabolic risk in subjects with schizophrenia spectrum disorders: A Delphi expert consensus study. Europ Psychiatry, 64, e7.

Galletly, C.A., Foley, D.L., Waterreus, A., Watts, G.F., Castle, D.J., et al., 2012. Cardiometabolic risk factors in people with psychotic disorders: The second Australian national survey of psychosis. Aust NZ J Psychiatry, 46, 753–761.

Gilbody, S., Peckham, E., Bailey, D., Arundel, C., Heron, P., et al., 2019. Smoking cessation for people with severe mental illness (SCIMITAR+): a pragmatic randomised controlled trial. Lancet Psychiatry, 6, 379–390.

Gilbody, S., Peckham, E., Man, M.-S., Mitchell, N., Li, J., et al., 2015. Bespoke smoking cessation for people with severe mental ill health (SCIMITAR): a pilot randomised controlled trial. Lancet Psychiatry, 2, 395–402.

Gogos, A., Skokou, M., Ferentinou, E. & Gourzis, P. 2019. Nicotine consumption during the prodromal phase of schizophrenia–a review of the literature. Neuropsychiatric Disease Treat, 15, 2943–2958.

Goldfarb, M., De Hert, M., Detraux, J., Di Palo, K., Munir, H., et al., 2022. Severe mental illness and cardiovascular disease: JACC state-of-the-art review. J Am Coll Cardiol, 80, 918–933.

Grajales, D., Ferreira, V. & Valverde, Á. M. 2019. Second-generation antipsychotics and dysregulation of glucose metabolism: Beyond weight gain. Cells, 8, 1336.

Greenhalgh, E.M., Brennan, E., Segan, C. & Scollo, M. 2022. Monitoring changes in smoking and quitting behaviours among Australians with and without mental illness over 15 years. ANZ J Pub Health, 46, 223–229.

Guembe, M.J., Fernandez-Lazaro, C.I., Sayon-Orea, C., Toledo, E. & Moreno-Iribas, C. 2020. Risk for cardiovascular disease associated with metabolic syndrome and its components: A 13-year prospective study in the RIVANA cohort. Cardiovasc Diabetol, 19, 1–14.

Hawes, M.R., Roth, K.B. & Cabassa, L.J. 2021. Systematic review of psychosocial smoking cessation interventions for people with serious mental illness. J Dual Diagnosis, 17, 216–235.

Heiberg, I.H., Jacobsen, B.K., Balteskard, L., Bramness, J.G., Næss, Ø., et al., 2019. Undiagnosed cardiovascular disease prior to cardiovascular death in individuals with severe mental illness. Acta Psychiatr Scand, 139, 558–571.

Hendry, A., Snowden, A. & Brown, M., 2018. When holistic care is not holistic enough: The role of sexual health in mental health settings. J Clin Nurs, 27, 1015–1027.

Howell, S., Yarovova, E., Khwanda, A. & Rosen, S.D. 2019. Cardiovascular effects of psychotic illnesses and antipsychotic therapy. Heart, 105, 1852–1859.

Institute of Medicine Committee on Sleep and Research 2006. The National Academies Collection: Reports funded by National Institutes of Health. In: Colten, H.R. & Altevogt, B.M. (eds), Sleep Disorders and Sleep Deprivation: An Unmet Public Health Problem. Washington (DC): National Academies Press (US) Copyright © 2006, National Academy of Sciences.

Jaén-Moreno, M.J., Rico-Villademoros, F., Ruiz-Rull, C., Laguna-Muñoz, D., Del Pozo, G.I. et al., 2023. A systematic review on the association between schizophrenia and bipolar disorder with chronic obstructive pulmonary disease. COPD 20, 31–43.

Kaskie, R.E. & Ferrarelli, F. 2020. Sleep disturbances in schizophrenia: What we know, what still needs to be done. Curr Opin Psychol, 34, 68–71.

Krieger, I., Bitan, D.T., Comaneshter, D., Cohen, A. & Feingold, D. 2019. Increased risk of smoking-related illnesses in schizophrenia patients: A nationwide cohort study. Schizophrenia Res, 212, 121–125.

Lambert, A.M., Parretti, H.M., Pearce, E.,Price, M.J., Riley, M., et al., 2022. Temporal trends in associations between severe mental illness and risk of cardiovascular disease: A systematic review and meta-analysis. PLoS medicine, 19, e1003960.

Lassale, C., Batty, G.D., Baghdadli, A., Jacka, F., Sánchez-Villegas, A., et al., 2019. Healthy dietary indices and risk of depressive outcomes: A systematic review and meta-analysis of observational studies. Molecular Psychiatry, 24, 965–986.

Lawley, M.E., Cwiak, C., Cordes, S., Ward, M. & Hall, K.S. 2022. Barriers to family planning among women with severe mental illness. Women's Reproduct Health, 9, 100–118.

Lawn, S., Kaine, C., Stevenson, J. & Mcmahon, J. 2021. Australian mental health consumers' experiences of service engagement and disengagement: A descriptive study. Int J Environ Res Pub Health, 18, 10464.

Lawrence, D. & Jablensky, A. Preventable physical illness in people with mental illness. Preventable physical illness in people with mental illness 2001. The University of Western Australia.

Liang, C.-S., Bai, Y.-M., Hsu, J.-W., Huang, K.-L., Ko, N.-Y., et al., 2020. The risk of sexually transmitted infections following first-episode schizophrenia among adolescents and young adults: A cohort study of 220 545 subjects. Schizophrenia Bull, 46, 795–803.

Lin, C.C., Yeh, L.L. & Pan, Y.J. 2023. Degree of exposure to psychotropic medications and mortality in people with bipolar disorder. Acta Psychiatr Scand, 147, 186–197.

Lister, J., Han, L., Bellass, S., Taylor, J., Alderson, S.L., et al., 2021. Identifying determinants of diabetes risk and outcomes for people with severe mental illness: A mixed-methods study. Health Serv Deliv Res, 9, 1–194.

Lluch, E. & Miller, B.J. 2019. Rates of hepatitis B and C in patients with schizophrenia: A meta-analysis. Gen Hosp Psychiatry, 61, 41–46.

Lockett, H., Bagnall, C., Cunningham, R. & Arcus, K. 2017. Cardiovascular disease risk and management in people who experience serious mental illness. Int J Integrat Care, 17.

Luciano, M., Sampogna, G., Del Vecchio, V., Giallonardo, V., Palummo, C., et al., 2021. The impact of clinical and social factors on the physical health of people with severe mental illness: Results from an Italian multicentre study. Psychiatry Res, 303, 114073.

Lum, A., Skelton, E., Wynne, O. & Bonevski, B. 2018. A systematic review of psychosocial barriers and facilitators to smoking cessation in people living with schizophrenia. Front Psychiatry, 9, 565.

Lundström, S., Jormfeldt, H., Hedman Ahlström, B. & Skärsäter, I. 2020. Mental health nurses' experience of physical health care and health promotion initiatives for people with severe mental illness. Int J Ment Health Nurs, 29, 244–253.

McCann, E., Donohue, G., De Jager, J., Nugter, A., Stewart, J. et al., 2019. Sexuality and intimacy among people with serious mental illness: A qualitative systematic review. JBI Evidence Synthesis, 17, 74–125.

McKee, J. & Brahm, N. 2016. Medical mimics: Differential diagnostic considerations for psychiatric symptoms. Ment Health Clin, 6, 289–296.

Mindgardens Positive Cardiometabolic Health Framework. Watkins, A., Gould, P., Fibbins, H., Morell, R., Samaras, K. et al., 2023a. Positive Cardiometabolic Health Resource: An early intervention framework for people on psychotropic medication (Adult version). doi.org/10.26190/2h3h kw57.

Mindgardens Tobacco Treatment Framework. Watkins, A., Gould, P., Fibbins, H., Morell, R., Metse, A. et al., 2023b, Tobacco Treatment Resource: An intervention framework for people on psychotropic medication. doi. org/10.26190/t259-mk60.

Molloy, R., Brand, G., Munro, I. & Pope, N. 2021. Seeing the complete picture: A systematic review of mental health consumer and health professional experiences of diagnostic overshadowing. J Clin Nurs.

Montejo, A.L., De Alarcón, R., Prieto, N., Acosta, J.M., Buch, B. et al., 2021. Management strategies for antipsychotic-related sexual dysfunction: A clinical approach. J Clin Med, 10, 308.

Morgan, V.A., Waterreus, A., Ambrosi, T., Badcock, J.C., Cox, K., et al.,. 2021. Mental health recovery and physical health outcomes in psychotic illness: Longitudinal data from the Western Australian survey of high impact psychosis catchments. ANZ J Psychiatry, 55, 711–728.

Morgan, V.A., Waterreus, A., Jablensky, A., Mackinnon, A., McGrath, J.J., et al., 2011. People living with psychotic illness in 2010: the second Australian national survey of psychosis. Aust N Z J Psychiatry, 46, 735–52.

Mukherjee, S., Skrede, S., Milbank, E., Andriantsitohaina, R., López, M. et al., 2022. Understanding the effects of antipsychotics on appetite control. Frontiers Nutrit, 8, 815456.

Mutwalli, H., Keeler, J.L., Bektas, S., Dhopatkar, N., Treasure, J. et al., 2023. Eating cognitions, emotions and behaviour under treatment with second generation antipsychotics: A systematic review and meta-analysis. J Psychiatric Res.

National Health and Medical Research Council (NHMRC) 2013. Australian dietary guidelines. Canberra (Australia): National Health and Medical Research Council. Online. Available at: www.nhmrc.gov.au/adg

Nielsen, R.E., Banner, J. & Jensen, S.E. 2021. Cardiovascular disease in patients with severe mental illness. Nature Rev Cardiol, 18, 136–145.

Nilsson, P.M., Tuomilehto, J. & Rydén, L. 2019. The metabolic syndrome – what is it and how should it be managed? Europ J Prevent Cardiol, 26, 33–46.

Ogunmoroti, O., Osibogun, O., Spatz, E.S., Okunrintemi, V., Mathews, L., et al., 2022. A systematic review of the bidirectional relationship between depressive symptoms and cardiovascular health. Prevent Med, 154, 106891.

Parletta, N., Zarnowiecki, D., Cho, J., Wilson, A., Bogomolova, S., et al., 2019. A Mediterranean-style dietary intervention supplemented with fish oil improves diet quality and mental health in people with depression: A randomized controlled trial (HELFIMED). Nutr Neurosci, 22, 474–487.

Pettey, D. & Aubry, T. 2018. Tobacco use and smoking behaviors of individuals with a serious mental illness. Psychiatric Rehab J, 41, 356.

Richmond-Rakerd, L.S., D'Souza, S., Milne, B.J., Caspi, A. & Moffitt, T.E. 2021. Longitudinal associations of mental disorders with physical diseases and mortality among 2.3 million New Zealand citizens. JAMA Network Open, 4, e2033448.

Rodrigues, M., Wiener, J.C., Stranges, S., Ryan, B.L. & Anderson, K.K. 2021. The risk of physical multimorbidity in people with psychotic disorders: A systematic review and meta-analysis. J Psychosomat Res, 140, 110315.

Sanz, M., Marco Del Castillo, A., Jepsen, S., Gonzalez-Juanatey, J.R., D'Aiuto, F., et al., 2020. Periodontitis and cardiovascular diseases: Consensus report. J Clin Periodontol, 47, 268–288.

Sara, G., Chen, W., Large, M., Ramanuj, P., Curtis, J., et al., 2021. Potentially preventable hospitalisations for physical health conditions in community mental health service users: A population-wide linkage study. Epidemiol Psychiatric Sci, 30.

Scheuer, S.H., Kosjerina, V., Lindekilde, N., Pouwer, F., Carstensen, B., et al., 2022. Severe mental illness and the risk of diabetes complications: A nationwide, register-based cohort study. J Clin Endocrinol & Metabol, 107, e3504–e3514.

Seminog, O.O. & Goldacre, M.J. 2013. Risk of pneumonia and pneumococcal disease in people with severe mental illness: English record linkage studies. Thorax, 68, 171–176.

Singh, R., Bansal, Y., Medhi, B. & Kuhad, A. 2019. Antipsychotics-induced metabolic alterations: Recounting the mechanistic insights, therapeutic targets and pharmacological alternatives. Europ J Pharmacol, 844, 231–240.

Smith, P. F., Smith, A., Miners, J., Mcneil, J. & Proudfoot, A. 2000. The safety aspects of dietary caffeine. Australia: Report from the expert working group 202–223.

Stubbs, B., Vancampfort, D., Hallgren, M., Firth, J., Veronese, N., et al., 2018. EPA guidance on physical activity as a treatment for severe mental illness: A meta-review of the evidence and Position Statement from the European Psychiatric Association (EPA), supported by the International Organization of Physical Therapists in Mental Health (IOPTMH). European Psychiatry, 54, 124–144.

Sweeney, K., Shui, H., Calder, R. & Duggan, M. 2016. The economic cost of serious mental illness and comorbidities in Australia and New Zealand. Royal Australian and New Zealand College of Psychiatrists, Melbourne.

Tanskanen, A., Tiihonen, J. & Taipale, H. 2018. Mortality in schizophrenia: 30-year nationwide follow-up study. Acta Psychiatr Scand, 138, 492–499.

Taylor, G.M., Lindson, N., Farley, A., Leinberger-Jabari, A., Sawyer, K., et al., 2021. Smoking cessation for improving mental health. Cochrane Database of Syst Rev, 3, 1465–1858.

Taylor, R. 2021. Type 2 diabetes and remission: Practical management guided by pathophysiology. J Intern Med, 289, 754–770.

Teasdale, S.B., Ward, P.B., Rosenbaum, S., Samaras, K. & Stubbs, B. 2017. Solving a weighty problem: Systematic review and meta-analysis of nutrition interventions in severe mental illness. Br J Psychiatry, 210, 110–118.

Teasdale, S.B., Ward, P.B., Samaras, K., Firth, J., Stubbs, B., et al., 2019. Dietary intake of people with severe mental illness: Systematic review and meta-analysis. Br J Psychiatry, 214, 251–259.

Teychenne, M., White, R.L., Richards, J., Schuch, F.B., Rosenbaum, S. et al., 2020. Do we need physical activity guidelines for mental health: What does the evidence tell us? Ment Health Phys Activ, 18, 100315.

Thornicroft, G., Sunkel, C., Aliev, A.A., Baker, S., Brohan, E., et al., 2022. The Lancet Commission on ending stigma and discrimination in mental health. Lancet, 400, 1438–1480.

Tobin, T. & Tobin, M. L. 2017. Staying Awake and aware: The importance of sleep in psychiatric nursing practice. Issues Ment Health Nurs, 38, 924–929.

Tyerman, J., Patovirta, A.-L. & Celestini, A. 2021. How stigma and discrimination influences nursing care of persons diagnosed with mental illness: A systematic review. Iss Ment Health Nurs, 42, 153–163.

Urry, K., Chur-Hansen, A. & Khaw, C. 2019. 'It's just a peripheral issue': A qualitative analysis of mental health clinicians' accounts of (not) addressing sexuality in their work. Int J Ment Health Nurs, 28, 1278–1287.

Vai, B., Mazza, M.G., Colli, C.D., Foiselle, M., Allen, B., et al., 2021. Mental disorders and risk of COVID-19-related mortality, hospitalisation, and intensive care unit admission: A systematic review and meta-analysis. Lancet Psychiatry, 8, 797–812.

Wium-Andersen, M.K., Jørgensen, T.S.H., Jørgensen, M.B., Rungby, J., Hjorthøj, C., et al., 2022. The association between birth weight, ponderal index, psychotropic medication, and type 2 diabetes in individuals with severe mental illness. J Diabetes Complicat, 36, 108181.

Wu, X., Gao, S. & Lian, Y. 2020. Effects of continuous aerobic exercise on lung function and quality of life with asthma: A systematic review and meta-analysis. J Thoracic Dis, 12, 4781.

Xie, Y., Xu, E. & Al-Aly, Z. 2022. Risks of mental health outcomes in people with covid-19: cohort study. BMJ, 376.

Yang, M., Chen, P., He, M.-X., Lu, M., Wang, H.-M., et al., 2018. Poor oral health in patients with schizophrenia: A systematic review and meta-analysis. Schizophrenia Res 201, 3–9.

Yeghiazarians, Y., Jneid, H., Tietjens, J.R., Redline, S., Brown, D.L., et al., 2021. Obstructive sleep apnea and cardiovascular disease: A scientific statement from the American Heart Association. Circulation, 144, e56–e67.

Zhang, D., Gabriel, K.P., Sidney, S., Sternfeld, B., Jacobs J.R., et al., 2021. Longitudinal bidirectional associations of physical activity and depressive symptoms: The CARDIA study. Preventive Medicine Reports, 23, 101489.

Zhang, L.-Y., Anderson, J., Higgins, N., Robinson, J., Francey, S., et al., 2022. Screening for obstructive sleep apnoea in patients with serious mental illness. Australas Psychiatry, 30, 615–618.

Psychopharmacology

Richard Lakeman and Irene Ngune

KEY POINTS

- Psychotropic medications are prescribed to alleviate symptoms of mental illness and distress. Nurses play pivotal roles in medication administration, promoting adherence, facilitating choice and educating service users about effects, interactions and side effects.
- Nurses need to have knowledge of the effects of medications and potential interactions and have responsibilities to monitor and intervene if medications cause adverse effects.
- Nurses need to maintain a curiosity about the lived experience of taking medications, and of abrupt cessation and tapering psychotropic medications.
- Many psychotropic medications contribute to physical health problems such as metabolic syndrome. Nurses need to be aware of these problems and assess service users prior to and during use of medications. Non-pharmaceutical or lifestyle interventions

can be prescribed to optimise the health and wellbeing of service users.
- Nurses must be aware of contraindications and dangers associated with the administration of medications to vulnerable groups such as children, pregnant women and the elderly.
- Polypharmacy is to be avoided where possible, especially the tendency to use medications from different classes at the same time.
- Nurses are often responsible for administering as-needed (prn) medications or stat doses of psychotropic medications in occasions of acute behavioural disturbance. Nurses need to be aware of non-pharmacological interventions to address these issues.
- Nurses need to understand and undertake assessment and interventions related to side-effects and adverse effects related to psychotropic drugs.

KEY TERMS

Agranulocytosis
Akathisia
Anticholinergic effects
Atypical antipsychotic medication
Collaborative prescribing
Discontinuation/withdrawal syndromes
Extrapyramidal side effects

Informed consent
Medication adherence
Metabolic syndrome
Mood-stabilising medication
Neuroleptic malignant syndrome
Neuroleptic medication
Polypharmacy

pro re nata (prn) medications
Psychopharmacology
Psychotropic medication
QT prolongation
Tardive syndromes
Typical antipsychotic medication

LEARNING OUTCOMES

The material in this chapter will assist you to:
- describe the nurse's role in administering psychotropic medications and related intervention including medication indications, expected effects, interactions, side effects and precautions
- identify the important classes of psychotropic medication and the conditions for which they are used
- understand the lived experience and issues of concern for people receiving psychotropic medications

- understand the actions, use and side effects related to antianxiety/sedative hypnotics, drugs used to address problems of mood, and antipsychotic medications
- understand the issues related to as-needed (prn) psychotropic medications and related interventions
- outline the relevant legal and ethical issues related to administering psychotropic medications
- understand the importance of monitoring and optimising physical health prior to and during treatment with psychotropic medications.

INTRODUCTION

This chapter provides an overview of how drugs are used in the field of psychiatry and mental health. *Psychopharmacology* is the study of how drugs affect the mind and behaviour, and, in particular, the effects of drugs on neurotransmitters, receptors and other molecular targets in the brain. If you take a "deep dive" into psychopharmacology you are

likely to discover that questions about how drugs work, and for whom, are far from settled (Stahl 2021). In order to inform and educate students and novice nurses on these drugs and their uses in practice, this chapter does not break with the tradition of classifying and discussing drugs according to the symptoms, syndromes or conditions they purport to treat. Thus, there are sections on antianxiety, anxiolytics, antidepressants, mood-stabilising medications, antipsychotic or neuroleptic medications, cognitive enhancers and stimulants. However, it is important to recognise that this is a problematic approach to considering drug treatments, as most drugs in psychiatry are used for multiple purposes. For example, diazepam is used for its muscle relaxant properties, in alcohol withdrawal, as an acute anticonvulsant, as a sedative, and sometimes in acute states of anxiety. Diazepam belongs to a drug class called benzodiazepines. A *drug class* is a group of medications with similarities in terms of mechanism of action, physiological effects and chemical structure.

In psychiatry, drugs from quite different classes may be used to treat the same problems. Rather than a disorder or disease-focused approach to psychopharmacology, which assumes that mental disorders are discrete diseases with specific biological causes, some have suggested a drug-centred approach to psychiatric drugs to be the most helpful (Moncrieff 2007). The drug-centred approach recognises that psychiatric drugs are powerful substances that have complex effects on the brain and body. Rather than assuming that a particular drug will be effective for a particular condition based on a diagnosis, the drug-centred approach looks at the specific properties of the drug, the effects of the drug, and how it interacts with the brain and body. From this standpoint one can rationally consider the effects of non-prescribed or illicit drugs. This approach also encourages consideration of all the effects of a drug and not simply dismissing some effects as side effects. Crucially for nurses, a drug-centred approach ought to provoke an interest in what it is like to take a particular drug (Lakeman et al 2023).

The readers of this chapter are urged to adopt a drug-centred approach to pharmacology. Nurses are uniquely placed to explore with individuals what the experience of taking a drug, tapering or ceasing a drug is like. Students of mental health nursing are urged to discuss with curiosity what the person experiences and how psychotropic drugs impact on their feelings, thought processes, motivation, behaviour, appetite and libido.

Using medications to alleviate mental distress and relieve some symptoms of psychiatric conditions has become widespread since the mid-1950s. Collectively, these medications are referred to as "psychotropic medications" and are the focus of this chapter. In Australia in recent years, more than 17% of the population filled a prescription for a psychotropic medication, making Australia one of the most medicated countries in the world (Lakeman et al 2022). Psychotropic medications can be administered using a variety of methods such as oral, sub-lingual, sub-cutaneous, intramuscular and intravenous routes.

Psychotropic medications are just one component of psychiatric treatment and on their own should not be considered a "quick fix" or cure-all. The first-line treatments for syndromes such as depression, for example, include diet, exercise, sleep hygiene, followed by psychotherapy, and only then should medications be considered (Malhi et al 2021). Although some people acknowledge that psychotropics have played a crucial role in their path to recovery, others report experiencing adverse emotional, cognitive and physical side effects of their medication, hindering their personal recovery. Some people experience medications as contributing to confusion and preventing them from attaining the mental clarity and stability necessary to achieve their recovery objectives (Mathew et al 2023).

Psychotropic medications do have the potential to improve quality of life for many people. However, these medications have the potential to cause a number of serious side-effects or adverse events. Mental health nurses need to be aware of these effects and develop the appropriate skills to assess and monitor for them, including physical health and related issues (see Chapter 20), and to educate people about potential problems related to psychotropic medications. For example, smoking cigarettes interferes with an enzyme pathway (cytochrome P450),

which leads to significantly reduced plasma concentrations of some commonly used psychotropic drugs (Miroshnichenko et al 2020). While nurses can encourage and assist people to quit smoking, the skilled mental health nurse will be mindful that abruptly ceasing smoking can lead to a rapid increase of drug concentrations to toxic and dangerous levels (Preskorn 2020).

Skillful mental health nursing therefore encompasses an understanding of the particular pharmacological actions of the psychotropic agents, as well as an empathic understanding of the potential issues for the person taking these medications (see Perspectives in practice: Nurse's Story 21.1). Regardless of the treatment setting, which can range from in-patient to community, mental health nurses play a pivotal role in working with service users and their families as they grapple with the issues surrounding these medications. Nurses require a comprehensive understanding of both the medications and their impact on an individual, as well as an understanding of the supportive and therapeutic nursing interventions that support medication adherence and effectiveness. Table 21.1 provides a list of commonly used terms related to psychopharmacology.

PERSPECTIVES IN PRACTICE
Nurse's Story 21.1: Diane

One day a consumer thanked me for looking after him and helping him to understand more about his medications and how they worked. This came as a surprise to me as I had never been thanked in this way before and thought it was my role to help consumers to better understand treatment options. While the older traditional antipsychotics were linked to many major side effects, the newer, second-generation treatments are better tolerated by consumers and have fewer reported side effects. However, it is easy to assume that, because of this, people no longer need to be informed and involved in their treatment decisions. It is important to recognise that the new antipsychotics do not provide a global effect for negative symptoms and in fact still have several unwanted side effects such as weight gain and metabolic disturbance. These side effects can be very distressing to the consumer and some have told me they think they are even worse off than before the treatment, even though it may have helped with their psychotic symptoms.

Reflecting on the incident described above I thought about how as nurses we often act in certain ways because of our own understanding or beliefs about an illness and its origins. For example, many nurses unwittingly propagate a pessimistic attitude to consumers with schizophrenia because of their belief that the disorder is caused by genetic factors. In such cases, nurses may engage with consumers minimally and seek instead to do activities such as medication rounds. For me, it is important to try to work with consumers in ways that are free of assumptions and to focus on the needs of the consumer at all times.

IMPORTANT PHARMACOLOGICAL PRINCIPLES

Supportive and therapeutic nursing interventions aim to foster understanding of the effective and safe use of medications and to negotiate and enhance adherence to the treatment plan. The most important predictor of adherence and treatment responsiveness is the quality of the relationship or alliance between the health provider and the individual (Bolsinger et al 2020). All medications are prescribed for particular effects or target symptoms that the prescriber and individual hope to change. Correctly identifying symptoms is a critical component of a thorough nursing assessment. On the other hand, side effects are the expression of effects for which the medication was not intended. Not all side effects are harmful,

TABLE 21.1 Commonly Used Terms

Term	Definition
Akathisia	Restlessness where the person cannot stay still
Agranulocytosis	Severely low neutrophil levels (less than 100 neutrophils per microlitre of blood). This is a potentially life-threatening adverse event which can lead to vulnerability to infection.
Anosognosia	Lack of insight
Antipsychotic medication	Medication prescribed to reduce psychotic symptoms
Ataxia	Lack of voluntary coordination of muscle movement
Atypical antipsychotic medication	Newer, second-generation antipsychotic medications
Cogwheeling rigidity	Type of rigidity seen in parkinsonism whereby the muscles respond with cogwheel-like jerks to the application of constant force in attempting to bend the limb
Dystonia	State of abnormal muscle tone
Extrapyramidal side effects	Drug-induced movement disorders
Efficacy	Medication efficacy refers to the ability of a medication to produce a desired therapeutic effect for its intended purpose. The efficacy of a medication is assessed through the clinical trials and is balanced against potential risks and side-effects. Medication efficacy can vary depending on the consumer characteristics such as gender, age and their overall health.
Half-life	The time until the serum level of a drug is reduced by half
Iatrogenic	An effect caused by a medication or by health personnel
Medication titration	Medication titration refers to the process of adjusting the medication dosage to get the minimum effective dose of a medication that produces the desired therapeutic effect and with the least side effects.
Neuroleptic malignant syndrome	Neuroleptic malignant syndrome (NMS) is a life-threatening neurological emergency associated with the use of antipsychotic (neuroleptic) agents and characterised by a distinctive clinical syndrome of mental status change, rigidity, fever, and dysautonomia.
Parkinson's syndrome	Imbalance between dopamine and acetylcholine, resulting in involuntary movements, reduced movements, rigidity and abnormal walking and posture
Polypharmacy	Use of multiple medications simultaneously
Pro re nata (prn)	As needed
Serotonin syndrome	A potentially life-threatening syndrome caused by excessive brain cell activity as a result of high levels of serotonin
Tardive dyskinesia	Involuntary movements of the tongue, lips, face, trunk and extremities related to taking antipsychotic medications
Tardive syndrome	Delayed-onset abnormal involuntary movement disorders caused by a dopamine-receptor blocking agent
Therapeutic dose	Therapeutic dose refers to the specific amount or range of a medication needed to attain the desired therapeutic effect.
Typical antipsychotic medication	Traditional type of antipsychotic medication

but some can be, so nurses need a sound working knowledge of this area of practice.

Nurses also need to be aware of polypharmacy. *Polypharmacy* involves the concurrent use of multiple psychotropic medications. Polypharmacy is generally not advisable because it can increase the chance of adverse medication side effects and interactions. It can make it difficult to determine which medications are causing which effects. Polypharmacy can be extremely problematic with specific groups of vulnerable people, including the elderly, who are commonly prescribed several different medications concurrently (Hubbard et al 2015; Li et al 2022).

An understanding of how psychotropic medications work in the brain can assist in understanding the overall effects of a drug. The neuron is the basic functional unit of the brain and the central nervous system (CNS), and all communication in the brain involves neurons communicating across synapses at receptors. Receptors are the targets for the neurotransmitters or chemical messengers necessary for communication between neurons. The neurotransmitters acetylcholine, noradrenaline (norepinephrine), dopamine, serotonin (5HT) and GABA (gamma-aminobutyric acid) are commonly impacted by psychotropic medication. Psychotropic medications produce their therapeutic action by altering communication among the neurons in the CNS. They alter the way neurotransmitters work at the synapse by modifying the reuptake of neurotransmitters into the presynaptic neuron, activating or inhibiting postsynaptic

receptors, or inhibiting enzyme activity (Goldberg & Stahl 2021). Psychotropic medications are believed to act by altering the activities of the receptors, enzymes, ion channels and chemical transporter systems.

IMPORTANT PSYCHOTROPIC MEDICATIONS

This section explores the most important groups of psychotropic medications in current use: the anxiolytics (antianxiety), antidepressants, mood-stabilisers and antipsychotics (neuroleptics). These groups of medications are listed in Table 21.2 along with their with commonly used trade names in the Australasian context. Understanding the effects of these drugs on human behaviour is an aim of behavioural pharmacology. Some selective effects of these drugs are illustrated in Box 21.1.

Antianxiety, Anxiolytic Medications and "Minor Tranquillisers"

Anxiety is a common human experience that is a normal reaction to a threat of some kind. It leads to a sympathetic nervous system response (sometimes known as fight-or-flight). Anxiety is also associated with many mental health problems. When anxiety becomes disabling or in states of acute distress, antianxiety medications may be useful (Bandelow et al 2023; Bandelow et al 2012). Antianxiety medications can be divided into benzodiazepines and non-benzodiazepines. Benzodiazepines (formerly called minor tranquillisers) are probably the

TABLE 21.2   Classification of Psychotropic Medications

Type	Medication Group	Examples
Antianxiety	Benzodiazepines	Chlordiazepoxide
		Diazepam
		Clonazepam
		Alprazolam
		Lorazepam
	Azapirones	Buspirone
	Beta-adrenergic blockers	Propranolol
Antidepressant	Tricyclic and related medications	Amitriptyline
		Lofepramine
		Trazodone
	Selective serotonin reuptake inhibitors (SSRIs) and related medications	Fluoxetine
		Paroxetine
	Noradrenaline serotonin reuptake inhibitors (NSRIs)	Venlafaxine
		Mirtazapine
	Monoamine oxidase inhibitors (MAOIs)	Isocarboxazid
		Phenelzine
		Tranylcypromine
Mood-stabilising	Lithium	Lithium carbonate
	Anticonvulsants	Carbamazepine
		Valproate
		Topiramate
		Lamotrigine
Antipsychotic	Phenothiazines	Thioridazine
Typical (traditional)	Thioxanthenes	Flupenthixol
	Butyrophenones	Haloperidol
	Diphenylbutylpiperidines	Pimozide
Atypical (second-generation)		Clozapine
		Risperidone
		Olanzapine
		Quetiapine
		Ziprasidone
Sedative-hypnotic	Benzodiazepines	Flurazepam
		Temazepam
	Cyclopyrrolones	Zopiclone
	Imidazopyridines	Zolpidem

BOX 21.1   How Psychiatric Drugs Work From a Behavioural Pharmacological/Drug-Centric Standpoint

A behavioural pharmacology approach examines directly how drugs affect human behaviour. Stated simplistically the major classes of drugs have the following effects:

1. Benzodiazepines are termed minor tranquillisers which dampen most emotions, and cognition, when used in a low dose.
2. SSRI/SNRIs can be called emotional tranquillisers which numb human feelings, both anxious, sad, happy and also more reliably, numb sexual sensations – which sometimes never come back even after treatment is ceased. Tricyclic antidepressants are largely SSRI/SNRIs in their actual functioning.
3. Mirtazapine/mianserin increase appetite and cause sleepiness.
4. "Antipsychotic" drugs (first and second generation) are major tranquillisers which more heavily dampen emotions, sometimes cognition, and often also motivation.
5. "Mood stabilisers", generally antiepileptics or antipsychotics, dampen emotions, sometimes cognition and often also motivation.
6. Stimulants narrow focus, also creativity, dampen appetite, often exacerbate anxiety, can cause psychosis and over the longer term do not significantly help attentional difficulties.

In certain clinical situations, particularly over the shorter to medium term, and sometimes longer, these behavioural effects can be quite helpful, but must always be carefully weighed against adverse effects.

Personal communication with the Australian Psychiatrist (Purssey 2023).

TABLE 21.3   Managing Benzodiazepine Side Effects

Side Effect	Intervention
Drowsiness	Encourage appropriate activity but warn against engaging in activities such as driving or operating machinery
Dizziness	Observe and take steps to prevent falls
Feelings of detachment	Encourage socialisation
Dependency, rebound insomnia/anxiety	Encourage short-term use
	Educate to avoid other medications such as alcohol
	Plan for withdrawal

most commonly prescribed medications in the world today. Although initially very effective in relieving anxiety symptoms, benzodiazepines are not recommended as first-line treatment for insomnia, panic disorders and anxiety (including anxiety with depression) (Bandelow et al 2023; Psychotropic Expert Group 2013). They are now recommended as second-line treatment (Bandelow et al 2023). This is due to the significant potential for tolerance and physical dependence to develop, especially in those with a history of substance use disorders. Treatment for longer than 2–4 weeks is not recommended in most cases (Brett & Murnion 2015; Champion 2021). Antidepressants are the primary pharmacological treatments for anxiety disorders in Australia and Aotearoa New Zealand. These are discussed later in this chapter.

Benzodiazepines

Indications for use. Benzodiazepines are thought to reduce anxiety because of their potentiation of the inhibitory neurotransmitter GABA, which results in a clinical decrease in the person's anxiety by inhibiting neurotransmission (Goldberg & Stahl 2021). Clinically they are used to treat anxiety, insomnia, akathisia, alcohol withdrawal, skeletal muscle rigidity, seizure disorders, anxiety associated with medical disease and psychotic agitation. Therefore, although the discussion here primarily relates to these medications as antianxiety agents, they also have a sedative effect and are often used for that purpose. Generally speaking, high potency short-acting drugs such as temazepam are used as sedative hypnotics (to aid sleep). Diazepam (which has a short time to peak effect, but a very long half-life) is more often used to treat acute and severe alcohol withdrawal (Weintraub 2017). For reasons that are not properly understood, the high-potency medication lorazepam (in relatively high doses) is an effective treatment for catatonia (Hirjak et al 2023).

Side effects. Side effects from benzodiazepines (see Table 21.3) are common, dose-related, usually short term and almost always harmless. They include drowsiness, reduced mental acuity and impaired motor performance. Other effects such as headache, dizziness, feelings of detachment, nausea, hypotension and restlessness may also be experienced. Therefore, people should be warned of the risk of accidents and cautioned about driving a car or operating dangerous machinery (there is usually a warning to this effect on the box or bottle of medication).

BOX 21.2 Symptoms of Benzodiazepine Withdrawal Syndrome

- Agitation
- Anorexia
- Anxiety
- Autonomic arousal
- Dizziness
- Hallucinations
- Insomnia
- Irritability
- Nausea and vomiting
- Seizures
- Sensitivity to light and sounds
- Tinnitus
- Tremulousness

These medications generally do not live up to their reputation of being strongly addictive, especially if they have been used for appropriate purposes, if their use has not been complicated by other factors such as the addition of other medications, and if their withdrawal is planned and gradual. However, a withdrawal syndrome can result (see Box 21.2) if ceased abruptly after long-term use. It is also important to remember that older adults are more vulnerable to side effects because the ageing brain is more sensitive to the action of sedatives (Lin et al 2019).

Contraindications/precautions. Benzodiazepines should not be taken in conjunction with any other CNS depressants, including alcohol (Champion 2021; Royal Australian College of General Practitioners (RACGP) 2015). If benzodiazepines are combined with other CNS depressants like alcohol and opioids, users may become vulnerable to respiratory depression, excessive sedation, coma, and even fatality. The concurrent consumption of alcohol and benzodiazepines can result in cross-tolerance, which exacerbates withdrawal symptoms and makes them more prolonged with frequent usage of both substances (RACGP 2015). Their safety in pregnancy is not established.

Interactions. Interactions may occur with alcohol, monoamine oxidase inhibitors (MAOIs), phenytoin, antacids and agents with anticholinergic activity (Champion 2021).

Service user education. People prescribed benzodiazepines should be educated about the following:

- Driving or operating machinery should be avoided until the consumer knows how they react to the medication.
- Alcohol and other CNS depressants potentiate the effects of benzodiazepines and, therefore, should be avoided.
- Benzodiazepines' use should not be stopped suddenly. Abrupt cessation can induce severe complications such as tremors, seizures, delirium and catatonia, especially in older adults (Reeves & Kamal 2019).
- The use of benzodiazepines during pregnancy is not recommended because of the potential that the child will experience adverse effects and toxicity (Champion 2021).

Non-Benzodiazepine Antianxiety Medications

Buspirone is a potent non-benzodiazepine anxiolytic medication with no addictive or sedative properties. It is effective in treating anxiety and has no muscle relaxant or anticonvulsant properties. It's efficacy in managing alcohol or other medication abuse or panic disorder has not been established (Soyka et al 2017). It generally takes 3–6 weeks before maximum anxiolytic effects are achieved.

Propranolol is a beta-blocker that is useful in treating anxiety. It blocks beta-noradrenergic receptors centrally as well as in the peripheral cardiac and pulmonary systems. Beta-blockers reduce some physiological symptoms of anxiety or sympathetic nervous system arousal such as increased heart rate.

Antidepressant Medications

Depression is a condition characterised by symptoms such as depressed mood, lack of pleasure or interest, appetite disturbance, sleep disturbance and fatigue. Depression was once thought to be associated with dysregulation of neurochemicals, particularly serotonin and noradrenaline. However, recent reviews have found little support for the hypothesis that depression is caused by lower serotonin activity or concentrations (Moncrieff et al 2022). Antidepressant medications enhance the transmission of these neurochemicals in several ways – they block the reuptake of the neurotransmitters at the synapse, inhibit their metabolism and destruction and/or enhance the activity of the receptors. The action of these medications at the synapse is immediate, but it takes several weeks for most people to report an improvement in mood (Cipriani et al 2018). Where rapid improvement in mood is desired, medications such as ketamine can have an immediate impact on mood on administration due to their dissociative and euphoric effects (Mandal et al 2019).

Indications for use. Antidepressant medications are indicated in treating persistent depressive disorders, major depression, depression (maintenance treatment and prevention of relapse) and anxiety disorders such as panic disorder and obsessive-compulsive disorder. The medications may elevate mood and alleviate other symptoms experienced as part of the syndrome, such as sleep disturbance. Choice of an antidepressant medication will depend on its effect profile, side effects, comorbid medical conditions, concurrent medications and risk of medication interactions, and the individual's medication history. If the person responds to the course of treatment with a particular medication, they should continue taking the medication at the same dosage for up to 9 months (Bauer et al 2015). If they remain symptom-free during this time, the medication dose ought to be gradually tapered down (often over several weeks or months), and the medication ceased (Bauer et al 2015). Particular care should be taken not to abruptly cease antidepressants, which often need to be tapered slowly to prevent withdrawal syndromes (which may be mistaken for a relapse).

Contraindications/precautions. Caution is warranted in the use of all antidepressant medications. Suicidal ideation and related risk can be increased with antidepressant treatment, both as an initial side effect and also once the medication starts to take effect and the consumer's mood lifts, potentially increasing their motivation to act on existing suicidal thoughts. Selective serotonin re-uptake inhibitors (SSRIs) should not be combined with monoamine amine oxidase inhibitors (MAOI) therapy. MAOIs should not be started within a week of discontinuing tricyclic therapy and, conversely, tricyclic medications should not be commenced within 2 weeks of stopping a MAOI. The tricyclics are a special risk with depressed people because of their severe cardiac toxicity if taken in large doses. Caution is warranted in older adults and people with cardiac disease. Tricyclics may also impair reaction times, especially at the beginning of treatment. Alcohol may increase the sedative effects of tricyclics (Soyka et al 2017). Monotherapy with antidepressants risks precipitating hypomania in people with a bipolar mood disorder can cause mood elevation for some people, even without a recognised history of mood instability.

Consumer education. Inform the person of the time it will take for a marked effect to be experienced from the medication and the importance of continuing to take the medication, even though they have not noticed an initial improvement in their condition. People need to be aware that long-term use of SSRIs can lead to a form of physiological dependence and the experience of withdrawal syndromes if the medication is abruptly stopped (Massabki & Abi-Jaoude 2021).

Other information:

- Warn the person that reaction time may be impacted and to take extreme caution when driving or operating machinery if sedation is experienced.
- Tell the person to discuss with their doctor if they become pregnant or intend to breastfeed.

BOX 21.3 Signs of Tricyclic Overdose

- Agitation
- Confusion, drowsiness, delirium
- Convulsion
- Bowel and bladder paralysis
- Disturbances with the regulation of blood pressure and temperature
- Dilated pupils

Treatment Protocol Project 2004.

- Warn the person about the effect that alcohol may have if combined with antidepressant medication.
- Inform the person about possible interactions with foods and other medications if taking MAOIs.

Tricyclic Antidepressants

Side effects. The tricyclic medications, which have been available on the market for many years now, are clinically similar, so their effects and side effects tend to vary only slightly between individual medications. They tend to have marked sedative effects. They work primarily by serotonin and noradrenaline reuptake inhibition. The blockade of reuptake leads to extra transmitters being available for receptor binding. Side effects include dry mouth, constipation, blurred vision and urinary retention (anticholinergic effects). They may also cause postural hypotension and serious cardiac problems, such as heart block and arrhythmias, and lower the seizure threshold in some people. Because of their serious side effects, these medications can lead to life-threatening consequences if taken in large quantities, such as in suicide attempts, and if this is suspected, immediate action to support life must be instigated (Box 21.3 lists signs of overdose). In the case of severe depression or suicidality, close supervision is required. When the person is not an in-patient, the dispensing of small, sub-lethal quantities is recommended. Personal Perspectives: Consumer's story - Julie relates some of the side effects of tricyclic medications.

PERSONAL PERSPECTIVES

Consumer's Story 21.1: Julie

When I began taking amitriptyline for severe depression, I felt overwhelmed by side effects. My energy level was comparable to having severe flu. I experienced blurred vision, difficulty waking in the morning and an incredibly dry mouth that woke me many times throughout the night. The health professional listened to my concerns and was very understanding, patient and collaborative. He asked me to be patient because the side effects should lessen with time, but explained that we could also experiment with adjusting the dosage, adding in other medications or, if necessary, changing the medication. Knowing of my anorexia diagnosis, he had also made me aware of the potential side effect of weight gain and allowed me to decide whether I could tolerate the risk of weight gain. It was good to feel heard and supported, and reassuring to know there were other options if the side effects continued to be unbearable. I don't think I should have to choose between living with terrible physical side effects or suffering from debilitating depression, but some health professionals don't appear to agree. It's important to me that they take the time and effort to find a good solution that minimises mental illness symptoms without creating unbearable physical side effects. Over time the side effects from amitriptyline decreased; however, they remained intolerable, so my health professional and I agreed that I would cease taking it. As I had made many lifestyle changes to support my physical and mental health, and since my depression had lessened, we decided I would try managing without medication. There is always an option to try a different medication if I need to; however, it has not been necessary.

BOX 21.4 Food and Medications to be Avoided by Consumers Taking MAOIs

Avoid:
- cheeses, especially matured cheeses
- pickled herrings, cured meats and beef extracts such as Marmite/Vegemite
- liver and chicken livers
- whole broad beans, avocados (especially if overripe), soybean paste
- figs, especially if overripe
- large numbers of bananas
- alcoholic drinks, especially chianti and red wine
- other antidepressant medications, nasal and sinus decongestants, narcotics, adrenaline (epinephrine)
- stimulants, hayfever and asthma medications.

Monoamine Oxidase Inhibitors (MAOIs)

MAOIs were the first group of antidepressant medications discovered. They remain very effective antidepressants; however, due to their potentially serious side effects, the newer antidepressant medications have mostly replaced their use. MAOIs work by inhibiting both types of the enzyme (MAO A and B) that metabolise serotonin and noradrenaline. People taking these medications must avoid noradrenaline agonists, which include its dietary precursor, tyramine. Adverse effects include drowsiness or insomnia, agitation, fatigue, gastrointestinal disturbances, weight gain, hypotension, dizziness, dry mouth/skin, sexual dysfunction, constipation and blurred vision.

Interactions. The major concern with using these medications is their potential to interact with specific foods that contain tyramine and other amine medications, such as those found in most cough preparations (see Box 21.4). Such an interaction can result in excessive and dangerous elevation in blood pressure, known as a *hypertensive crisis*.

Selective Serotonin Reuptake Inhibitors (SSRIs)

The SSRI group of antidepressant medications inhibits the reuptake of serotonin at the presynaptic membrane. This leads to an increased availability of serotonin in the synapse and, therefore, at the receptors, thereby promoting serotonin transmission. These medications are as effective as tricyclic antidepressants, but safer because they cause less serious side effects and have decreased risk of death by overdose.

HISTORICAL ANECDOTE 21.1

The Evolution of Methamphetamine

One of the earliest antidepressant medications of the 20th century was the amphetamine Benzedrine, launched by the pharmaceutical company Smith, Kline & French in 1936. The company began advertising Benzedrine for treating mild depression in 1942 and by 1948 they were promoting the amphetamine as the "antidepressant of choice". In 1950, Smith, Kline & French released a hybrid amphetamine and barbiturate medication called Dexamyl, which was a combination of dextroamphetamine and the barbiturate amobarbital. The medication was promoted for its "smooth and profound antidepressant effect". By 1950, several pharmaceutical companies were marketing methamphetamine for its antidepressant qualities. The firm Burroughs Wellcome named its product "Methedrine", while the company Endo Products called theirs "Norodin". Few people in the 1950s could have predicted that methamphetamine would go on to become one of the most tightly regulated and stigmatised drugs of the early 21st century – colloquially referred to as "ice".

Read More About It:
Hirschfeld 2000, History and evolution of the monoamine hypothesis of depression. J Clin Psychiatry, 61(Suppl6), 4–6.

While the actions and effectiveness of these medications are similar, they are all structurally different from each other, resulting in differences in their side effects. Side effects are similar to those of the tricyclic group, except that they do not have cardiovascular, sedative and anticholinergic side effects. Nausea, diarrhoea, anxiety and restlessness, insomnia, sexual dysfunction (numbing), loss of appetite, weight loss and headache are the most common side effects. They should not be stopped abruptly; the withdrawal syndrome includes symptoms such as dizziness, paraesthesia, anxiety, sleep disturbance, agitation and tremor. They should not be combined with MAOIs.

Interactions. Alcohol may potentiate the effect of SSRIs. Use with cimetidine may result in increased concentrations of SSRIs in the bloodstream. Hypertensive crisis may occur if taken within 14 days of MAOIs. *Serotonin syndrome* is an uncommon but potentially serious set of adverse effects linked to SSRIs when the levels of serotonin become too high. This may be a result of taking other medications which also elevate serotonin levels (e.g. St John's Wort). Symptoms of serotonin syndrome include: confusion, agitation, muscle twitching, sweating, shivering, diarrhoea. Serotonin syndrome should be treated as a medical emergency.

Noradrenaline Serotonin Reuptake Inhibitors

Noradrenaline serotonin reuptake inhibitors (NSRIs) are a newer class of antidepressant medications. They are considered more effective than SSRIs in some people. NSRIs block the reuptake of serotonin and noradrenaline, thus increasing the amount of these neurotransmitters available at the synapse. Common side effects associated with NSRIs include nausea, dry mouth, dizziness, excessive sweating, agitation and constipation.

Mood-Stabilising Medications

Mood-stabilising medications are primarily used for treating bipolar disorder. Bipolar disorder is characterised by periods of major depressive disorder or dysthymia, as well as periods of mania or hypomania. Treatment aims to stabilise a person's mood between these two "poles". Lithium, a naturally occurring salt, has been and largely remains the medication of choice for treating acute mania and for the ongoing maintenance of consumers with a history of mania. An Australian, John Cade (Cade 2000), discovered its effectiveness as a treatment for mania in 1949 (see also Chapter 12). Cade observed that lithium was highly sedative in doses which were close to toxic levels. Just how lithium works is not clear, but it is known to mimic the effects of sodium, thereby compromising the ability of neurones to release, activate or respond to neurotransmitters. It does appear to reduce the sodium content of the brain and increase central serotonin synthesis and noradrenaline reuptake (Goldberg & Stahl 2021). Lithium use has been decreasing in recent years due to concerns about side effects and long-term health impacts (particularly on kidney function), as well as an increasing number of other medications being used successfully, either alone or in combination with lithium, to control the symptoms of mania. A number of anticonvulsant medications are used successfully to reduce mania and manage depression in bipolar affective disorder. Antipsychotics and particularly atypical antipsychotics are increasingly used to manage both acute mania and prophylactically to prevent relapse. Some atypical antipsychotics are also effective in treating bipolar depression. Antipsychotic medications are discussed later in this chapter.

Lithium

Indications for use. Lithium is the medication of choice for treating acute mania and the ongoing maintenance of people with bipolar disorder (Grunze et al 2018; Malhi et al 2021; Malhi et al 2017). It is also used in the treatment of unipolar depression, aggressive behaviour, conduct disorder and schizoaffective disorder.

Side effects. Most side effects of lithium depend on the plasma level and are widely recognised. However, individuals frequently experience mild neurological symptoms with higher plasma lithium levels. Around 75% of individuals who use lithium experience some side effects, but most are minor. These may include temporary metallic taste in the mouth, nausea/vomiting, polyuria and thirst, mild swelling, fine hand tremor, hypotension, difficulty concentrating and drowsiness. Fortunately, these side effects can be minimised or eliminated by adjusting the dose or dosage schedule. Aside from the previously mentioned adverse effects, patients may find the risks of weight gain and mental side effects (such as cognitive impairment or reduced intensity of perceptions and emotions) important (Livingstone & Rampes 2006).

The long-term use of lithium can impact kidney function, and it is crucial to closely monitor the estimated glomerular filtration rate (eGFR) as part of safety measures, especially in older people. Hypothyroidism is also common with lithium treatment, and substitution therapy may be necessary (Livingstone & Rampes 2006). Women are at a higher risk than men, with 14% of women being affected versus 4.5% of men (Grunze et al 2018). In some cases, the first signs of deterioration in thyroid or kidney function due to lithium treatment may be detectable within the first 3 months of use. Although lithium has a teratogenic effect, it is rarely a reason to avoid treatment, since the risk is well understood and relatively low in absolute terms. Nonetheless, specific management is required during pregnancy.

Contraindications/precautions. Lithium is contraindicated with cardiac or renal disease, dehydration, sodium depletion, brain damage, pregnancy and lactation. Care should be taken with thyroid disorders, diabetes, urinary retention and in people with a history of seizures. The therapeutic range for lithium in Australia is 0.6–1.2 mmol/L for acute mania and 0.4–0.8 mmol/L for maintenance, while the recommended levels in Aotearoa New Zealand are 0.6–0.8 mmol/L, but lower in maintenance and up to 1 mmol/L for severe symptoms (Gay et al 2019; Malhi et al 2021). A lower therapeutic range is recommended for maintenance therapy because long-term administration of lithium can be associated with serious side effects, such as renal and thyroid dysfunction. Symptoms of lithium toxicity rarely appear at levels below 1.2 mmol/L, but are common above 2.0 mmol/L (Megarbane et al 2014). Therefore, as the therapeutic and toxic levels are so close, extreme care must be taken in monitoring the consumer's blood level regularly, especially during early phases of the treatment. If the level exceeds 1.5 mmol/L, the next dose should be withheld and the doctor notified. Levels are usually monitored weekly until stable and then monthly. The blood samples for testing should be taken 12 hours after the last dose when lithium has been taken for at least 5–7 days (Malhi et al 2017; Psychotropic Expert Group 2013).

Interactions. Diuretics, ACE (angiotensin-converting enzyme) inhibitors, neuroleptics, non-steroidal anti-inflammatory medications, alcohol and caffeine may interfere with lithium absorption.

Consumer education

- Educate the person about the side effects and signs of toxicity (see Box 21.5 and Perspectives in practice: Nurse's story 21.2) and the need for regular blood level checks.
- Encourage the person to avoid dehydration and include a regular intake of approximately 10 glasses of water every day.
- Remind the person to take their medication regularly, even when they are feeling well.

BOX 21.5 Signs of Lithium Toxicity

- **Early stages** – anorexia, nausea, vomiting, diarrhoea, coarse hand tremor, twitching, lethargy, dysarthria, hyperactive deep tendon reflexes, ataxia, tinnitus, vertigo, weakness, drowsiness
- **Later stages** – fever, decreased urinary output, decreased blood pressure, irregular pulse, ECG changes, impaired consciousness, seizures, coma, death

Note: Lithium toxicity is a medical emergency.

- Advise the person not to operate machinery until the initial drowsiness subsides.
- Discuss the risks of taking lithium during pregnancy or when considering pregnancy.
- Advise the person of the potential dangers of only taking lithium prior to a blood test and to discuss their concerns about taking the medication with their prescriber.

PERSPECTIVES IN PRACTICE

Nurse's Story 21.2: Marnie

An older consumer was admitted to an in-patient unit for an episode of manic behaviour. She had experienced mania before and was on continuous treatment with lithium. The lithium dose was increased during the admission. The nurse returned to the ward after 2 days' leave and noticed that the consumer appeared unwell, had a coarse tremor, was confused, ataxic and had myoclonic jerks. She called the doctor on call, expressed her concern and told him she would withhold the evening dose of lithium. She asked him to see the consumer as soon as possible and to organise to have blood taken for a lithium level. The doctor refused to come to the ward and disagreed with the nurse's concern about the consumer. He insisted she give the evening dose of the medication and said he would see the consumer the next morning. The nurse refused to accept his decision and called her immediate supervisor and explained her concern for the consumer's wellbeing. The medication was withheld, and an urgent blood request determined that the consumer's lithium level was 2.2 mmol/L. The nurse had correctly diagnosed lithium toxicity and taken the correct action to advocate best care for the consumer.

Anticonvulsants

Indications for use. Several anticonvulsant medications have been used to treat mania, especially when lithium is ineffective. Carbamazepine, valproate, lamotrigine and topiramate are examples of commonly used anticonvulsants. These medications have been found to have acute antimanic and mood-stabilising effects. Carbamazepine, sodium valproate, topiramate (Fountoulakis et al 2020) and lamotrigine (Fountoulakis et al 2020) are recommended treatments for mixed or bipolar states, secondary mania, rapid cycling bipolar affective disorder, and lithium refractoriness. Lamotrigine is identified as an effective alternative to antidepressants in treating bipolar depression, particularly in relation to concerns about antidepressant-induced mania.

Side effects

- **Carbamazepine** – blood dyscrasias, drowsiness, nausea, vomiting, constipation or diarrhoea, hives or skin rashes, hepatitis
- **Sodium valproate** – prolonged bleeding time, gastrointestinal upset, tremor, ataxia, weight gain, somnolence, dizziness, hepatic failure, polycystic ovary syndrome in women
- **Topiramate** – cognitive impairment, sedation, nausea, weight loss, dizziness, vomiting, rash, agitation, paraesthesia
- **Lamotrigine** – blurred vision, rash, nausea, ataxia, drowsiness

Contraindications/precautions. Anticonvulsants are contraindicated with MAOIs and during lactation. Caution is required in older adults, people with cardiac/renal disease and during pregnancy. Before commencing carbamazepine, a range of tests should be performed, including blood film examination, electrolytes, liver and kidney function and an ECG. Carbamazepine may also interfere with the metabolism and blood concentrations of other medications, so care is needed with oral contraceptives and other medications. There is a risk of fetal malformation, so it should not be taken during pregnancy.

Sodium valproate should not be taken with aspirin and some antipsychotics. It may enhance the effects of alcohol and other CNS depressants. Polycystic ovary syndrome is more common among women

treated with valproate; symptoms tend to emerge early, often within the first few months of treatment (Li et al 2021). Women should be informed of this risk before starting treatment.

Interactions

- **Carbamazepine** – erythromycin, isoniazid, oral contraceptives, theophylline, fluoxetine
- **Valproate** – may potentiate alcohol, carbamazepine, barbiturates; should not be taken with aspirin or antipsychotics
- **Topiramate** – concomitant use with lithium and valproate can cause cognitive impairment

Consumer education

- Inform the person about avoiding sudden cessation of the tablets.
- Encourage the person to report unusual symptoms to their doctor: spontaneous bruising, unusual bleeding, sore throat, fever, malaise, or yellow skin or eyes.
- Remind the person to take medications with meals if gastrointestinal upset occurs.
- Advise the person to avoid taking alcohol or non-prescription medications without consulting a doctor.
- Explain that pregnancy must be avoided while taking the medication. Alternative methods of contraception may be required if taking sodium valproate, as oral contraception may not be effective.

Antipsychotic or Neuroleptic Medications

The traditional neuroleptic or antipsychotic medications (also known as the typical antipsychotics, major tranquillisers, or first generation antipsychotics) have played an important role in the treatment of people with psychotic disorders since their discovery in the 1950s. Each group of the typical antipsychotics appears to be equally effective for reducing or eliminating the positive symptoms of psychosis (e.g. delusions, hallucinations, motor disturbances). However, these drugs were often administered in doses that led to stigmatising side effects. The newer, second-generation antipsychotics, commonly referred to as the "atypical" or "novel" antipsychotics, were introduced in the 1990s and have quickly become the medications of choice for psychotic symptoms. These medications tend to be better tolerated and less likely to lead to problems with medication adherence (Goldberg & Stahl 2021). Apart from clozapine, which has superior efficacy to the typical antipsychotics, their efficacy appears to be equal to that of the typical antipsychotics (Myles et al 2019; Psychotropic Expert Group 2013), but they are believed to be more effective in reducing the negative symptoms of psychosis. Clozapine, risperidone, paliperidone, amisulpride, olanzapine and quetiapine remain the most widely used examples of the second-generation antipsychotics.

HISTORICAL ANECDOTE 21.2

The Evolution of Phenothiazines

In the 1950s a French surgeon, Henri Laborit, used the antihistamine drug chlorpromazine to reduce the amount of general anaesthesia required by patients during surgery. Later, the calming effect of chlorpromazine was applied to psychiatric patients and, thanks to its tranquillising effect, it grew a reputation as the first "typical antipsychotic" or "major tranquillisers" belonging to the phenothiazine group, which includes thioridazine, trifluoperazine and fluphenazine. These drugs revolutionised management of the disruptive positive symptoms of schizophrenia. Although in recent years their use has been associated with problematic adverse reactions, back in the mid-20th century the phenothiazines provided new hope of successful illness management and even the prospect of independent living outside of the hospital setting.

Read More About It
Lopez-Munoz et al. 2005. History of the discovery and clinical introduction of chlorpromazine. Ann Clin Psychiatry, 17(3), 113–135.

The typical antipsychotics are dopamine antagonists. They primarily block the postsynaptic D_2 receptors but also exert other synaptic effects. They reduce the positive symptoms of schizophrenia. Atypicals, on the other hand, have dopamine receptor subtype 2 (D_2) and serotonin receptor subtype 2 ($5HT_2$) blocking actions.

Indications for use. Antipsychotics are indicated for treating acute and chronic psychoses, delusional disorder and severe depression where psychotic symptoms are present. Schizophrenia and schizoaffective disorders are the most common indications for antipsychotic medications. Some of the phenothiazine group have other uses, such as being an antiemetic in the case of prochlorperazine and treating intractable hiccups in the case of chlorpromazine (Srinivasan et al 2022). Many of the antipsychotic medications, especially chlorpromazine and haloperidol, have profound sedative effects (Meng et al 2018). This effect is particularly conspicuous early in treatment, although tolerance usually develops quickly.

Side effects. The side effects of the typical antipsychotics are varied. They can affect every system of the body and range from effects on the CNS – including movement disorders, sedation and seizures – through to potentially life-threatening side effects such as neuroleptic malignant syndrome (NMS) (see Table 21.4 for an overview of the side effects of the typical antipsychotics). The most troubling of the side effects are the *extrapyramidal reactions*. These result from the effects of the antipsychotic medications on the extrapyramidal motor system. This is the same system responsible for the movement disorders of Parkinson's disease. Acute dystonia, parkinsonism and akathisia occur early and can be managed by a variety of medications, including antiparkinsonian and benzodiazepine medications. *Tardive dyskinesia* generally occurs later and has no known effective treatment (NewsRx LLC – Clinical Trials 2021; Soares & McGrath 1999). The Abnormal Involuntary Movements Scale (AIMS) (see Box 21.6) is useful for nurses to detect movement disorders in consumers. Neuroleptic malignant syndrome (NMS), an idiosyncratic hypersensitivity to antipsychotic medications, is a rare but serious reaction that is potentially life threatening (see Box 21.7). Perspectives in Practice: Nurse's story: Lesley (overleaf) relates the experiences of a patient who contracted oculogyric crisis (OGC).

Contraindications/precautions. Caution should be taken in administering antipsychotics to older people and to those who are medically ill or diagnosed with diabetes. Safety in pregnancy and lactation is not clear. They are contraindicated in people with a known sensitivity to one of the phenothiazines as a cross-sensitivity is possible. People taking typical antipsychotics should avoid extremes of temperature because of potential photosensitivity, hypothermia and heatstroke. Typical antipsychotics may affect the body's ability to regulate temperature, primarily by inhibiting sweating. The medications may also cause photosensitivity.

TABLE 21.4 Side Effects of the Typical Antipsychotics

Side Effects	Key Features	Time of Maximal Risk	Interventions
CNS Extrapyramidal Side Effects			
Acute dystonic reaction	Painful muscle spasms in the head, back and torso; can last minutes to hours, occur suddenly; can cause fear	1–5 days	Administer antiparkinsonian medication quickly; respiratory support if needed; reassure and remain with the consumer
Akathisia	Restlessness, leg aches, person cannot stay still	5–60 days	Administer antiparkinsonian medication; change medication
Neuroleptic malignant syndrome	Potentially fatal with hyperthermia, severe extrapyramidal side effects, sweating, muscle rigidity, clouding of consciousness, elevated creatine phosphokinase	Usually hours or days after a dose increase	Supportive therapy; cease all medications; treat with bromocriptine or dantrolene
Parkinsonism	Rigid, mask-like facial expression; shuffling gait; drooling	5–30 days; can recur even after a single dose	Administer dopamine agonist; support the consumer
Seizures	Typical antipsychotics reduce seizure threshold, risk about 1% but greater with rapid titration or history of seizures	Early in treatment	May need to stop the medication, observe the consumer or manipulate the medication dose
Tardive dyskinesia	Usually results from prolonged use of typical antipsychotics; stereotyped involuntary movements (tongue, lips, feet)	After months or years of treatment (worse on withdrawal)	Assess the consumer often; change to atypical medications; no other treatment available
Other			
Anticholinergic	Dry mouth, blurred vision, orthostatic hypotension, tachycardia, urinary retention, nasal congestion		Observe, educate the consumer; provide support where needed; may need to change medication
Endocrine	Weight gain, diminished libido, impotence, amenorrhoea, galactorrhoea		Educate the consumer; reduce kilojoule intake; may need to change medication
Photosensitivity	Skin hyperpigmentation		Educate the consumer to avoid sun and wear protective clothing, sunscreen and sunglasses
Sedation	May be beneficial in agitated consumers; can be mistaken for cognitive slowing		Educate the consumer to avoid driving or operating machinery; rest periods; adjust dose

BOX 21.6 Useful Tools for Assessing Medication Side Effects

LUNSERS

The LUNSERS (Liverpool University Neuroleptic Side Effect Rating Scale) is a useful tool for assessing side effects. It is designed for self-administration but can also be a useful tool for nurses to help detect consumer reactions to changes in treatment (Morrison et al 2000).

To access the scale, see: Day JC, Wood G, Dewey M et al. 1995 A self-rating scale for measuring neuroleptic side effects: Validation in a group of schizophrenic patients. Br J Psychiatry 166(5), 650–653.

AIMS

The AIMS (Abnormal Involuntary Movements Scale) is a widely used tool for use with people on long-term antipsychotic medications. It is designed to assess for signs of tardive dyskinesia.

To access the scale, see: Munetz MR, Benjamin S 1988 How to examine patients using the Abnormal Involuntary Movements Scale. Hospital and Community Psychiatry 39(11), 1172–1177.

BOX 21.7 Neuroleptic Malignant Syndrome

NMS is a rare disorder that resembles a severe form of parkinsonism with coarse tremor and catatonia, fluctuating in intensity, accompanied by signs of autonomic instability (labile pulse and blood pressure, hyperthermia), stupor, elevation of creatinine kinase in serum, and sometimes myoglobinaemia. In severe forms it may persist for more than a week after ceasing the medication. The risk of death from this syndrome is high (more than 10%); therefore, immediate medical intervention is required if suspected. NMS is associated with higher number of antipsychotics used, use of first-generation agents (typical antipsychotics), and higher maximum doses. In particular, NMS is associated more highly with haloperidol, aripiprazole, depot flupenthixol decanoate and benzodiazepines.

Su et al 2014.

PERSPECTIVES IN PRACTICE

Nurse's Story 21.3: Lesley

Oculogyric crisis (OGC) is an acute dystonic reaction that is a side effect of some of the neuroleptic medications prescribed for psychosis. It is a distressing side effect characterised by prolonged involuntary upward deviation of the eyes.

Phil was a young man who had been admitted to an acute in-patient mental health unit as an involuntary patient to treat a first presentation psychosis. He was prescribed a neuroleptic medication (risperidone) by the psychiatrist. On the third day of pharmacological treatment, Phil was sitting in the unit corridor when I arrived for my shift. I noted him sitting stiffly in the chair with his eyes turned towards the ceiling, his neck flexed and his mouth open wide. These are classic symptoms of OGC and require immediate intervention.

Speaking with Phil, I realised he was distressed by the symptoms. Working quickly and quietly so as not to cause further anguish, benztropine was administered by intramuscular route as prescribed with the symptoms abating within 15 minutes. I sat with Phil for the next 30 minutes to ensure the efficacy of the prescribed medication, to describe in detail what had occurred and to allay his fears. During his 3-week admission to the mental health unit, Phil experienced further OGC episodes, all treated in the same manner.

Offering immediate assistance, support and ongoing education is imperative to ensure that appropriate treatment is provided. While OGC is not a common side effect from neuroleptic medications, it is experienced by young men in particular. As mental health nurses, we need to be able to recognise medication side effects and manage them effectively.

Interactions. Concurrent use with antidepressants, antihistamines and antiparkinsonian agents may result in additional anticholinergic effects. Antacids and antidiarrhoeals may disrupt absorption of the antipsychotic. Alcohol may cause additional CNS depression.

Consumer education. The person will need education about the medication side effects and assistance with managing these effects and recognising problematic adverse events. People taking typical antipsychotics should be careful in the sun (wear hats, sunglasses and sunscreen) and in extremes of temperature (remaining cool and hydrated).

Atypical Antipsychotics

Atypical antipsychotics are not all pharmacologically alike, so they tend to have different effect profiles. They do, however, have some similar side effects, such as weight gain, constipation and dizziness, and are also linked to the development of metabolic syndrome and diabetes (Hasan et al 2017; McDaid & Smyth 2015). Some may cause extrapyramidal side effects at higher doses (e.g. risperidone), but they are not uniformly associated with parkinsonian symptoms, akathisia, dystonia or dyskinesia (Hasan et al 2017; Remington et al 2013). Seizures may also occur with too rapid a titration associated with an increase in dosage. In addition, cardiac problems such as atrial fibrillation, atrial flutter or myocarditis early in treatment, although uncommon, may occur.

Some of the side effects of individual medications include:

- **clozapine** – more safety concerns than any other antipsychotic medication (Hasan et al 2017; Remington et al 2013). A serious adverse effect is agranulocytosis, which is reduced white blood cell count in the body, and it occurs in 1–2% of consumers. Precautions must be taken to ensure swift detection of agranulocytosis (which may manifest in an acute cough or infection). Other adverse effects include constipation and paralytic ileus, hypersalivation (especially annoying during sleep) and tachycardia. Clozapine is one of the two most obesogenic antipsychotic medications (along with olanzapine).
- **ziprasidone** – dizziness, tremor, dry mouth, hypotension
- **risperidone** – insomnia, agitation, anxiety, headache, postural hypotension particularly at the start of treatment, drowsiness, weight gain, gastrointestinal upset, sexual dysfunction and extrapyramidal symptoms
- **olanzapine** – drowsiness, weight gain, postural hypotension, peripheral oedema, extrapyramidal symptoms and anticholinergic side effects (dry mouth, hypotension, tachycardia)
- **quetiapine** – mild somnolence, mild asthenia, dry mouth, limited weight gain, postural hypotension, tachycardia and occasional syncope.

Weight Gain and Metabolic Syndrome

Weight gain and the development of *metabolic syndrome* associated with the atypical antipsychotics is a serious health concern (Hasan et al 2017; McDaid & Smyth 2015). All commonly-used antipsychotics can contribute to rapid and clinically significant weight gain (Barton et al 2020). The weight gain usually occurs during the first 4–12 weeks of treatment. After the initial period the weight gain continues at a lower level over a prolonged period (Rotella et al 2020). Weight gain linked to atypical antipsychotics is typically associated with abdominal obesity and enhanced adiposity, which is linked with increased morbidity and mortality, as well as reduced quality of life (Rotella et al 2020). Together these changes make up what is referred to as "metabolic syndrome", a cluster of metabolic abnormalities, including hypertension, hyperlipidaemia, hyperglycaemia and abdominal obesity, which, when experienced together, lead to an increased risk of diabetes and cardiovascular disease.

Previous Australian studies have found the prevalence rates of metabolic syndrome in people with schizophrenia to range between 51% and 68% (John et al 2009; Tirupati & Chua 2007). Another Australian cohort study of people prescribed clozapine (Hyde et al 2015) found higher prevalence rates for cardiovascular and metabolic events than previous Australian studies. The most common cardiovascular condition revealed was ECG-defined abnormalities (60%), while low high-density lipoprotein (HDL) cholesterol levels (69%) and high triglyceride levels (77%) were the most common metabolic abnormalities.

The weight gain and high rate of metabolic disturbance with the atypical antipsychotics is linked to several factors, including impairment of the glucose metabolism system, which regulates appetite and weight management. Impairment of this system appears to be linked to developing type 2 diabetes and dyslipidaemia (Hepburn & Brzozowska 2016; Rotella et al 2020). However, while weight gain and cardiovascular risk have been attributed to modifiable risk factors, including smoking, sedentary lifestyles, lack of exercise and substance misuse, there is evidence to suggest that autonomic dysfunction exists, even in medication-free individuals, and that some of the psychotropic medications can exacerbate cardiac risk in these individuals (Alvares et al 2016; Rotella et al 2020).

Metabolic syndrome is diagnosed when a person has a girth measurement higher than recommended and any two of the following: Raised triglycerides, reduced HDL cholesterol, raised blood pressure and raised fasting plasma glucose. Management of the syndrome includes lifestyle changes (improving nutrition and increasing exercise), ongoing monitoring and medication for dyslipidaemia, hypertension and glucose intolerance if required. Guidelines for assessing metabolic syndrome include baseline screening that includes girth measurement, weight, height, body mass index (BMI), blood chemistry and family and personal history, followed by regular monitoring. Thus, attention to the physical health of people prescribed antipsychotics is an important nursing role (discussed in more detail in Chapter 20).

Early intervention for weight gain with the atypical antipsychotics should occur when the person begins taking the medication or when medication changes are made and should target reduced kilojoule intake and increased exercise, as these have been shown to have a positive ameliorating effect on weight gain. Several interventions have been introduced to manage the weight gain linked to these medications. For example, lifestyle interventions, education, weight loss medications and exercise have all been implemented and evaluated. Research to date indicates significantly greater weight reduction in lifestyle intervention groups than in pharmacological intervention groups or standard care groups (Bradley et al 2022; Park et al 2011).

Nurses should ensure consumers are regularly screened for weight gain, diet and exercise. Indeed, nurses are well placed to educate people to make healthy choices to prevent weight gain and associated complications (Watkins et al 2020). It is important for nurses to be aware of the potential for weight gain with the atypical antipsychotics and to work with people when the medication is first introduced, rather than waiting until the weight gain becomes problematic (Park et al 2011), as the weight gain associated with these medications is known to cause significant distress (Goldberg & Stahl 2021).

Contraindications/precautions.

Clozapine. People taking clozapine must be made aware of the potential risk of agranulocytosis and be monitored regularly. Because of the medication's link to agranulocytosis, it is restricted to those who have not responded to at least two other antipsychotics. Clozapine can be prescribed through the Clozaril Patient Monitoring

---

BOX 21.8 Managing Constipation Side Effects Caused By Psychotropic Medications

Assess for:
- regular bowel movements
- current diet, exercise
- other medications

Advise to:
- drink 10 glasses of water per day
- increase fibre in diet
- increase exercise
- use available pharmacological products as needed.

System program only. The person's blood (specifically white blood cell counts) should be monitored weekly for 18 weeks and monthly thereafter. An immediate differential blood count must be ordered if the consumer reports flu-like symptoms. If during treatment an infection occurs and/or the white blood cell (WBC) count drops below 3500/mm^3, or drops by a substantial amount from baseline, a repeat WBC and differential count should be completed. If the results confirm a WBC count below 3500/mm^3 and/or reveal an absolute neutrophil count (ANC) of between 2000 and 1500/mm^3, the WBC and ANC must be checked at least twice weekly. If the WBC count falls below 3000/mm^3 and/or the ANC count drops below 1500/mm^3, clozapine must be withdrawn at once and the consumer closely monitored. Care should be taken when using these medications with older people.

Interactions. Medications known to have substantial potential to depress bone marrow function should be avoided concurrently with clozapine. Atypical antipsychotics may enhance the effect of alcohol and other CNS depressants.

Consumer education. Advice about having regular blood tests when taking clozapine should be provided. People should also be told the importance of seeing a doctor immediately for any flu-like symptoms while taking clozapine. Information on possible side effects and medication interactions related to atypical antipsychotic medications should be provided.

While constipation is often considered a minor medication side effect, it is a potentially serious side effect of clozapine. There have been several deaths associated with constipation resulting from clozapine. Other serious outcomes include paralytic ileus, bowel obstruction and toxic megacolon (Every-Palmer & Ellis 2017; Jessurun et al 2013). It is essential for people to be warned of the potential for constipation, be educated about the need to monitor bowel habits and use interventions to manage constipation (e.g. drinking 6–8 glasses of water per day). See Box 21.8 for more interventions.

Antiparkinsonian Medications Used to Treat Tardive Symptoms

Antiparkinsonian medications, also referred to as anticholinergics, are used to reduce the extrapyramidal side effects or tardive side effects of antipsychotic medications. Antiparkinsonian medications with a central anticholinergic action act to reduce the symptoms associated with parkinsonism, acute dystonia and akathisia (which together make up the tardive symptoms experienced by some who take antipsychotic medications). They inhibit the action of acetylcholine and are presumed to decrease cholinergic influence in the basal ganglia and thereby help balance the effects of antipsychotic medication reduction of dopaminergic influence (Cornett et al 2017; Psychotropic Expert Group 2013). See Table 21.5 for examples of antiparkinsonian medications, action and side effects.

TABLE 21.5 Antiparkinsonians: Action and Side Effects

Name	Action	General Side Effects (Dose-Related)
Benztropine mesylate	Antihistamine and sedating qualities, long acting	(Anticholinergic) Dry mouth, dilated pupils, urinary hesitancy, constipation, blurred vision, nausea
Benzhexol (trihexyphenidyl)	Specific anticholinergic action; stimulant properties	Dizziness, hallucinations
Biperiden	Anticholinergic action	Euphoria, hyperpyrexia
Orphenadrine	Anticholinergic action	Delirium in older people

SPECIAL ISSUES WITH PSYCHOTROPIC MEDICATIONS

Anticholinergic Psychosis

Caution should be used with the anticholinergic drugs because many other medications have anticholinergic effects (e.g. over the counter cold and flu remedies) and the effects can be cumulative and lead to anticholinergic toxicity. The anticholinergic toxidrome can be remembered by the mnemonic, "red as a beet, dry as a bone, blind as a bat, mad as a hatter, hot as a hare, full as a flask" (Feinberg 1993). This refers to dry, red flushed skin and mucus membranes, blurred vision, symptoms of delirium, hyperthermia and urinary retention.

Serotonin Syndrome

Serotonin is a chemical involved in communication between nerve cells in the brain. Too much serotonin can cause excess cell activity, leading to a potentially serious expression of symptoms known as "serotonin syndrome". Serotonin syndrome may occur within hours of taking a new medication (Werneke et al 2016). Medications that affect any step in the serotonin metabolism or regulation pathways can provoke the syndrome. Antidepressants, especially SSRIs, are the most implicated. Symptoms of serotonin syndrome include confusion, agitation, dilated pupils, headache, nausea/vomiting, rapid heart rate, tremors, shivering, loss of muscle coordination and heavy sweating. Prompt treatment and discontinuation of the offending medications is vital. Most situations are self-limiting if the medication is ceased quickly; however, supportive care is required until the crisis is over.

Cognitive Enhancers/Stimulants

Cognitive enhancers improve memory, boost energy and alertness levels, and increase concentration. These medications have been studied extensively over the last decade to improve cognitive function across a number of clinical conditions. Developmental conditions such as attention deficit/hyperactivity disorder are treated with methylphenidate and atomoxetine (Husain & Mehta 2011; Kowalczyk et al 2019). Side effects include high body temperature; increased activity; dry mouth; euphoria; decreased fatigue, drowsiness and appetite; nausea and headaches; and increased blood pressure and respirations (Liang et al 2018). Neurodegenerative disorders such as Alzheimer's disease and Parkinson's disease are commonly treated with acetylcholinesterase inhibitors and memantine as standard practice. However, it is hard to determine whether these improve memory or alertness (Husain & Mehta 2011; Kowalczyk et al 2019). Side effects include nausea and other gastrointestinal upsets, and impairment of verbal and visual memory (Husain & Mehta 2011; Kowalczyk et al 2019).

PRO RE NATA (PRN) ANTIPSYCHOTIC MEDICATION ADMINISTRATION

The need to rapidly reduce agitation, distress or aggression often results in the prescription and administration of a prn antipsychotic medication in in-patient mental health facilities and emergency departments. Antipsychotics (major tranquillisers) and benzodiazepines (minor tranquillisers) are the main groups of medications used in this way. Generally, most prn medications are given in the first few days after admission and are most frequently administered during the evening shift, from 6.00 pm onwards, and at weekends (Goldberg & Stahl 2021). It appears that peaks in prn administration coincide with regular medication and mealtimes.

Reasons given for administering prn medications include agitation, threatening behaviour, irritability, abusiveness, insomnia, disruptiveness, physical reasons, nicotine craving or drug withdrawal, assaultive behaviour and request by the service user (Barr et al 2018). Nursing variables, such as skill mix and workloads, have also been identified as factors contributing to increased prn administrations (Mardani et al 2022; Ngune et al 2023).

When nurses give prn medications, they are often required to decide what to give from a range of medications, as well as the amount to give and when to administer them (Mardani et al 2022). This allows nurses to administer psychotropic medications rapidly in acute situations. Unfortunately, while this is an area of relative autonomy for nurses, it is also an area of practice that has been criticised, with concerns raised about over-reliance on psychotropic medications, the additive impacts of medications and polypharmacy (Barr et al 2018). Researchers have suggested that mental health facilities should offer a range of therapeutic options and ensure that prn medications are used sparingly, and that their use is monitored regularly (Mardani et al 2022; Mullen & Drinkwater 2011).

The medications most often prescribed for prn administration include olanzapine, which can be administered in a wafer form (sublingually). Olanzapine is particularly sedating when given to an otherwise drug naive person. In emergency settings, droperidol (which is a short-acting and potent D_2 antagonist) is often prescribed and administered intramuscularly to induce rapid sedation. The typical antipsychotics, particularly medications like haloperidol, have a long history of use. There is evidence to suggest that the benzodiazepines are just as effective as the typical antipsychotics in managing acute agitation and disturbed behaviour and should therefore be the medications of choice (Taylor et al 2021).

ADHERENCE AND CONCORDANCE WITH MEDICATIONS

Effective treatment for people with schizophrenia often requires a commitment to taking medications on a regular basis. Adherence to a prescribed antipsychotic medication regimen is often an ongoing problem for many service users. In the past, this issue has been referred to in the literature as non-compliance. However, the term "compliance" implies a power differential between the consumer and the healthcare provider, as well as passive rather than active participation by the person in the management of their mental health, so the accepted term is now "adherence".

The issue of medication adherence is complex and multifaceted and commentary rarely makes reference to the perceptions or experiences of service users (Shields et al 2019). When a person does not take their medication as prescribed, their symptoms may not improve at the rate expected, and they may be prone to cessation syndromes. Non-adherence may also be a signifier of a poor alliance with or lack of

BOX 21.9 Interventions to Help With Adherence to Medication

- Get to know the consumer well.
- Help the consumer to develop an understanding of why the medications have been prescribed.
- Spend time talking about medications and the decisions related to adherence.
- Ask about the side effects being experienced and offer strategies to manage side effects where possible.
- Help the consumer to discuss issues related to their medications with their doctor or nurse.
- Offer dispensers to assist with organising medications.
- Provide education sessions for family or significant others.

CASE STUDY 21.1

Discontinuation Leading to Neuroleptic Malignant Syndrome

A woman in her 40s diagnosed with paranoid schizophrenia attended the emergency department. She reported recently discontinuing antipsychotic and antidepressant medication she had been taking for eight years (clozapine 225 mg daily and venlafaxine XL 225 mg daily). On presentation she was perplexed, sweaty and shaking, and told the nurse she was hearing "voices". Assessment revealed WBC count 20,600/mL (20,600 mm³) and CPK 17361U, temperature 37.7°C, pulse 80–122 beats per minute and respirations 18–40 breaths per minute. She was diagnosed with NMS as a result of cholinergic rebound from clozapine and venlafaxine. She was transferred to the mental health unit and treatment included regular oral diazepam 20 mg and lorazepam 4 mg daily as needed. Her mental and physical state improved gradually over the following 2 weeks. She was then recommenced gradually on clozapine and venlafaxine and her mental state improved.

Adapted from Kurien & Vattakatuchery 2013.

engagement by health providers with the person. This can lead to assumptions by health professionals that the medication is not effective. In the long run, this can cause unnecessary treatment changes. However, taking these medications as prescribed can facilitate functional recovery and help prevent illness-related complications.

Causes of non-adherence are related to issues such as:
- medication side effects (the different side effects of the typical and atypical antipsychotic medications impact adherence differently), where the antipsychotic medication may have an adverse impact on the person's quality of life and may even cause more distress than the symptoms of the illness (Mathew et al 2023).
- anosognosia, or lack of insight into the illness and the relationship between the illness and the need to take medications (believed by some to be associated with some psychotic illnesses)
- personal preference.

Against advice, people sometimes stop taking their medications and, because they do not relapse immediately, fail to see the connection between the medications and their health. To help overcome lack of adherence with antipsychotic medications, several strategies have been explored (see Box 21.9). Evidence suggests that an active relationship between the nurse and the consumer is essential for improving adherence (Shields et al 2019). Other helpful strategies to aid adherence include education about the medications and their side effects, providing medication dispensers (Clyne et al 2011), frequent follow-up and support, and motivational interviewing strategies (Ertem & Duman 2019). It appears that no strategy is sufficient on its own, and a mixed approach to adherence may in fact be best. A recent study (Mathew et al 2023) sought to explore the views of mental health staff regarding adherence. The authors report a lack of clarity about who is responsible for adherence and a focus on personal belief rather than evidence when considering adherence strategies.

"Concordance" is a term now used to indicate an agreement between the consumer and a clinician regarding medication plans and choice. The key aspects of concordance are working together collaboratively and flexibly, understanding the consumer's beliefs about their condition and medications plans, and working towards agreed goals that end in shared decision-making (Edward & Alderman 2013; Fiorillo et al 2020; Mathew et al 2023).

Discontinuation Syndromes

Discontinuation syndrome can result from switching between or rapid withdrawal of one of the antidepressant or antipsychotic medications. Common symptoms of withdrawal include dizziness, paraesthesia, numbness, electric-shock-like sensations, lethargy, headache, tremor, nausea, sweating, anorexia, insomnia, nightmares, vomiting,

diarrhoea, rhinorrhoea, irritability, anxiety, restlessness, agitation and low mood (Reeves & Kamal 2019), as well as hyperthermia related to clozapine withdrawal (Cerovecki et al 2013). Rapid-onset psychosis (also called "hypersensitivity psychosis") occurs in some cases of discontinuation. As well as relapse of illness, sudden withdrawal of antipsychotic medications has been linked to rare but potentially life-threatening events, including NMS (Horowitz et al 2021; Kurien & Vattakatuchery 2013) and withdrawal catatonia (Horowitz et al 2021; Thanasan & Jambunathan 2010). Case study 21.1 overviews a case of discontinuation leading to NMS and demonstrates the importance for mental health nurses to be educated and aware of the physical conditions that can occur as a result of the withdrawal of psychotropic medications.

Exactly why discontinuation syndrome occurs is unclear (Salomon & Hamilton 2014), but it is thought to be linked to cholinergic and/or dopaminergic blockade and subsequent rebound (Cerovecki et al 2013). To avoid discontinuation syndrome, mental health nurses can facilitate open and ongoing conversations about this phenomenon and explore the lived experience of taking psychotropic medications. The important principle of education is to gradually reduce the dose (sometimes extremely slowly) before withdrawal or switching of medications. See Box 21.10 for more ways to minimise the occurrence of discontinuation syndrome.

Cardiac Risks Related to Psychotropic Medications

Mental health disorders are associated with an increased risk of all-cause mortality, most commonly related to cardiovascular disease, where an estimated two- to three-fold increased risk of cardiovascular disease has been noted across disorders, resulting in a reduction in life expectancy greater than that associated with heavy smoking (Alvares et al 2016).

BOX 21.10 How to Avoid and Manage Discontinuation Syndrome

- Switch between or withdraw from medications slowly – taper doses.
- Plan withdrawal and monitor closely.
- Prescribe hypnotics for insomnia.
- Prescribe antianxiety agents for other symptoms.

Cerovecki et al 2013

Several psychotropic medications have been associated with prolongation of the electrocardiograph QT interval, which is linked to lethal arrhythmias such as torsades de pointes, especially in individuals with underlying medical issues. Torsades de pointes, an uncommon ventricular tachycardia, is associated with QT prolongation, which can lead to sudden death.

Clinicians need to be vigilant regarding the emergence of cardiovascular symptoms, and a cardiovascular assessment of at-risk patients ought to be undertaken before treating with psychotropic medications or before an increase in dosage is considered. In particular, ECG monitoring, and a careful analysis of other QT risk factors, such as the consumer's other medications (other drugs may prolong the QT interval, such as some antibiotics and methadone) is required. Collaboration with other members of the healthcare team can often identify simple solutions to allow for optimal medical and mental health treatment (Beach et al 2018). Those drugs implicated in this problem include antidepressants such as citalopram and escitalopram, as well as antipsychotics ziprasidone, haloperidol (particularly intravenous infusion medications) and iloperidone (Beach et al 2018).

Consumer Education

Education about the need to take medications as prescribed has been identified as a key role for nurses. However, nurses report feeling inadequately prepared to educate others about psychotropic medications and many express concerns about their own knowledge deficit about these medications (Sanjeevi & Cocoman 2020). While education about medication has been proposed as an important strategy for improving adherence, education alone is not always effective. Education programs designed for improving adherence with psychotropic medications are more effective when combined with behavioural aspects of taking medication or motivational approaches, family therapy, psychological therapy or counselling, and enhancing the therapeutic alliance between the person and the treating team.

See Case studies 21.2 and 21.3 for examples of non-adherence and nursing responses.

CASE STUDY 21.2

Non-Adherence to Psychotropic Medications (Part A)

Tony was first diagnosed with paranoid schizophrenia 5 years ago. His symptoms were exacerbated by poor adherence to prescribed medications and "self-medication" with cannabis. Despite it being objectively clear that cannabis use made him more paranoid, Tony felt it helped him relax and was dismissive of education about harm-minimisation or abstaining.

The main hurdle to adherence with prescribed medication for Tony was denial. Tony did not accept his diagnosis; consequently, he did not accept his treatment. If we accept that a diagnosis of schizophrenia would provoke a sense of loss (e.g. normalcy, altered levels of independence, re-evaluated life goals, decreased acceptance), we may be able to understand the denial as a component of grief. Tony certainly displayed other classic stages of grief, most notably anger (at his treating psychiatrist) and bargaining (with his community case manager about postponing or cancelling administration of depot medications).

Other contributing factors to Tony's non-adherence were: the illness itself – paranoia is a barrier to building trust and rapport with clinicians; lack of education/understanding about the illness and its treatment; and the side effects of the prescribed medications.

CASE STUDY 21.3

Non-Adherence to Psychotropic Medications (Part B)

A management plan was developed to address the factors contributing to Tony's non-adherence. Tony's outpatient care was assigned to a clinical nurse in the role of case manager. This nurse administered and monitored prescribed medications and worked to build a therapeutic alliance with Tony. When Tony was an in-patient, as occurred frequently during the first 3 years of diagnosis, he was assigned a primary nurse on the mental health unit, who collaborated with the case manager to provide continuity of care and another avenue for Tony to develop rapport.

Over time, Tony began to engage with his two primary carers, which provided an opportunity for education about his diagnosis and treatment options. In time, Tony became more accepting of the treating team as a whole and would discuss medication issues freely with his treating psychiatrist.

As Tony's acceptance improved, medication options were no longer restricted to depot injections, and oral medications were trialled. Tony was very sensitive to typical antipsychotics and developed extrapyramidal side effects at sub-therapeutic doses. Trials of other atypical antipsychotic medications also had problems – poor symptom control and marked weight gain. Twelve months ago, a trial of clozapine began. It took 4 months to stabilise the dose at 450 mg nocte (at night). In doing so, Tony's mental state also stabilised. He developed considerable insight into his condition and treatment and has developed a good degree of acceptance.

Nine months later, with encouragement from the treating team, Tony undertook a trial of abstinence from cannabis. Tony says he has used cannabis only twice since. This hasn't been objectively checked through urine samples, but his case manager has noted further improvement in symptom control and motivation to undertake activities of daily living and social interaction.

Tony has not required admission to the mental health unit for over 8 months now. If he remains stable until the new year, his case manager intends to assist Tony in seeking work.

(The authors acknowledge this contribution from Paul McNamara, CNC, Consultation Liaison Team, Cairns Base Hospital, to this case study.)

? CRITICAL THINKING EXERCISE 21.1

1. Denial is a commonly used defence mechanism when a person is faced with issues they are not yet able to cope with on a conscious level. Discuss the concept of denial as a component of grief and loss in relation to the diagnosis of a chronic mental illness. How does the concept of denial differ from that of insight? In part A of the case study (Case study 21.2), how could the nurse manage Tony's non-adherence while recognising the importance of denial as a coping mechanism?
2. Explore relevant strategies to address the other factors contributing to Tony's non-adherence, such as his paranoia, lack of education and understanding and unwanted medication side effects.

? CRITICAL THINKING EXERCISE 21.2

1. In part B of the case study (Case study 21.3), Tony was trialled on atypical antipsychotics. How does this group of medications differ from typical antipsychotics? Identify the benefits and disadvantages of each of these medication groups.
2. The incidence of extrapyramidal side effects varies according to the particular antipsychotic medication used. Identify the various extrapyramidal side effects and explore the most effective management for these.
3. Tony was trialled on clozapine. What are the benefits and disadvantages of using this medication? Why is it not necessarily the first medication of choice for consumers with psychosis?

CRITICAL THINKING EXERCISE 21.2—cont'd

4. Cannabis is commonly used by consumers with a mental illness. What are the reasons for this? What does the term "self-medicating" mean? Explore the effect(s) of cannabis when a person has a psychosis.
5. Critically analyse the strategies in the management plan used for Tony's non-adherence. In your opinion, was the plan successful? If so (or not) explain the reason(s) for this.

Collaborative Prescribing

In some countries, including Australia and Aotearoa New Zealand, medications that could once only be prescribed by medical practitioners are being legally prescribed by other members of the multidisciplinary team including nurses, pharmacists and psychologists. In Australia and Aotearoa New Zealand, mental health nurse practitioners can legally prescribe medications to mental health consumers in both in-patient and community settings in collaboration with other members of the multidisciplinary team. Collaborative practice is said to occur when multiple health professionals from different discipline areas work together with consumers, their families and others to deliver the highest quality care across diverse settings (Fiorillo et al 2020). Collaborative practice has a positive impact on consumer outcomes. It rests on the principle of involving consumers in all aspects of mental health service delivery to support them in making informed decisions (Fiorillo et al 2020), in this case, about medication prescription.

Informed Consent and the Ethics of Psychotropic Medications

The right of a consumer to determine their own treatment underpins the underlying values of beneficence and respect for an individual's autonomy and wellbeing. The elements of a valid informed consent include that the person has the capacity to consent, has received adequate information to consent and has given consent voluntarily and freely. It is not enough to assume a person lacks the capacity to give consent based on their age, disability, appearance, behaviour, medical condition (including the presence of a mental disorder), beliefs or apparent inability to communicate, or because the consumer does not agree with the clinician's decision. Competent people have the right to refuse treatment for any reason. At times, substitute decision-makers, including family and carers, may consent on behalf of an individual when that individual is deemed to lack the capacity to make an authoritative decision (Law et al 2023). Informed consent regarding psychotropic medications can be very challenging. A consumer's mental illness may make it difficult for them to make a competent decision regarding treatment and the clinician may be concerned about their ability to make appropriate decisions about the need to continue medication.

This brings us to the issues of coerced or covert medication administration. Making consumers feel they have no option but to take a medication, or covertly (hiding the fact the consumer is being given a medication) administering a medication, is entirely unethical because it violates an individual's right to autonomy. However, if a consumer is deemed to lack the capacity to make a decision, the principle of autonomy is not violated as long as the treatment is deemed to be in the best interests of the consumer. Generally speaking, for such practices to be legal the person must be placed under relevant State guardianship laws or Mental Health Acts (which specify the conditions and circumstances under which a person can be administered medication against their expressed wishes or without their consent). It is therefore important that the clinician assesses whether the consumer has the capacity to agree to, or refuse, treatment as a matter of urgency, especially in emergency situations. An advance directive should be consulted if one is in place (Braun et al 2022). Case Study 21.4 examines some of the issues related to consent for these medications.

CASE STUDY 21.4

Ethical Issues Related to Consent to Psychotropic Medication

Jill, a registered nurse, commences her medication round and enters the bay of four consumers with the drug trolley.

She approaches consumer A, who is lying down in long-sleeve pyjamas. Having drawn up the injection, she approaches A, who sits up in bed and rolls up his sleeve to expose the injection site. Jill administers the injection without saying anything.

Jill moves to consumer B, aged 10, who is "groggy" from an anaesthetic and swallows his medication after Jill asks him to take his tablets.

Jill moves to consumer C and as she hands over the tablets the consumer asks what the various tablets are for. Jill says she does not know, but answers, "You'd better take them because that's what the doctor ordered".

Jill then moves to consumer D, and when handing the tablets to D the consumer says, "I'm not taking them." Jill replies: "If you don't, then don't expect dinner." D reluctantly takes the tablets.

Consent for these four consumers:

A. Consent can be expressed or implied. Rolling up the sleeve, for example, is an act consistent with giving *implied consent*. However, there should be some interpersonal engagement.

B. No consent for two reasons. First the consumer does not have *legal capacity* due to being minor (under 18); and second, no mental capacity to make a decision due to the anaesthetic.

C. Consent needs to be informed consent. C does not have the necessary information to make an *informed decision*.

D. Consent must be *freely* given without threat, inducement or coercion. Threatening to withhold a meal overrides the "free will" of D.

Remember the four elements of a valid consent. To take medication the consumer must have:

1. competence/capacity (age and cognitive ability)
2. the consent is given voluntarily
3. the consent covers the medication in question
4. that the consumer was fully informed in making that decision.
   (The authors acknowledge this contribution from Scott Trueman).

DEPOT OR LONG-ACTING INTRAMUSCULAR INJECTABLE ANTIPSYCHOTICS

Depot, or long-acting injectable antipsychotic preparations, introduced in the 1960s, are useful when there might be problems with adherence with oral medications, when the person is unable to take oral medications, if intestinal absorption is questioned or where accidental overdose is a possibility. Importantly, this strategy offers a more consistent treatment option (Smith & Herber 2015). There are also occasions where consumers express a preference for this form of treatment (Mathew et al 2021). These long-acting, injectable forms of antipsychotic medications, produced mostly in decanoate esters dissolved in an oily base, are prescribed for up to 33% of people with a diagnosis of schizophrenia (Taylor et al 2021). Mental health nurses are most commonly responsible for administering injectable antipsychotic medications, which may be delivered in both in-patient and community settings (Smith & Herber 2015). When administered by deep intramuscular injection, the medication is de-esterified to release the active medication, which slowly diffuses into the circulation. The injections are usually given every 2–4 weeks (Psychotropic Expert Group 2013) (see Table 21.6), and generally the release of medication must last at least 1 week to be considered a depot preparation. As depot injections involve large amounts of fluid, they should be injected into

TABLE 21.6   Long-Acting Injectables (Depot Medications)

Drug	Trade Names	Test Dose	Dose Range	Injection Interval	Comments
First-Generation Antipsychotics					
Flupenthixol decanoate	Depixol	5–20 mg injection	Usual dose range 20–40 mg every 2 to 4 weeks Higher doses of > 100 mg are used for treatment resistance	2–4 weekly	
Haloperidol	Haldol	Suggested 25 mg injection	50–300 mg	2–4 weekly	High prevalence of extrapyramidal side effects
Zuclopenthixol decanoate	Clopixol	100 mg injection	200–400 mg Higher doses are used for treatment resistance	Usually 2–4 weekly, although frequency can be increased	High prevalence of extrapyramidal side effects
Second-Generation Antipsychotics					
Aripiprazole monohydrate	Abilify Maintena	Establish tolerability with oral aripiprazole	300–400 mg	Usually 4 weekly Minimum of 26 days between injections	Requires 2 weeks of overlap with oral aripiprazole
Olanzapine pamoate	Zyprexa Relprevv	Establish tolerability with oral olanzapine	210 or 300 mg fortnightly or 405 mg monthly	2–4 weekly	Risk of post-injection syndrome Monitoring needed for at least 2 hours after administration
Paliperidone palmitate	Invega Sustenna	Establish tolerability with oral paliperidone or oral risperidone	25–150 mg	Monthly (after loading dose)	Loading dose schedule at initiation of treatment, 2 injections in first 8 days
Paliperidone palmitate	Invega Trinza	Only initiate after 4 months of treatment with Invega Sustenna (1-month paliiperidone palmitate)	175 mg, 263 mg, 350 mg or 525 mg	Every 3 months	
Paliperidone palmitate	Invega Hafyera	Only initiate after 4 months of treatment with Invega Sustenna (1-month paliperidone palmitate) or at least one 3-month injection cycle of Invega Trinza (3-month paliperidone palmitate)	700 mg or 1000 mg	Every 6 months	Administer the dose in a single injection; do not administer the dose in divided injections. Inject slowly, deep into the deltoid or gluteal muscle. For gluteal intramuscular use only. Do not administer by any other route. If the last dose of 1-month paliperidone was 100 mg the initial 6-month dose ought to be 700 mg, and 1000 mg where the last 1-month dose was 150 mg. If the last 3-month dose of paliperidone palmitate was 350 mg initiate the 6-month dose at 700 mg, and 1000 mg where the 3-month dose was 525 mg.
Risperidone	Risperdal Consta	Establish tolerability with immediate release oral risperidone	25–50 mg	Every 2 weeks	Initiation needs to overlap with oral treatment due to delayed action

Note: Please refer to current TGA information online for further information.
TGA 2024.

a large muscle using the Z-track technique (Yilmaz et al 2016). While this strategy is one way to manage adherence issues, it is important to remember that a strong therapeutic relationship can help promote medication adherence and that the consumer has a right to be involved in choosing the route of administration of prescribed medications wherever possible.

Medication for Acute Agitation

Acute agitation that may escalate to violence and aggression depends on a combination of personal factors (e.g. personality characteristics and intense mental distress) and external factors (e.g. the attitudes and behaviours of surrounding staff and service users, the physical setting and any restrictions that limit a person's freedom (National Collaborating Centre for Mental Health 2015). Acute agitation can occur in many different contexts, from a medical ward to a psychiatric intensive care unit, and is not necessarily related to a mental illness or disorder. Initial approaches to managing agitation should be psychosocial, particularly because medication interventions are often coercive, involve restraint and can be traumatising (Chieze et al 2019). However, at times when psychosocial intervention is unsuccessful, medication may be needed to prevent harm occurring to the person themselves or to others, including staff, family/carers and other patients.

Medications for acute agitation generally work as a result of their sedating, anxiolytic and tranquillising effects as opposed to treating

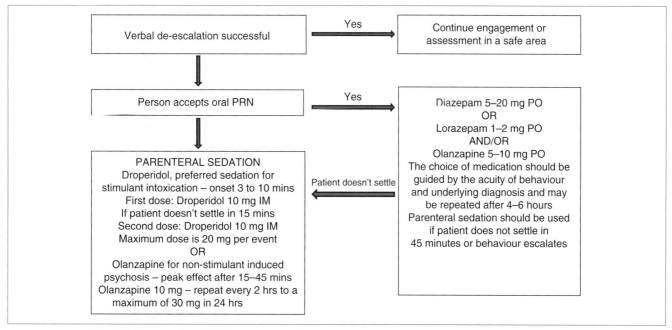

Fig. 21.1 Pharmacological Management of Acute Agitation and/or Aggression: Adults (Under 65 Years and/or no Diagnosis of Organic Cognitive Impairment). (Adapted from Galletly et al 2016 and Ministry of Health 2015.)

an underlying cause. First-line intervention should be to offer oral medications with benzodiazepines due to the favourable and broader effect profile (having muscle relaxant, anxiolytic, anticonvulsant and sedative effects) (Stahl 2021). Antipsychotics are very effective for managing agitated behaviour due to the neuroleptic effect of D_2 blockade, as well as strong histamine binding (that causes sedation) with first-generation medications (e.g. haloperidol and droperidol) and second-generation medications such as olanzapine (Stahl 2021). Antipsychotic medications may also have the benefit of helping to treat underlying psychotic symptoms when agitation is related to psychotic processes. Fig. 21.1 outlines the choices of medications in different circumstances.

PSYCHOTROPIC MEDICATION USE IN SPECIAL POPULATIONS

Pregnant and breastfeeding women

The management of women who are pregnant or breastfeeding poses a significant challenge for mental health nurses. The prescription and administration of psychotropic medications, if required during pregnancy and breastfeeding, presents many risks to the unborn fetus or the newborn child. Antipsychotic medications, especially the atypical antipsychotics, commonly prescribed for women who experience psychoses during pregnancy or in the immediate postpartum period, have not been proven safe in pregnancy, and their use in pregnancy is not based on evidence from randomised clinical trials (Goldberg & Stahl 2021). However, the consequences of untreated psychiatric disorders during pregnancy must be weighed against the risk of prenatal exposure to medications, as antenatal psychological distress is known to be linked to premature labour, low birth weight, smaller head circumference and inferior functional assessments in newborns (Kieviet et al 2017).

The evidence of the teratogenic effects of psychotropic medications is mixed, and their use during pregnancy can expose the fetus to an increased risk of congenital malformation. Several psychotropic medications are known to have teratogenic effects in early pregnancy, as

well as probable adverse effects on neonates late in pregnancy (Kicviet et al 2017). Most antidepressants appear to be safe during pregnancy. However, as antidepressants and lithium are excreted in breast milk, at least in small quantities, the babies of mothers who choose to breastfeed should be monitored closely, especially in the first few weeks after birth (Imaz et al 2021). Larsen and colleagues (2015) synthesise the evidence on safety of psychotropic drugs in pregnancy and breastfeeding and conclude:

Sertraline and citalopram are first-line treatment among selective serotonin reuptake inhibitors for depression. It is recommended to use lithium for bipolar disorders if an overall assessment finds an indication for mood-stabilising treatment during pregnancy. Lamotrigine can be used. Valproate and carbamazepine are contraindicated. Olanzapine, risperidone, quetiapine and clozapine can be used for bipolar disorders and schizophrenia.

Children and Adolescents

Although psychotropic medications have been used with children and adolescents for several decades, the use of these medications with this group should be monitored carefully. Psychotropic medications can be used to manage symptoms of numerous conditions such as autism spectrum disorder, Tourette's syndrome and tic disorders. Non-pharmacological options are the preferred treatments. If pharmacological agents are used, the atypical antipsychotics are usually chosen because they have less serious side effects in children and adolescents (Goldberg & Stahl 2021).

Antidepressants should be prescribed only with extreme caution in this group, as children are particularly vulnerable to the cardiotoxic and seizure-inducing effects of high doses of tricyclic compounds. Deaths have been reported in children after accidental or deliberate overdosage with as little as a few hundred milligrams of a tricyclic medication. A recent review of the safety of commonly prescribed medication in children and adolescents (Solmi et al 2020) found a safer profile for escitalopram and fluoxetine among antidepressants, lurasidone for antipsychotics, methylphenidate among anti-ADHD medications, and lithium among mood stabilisers. Nurses must be particularly vigilant if working with children who are prescribed psychotropic medications.

Older People

Psychotropic medications are prescribed for older people for conditions such as mood and anxiety disorders, bipolar affective disorder, depression and dementia. Particular care must be taken when psychotropic medications are considered for older adults as they are likely to experience more adverse effects from psychotropic medication use, especially people over the age of 70, due to slower medication metabolism and excretion. For example, benzodiazepines are more likely to cause dizziness, which can lead to falls and serious injury. Antidepressants in older people can be problematic and are more likely to cause dizziness, postural hypotension, constipation, delayed micturition, oedema and tremor (Goldberg & Stahl 2021). There is also evidence that psychotropic medication prescription in the older person is linked to cognitive impairments such as delirium (Geyer et al 2022). Polypharmacy may have dire consequences for this group and should be avoided wherever possible. Older people are known to take more medications than younger people and often take more than one medication.

The use of psychotropic medications to manage agitation in dementia is common, but has been reported as being of little benefit and with considerable attendant risks (Geyer et al 2022). The Aged Care Quality and Safety Commission (2020) notes particular concern over the use of psychotropic drugs to manage behavioural and psychological symptoms in people living with dementia. Their recommendation is that the first treatment options should not be pharmaceutical and, when prescribed, psychotropics should be the lowest effective dose and used for the shortest period of time, reviewed at least every 3 months and ceased at the earliest opportunity.

EMERGING PSYCHOTROPICS: KETAMINE

Ketamine is a new emerging treatment in psychiatry, primarily for treatment-resistant depression (Swainson et al 2021). Ketamine is approved as an anaesthetic drug in Australia and Aotearoa New Zealand, but only intranasal ketamine (Spravato) is approved for use in treatment-resistant depression. Its use in treating mental disorders is considered off-label and requires adherence to Royal Australian and New Zealand College of Psychiatrists (RANZCP) guidelines and models of care. According to Malhi and colleagues (2021), its use should only be initiated after consideration of published evidence and assessment by a psychiatrist familiar with its effects. Ongoing research and monitoring are encouraged, and psychiatrists should establish appropriate clinical infrastructure and guidelines for its use in clinical practice (Malhi et al 2021).

The growing evidence for the efficacy of ketamine in rapidly relieving symptoms of depression has increased interest in its use, and its approval for use in treatment-resistant depression has led to its transition to clinical practice in various countries. However, there are concerns regarding long-term efficacy, safety, patient selection and appropriate administration (Bahji et al 2021). Ketamine has been shown to be effective in treating treatment-resistant depression, with response rates of 50–70% and remission rates of 30% (McIntyre et al 2021; Swainson et al 2021). It has advantages over standard antidepressants in terms of speed of onset, but its effects generally last less than a week following a single dose (Swainson et al 2021). Serious adverse effects have been reported in the recreational context, but not in clinical trials where treatments have been carefully monitored. Consensus has not been reached on the appropriate use of ketamine and esketamine

in treatment algorithms (Bahji et al 2021; Bayes et al 2021; Swainson et al 2021). There are limited studies for its use in refractory bipolar depression, anxiety disorders and older people. Further research is needed to determine the relative benefits and risks of the different modes of administering ketamine and how dosing should be optimised (Bahji et al 2021).

Specific regulations govern the prescription of ketamine and it is considered a controlled substance due to its potential for abuse and addiction. Practitioners, including nurses, must comply with regulations regarding prescription periods, prescribing to substance-dependent patients, storage, disposal and record-keeping.

ALTERNATIVE THERAPIES AND PSYCHOPHARMACOLOGY

Complementary medicines or alternative therapies refer to non-conventional approaches to treating mental illnesses that some people may use in conjunction with prescription-only psychotropics. Some examples of complementary approaches that may interact with psychotropics when used concurrently include nutritional supplements, diets, cannabis and psychedelics. In relation to cannabis, population-based studies have found associations between use of cannabis in adolescence and the development of certain psychotic disorders (Zeraatkar et al 2022). Other studies have reported some benefits for sleep disorders (Bhagavan et al 2020), while some have reported mixed results on its benefits for anxiety and mood disorders (Hindocha et al 2020; Whiting et al 2015). While cannabis can be medically prescribed in Australia and Aotearoa New Zealand for chronic health conditions, there has been no endorsement of cannabis use for serious mental health problems. However, nurses will increasingly encounter people who have used cannabis products to manage anxiety, depression, stress, chronic pain and other health conditions.

In 2023 the Therapeutic Goods Administration (TGA) in Australia approved the prescription of 3,4-methylenedioxymethamphetamine (MDMA) for the treatment of PTSD, and psilocybin (the psychoactive ingredient of "magic mushrooms") for treatment-resistant depression by psychiatrists in limited circumstances. This controversial decision was based on a limited number of trials of these substances for a range of conditions in the context of "psychedelic assisted psychotherapy" (Lakeman et al 2020). Similar to the use of ketamine (administered primarily in private psychiatric practice), it is unclear when or how these treatments may be available in public mental health services. What is clear is that the therapeutic impact of these drugs is highly contingent on the psychotherapy component of the drug, which in trials to date have included lengthy preparation, attendance during the dosing period by two competent therapists and often lengthy post-dosing integration of the experience (Lakeman et al 2020). Self-administered "recreational use" of these substances may lead to desirable effects, but rarely the profound therapeutic experiences reported in the trial literature (Crowe et al 2023). Crowe and colleagues (2023) note that appropriately trained mental health nurse psychotherapists are well placed to play lead roles in the administration of psychedelic assisted psychotherapy in future.

CONSUMER EDUCATION

Discuss with the person the potential interaction of these alternative therapies with their prescribed medication, as some supplements or therapies may interact with psychotropics or have adverse effects. Encourage consumers to openly discuss the type of alternative therapy they are using with their prescribing clinician.

CHAPTER SUMMARY

This chapter has presented an overview of the issues related to psychopharmacology, including the use of prn psychotropic medications, adherence with medications as prescribed and their use with special populations. Alternative therapies have also been outlined. To be effective practitioners, mental health nurses need to be equipped with knowledge and understanding of the distinct medication indications, interactions, side effects and precautions related to the four major psychotropic medication groups (anti-anxiety, antidepressant, mood-stabilising and antipsychotic). Mental health nurses need to have a working knowledge of psychopharmacology and related issues because administering these medications is a common but important nursing intervention. The information presented here will help to prepare mental health nurses to make well-informed treatment decisions and engage in successful consumer assessment and education. It will also help the nurse to detect and manage side effects from psychotropic medications, many of which can be harmful or even life-threatening.

REVIEW QUESTIONS

1. In a small group, discuss the legal and ethical issues that a mental health nurse needs to consider when administering psychotropic medications. In particular, consider the issues related to consent regarding emergency situations.

2. In a small group, outline what you believe are the important issues related to medication adherence. How might your beliefs differ from those of consumers? Discuss your findings with the larger group.

3. In a small group, debate and respond to the following questions:
   a. Discuss how you would manage a situation where you believed a consumer was being prescribed and administered a toxic level of a medication.
   b. Describe how polypharmacy can be a problem for people taking antipsychotic medications and for members of vulnerable groups such as older people.
   c. Describe the signs of a tricyclic overdose and list those who might be at high risk of such an outcome.
   d. Anticonvulsant medications are used in the management of people with bipolar disorder. Describe the action of these medications and list their potential side effects.
   e. Lithium is commonly used as a mood-stabilising medication. Outline why it is important to obtain regular blood tests for people taking this medication and outline the therapeutic range and signs of lithium toxicity.
   f. Discuss the physical issues of importance when working with consumers taking psychotropic medications.

USEFUL WEBSITES

Australian Prescriber – useful information on drugs: www.nps.org.au/australian-prescriber/

Glasgow Antipsychotic Side-effect Scale (GASS): rightdecisions.scot.nhs.uk/mypsych-app/working-in-greater-glasgow-clyde/

Healthline – drug interactions: www.healthline.com/health/what-is-a-psychotropic-drug#drug-interactions

Medsafe (New Zealand Medicines and Medical Devices Safety Authority): www.medsafe.govt.nz/

National Prescribing Authority (Australia): www.nps.org.au/

Pharmaceutical Management Agency of New Zealand (PHARMAC): www.pharmac.govt.nz/

REFERENCES

Aged Care Quality and Safety Commission 2020. Psychotropic medications used in Australia: Information for aged care. Online. Available at: www.agedcarequality.gov.au/sites/default/files/media/acqsc_psychotropic_medications_v10_hr.pdf

Alvares, G.A., Quintana, D.S., Hickie, I.B. & Guastella, A.J. 2016. Autonomic nervous system dysfunction in psychiatric disorders and the impact of psychotropic medications: A systematic review and meta-analysis. J Psychiatry Neurosci, 41(2), 89–104.

Bahji, A., Vazquez, G.H. & Zarate Jr, C.A. 2021. Comparative efficacy of racemic ketamine and esketamine for depression: A systematic review and meta-analysis. J Affect Disord, 278, 542–555.

Bandelow, B., Allgulander, C., Baldwin, D.S., Costa, D.L.d.C., Denys, D., et al. 2023. World Federation of Societies of Biological Psychiatry (WFSBP) guidelines for treatment of anxiety, obsessive-compulsive and posttraumatic stress disorders – Version 3. Part I: Anxiety disorders. World J Biol Psychiatry, 24(2), 79–117.

Bandelow, B., Sher, L., Bunevicius, R., Hollander, E., Kasper, S., et al., 2012. Care, WFSBP Task Force on Mental Disorders in Primary Care & WFSBP Task Force on Anxiety Disorders, OCD and PTSD. Guidelines for the pharmacological treatment of anxiety disorders, obsessive–compulsive disorder and posttraumatic stress disorder in primary care. Int J Psychiatry Clin Pract, 16(2), 77–84.

Barr, L., Wynaden, D. & Heslop, K. 2018. Nurses' attitudes towards the use of PRN psychotropic medications in acute and forensic mental health settings. Int J Ment Health Nurs, 27(1), 168–177.

Barton, B.B., Segger, F., Fischer, K., Obermeier, M. & Musil, R. 2020. Update on weight-gain caused by antipsychotics: A systematic review and meta-analysis. Expert Opin Drug Saf, 19(3), 295–314.

Bauer, M., Severus, E., Kohler, S., Whybrow, P.C., Angst, J., et al., 2015. Task Force on Treatment Guidelines for Unipolar Depressive, D. World Federation of Societies of Biological Psychiatry (WFSBP) guidelines for biological treatment of unipolar depressive disorders. Part 2: maintenance treatment of major depressive disorder – update 2015. World J Biol Psychiatry, 16(2), 76–95.

Bayes, A., Dong, V., Martin, D., Alonzo, A., Kabourakis, M. et al., 2021. Ketamine treatment for depression: A model of care. Aust N Z J Psychiatry, 55(12), 1134–1143.

Beach, S.R., Celano, C.M., Sugrue, A.M., Adams, C., Ackerman, M.J., et al., 2018. QT Prolongation, Torsades de Pointes, and psychotropic medications: A 5-year update. Psychosomatics, 59(2), 105–122.

Bhagavan, C., Kung, S., Doppen, M., John, M., Vakalalabure, I., et al., 2020. Cannabinoids in the treatment of insomnia disorder: A systematic review and meta-Analysis. CNS Drugs, 34(12), 1217–1228.

Bolsinger, J., Jaeger, M., Hoff, P. & Theodoridou, A. 2020. Challenges and opportunities in building and maintaining a good therapeutic relationship in acute psychiatric settings: A narrative review [Systematic Review]. Front Psychiatry, 10.

Bradley, T., Campbell, E., Dray, J., Bartlem, K., Wye, P., et al., 2022. Systematic review of lifestyle interventions to improve weight, physical activity and diet among people with a mental health condition. Systematic Rev, 11(1), 198.

Braun, E., Gaillard, A.-S., Vollmann, J., Gather, J. & Scholten, M. 2022. Mental health service users' perspectives on psychiatric advance directives: A systematic review. Psychiatric Services, 74(4), 381–392.

Brett, J. & Murnion, B. 2015. Management of benzodiazepine misuse and dependence. Aust Prescr, 38(5), 152–155.

Cade, J.F.2000. Lithium salts in the treatment of psychotic excitement. 1949. Bull WHO, 78(4), 518–520.

Cerovecki, A., Musil, R., Klimke, A., Seemuller, F., Haen, E., et al., 2013. Withdrawal symptoms and rebound syndromes associated with switching and discontinuing atypical antipsychotics: Theoretical background and practical recommendations. CNS Drugs, 27(7), 545–572.

Champion, C., Kameg, B. 2021. Best practices in benzodiazepine prescribing and management in primary care. Nurse Pract, 46(5), 1.

Chieze, M., Hurst, S., Kaiser, S. & Sentissi, O. 2019. Effects of seclusion and restraint in adult psychiatry: A systematic review. Front Psychiatry, 10, 491.

Cipriani, A., Furukawa, T.A., Salanti, G., Chaimani, A., Atkinson, L.Z., et al., 2018. Comparative efficacy and acceptability of 21 antidepressant drugs for the acute treatment of adults with major depressive disorder: A systematic review and network meta-analysis. Lancet, 391(10128), 1357–1366.

Clyne, W., Mshelia, C., Hall, S., McLachlan, S., Jones, P., et al., 2011. Management of patient adherence to medications: Protocol for an online survey of doctors, pharmacists and nurses in Europe. BMJ open, 1(1), e000355.

Cornett, E.M., Novitch, M., Kaye, A.D., Kata, V. & Kaye, A.M. 2017. Medication-induced tardive dyskinesia: A review and update. Ochsner J, 17(2), 162–174.

Crowe, M., Manuel, J., Carlyle, D. & Lacey, C. 2023. Experiences of psilocybin treatment for clinical conditions: A qualitative meta-synthesis. Int J Ment Health Nurs, 32(4), 1025–1037.

Edward, K.-L. & Alderman, C. 2013. Psychopharmacology: Practice and Contexts. Oxford University Press, Melbourne.

Ertem, M.Y. & Duman, Z. C. 2019. The effect of motivational interviews on treatment adherence and insight levels of patients with schizophrenia: A randomized controlled study. Perspect Psychiatr Care, 55(1), 75–86.

Every-Palmer, S. & Ellis, P.M. 2017. Clozapine-induced gastrointestinal hypomotility: A 22-year bi-national pharmacovigilance study of serious or fatal "slow gut" reactions, and comparison with international drug safety advice. CNS Drugs, 31(8), 699–709.

Feinberg, M. 1993. The problems of anticholinergic adverse effects in older patients. Drugs Aging, 3, 335–348.

Fiorillo, A., Barlati, S., Bellomo, A., Corrivetti, G., Nicolo, G., et al., 2020. The role of shared decision-making in improving adherence to pharmacological treatments in patients with schizophrenia: A clinical review. Ann Gen Psychiatry, 19, 43.

Fountoulakis, K.N., Yatham, L.N., Grunze, H., Vieta, E., Young, A.H., et al., 2020. The CINP guidelines on the definition and evidence-based interventions for treatment-resistant bipolar disorder. Int J Neuropsychopharmacol, 23(4), 230–256.

Gay, S., Sikaris, K. & Badrick, T. 2019. Reporting critical pathology results – what is the current state of play in Australian laboratories?: An opinion based on findings of a KIMMS audit. Aust J Med Sci, 40(4), 126–130.

Geyer, H., Kaufman, D.M., Milstein, M.J. & Rosengard, J. 2022. Kaufman's Clinical Neurology for Psychiatrists-E-Book. Elsevier Health Sciences.

Goldberg, J.F. & Stahl, S.M. 2021. Practical Psychopharmacology. Cambridge University Press.

Grunze, H., Vieta, E., Goodwin, G.M., Bowden, C., Licht, R.W., et al., 2018. The World Federation of Societies of Biological Psychiatry (WFSBP) guidelines for the biological treatment of bipolar disorders: Acute and long-term treatment of mixed states in bipolar disorder. World J Biol Psychiatry, 19(1), 2–58.

Hasan, A., Falkai, P., Wobrock, T., Lieberman, J., Glenthoj, B., et al., WTFo TGf, 2017. World Federation of Societies of Biological Psychiatry (WFSBP) guidelines for biological treatment of schizophrenia – a short version for primary care. Int J Psychiatry Clin Pract, 21(2), 82–90.

Hepburn, K. & Brzozowska, M.M. 2016. Diabetic ketoacidosis and severe hypertriglyceridaemia as a consequence of an atypical antipsychotic agent. Case Reports 2016, bcr2016215413.

Hindocha, C., Cousijn, J., Rall, M. & Bloomfield, M.A.P. 2020. The effectiveness of cannabinoids in the treatment of posttraumatic stress disorder (PTSD): A systematic review. J Dual Diagnosis, 16(1), 120–139.

Hirjak, D., Fricchione, G., Wolf, R.C. & Northoff, G. 2023. Lorazepam in catatonia – Past, present and future of a clinical success story. Schizophrenia Res, S0920-9964.

Hirschfeld, R.M.2000. History and evolution of the monoamine hypothesis of depression. J Clin Psychiatry, 61 Suppl 6(6), 4–6.

Horowitz, M.A., Jauhar, S., Natesan, S., Murray, R.M. & Taylor, D. 2021. A method for tapering antipsychotic treatment that may minimize the risk of relapse. Schizophrenia Bull, 47(4), 1116–1129.

Hubbard, R.E., Peel, N.M., Scott, I.A., Martin, J.H., Smith, A., et al., 2015. Polypharmacy among inpatients aged 70 years or older in Australia. MJA 202(7), 373–377.

Husain, M. & Mehta, M.A 2011. Cognitive enhancement by drugs in health and disease. Trends Cogn Sci, 15(1), 28–36.

Hyde, N., Dodd, S., Venugopal, K., Purdie, C., Berk, M., et al., 2015. Prevalence of cardiovascular and metabolic events in patients prescribed clozapine: A retrospective observational, clinical cohort study. Curr Drug Saf, 10(2), 125–131.

Imaz, M.L., Soy, D., Torra, M., Garcia-Esteve, L., Soler, C., et al., 2021. Case report: Clinical and pharmacokinetic profile of lithium monotherapy in exclusive breastfeeding. A follow-up case series. Front Pharmacol, 12, 647414.

Jessurun, J.G., van Harten, P.N., Egberts, T.C., Pijl, B.J., Wilting, I., et al., 2013. The effect of psychotropic medications on the occurrence of constipation in hospitalized psychiatric patients. J Clin Psychopharmacol, 33(4), 587–590.

John, A.P., Koloth, R., Dragovic, M. & Lim, S.C.B. 2009. Prevalence of metabolic syndrome among Australians with severe mental illness. MJA, 190(4), 176–179.

Kieviet, N., de Jong, F., Scheele, F., Dolman, K.M. & Honig, A.2017. Use of antidepressants during pregnancy in the Netherlands: Observational study into postpartum interventions. BMC Pregnancy Childbirth, 17, 1–9.

Kowalczyk, O.S., Cubillo, A.I., Smith, A., Barrett, N., Giampietro, V., et al., 2019. Methylphenidate and atomoxetine normalise fronto-parietal underactivation during sustained attention in ADHD adolescents. Eur Neuropsychopharmacol, 29(10), 1102–1116.

Kurien, R. & Vattakatuchery, J.J. 2013. Psychotropic discontinuation leading to an NMS-like condition. Progress Neurol Psychiatry, 17(5), 8–10.

Lakeman, R., Cashin, A., Hurley, J. & Ryan, T. 2020. The psychotherapeutic practice and potential of mental health nurses: An Australian survey. Aust Health Rev, 44(6), 916–923.

Lakeman, R., Foster, K., Hazelton, M., Roper, C. & Hurley, J. 2022. Helpful encounters with mental health nurses in Australia: A survey of service users and their supporters. J Psychiatric Ment Health Nurs, 30(3), 515–525.

Lakeman, R., Ryan, T. & Emeleus, M. 2023. It is not and never has been just about the drug: The need to emphasise psychotherapy in psychedelic-assisted psychotherapy. Int J Ment Health Nurs, doi.org/10.1111/inm.13147.

Larsen, E.R., Damkier, P., Pedersen, L.H., Fenger-Gron, J., Mikkelsen, R.L. et al., 2015. Use of psychotropic drugs during pregnancy and breastfeeding. Acta Psychiatrica Scandinavica, 132(S445), 1–28.

Law, S., Stergiopoulos, V., Zaheer, J. & Nakhost, A. 2023. "Everyone means well but the one person who's really going to go to bat"– experiences and perspectives of substitute decision makers in caring for their loved ones with serious mental illness. Int J Law Psychiatry, 88, 101873.

Li, S., Zhang, L., Wei, N., Tai, Z., Yu, C., et al., 2021. research progress on the effect of epilepsy and antiseizure medications on PCOS through HPO axis. Front Endocrinol (Lausanne), 12, 787854.

Li, Y., Zhang, X., Yang, L., Yang, Y., Qiao, G., et al., 2022. Association between polypharmacy and mortality in the older adults: A systematic review and meta-analysis. Arch Gerontol Geriatr, 100, 104630.

Liang, E.F., Lim, S.Z., Tam, W.W., Ho, C.S., Zhang, M.W., et al., 2018. The effect of methylphenidate and atomoxetine on heart rate and systolic blood pressure in young people and adults with attention-deficit hyperactivity disorder (ADHD): systematic review, meta-analysis, and meta-regression. Int J Environ Res Pub Health, 15(8), 1789.

Lin, C., Darling, C. & Tsui, B.C.H. 2019. Practical Regional Anesthesia Guide for Elderly Patients. Drugs Aging, 36(3), 213–234.

Livingstone, C. & Rampes, H. 2006. Lithium: A review of its metabolic adverse effects. J Psychopharmacol 20(3), 347–355.

Lopez-Munoz, F., Alamo, C., Cuenca, E., Shen, W.W., Clervoy, P., et al., 2005. History of the discovery and clinical introduction of chlorpromazine. Ann Clin Psychiatry, 17(3), 113–135.

Malhi, G.S., Bell, E., Bassett, D., Boyce, P., Bryant, R., et al., 2021. The 2020 Royal Australian and New Zealand College of Psychiatrists clinical practice guidelines for mood disorders. Aust N Z J Psychiatry, 55(1), 7–117.

Malhi, G.S., Gessler, D. & Outhred, T. 2017. The use of lithium for the treatment of bipolar disorder: Recommendations from clinical practice guidelines. J Affect Disord, 217, 266–280.

Mandal, S., Sinha, V. K. & Goyal, N. 2019. Efficacy of ketamine therapy in the treatment of depression. Ind J Psychiatry, 61(5), 480–485.

Mardani, A., Paal, P., Weck, C., Jamshed, S. & Vaismoradi, M. 2022. Practical considerations of PRN medicines management: An integrative systematic review. Front Pharmacol, 13, 759998.

Massabki, I. & Abi-Jaoude, E. 2021. Selective serotonin reuptake inhibitor "discontinuation syndrome" or withdrawal. Br J Psychiatry, 218(3), 168–171.

Mathew, S.T., Nirmala, B.P. & Kommu, J.V.S. 2023. Personal meaning of recovery among persons with schizophrenia. Int J Soc Psychiatry, 69(1), 78–85.

McDaid, T.M. & Smyth, S. 2015. Metabolic abnormalities among people diagnosed with schizophrenia: A literature review and implications for mental health nurses. J Psychiatric Ment Health Nurs, 22(3), 157–170.

McIntyre, R.S., Rosenblat, J.D., Nemeroff, C.B., Sanacora, G., Murrough, J.W. et al., 2021. Synthesizing the evidence for ketamine and esketamine in treatment-resistant depression: An international expert opinion on the available evidence and implementation. Am J Psychiatry, 178(5), 383–399.

Megarbane, B., Hanak, A.S. & Chevillard, L. 2014. Lithium-related neurotoxicity despite serum concentrations in the therapeutic range: Risk factors and diagnosis. Shanghai Arch Psychiatry, 26(4), 243–244.

Meng, Q., Li, R., Hou, F. & Zhang, Q. 2018. Effects of chlorpromazine on sleep quality, clinical and emotional measures among patients with schizophrenia. Clin Neurol Neurosurg, 165, 134–138.

Miroshnichenko, I.I., Pozhidaev, I.V., Ivanova, S.A. & Baymeeva, N.V. 2020. Therapeutic drug monitoring of olanzapine and cytochrome P450 genotyping in nonsmoking subjects. Therapeut Drug Monitor, 42(2), 325–329.

Moncrieff, J., Cooper, R.E., Stockmann, T., Amendola, S., Hengartner, M.P. et al., 2022. The serotonin theory of depression: A systematic umbrella review of the evidence. Molecular Psychiatry, 28(3157), doi.org/10.1038/s41380-023-02091-2.

Moncrieff, J.2007. The myth of the chemical cure: A critique of psychiatric drug treatment. Palgrave Macmillan, London.

Morrison, P., Gaskill, D., Meehan, T., Lunney, P., Lawrence, G., et al., 2000. The use of the Liverpool University Neuroleptic Side-Effect Rating Scale (LUNSERS) in clinical practice. Aust N Z J Ment Health Nurs, 9(4), 166–176.

Mullen, A. & Drinkwater, V. 2011. Pro re nata use in a psychiatric intensive care unit. Int J Ment Health Nurs 20(6), 409–417.

Myles, N., Myles, H., Xia, S., Large, M., Bird, R., et al., 2019. A meta-analysis of controlled studies comparing the association between clozapine and other antipsychotic medications and the development of neutropenia. Aust N Z J Psychiatry, 53(5), 403–412.

National Collaborating Centre for Mental, National Institute for Health and Care Excellence (NICE) 2015. Guidelines. In: Violence and Aggression: Short-Term Management in Mental Health, Health and Community Settings: Updated edition. British Psychological Society (UK).

NewsRx LLC– Clinical Trials, 2021. Reports Outline Dyskinesias Findings from University of Pennsylvania (A Modified Delphi Consensus Study of the Screening, Diagnosis, and Treatment of Tardive Dyskinesia). 5075.

Ngune, I., Myers, H., Cole, A., Palamara, P., Redknap, R., et al., 2023. Developing nurse-sensitive outcomes in acute in-patient mental health settings–A systematic review. J Clin Nurs, 32(17–18), 6254–6267.

Park, T., Usher, K., & Foster, K. 2011. Description of a healthy lifestyle intervention for people with serious mental illness taking second-generation antipsychotics. Int J Ment Health Nurs, 20(6), 428–437.

Preskorn, S.H. 2020. Drug–Drug Interactions (DDIs) in psychiatric practice, part 9: Interactions mediated by drug-metabolizing cytochrome P450 enzymes. J Psychiatric Prac, 26(2).

Psychotropic Expert Group 2013. Therapeutic guidelines: Psychotropic. Therapeutic Guidelines Limited, Melbourne.

Purssey, R. 2023. Personal Communication with Richard Lakeman (24/5/23).

Reeves, R.R. & Kamal, A. 2019. Complicated withdrawal phenomena during benzodiazepine cessation in older adults. J Am Osteopath Assoc, 119(5), 327–331.

Remington, G., Agid, O., Foussias, G., Hahn, M., Rao, N., et al. 2013. Clozapine's role in the treatment of first-episode schizophrenia. Am J Psychiatry, 170(2), 146–151.

Rotella, F., Cassioli, E., Calderani, E., Lazzeretti, L., Ragghianti, B., et al., 2020. Long-term metabolic and cardiovascular effects of antipsychotic drugs. A meta-analysis of randomized controlled trials. Eur Neuropsychopharmacol, 32, 56–65.

Royal Australian College of General Practitioners (RACGP) 2015. Prescribing drugs of dependence in general practice, Part B – Benzodiazepines. RACGP. Online. Available at: www.racgp.org.au/getattachment/1beeb924-cf7b-4de4-911e-f7dda3e3f6e9/Part-B.aspx

Salomon, C. & Hamilton, B. 2014. Antipsychotic discontinuation syndromes: A narrative review of the evidence and its integration into Australian mental health nursing textbooks. Int J Ment Health Nurs, 23(1), 69–78.

Sanjeevi, S. & Cocoman, A. 2020. Mental health nurses' confidence in applying pharmacological knowledge: A survey. Br J Ment Health Nurs, 9(4), 1–9.

Shields, M., Scully, S., Sulman, H., Borba, C., Trinh, N.H., et al., 2019. Consumers' suggestions for improving the mental healthcare system: Options, autonomy, and Respect. Community Ment Health J, 55(6), 916–923.

Smith, J.P. & Herber, O.R. 2015. Ethical issues experienced by mental health nurses in the administration of antipsychotic depot and long-acting intramuscular injections: A qualitative study. Int J Ment Health Nurs, 24(3), 222–230.

Soares, K.V. & McGrath, J.J. 1999. The treatment of tardive dyskinesia – a systematic review and meta-analysis. Schizophr Res, 39(1), 1–16; discussion 17–18.

Solmi, M., Fornaro, M., Ostinelli, E.G., Zangani, C., Croatto, G. et al., 2020. Safety of 80 antidepressants, antipsychotics, anti-attention-deficit/hyperactivity medications and mood stabilizers in children and adolescents with psychiatric disorders: A large scale systematic meta-review of 78 adverse effects. World Psychiatry, 19(2), 214–232.

Soyka, M., Kranzler, H.R., Hesselbrock, V., Kasper, S., Mutschler, J. et al. & Disorders, W.T.F.o. T.G.f. S.U. 2017. Guidelines for biological treatment of substance use and related disorders, part 1: Alcoholism, first revision. World J Biol Psychiatry, 18(2), 86–121.

Srinivasan, M., Yadav, G., Singh, Y., Sahu, A., Kumari, S., et al., 2022. Comparison of efficacy of combination therapy with chlorpromazine and olanzapine with chlorpromazine alone for treatment of hiccups in traumatic brain injury patients: A randomised control trial. J Clin Diagnost Res, 16(9), UC28–UC31.

Stahl, S.M. 2021. Stahl's Essential Psychopharmacology: Neuroscientific Basis and Practical Applications. 5th ed. Cambridge University Press.

Su, Y.P., Chang, C.K., Hayes, R.D., Harrison, S., Lee, W., et al., 2014. Retrospective chart review on exposure to psychotropic medications associated with neuroleptic malignant syndrome. Acta Psychiatr Scand, 130(1), 52–60.

Swainson, J., McGirr, A., Blier, P., Brietzke, E., Richard-Devantoy, S. et al., 2021. The Canadian Network for Mood and Anxiety Treatments (CANMAT) Task Force Recommendations for the Use of Racemic Ketamine in Adults with Major Depressive Disorder: Recommandations Du Groupe De Travail Du Réseau Canadien Pour Les Traitements De L'humeur Et De L'anxiété (Canmat) Concernant L'utilisation de la Kétamine Racemique Chez Les Adultes Souffrant De Trouble Depressif Majeur. Can J Psychiatry, 66(2), 113–125.

Taylor, D.M., Barnes, T.R. & Young, A.H. 2021. The Maudsley Prescribing Guidelines in Psychiatry. 14th ed. John Wiley & Sons, London.

Thanasan, S. & Jambunathan, S. 2010. Clozapine withdrawal catatonia or lethal catatonia in a schizoaffective patient with a family history of Parkinsons disease. Afric J Psychiatry, 13(5), 402–404.

Tirupati, S. & Chua, L.E. 2007. Obesity and metabolic syndrome in a psychiatric rehabilitation service. A N Z J Psychiatry, 41(7), 606–610.

Watkins, A., Stein-Parbury, J., Denney-Wilson, E., Ward, P.B., Rosenbaum, S. 2020. Upskilling mental health nurses to address the burden of poor metabolic health: A mixed method evaluation. Iss Ment Health Nurs, 41(10), 925–931.

Weintraub, S.J. 2017. Diazepam in the treatment of moderate to severe alcohol withdrawal. CNS Drugs, 31(2), 87–95.

Werneke, U., Jamshidi, F., Taylor, D.M. & Ott, M., 2016. Conundrums in neurology: Diagnosing serotonin syndrome – a meta-analysis of cases. BMC Neurol, 16(1), 97.

Whiting, P.F., Wolff, R.F., Deshpande, S., Di Nisio, M., Duffy, S., et al., 2015. Cannabinoids for medical use: A systematic review and meta-analysis. JAMA, 313(24), 2456–2473.

Yilmaz, D., Khorshid, L. & Dedeoglu, Y. 2016. The effect of the Z-track technique on pain and drug leakage in intramuscular injections. Clin Nurse Spec, 30(6), E7–E12.

Zeraatkar, D., Cooper, M.A., Agarwal, A., Vernooij, R.W.M., Leung, G., et al., 2022. Long-term and serious harms of medical cannabis and cannabinoids for chronic pain: A systematic review of non-randomised studies. BMJ open, 12(8), e054282.

Contexts of Practice

22

Mental Health in Every Setting

Peta Marks

KEY POINTS

- People experiencing mental health issues, mental illness and mental distress present to all health settings.
- Mental health service delivery occurs across the service spectrum in a stepped-care model that is person-centred and recovery-oriented.
- The stepped care model matches interventions to meet the person's needs.

- In a stepped care model, generalist nurses use fundamental mental health knowledge and skills, and mental health nurses use specialised mental health knowledge and skills.
- All nurses need to develop their mental health nursing knowledge and skills relevant to their clinical setting and scope of practice.

KEY TERMS

Holistic care

Mental distress

Mental health issues

Mental health service delivery

Mental illness

Stepped care

LEARNING OUTCOMES

The material in this chapter will assist you to:

- orientate yourself to Part 3 of this textbook, which describes how mental health nursing skills can be applied across all care settings and services

- describe how mental health service delivery is integrated across the health service spectrum in Australia and Aotearoa New Zealand.

LIVED EXPERIENCE COMMENT BY JARRAD HICKMOTT
The reflection points in this chapter provoke thought about what the consumer may be experiencing when they are engaging with the healthcare system. Such thoughts help to promote the therapeutic relationship, which is of utmost importance, and speaks to the importance of strengths-based and trauma-informed care.

INTRODUCTION

As described in Part 1 of this text, a person's health, mental health and wellbeing are linked to their biology, lifestyle, socio-economic and societal factors – and how these factors interact. From a socio-ecological perspective, a person's individual circumstances (including social connections, parenting and family), their experience of a range of social determinants (e.g. housing security, educational opportunities, employment and income), their identities (cultural, spiritual, gender) and their environment all influence health and wellbeing. Importantly, people's beliefs and the meanings they attribute to health, illness and wellbeing, are individually defined – by age, gender, education, personal experiences and cultural perspectives, which are diverse (McGough et al 2022; Marks 2023). What this means for us as nurses is that regardless of the clinical setting we choose to work in, we will encounter people experiencing a mental illness or who are in crisis and experiencing mental distress. We will work with people who may be struggling with any

number of issues related to the social determinants and other factors outlined above, or who have a life-changing experience as the result of physical or mental illness, who are gravely ill, or who die from disease or injury. We will interact with people, their families and friends, and from a social ecological perspective, if we are to practise in a holistic way, we will attempt to make meaning of and understand their experience – taking into consideration the individual circumstances that may have impacted on or influenced the person's health and wellbeing. Box 22.1 includes some questions that will help you to reflect on what the role of the nurse might be regarding a person's emotional or mental wellbeing in a range of different circumstances.

This chapter introduces and sets the scene for Part 3, Chapters 23–29, and introduces the concepts that will be expanded upon and addressed in these chapters. This chapter will briefly overview how mental health care is integrated across the healthcare system and how nurses provide mental health care in a stepped care model. You will notice that chapters in this section are quite different in style to Parts 1 and 2 of the text; they have been written by clinicians who describe common scenarios relevant to their area of practice as they relate to mental health. They explore a range of presentations, a range of healthcare contexts, and demonstrate a range of effective nursing practices in mental health related to the person's story. These chapters are practical rather than theoretical and are designed to demonstrate how mental health skills can be applied in various clinical settings, at times describing the role of the mental health nurse working within a particular mental health setting using advanced mental health nursing skills, at other times describing the fundamental mental health related knowledge and skills required of nurses working in other areas. Some new elements that you will encounter in this section include "scenarios" and "red flags".

SCENARIOS

Chapters in Part 3 include two scenarios developed by the authors that demonstrate typical presentations they might encounter in the respective healthcare setting. The scenario may demonstrate the physical health needs of a person with mental illness (which are often overlooked and contribute to the poor physical health outcomes of people with mental illness) or the mental health needs of a person with a physical illness (which are often ignored and impact on physical and mental health outcomes).

RED FLAGS

With each scenario you will find a section outlining the "red flags" that the scenario presents. These are elements of the person's background or clinical presentation that would highlight that a mental health issue may be present. They demonstrate the type of issues that should prompt you to consider the mental health needs of the individual concerned and the mental health nursing knowledge and skills you might need in order to provide comprehensive nursing care in these situations.

In demonstrating how you think about "mental health" across a range of clinical scenarios in a range of settings, Part 3 aims to support you to provide more holistic nursing care to *all* people you come in contact with during your nursing career – whether they have a diagnosed mental illness or not. As you read through these chapters, identify any knowledge or skill gaps that you may have that relate to the scenarios presented, then review the chapters from Parts 1 and 2 to help you to develop your practice. In addition, Chapter 23 will help you to prepare for your mental health clinical placement.

INTEGRATING MENTAL HEALTH ACROSS THE SERVICE SPECTRUM

Mental health promotion and illness prevention occurs in the community, in schools and in primary care settings. For example, the reciprocal relationship between physical and mental health is well known, so if someone presents to general practice with a physical condition that places them at high risk for developing mental health issues, then raising that potential with the person, discussing how they might maintain good mental health in the face of the healthcare challenge, and encouraging them to talk about any symptoms they may experience will increase the chances that the person will present early with any mental health issues. Once a person has identified that they are experiencing mental distress, or that they have a mental health issue, intervention at the person's level of need is required.

Mental health service delivery in Australia and Aotearoa New Zealand occurs in primary, community and hospital settings. While hospital and bed-based services have dominated mental health care in the past, deinstitutionalisation and a focus on recovery mean community-based services are the preferred site for contemporary mental health service delivery.

Services are provided by government (public), non-government and private organisations; they can be generalist or specialist mental health services and provide mental health assessment, management and treatment across the lifespan, from the perinatal and infant period, through to childhood and adolescence and on to adulthood and older age. It is also essential to consider the mental health and emotional needs of families, carers and significant others when supporting a loved one in any healthcare setting; they may be frightened, distressed, angry or upset (or all of those).

At all times and in all settings, a "least restrictive" model of care in relation to mental health is required; that is, one which enhances the person's autonomy, respects their rights, individual worth, dignity and privacy, and where any limitations placed on the person are the minimum necessary, enabling the person to participate as much as possible regarding all decisions that affect them. The philosophy of providing the least restrictive treatment option guides the choice of clinical setting and is one of the World Health Organization's Ten Basic Principles of Mental Health Care Law (1996). It requires that, in determining where a person will be treated, the health professional considers the symptoms the person is experiencing, the treatments available, their level of autonomy, acceptance and cooperation with treatment, and the potential for harm to be caused to themselves or to any others (WHO 1996).

As we have discussed in this textbook, in a person-centred healthcare system services should be organised around the needs of people rather than people having to organise themselves around the system. As a person's needs increase, the healthcare team should expand to include different support providers; and as people's needs decrease, the number of people involved will also decrease, with connection being maintained throughout by a general practitioner, the person's family and other key supports.

A STEPPED CARE APPROACH

As described in Chapter 1, in Australia and Aotearoa New Zealand, a "stepped care" model of matching an individual's needs with evidence-based staged interventions (from least restrictive to most intensive) forms the framework of mental health service delivery. The model helps organise services, matches the person to the intervention level that most suits their current need and helps consumers, family/carers/kin and healthcare professionals to identify and use interventions that will be the most effective to recovery (Rivero-Santana et al 2021). Stepped care services range from no-cost and low-cost options for people with common mental health issues such as anxiety and depression, through to support and wraparound services for people with severe and persistent mental illness, such as psychotic illness. In a stepped care approach people don't have to start at the lowest, least intensive level of intervention in order to progress to the next "step"; rather, they enter the system and have their service level aligned with their requirements.

You can see how the stepped care approach integrates well with a person-centred and least-restrictive model of care. The stepped mental health care model also aligns with providing a continuum of mental health care services – across primary, community, sub-acute, acute and extended care (rehabilitation) settings – that respond to the person's level of need. Table 22.1 demonstrates how these concepts integrate and the nurse's role regarding mental health care and managing mental

TABLE 22.1 Nursing, Mental Health and a Stepped Care Response

Person's Mental and Emotional Distress	Person's Need for Support	Elements of Care	Care Setting	Nurses Involved
Severe distress	*Very high level of need* Risk to life; severe self-neglect	Assessment Risk assessment Manage critical incidents Acute mental health care Medication Treatment	Acute mental health services Acute care teams	Mental health nurse practitioners Credentialled mental health nurses Mental health nurses
		Assessment Risk assessment Manage critical incidents Medication Arrange admission	Emergency departments	Consultation–liaison mental health nurses Mental health nurse practitioners ED nurses
Moderate to severe distress	*High level of need for support* Recurrent, atypical and those at significant risk; complex care needs	Assessment and risk assessment Brief psychological interventions Psychological therapy Medication education and management Social support and care coordination	In-patient mental health Acute care teams Community mental health Primary health	Mental health nurse practitioners Credentialled mental health nurses Mental health nurses Mental health nurse practitioners Credentialled mental health nurses
		Assessment Risk assessment Brief interventions Medication education and management Referral	Emergency departments Acute alcohol and other drug services	Consultation–liaison mental health nurses Mental health nurse practitioners ED nurses Alcohol and other drug nurses
Moderate distress	*Moderate level of need for support* Moderate or severe mental health problems	Brief psychological interventions Psychological therapy Medication education and management Rehabilitation services	Community mental health Primary health Forensic mental health	Mental health nurse practitioners Credentialled mental health nurses Mental health nurses Forensic mental health nurses
		Identifying distress Appropriate referral Social support	Medical settings Primary health General practice	ED nurses and general nurses Alcohol and other drug nurses Nurses working in chronic disease Nurses working in primary health General practice nurses
Mild to moderate distress	*Low level of need for support* Mild mental health problems	Guided self-help Brief psychological interventions Assessment and Risk assessment	Primary health headspace General practice	Mental health nurse practitioners Credentialled mental health nurses
		Identifying distress Raising awareness Flagging risk Watchful waiting	Medical settings Primary health General practice	ED nurses Alcohol and other drug nurses Nurses working in chronic disease Nurses working in primary health General practice nurses
Minimal to mild distress	*Need for wellbeing and resilience promotion*	Recognition of risk and distress Mental health literacy Mental health promotion	All healthcare settings	All nurses in all settings

Legend
  Blue: generalist nurses, who use fundamental mental health knowledge and skills
  Green: mental health nurses, who use specialised mental health knowledge and skills

and emotional distress at each point in the mental health service continuum. Of course, these are not the only care settings or nurses that need to respond to a person's mental health needs; these are merely some of the most common.

CARE SETTINGS AND NURSES' ROLES

Primary Care Services

Primary care services include general practice and mental health clinicians working in private practice (e.g. credentialled mental health nurses and mental health nurse practitioners, psychiatrists and psychologists). They also include services such as the Royal Flying Doctor Service (RFDS), Aboriginal and Torres Strait Islander and Māori health services, correctional health settings and rural and remote mental health services.

In Australia, primary health-based mental health services are funded by the Commonwealth Government, either through services commissioned by Primary Health Networks and rolled out within a particular geographical area or provided nationally through Medicare-funded psychological services. These services include models of practice that incorporate peer workers as multidisciplinary team members providing person-centred, recovery-oriented and trauma-informed stepped care in mental health and suicide prevention services (Department of Health 2021). In Aotearoa New Zealand, local private primary health organisations provide overall management of primary health services, including general practice, and are largely funded or subsidised by the Ministry of Health. In both Australia and Aotearoa New Zealand, nurses are also employed in school-based settings with a focus on improving the mental health of students and responding to mental health crises.

Community Health, Community Mental Health and Acute Care Services

Community health, community mental health and acute care services (e.g. crisis teams, mobile assessment teams) are funded and managed by state-based mental health services. Non-government community-based services are often grant-based (state or Commonwealth) or funded through religious or philanthropic organisations.

One of the major ways in which nurses working in primary and community health settings promote optimal mental health and wellbeing is to engage with the person around the environment in which they live, work, play and interact, and to support them to connect with services or supports within the community that can provide culturally appropriate assistance or support where required. Nurses in these settings need to be able to identify clients who are particularly at risk for developing mental health problems and to recognise and intervene appropriately when people present with mental health symptoms, chronic disease or other comorbid mental health needs and physical illnesses. They need to be able to collaborate with and refer to mental health clinicians to ensure people experiencing mental health conditions receive the level of specialist care they require. They can also work with a person's family or other support network to help identify and respond to unmet needs, which may be financial, emotional or practical/physical (McInnes et al 2022). Chapter 24 will help you recognise how to adequately consider a person's mental health when delivering care in the primary care and community setting and help you to identify how to apply mental health nursing skills to improve the overall health and quality of life of all clients.

Bed-Based Services

Bed-based services include emergency departments (EDs), general hospitals and in-patient mental health units, as well as rehabilitation units. EDs are the key access point for health emergencies of all types,

including psychiatric emergencies. People may present with mental health problems or mental illness, which could be mild, moderate or severe. Those who require attention after self-harm, or who are suicidal, commonly present for care to EDs and may require ongoing care in a general hospital or acute mental health unit. Their management will be in response to a triage process and respond to essential elements of care.

In an ED or in a general medical setting, a nurse may use a mental health screening or a risk assessment tool, or identify the possibility that mental health symptoms are present and make the appropriate referral within their service context. Nurses provide person-centred and consumer-focused therapeutic approaches and deliver specialised, recovery-oriented, evidence-based care to people across diverse life stages, cultures and settings. Targeted, integrated clinical and social support helps people to maintain connections with family and community. The focus is on keeping people out of acute care (or getting them back to their community as rapidly as possible) by working with them to identify what it is they are experiencing and assisting in providing engagement with the level of mental health services and treatments that they need.

The co-location of mental health units into mainstream general hospitals has resulted in staff who are working in general hospitals having increased contact with service users and clinicians from mental health services, and, of course, people with mental illness experience the same physical illnesses as the rest of the population and require treatment in general medical settings. Chapters 25 and 26 will give you some insight into the mental health needs of people you are likely to come across in emergency and general medical settings and, in particular, about assessing and responding to alteration in a person's mental state to promote optimal wellbeing.

In-Patient Mental Health Units

In-patient mental health units provide a range of services relevant to a person's care needs, presenting circumstances and age. For example, they might focus on children and adolescents, adults or older adults, or they may be considered suitable for acute or subacute presentations, and will provide varying levels of observation, supervision and restriction. They may only accept admissions of people who present voluntarily for treatment, or they may see people who are being detained and treated under mental health legislation; they might be locked or open units. Chapters 27 and 28 provide scenarios that describe some of these variations, and Chapter 29 overviews forensic mental health services for people requiring a secure care setting. Mental health rehabilitation units, which can be provided in hospital or community settings, provide longer term admission (e.g. 3–12 months) for people with complex needs or enduring mental health symptoms, who require intensive treatment and support to develop skills that will support recovery, independent living and improve quality of life.

Increasingly, healthcare is provided in community settings, so it is the person's family, partner and/or friends who often take on an informal carer role. Regardless of whether the person they are caring for has a physical or mental health concern (or both), the caring role has adverse health and mental health impacts on carers themselves (Liu et al 2020). Research shows that carers of people experiencing a mental health crisis describe feeling rejected and overlooked by health professionals and that they can become socially isolated by trying to protect others in their social network from the burden they perceive in sharing their stress and distress (Labrum & Newhill 2021). As such, it is essential that nurses in all service settings provide families and carers with support. This can take the form of acknowledging and validating carers' role, providing advice and education about mental health and illness and its management, making linkages with resources in the community to assist carers with day-to-day issues, and encouraging carers to monitor and respond to their own health and mental health needs (Albert & Simpson 2015). Families also require information about relevant services and payments they may be entitled to if they are providing care for their loved one, including voluntary and non-government services that might assist them. Often, it is a person's family or carers who will be providing the individual with the most infor-

mal care and support, and who will be the ones liaising with health and other services on behalf of the person, especially when the person is acutely unwell. As such, to be able to provide families and carers with all the information they require, an awareness of what these services are in your local community should be part of every nurse's local knowledge. For more detailed information about working with families and carers, see Chapter 5.

CHAPTER SUMMARY

The social ecological or holistic approach to mental health nursing requires that nurses are as competent in recognising and responding to emotional distress and the mental health needs of a person as they are in identifying signs of physical deterioration or a treatment side effect, and that acknowledging the impact of a person's environment and experiences on their health and health outcomes is an important part of understanding their overall health.

The interdependence between all aspects of personhood – including biological, psychological, social and spiritual dimensions – requires that

all nurses consider a person's mental health as part of their core business. The chapters in this section have been designed to provide you with some insight into how fundamental mental health nursing skills are required and can be used across common clinical care settings, as well as to describe the specialist role that mental health nurses might take in a given clinical situation, and provide information relevant to undertaking a mental health clinical placement.

USEFUL WEBSITES

Australian College of Mental Health Nurses: www.acmhn.org/
headspace: headspace.org.au/
Mental Health Australia: mhaustralia.org/
Primary Health Network mental health tools and resources: www.health.gov.au/resources/collections/primary-health-networks-phn-collection-of-primary-mental-health-care-resources?utm_source=health.gov.au&utm_medium=callout-auto-custom&utm_campaign=digital_transformation
SANE Australia: www.sane.org/
Te Ao Maramatanga (New Zealand College of Mental Health Nurses): www.nzcmhn.org.nz/

REFERENCES

Albert, R., Simpson, A., 2015. Double deprivation: A phenomenological study into the experience of being a carer during a mental health crisis. J Adv Nurs, 71 (12), 2753–2762.

Department of Health, 2021. Peer workforce role in mental health and suicide prevention. Online. Available at: www.health.gov.au/sites/default/files/documents/2021/04/primary-health-networks-phn-mental-health-care-guidance-peer-workforce-role-in-mental-health-and-suicide-prevention.pdf

Labrum, T., Newhill, C.E. 2021. Perceived isolation among family caregivers of people with mental illness. Social Work, 66(3), 245–253.

Liu, Z., Heffernan, C., Tan, J. 2020. Caregiver burden: A concept analysis. Int J Nurs Sci. 7(4), 438–445.

Marks, P., 2023. Practice Setting Scenarios: Introduction to the practice-based scenarios. In: Marks, P. Mental Health in Emergency Care. Elsevier, Sydney.

McGough, S., Wynaden, D., Gower, S., et al., 2022. There is no health without cultural safety: Why cultural safety matters. Contemp Nurse 25, 1–10.

McInnes, S., Halcomb, E., Ashley, C., Keann A., Moxham, L., et al., 2022. An integrative review of primary health care nurses' mental health knowledge gaps and learning needs. Collegian, 29(4), 540–548.

Rivero-Santana, A., Perestelo-Perez, L., Alvarez-Perez, Y., Ramos-Garcia, V. et al., 2021. Stepped care for the treatment of depression: a systematic review and meta-analysis. J Affect Disord, 294, 391–409.

World Health Organization (WHO), 1996. Mental health care law: Ten basic principles, WHO, Geneva. policycommons.net/artifacts/468662/mental-health-care-law/1442420/

23

Preparing for Mental Health Clinical Placement

Stephen Van Vorst and Nicole Graham

KEY POINTS

- Mental health nursing is a complex and challenging area of practice that requires students to have an adequate level of preparation. Society still holds many misconceptions about mental illness, and nursing students, as members of society, often share these misconceptions.
- Developing appropriate interpersonal communication and the "therapeutic use of self" is key to establishing therapeutic relationships with the mental health consumer. The relationship should be collaborative and include the consumer's family/ significant others.
- Mental health settings are often less formal than other nursing settings. This can sometimes cause confusion for the student

nurse, who may have difficulty understanding the difference between a social and a therapeutic relationship. Establishing clear professional boundaries is essential to begin to understand the difference.
- Mental health nursing is a highly specialised and rewarding area of nursing practice. While your experience in your mental health placement will help you care for individuals with mental illness in all areas of nursing, we hope that you have a positive placement experience and will consider mental health nursing as a new graduate.

KEY TERMS

Areas of mental health practice	Safety	Therapeutic communication
Goal setting	Safewards	
Professional boundaries	Student attitude and placement concerns	

LEARNING OUTCOMES

The material in this chapter will assist you to:
- understand the uniqueness of a mental health nursing placement and some specific issues that need to be addressed prior to your placement
- identify with, and relate to, the expectations and concerns of other nursing students prior to your first mental health nursing placement
- develop strategies to address your concerns prior to and during your mental health nursing placement

- appreciate the unique contribution all nurses can make in a person's recovery journey
- understand professional boundaries in the mental health setting
- identify the need to care for self in the mental health setting
- achieve the most from the limited time on your mental health nursing placement.

INTRODUCTION

The first clinical placement in a mental health setting can be both daunting and exciting for nursing students. Many students have never experienced a serious mental health issue or illness or entered a mental health service setting. However, most students will know someone who has gone through significant anxiety, depression, substance-related issues, an eating disorder or even a psychotic disorder. While you may have had some solid theoretical preparation for this placement, for most it is the unknown nature of a wide variety of clinical presentations that may make your first day of placement one that is anxiety provoking. As you may have already learnt, having a mild to moderate level of anxiety can be healthy in focusing your preparation for placement and

for ensuring you are giving your best when you begin your placement. It is the aim of this chapter to assist you to manage any anxieties you have about your mental health clinical placement.

While societal attitudes towards mental illness have changed significantly over the last few decades, it is still well documented that student nurses report some misconceptions and stigma, before their first mental health nursing placement (Foster et al 2019; Happell & Gaskin 2013).

This chapter will work through the issues that have been identified by previous nursing students and will provide evidence-based suggestions to enable you to feel more comfortable before and during your first mental health nursing placement. This chapter will also provide you with some strategies to keep yourself safe, care for yourself, and to maximise learning opportunities from your placement.

CHOOSING A STUDENT PLACEMENT

1. It is inappropriate for students to be placed in a mental health service where they currently work (e.g. as an assistant in nursing (AIN) or enrolled nurse (EN)) as this causes role confusion. You are there to be assessed as a student nurse and being placed with your work colleagues may cause bias for or against the assessment of your practice.
2. It is also inappropriate for students to be placed in a mental health service where they have been admitted for mental health treatment at any time. You must notify the university before placements are allocated to ensure this does not occur.

WHAT TYPE OF MENTAL HEALTH SETTING WILL I BE PLACED IN FOR MY MENTAL HEALTH PLACEMENT?

Mental health nursing is a much larger nursing field than most people realise. Mental health nursing provides many subspecialty areas to choose from if you decide to pursue a mental health nursing new graduate program following registration. Here is a list of some of the areas/sub-specialties where you could be placed for your mental health nursing placement:

- Acute – adult in-patient, high dependency, intensive psychiatric care (IPCU/PICU), psychiatric emergency centre (PEC)
- Community (crisis, intake, case management, rehabilitation/living skills)
- Primary care mental health
- Rural and remote
- Forensic (units or in a prison)
- Child and adolescent
- Early intervention
- Mood disorders
- Eating disorders
- Perinatal (antenatal through to postnatal)
- Consultation-liaison – to support non-mental health wards (e.g. – emergency departments (EDs), wards within hospitals "on call")

- Psychogeriatric (specialised aged care in hospitals and the community).

While "Alcohol & Other Drug" (AOD) placements are often utilised for a mental health nursing placement, AOD is a specialty in its own right, and specific preparation for an AOD placement should be provided before such a placement. AOD knowledge and skills (including screening, assessment and treatment) are important for mental health nurses, given the high levels of co-occurring mental health and AOD conditions. Box 23.1 lists some of the common thoughts and concerns of student nurses prior to their first placement in a mental health setting.

ADDRESSING CONCERNS AND SOME TIPS FOR PREPARING FOR PLACEMENT

I'm concerned that I will say something that will make the person more unwell or annoyed.

Remember, mental health consumers are first and foremost people. The consumers you will be placed with and caring for will respond primarily to your intentions. While your intentions will be informed by what you have learnt theoretically in class and within this text, even the most experienced clinician does not always engage in "perfect" communication. There is no perfect communication or response to every situation you face. What is most important is that you always approach and speak genuinely and respectfully. The consumer will recognise a respectful approach in your tone of voice and your willingness to engage. See therapeutic communication below.

I'm concerned it will be difficult to initiate conversations with consumers.

This is another common concern that usually disappears quite early on in the placement, and often on the first day. This is because several consumers will probably approach you to find out what you are doing there. This provides you with the perfect opportunity to introduce yourself and begin a conversation. It is vital that you inform everyone you meet that you are a student nurse and that this is your first placement in a mental health setting. This lets consumers know that you are inexperienced. This is important as some consumers would prefer to

---

BOX 23.1   Common Student Thoughts and Concerns Prior to Placement in a Mental Health Setting

Common Positive Thoughts Prior to Their First Placement	Common Concerns Prior to First Placement in a Mental Health Setting
Looking forward to meeting individuals with significant mental health issues. Engaging with them and learning from them.	I'm concerned that I will say something that will make the person more unwell or annoyed. (This is probably the most common concern expressed by nursing students prior to a mental health nursing placement.)
Looking forward to meeting nursing staff who are good role models and learning from them.	I'm concerned it will be difficult to initiate conversations with consumers.
I'm excited to experience such a different area of nursing.	I'm concerned about seeing aggression/violence in this setting.
I'm keen to understand the impact of past experiences, particularly any history of trauma.	I'm concerned I don't know what type of nursing skills I will be able to demonstrate in this type of clinical setting.
I'd like to gain a better understanding of the *Mental Health Act* and how the rights of an individual are protected when being held involuntarily.	I'm worried about someone talking to me about suicide or self-harm. What should I say? What if I make the situation worse?
I'm interested in better understanding therapeutic interventions in mental health nursing – interpersonal, diversional, pharmacological, and other treatments like electroconvulsive therapy (ECT) and transcranial magnetic stimulation (TMS).	I'm worried about what to do if someone tells me something they haven't told anyone else or asks me not to tell? What if they reveal trauma? What if I can't cope with hearing other people's traumatic stories?
See "Useful Websites" at the end of this chapter.	

engage with a more experienced staff member, depending on what stage they are at with their recovery. This is something you shouldn't take personally. Empathy is key to understanding what stage of recovery each consumer is at. On the other hand, some consumers may see your lack of experience as an opportunity to assist you with your learning by giving you more of their time and sharing their experiences of illness and recovery. This is a perfect time to ask questions such as: "When you are unwell, what can nurses do to help you?" "What do they do that you find unhelpful?"

I'm concerned about seeing aggression/violence in this setting.

This is a concern that comes primarily from media representations of mental illness or from movies that, historically, have exaggerated or misrepresented mental illness due to a lack of understanding and/or for dramatic purposes. While the media and movies have become increasingly accurate in recent times, you will quickly realise that the reality remains far from these representations. However, depending on where you are placed, you may witness some consumers with significant anxiety, agitation and restlessness. To the inexperienced nurse, these behaviour states may incorrectly be interpreted as aggression. Regarding actual aggression, you are most likely to encounter verbal aggression or physical aggression where someone may punch a wall or damage furniture. This should be explained at the beginning of your placement by your facilitator and the staff in the facility.

The key in these situations is to talk with your "buddy" nurse or your clinical teacher if you feel uncomfortable or out of your depth. Experienced nurses remember what it was like to be new to the mental health setting and will help you with specific tips for the individual and the situation. This is one of the reasons why attending orientation is essential. If you are in an acute setting, you will be advised of any consumers who are "at risk" for several reasons, including self-harm, vulnerabilities, risk for absconding and risk for harm to others. In the acute settings, you will probably be provided with a duress alarm and instructed on when and how to use it. **It is important to remember that student nurses are not to be involved in intervening in aggression. Please seek help from staff if a situation is escalating**.

I'm worried about someone talking to me about suicide or self-harm. What should I say? What if I make the situation worse?

We have a duty of care to ask consumers if they are having suicidal thoughts. This may be one of the most challenging conversations for a student nurse or anyone who is new to mental health nursing. While asking someone if they are suicidal can cause you anxiety, most people will be relieved that you are willing to discuss suicide and they may start to share quite openly and deeply. Depending on your experience, this may soon cause you to feel anxious and out of your depth. Don't stress; this is normal. As soon as possible, inform the person that you are feeling out of your depth as you are a student nurse (or new to the setting) and have not had experience with helping people who have suicidal thoughts. You could also suggest that they speak to someone with more experience. This will not make the situation worse. In fact, the consumer will respect you for informing them of your inexperience and discomfort. They will either wait to speak with someone else or, from our experience, might choose to help you by offering to educate you about how to help someone in their position.

I'm worried about what to do if someone tells me something they haven't told anyone else, or asks me not to tell. What if they reveal trauma? What if I can't cope with hearing other people's traumatic stories?

As you may already know, developing a rapport and maintaining confidentiality are key components for the development of a therapeutic relationship. In the mental health setting, the mental health team is part of the therapeutic relationship, and it is inappropriate to promise that you can hold a secret from other members of the team. This could leave gaps in the care delivered by others in the team and could create circumstances where staff could be played off against each other. Therefore, it is vital that you inform the person that everything that is shared will be discussed with the wider mental health team. See the section on "The importance of maintaining confidentiality" below. If the person reveals past trauma, this should also be shared with other members of the team. Following these principles will ensure that comprehensive and consistent care is delivered, while ensuring that you are supported by senior staff to assist you to cope with hearing stories of trauma as a nursing student.

Someone I know, or in my family, has a mental illness and I'm concerned that I might feel uncomfortable talking about or hearing about other people's mental health problems.

This situation can go two ways. Your personal experience with mental illness may place you in an advantageous position as you may have a better ability to place yourself in someone else's shoes and therefore be more helpful. The temptation will be to overshare from your own experience, potentially burdening the consumer with your story. For this reason, it is not advised that you share your personal stories with consumers. On the other hand, hearing other people's stories may make you feel uncomfortable, especially if you have not come to a clear understanding of how best to help your loved one. This is a situation that you should raise with your clinical teacher/facilitator early in the placement as they are there to guide you through such situations.

I'm concerned that I don't know what type of nursing skills I will be able to demonstrate in this type of clinical setting.

There are many clinical tasks in mental health settings that are shared with other clinical environments. For example, the mental health nursing staff will need to attend to the individual physical health care needs of each consumer. These tasks vary depending on the type of clinical setting and consumer cohort and can include the following: physical observations, medication administration, perioperative checklists, postoperative observations, wound management, food and fluid monitoring, nasogastric tube insertion and management, A–G assessments, assisted daily living skills, and in some cases, management of indwelling catheters and intravenous therapy. Nursing students will also be expected to have current skills in cardiopulmonary resuscitation.

The tasks above also offer opportunities for the nurse to develop and maintain the therapeutic relationship and conduct assessments of mental state in a more natural and informal interaction. There are also additional learning and practice opportunities in many of the mental health clinical environments, such as:

- comprehensive mental health assessments
- mental state assessments
- risk assessments
- attending and observing electroconvulsive therapy (ECT)
- attending and observing transcranial magnetic stimulation (TMS)
- participating in consumer therapy and activity groups
- attending and contributing to case reviews
- attending and contributing to reviews, assessments and interventions with different members of the multidisciplinary team
- becoming familiar with the Mental Health Act and associated requirements
- participating in staff and consumer debrief sessions
- attending home visits and/or therapeutic social outings.

Active participation in the team and engaging with consumers is highly valued and often helps to break down preconceived ideas and notions. It allows you to develop a comprehensive understanding of the role of the mental health nurse. It is important to remain under the supervision of your "buddy" or practice partner and to alert the team to any concerns you may have as you develop your confidence and skills in this new area.

THERAPEUTIC COMMUNICATION AND SETTING PROFESSIONAL BOUNDARIES

Empathetic understanding, unconditional positive regard and congruence form the foundations for building effective therapeutic relationships (Moreno-Poyato & Rodriquez-Nogueira 2019; Rogers 1959). In mental health nursing, emphasis is placed on the nurse's therapeutic use of self, with communication as a core skill. Activities such as taking physical observations as part of the nursing role provide the opportunity to develop or build engagement, at the same time as addressing physical health needs.

A model of reducing conflict and containment known as the Safewards model is widely implemented in mental health wards/units and has been adapted for community settings. The model recognises that there are social, emotional or environmental stressors (originating domains) that can lead to conflict (flashpoints), resulting in containment which can seriously impede therapeutic relationships between consumers and the team who support their recovery (Bowers 2014; Fletcher et al 2019). Strategies are suggested within the model that can improve consumer experience and help develop and maintain therapeutic relationships. With an awareness of common flashpoints, modifiers can be implemented through a variety of Safewards interventions. Even without the model being implemented in the clinical setting, the following interventions can be easily applied.

Soft Words

Be respectful and polite, verbally express your understanding of frustration and difficulty for the person, monitor body language, and ensure you are not presenting as authoritarian. Be attentive, listen and hear a consumer's request, and provide reasons why they may not be able to be fulfilled, with a willingness to negotiate.

Positive Words

Saying something positive about a person in handover promotes appreciation of the person. This could include highlighting a positive quality of the person or something positive that the person has been doing today. If this is not possible, sharing something positive about how staff have supported the consumer should be offered. Detailed reasons for difficult or disruptive behaviour should also be included to help better understand the person's behaviour.

Bad News Mitigation

When a consumer receives unwelcome or bad news either from within or external to the place of treatment, it can lead to a desire to leave the facility impulsively or be a leading factor in escalating behaviour. It is important to be aware of occasions or events that might generate strong emotional reactions and allow a quiet place for the person to express their feelings, while acknowledging frustrations. Answer questions honestly and give the person time, sympathy and empathy.

Reassurance

Adverse events such as aggression, containment or medication coercion can impact everyone in the clinical area. Consumers can react with fear or anger, which can increase the risk of a contagion effect occurring between consumers. Following adverse events, a debrief and opportunity to consider psychological explanations should be offered to all consumers, either alone or in small groups. This will provide a chance to help reduce stereotypes and stigma often portrayed in the media (Bowers 2014; Bowers et al 2014; Fletcher et al 2019).

In summary, being kind, empathetic and respectful in your communication, along with being present and allowing a person to express their concerns or fears without judgement, are the key attributes required to be helpful and to build therapeutic relationships. The Safewards model is becoming more popular as it is proven to reduce conflict and containment. You may find the UK website helpful to expand your knowledge of the model in more detail (see Useful websites at the end of the chapter), as well as find additional interventions not mentioned above.

THE IMPORTANCE OF MAINTAINING CONFIDENTIALITY

Confidentiality is a legal and legislative requirement, as well as an ethical and registration requirement for registered health practitioners and students (Nursing and Midwifery Board of Australia (NMBA) 2022). It is vital that the care of a consumer is only discussed among the staff involved in their care. This includes avoiding conversations about consumers outside of the service setting, on public transport, or with family or friends. This is to protect the privacy of the consumer and any breach of this will be considered a serious disciplinary matter.

Occasionally a student turns up to placement and finds that someone they know is in the unit or facility and is therefore, potentially in their care. This is a situation that the nurse in charge and your clinical teacher/facilitator must immediately be made aware of. As you would appreciate, there are many variables that could influence such a situation. Depending on these variables, you may be able to stay in the facility if you are not involved in direct care of the person. In some circumstances, however, you may need to be moved to another facility for your placement.

Despite the evidence that bedside handover is best practice, there has been research to indicate that some nurses have concerns about implementation of bedside handover in the mental health setting. The research found that the nurses strongly identified the importance of confidentiality and privacy of the consumers they are caring for (Mullen et al 2020). Confidentiality is an incredibly important element in maintaining the therapeutic relationship. A person will feel safe to seek help and open up if they are aware of your requirements and commitment to maintain confidentiality. The development of trust enables a person to feel safe in sharing their experiences, thoughts and symptoms. This level of communication will facilitate the completion of a holistic assessment and better align support and interventions.

There are very few circumstances that allow for information sharing outside of the one-to-one nurse–consumer relationship, the most common being related to disclosure by the consumer of the intention of serious harm to self or others. In this instance, it is highly recommended that the nurse, including students, discuss their concerns with the nurse in charge and the treating team.

PROFESSIONAL BOUNDARIES AND PERSONAL SAFETY

Students often inquire about maintaining personal safety and professional boundaries. The nurse intentionally works to remove barriers and reduce power imbalances, with emphasis placed on the consumer's autonomy and control over their life and treatment (Thomson et al 2022). These actions may result in what appears to be more of a social relationship. However, the professional nursing relationship is not a social relationship.

Maintaining professional boundaries is the key to ensuring that the relationship remains professional and goal-directed, and complies with the Nursing and Midwifery Board of Australia Code of Conduct for Nurses (2022) Principle 4: Professional behaviour. There is a variety of different professional boundary considerations. There are boundaries related to role, time, place and space, money, gifts and services, clothing, language, self-disclosure and physical contact. See Box 23.2 for details.

BOX 23.2   Boundary Considerations

Clothing Boundaries	Some placement providers request that students wear civilian clothing instead of uniforms to help reduce the power imbalance. In this case, it is the nurse's obligation to ensure that their dress is professional, well-fitting with appropriate coverage, and with no motifs that may convey confusing messages or be offensive.
Gifts and Services	Receiving gifts can compromise the professional relationship. This includes what are considered small token gifts, such as paying for coffee when out on a social outing. Gift-giving may be motivated by a consumer's sense of obligation and may lead to an inappropriately personal relationship. In addition, giving gifts to consumers is inappropriate as it is not part of the professional relationship and can impact on recovery.
Language Boundaries	Informal language is often used by nursing staff when communicating with consumers. The use of abusive language and swearing is not appropriate and is considered unprofessional.
Money Boundaries	There may be a situation where a consumer may be short on money or not have immediate access to money. Lending or gifting money, even small amounts, impedes independence and recovery goals, and impacts on professional relationships.
Physical Contact Boundaries	Often consumers lack connection or have a history of trauma. When someone is upset, natural instincts may be to provide physical contact, such as a hug. Physical contact may cause unintended re-traumatisation and/or be misinterpreted. On the other hand, therapeutic touch is also beneficial. It is best to be guided by a clinical supervisor and included in a reflection. The nature of an informal relationship can also present challenges such as physical and emotional attraction for the consumer or their carer. Sexual behaviours, contact or relationships between health professionals and consumers is a clear boundary violation.
Place and Space Boundaries	Social and recreational outings are often integrated into recovery plans. It is important to recognise the difference between professional and social relationships. The outing should be goal-directed and focused on the recovery plan for the consumer.
Role Boundaries	Holistic care plays a vital role within mental health nursing. Your role is to support the physical, social and emotional wellbeing and recovery of the consumer. The broader role of a mental health nurse is at risk of being misinterpreted as a social relationship. It is essential to ensure you communicate clearly with the consumer and reflect on your own emotions.
Self-Disclosure Boundaries	When developing relationships, it is often a shared transaction of information. There is a Safewards intervention, "Get to know each other," whereby the nurse will provide some general information about themselves, such as favourite food, movies and broad hobbies. It is inappropriate for nurses to discuss personal problems, feelings or aspects of intimate or personal life with a person in their care.
Time Boundaries	As with all relationships, there are times when a nurse may feel a more comfortable connection with a particular consumer. This can result in the nurse spending more time with this consumer than other allocated consumers. It is essential to monitor such occurrences, so as not to impact on your relationship and the care of other consumers being cared for. It is also inappropriate to spend time with a person when off-duty or if the person is no longer in their direct care.

Bowers 2014; NMBA 2010, 2016, 2019, 2022.

Professional boundaries are at a higher risk of being confused in the more informal setting of mental health. Considering these in more detail will help to identify any issues that may need to be addressed.

PERSONAL SAFETY

In all areas of health care, personal safety and caring for self are important aspects of nursing. Depending on the clinical area that you are attending for placement, the strategies implemented to reduce risk will vary. It is important to identify the local procedures in place to manage risk. In the community setting, it is common to complete an environmental risk assessment, and there are processes to monitor the movement of staff. In a hospital setting, duress systems are often in place, which alert the team if a risk presents to a consumer or staff, such as a person experiencing a significant behavioural disturbance or absconding. If you are given a duress alarm device, please ensure you are aware of the processes to activate it, under what circumstances and how to deactivate an accidental alarm. Please ensure your device is suitably attached to your person.

If an incident occurs, it is important to engage in debriefing activities, even if you did not participate or directly witness the event. Care providers are recognised as second victims and incidents can have considerable emotional distress or can contribute to trauma and burnout (Morris 2022).

Nursing requires listening to consumers' experiences, including trauma, and witnessing distress and pain with empathy. While compassion is considered a core skill, this quality can contribute to the experience of vicarious trauma (Isobel & Thomas 2022). It is also important to acknowledge that many healthcare professionals have also experienced trauma, which can lead to re-traumatisation. Self-care strategies are essential for healthcare professionals regardless of their discipline or which clinical setting they practice in (Murphy et al 2022). Here are some suggested helpful activities:

- Engaging in activities such as mindfulness, exercise, relaxation, hobbies
- Engaging in reflective practices, clinical supervision or debriefing
- Psychological first aid or employee/student assistance programs or spiritual support
- Support by practice partners, team leaders or clinical educators (Isobel & Thomas 2022; Morris et al 2022).

SAFETY AND SUPERVISION

- Students must be orientated to code responses and any personal duress alarm system. **Students are not to participate in any part of a physical restraint of or seclusion and must remove themselves to a safe location.**
- Students are to be directly supervised by a registered nurse when administering medications.
- Communicate to "buddy" nurse or nurse in charge when leaving the clinical area for any period of time.
- If the unit is locked it is important to confirm with the nurse in charge before letting consumers leave. Be mindful of a person's status under the Mental Health Act and any leave provisions that may be in place.

In summary, professional boundaries are essential when working in mental health settings. Many people accessing mental health services are vulnerable, and the onus is on the student nurse to ensure that they maintain and promote professional relationships. There are often safety procedures and protocols in the local healthcare environments. It is essential to become familiar with these. Self-care is a crucial element of nursing practice and is highly recommended when completing placement.

GOAL SETTING PRIOR TO PLACEMENT

Setting goals for placement is essential, both personal and professional. While it is your choice what goals you want to set, here are some examples to get you started:

- Become comfortable being with the consumers within a mental health service setting.
- Better understand the influence of past trauma on current mental states.
- Better understand the impact of other past influences and experiences (genetics, environmental, developmental, etc.).
- Better understand the influence of current social factors on mental state (isolation, accommodation/homelessness, significant loss – loved one, employment, financial independence, relationship/s, etc.)
- Overcome fears of challenging behaviour. Identify what behaviours are challenging, understand why these behaviours may occur and observe how others manage these behaviours. Follow local safety protocols.
- Understand the key role a mental health nurse plays within the multi-disciplinary team.
- Make deliberate efforts to stay self-aware. For example, how is the placement affecting me and how is my behaviour effecting others?
- Understand the potential for a medical condition to impact mental health (e.g. chronic pain, cancer, terminal illness, brain injury, substance dependency, etc.).
- Pursue opportunities to reduce stigma.
- Sit in on an assessment with one of the registered nurses or doctors.
- Get to know the common medications that are administered (indications, side effects, and side effect management) and feel confident in medication administration (**always and only when accompanied by a registered nurse**).

- Better understand the components and importance of a mental state assessment.
- Develop confidence in descriptive report writing.
- Feel confident to present a handover of allocated consumers.
- Attend a Mental Health Review Tribunal if possible.
- Attend at least one case review.
- Attend any education sessions.

To assist with your goal setting, you could frame your goals using the SMART technique (Doran 1981); that is, ensuring that each goal is:

Specific
Measurable
Achievable
Relevant
Time-bound

We recommend that you create these goals prior to placement, discuss them with your clinical teacher/facilitator at the commencement of your placement, and review them after a couple of days or at the end of your first week of placement. Also, be prepared to reset some of these goals by the end of your first week, as you will probably find that you settle into your mental health placement more quickly than you expect.

OCCUPATIONAL SCREENING AND VACCINATIONS (OSV)

If your mental health nursing placement is not your first professional experience placement, you will have already completed the necessary occupational screening and vaccination requirements. Otherwise, all requirements of your state or territory Department of Health for nursing apply to mental health. In most cases, this includes vaccinations against COVID-19, hepatitis B, varicella, DTPa, influenza, tuberculosis, measles, mumps and rubella (MMR), a National Police Check (NPC), and a Working with Children Check (WWCC). Some universities may also require a first aid and CPR qualification.

Remember, some of the above are time-limited and will require an annual or three-yearly update. For example, some states and territories require you to have an annual flu vaccine prior to June. Some universities may require an annual first aid and CPR update. You will need to find out whether your NPC or WWCC is due to expire before the completion of your nursing program. Not keeping on top of these requirements could mean you will not be able to attend your placement.

? CRITICAL THINKING EXERCISE 23.1

1. Kirsty is a second-year nursing student who is on placement on a mental health in-patient ward and has been working with her clinical supervisor on developing interpersonal skills and maintaining professional boundaries. One of the consumers Kirsty is caring for is Marissa, a young woman close to Kirsty's age. In talking with Marissa, Kirsty becomes aware that they share certain life issues. These are to do with trust, forming intimate relationships and a fear of being abandoned if they let anyone get too close to them. Because they have so much in common Kirsty feels able to help Marissa more than the other nurses on the ward. Kirsty's friends are having a party next weekend and she decides to invite Marissa so that Marissa can meet some new people and perhaps form some friendships. Kirsty decides to discuss this with her supervisor after the party, when she will be able to report on how the intervention has worked.

Q. Do you think Kirsty is at risk of breaking professional boundaries? What suggestions can you make that would help Kirsty to develop safe and positive interpersonal relationships?

2. Robert is a nursing student who has just finished the first week of his mental health nursing placement. Robert has been surprised how much he has enjoyed the placement so far and shares some of his experiences on Facebook, including the name of the facility where he is placed and some information about one of the consumers. He wrote about a woman in a manic state who was "sexually disinhibited and was dancing on a table in the middle of the ward". He also wrote how great the nurses were, except for one who he described as "a real dragon who should have retired twenty years ago". His post is seen by someone at the facility and he is reported to the university. Robert's placement is cancelled, and he is given a fail grade for the unit. The facility has stated that they will not have Robert back, ever!

Q. What are the key concerns in this scenario?

3. Sally is nearing the end of her clinical placement and is happy that she has, as she describes, "developed some good relationships". In particular, Sally feels quite close to a 21-year-old man Bill, who is about to be discharged from the acute unit after a lengthy admission for drug-induced psychosis.

Continued

❓ CRITICAL THINKING EXERCISE 23.1—cont'd

Bill asks if they could catch up in the future for a coffee and a chat. They exchange phone numbers and begin texting each other.

Q. Has Sally crossed any professional boundaries?

4. After a couple of weeks, Sally and Bill catch up for a coffee and pretty soon their connection changes to a romantic relationship. Bill starts smoking cannabis again and soon starts to develop psychotic symptoms, hearing voices and experiencing paranoid delusions. Part of his paranoid beliefs include ideas that Sally is trying to influence his thinking and that she has been instrumental in causing him to lose his part-time job as a barista. Bill is also struggling with his university studies and eventually, he requires re-admission to the acute unit. Sally truly thought she could help Bill to stay well, but now she is confused and scared as he is blaming her for everything that is going wrong in his life. Sally makes an appointment with her mental health nursing lecturer to discuss the situation as she is afraid that Bill will physically harm her.

Q. How do you think her lecturer will respond?

CHAPTER SUMMARY

In this chapter we have explored key issues that will provide assistance in planning and preparing for an initial placement in the mental health setting. We have identified the wide range of areas that you may be sent to for your mental health placement and hope that you appreciate how extensive the field of mental health nursing is. We shared some common student thoughts and concerns prior to a first mental health placement and provided some tips to manage these concerns. We have revisited the importance of the therapeutic relationship and the therapeutic use of self in mental health nursing. We have also included Safewards as a clinical model to help nurses reduce conflict and containment. We hope that you appreciate the importance of managing professional boundaries, safety concerns and caring for self in the mental health setting. We have also provided you with some tips for setting goals in preparation for your placement and hope you see the importance of renewing these goals on a regular basis and that you utilise the model of reflection provided to you by your institution of study to continue to improve your clinical practice. We wish you all the best for an enjoyable and fruitful mental health nursing experience.

USEFUL WEBSITES

ECT – The Whole Story, Gold Coast Health (8 min 13s): www.youtube.com/watch?v=IjoS31JC0As

The ECT Journey, Gold Coast Health (6 min 4s): www.youtube.com/watch?v=HEot7ow3yfk

Nursing and Midwifery Board of Australia: www.nursingmidwiferyboard.gov.au/

Safewards: www.safewards.net

Transcranial Magnetic Stimulation (ABC) (2 min 24s + article): www.abc.net.au/news/2021-07-06/transcranial-magnetic-stimulation-added-to-medicare/100170484

REFERENCES

Bowers, L. 2014. Safewards: A new model of conflict and containment on psychiatric wards. Journal of Psychiatric and Mental Health Nursing, 21(6), 499–508.

Bowers, L., Alexander, J., Bilgin, H., Botha, M., Dack, C., et al., 2014. Safewards: The empirical basis of the model and a critical appraisal. J Psychiatric Ment Health Nurs, 21(4), 354–364.

Doran, G.T. 1981. There's a S.M.A.R.T. way to write management's goals and objectives. Manage Rev, 70, 35–36.

Fletcher, J., Hamilton, B., Kinner, S.A., & Brophy, L. 2019. Safewards impact in inpatient mental health units in Victoria, Australia: Staff perspectives. Frontiers Psychiatry, 462.

Foster, K., Withers, E., Blanco, T., Lupson, C., Steele, M., et al., 2019. Undergraduate nursing students' stigma and recovery attitudes during mental health clinical placement: A pre/post-test survey study. Int J Ment Health Nurs, 28, 1068–1080.

Happell, B. & Gaskin, C.J. 2013. The attitudes of undergraduate nursing students towards mental health nursing: A systematic review. J Clin Nurs, 22, 148–158.

Isobel, S. & Thomas, M. 2022. Vicarious trauma and nursing: An integrative review. Int J Ment Health Nurs, 31(2), 247–259.

Moreno-Poyato, A.R., & Rodríguez-Nogueira, Ó. 2021. The association between empathy and the nurse–patient therapeutic relationship in mental health units: a cross-sectional study. J Psychiatric Ment Health Nurs, 28(3), 335–343.

Morris, D., Sveticic, J., Grice, D., Turner, K., & Graham, N. 2022. Collaborative approach to supporting staff in a mental healthcare setting: "Always There" Peer Support Program. Iss Ment Health Nurs, 43(1), 42–50.

Mullen, A., Harman, K., Flanagan, K., O'Brien, B., & Isobel, S. 2020. Involving mental health consumers in nursing handover: A qualitative study of nursing views of the practice and its implementation. Int J Ment Health Nurs, 29(6), 1157–1167.

Murphy, J., Farrell, K., Kealy, M.B., & Kristiniak, S. 2023. Mindfulness as a self-care strategy for healthcare professionals to reduce stress and implicit bias. J Interprofess Ed Prac, 30, 100598.

Nursing and Midwifery Board of Australia (NMBA), 2022. Code of Conduct for Nurses. Australian Health Practitioner Regulation Agency. Victoria.

Nursing and Midwifery Board of Australia (NMBA), 2019. Social media: How to meet your obligations under the National Law. Online. Available at: www.nursingmidwiferyboard.gov.au/Codes-Guidelines-Statements/Codes-Guidelines/Social-media-guidance.aspx

Nursing and Midwifery Board of Australia (NMBA), 2016. Registered Nurse Standards of Practice. Australian Health Practitioner Regulation Agency, Victoria.

Nursing and Midwifery Board of Australia (NMBA), 2010. A nurse's guide to professional boundaries. Australian Health Practitioner Regulation Agency, Victoria.

Rogers, C.R. 1959. A theory of therapy, personality and interpersonal relationships as developed in the client-centered framework. In: Koch, S. (ed.), Psychology: A study of a science. Vol. 3: Formulations of the person and the social context. McGraw-Hill, New York.

Thomson, A.E., Smith, N. & Karpa, J. 2022. Strategies used to teach professional boundaries psychiatric nursing education. Iss Ment Health Nurs, 43(10), 895–902.

24

Primary Care and Community

Elizabeth Halcomb, Elissa-Kate Jay and Taylor Yousiph

KEY POINTS

- Mental health issues arise in all clinical settings. Primary and community care settings provide an important opportunity for the early identification of mental health symptoms and the implementation of appropriate therapeutic interventions.
- While nurses need to perform within their individual scope of practice, primary care and community nurses should be confident in talking to clients about their mental health, competently undertake an initial assessment of mental health and identify where referral to specialist services is required.
- Primary care and community nurses need to be vigilant in identifying mental health issues opportunistically when providing care for physical health issues, as well as in those with established mental illness.

- People living with mental health issues also have a high risk of poor physical health. Primary care and community care nurses can improve health outcomes by ensuring people have adequate access to physical health services, including metabolic and preventative health screening.
- Stigma still plays a substantial role in people accessing mental health services. Non-judgmental care and value-free language are important to reduce stigma.
- Primary care and community nurses should talk openly with people about their mental health to build a relationship of trust upon which to share symptoms or concerns.

KEY TERMS

Communication	Counselling	Primary care
Community care	General practice	Stigma

LEARNING OUTCOMES

The material in this chapter will assist you to:
- understand the importance of a person-centred approach to both physical and mental health within Primary care and community settings
- recognise the need to ensure mental health is adequately considered when delivering nursing care in the community

- consider how primary care and community nurses can influence the recovery of people with enduring mental health conditions and short-term mental health issues
- appreciate that support for mental health can improve overall health, wellbeing and quality of life.

LIVED EXPERIENCE COMMENT BY JARRAD HICKMOTT
The scenarios in this chapter acknowledge the difficulty that people experiencing mental health concerns can have in putting forward their concerns and perspectives. Pharmacology is not the be-all and end-all, but rather a cog in the wheel that makes up the mental health sector. Providing consumers with the breadth of services and options out there is of the greatest benefit. Identifying the role the media plays in the portrayal and perpetuation of mental health stigma is extremely important.

INTRODUCTION

This chapter provides an overview of the key considerations regarding mental health in the primary care and community setting. In reading this chapter, you will explore mental health as an important aspect of holistic health care for everyone. While for some people mental health problems are enduring, for others mental health issues occur at various points in their life and are often related to situational crises. Regardless of the nature or severity of the mental health issue, early identification, assessment and intervention are likely to offer the best outcomes. This chapter will help you to understand that although every nurse may not choose to develop specialist mental health nursing skills, all nurses have an important role to play in supporting mental health in our community.

Specialist mental health nurses have expert skills and knowledge in mental health that extends their scope of practice in this area. However, every nurse has a responsibility to practise safely, within their scope of practice, to deliver mental health screening, assessment, referral and support (Halcomb et al 2018). A recent review of randomised trials of primary care, nurse-delivered interventions for adults with a mental illness reported that these interventions were acceptable to consumers and health professionals (Halcomb et al 2019). This review also found that participants experienced significant improvement in symptoms, while also reporting higher levels of satisfaction when engaging in the general practice nurse-led intervention (Halcomb et al 2019). This highlights the important role of primary care and community nurses in supporting mental health.

PRESENTATIONS TO PRIMARY CARE AND COMMUNITY SETTINGS

Although there are differences in access to primary care and community services across metropolitan and rural areas, and barriers exist for some population groups, most people in Australia and Aotearoa New Zealand attend primary care and community settings for healthcare services. Some 83.6% of Australian adults see a general practitioner (GP) each year (Australian Bureau of Statistics (ABS) 2022c). In 2021, 70% of GPs reported psychological presentations to be the most common presentation in Australia (Suetani et al 2022). During the COVID-19 pandemic, primary care nurses reported an increase in mental health presentations (Halcomb et al 2020). For this reason, primary care and community settings are important, particularly in terms of mental health promotion for all, identifying those at risk of mental ill health and early identification of those with symptoms (see Chapters 1 and 3, which provide more information about a stepped care approach in mental health and what this means for mental health care across the spectrum of experiences). In addition, we know that primary care and community settings are essential to supporting the physical health of people with enduring mental illness.

While many people who live with mental illness experience good physical health and long, productive lives, there is significant evidence linking mental illness diagnoses and poor physical health (Spooner et al 2022). People living with severe mental illnesses have been demonstrated to have, on average, a life expectancy up to 20 years shorter than people in the general community (Spooner et al 2022). The majority of deaths that occur in people with mental illness are preventable physical illnesses, such as cardiovascular disease and diabetes (Spooner et al 2022). Antipsychotic medications, lifestyle risk factors and socioeconomic status are all factors that contribute to the higher prevalence of physical ill health (Hackett & Fitzgerald 2020). The Australian Institute of Health and Welfare (AIHW) (2022b) reports that 71.1% of individuals with a severe mental illness have at least one physical health condition.

An international meta-analysis has demonstrated that people with mental illness have a mortality rate 2.2 times greater than those living without mental health conditions (Walker et al 2015). Among those with mental health conditions, there is a median of 10-year potential life lost due to premature death (Walker et al 2015). It has been reported that this gap continues to increase (Firth et al 2019). In Australia, 10 people living with a mental illness die prematurely as a consequence of a physical illness such as cancer or cardiovascular or respiratory diseases for every one person living with a mental illness who dies as a result of suicide (ABS 2017). There is a similar situation in Aotearoa New Zealand, where an estimated two-thirds of premature mortality in those with mental illness is attributable to preventable and manageable physical health issues (Ministry of Health 2019b). Optimising physical health in people experiencing mental illness is becoming a priority area for governments and policymakers (Ministry of Health 2019b).

There is a fundamental role for nurses in supporting people living with mental illness to manage their physical health as well as their mental health. Importantly, nurses should believe people with mental illness when they talk about their physical and emotional symptoms. People with mental illnesses often have their opinions disregarded and their voices silenced (Cutler et al 2020; Ellegaard et al 2020). Further,

it is recognised that a historical or current diagnosis of mental illness may overshadow coexisting physical conditions, potentially leading to inadequate treatment of the presenting problems.

Nurses can make a valuable contribution by educating individuals living with mental illness, their families, carers and kin, to understand the medications that they are taking, their side effects and ways to manage any adverse reactions (Ameel et al 2019). Nurses have an important role in supporting people to engage in and maintain a healthy lifestyle (Lundstrom et al 2020). Lifestyle risk factors such as inadequate diet, limited physical activity and smoking are higher in this population (Spooner et al 2022), and add to the higher risk of chronic physical conditions in this group. Nurses can help evaluate a person's readiness to change lifestyle risk factors, support people to identify and implement change actions and reinforce the benefits of sustaining even small changes. The value of positive reinforcement, encouragement and emotional support should never be underestimated.

It is also essential for nurses to consider the mental health of people presenting to primary care and community settings with physical health problems and to keep alert to the fact that the person may be experiencing a mental health issue. For example, when people visit their primary care practitioner for a physical health issue, they could report many symptoms and manifestations of a mental health issue, including describing physical symptoms or talking about lifestyle stressors (McInnes et al 2022). Indeed, pain is one of the most frequent initial complaints among mental health presentations in primary care. Compared with the wider population, people with chronic diseases such as diabetes and cardiovascular disease are significantly more likely to experience major depression (Bucciarelli et al 2020). Keep in mind too that men are less likely than women to seek help for mental health concerns, with one in eight males compared to one in five females seeking advice from a health professional for their mental health (ABS 2022b).

More than 30% of individuals saw their primary care provider during the month before suicide and almost 90% of people who died by suicide had reported at least one "red flag" (ABS 2022a). Primary care presents a valuable potential intervention point for identifying people at risk of suicide and offering help (Pedersen et al 2021). It is incumbent upon nurses to notice and act on "red flags" and to open conversations about mental health to help people communicate their mental health needs. Nurses should not only seek to pick up on cues and ask appropriate and effective probing questions, but also initiate conversations about mental health – in the same way that nurses should explore the physical health of people with mental illness. It is also imperative that nurses seriously consider the presence of suicidal ideation and intent and ask people directly. Many people worry that asking about suicide will cause people to act. That attitude and belief is a myth. Suicide can be a real concern across the lifespan regardless of a person's background, education or financial status. Ignoring the topic of suicide won't make it go away, but having an honest and respectful conversation about how a person is feeling might just save their life. To read more about suicide and risk assessment see Chapter 9.

The Australian College of Mental Health Nurses' *Mental Health Practice Standards for Nurses in Australian General Practice* (Halcomb et al 2018) are aligned with (and follow the same domains as) the Australian Nursing and Midwifery Federation's *National Practice Standards for Nurses Working in Australian General Practice* (Halcomb et al 2017). This document provides a broad framework that articulates how nurses working in primary care and community settings can contribute to the mental health and wellbeing of Australians.

The following scenarios (24.1 and 24.2) describe how the application of a "mental health" lens can be applied to people presenting to primary care and community settings.

EVIDENCE-BASED PRACTICE

Scenario 24.1: Jack

Jack is a 70-year-old man with a long history of hypertension and cardiovascular disease. He has come into the general practice for his routine health assessment and care plan review. Last year, while playing golf, Jack had a significant heart attack that necessitated bypass surgery and left him in the hospital for several weeks. Even though it has been more than 8 months since he came home, Jack hasn't played golf since his heart attack and says he does not see his golfing mates much anymore. The nurse observes that Jack looks tired and, when asked, he says that he isn't sleeping well and that he lacks energy. Jack describes how everything seems to take so much more effort than it used to. He says he just can't get going. The nurse notes that Jack has lost 8 kg since last year and looks dehydrated. Jack says that his weight loss is good because the nurses at the hospital told him that he needed to watch his weight to improve his heart health. He then jokes that it has been easy to lose weight as he doesn't really have much of an appetite or even desire to eat or drink much these days.

! RED FLAGS

- Everyone has periods of low mood from time to time. However, when low mood affects a person's usual functioning or lasts longer than 2 weeks, the nurse needs to think about depression being present.
- Not engaging in usual activities, experiencing a lack of energy, having difficulty sleeping and poor food and fluid intake related to Jack's diminished desire to eat should prompt the nurse to ask some probing questions about Jack's mental health and emotional wellbeing.
- The fact that Jack is not engaging with his friends at golf and not seeing them much should also prompt consideration of whether Jack has become socially isolated. Social isolation and loneliness are risk factors for suicide in older males, with suicide rates alarmingly high for this population (De Leo 2022).
- Because it is unclear whether Jack has much family support, the nurse should also explore this further.

Protective Factors

- Social support can reduce the symptoms of depression in individuals with cardiovascular disease, as well as improving the person's coping ability and promoting the uptake of positive health behaviours (Halcomb et al 2022). Conversely, a lack of social support and depression, are independent risk factors for poor cardiac prognosis, diminishing quality of life and increasing morbidity (Czajkowski et al 2022; Freak-Poli et al 2021).
- Social support can include practical or emotional support and can be provided by a range of people, including family members, friends, neighbours and acquaintances. People with cardiovascular disease who live with a spouse or partner perceive higher levels of social support and fewer instances of depression than those living alone (Halcomb et al 2022; Thompson et al 2023). Unfortunately, as the population ages, many people no longer have a spouse or partner and are left to rely on other sources of social support. See Chapter 5 for more information about working with families in mental health.
- Primary care and community nurses have an important role in assessing social support and linking individuals who have social support needs with social groups and community services that can assist in building networks (Thompson et al 2023). Notably, primary care and community nurses can also provide social support in the form of emotional support.
- While he hasn't been in contact for a while, Jack does have a social network within the golfing community he may be able to reconnect with.

Knowledge

- As many as one in five people are affected by depression after a cardiac bypass, acute coronary syndrome or chronic heart failure (Yuan et al 2019).

- The presence of depression can have significant consequences following a myocardial infarction because of its impact on the recovery process, use of social support and behavioural modification by decreasing motivation and interest, reducing energy, lessening enjoyment of life, and causing poor sleep and appetite (Silverman et al 2019; Upadhyay et al 2022).
- Someone who is depressed may lack the desire to engage in physical rehabilitation and participate in programs such as cardiac rehabilitation, which will improve long-term physical and mental health outcomes (Pedersen et al 2021). One in five patients with cardiac disease has depression or anxiety, which increases mortality and has a negative impact on quality of life (Pedersen et al 2021; Silverman et al 2019).
- Depression in people with cardiovascular disease increases healthcare costs and precipitates more unscheduled episodes of care (Tápias et al 2021).
- Detecting and appropriately managing depression in people with cardiovascular disease is an important strategy to optimise cardiac rehabilitation (Rao et al 2020).
- Many people still do not receive enough support and treatment to effectively manage depression following a cardiac event, despite recognising the importance and the availability of interventions based on robust evidence (Wiesmaierova et al 2019).
- While some interventions can be delivered via cardiac rehabilitation and hospital outreach programs, these programs do not reach all potential people who would benefit. Therefore, individuals presenting to primary care and community healthcare providers following cardiovascular events need to be carefully screened and assessed to ensure timely referral to the most appropriate health professionals to provide effective depression management for those who require it.

Attitudes

- Attitudes towards people with mental illness remain poor, and consequently, people with mental illness are among the most marginalised and vulnerable people in society. Although this has changed over the years, stigma is still very prevalent (Adu et al 2022).
- Experiencing stigma, whether from members of the broader community, health professionals or self-stigma, is often a barrier to people seeking help (Adu et al 2022). It is often because of these widely held negative attitudes that people like Jack don't seek help for mental health symptoms.
- The attitude of the nurse is vitally important. People with mental health issues describe feeling judged by health professionals and are often highly attuned to health professionals holding negative attitudes.
- All people should be treated with unconditional positive regard, and the care and treatment provided by nurses should be value- and judgement-free.

Mental Health Skills
A Basic Mental Health Assessment

While clients with cardiovascular disease may receive psychological assessment and/or intervention from cardiovascular services following an acute cardiac event, many do not. In many cases, mental health symptoms appear after the person has left the acute hospital setting. Additionally, some people may feel more comfortable seeking help from community-based care providers, who they trust and have long-established relationships with (Stephen et al 2022).

It is vital that primary and community nurses feel confident in talking to clients about their mental health and that they can competently undertake a basic assessment of mental health issues using a validated assessment tool (Halcomb et al 2018).

Standardised screening tools, such as the Kessler Psychological Distress scale (K10) (Kessler et al 2003) and the Primary Care PTSD Screen (PC-PTSD) (Prins et al 2016) can help primary care and community nurses to undertake initial mental health

Continued

Scenario 24.1: Jack

screening. The K10 is widely used to measure clients' mental state and to identify people who potentially require further assessment for depression and anxiety. However, it is also important for nurses to recognise their individual scope of practice, its limitations, and when referral to specialist services is required (Halcomb et al 2018).

Establish Trust and a Therapeutic Relationship

When working with someone like Jack, nurses must do the following:

- Listen! Listening helps to identify the person's concerns about symptoms and their possible impact on daily life.
- Open up the conversation in a matter-of-fact way, to show that the person's mental health is of equal importance to their physical health and that it can be discussed.
- Be open, factual and speak without negative judgement or using value-laden statements (e.g. telling people they have nothing to be anxious about or telling people they have no reason to be depressed). This demonstrates that the nurse can help to address the issues they are currently facing and that doing so will optimise their mental and physical health and recovery.
- Demonstrate a manner that facilitates an ongoing trustful and therapeutic relationship to be maintained between the patient and the nurse. For example, the nurse might ask Jack about why he isn't playing golf or seeing his mates to understand what his concerns are.
- In Jack's case, if appropriate, offer a referral to cardiac rehabilitation, which may include opportunities to review his diet and nutrition and link him to social supports such as the local men's shed or a seniors walking group.

Relevant Treatment Modalities and Considerations
Talking Therapy

- Not everyone who has depression needs medication.
- Counselling or talking/psychotherapy is very effective for many people and a referral to a mental health specialist to provide such services may be all that is required. See Chapter 12 for a detailed description of the type of therapies that can be useful for people with mood disorders.
- E-mental health internet treatment programs can be helpful for common mental health conditions – these might be offered in a pure self-help or guided self-help (with a mental health clinician) format (Lattie et al 2022). While these may often be considered most appropriate for younger people,

older people should be individually assessed to determine if an online intervention is appropriate.

Medication

Medication is often prescribed for people who are experiencing depression (see Chapter 21 for more information about psychopharmacology).

The role of the primary and community care nurse regarding medication management will be to speak with Jack and ask him:

- how he is managing his medication
- whether he is taking medications as prescribed
- importantly, about any side effects he may be experiencing. Understanding side effects is important because if these are unpleasant, or embarrassing, they may result in Jack not taking his medication.

If Jack is experiencing side effects, work with him to establish effective strategies to manage these. Jack must be part of goal-setting and identifying the solution.

Working *with* people in managing their mental health issues will elicit better outcomes than taking a paternalistic approach and telling them what to do.

Social and Emotional Support

- Primary care nurses can provide social support and offer emotional support. This is also an effective treatment modality.
- Providing emotional support to Jack includes validating his feelings and actively listening to what he has to say.
- Talk with Jack about ways he can improve his mood and work with him to set attainable goals.
- Demonstrate to Jack the difference between negative self-talk and constructive self-talk.
- Talk to Jack about relaxation or mindfulness activities and let him know that physical activity can help lift his mood. Help Jack to develop a schedule for these kinds of activities, incorporating activities he enjoys, such as golf, and identify who might support him to undertake these activities.
- Most importantly, do not dismiss his concerns nor diminish their impact. This involves not offering simplistic narratives or solutions, or comments such as "Everything will be fine" or "You've got nothing to worry about".

Scenario 24.2: Fiona

Fiona is a 45-year-old Aboriginal woman who was diagnosed with paranoid schizophrenia in her mid-20s. She is currently working with a care coordinator from the community mental health team, but receives her monthly paliperidone palmitate depot injection through the general practice. She lives in a rented house with her mother, after her father died 5 years ago. Since her father died, Fiona hasn't left the house much and has been admitted to the hospital twice due to experiencing thoughts of self-harm, thought disorder and increasing paranoia. Her admissions lasted for several months each time because she had the fixed belief that police were tracking her through the television and she took some time to respond to medication.

Over previous visits to the Aboriginal Medical Service, Fiona's symptoms of thought disorder, auditory hallucinations and paranoia have been fairly well under control and she has regularly taken prescribed antipsychotic medications. In the past, Fiona has been on a community treatment order, but is not anymore. She successfully stopped drinking alcohol a year ago, but continues to smoke a packet of 30 cigarettes each day – although she has tried to give up three times. While she was previously working in a

supermarket, recurring mental health symptoms have meant she is currently unemployed.

Physical observations reveal that Fiona's blood pressure is elevated (150/90), her random blood glucose is 9.8 mmol/L and she has put on 6 kilograms in the past 4 months.

Fiona is quite guarded when she speaks and fears that she may end up back in the hospital. She does not describe hospital admission in a positive way. She is reluctant to speak to anyone about her thoughts until she has built up a rapport and feels as though she can trust the person. Fiona has been ridiculed about her mental health in the past.

Fiona's current mental state is stable, and she describes herself as being in a good stage of her personal recovery. She continues to hear voices, but her beliefs about being tracked by the police have subsided. Fiona says the voice she hears says nice things, but she wishes sometimes the voice – who is called "Tim" – would be quiet. She has to shout at him sometimes to "shut up" and that upsets her mother.

When asked, Fiona says she is not thinking about self-harm or suicide.

EVIDENCE-BASED PRACTICE—cont'd

Scenario 24.2: Fiona

> **! RED FLAGS**
>
> - The physical examination revealed several red flags. The combination of hypertension, raised random blood glucose and increased body weight all highlight a need for further investigation of Fiona's physical health status and cardiometabolic health.
> - Further investigation of lifestyle risk factors, such as smoking, alcohol, nutrition (dietary intake) and physical activity is required to identify additional risks to physical health.
> - Antipsychotic medication will also contribute to the risk of developing metabolic syndrome.

Protective Factors

- Despite the growing recognition of the importance of monitoring for metabolic syndrome among mental health professionals, this remains inconsistently applied in clinical practice. Rates of metabolic monitoring have been reported as low as 5% at baseline in some studies; however, a systematic review of monitoring strategies reported achieving monitoring rates of 40–80% following intervention (Poojari et al 2022). This highlights the need for primary care providers to be alert and ensure that this monitoring is occurring. Low-cost educational interventions have been shown to increase monitoring rates and so should be considered for primary care and community health professionals (O'Brien & Abraham 2021; Soda et al 2021).
- Regular monitoring provides opportunities for early detection of abnormalities and treatment to reduce risk and is a demonstration to the person that the primary care nurse cares about their health.
- People like Fiona, who take antipsychotic medications, should undergo regular metabolic screening including:
  - an annual electrocardiograph
  - 3-monthly blood tests (full blood count, urea, electrolytes, fasting blood glucose and lipids, liver function tests and prolactin)
  - monitoring of physical parameters, such as weight, waist circumference, blood pressure and body mass index (O'Brien & Abraham 2021).
- Monitoring a person's physical health also provides a good opportunity to discuss their mental health in a non-threatening way. A person-centred, holistic and culturally appropriate approach would indicate that the two should always be undertaken together.

Knowledge

- GPs manage mental health problems for First Nations Australians at 1.2 times the rate of non-Indigenous Australians (National Indigenous Australians Agency 2020).
- Some 24% of Aboriginal and Torres Strait Islander Australians report having a diagnosed mental health or behavioural condition. Additionally, 31% of these individuals have reported high or very high levels of psychological distress (AIHW 2022a).
- Rates of suicide among Aboriginal and Torres Strait Islander Australians are twice as high as for non-Indigenous Australians (AIHW 2021). A similar picture can be seen in Aotearoa New Zealand, with Māori people 1.6 times more likely to experience a mental health issue than non-Māori (Ministry of Health 2019a).
- We know that Aboriginal and Torres Strait Islander women have an average life expectancy of 75.6 years – around 7 years less than a non-Indigenous Australian woman (AIHW 2015).

Metabolic Syndrome

- A key marker of physical health in people with mental illness is metabolic syndrome.
- Metabolic syndrome is a cluster of symptoms that include hypertension, central obesity, dyslipidaemia and impaired fasting blood glucose (O'Brien &

Abraham 2021). When clustered together, these symptoms significantly increase a person's risk of developing diabetes, stroke and cardiovascular disease, and lead to high rates of morbidity and mortality (Sud et al 2021).
- The risk of metabolic syndrome is increased by the prescription of antipsychotic medications, predominantly secondary to weight gain and other metabolic disturbances.
- The positive and negative symptoms experienced by people living with schizophrenia (see Chapter 12 for a description of signs and symptoms), as well as stigma and social isolation, can impair the person's ability to participate in activities that would enhance their physical health and reduce the risk of metabolic syndrome (Ward et al 2018).

Modifiable Risk Factors

- As the severity of negative symptoms of schizophrenia increases, there is likely to be weight gain (which may be related to medication), as well as reductions in engagement with activities that would promote good health, such as healthy diet and exercise.
- Recent studies have shown that smoking rates have decreased among those living with mental illness; however, they are three times more likely to smoke compared to the general population (Greenhalgh et al 2022). It is important to remember that smoking also decreases the efficacy of some medications for mental health. Thus, if the person ceases or increases smoking, their medication may need to be adjusted (Hermann et al 2023).

Attitudes

- People living with mental illness, and psychotic disorders in particular (especially paranoid schizophrenia), are often portrayed negatively in movies and the media. Additionally, people without mental illness, but who commit violent crimes and take out their anger on others, are often described as "psycho" or even "schizo". This kind of stereotyping, as well as discriminatory and stigmatising language, serves to alienate people with mental illnesses even further.
- People with mental illness are more likely to be victims of crime than they are to be perpetrators, with this myth being an ongoing way that people living with mental illness are being stigmatised (Holland 2018; US Department of Health & Human Services 2017).
- As a result of pervasive stigmatising attitudes and inaccurate and sensationalist media portrayal in the community, nurses can also be fearful of people who experience psychotic disorders such as schizophrenia (Stuhlmiller & Tolchard 2019).
- Nurses who subscribe to negative beliefs can provide care underpinned by stigmatising or discriminatory attitudes, leading to less-than-ideal nursing care.
- It is important that primary care nurses engage in self-reflection and self-awareness, reflecting on the attitudes that they hold towards people with mental illness.
- In a relatively professionally isolated environment, such as primary care and community health care settings, nurses might benefit from mentoring and clinical supervision to help them develop professional skills in this area of practice.

Mental Health Skills
The Therapeutic Relationship

- Develop and maintain a positive rapport with Fiona, building a therapeutic relationship based on trust and mutual respect. Fiona is far more likely to speak truthfully if she trusts and respects the nurse.
- Speaking freely to Fiona about her experience of auditory hallucinations in a curious and matter-of-fact way will help build trust.
- Ask Fiona about "Tim". What is he saying? When does he stop talking? Does he command her to do things? Can she resist his commands?
- Even though Fiona denies having thoughts of suicide or self-harm, ask her again about this. Creating a safety plan with her might be appropriate (see Chapter 9 and the Useful websites link at the end of this chapter).
- Ask Fiona if she thinks anyone wants to harm her.

Continued

Scenario 24.2: Fiona

- Ask Fiona if she feels there is anything she needs help with regarding her mental health or other aspects of her life that relate to her health and emotional well-being more broadly.
- Open honest communication is always best.

Nursing Actions and Interventions
Collaborative Care Planning

- Where it is decided that Fiona would benefit from referral to other health professionals, such as exercise physiology, dietetics or a credentialled diabetes educator to help her to address the various health issues that she is facing, a care plan will be developed.
- Care should be taken to negotiate such a plan with Fiona to build trust with her rather than appear paternalistic or demanding as uptake of the plan is promoted.
- Fiona may need ongoing support from the nurse to encourage the uptake of these referrals and continued engagement with other health providers because barriers to engagement with health professionals may be present.
- With her permission, discuss Fiona's history with the other healthcare providers to ensure she receives appropriate interventions that meet her needs.

Physical Health Assessment and Monitoring

- The nurse should conduct a full physical health assessment, including an electrocardiograph (ECG) if one has not been done in the preceding year.
- In addition to assessing physical parameters, such as blood pressure, waist circumference, serum lipids, blood glucose level, oxygen saturation, weight and body mass index, the nurse should carefully assess lifestyle risk factors and Fiona's readiness to change.
- An assessment of Fiona's nutrition and physical activity will also be crucial considering the elevated blood glucose and hypertension.
- With Fiona's permission, contact with the community health team will be valuable.
- The nurse should also refer Fiona to a GP for appropriate blood tests and pharmacology review.

Relevant Treatment Modalities and Considerations
Talking Therapy

- Clinicians used to think that talking about symptoms with people who had a psychotic illness such as schizophrenia should be avoided. These days, evidence suggests that verbal and social interventions are showing some promise when used with an appropriate medication regimen.

- The efficacy of family interventions for schizophrenia has been associated with reduced rates of relapse and enhanced social functioning. One to two sessions of family psychoeducation can significantly reduce the rate of relapse for individuals with schizophrenia in a 12-month period (Rodolico et al 2022).
- Further education might be needed for Fiona's mother about her daughter's need to talk to her when experiencing symptoms. At these moments, it would be helpful for her mother to show empathy and compassion.
- Adapted cognitive behaviour therapy (CBT) can be a positive treatment for people experiencing positive psychosis symptoms, decreasing delusions over time (Sitko et al 2020).
- When aimed at improving memory and attention, interventions such as social skills training and cognitive remediation can assist in managing negative symptoms (Mahmood et al 2019).
- These treatment modalities can help improve motivation or poor confidence, which can help to improve social and workplace skills.
- See Chapter 14 for detailed information about treatment relevant to people who experience psychosis.

Physical Health and Lifestyle

- Monitoring Fiona's physical health and metabolic risk factors, as outlined above, will be essential.
- Fiona should be supported to consider lifestyle changes, at her own pace, using a motivational approach.
- Supporting people to quit smoking is an ongoing process and often requires prescription pharmacotherapy. However, interventions by primary care and community nurses using motivational interviewing can effectively assist in supporting smoking cessation and lifestyle risk factor reduction (Greenhalgh et al 2022; Stephen et al 2022).
- Community psychosocial support programs provide short-term help, including one-on-one training and group activities, helping to increase vocational skills, improve social skills and to connect with clinical care services. In Australia, Primary Health Networks (PHNs) work with state and territory governments to help meet these needs through commissioning community-based services such as NGOs, including getting back to work (Australian Government Department of Health and Aged Care 2020). Psychosocial support may also be provided through NDIS providers for those who are eligible.

CHAPTER SUMMARY

This chapter has provided some information about mental health within the primary care and community context by exploring two clinical scenarios. Several actions and interventions have been described that will assist you in developing confidence in working with people who experience mental illness. Some of these strategies apply to specific situations; however, there is always a way of effectively working with people who are experiencing challenging mental health issues. Some are more technical than others and require further education and practice to master, but many of the skills outlined here can be learnt and applied to the interactions you will experience as a novice nurse and as your clinical experience develops. The main thing to remember is to be caring and authentic, and to listen to the people you are working with. See Chapter 2 for more detailed explanations of the interpersonal skills and mental health interventions that should be applied by nurses in all clinical settings.

Nurses frequently express concern that they might "say the wrong thing" and make the situation more challenging for the person receiving care. If you take a caring and thoughtful approach that avoids the generous delivery of advice, it is unlikely that you will cause harm. Be genuine and authentic – people can tell when you aren't – and always come from a place of "naive enquirer". However, if you practise specific skills, such as active listening and validating feelings, and understand the models underpinning your practice, you are likely to feel more confident and understand the goals of your interaction. It is also hoped that through reading this chapter you have developed a sense of the importance of responding to people with mental health concerns with unconditional positive regard and respect. Value them as people and plan care *with* them, not *on* or *for* them. Take note of their lived experience; after all, they are the experts of their own life, including their experience of health and illness. One in four people live with a mental health issue (Moxham et al 2018), and everyone experiences challenges to their emotional wellbeing at times, so it is wise to develop your mental health knowledge and skills to be able to provide truly holistic nursing care.

USEFUL WEBSITES

Australian College of Mental Health Nurses Mental Health Practice Standards for Nurses in Australian General Practice: acmhn.org/Web/Resources/Best-practice-resources.aspx

Beyond Blue Safety Planning: www.beyondblue.org.au/get-support/beyond-now-suicide-safety-planning/create-beyondnow-safety-plan

Black Dog Institute: www.blackdoginstitute.org.au/

Blue Knot Foundation: National Centre of Excellence for Complex Trauma: www.blueknot.org.au/

eMHprac – e-mental health in practice: www.emhprac.org.au/

headspace youth mental health: headspace.org.au/

Primary Health Network collection of mental health care resources: www.health.gov.au/resources/collections/primary-health-networks-phn-collection-of-primary-mental-health-care-resources?utm_source=health.gov.au&utm_medium=callout-auto-custom&utm_campaign=digital_transformation

SANE Australia: www.sane.org/

Te Oranga Hinengaro Māori Mental Wellbeing (2018): www.hpa.org.nz/sites/default/files/Final-report-TeOrangaHinengaro-M%C4%81ori-Mental-Wellbeing-Oct2018.pdf

UK Mental Health Triage Scale: ukmentalhealthtriagescale.org/

University of Melbourne Recovery Library: recoverylibrary.unimelb.edu.au/

REFERENCES

Adu, J., Oudshoorn, A., Anderson, K., Marshall, C.A. & Stuart, H. 2022. Social contact: Next steps in an effective strategy to mitigate the stigma of mental illness. Iss Ment Health Nurs, 43, 485–488.

Ameel, M., Kontio, R. & Valimaki, M. 2019. Interventions delivered by nurses in adult outpatient psychiatric care: An integrative review. J Psychiatr Ment Health Nurs, 26, 301–322.

Australian Bureau of Statistics (ABS) 2022a. Causes of Death, Australia: Statistics on the number of deaths, by sex, selected age groups, and cause of death classified to the International Classification of Diseases (ICD). ABS, Canberra.

Australian Bureau of Statistics (ABS) 2022b. National Study of Mental Health and Wellbeing: Summary statistics on key mental health issues, including the prevalence of mental disorders and the use of services. ABS, Canberra.

Australian Bureau of Statistics (ABS) 2022c. Patient Experiences: 2021–2022 financial year. ABS, Canberra.

Australian Bureau of Statistics (ABS) 2017. Mortality of People using Mental Health Services and Prescription Medications. Analysis of Data 2011. ABS, Canberra.

Australian Government, Department of Health and Aged Care. 2020. Psychosocial support programs for people with severe mental illness. Australian Government, Canberra. Online. Available at: www.health.gov.au/our-work/commonwealth-psychosocial-support-programs-for-people-with-severe-mental-illness

Australian Institute of Health and Welfare (AIHW) 2022a. Indigenous Health and Wellbeing. AIHW, Canberra. Online. Available at: www.aihw.gov.au/reports/australias-health/indigenous-health-and-wellbeing

Australian Institute of Health and Welfare (AIHW) 2022b. Mental health services in Australia: Physical health of people with mental illness. AIHW, Canberra.

Australian Institute of Health and Welfare (AIHW) 2021. Aboriginal and Torres Strait Islander Stolen Generations aged 50 and over: Updated analyses for 2018–19. Cat. no: IHW257. AIHW, Canberra.

Australian Institute of Health and Welfare (AIHW) 2015. The health and welfare of Australia's Aboriginal and Torres Strait Islander peoples: 2015. Cat. no: IHW 147. AIHW, Canberra.

Bucciarelli, V., Caterino, A.L., Bianco, F., Caputi, C.G., Salerni, S., et al., 2020. Depression and cardiovascular disease: The deep blue sea of women's heart. Trends Cardiovasc Med, 30, 170–176.

Cutler, N.A., Sim, J., Halcomb, E., Moxham, L. & Stephens, M. 2020. Nurses' influence on consumers' experience of safety in acute mental health units: A qualitative study. J Clin Nurs, 29, 4379–4386.

Czajkowski, S.M., Arteaga, S.S. & Burg, M.M. 2022. Social support and cardiovascular disease. Handbook of Cardiovascular Behavioral Medicine. Springer, New York.

De Leo, D. 2022. Late-life suicide in an aging world. Nature Aging, 2, 7–12.

Ellegaard, T., Bliksted, V., Mehlsen, M. & Lomborg, K. 2020. Feeling safe with patient-controlled admissions: A grounded theory study of the mental health patients' experiences. J Clin Nurs, 29, 2397–2409.

Firth, J., Siddiqi, N., Koyanagi, A., Siskind, D., Rosenbaum, S., et al., 2019. The Lancet Psychiatry Commission: A blueprint for protecting physical health in people with mental illness. Lancet Psychiatry, 6, 675–712.

Freak-Poli, R., Ryan, J., Neumann, J.T., Tonkin, A., Reid, C.M. et al., 2021. Social isolation, social support and loneliness as predictors of cardiovascular disease incidence and mortality. BMC Geriatr, 21, 711.

Greenhalgh, E.M., Brennan, E., Segan, C. & Scollo, M. 2022. Monitoring changes in smoking and quitting behaviours among Australians with and without mental illness over 15 years. ANZ J Pub Health, 46, 223–229.

Hackett, D. & Fitzgerald, C. 2020. Improving and standardizing metabolic screening for people prescribed antipsychotic medication who are at risk of developing metabolic syndrome within the community mental health setting. Int J Ment Health Nurs, 29, 935-941.

Halcomb, E.J., McInnes, S., Moxham, L., & Patterson, C. 2019. Nurse-delivered interventions for mental health in primary care: A systematic review of randomised controlled trials. Family Practice, 36(1), 64–71.

Halcomb, E., McInnes, S., Moxham, L. & Patterson, C. 2018. Mental Health Practice Standards gor Nurses in Australian General Practice. Australian College of Mental Health Nurses, Canberra, ACT.

Halcomb, E., McInnes, S., Williams, A., Ashley, C., James, S., et al., 2020. The experiences of primary healthcare nurses during the COVID-19 pandemic in Australia. J Nurs Scholarship, 52, 553–563.

Halcomb, E., Thompson, C., Tillott, S., Robinson, K. & Lucas, E. 2022. Exploring social connectedness in older Australians with chronic conditions: Results of a descriptive survey Collegian, 29, 860–866.

Halcomb, E. J., Stephens, M., Bryce, J., Foley, E. & Ashley, C. 2017. The development of professional practice standards for nurses working in Australian general practice. J Adv Nurs, 73, 1958–1969.

Hermann, R., Rostami-Hodjegan, A., Zhao, P. & Ragueneau-Majlessi, I. 2023. Seeing what is behind the smokescreen: A systematic review of methodological aspects of smoking interaction studies over the last three decades and implications for future clinical trials. Clin Transl Sci.

Holland, K. 2018. Lay theories and criticisms of mental health news: Elaborating the concept of biocommunicability. Disabil Soc, 33, 1327–1348.

Kessler, R.C., Barker, P.R., Colpe, L.J., Epstein, J.F., Gfroerer, J.C., et al., 2003. Screening for serious mental illness in the general population. Arch Gen Psychiatry, 60, 184–189

Lattie, E.G., Stiles-Shields, C. & Graham, A.K. 2022. An overview of and recommendations for more accessible digital mental health services. Nature Rev Psychol, 1, 87–100.

Lundstrom, S., Jormfeldt, H., Hedman Ahlstrom, B. & Skarsater, I. 2020. Mental health nurses' experience of physical health care and health promotion initiatives for people with severe mental illness. Int J Ment Health Nurs, 29, 244–253.

Mahmood, Z., Clark, J.M. & Twamley, E.W. 2019. Compensatory cognitive training for psychosis: Effects on negative symptom subdomains. Schizophrenia Res 204, 397–400.

McInnes, S., Halcomb , E., Ashley, C., Keane, A., Moxham, L. et al., 2022. An integrative review of primary health care nurses' mental health knowledge gaps and learning needs. Collegian, 29, 540–548.

Ministry of Health. 2019a. NZ Health Survey 2017–18 annual data. MOH, Wellington.

Ministry of Health. 2019b. Office of the Director of Mental Health and Addiction Services. Annual Report 2017. MOH, Wellington.

Moxham, L., Hazelton, M., Muir-Cochrane, E., Heffernan, T., Kneisel, C.R. et al., 2018. Contemporary Psychiatric-Mental Health Nursing: Partnerships in Care. Pearson Australia, Sydney.

National Indigenous Australians Agency 2020. Access to mental health services [Online]. AIHW, Canberra, ACT. Available: www.indigenoushpf.gov.au/measures/3-10-access-mental-health-services

O'Brien, A.J. & Abraham, R.M. 2021. Evaluation of metabolic monitoring practices for mental health consumers in the Southern District Health Board Region of New Zealand. J Psychiatric Ment Health Nurs, 28, 1005–1017.

Pedersen, S.S., Andersen, C.M., Ahm, R., Skovbakke, S.J., Kok, R., et al., 2021. Efficacy and cost-effectiveness of a therapist assisted web-based intervention for depression and anxiety in patients with ischemic heart disease attending cardiac rehabilitation [eMindYourHeart trial]: A randomised controlled trial protocol. BMC Cardiovasc Disord, 21, 1–10.

Poojari, P.G., Khan, S., Shenoy, S., Shetty, S., Bose, S., et al., 2022. A narrative review of metabolic monitoring of adult prescribed second-generation antipsychotics for severe mental illness. Clin Epidemiol Global Health, 15, 101035.

Prins, A., Bovin, M.J., Smolenski, D.J., Marx, B.P., Kimerling, R., et al., 2016. The primary care PTSD screen for DSM-5 (PC-PTSD-5): Development and evaluation within a veteran primary care sample. J Gen Intern Med, 31, 1206–1211.

Rao, A., Zecchin, R., Newton, P., Phillips, J., DiGiacomo, M., et al., 2020. The prevalence and impact of depression and anxiety in cardiac rehabilitation: A longitudinal cohort study. Euro J Prevent Cardiol, 27, 478–489.

Rodolico, A., Bighelli, I., Avanzato, C., Concerto, C., Cutrufelli, P., et al., 2022. Family interventions for relapse prevention in schizophrenia: A systematic review and network meta-analysis. Lancet Psychiatry, 9, 211–221.

Silverman, A.L., Herzog, A.A. & Silverman, D.I. 2019. Hearts and minds: Stress, anxiety, and depression: unsung risk factors for cardiovascular disease. Cardiol Rev, 27, 202–207.

Sitko, K., Bewick, B.M., Owens, D. & Masterson, C. 2020. Meta-analysis and meta-regression of cognitive behavioral therapy for psychosis (CBTP) across time: The effectiveness of CBTP has improved for delusions. Schizophrenia Bulletin Open, 1, https://doi.org/10.1093/schizbullopen/sgaa023

Soda, T., Richards, J., Gaynes, B.N., Cueva, M., Laux, J., et al., 2021. Systematic quality improvement and metabolic monitoring for individuals taking antipsychotic drugs. Psychiatr Serv, 72, 647–653.

Spooner, C., Afrazi, S., de Oliveira Costa, J. & Harris, M.F. 2022. Demographic and health profiles of people with severe mental illness in general practice in Australia: A cross-sectional study. Aust J Prim Health, 28(5), 408–416.

Stephen, C., Halcomb, E., Fernandez, R., McInnes, S., Batterham, M. et al., 2022. Nurse-led interventions to manage hypertension in general practice: A systematic review and meta analysis. J Adv Nurs, 78, 1281–1293.

Stuhlmiller, C. & Tolchard, B. 2019. Understanding the impact of mental health placements on student nurses' attitudes towards mental illness. Nurse Ed Pract, 34, 25–30.

Sud, D., Laughton, E., McAskill, R., Bradley, E. & Maidment, I. 2021. The role of pharmacy in the management of cardiometabolic risk, metabolic syndrome and related diseases in severe mental illness: A mixed-methods systematic literature review. Syst Rev, 10, 92.

Suetani, S., Sardinha, S. & Gill, N. 2022. Improving the mental health of Australians: A renewed call for primary care psychiatry. Australasian Psychiatry, 10398562221104418.

Tápias, F.S., Otani, V.H.O., Vasques, D.A.C., Otani, T.Z.S. & Uchida, R.R. 2021. Costs associated with depression and obesity among cardiovascular patients: Medical expenditure panel survey analysis. BMC Health Serv Res, 21, 433.

Thompson, C., Halcomb, E. & Masso, M. 2023. The contribution of primary care to interventions to reduce loneliness and social isolation in older people: An integrative review. Scand J Caring Sci, 37(3), 611–627.

Upadhyay, V., Bhandari, S.S., Rai, D.P., Dutta, S., García-Grau, P. et al., 2022. Improving depression and perceived social support enhances overall quality of life among myocardial infarction survivors: Necessity for integrating mental health care into cardiac rehabilitation programs. Egypt J Neurol, Psychiatry Neurosurg, 58, 1–9.

US Department of Health & Human Services 2017. Mental health myths and facts. Online. Available at: www.mentalhealth.gov/basics/mental-health-myths-facts

Walker, E.R., McGee, R.E. & Druss, B.G. 2015. Mortality in mental disorders and global disease burden implications: A systematic review and meta-analysis. JAMA Psychiatry, 72, 334–341.

Ward, T., Wynaden, D. & Heslop, K. 2018. Who is responsible for metabolic screening for mental health clients taking antipsychotic medications? Int J Ment Health Nurs, 27, 196.

Wiesmaierova, S., Petrova, D., Arrebola Moreno, A., Catena, A., Ramírez Hernández, J.A. et al., 2019. Social support buffers the negative effects of stress in cardiac patients: A cross-sectional study with acute coronary syndrome patients. J Behav Med, 42, 469–479.

Yuan, M.-Z., Fang, Q., Liu, G.-W., Zhou, M., Wu, J.-M. et al., 2019. Risk factors for post-acute coronary syndrome depression: A meta-analysis of observational studies. J Cardiovasc Nurs, 34, 60–70.

25

Emergency Care

Justin Chia

KEY POINTS

- Many people presenting to emergency departments have mental health issues, either as the primary reason for their presentation or in conjunction with a physical health issue for which they have presented.
- Physical symptoms, such as chest pain and breathlessness, should be medically investigated before assuming they are due to anxiety or panic.

- The nursing skills required for responding to mental health presentations are the skills of therapeutic engagement.
- Therapeutic interventions, such as solution-focused therapy, are useful in helping consumers to identify previous stressful situations they have managed successfully.
- The importance of adjunctive interventions, such as exercise and exposure to nature, should not be underestimated.

KEY TERMS

Anxiety

Assessment

Engagement

Self-harm

Therapeutic relationships

Trauma

LEARNING OUTCOMES

The material in this chapter will assist you to:

- identify mental health assessment skills for use in emergency departments (EDs)
- understand the need for therapeutic engagement with people presenting to an ED

- understand the relationship between acute physical symptoms and psychological distress
- identify useful nursing approaches and therapeutic interventions for responding to people presenting with acute distress.

LIVED EXPERIENCE COMMENT BY JARRAD HICKMOTT
The prevalence of trauma in those who experience mental health concerns is extremely high. Acknowledging and discussing trauma-informed care and supporting the person to develop coping strategies are important elements of strength and recovery models. It's important to consider an alternative to the term "patient". General consensus among lived experience circles is that "consumer" is the preferred term. Noting this, everyone will have their own perspectives and options about how they prefer to be referred to.

INTRODUCTION

Presentation rates for people with mental health problems to emergency departments (EDs) are increasing, and this is an international phenomenon. General hospital EDs are frequently the first point of contact for people accessing mental health services. This necessitates a change in thinking and practice and a re-orientation of resources to meet this change in demand. While it is important for EDs to have access to additional specialist resources on-hand to provide timely care and support ED staff, the knowledge and skills of ED nursing and medical staff also need to expand to address this clinical need.

Using two clinical examples, this chapter provides an overview of the key considerations in responding to people presenting to an ED in a state of agitation or mental distress. What classifies as a "mental health" presentation in the ED context is not clearly defined, and the mental health of all people accessing health care should always be considered. For example, the incidence of depression is generally higher for people with medical illnesses such as heart disease, hypertension, cancer and diabetes. There are common types of mental health-related presentations in EDs, including:

- anxiety and panic
- self-harm
- suicidal ideation and suicide attempts
- depression
- psychosis
- physical health issues causing mental distress
- pain (acute and/or chronic)
- situational crisis
- cumulative stress
- drug- and alcohol-related issues.

APPROACHES TO MENTAL HEALTH PRESENTATIONS IN THE EMERGENCY SETTING

In mental health, assessment is considered a central clinical activity. For nurses, assessment is a continuous process integrated within routine interactions with consumers. While the word "assessment" carries a fairly procedural connotation, it is important to remember that effective assessment and data gathering hinges on effective therapeutic engagement (Shea 2017), and that holistic, person-centred engagement is central to the practice of nursing (Santangelo et al 2018). See Chapter 9 for more detailed information about mental health assessment in nursing.

Conducting formalised risk assessments dominated mental health services until recently. However, there is now recognition that a focus on these assessments and risk stratification (high, medium, low) should not form the basis for allocation of clinical services or follow-up (Carter et al 2016; Large 2018). While suicidal thoughts and plans are common, the act of suicide is statistically rare, with a recognition that these formalised assessments have limited accuracy in predicting suicide (Large 2018). Importantly, intervention based on risk stratification (high, medium, low) carries significant potential for harm from unnecessary coercive interventions for "high"-risk individuals, and from a lack of care allocated to those at "low" risk (Large 2018).

Rather than a focus on risk assessment and stratification, there is an emphasis on the importance of therapeutic rapport building to foster hope and reduce distress, while an assessment of the consumer's individual needs is also crucial, in order to target specific interventions where they are most needed by the individual (Carter 2016; Large 2018; Wand et al 2022). Specific to mental health care in the ED, it has been found that consumers value therapeutic interactions highly where they feel listened to and understood (Wand et al 2022). This does not have to constitute a lengthy interaction. Listening to a person and conveying that you appreciate the challenges they are facing can be achieved in a short exchange. Shea (2017) points out that for some people experiencing suicidal ideation, feeling comfortable to share this painful experience with a fellow human being who cares may represent hope that the person has not experienced recently, if ever. Similarly, Wand and colleagues (2022) emphasise that a focus on therapeutic engagement is, and should remain, the focus of mental health nursing.

Additionally, simple gestures, such as providing information and reassurance, as well as basic comforts, such as seating, food and drink, can ameliorate anxiety and distress, and improve engagement between clinicians and consumers. The following scenario illustrates the importance of appreciating that most people with mental health challenges have experienced some form of trauma or adversity, particularly in early childhood, and this is common in people who frequently attend EDs. This perspective also recognises that people who have experienced trauma are more likely to experience distress and re-traumatisation as a result of encountering the healthcare system (Ranjbar et al 2020). See Chapter 2 for more information about a trauma-informed approach in mental health.

EVIDENCE-BASED PRACTICE

Scenario 25.1: Rachel

Rachel is a 27-year-old woman who has been brought in by ambulance to the ED having called a telephone counselling crisis line. She said she was having thoughts of killing herself by taking an overdose of her prescribed medication, so the crisis line worker called emergency services.

Rachel is well known to the ED, the toxicology service at the hospital and to the local mental health service. She carries a diagnosis of complex post-traumatic stress disorder secondary to childhood trauma and has a history of longstanding suicidal ideation, difficulty managing her emotions and frequent episodes of both deliberate self-harm and serious suicidal behaviour. She has previously taken large overdoses requiring intubation and intensive care admissions. While Rachel's care is coordinated by the local community mental health service, she presents regularly to the ED under similar circumstances and frequently accesses the local mental health acute care team after hours.

Rachel also has significant medical comorbidities. These include morbid obesity (weight of 147 kg and a body mass index of 57), type 2 diabetes, obstructive sleep apnoea, sinus tachycardia and chronic knee and back pain.

On arrival at the ED, Rachel is lying on the ambulance stretcher swearing at staff, screaming, "Let me the fuck out of here!" She is agitated and thrashing her arms and legs against the stretcher's seatbelt restraints. Rachel has been transported under the Mental Health Act due to her reluctance to attend hospital and the suicidal thoughts she has continued to voice in the ambulance.

> ### ⚠ RED FLAGS
>
> - Significant trauma history and risk of the hospital experience causing further psychological harm
> - Bariatric/obese individual with respiratory and cardiac comorbidities
> - Aggression risk
> - Risk of harm to herself (potential future harm and possible harm already inflicted, such as an as-yet undisclosed overdose)
> - Absconding risk.

Protective Factors
- While this is not an uncommon scenario for Rachel, she has previously responded well to verbal de-escalation strategies using a trauma-informed approach from clinicians she is familiar with.

- While not always the case, she has also previously responded well to clinicians reminding her of the various distress tolerance and other psychological strategies she speaks to her psychologist about.
- While Rachel has an extensive history of deliberate self-harm and suicidal behaviour, she also has a history of seeking help, either when feeling at risk of engaging in these behaviours or shortly after engaging in these behaviours. It is important to note that for some consumers, accessing help shortly after engaging in self-harm or suicidal behaviour may represent a significant improvement in coping compared with their past patterns of behaviour.

Knowledge
General knowledge
- General principles of a trauma-informed care approach
- Contribution of physical health problems to a consumer's mental health.

Managing Agitation and Distress
- Verbal de-escalation knowledge and skills to manage Rachel's clear agitation and distress
- Possible need for sedation in response to Rachel's behaviour if verbal de-escalation is ineffective (in this instance, it is important to consider obesity-related risk of respiratory, airway or other complications from sedation).

Protocols
- Knowledge of protocols around medications used for acute sedation of behavioural disturbances – for example, the New South Wales Guidelines for management of patients with acute severe behavioural disturbance for adults under 65 years old (NSW Ministry of Health 2015):
  - First preference – offer oral sedation (diazepam 5–20 mg PO or lorazepam 1–2 mg PO and/or olanzapine 5–10 mg PO)
  - If not accepting of oral sedation, move to parenteral sedation (first dose droperidol 5–10 mg IM)
  - If not settled in 15 minutes, then a second dose of droperidol (10 mg IM/IV), with a maximum dose of 20 mg per event
- Knowledge of COVID-19 specific considerations (NSW Ministry of Health 2021):
  - All staff involved should be dressed in appropriate PPE (contact, droplet and airborne precautions)

Scenario 25.1: Rachel

- Consider potential drug interactions between COVID-19 treatments and medications used for sedation
- Obtain baseline physical observations prior to (or immediately after) sedation, with a focus on oxygen saturation and ECG
- Be alert to potential with COVID-19 infection for respiratory status to drop precipitously
- Post-sedation: Monitor vital signs, with especially stringent focus on oxygen saturation.
- Knowledge of the record-keeping requirements for restraint and sedation mandated by the facility or health department policy, and by the relevant jurisdiction's legislation
- Knowledge of the service protocols related to:
  - the legal procedure for reviewing people detained under the Mental Health Act
  - whether the ED makes provisions for senior ED medical officers to review and discharge someone detained under the Mental Health Act where they consider psychiatry consultation is not required (this may be the preferred option if the person is adamant they want to leave and will require significant physical restraint and sedation to ensure they stay).

The risks of engaging in further coercive treatment and complications of sedation should be weighed against the benefits of keeping Rachel in hospital for further review, and the risks associated with discharge from ED without waiting for psychiatry review. While it may not apply directly to Rachel in this instance, it has been asserted that, contrary to some published guidelines, not every consumer who presents to an ED with suicidal thinking needs to be seen by a mental health professional. In some cases, a senior ED clinician can decide to discharge the person without a formal psychiatric assessment (Ryan et al 2015).

Staffing

- Capacity of the ED to provide the high level of care Rachel requires given the resources available and competing workload/acuity demands on the department as a whole. For example:
  - Rachel may respond to verbal de-escalation and low-dose oral sedation, so could be cared for in a more open space with a 1:1 nurse.
  - If sedation is indicated, Rachel may require a resuscitation bay level of observation, given the increased risk of complications.
- Access to psychiatry staff:
  - On-site psychiatry staff can provide a quick response for a psychiatrist review.
  - If psychiatry staff are on site but limited (few in number or because of a high demand for service) there could be delays in conducting a psychiatry review.
  - If psychiatry staff are off-site but contactable via phone or videoconference, this could result in delays.

Attitudes

- A calm, non-judgemental, empathetic, validating approach is required. Consider Rachel's trauma history, including possible trauma she may have experienced in the hospital environment when accessing health care previously.
- Rachel's presentation may be the psychological equivalent of a serious medical emergency and her care should be prioritised as such.
- Be mindful that Rachel has several medical comorbidities that also require consideration in the emergency/acute setting. Neglecting the physical health of people with mental illness is common.

Skills

Engagement and a Person-Centred Approach

Engage with Rachel from a person-centred approach: "In person-centred interviewing, the patient is not viewed as the problem but as a unique individual filled with solutions to the many problems that life invariably brings to all of us. There is a humbleness to a person-centred interviewer. It is the wisdom that, even at our best, we do not know all the answers, for we do not even know all the questions. Thus, it is intensely important to listen to what our patients have to teach us and the questions that they bring us" (Shea 2017, p. 9).

Verbal De-escalation

- Use a trauma-informed approach to minimise the chance of re-traumatisation.
- Engage verbal de-escalation skills with Rachel.
- Convey empathy and validation to start building a therapeutic rapport.
- Convey a genuine interest in hearing what Rachel has to say in an effort to understand what her experiences mean for her.
- Be mindful of non-verbal communication (posture, gestures, eye contact, facial expression and rate, pitch and tone of voice) – your own and the person's.

Safety

- Consider variables in the physical environment, such as ready access to IV lines/poles, sharps or other implements that Rachel could use to cause harm to herself or others. Generally, EDs are noisy, busy places. Is there a suitable place in the ED that is lower stimulus and clinically appropriate to care for Rachel?
- Using the above considerations to positively affect our bedside manner facilitates an environment that is both physically and psychologically safe. This enables a person's neurologically-based fear response to be calmed, thereby maximising engagement and promoting recovery (Parnas & Isobel 2017).
- Use your knowledge and skills to engage in the process of safe physical restraint and administration of parenteral sedation where required and when verbal de-escalation and therapeutic engagement have been insufficient to reduce the risk of harm associated with Rachel's current behaviour.

Treatment Modalities and Considerations

Solution-Focused Brief Therapy

A person-centred, strengths-based approach to engage Rachel and attempt to verbally de-escalate her initial agitation and distress can be used. Once calmed, a solution-focused brief therapy (SFBT) approach may be useful in engaging Rachel and collaboratively working out a reasonable outcome to her presentation. SFBT is a strengths-based approach that has a strong evidence base. The approach empowers the consumer by inviting them to explore their own resources and past success as solutions to achieve their identified future hopes and goals, with a recent review of the evidence base supporting SFBT as helpful for the right consumer and clinical context (Kim et al 2019).

SFBT assumes the consumer is their own expert on what is helpful for them. The SFBT approach draws attention to those occasions in the past where individuals have successfully coped with a challenging or stressful situation and assists them in articulating, to clinicians and themselves, how they achieved that. It also assists the individual to build a positive picture of what their life will look like without their current problems and the ways their current life is even a bit like that preferred future.

A Consistent, Coordinated Approach

A consistent, coordinated approach across all service delivery locations and teams involved in Rachel's care are crucial aspects of her treatment, given the multitude of services she accesses concurrently. This could take the form of an inter-service agreement document briefly outlining her background history, a consistent approach to be taken by all teams/clinicians, and specific strategies to use in each setting.

Examples of possible agreed aims or general principles for the plan could be:
- supporting Rachel to develop safe ways of coping with stress as opposed to her current ones that put her at significant risk of harm

Continued

EVIDENCE-BASED PRACTICE—cont'd

Scenario 25.1: Rachel

- supporting Rachel's recovery within the community
- facilitating psychotherapy within the community to support recovery
- reducing hospital and ED presentations and admissions
- providing a consistent and coordinated approach between services if admission is required
- allocating a lead clinician who is readily accessible for consultation by other clinicians to discuss Rachel's care.

  Examples of a strategy specific to the ED context might be:
- prompt review by an ED medical officer (senior medical officer only) on arrival, with or without a mental health nurse

- early liaison with the lead clinician on every presentation to ED during the lead clinician's operating hours
- a reminder of the importance of using a calm, empathetic, validating approach when engaging with Rachel
- using examples of treatment strategies from other services aimed to assist in the ED setting
- having the lead clinician support the acute care team and the ED mental health clinicians in providing a consistent approach to Rachel.

EVIDENCE-BASED PRACTICE

Scenario 25.2: Yasmina

Yasmina is a 40-year-old woman of Turkish background. She has presented to the ED several times over a 2-week period reporting dizziness, palpitations, shortness of breath, dry mouth, tingling in the fingers and gastrointestinal discomfort. She has undergone numerous investigations during her ED visits, including vital signs, ECGs, a chest X-ray, full blood count and thyroid function. Yasmina has also been referred to the neurology outpatient "dizzy clinic".

Yasmina is a non-smoker and does not consume alcohol or any illicit substances such as cannabis or amphetamines. She drinks minimal coffee and tea and doesn't consume "energy drinks", which also have a high caffeine content. Yasmina is referred to the mental health nurse in the ED for a review.

With little prompting, Yasmina recognises that stress has played a role in her symptoms. She has a supportive husband, two small children and works full-time as a community pharmacist. Yasmina acknowledges that she tends to worry, especially about her children. She often fears that something bad, such as an illness or accident, will happen to them. Yasmina explains that her mother died from cancer when she was 10 and that her father died from a heart attack when she was 16. Yasmina was essentially raised by her grandmother, who she describes as highly anxious and "overprotective". Recently Yasmina's grandmother was admitted to intensive care in a hospital in Turkey and was not expected to survive. Yasmina flew to Turkey to see her grandmother; however, she had panic symptoms on the flight over. She has not experienced any difficulty flying in the past. The hospital where she visited her grandmother was the same hospital in which her mother was treated and died. Returning to that hospital and seeing her grandmother in the ICU caused great distress for Yasmina. She also missed her husband and children and decided to fly home only 2 days after arriving in Turkey.

> ### ⚠ RED FLAGS
>
> - Panic symptoms can mimic many medical conditions, including cardiovascular and respiratory conditions, hyperthyroidism and others.
> - Comorbid cardiac and respiratory conditions also increase with panic.
> - Many of the symptoms associated with coronary artery disease are common with panic.
> - Even if a history of anxiety is known, clinicians should not discount the potential for comorbid coronary disease.
> - For people presenting with chest pain, a focused history, physical examination, ECG and judicious use of diagnostic tests should occur to rule out acute life-threatening conditions.

Protective Factors

- Yasmina has a supportive husband and family.
- She is educated, has full-time employment, has stable housing and no financial stress.

- Her diet and lifestyle do not predispose her to any serious physical conditions.
- Yasmina is seeking help and recognises that stress plays a role in her symptoms.

Knowledge

Anxiety and panic symptoms are widespread in the general population. Australian data from the most recent National Survey of Mental Health and Wellbeing shows anxiety disorders were the most common group of mental disorders experienced in the previous 12 months, with a prevalence of 16.8% for any anxiety disorder, and 3.7% for panic disorder specifically (Australian Bureau of Statistics (ABS) 2020–21). This equates to 3.3 million Australians experiencing anxiety in the previous 12 months. See Chapter 11 for a more detailed discussion of anxiety.

The Nature of Anxiety and Panic Symptoms

The acute symptoms of anxiety and panic are manifestations of the fight-or-flight response. These symptoms are the result of both an increase in release of catecholamines and a consequence of hyperventilation, which have overlapping symptom profiles. During the fight-or-flight response, catecholamines are released from the adrenal medulla and the sympathetic nerve terminals, which precipitates behavioural and physiological changes that prepare the body to overcome a stressor.

The catecholamines adrenaline and noradrenaline play a vital role in the fight-or-flight response, acting as both neurotransmitters and hormones, producing cardiovascular, respiratory and metabolic effects. They increase two- to tenfold during times of stress and act as powerful cardiac stimulants, raising the heart rate and increasing the force of myocardial contraction and coronary blood flow. Another manifestation of the fight-or-flight response is increased respiration, which occurs via connections between the limbic system and hypothalamus to the brainstem respiratory centre. Hyperventilation is one of the physiological responses most frequently seen in panic attacks. During hyperventilation, individuals exhale excessive carbon dioxide precipitating an acute respiratory alkalosis with a drop in arterial partial pressure of carbon dioxide ($PaCO_2$) and an elevation in pH. Patients who chronically over-breathe may develop a compensated respiratory alkalosis with near normal pH and a decrease in bicarbonate (HCO_3^-).

Alkalosis increases calcium binding to albumin and a decreased ionised calcium, as well as shifting potassium into cells leading to serum hypokalaemia. This hypocapnia-induced respiratory alkalosis produces a variety of symptoms. Increased neuro-excitability as a result of hypocalcaemia causes paraesthesia (tingling in lips and extremities) and carpopedal spasm. Tachycardia can result from the physiological changes that occur in respiratory alkalosis, including hypokalaemia and increased sympathetic activity. Chest pain may be caused by

EVIDENCE-BASED PRACTICE—cont'd

Scenario 25.2: Yasmina

coronary vasospasm or decreased myocardial oxygen delivery and may also be the result of overuse of chest wall muscles in over-breathing, rather than using the diaphragm, as in normal breathing. Feeling hot, flushed and sweaty is attributed to hyperventilation, leading to increased work in breathing. Gastrointestinal symptoms occur in acute respiratory alkalosis, including nausea, vomiting and increased gastrointestinal motility. Peripheral and central nervous system symptoms include dizziness, vertigo, anxiety, forgetfulness and clumsiness.

Attitudes

* It is important that symptoms are not dismissed, even if due to psychological stress.

Skills

Psychoeducation

* Information on the nature of anxiety, the fight-or-flight response, the role of hyperventilation and fears and cognitive reactions commonly held by those who panic are the first steps in supporting people to address anxiety and panic symptoms.
* Hearing of common fears associated with anxiety and panic can provide reassurance and normalise the person's experience. For example, people who experience panic attacks often report that they are "going mad" or "losing control". Reassurance that this is a fear held by many people who experience panic attacks can be immensely therapeutic.

Screening

* Screen for substances and medications that are associated with anxiety and panic symptoms, such as alcohol, nicotine, caffeine (including energy drinks), cannabis, amphetamines, cocaine, antidepressants, steroids, thyroxine and phenytoin.

Treatment Modalities and Considerations

* The recommended approaches for resolving anxiety and panic symptoms are non-pharmacological.
* People should be encouraged to engage in activities and interests that they find relaxing and shift attention from their physical and cognitive symptoms – for example, yoga, meditation or gardening.
* Metabolism-altering exercise (e.g. brisk walking, running, swimming or cycling) has proven effectiveness for discharging the nervous energy associated with anxiety and panic, thereby reducing symptoms.
* There is mounting evidence that walking in nature, or simply exposure to natural settings, has a positive impact on mental and emotional wellbeing (Bratman et al 2019; Cartwright et al 2018; Schertz & Berman 2019; White et al 2019). The practice of actually prescribing nature, and exercise in nature, has been adopted in an increasing number of countries, including the United States, the United Kingdom and New Zealand.

CHAPTER SUMMARY

Working effectively in a busy ED setting requires consideration of the inextricable interrelationship between physical and mental health and sensitivity to the heightened states of physical and emotional arousal in people presenting. Therapeutic care in the ED need not entail lengthy and in-depth discussions with consumers. Indeed, an approach that is mindful of non-verbal responses, that conveys an attitude of humility and respect and is focused on providing reassurance and support can be immensely therapeutic. While risk issues do need to be considered, the underlying philosophy of person-centred therapeutic engagement is the key to maximising positive outcomes for consumers accessing care in an ED. A solution-focused perspective provides a practical framework in the emergency setting for engaging consumers in conversations that surface current strengths, coping skills and assist in orienting people towards a future focus.

USEFUL WEBSITES

Blue Knott Foundation – support for adults traumatised as children: www.blueknot.org.au/

Breathe App by Reach Out – free app for iOS that provides coaching for deep-breathing exercises: au.reachout.com/tools-and-apps

Head to Health – information on anxiety disorders, with useful information and links to other useful websites and apps: www.headtohealth.gov.au/

REFERENCES

Bratman, G.N., Anderson, C.B., Berman, M.G., Cochran, B., de Vries, S., et al., 2019. Nature and mental health: An ecosystem service perspective. Science Advances, 5(7), eaax0903.

Carter, G., Page, A., Large, M., et al., 2016. Royal Australian and New Zealand College of Psychiatrists clinical practice guidelines for the management of deliberate self-harm. A N Z J Psychiatry 50, 939–1000.

Cartwright, B.D.S., White, M.P., & Clitherow, T.J. 2018. Nearby nature "buffers" the effect of low social connectedness on adult subjective wellbeing over the last 7 days. Int J Environ Res Pub Health, 15(6), 1238.

Kim, J.S., Akin, B.A., & Brook, J. 2019. Solution-focused brief therapy to improve child well-being and family functioning outcomes with substance using parents in the child welfare system. Dev Child Welfare, 1(2), 124–142.

Large, M. 2018. "The role of prediction in suicide prevention", Dialogue Clin Neurosci, 20(3), 197–205.

NSW Ministry of Health 2021. Safe sedation of acute severe behaviourally disturbed patients known or suspected to have COVID-19 infection. Online. Available at: www.health.nsw.gov.au/Infectious/covid-19/communities-of-practice/Pages/mh-sedation.aspx

NSW Ministry of Health 2015. Management of patients with acute severe behavioural disturbance in emergency departments. Ministry of Health, North Sydney. Online. Available at: www1.health.nsw.gov.au/pds/ActivePDSDocuments/GL2015_007.pdf

Parnas, S., Isobel, S. 2017. Navigating the social synapse: The neurobiology of bedside manner. Australas Psychiatry 26(1), 70–72.

Ranjbar, N., Erb, M., Mohammad, O., Moreno, F.A., 2020. Trauma-informed care and cultural humility in the mental health care of people from minoritized communities. Focus, 18(1):8–15.

Ryan, C.J., Large, M., Gribble, R., et al., 2015. Assessing and managing suicidal patients in the emergency department. Australas Psychiatry, 23, 513–516.

Santangelo, P., Procter, N., Fassett, D. 2018. Mental health nursing: Daring to be different, special, and leading recovery-focused care? Int J Ment Health Nurs, 27(1), 258–266.

Schertz, K.E., & Berman, M.G. 2019. Understanding nature and its cognitive benefits. Curr Dir Psychol Sci, 28(5), 496–502.

Shea, S.C. 2017. Psychiatric Interviewing: The Art of Understanding, 3rd ed. Elsevier, Edinburgh.

Wand, T., Glover, S., Paul, D., 2022. What should be the future focus of mental health nursing? Exploring the perspectives of mental health nurses, consumers, and allied health staff. Int J Ment Health Nurs 31(1), 179–188.

White, M.P., Alcock, I., Grellier, J., Wheeler, B.W., Hartig, T., et al., 2019. Spending at least 120 minutes a week in nature is associated with good health and wellbeing. Sci Rep, (9), 7730.

26

Generalist In-patient Settings

Catherine Daniel and Cynthia Delgado

KEY POINTS

- People who experience ill-health physically, mentally, emotionally and/or socially are likely to experience alterations of varying degrees of severity and duration to their mental state.
- Manifestations of ill-health and alterations in mental state present as changes in the person's usual behaviour, emotional expression, thinking and/or cognitive state.
- Early assessment, monitoring, and reporting of any alteration in a person's mental state is key to early identification of potential deterioration in a person's overall health state and to early intervention.

- As the experience of ill-health improves, a person's mental state will return to its usual state (biopsychosocial homeostasis).
- In-patient care in generalist settings should include mental health care and promotion of optimal wellbeing.
- All nurses working in generalist in-patient settings have a role in providing quality care for patients. This comprises a biopsychosocial focus in care, including assessment and nursing interventions for people experiencing alterations in mental state due to physical and/or mental ill-health.

KEY TERMS

Alteration in mental state
Biopsychosocial
Consultation-liaison psychiatry

Holistic care
Mental ill-health
Mental illness

Mental state
Optimal wellbeing
Physical ill-health

LEARNING OUTCOMES

The material in this chapter will assist you to:
- identify, describe and discuss contributing factors for a person experiencing alterations in their mental state
- discuss the complexity of care in co-associated physical and mental-ill health conditions
- identify the role of nurses in assessing alterations in mental state
- describe interpersonal strategies to assist a person experiencing alterations to their mental and emotional state, such as

experiencing mental–emotional distress and related changes in their behaviour
- differentiate the clinical features of mental illness and/or organic disorders and identify principles of management
- identify the role of consultation–liaison psychiatry in providing consultation to, collaboration with and support of colleagues to assess and work with people experiencing alterations in their mental state.

INTRODUCTION

A physical health condition is usually the primary reason for people presenting or being admitted to a general hospital. The physical ill-health experience and condition can significantly affect a person's thoughts, as well as their emotional, behavioural and cognitive state. For example, a usually calm person who experiences pain can also experience mental–emotional distress. This may manifest as fear, frustration or anger (alteration in emotional state), hypermotor activity and verbal abuse (alteration in behavioural state) and an inability to focus or concentrate (alteration in cognitive state). That is, the person experiences an alteration in their mental state.

There is a complex bi-directional relationship between mental and physical ill-health. Declining health and physical ill-health are associated with increased risk and vulnerability for experiencing co-associated mental ill-health across the lifespan (Bergmans & Smith 2021; Jansen et al 2022). Mental ill-health is also associated with higher risk of physical ill-health. Mental illnesses, including psychotic, mood, anxiety

and personality disorders, have a high prevalence of co-associated serious physical health conditions including cardiovascular disease, diabetes, chronic obstructive pulmonary disease, cancer and dental problems (Launders et al 2022; Mansour et al 2020). Consequently, people who have a mental illness are likely to have physical ill-health conditions that will require hospitalisation and treatment in general in-patient settings. A person with a mental illness who is hospitalised for a physical health condition may experience an exacerbation of symptoms related to their mental illness, due to, or in conjunction with, their physical health condition. This does not automatically mean they will require input from psychiatric–mental health services. It is important to consider that a person with a past or present diagnosis of mental illness may not experience active symptoms of their mental illness during hospitalisation. Additionally, people with a mental illness often achieve optimal overall wellbeing while continuing to experience some symptoms of mental ill-health, but do not experience adverse impacts from these.

THE ILL-HEALTH EXPERIENCE

A person's ill-health experience often signifies an episode of diminished wellbeing that may have an impact on the whole person. As described in Chapters 1 and 2 of this text, this includes disruptions to any of the biopsychosocial domains – that is, the person's physical, developmental, psychological, social, cultural and/or spiritual experience (Fig. 26.1). An experience of ill-health may affect a person's relationships, ability to study or work, or the way they cope. Conversely, factors closely aligned with the social determinants of health and the conditions in which people grow, live and age can also affect and influence a person's overall health and wellbeing (World Health Organization (WHO) 2022). Depending on the person's individual experiences, supports and ability to develop, maintain or access resources, these factors may protect against or increase their risk and vulnerability for developing or recovering from ill-health. In addition to assessing and identifying the signs and symptoms of illness, conditions or risk factors (Box 26.1) that may contribute to the person's experience of ill-health, protective factors should also be identified. Protective factors can impact positively on the person, improve their mental state and contribute to their recovery, and therefore should also be assessed for, identified and incorporated into their care, treatment and discharge plan. For example, a supportive family can provide financial and emotional support and resources to aid recovery. In contrast, families may also contribute to risk if there is a history of family violence, substance misuse or conflict.

Mental State

A person's mental state reflects their overall state of being. Mental state is closely linked to biopsychosocial aspects of the person's experience. Fluctuations in mental state are a normal aspect of a person's individual adaptation to changes in their internal or external experience, environment and circumstance. Every person's mental state is demonstrated differently through their verbal and non-verbal communication at various points in time based on their overall functioning and (positive or negative) experiences. A person's thoughts, cognitive and

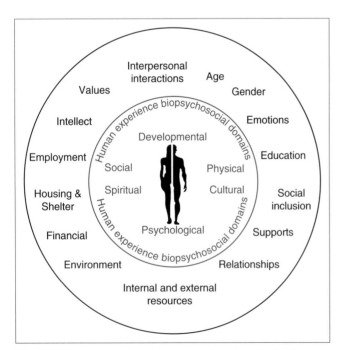

FIG. 26.1 Biopsychosocial Domains and Factors that Affect and Influence Health and Wellbeing.

BOX 26.1   Defining Risk and Protective Factors in Health and Wellbeing

In everyday life, we all experience situations, interactions and events that may impact positively or negatively on our whole being. Across the lifespan there are risk and protective factors that may be present, develop or occur that can affect and influence our health and wellbeing. Risk and protective factors are also discussed in the chapters in Part 1 of this book.

Risk factors may increase the likelihood that:
- mental health problems, physical/mental illness or diminished overall biopsychosocial health and wellbeing will occur in the short or long term
- existing issues may become more severe and last longer (Everymind 2022).

Examples of risk factors may include chronic physical illnesses and conditions, psychological trauma, lack of social support, poor interpersonal relationships, loss, stigma, stress and homelessness.

Protective factors may:
- enhance and protect a person's biopsychosocial health and wellbeing
- be preventative against, or reduce the likelihood of, developing a mental illness
- minimise the impact of ill-health
- enhance a person's capability to manage stressful life events and improve their resistance to risk factors (Everymind 2022).

Examples of protective factors include supportive close personal relationships, employment, positive interpersonal interactions, sense of humour and engagement in hobbies and interests.

Risk and protective factors are closely linked to the social determinants of health and can occur or exist in individual, biopsychosocial, cultural or environmental contexts.

Commonwealth Department of Health and Aged Care 2000.

---

emotional experience are expressed through their behaviour. The way a person responds to others, conducts themselves or acts is therefore directly reflective of their mental state.

Alteration in Mental State

An alteration in mental state occurs when a person's mental state – that is, their behaviour, emotional expression, thinking and cognitive capacity – has deviated or changed from their usual ways of being within their cultural/social norms. In the healthcare context, changes to a person's mental state signify a disruption to their biopsychosocial homeostasis and can often be the first sign of ill-health. Often, this presents as, and/or results in, mental–emotional distress. The type, severity and duration of alteration in mental state are highly dependent on the individual; for example, their ill-health condition and symptoms (physical/mental or both), treatments and existing biopsychosocial contributing factors, such as coping style, internal/external resources and supports, personal circumstances and acuity in their existing condition and situation. Every person is different and therefore changes to mental state may develop slowly and subtly, or very quickly and suddenly. Depending on the person's ill-health experience, changes to mental state may resolve very quickly or intermittently, last for days, weeks or months, and fluctuate or remain the same for the duration of the episode of care. As a person's health condition and situation improves, however, their mental state also improves (at varying rates) and should return to their usual baseline (homeostasis).

In general healthcare settings, a commonly observed condition that causes significant fluctuating alteration in mental state, particularly in older people, is delirium. Delirium is an acute confusional state characterised by disturbed consciousness, cognitive function and sleep–wake cycle, altered perception and changes to a person's emotional state (Australian Commission on Safety and Quality in Health Care

2016; Oliveira et al 2022). For example, an older person whose emotional expression and behaviour (emotional state) are usually very calm and pleasant, and who is able to have a coherent conversation, may suddenly become confused, fearful and irritable when experiencing delirium. These cognitive and emotional changes may lead to changes in behaviour, such as becoming hyperalert, restless, aggressive or, conversely, completely withdrawn. The changes are usually sudden and episodic; a person could return to their usual mental state during one shift and change in the next. This fluctuating alteration in mental state could last for days or weeks, depending on the cause and how long treatment begins to work. Delirium in older people can often be caused by a urinary tract infection. As the infection is treated, the person's mental state returns to their usual baseline.

Assessing for Deterioration in Mental State

In any general hospital setting, you are likely to be working with people of all ages (and their families) experiencing an alteration in their mental state. As part of holistic care, it is good practice to assess and document your observations of a person's mental state (thoughts, cognition, emotional and behavioural state) when they first arrive and as part of your observations on a shift-to-shift basis. There is potential to incorporate monitoring for deterioration in mental state into usual nursing practice by using a response chart to identify changes (Forster et al 2022). When able, it is also helpful to gain an understanding about what the person's premorbid mental state is usually like (by asking the person or obtaining corroborative information from family and/or other care providers). This enables you as a nurse to accurately detect any fluctuations and changes in mental state that could indicate a deterioration or improvement to the person's health condition. Regular assessment of mental state is also helpful in noting and monitoring for triggers or patterns that may be contributing to changes in a person's mental health condition.

Like every person admitted to or receiving treatment in general health care, people with a pre-existing mental illness who have physical ill-health may also experience some deterioration in their mental state. This does not necessarily mean the person will experience a relapse of their mental illness or experience deterioration in their overall mental health and wellbeing. In every instance, initial and

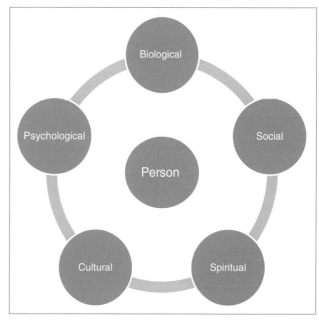

FIG. 26.2 Biopsychosocial Domains of Assessment.

ongoing biopsychosocial assessment of the individual person's experience, severity and duration of symptoms and impacts on the person's healing and recovery in the context of their physical health condition and treatment, is needed (see Fig. 26.2).

For any person experiencing a marked and/or prolonged alteration in mental state, or who is experiencing deteriorating symptoms of a mental illness, consultation–liaison psychiatry services (Box 26.2) or another mental health service that provides a service to the general hospital can be contacted for further assessment and consultation about care planning, intervention or treatment.

In the following scenarios, the principles of a holistic approach to care in conducting a biopsychosocial nursing assessment, mental state assessment and recommended nursing actions and interventions have been illustrated.

BOX 26.2 Consultation–Liaison Psychiatry – A Resource for General Health Settings

Consultation–liaison psychiatry is a subspecialty of psychiatry mental health. Consultation–liaison psychiatry multidisciplinary teams include psychiatrists, psychiatric registrars, mental health nurses and allied mental health staff, who provide mental health services to and within a general health setting (Sharrock et al 2022; The Royal Australian & New Zealand College of Psychiatrists (RANZCP) 2016). The services provided by the consultation–liaison psychiatry team (see Box 26.3 on p. 377 for examples) include assessment, education, consultation, care and treatment planning support.

These services are offered to non-mental health staff and treating teams in relation to the care and treatment of people who may be experiencing mental ill-health in a general hospital setting. This includes people who experience alteration of their mental state due to a physical ill-health condition and who may or may not have a comorbid mental illness.

Consultation–liaison psychiatry teams work in partnership with the patient's treating team(s) and provide consultation through direct involvement with the patient (e.g. assessment or psychological support and counselling), or indirectly by liaising, educating and working with general health staff involved in the patient's care, with the aim of enhancing and providing the best patient-centred care (RANZCP 2016; Sharrock et al 2022).

Consultation–liaison psychiatry nurses often provide a significant component of liaison, assisting staff at the local and wider health service level in developing and providing education, quality improvement projects and policy development for safe holistic practice (Sharrock et al 2022). Due to individual complexities and those of the working environment, consultation, assessment and intervention processes can be provided at any time of a person's admission. For example, obtaining collateral information, providing support to family/carers, and health staff advice and education on treatment and intervention related to the patient's care can be given, even in instances where the person receiving care may not be fully conscious.

The role of consultation–liaison psychiatry nurses has been articulated by the Australian College of Mental Health Nurses (2018) Consultation–Liaison Nurse Special Interest Group and includes:

- working with patients and their relatives, providing expert mental health assessment and intervention
- providing guidance, education and support to generalist staff caring for the patient and collaborating with them to develop a care plan
- being a positive role model to generalist staff in mental health care and practice
- working with the organisation or department as a mental health resource on mental health–related projects, education and policy development
- providing a link between generalist and mental health services (public and private, hospital and community).

EVIDENCE-BASED PRACTICE

Scenario 26.1: Jane

Jane is a 38-year-old woman with breast cancer, who has recently been diagnosed with secondary brain cancer. She had been home when her family noted sudden changes in her behaviour and emotional state such as staying awake all night, increased amount of speech and irritability, and becoming focused on charity work, which is something she has not done previously. Jane has also had surgery for a wound that was not healing (previous breast surgery) and has been on high doses of prednisolone. Once she was transferred to the ward, staff noted signs of mental–emotional distress, being irritable and abusive towards her family and staff.

You have been allocated to take a handover from ICU. Jane is present and orientated to person, time and place. She is observed to be irritable and arguing with every comment the ICU nurse is making. Jane appears to become hostile when comments are made about her mood. In front of her, the ICU nurse says, "Psych need to be involved", and this increases Jane's distress and her level of agitation considerably. Now she wants to leave hospital.

> ### ⚠ RED FLAGS
> - ICU admission is known to increase the risk of delirium.
> - The use of prednisolone may precipitate changes in behaviour including features of mania.
> - There is a risk Jane may leave hospital and not get the required treatment.
> - Irritability, agitation and using abusive language is not Jane's usual manner.

Protective Factors
- Jane has a supportive family.
- Jane is alert and orientated.
- Jane is well known to the oncology team.
- Since transfer to the ward Jane will be cared for by staff who she is well engaged with.

Knowledge
- There are risks of behavioural changes with prednisolone.
- Mental–emotional distress can be due to the person's current situation, ill-health condition and organic factors.
- Establish the person's rights and responsibilities/ethical care.
- Consider the escalation pathway if supportive nursing care does not alleviate the person's mental–emotional distress and agitation. This includes when to seek medical review, medications that may be used to manage clinical agitation and any further investigations.
- Potential organic causes such as hypoxia, urinary tract or respiratory infections that contribute to reversible changes to behaviour on transfer from ICU to ward bed should be investigated.

Skills
- Assessment of mental state
- Assessment of risk (leaving hospital, missing required treatment)
- Assessment of safety and care planning (minimise invasive lines, such as indwelling urinary catheters, early escalation for review)
- Interpersonal skills (e.g. introduce yourself, respect privacy, use Jane's preferred name when referring to her, respect personal space, explain care to Jane prior to commencing nursing care)

- Empathy about Jane's situation
- Emotional intelligence (recognising emotions in self and others, and emotional self-regulation)
- Assessment of Jane's capacity to understand what is happening to her, provide informed consent and make sound decisions in relation to her care, interventions and treatment

Nursing Actions and Interventions
In the first instance:
- Respond to Jane's mental–emotional distress and listen to her content and concerns.
- Speak in a calm and soft manner.
- Avoid staff clinical conversations near Jane if this is distressing her, but include her in handover communication.
- Do not debate, justify or argue.
- Allow time for communication and explain all care before it is provided.

Once handover is completed:
- Attend to orientation to the ward (Who will care for Jane? What will happen next?), ensuring she is comfortable.
- Conduct observations (pain, vital signs, review medications).
- Prioritise nursing care and group together tasks to avoid multiple interruptions.
- Consider current cognitive, behavioural and emotional state against Jane's usual behaviour, emotional expression and cognitive functioning. (What is the alteration/deterioration in the patient's mental state?)
- Seek clinical review given her change in behaviour.

Involving the family:
- Prepare Jane's family for the change in her behaviour.
- Prepare the family to respond to Jane by providing education (e.g. listen, don't argue, don't collude or agree with the content, but acknowledge Jane's distress, focus conversation on simple concepts, limit demands and decision-making being placed on Jane).
- Review nursing resources required to care for Jane (Are there staff on shift who know her? Is there flexibility in the allocation of staff if Jane needs some additional time for reassurance?)

Assessment of potential contributing factors for alteration in mental state:
- Pain
- Sleep deprivation in ICU
- Dehydration
- Urinary tract infection (had an indwelling catheter in ICU)
- Emotional distress/fear (diagnosis and deterioration)
- Biochemical imbalance (review bloods)
- Potential for infection/collection at surgery site
- Delirium

Documentation:
- Observed behaviour and Jane's concerns
- Description of what happened and what helped
- Diet/food intake
- Nursing care plan
- Investigations pending such as results of blood tests for infections

BOX 26.3   When to Contact the Consultation–Liaison Psychiatry Team for Jane

Sometimes changes in a person's behaviour may lead the treating team to query if the person has a history of, or is experiencing an episode of, mental ill health. In this instance, it is highly likely that the consultation–liaison psychiatry team would be contacted with a request for a more comprehensive mental health assessment and/or recommendations for care planning, interventions and treatment. The consultation–liaison psychiatry team could support the medical team to confirm there is no history of mental illness by presenting assessment findings and providing a possible differential diagnosis or other reasons for the person's change in mental state. Given Jane's symptoms, the most plausible differential diagnosis would be delirium.

The consultation–liaison psychiatry team would liaise with the relevant members of Jane's treating team (doctors, nursing staff and allied health) and recommend that delirium care pathways and management principles are applied. These include establishing if there are reversible causes, such as urinary tract infections or side effects of medication, and providing ongoing review and liaison to the medical team. The consultation–liaison psychiatry team has expertise in managing agitation and can provide information on medications that can be used for agitation and also explore contributing factors to the change in a person's mental state.

EVIDENCE-BASED PRACTICE

Scenario 26.2: John

John is a 48-year-old overweight man with a history of bipolar 1 disorder who is admitted to a general ward after collapsing at home. John's partner, Rita, found him unconscious on their living room floor and called an ambulance. Rita reported that John had been "fine" up until then. John is prescribed and is adhering to his medication regimen of quetiapine 300 mg and sodium valproate 600 mg PO twice daily. John also has type 2 diabetes treated with metformin 500 mg twice daily and consistently monitors his own blood sugar levels. John received intravenous fluids in the emergency department for rehydration and was commenced on intravenous antibiotics for a urinary tract infection. John is now on the ward in a four-bed bay for further observation and treatment.

You introduce yourself to John and explain you will be taking basic observations to monitor his pulse, blood pressure and blood sugar levels. John verbally responds by talking rapidly and incoherently. He is confused and disoriented to time and place. You note he has been incontinent of urine. He is fidgeting with his fingers, pulling at the bed sheet and looking around him. He starts repeatedly screaming "Help me! Help me!" and suddenly jumps out of bed.

! RED FLAGS

- Incontinent of urine
- Diabetes
- Dehydration
- Rapid, incoherent speech
- Fidgeting and pulling at sheets
- Screaming "Help me"
- Confused and disoriented
- Recent loss of consciousness
- Prescribed sodium valproate
- Suddenly jumps out of bed

Protective Factors
- Prior wellbeing
- Has a significant relationship (lives with his partner)
- Responds to his name
- Is adherent with usual medication regimens
- Usually monitors his own blood sugar levels

Knowledge
- John's usual/baseline behaviour, emotional expression, cognitive functioning (mental state homeostasis)
- Differentiation between physical and mental ill-health conditions and their expected/potential manifestations (signs and symptoms of bipolar 1 disorder, diabetes, urinary tract infection, dehydration and how these may affect a person's mental state)
- Medications (interactions, indications, side effects)
- Recognising mental–emotional distress
- Co-associated conditions
- Ward processes and alerts
- Contacts and escalation of care pathways
- Referral processes and pathways
- Patient's rights and responsibilities, ethical care

Skills
- Mental state and related risks and protective factors assessment
- Interpersonal communication (verbal and non-verbal)
- Empathy
- Emotional intelligence (recognising emotions in self and others, and emotional self-regulation)
- Safety and care planning (physical and mental)
- Performing procedures and administering treatment safely and sensitively
- Reporting and documentation
- Ability to prioritise needs
- Assessing John's capacity to understand what is happening to him, to provide informed consent and make sound decisions in relation to his care, interventions and treatment
- Recognising abnormal blood pathology (deviation from John's usual/baseline)

Attitudes
Behaviours and understandings that help to promote and maintain safety for the patient and others include:
- a non-judgemental approach
- professional curiosity
- objectivity
- empathy

Nursing Actions and Interventions
In the first instance:
- Assess for levels of safety in relation to John, other patients and yourself/staff members.
- Remain calm (role-modelling desired behaviour) and attempt to engage John by providing him with a little space, speaking in a soft, calm voice and addressing John by his preferred name. Acknowledge his distress, ask him what happened and let him know you are there to help. Use short sentences and provide brief information to re-orient him, asking what he feels he needs and inviting

Continued

EVIDENCE-BASED PRACTICE—cont'd

Scenario 26.2: John

him to sit down or, if able, to have a shower before returning to bed (because he has been incontinent and this could be a source of embarrassment).

- Ask for help from another nurse if needed.

When John is less distressed:

- Attend to basic observations. Observe his breathing, colour and level of consciousness and explain that his pulse, blood pressure and blood sugar levels need to be taken.
- Ensure that before each procedure (before touching the patient), you explain what the procedure will involve (e.g. "I am going to put this cuff around your arm to take your blood pressure. It will feel a little tight on your arm for a bit but will pass quickly"). This is important to ensure John is given due respect and his dignity is maintained. It also minimises the possibility for him to become startled. Proceeding in this way will give John the opportunity to ask any questions if he's able, and you the opportunity to observe for safety concerns and cues.
- If safe to do so, encourage John's self-efficacy by inviting him to attend to his own blood sugar level (he does this regularly at home) and assess his current capacity to understand what is happening to him and his ability to make sound/relevant decisions about his care.
- Consider John's current thinking, cognitive capacity, behaviour and emotional state against his usual known and reported behaviour, emotional expression and cognitive functioning (What is the alteration/deterioration in John's mental state?).
- Consider John's current physical health status and any deviations from his usual experience of his physical health condition.

- Plan with and offer John assistance with toileting if needed and take a urine sample for urinalysis.
- Change the bed or ask someone to assist with changing the bed linen if you are attending to John.

Assessment of potential contributing factors for alteration in mental state:

- Blood sugar level
- Dehydration
- Sodium valproate overdose
- Urinary tract infection
- Mental–emotional distress/fear
- Active symptoms of bipolar disorder
- Unknown potential another infection or a related physical condition – look at blood pathology results (or ensure bloods are ordered)
- Delirium

Documentation:

- Observations of specific behaviour, emotional expression, thinking and physical assessments (including fluid input/output; food intake)
- Note what interventions and actions were taken and the outcomes from these
- Details of what and to whom referrals were made
- A clear and updated care plan

Referral:

- Refer John to the treating team for further medical review.
- Given John's history of mental illness and change in level of mental state alteration and deterioration, a referral to the Consultation–liaison psychiatry team could be considered (Box 26.4).

BOX 26.4   Referring John to the Consultation–Liaison Psychiatry Team

John has a known comorbid physical (type 2 diabetes) and mental illness (bipolar 1 disorder). Given that John's partner said he was "fine" before his hospitalisation, it is likely that John's current alteration in his mental state, demonstrated predominantly as emotional and behavioural distress, is not due to his pre-existing mental illness. There is, however, a marked deterioration in John's mental state from his baseline. In this case, the consultation–liaison psychiatry team may be contacted to provide staff support and education about:

- John's mental illness – this would help the treating team and nursing staff become aware of how and what bipolar 1 disorder symptoms John experiences, and may be differentiated from a physical cause
- psychotropic medication
- interpersonal interventions and strategies in effectively communicating and attending to John when he's experiencing high levels of distress
- care planning strategies aimed at engaging John and promoting his self-efficacy and recovery while he is hospitalised.

If John's mental state continues to deteriorate (see Box 26.5), the consultation–liaison psychiatry team may complete a further comprehensive mental health assessment of John, review his current psychotropic medication and may provide recommendations about any changes or additions to his current treatment. In this instance, the consultation–liaison psychiatry team may become regularly involved in more formalised care processes (such as case reviews) and may also take a role if needed in coordinating John's care and discharge planning (including advocacy and referral to the relevant care provider upon discharge).

If John's deterioration in mental state was caused by a physical health condition, it is important to note that, as his physical health improves, his mental state will also improve and return to baseline. If this happens quickly, the consultation–liaison psychiatry team may not need to be involved.

BOX 26.5   Useful Tips to Engage With Patients Who Have a Deterioration in Mental State

- As soon as possible in their admission, explore and discover what the person's usual way of being is (What is their usual baseline mental state?) and clearly document this.
- Develop an awareness of the person's usual functioning (Do they live alone? Are they independent? Are any regular healthcare services involved? What are their personal preferences for food, fluid and personal items?).
- Speak to the patient, even if they are experiencing alteration in their mental state. Ask direct questions and try to talk to them rather than about them.
- Monitor for patterns or triggers that may contribute to changes in a person's mental state. Don't assume the behaviour is due to mental illness. It can often

be the first or main feature or sign of ill-health (Could it be due to pain, delirium, or other reversible causes?).

- Don't focus on the diagnosis but ask yourself: "What care is required here?" Patients depend on healthcare staff to advocate for evidence-based care.

The patient's capacity to consent and refuse treatment may need to be determined. Be aware that a person with capacity will not necessarily make decisions you agree with.

CHAPTER SUMMARY

In this chapter we have explored and identified examples of contributing factors to a person's alteration in mental state. The nursing care and interpersonal interventions to assist a person experiencing mental–emotional distress and related changes in their behaviour have been described and applied to examples from practice. Nursing assessment to differentiate features or signs and symptoms of mental illness and/or organic disorders and identify the key principles of nursing management has been described. The role of consultation–liaison psychiatry in assessing and supporting people who experience deterioration in their mental state has been outlined.

USEFUL WEB RESOURCES

Australian College of Mental Health Nurses – Consultation Liaison Nurses Special Interest Group: acmhn.org/Web/Resources/SIG-Documents-Public/Consultation-Liaison-Special-Interest-Group.aspx

Australian Commission of Safety and Quality in Health Care (ACSQHC) 2021. National Safety and Quality Health Service Standards: Standard 8 – Recognising and responding to acute deterioration standard: www.safetyandquality.gov.au/standards/nsqhs-standards/recognising-and-responding-acute-deterioration-standard#:,:text=The%20Recognising%20and%20Responding%20to,in%20cognition%20and%20mental%20state

Victorian Department of Health:
Physical health framework for specialist mental health services: www.health.vic.gov.au/chief-psychiatrist-guidelines/equally-well-in-victoria-physical-health-framework-for-specialist-mental-health-services

Victorian nursing observation guidelines: www.health.vic.gov.au/practice-and-service-quality/nursing-observation-through-engagement-in-psychiatric-in-patient-care

REFERENCES

Australian College of Mental Health Nurses 2018. Consultation Liaison Special Interest Group. Online. Available at: acmhn.org/Web/Resources/SIG-Documents-Public/Consultation-Liaison-Special-Interest-Group.aspx

Australian Commission on Safety and Quality in Health Care (ACSQHC), 2016. Delirium Clinical Care Standard. ACSQHC, Sydney. Online. Available at: www.safetyandquality.gov.au/our-work/clinical-care-standards/delirium-clinical-care-standard

Bergmans, R.S., & Smith, J. 2021. Associations of mental health and chronic physical illness during childhood with major depression in later life. Aging Ment Health, 26(9), 1813–1820.

Commonwealth Department of Health and Aged Care 2000. National Action Plan for Promotion, Prevention and Early Intervention for Mental Health. Mental Health and Special Programs Branch. Commonwealth Department of Health and Aged Care, Canberra.

Everymind 2022. Prevention First Frameworks: A Prevention and Promotion Framework for Mental Health. Everymind, New South Wales Ministry of Health, Newcastle. Online. Available at: https://everymind.org.au/prevention-and-promotion-approaches/prevention-first-frameworks

Forster, J.A., Coventry, A., Daniel, C. 2022. Optimizing the response to mental health deterioration: Nurses' experiences of using a Mental Health Observation Response Chart. Int J Mental Health Nurs, 32(1), 95–105.

Jansen, M., Chapman, C., Richardson, T., Elliott, P., & Roberts, R. 2022. The relationship between mental and physical health: A longitudinal analysis with British students. J Pub Ment Health, 21(3), 218–225.

Launders, N., Kirsh, L., Osborn, D.P.J. & Hayes, J. F. 2022. The temporal relationship between severe mental illness diagnosis and chronic physical comorbidity: A UK primary care cohort study of disease of burden over 10 years. Lancet Psychiatry, 9, 725–735.

Mansour, H., Mueller, C., Davis, K.A., Burton, A., Shetty, H., et al., 2020. Severe mental illness diagnosis in English general hospitals 2006–2017: A registry linkage study. PLoS Medicine, 17(9), e1003306.

Oliveira J. e Silva, L., Stanich, J.A., Jeffery, M.M., Lindroth, H.L., et al., 2022. Association between emergency department modifiable risk factors and subsequent delirium among hospitalized older adults. Am J Emerg Med, 53, 201–207.

Sharrock, J., Happell, B., & Jeong, S.Y. 2022. The impact of Mental Health Nurse Consultants on the care of general hospital patients experiencing concurrent mental health conditions: An integrative literature review. Int J Ment Health Nurs, 31(4), 772–795.

The Royal Australian & New Zealand College of Psychiatrists (RANZCP) 2016. Service Model for Consultation–liaison psychiatry in Victoria. RANZCP Victorian Branch, Melbourne. Online. Available at: www.ranzcp.org/files/resources/reports/10-20-1-service-model-for-consultation-liaison-wor.aspx

World Health Organization (WHO) 2022. World mental health report: Transforming mental health for all. WHO, Geneva.

27

Care of Older Adults

Sharon Rydon and Jane Ferreira

He aha te mea nui o te ao?
He tāngata, he tāngata, he tāngata.
What is the most important thing in the world?
The people, the people, the people.

KEY POINTS

- Mental health and wellbeing in older adults is impacted by issues related to frailty, longevity and ageing, as well as pre-existing or new mental health disorders.
- Ageing affects all the health dimensions, although all people age differently. Physical changes can lead to poorer health outcomes and have the potential to impact the mental health and wellbeing of older adults.
- Caring for older adults requires nurses to have an awareness of issues associated with frailty, longevity and ageing.

- Nurses need to be able to identify factors that contribute to changes in an older person's health and wellbeing, and respond effectively to these with a range of interventions, including culturally appropriate holistic assessment tools.
- Nurses caring for older people are well situated to promote meaning, purpose and connectedness in the life of the older person through the therapeutic relationship.

KEY TERMS

Ageing
Assessment
Connectedness

Frailty
Longevity
Meaningfulness

Therapeutic relationships
Wellbeing

LEARNING OUTCOMES

The material in this chapter will assist you to:
- understand the relationship between health, wellbeing and the ageing process
- consider the implications of living longer and the potential challenges or limitations that may impact on mental health and wellbeing, including health literacy and knowing how and where to seek help

- identify strategies to support an older person to maximise their level of wellbeing
- reflect on nursing practice to deliver care that promotes quality of life for the older person.

INTRODUCTION

Older people generally report higher levels of mental health and wellbeing compared to the rest of the population. Caring for older adults is multifaceted and can be complicated by factors such as frailty, longevity and ageing. Events and experiences that have impacted on a person's life can also influence health and wellbeing.

Although a person may have a strong awareness of their mortality, this is influenced by their individual life circumstances, as you will read in the two case scenarios presented in this chapter. Health knowledge, understanding and decision-making are influenced by the person's level of health and wellbeing, and their previous life experiences. Loss of physical independence, social support or financial changes can contribute to how an older person perceives their value in the community. There are many transition points in life that are relevant to older adults, which include loss related to physical, psychological, social or environmental changes. Loss of significant people in their lives, along with financial, social and intimacy losses, are common for the older adult. This chapter builds on the key considerations discussed in Chapter 18 regarding mental health care of older people and disorders associated with older age.

While working though the two scenarios provided in this chapter, consider the clinical assessment skills and tools that may assist in assessing an older person in your care. A variety of screening and assessment tools is available, so it is important to ensure the tool chosen is appropriate for the assessment and your level of experience. Be sure to discuss this further with your placement preceptor, clinical adviser or senior nurse.

Having an awareness of the factors contributing to an older person's behaviour and an understanding of the underlying circumstances surrounding the behaviour is the initial approach to care. Gathering all the relevant information contributes to a holistic assessment and informs the management/interventions to be undertaken to provide the best outcome for the person. Interventions may include increased social support, brief psychological interventions and health promotion. It is important to be aware of local organisations and specialist health teams that can support an individual needing higher levels of care to restore or maintain health and wellbeing and there is an option for referral to a specialist mental health team as part of primary care and a stepped care strategy.

EVIDENCE-BASED PRACTICE

Scenario 27.1: Bill

Bill is an 80-year-old man who cares for his wife at home. Bill was previously a mechanic working seven days a week and rarely took holidays. His working life ended after an industrial accident 16 years ago, where he sustained a right shoulder injury (the proximal humerus was fractured causing irreversible nerve damage), and despite multiple surgeries he has never regained full function of his right arm. Bill often contemplates leaving his home or hopes for his life to end, given the impact of his physical disabilities and health needs, loss of income since retirement and the stress of maintaining the household. He drives his wife, who has a chronic illness, to her appointments three times a week. and supports her to meet her activities of daily living.

Bill refuses home help. He tries to keep order in his day and feels external interference in the home would interrupt his routine. At times, his health deteriorates because he cannot afford his prescribed medications that he feels "do not help anyway". Bill is struggling to manage the household finances and becomes tearful and distressed when asking others for help. He tries to have enough money available for scheduled household expenses, but his pension falls out of sequence with due payment dates. Any unexpected expenses affect his budget and create additional financial pressures.

Bill feels his general practitioner (GP), who is aware of his personal circumstances, is often dismissive of the symptoms he describes, even when he says his mood is low, he has thoughts of wanting to leave his current living situation, his weight fluctuates, his sleep is of poor quality, or that he has unusual feelings of having no physical strength.

! RED FLAGS

- Ageism and longevity: Life is ever-changing and living longer (longevity) can impact a person's role and sense of purpose. Not all older people experience the same issues, although some may experience circumstances that cause stress or distress, and affect their ability to function as they had previously. In a person-centred approach, always beware of assuming that Bill's issues are the same as other older people's.
- Quality of life: Bill is experiencing significant loss in his life. His retirement may feel like a burden rather than a rewarding time after many years of hard work. The loss of income and reduced social contact, health problems being experienced by himself and his wife, loss of identity associated with work and therefore his perceived value in society, are having a detrimental effect on Bill's mental health and wellbeing.
- Wellbeing: Bill is struggling with his life circumstances and is likely to be experiencing depression. Bill is voicing thoughts or ideas which may be assessed as potentially at-risk behaviour and a sign that he needs help. The contributing factors that are affecting him may not be obvious to Bill or those around him (Harmer et al 2022).

- Context: Several issues are influencing how Bill is coping. It is important to understand and explore these issues with Bill, as feelings of low mood and expression of passive suicidal thoughts raise the potential risk of self-harm. The cumulative impact of the difficulties he describes in caring for his wife, being responsible for all the household chores, trying to manage on his pension, in addition to experiencing his own health issues, are indicators that raise safety concerns.
- Age: Bill's presentation in the context of healthy ageing raises points of concern. Studies show that risk factors such as loneliness, poverty, declining abilities due to the ageing process or a change in living circumstance can contribute to an increased incidence of low mood, self-harm and suicidality in older people, particularly in males over the age of 85 years (Australian Bureau of Statistics (ABS) 2022; Barak et al 2022). Bill's social isolation, financial stress, difficult home life and limited ability to attend to his own health issues should prompt further assessment of his mental health, wellbeing, care and safety needs.

Protective Factors

- It is important to identify Bill's current supports, including his wife or any other family members or friends who might help. Consider identifying the appropriate services to assist him to feel a greater sense of empowerment, and to support his recovery.
- Although he has described his GP as dismissive, Bill is still connected to the health practice. There may be an opportunity to support Bill to see a different GP in the same practice or there may also be a mental health practitioner associated with the health centre.
- Bill has limited time to develop or engage in his own interests. Assisting him to plan for something that he enjoys regularly and making it a priority would support him in overcoming some of the contextual issues he faces, such as social isolation, feeling undervalued and stressed, and perhaps being unsure of his identity and value. Community support services would be an integral part of this intervention to allow him time for himself, while feeling reassured that the needs of his wife are being met.
- It would be helpful to understand how Bill has coped before when experiencing stress during his life, and to discuss with him if some of these strategies may be useful in the current situation.

- Bill's current low mood may potentially influence his ability to engage in meaningful conversation, so exploring supportive interventions such as the application of talking therapies may be useful.

Knowledge

Older People at Risk of Suicide

- Related factors that contribute to increased suicide risk in older adults include being male, poor socioeconomic standing, chronic pain and illness (ABS 2022; Barak et al 2022).
- Suicidal ideation and behaviour in individuals over the age of 65 years has been attributed to changes in health and wellbeing factors, such as loneliness, loss of a partner, environmental changes, physical illness or declining functional abilities (Barak et al 2022; Fässberg et al 2016).
- Research also suggests caregivers may be in the high-risk group related to factors such as carer stress (Abey-Nesbit et al 2021; Anderson et al 2019; Joling et al 2018; Solimando et al 2022).
- Although risk factors for suicide may include feelings of loneliness or hopelessness, lack of social supports, or living with a limiting physical or mental

Continued

Scenario 27.1: Bill

- health condition, it is important to consider applying a holistic nursing assessment to identify areas of actual or potential risk.
- Studies identify that older people often consult their GP within weeks before their death (Ahmedani et al 2017; Barak et al 2022; Fässberg et al 2016).

Age-Related Considerations
- Cognitive function, health knowledge and understanding form part of the holistic nursing assessment of an older person. Identified changes in cognitive abilities may affect a person's decision-making and problem-solving skills, and impact on their health outcomes (Conejero et al 2018; Wand et al 2021).
- Studies indicate that symptoms of depression in older people are common and often underdiagnosed. If untreated, depression may negatively impact on the older person's wellbeing and ability to enjoy their later years of life (Conejero et al 2018; Wand et al 2021).
- There is also evidence that older males, aged 85 and over with a diagnosis of depression co-existing with suicidal ideation, are at increased risk of self-harm events (Barak et al 2022; Joling et al 2018; Solimando et al 2022).

Physical Health
- Screening for thyroid dysfunction and vitamin B12 deficiency is recommended to rule these out as causal factors for depression, as a low-functioning thyroid has been implicated in depressive symptoms (Wildisen et al 2019), and vitamin B12 deficiency can be a contributing factor to depression and cognitive decline in older adults (da Rosa et al 2019).

Carer Responsibilities
- A carer's quality of life is impacted by the increased responsibility needed to care for the family member, which can become challenging and burdensome (Abey-Nesbit et al 2021; Gilbertson et al 2019; Joling et al 2018; Solimando et al 2022).
- Independent risk factors, such as family conflict and loss of employment, can reduce social integration and the feeling of belonging (Conejero et al 2018; Solimando et al 2022; Wand et al 2021).

Attitudes
- Stereotyping older people as "frail, incompetent or impaired" is ageist, and represents the use of assumption, bias and stigma (Health Quality and Safety Commission (HQSC) 2019). This messaging, or perceived view by older people, may contribute to their inability or reluctance to seek help (HQSC 2019; Wand et al 2021).
- There is an assumption that older people living independently have a higher level of functioning compared to those who may be living in the aged residential care environment because people in aged care facilities require additional support.
- There is an assumed view that the role of caring for predominantly frail, unwell older people is a less important, skilled or valued occupation. This view is associated with negative stereotyping of older adults, bias and stigma (HQSC 2019; Ross et al 2019). To gain an understanding of what it is like to be an older person, consider how you would like to be treated as you age. Or ask yourself how would you like your parents, grandparents or other significant people in your life cared for as they age?
- Too often, for example, as clinicians are talking with older people, their voices are raised and they use slowed, simple speech that can feel patronising to the recipient. This contributes to the maintenance of stereotypical attitudes that infer that older people are hearing impaired or have difficulties understanding and contributes to lowering a person's self-esteem (Schroyen et al 2018).
- Older people living with a diagnosis such as depression or cognitive impairment may be considered incompetent, with assumptions made that they will be unable to complete their activities of daily living due to frailty or make choices or rational decisions related to their care (Aronson 2020; Fullen et al 2018).

- Our attitudes about older people, particularly if developed at an early age, potentially remain with us throughout our nursing career. Understanding of, or exposure to, traditional cultural and social models of extended family/whānau living in Aotearoa New Zealand and Australia, and the contribution of older people within these relationships may be limited, contributing to a lens of unconscious bias (HQSC 2019).
- It is also suggested that negativity towards becoming old is impacted by the assumption that ageing means a person will experience illness, become isolated from lifelong friends and family, and lose independence (Gale & Cooper 2018; Parr-Brownlie et al 2020). Studies indicate that overcoming loneliness may positively influence older people's physical and mental health, and this is evidenced by the increased demand for the retirement village lifestyle, which promotes independence, social interaction and companionship within a supportive community (Boyd et al 2021; Chen et al 2022).

As you read in Chapter 18, mental health of the older adult is affected by the person's life trajectory and interrelated with physical changes and loss. If Bill is viewed with a negative attitude and seen in a stereotypical way because of his age and his presentation, this increases the risk of poor management of his needs. Early exploration of warning signs is a proactive approach, including knowing and addressing your own beliefs and bias towards caring for older people. This can prevent an unconscious belief that Bill can't recover from his present poor state of mental health and wellbeing. A nurse's positive attitude and a willingness to demonstrate care will influence their behaviour and will support actions that will assist older people in managing their mental health issues.

Skills
Assessment
- Health and wellbeing assessments for older adults need to be structured and comprehensive to inform appropriate care planning. The clinical assessment tool interRAI provides questions from multiple health and social domains to identify abilities, areas of risk or need for increased support. Factors such as living arrangements, loneliness, social interactions and social isolation are assessed and scored (Jamieson et al 2019).
- Exploring the individual's history and current plan of care in collaboration with the older person and with other health professionals such as in a multidisciplinary team will help inform the most appropriate person-centred approach to care management.
- Comprehensive assessment includes a full understanding of the health history, a detailed physical and mental health assessment that collects objective and subjective information, and evaluation of care interventions to date. The assessment includes a review of the medications the person has been prescribed, their understanding of the therapeutic effects and whether they adhere to the prescribed plan to ascertain if the agreed outcomes have been achieved.

Therapeutic Relationship
- Establishing a rapport and gaining trust is vital to ensuring the person is comfortable disclosing personal information and will facilitate an open discussion.
- Using a person-centred approach will improve the person's confidence and have a positive impact on the relationship and on health outcomes (Ross et al 2019).
- Listening is the simplest and yet one of the most important skills a nurse can utilise. Listening in an open and non-judgemental way to the stories or experiences shared by the person in our care enables us to collect information that will guide us with interventions and management. By listening, we are gaining an understanding of how the person feels and how they experience the environment they live in. As the receiver of this personal information it's important to acknowledge the person's vulnerability in sharing their thoughts, memories, feelings or experiences, and for the nurse to show kindness, validation and understanding.

EVIDENCE-BASED PRACTICE—cont'd

Scenario 27.1: Bill

- The way you communicate is equally important to ensure the older person feels valued. Using a patronising tone or condescending terms of endearment such as "lovey", "darl" or "dear" ignores the person's individuality. Ask the person how they wish to be addressed and ensure you use their preferred name as part of a respectful approach to the older person.
- By listening, observing and communicating appropriately, you are building rapport and trust which are essential elements of the therapeutic relationship. It is important to ensure that the person's wishes and needs are central to the care planning process before any strategies are introduced.

Promoting Health and Wellbeing

Promoting wellness, resilience and a sense of belonging is an important part of delivering care and improving our own knowledge and skills in these approaches will improve our confidence when interacting with older people. It is always appropriate for you to seek professional support, or to refer the person to a more experienced clinician or service if you feel out of your depth (Aronson 2020; Fullen et al 2018).

Observation

- Observing the person's surroundings and the interactions they have with others can help to build a picture of what may be occurring or contributing to how they are feeling.
- Inquiring about who the person's supports are and whether/how they are managing in the community will also inform management.

There are validated screening and assessment tools available that can be incorporated into your nursing care and can help you to identify what the focus of nursing interventions might be. Seek assistance and develop your skills if you are not familiar with any tools. For example:

- The UCLA Loneliness Scale is recommended when you suspect the person is experiencing loneliness, which may be contributing to the behaviours displayed (Akpan et al 2018; Matthews et al 2022). This tool has three questions and can be easily incorporated into your discussion without needing a tickbox sheet for the person to complete. Inquiring about how often they feel (1 = lonely; 2 = left out; 3 = isolated from others) can enable the person to respond, with "hardly ever" scoring 1, "sometimes" scoring 2, or "often" scoring 3. A total score of 6–9 indicates the person is "lonely".
- Once you have established this or ruled out loneliness, other tools such as the Depression Rating Scale within the InterRAI Clinical Assessment tool or Geriatric Depression Scale short form (GDS-15 or GDS 5/15) can be used to assess mood in cognitively intact people (Heerema 2022; Sheikh & Yesavage 1986).
- Screening or assessing for suicide intent can be based on the Patient Health Questionnaire (PHQ), although people can answer the questions with a "no"

and still have thoughts of suicide, so it is important for the nurse to sensitively inquire about the nature of suicidal thoughts. Any indication by the older person of suicidal ideation should be considered as an indication of increased risk.

Relevant Treatment Modalities

Once all the assessments have been conducted and information gathered, a decision can be made on the most appropriate support strategies or treatment modalities for the person. For example, identifying loneliness as an issue then prompts interventions and actions that increase social connection and reduce the risk of isolation. The assessment will also determine if care needs require referral to support services. For Bill, getting a sense of how he understands his own health and healthcare needs is the first action.

- Talking to Bill and ascertaining what he wants and needs can help identify the goals of care.
- Bill's GP or primary care nurse should also be engaged early in determining how Bill's health is currently being managed and if there are any other underlying health issues.
- Understanding his current medications and whether he is adhering to the treatment plan will help to identify whether any changes need to be made or if any additional interventions are required.
- Non-pharmacological strategies – for example, cognitive behaviour therapy (CBT) or acceptance and commitment therapy – should be used as a first-line approach, with consideration of prescribed medication if psychological therapy alone is not effective. Research has shown that older people respond better to psychological intervention than working age people (Saunders et al 2021).
- Antidepressant medication is a commonly used treatment for people who are depressed. Prescribing for older adults must be planned and monitored carefully because of age-related physical changes that occur, such as increased risk of falls or renal function impairment (Australian Medicines Handbook 2023), which can impact on therapeutic effects and side effects. Bill will require support if commencing antidepressant medication and should be started at the lowest dose to minimise any adverse effects, such as dizziness, nausea, blurred vision or hyponatraemia, and the associated risk of falls (Australian Medicines Handbook 2023).
- Considering the initial identified concerns, it is important to understand Bill's goals for care. Strategies, such as involving Bill's immediate family and friends as a primary support network, can be positive interventions to achieve his care goals. Additional aspects for consideration may include the involvement of community support services, such as social work input, counselling, homecare or respite options with an aged care service provider. Based on professional health assessment, a referral to specialist health services may be indicated for further assessment of Bill's wellbeing and provision of ongoing care.

EVIDENCE-BASED PRACTICE

Scenario 27.2: Mabel

Mabel is an 85-year-old woman who has been living in residential care for 3 months. She has complex medical disorders, including congestive heart failure and osteoarthritis in her left knee. She has been treated for hypertension, hyperlipidaemia and gastric reflux for some years. The diversional therapist at the care home has worked with Mabel to provide a life story to help the healthcare team to get to know and understand her as a person. Mabel never married after her fiancé was killed in a farming accident when he was 22 years old, a year before their planned wedding. As a young woman needing to support herself in the 1950s, when options for women were limited, Mabel

became a hairdresser and over time acquired her own salon, which she owned and managed until she retired fully at 75 years of age. She has one brother, who is married with three adult children, all of whom have been an important part of Mabel's life.

Mabel also has a companion, Betty, who lived with her for 25 years before her admission to the aged care facility. Betty is 10 years younger than Mabel and provided Mabel with daily care for about the past 7 years; she is now a daily visitor to the care centre. Betty continues to live independently in the home she previously shared with Mabel in a neighbouring area, although she now takes

Continued

Scenario 27.2: Mabel

the bus to visit because she no longer feels confident driving. Mabel experiences daily pain from her osteoarthritis and requires the registered nurses to help manage this through pharmacological and non-pharmacological interventions. A multidisciplinary team review is coming up for Mabel because she has been in care for 3 months. Since admission to the care home Mabel has struggled with multiple losses; her mobility is becoming increasingly limited, her independence regarding activities of daily living has been affected with her increasing pain on movement and her sleep is often of poor quality. She expresses a great sense of loss having been physically parted from Betty, despite her almost daily visits. She misses the privacy of the home they shared, their dog Scamp and two cats, along with the meals they enjoyed cooking together and the friends who visited. Mabel remains cognitively unimpaired; however, since admission she has become increasingly anxious – partially related to financial and family pressures because her brother and nephew believe Betty should leave the home they shared so it can be sold to support Mabel's care. The staff have also noticed Mabel is increasingly reluctant to leave her room for meals or activities. Her disinterest in food has led to a 4 kg weight loss since admission, despite her diet being adjusted to provide her with more calories.

During the assessment, the registered nurse spent time with Mabel to undertake some advance care planning. During this conversation, Mabel expressed feelings of sadness and despair – particularly about her relationship with Betty, as she has confided that they were more than companions and were in an intimate relationship for many years. She desperately misses the intimacy of the relationship and dreads that it won't remain private now she is in care. She does not feel confident telling her brother and nephews that this is the reason she does not wish to sell the house Betty lives in. However, they have been increasingly pressuring her about this, wanting to ensure that Mabel has a valid will and an advance care directive. They are making assumptions that they will be the primary recipients and executors of Mabel's will and that her brother will be the person she nominates as her enduring power of attorney when the needs arises. While Mabel is frail, she continues to retain the right to make her own decisions as she is cognitively unimpaired. Betty cannot easily take Mabel to their home because of her limited mobility and Betty's inability to drive.

❗ RED FLAGS

- Mabel is increasingly frail, and her complex issues are affecting her quality of life and her resilience as she copes with the transition to the care home. For an older person, this may include a loss of identity, independence and autonomy.
- In the face of feelings of helplessness, social isolation and loneliness, it is difficult for Mabel to develop new fulfilling relationships with team members and other residents.
- The sensitive issues of love, intimacy and sex attract a great degree of stigma and discrimination in relation to older people (Henrickson et al 2022). Mabel fears she will be unable to keep her relationship with Betty private and her expectation is that having the relationship exposed to staff and other residents will mean she will not be accepted by others and that tensions will increase with her brother and his family.
- Mabel is at risk of being compromised nutritionally because of her reduced appetite and isolation. Her food preferences are very different to what is offered in the care home as she has previously enjoyed cooking and entertaining with friends.
- Chronic pain affects her sleep quality and contributes to her feeling tired and less willing to socialise with other residents at mealtimes.
- A primarily pharmacological approach to supporting Mabel may contribute to a situation of polypharmacy and poorer health outcomes such as the unintended consequence of increasing her risk of falls (Nguyen et al 2020; Toh et al 2022).

Knowledge

Ageing

- Underpinning an effective toolbox of skills is knowledge of anatomy and physiology and an understanding of the process of ageing.
- Developing comprehensive assessment skills requires knowledge about specific physical systems (e.g. integumentary, oral, urinary, cardiovascular, respiratory, musculoskeletal), as well as knowledge about clinical reasoning, psychosocial assessment and ethico-legal and professional considerations (Bauer et al 2018).
- Frailty is an important concept linked to the increasing impact of ageing from disease processes on a person's functional and physical abilities, along with the potential decline in cognitive functioning and physical strength (HQSC 2019).
- In residential aged care facilities, care to ensure quality of life must not be constrained by a person's physical or mental decline. Frailty should not be a barrier to providing interventions with the goal of improving the older person's health and quality of life (Burn et al 2018).

Loss, Grief and Social Isolation

- Loss is a significant issue for people admitted to residential aged care facilities, with the loss of relationships, independence, privacy and the ability to make decisions about daily routines, personal care and meals, belongings and pets.
- Experienced as sometimes the most difficult transition they have had to make, older people moving into a residential aged care facility experience significant mental health and wellbeing issues, with loneliness being prevalent among this population. In practical terms, a person-centred model of care can support the person to engage in individualised meaningful activities. While maintaining relationships with family and friends is key (Chen et al 2022), healthcare providers need to recognise that those living in aged residential care can form new friendships and relationships if they provide opportunities for their social interaction with others (Siette et al 2021).
- The decision to live in an aged care facility may be the result of increasing frailty and is sometimes preceded by a hospital admission for complex medical issues that may also mask emotional issues. It may also be related to the inability of a carer to continue providing adequate levels of care in the community setting. Older people may experience distress related to the suddenness or unexpectedness of the need to move to residential aged care and the accompanying sense of loneliness that may ensue (Chen et al 2022).

Sexuality and Relationships

- Increasingly, the population of residential aged care facilities will reflect the diversity of the communities they serve.
- The issues faced by heterosexual residents are amplified for residents from the LGBTIQA+ community. Studies identify that LGBTIQA+ people fear ageing and admission to residential aged care. They are subject to ageist attitudes around sexuality and intimacy and additionally are at risk of experiencing stereotypical and negative attitudes towards their sexuality.
- There is also a high degree of invisibility in residential aged care for anything other than heterosexual relationships, leaving those not in heterosexual relationships feeling vulnerable, even when they have been comfortable and confident in their relationships outside this setting (Mahieu et al 2019).

Nutrition

- Nutritional needs are not always easily met for people living in residential aged care as residents will have a range of food practices prior to admission and have enjoyed, eaten and cooked for family and friends in diverse ways.

Scenario 27.2: Mabel

- Food choice and food service satisfaction affect nutritional status and, conversely, dissatisfaction with food has been linked with poor food intake and a negative impact on quality of life.
- Accommodating personal preferences is challenging when some residents will appreciate fresh food, some will enjoy unhealthy food, some will only consume a narrow range of foods and others will enjoy diversity (Govindaraju et al 2022).
- Individuals eating the same food and portions will still experience the taste and fulfilment from the food differently, so while some may find food too salty, for others the food will seem to lack enough salt.
- Person-centred care requires residents to have choice when it comes to the food and drink they consume by identifying their preferences, so the challenge is to cater to the diverse individual preferences of residents who all prefer food they are familiar with and have consumed before living in an aged care facility.

Attitudes

- For many students and registered nurses, the aged care environment is not considered an attractive option in nursing, making recruitment for aged care providers problematic. Historically, nurses working in aged residential care have arguably been valued less than those working in other settings, and this, along with the lack of a focus on gerontology and the lack of an aged care specialisation in nursing degrees, has contributed to recruitment and retention issues in residential aged care (Rababa et al 2021).
- The experience of nursing students in aged care needs to be developed and improved; however, nursing students have been shown to have a more positive attitude to ageing than other health professionals (Jester et al 2021). Nurses should be well prepared in physical care (such as wound dressings and more intimate tasks such as showering) and in mental health nursing skills, such as developing a good rapport with someone, mental health assessment in the context of older people, communication skills and building relationships with residents including those living with dementia.

Ageism, Sexuality and Intimacy

- Ageist attitudes lead to assumptions from nurses and families when addressing sexuality and intimacy for the older person in residential aged care. Nurses will be working with older adults who are diverse in cultural aspects, such as age, gender, sexual orientation, religious or spiritual beliefs, disability, occupation and socioeconomic status, ethnic origins or migrant experience. Nurses need to be self-aware and prepared to examine and challenge their own attitudes, values and beliefs related to the social and cultural determinants of mental health and wellbeing as part of the social ecological approach (Chapter 2).
- Older people continue to see sexuality and intimacy as important and contributing to their quality of life. Mabel's increasing anxiety, low mood and social isolation can be viewed in the context of cultural, sexual and spiritual identities (Chapter 2). Broaching these issues requires empathy and compassion (Laramie 2021).
- An older person may experience negative and discriminatory responses from team members, residents and family, related to their intimate relationships and other expressions of sexuality, resulting in the older person's sexuality and intimacy needs being constrained by the attitudes and expectations of how older people "should" be.
- An ethical decision-making process that focuses on the privacy, wellbeing and quality of life of the resident in relation to their needs around sexuality and intimacy is required to navigate the barriers that exist to sexuality and intimacy needs being met (Henrickson et al 2020).
- The first action point for staff would be to engage in training that is focused on increasing staff awareness of their own attitudes and how they can provide culturally safe care for LGBTIQA+ residents (Mahieu et al 2019).

- Establishing a therapeutic relationship and utilising tools for knowing the person and ensuring care is person-centred helps prevent the nurse from making assumptions about what interventions will support the person. For example, it might seem like an obvious choice for Mabel to be involved in animal therapy through an animal visiting program because of her affinity with her own dog and cats. Yet recent research from Wong and Breheny (2021) suggests that people in aged residential care may experience only "fleeting pleasure" from animal visits. Alternatively, the nurse can explore with Mabel whether she would enjoy her own pets visiting her in the care home and work with Betty to facilitate this by looking at options that mean she can go to her own home to spend time in her familiar environment with her pets.

Skills
Communication

- Highly developed communication skills are essential for nurses to effectively manage their healthcare team, work with residents, participate in the multidisciplinary team and interact with families.
- Ensuring privacy and the ability to have private space for interactions with family, friends and pets and to engage with children and animals in activities helps promote communication, prevent boredom and provides the opportunity to develop and engage in meaningful social relationships.

Individualised and Culturally Appropriate Care

- Getting to know a resident by reading their notes or a life story helps to grow an understanding of the person. A life story may contribute more detail in terms of person-centred care, such as preferences, their life journey, and family and social history; however, both provide a richer understanding of the person and improve attitudes towards residents (Dennerstein et al 2018).
- Some cultural aspects of Mabel have been identified related to her occupation, age, gender and sexuality. Consider how your responses to Mabel would differ if she was described as being aligned to a specific ethnic culture, migrant group, religious group or had a disability related to a mental illness or intellectual disability and what this helps you to understand about yourself.
- Assessing whether Mabel would benefit from additional support from an LGBTIQA+ community organisation needs to be determined in discussion with Mabel and Betty. While residents in aged residential care may not be sexually active, experiencing love and intimacy are important to wellbeing (Roelofs et al 2021)
- For residents, feeling cared for, having the opportunity to reminisce about treasured memories and having professional support so they can safely express their grief and loss, as well as being affirmed for their personal strengths, allows them to still set goals and engage in opportunities that continue to expand their life experiences. Digital reminiscence therapy for people with cognitive impairment has been shown to have some positive effects (Moon et al 2022).

Therapeutic Relationship

Mental health nursing knowledge, skills and attitudes will help develop the therapeutic relationship between nurses and older people in long-term care. Therapeutic use of self will enable the nurse to empathise with Mabel to establish an emotional connection and to demonstrate caring to support courageous conversations, such as those required during the process of advance care planning and the discussion of wills, executors, enduring power of attorney and the sale of assets such as a house.

In view of Mabel's increasing anxiety around her anticipation that her brother and his family will react in a negative way if she clarifies with them the nature

Continued

Scenario 27.2: Mabel

of her relationship with Betty, the nurse can provide support for Mabel to initiate conversations with her whānau about these sensitive issues.

The ability of the nurse to be self-aware, to recognise verbal and non-verbal cues and to be compassionate and caring will support Mabel to express her immediate and long-term anxieties and concerns in developing approaches to sensitive issues, such as her will, the enduring power of attorney, the tensions in her relationship with her brother and his family, and her fear of being stigmatised and discriminated against because of her sexuality.

Relationships with staff have been found to be significant in ameliorating loneliness in people in aged residential care; however, there are many time constraints for staff that impact on their ability to have meaningful conversations with those in their care. The presence of students in a care home is an opportunity for people living there to engage with a different generation, to support student learning and to feel helpful in doing so (Jester et al 2021).

Nursing Actions and Interventions
Assessment and Care Planning

- Because of the increasingly complex care needs of older people, nurses working in aged care need to exhibit a high level of nursing skills, especially in assessment, an understanding of the concept of frailty and the ability to recognise when residents are deteriorating and to respond effectively.
- Assessment, including physical health assessment, mental health assessment and cognitive assessment, is key to delivering quality care to residents and nurses working in residential aged care. Nurses need to call on an extensive range of assessment skills that support a person-centred approach to care within a multidisciplinary team.
- Residents need an initial assessment to inform a care plan and then, for a longer term care plan, ongoing assessment is essential because the health status of older people changes related to frailty. In addition, there will be times when a focused assessment and plan of care is required for a specific problem such as delirium, a pressure injury or an infection.
- There will also be a need for urgent assessment when the resident experiences a specific event such as a fall or health deterioration from another disease process that requires additional levels of care.

Observation and Monitoring

- Monitoring intake is important because malnutrition in older people will impact on wound healing and increase their susceptibility to infection, anaemia, fractures and pressure ulcers, hypotension and deterioration in mental acuity.

- Nutritional assessment tools (such as the MUST screening tool (Sharma et al 2022)) need to be utilised to assess and prevent complications.
- Dehydration will have a similar impact and additionally increase the risk of urinary tract infection or acute kidney injury (Health Quality Safety Commission 2019).

Relevant Treatment Modalities
Person-Centred Care

- A person-centred model of care allows those in residential aged care to exert as much choice over their lives as possible.
- Placing the resident at the centre of care facilitates their involvement in activities that contribute to them forming relationships with other residents and staff and attaining a sense of belonging.
- Promoting autonomy and independence for residents through choice (food, activities, clothing, personalising their own space with plants and personal effects) and facilitating the person's ability to be involved in decision-making in a wide range of aspects of daily life encourages a feeling of control.
- A holistic assessment provides the basis for deciding on relevant treatment modalities for Mabel, along with the involvement of the multidisciplinary team. While Mabel's GP will be an integral part of the multidisciplinary team in the review process, other health professionals have much to offer, as well as those nurses with specialties in gerontology and mental health of older people.

Pharmacological and Non-Pharmacological Interventions

- Non-pharmacological interventions, including diversional therapy, will be beneficial for Mabel's emotional and social wellbeing in the same way that non-pharmacological interventions for her pain and poor sleep will promote wellbeing.
- Because she is significantly concerned with the issues to do with her life partner and her family, it is likely that supporting Mabel to resolve some of her fears and concerns about this will help improve her mental health and emotional wellbeing.
- For the reasons explained in Scenario 27.1 and Chapter 21, minimising polypharmacy is an objective for those in aged residential care and careful prescribing is critical because of the decreasing resilience of the older person to the impact of multiple disease processes.
- While Mabel may be exhibiting symptoms of anxiety and a mild depressive disorder, in the short term this is best understood as an understandable response to life circumstances rather than within a diagnostic framework. While additional medication could be considered if non-pharmacological approaches are not effective, benefits need to be weighed up against the increased risk of falls, as well as other physical complications (Nguyen et al 2020).

CHAPTER SUMMARY

Every nurse will work with older people, regardless of the clinical setting. The two scenarios highlight the importance of you developing knowledge, skills and confidence in providing nursing care to older people and the importance of person-centred care when supporting people at this life stage. There are differences in providing care for older people independently in their own home, in contrast to older people with support in a care home, who require a higher level of care. Both contexts present challenges that need to be approached with consideration and respect for the person as an individual. Healthcare which embodies an interdisciplinary approach that brings a collaboration of skills together supports the best health outcome for the older person in both community and residential contexts. Working in a person-centred way with the older person will support identifying the goals of care based on what they want and need. Working with mental

health and wellbeing issues in older people requires reflection on our personal beliefs, attitudes and values related to ageing. This work can also help develop effective interpersonal communication as part of developing mental health nursing skills. Utilising reflection is also a strategy for developing self-confidence and to ensure that professional boundaries are considered and maintained within the therapeutic relationship.

Caring for the older adult involves recognition of changes in wellbeing, such as those associated with acute or gradual deterioration, the need for palliative care or individualised care during the last days of life. Developing the skills and knowledge to recognise that the older person in your care is experiencing changes in their health and wellbeing facilitates your ability to effectively intervene in a clinically competent and culturally safe way within your scope of practice.

REFERENCES

Abey-Nesbit, R., Van Doren, S., Ahn, S., Iheme, L., Peel, N., et al., 2021. Factors associated with caregiver distress among home care clients in New Zealand: Evidence based on data from interRAI Home Care assessment. Australas J Nurs, 41(2), 237–246.

Ahmedani, B.K., Peterson, E.L., Hu, Y., et al., 2017. Major physical health conditions and risk of suicide. Am J Prev Med, 5 (3), 308–315.

Akpan, A., Roberts, C., Bandeen-Roche, K., et al., 2018. Standard set of health outcome measures for older persons. BMC Geriatr, 18(1), 36.

Anderson, J.G., Eppes, A., O'Dwyer, S.T., 2019. "Like death is near": Expressions of suicidal and homicidal ideation in the blog posts of family caregivers of people with dementia. Behav Sci Basel, 9 (3), 22.

Aronson, L. 2020. Healthy aging across the stages of old age. Clin Geriatr Med, 36(4), 549–558.

Australian Bureau of Statistics (ABS), 2022. Australian demographic statistics, June 2022. Online. Available at: www.abs.gov.au/statistics/people/population/national-state-and-territory-population/latest-release#key-statistics

Australian Medicines Handbook, 2023. Australian Medicines Handbook. Online. Available at: amhonline.amh.net.au/

Barak, Y., Fortune, S., Hobbs, L., Cheung, G., Johari, N., & Zalsman, G. 2022. Strategies to prevent elderly suicide: A Delphi consensus study. Australas Psychiatry, 30(3), 298–302.

Bauer, M., Fetherstonhaugh, D., Winbolt, M., 2018. Perceived barriers and enablers to conducting nursing assessments in residential aged care facilities in Victoria, Australia. Aust J Adv Nurs, 36(2), 14–22.

Boyd, M., Calvert, C., Tatton, A., Wu, Z., Bloomfield, K., et al., 2021. Lonely in a crowd: Loneliness in New Zealand retirement village residents. Int Psychogeriatr, 33(5), 481–493.

Burn, R., Hubbard, R.E., Scrase, R.J., et al., 2018. A frailty index derived from a standardized comprehensive geriatric assessment predicts mortality and aged residential care admission. BMC Geriatr 18 (1), 319.

Chen, C., Shannon, K., Napier, S., & Neville S. 2022. Loneliness among older adults living in aged residential care in Aotearoa New Zealand and Australia: An integrative review. Nurs Prax Aotearoa NZ, 38(1), 5015.

Conejero, I., Olie, E., Courtet, P., et al., 2018. Suicide in older adults: Current perspectives. Clin Interv Aging 13, 691–699.

Da Rosa, M.I., Beck, W.O., Colonetti, T., et al., 2019. Association of vitamin D and vitamin B12 with cognitive impairment in elderly aged 80 years or older: A cross-sectional study. J Hum Nutr Diet, 32(4), 518–524.

Dennerstein, M., Bhar, S.S., Castles, J.J., 2018. A randomised controlled trial examining the impact of aged care residents' written life-stories on aged care staff knowledge and attitudes. Int Psychogeriatr, 30(9), 1291–1299.

Fässberg, M.M., Cheung, G., Canetto, S.S., et al., 2016. A systematic review of physical illness, functional disability, and suicidal behaviour among older adults. Aging Ment Health 20(2), 166–194.

Fullen, M.C., Granello, D.H., Richardson, V.E., et al., 2018. Using wellness and resilience to predict age perception in older adulthood. J Couns Dev, 96(4), 424–435.

Gale, C.R., Cooper, C., 2018. Attitudes to ageing and change in frailty status: the English longitudinal study of ageing. Gerontol, 64 (1), 58–66.

Gilbertson, E.L., Krishnasamy, R., Foote, C., et al., 2019. Burden of care and quality of life among caregivers for adults receiving maintenance dialysis: A systematic review. Am J Kidney Dis, 73(3), 332–343.

Govindaraju, T., Owen, A., & McCaffrey, T. 2022. Past, present and future influences of diet among older adults – A scoping review. Age Res Rev(77), 101600.

Harmer, B., Lee, S., Duong, T.V.H., & Saadabadi, A. 2022. Suicidal ideation. StatPearls. StatPearls Publishing.

Health Quality Safety Commission. 2019. Frailty Care Guides: Ngā Aratohu Maimoa Hauwarea. HQSC, Auckland.

Health Quality and Safety Commission, 2019. Understanding unconscious bias. Online. Available at: www.hqsc.govt.nz/our-work/system-safety/aotearoa-patient-safety-day/previous-patient-safety-week-campaigns/patient-safety-week-2019-understanding-bias-in-health-care/

Heerema, E. 2022. Overview of the Geriatric Depression Scale (GDS), content, scoring, and accuracy of the GDS. Online. Available at: www.verywellmind.com/geriatric-depression-scale-98621

Henrickson, M., Cook, C.M., & Schouten, V. 2022. Culture clash: Responses to sexual diversity in residential aged care. Cult, Health Sexual, 24(4), 548–563.

Henrickson, M., Cook, C., Schouten, V., McDonald, S. & Atefi, N. 2020. What counts as consent? Sexuality and ethical deliberation in residential aged care. Massey University, Auckland. Online. Available at: mro.massey.ac.nz/handle/10179/15720

Jamieson, H., Abey-Nesbit, R., Bergler, U., Keeling, S., Schluter, P., et al., 2019. Evaluating the influence of social factors on aged residential care admission in a national home care assessment database of older adults. J Am Med Dir Ass, 20(11), 1419–1424.

Jester, D, Hyer, K., Wenders, A., & Ross Andel, R. 2021. Attitudes toward aging of health professions students: Implications for geriatrics education, Gerontol Geriatr Ed, 42(4), 589–603.

Joling, K.J., O'Dwyer, S.T., Hertogh, C.M., et al., 2018. The occurrence and persistence of thoughts of suicide, self-harm and death in family caregivers of people with dementia: A longitudinal data analysis over 2 years. Int J Geriatr Psychiatry 33(2), 263–270.

Laramie, J. 2021. Issues in the lives of older lesbian, gay, bisexual, transgender, and/or queer women. Clin Geriatr Med, 37(4), 579–591.

Mahieu, L., Cavolo, A., & Gastmans, C. 2019. How do community-dwelling LGBT people perceive sexuality in residential aged care? A systematic literature review, Aging Ment Health, 23, 5, 529–540.

Matthews, T. Bryan, B.T. Danese, A. Meehan, A.J. Poulton, R. et al., 2022. Using a loneliness measure to screen for risk of mental health problems: A replication in two nationally representative cohorts. Int J Environ Res Pub Health, 19, 1641.

Moon Gautam, S., Park, K., Montayre, J., & Neville, S. 2022. Making meaning of digital reminiscence therapy on people with dementia: A pilot randomized controlled trial. BMC Geriatr 20, 166.

Nguyen, T., Wong, E., & Ciummo F.l., 2020. Polypharmacy in older adults: Practical applications alongside a patient case. J Nurse Pract, 16(3), 205–209.

Parr-Brownlie, L., Waters, D., Neville, S., Neha, T., Muramatsu, N. 2020. Aging in New Zealand: Ka haere ki te ao pakeketang. Gerontologist, 60(5), 812–820.

Rababa, M., Al-Dwaikat, T. & Almomani M. 2021 Assessing knowledge and ageist attitudes and behaviors toward older adults among undergraduate nursing students. Gerontol Geriatr Ed, 42(3), 347–362.

Roelofs, T., Luijkx, K., & Embregts, P. 2021. Love, intimacy and sexuality in residential dementia care: a client perspective. Clin Gerontol, 44(3), 288–299.

Ross, L.J. 2019, Improving health care student attitudes toward older adults through educational interventions: A systematic review. In: J.L. Howe & T.V. Caprio (eds), Clinical Education in Geriatrics: Innovative and Trusted Approaches Leading Workforce Transformation in Making Health Care More Age-Friendly. Routledge, Oxon.

Saunders, R., Buckman, J.E.J., Stott, J., Leibowitz, J., Aguirre, E., & NCEL Network. 2021. Older adults respond better to psychological therapy than working-age adults: Evidence from a large sample of mental health service attendees. J Affect Disord, 294, 85–93.

Schroyen, S., Adam, S., Marquet, M., et al., 2018. Communication of healthcare professionals: Is there ageism? Eur J Cancer Care Engl, 27(1), e12780.

Sharma, Y., Avina, P., Ross, E., Horwood, C., Hakendorf, P., et al., 2022. Validity of the malnutrition universal screening tool for evaluation of frailty status in older hospitalised patients. Gerontol Geriatr Med, 8, 23337214221107817.

Sheikh, J.I., Yesavage, J.A., 1986. Geriatric Depression Scale (GDS): Recent evidence and development of a shorter version. Clin Gerontol, 5 (1–2), 165–173.

Siette, J., Jorgensen, M., Nguyen, A. et al., 2021. A mixed-methods study evaluating the impact of an excursion-based social group on quality of life of older adults. BMC Geriatr 21, 356.

Solimando, L., Fasulo, M., Cavallero, S. et al., 2022. Suicide risk in caregivers of people with dementia: A systematic review and meta-analysis. Aging Clin Exp Res, 34, 2255–2260.

Toh, J., Zhang, H., Yang Y., Zhang, Z., & Wu, X. 2022. Prevalence and health outcomes of polypharmacy and hyperpolypharmacy in older adults with frailty: A systematic review and meta-analysis. Ageing Res Rev, 83, doi.org/10.1016/j.arr.2022.101811.

Wand, A; Verbeek, H., Hanon, C., Augustode Mendonça Lima, C. et al., 2021. Is suicide the end point of ageism and human rights violations? Am J Geriatr Psychiatry, 29(10), 1047–1052.

Wildisen, L., Moutzouri, E., Beglinger, S., et al., 2019. Subclinical thyroid dysfunction and depressive symptoms: Protocol for a systematic review and individual participant data meta-analysis of prospective cohort studies. BMJ Open 9 (7), e029716.

Wong, G., & Breheny, M. 2021. The experience of animal therapy in residential aged care in New Zealand: A narrative analysis. Ageing Soc, 41(11), 2641–2659.

28

Perinatal and Infant Mental Health

Julie Ferguson

KEY POINTS

- The perinatal period is a time of rapid physical and mental change.
- During the perinatal period, mental health disorders can surface for the first time.
- Changes during the perinatal period can trigger exacerbation of a pre-existing mental health problem.
- The perinatal period is an opportunity for mental health promotion, early identification, intervention and mental health treatment.
- A variety of therapies are regarded as very effective during this period, including cognitive behaviour therapy, interpersonal psychotherapy, couples therapy, parent–infant psychotherapy and attachment-focused psychotherapy.
- Antidepressants and mood stabilisers are major classes of medication used during the perinatal period.

KEY TERMS

- Antenatal
- Care planning
- Ethics
- Lithium
- Medication
- Parent–infant dynamic
- Perinatal
- Postnatal
- Prenatal

LEARNING OUTCOMES

The material in this chapter will assist you to:

- describe the incidence of perinatal depression and anxiety
- identify who is vulnerable within the population at risk of developing perinatal difficulties
- identify risk factors to look for when screening women during the perinatal period
- describe the care-planning process when working with women with severe mental illness during the perinatal period
- describe risk assessment for the parent–infant dynamic
- understand the risk–benefit dynamic process used when deciding on medication options for women during the perinatal period
- understand the importance of working within an interprofessional collaboration framework in the perinatal period
- understand the importance of including the partner when assessing and treating a woman experiencing perinatal difficulties
- examine some of the therapeutic modalities used when working with women and their families during the perinatal period.

> **LIVED EXPERIENCE COMMENT BY JARRAD HICKMOTT**
> Acknowledging trauma and the role it may play in someone's life, and the importance of interacting with this in a trauma-informed way that leads to a positive and safe outcome for those involved, is essential.

INTRODUCTION

The perinatal period is defined as the time from conception until the first year after birth (postnatal) (Highet et al 2023). It is a time of great change both physically and mentally for women and their partners. For most women and their families it is a time of great joy. As described by Scioli and Biller (2009), the arrival of a new baby is like a "dance of hope" – the new child bringing promise and possibility that can re-energise parents, allowing them to reinvest in themselves and their family.

While many women feel joy about their pregnancy, not all women experience pregnancy and parenthood as a positive time. The experience of pregnancy is different for each woman, and her relationships and psychosocial circumstances need to be considered. For some pregnant women, their previous experiences of miscarriage, traumatic delivery or the loss of a child can cause great distress. An unwanted or unplanned pregnancy, a teenage pregnancy, a difficult relationship with her partner (including domestic violence) or lack of support from her family can also cause increased stress. A history of trauma, sexual abuse or drug and alcohol dependence can also cause considerable impact during pregnancy and increase a person's vulnerability to developing a mental health concern during the perinatal period.

The perinatal period is also associated with increased risk of mental health conditions including antenatal depression/anxiety, the "baby blues", postpartum depression and postpartum psychosis (see Chapter 12 for more detailed information), or the exacerbation of pre-existing mental health problems including anxiety disorders, bipolar disorder, psychosis and schizophrenia (Austin et al 2017). In Australia, perinatal depression and anxiety affects one in five mothers (PwC Consulting Australia 2019). This means around 60,000 women will experience perinatal depression and anxiety annually (PwC Consulting

Australia 2019). Some women are at higher risk of developing mental health problems during the perinatal period (Highet et al 2023); see Box 28.1. For example, women who experience moderate or high risk maternal and fetal complications are at five to seven times greater risk of developing prenatal onset anxiety disorders (Fairbrother et al 2016).

The perinatal period offers a window of opportunity for intervention. Many women see more health professionals during pregnancy and early parenting than at other times in their lives. As suggested by Bowlby (1979), because relationships at this stage of the parent's development are in a state of change, it is a time when families will seek help and accept it. So, the perinatal period provides an important opportunity for intervention, not only for the parents but for the long-term outcomes of the child. Nurses from many areas of the healthcare system come into contact with a woman and her family during the perinatal period – including midwives, child and family nurses, mental health nurses (inpatient, community, primary care), primary health and general practice nurses, nurses in all generalist settings including the emergency department and, of course, specialist perinatal and infant mental health nurse specialists. All nurses and midwives, in all clinical settings, can make a significant difference to the mental health outcomes of women in the perinatal period, providing we are aware of the early warning signs and risk factors.

In this chapter we will explore two clinical scenarios to understand the complex presentations that can occur during the perinatal period and examine the nursing responses, medication treatments and psychological interventions that can help facilitate better mental health outcomes for women, their offspring and families.

BOX 28.1   Women at Increased Risk of Perinatal Mental Health Problems

- **Indigenous women** are more likely to experience mental health problems during the perinatal period. In a service in New South Wales up to 40% of First Nations women accessing the service had a history of mental health problems. In an area of New Zealand one in three Māori women accessing the service experienced at least one mental health problem. In Canada, Aboriginal women are twice as likely to be depressed as non-Aboriginal women.
- **Migrant women** are at higher risk of developing perinatal depression, with refugee women at heightened risk of psychological morbidity.
- **Women experiencing intimate partner violence** are four times more likely to develop depressive symptoms and 10 times more likely to experience anxiety than the general perinatal population.
- **Women who experience life stressors** such as family problems, violence or loss are at higher risk of developing mental health problems postpartum.
- **Women from lesbian, gay, bisexual, trans and/or intersex groups** are more likely to face discrimination and have their parenting abilities questioned.
- **Women who have experienced mental illness previously** and those with a family history of mental illness are more likely to be affected during the perinatal period.

Hartz & McGrath 2017; Highet et al 2023

EVIDENCE-BASED PRACTICE

Scenario 28.1: Jane

Jane was a 30-year-old woman referred to a perinatal and infant mental health service following her 6-week postnatal appointment with a child and family nurse. During that appointment, the nurse asked Jane to complete an Edinburgh Perinatal Depression Scale (EPDS) (Cox et al 1987). The EPDS is an important aspect of the routine 6-week postnatal check-up that child and family nurses conduct (and is also used during the antenatal period by midwives, which can alert them to the risk of the woman developing perinatal depression or anxiety). Jane scored 18, with a 2 on question 10 (which relates to self-harm), both of which indicate a risk of depression. The child and family nurse arranged a referral to the perinatal and infant mental health service.

This was Jane's first baby (a daughter) to her partner, Chris. It was not a planned pregnancy, but was wanted once the couple had become accustomed to the idea of being parents. Jane had previously had two terminations of pregnancy

to Chris due to her anxiety about not being ready to be a parent and worrying how she would cope with a child of her own.

Jane had a complex family history. She was the youngest child of five and her father died when she was only 3 years old. Jane's mother struggled to cope with the loss of her husband; she was diagnosed with bipolar disorder and hospitalised on many occasions throughout Jane's childhood. Over the past 30 years we have come to understand the important role that fathers play in assisting children to modulate intense affect (Fischer 2012). Jane was often without enough adult emotional input to help her make sense of her world. Jane experienced difficulties during adolescence; she dropped out of school early and often had challenging relationships with her peer group. Jane had, however, experienced a positive, supportive relationship with a counsellor during adolescence.

❗ RED FLAGS

- Jane somehow slipped through the net of psychosocial screening in the antenatal stage of pregnancy, despite her history ticking many boxes for risk factors that would indicate struggles in the perinatal period.
- An EPDS score above 13 can indicate possible depression, and any score on question 10 (self-harm) will require further risk assessment. Jane scored 2 on question 10, which asks, "The thought of harming myself has occurred to me …" Jane answered "Sometimes". When a person responds positively to this question, it is important to explore feelings of self-harm. In this circumstance Jane was able to describe her feelings of wanting to flee when her baby was distressed. She often felt overwhelmed, but not suicidal.

- Jane scoring 18 overall on the EPDS was a trigger for her being referred to a specialist mental health service, indicating that she was possibly experiencing depression and required further assessment.
- A complex family history, with her mother having a diagnosed mental health problem (bipolar disorder) and regular hospital admissions, and the death of her father in early childhood, is another red flag.
- Jane had two previous terminations of pregnancy due to ambivalence about becoming a parent.
- If Jane is struggling, how is her partner coping?

Knowledge
Psychosocial Screening During Pregnancy

- All pregnant women should be routinely screened for depression and anxiety symptoms using the EPDS scale, as well as screening for psychosocial risk factors as early as possible in the pregnancy.

- The EPDS has been used extensively throughout the perinatal period since its development in 1987 (Cox et al 1987).
- When a person scores above 13 on the EPDS, depression is indicated. When working with women from different cultural backgrounds, it is important to keep in mind that across studies of different cultural groups, this cut-off

Scenario 28.1: Jane

score varies considerably. This is because people from different cultural backgrounds report symptoms differently (Smith-Nielsen et al 2018).

○ Any score on question 10 (self-harm) requires further assessment. Most people use self-harm as a way of coping with overwhelming feelings, not because they are experiencing suicidal thoughts (Hungerford et al 2021).

Barriers to Screening

Barriers to screening include:

- a woman's experience of stigma (e.g. feeling worried about being judged)
- normalising emotional difficulties as being related to "hormones", or the situation
- preferring to manage feelings themselves
- not knowing what "normal" feelings during the perinatal period are (Highet et al 2023).

It is also important to consider the cultural background of a woman and her family, and their beliefs about pregnancy, birth and parenthood, as well as about mental health and illness. Consider, too, how experiences of women and families from marginalised groups may impact on help-seeking or increase the fear of being judged as an unfit parent, or of having children removed (Anderson & Tilton 2017).

Reflection

Jane delivered her baby in a large public hospital, so did have psychosocial screening early in her pregnancy. (Many private hospitals have not offered routine psychosocial screening until recently (Highet et al 2023).) So how did she slip through the net during the antenatal period? When Jane was contacted to make a follow-up appointment, she played down what was happening for her, saying she was okay, which is not uncommon for women who have had a difficult childhood and have learnt to cope on their own.

Safety, Risk Assessment and Protective Factors

- Risk factors, which are described as vulnerabilities, are adverse factors that are present in a woman's life (Jomeen et al 2017). The presence of risk factors may be used to highlight the possibility of a woman developing postnatal depression.
- Research has also explored the impact of protective factors that influence an individual's adaptation to life stressors. Evidence has suggested that there is an association between resilience and avoidance of postnatal depression (Jomeen et al 2017). This raises questions about the possibility of treatment strategies for supporting women to increase their resilience during the perinatal period.

Assessing Risk to the Baby

When assessing the level of risk of suicide for a woman in the postnatal period, it is also important to assess any risk to her baby (Highet et al 2023).

- The mother–infant interaction can be a valuable aspect of the risk assessment. If difficulties in the interaction are observed and if the woman has a significant mental health condition, further assessment will be required (Highet et al 2023).
- Sometimes the risk of harm to the infant is related to the mother's suicide risk, but this is not always the case, and needs to be further assessed.
- This assessment would include psychosocial risk factors (see Box 28.2), infant factors, infant behaviours of concern (observed or reported), relationship factors (observed or reported), maternal factors and protective factors (Highet et al 2023).
- If there is a risk to the baby, then the care planning will need to include other important supports from within the family or close friends, and referral to the relevant child protection agency may be necessary.

- A safety plan is essential to ensure that both the mother and the baby are kept safe during this difficult time. Jane indicated no immediate risk to her baby during the assessment.

Perinatal Mental Health in Partners

- The transition to parenthood occurs for both the mother and her partner. The change in relationship from a couple to a trio can be a difficult transition.
- Whenever a woman is diagnosed with a perinatal mental health disorder, it is important to assess how her partner is coping. Research in Australia has shown that one in 10 men experience paternal depression between the first trimester of pregnancy and 1 year postpartum, and one in six fathers experience anxiety during the perinatal period (Highet et al 2023). Studies have shown that 50 per cent of fathers are unaware that they can experience depression and anxiety (Beyond Blue 2023). This lack of awareness means that this group is less likely to reach out to appropriate support networks or be diagnosed. Other risk factors for non-birthing parents can include financial stress, particularly as they may be the main income earner following the birth of a child, as well as attitudes towards perinatal depression and anxiety and fear of being seen as a "failure" if they are not coping with parenting as they expected (Beyond Blue 2023).
- Untreated depression and anxiety in fathers during the perinatal period can have long-term effects on their relationships with their children, as well as their partners (Scarff 2019).
- There is limited research (Darwin & Greenfield 2019) available for same-sex partners; suffice to say that all partners need to be included in the same way a father would be included in the assessment.

Treatment Modalities and Considerations

Over the past 30 years we have gained a greater understanding of intergenerational trauma. Fallon and Brabender (2012) highlighted the importance of a woman working through her trauma history to develop a coherent narrative of her own childhood experiences, such that it allows her to go on to provide care for her baby and children. Highet and colleagues (2023) highlight that women with a history of trauma experience higher incidents of psychological distress during the perinatal period.

Treatment in the perinatal period is usually similar to that used to treat any depressive episode or significant anxiety problem, including cognitive behaviour therapy (CBT), interpersonal therapy and dialectical behaviour therapy, and are associated with good outcomes (Stephens et al 2016). In addition, there are a few treatments specific to the perinatal period.

Parent–Infant Psychotherapy

There are many forms of parent–infant therapy available. When there has been relational trauma in the early relationship due to mental health problems such as depression, this repair work helps to develop a secure relationship between the mother, partner and their child. The therapy addresses a range of conscious and unconscious factors that shape the individual parent's and infant's specific modes of being with each other, which focuses on the attachment relationship (Baradon & Joyce 2016).

Parenting Training Programs

A wide range of parenting programs are available. These are often run in the community by specialist parenting support services, such as Tresillian and Karitane, as well as other non-government services. Organisations and programs such as Circle of Security (Powel et al 2016) and Triple-P (Sanders & Mazzucchelli 2018) focus on supporting positive parenting strategies.

Couples Therapy

The transition from couple to trio can be a challenging time for parents. Couples therapy can provide a valuable space to process this change.

Continued

EVIDENCE-BASED PRACTICE—cont'd

Scenario 28.1: Jane

Medication During Pregnancy and Breastfeeding

There is a great deal of misinformation circulating about antidepressant medication use during the perinatal period. It is vital for clinicians to be well informed about the research on antidepressant use during this period to accurately convey and translate the latest findings to women and their families (Grigoriadis & Peer 2019). Sudden discontinuation of pharmacological treatments leads to higher risk for relapse.

- When working with mothers who are pregnant or breastfeeding, it is important to weigh up the risks and benefits of medication (Kendall-Tackett 2017). A mother who is experiencing moderate to severe depression or anxiety would most likely benefit from continuing antidepressant medication.
- It is important to consider the types of symptoms she is experiencing (or experiences when she is unwell), such as the symptoms of depression and her attitude towards taking medication.
- Women often worry about becoming addicted to medication or that the antidepressant medication could have a negative effect on their fetus or infant (Kendall-Tackett 2017). Studies have shown that many women cease antidepressant medication upon becoming pregnant due to concerns about fetal wellbeing (Grigoriadis & Peer 2019).
- Clinicians need to discuss with women the risk of ceasing antidepressant medication abruptly and that, if a medication is ceased, this needs to be done gradually with advice from a mental health professional (Highet et al 2023). Depression and other psychiatric disorders are not benign – there are consequences for the baby, mother and family – so women with psychiatric illness must be given the same consideration and be treated with the same seriousness as would a woman with any other medical disease during pregnancy. A thorough review of all the potential risks with the mother and her family is paramount, in order for a mutual decision to be reached and to prioritise the mother's health (Grigoriadis & Peer 2019).
- For many women with moderate to severe anxiety or depressive disorders, the first-line treatment is likely to be pharmacological, with psychological treatments introduced once medications have become effective (Highet et al 2023). They suggest using a selective serotonin reuptake inhibitor (SSRI) as first-line treatment for depression and/or anxiety in pregnant women. The risk of transmitting SSRIs and tricyclic antidepressants through breastmilk is very low; the rate of transmission of larger molecule medication through the alveolar cells (milk ducts) reduces after the first three days postpartum when the milk matures (Hale 2019).
- In most instances, the most important determinant of drug penetration into milk is the mother's plasma level. This means that being aware of peak plasma levels (when the amount of medication in the plasma is at its highest) can help to reduce the infant ingesting the small amounts of medication found in breastmilk (Kendall-Tackett 2017).

Attitudes

- Sometimes nurses struggle to understand a woman's choice to have a baby when she has a mental illness. Nurses need to consider our attitudes towards the decisions that clients make and any stereotypes or biases we may hold about this. Using clinical supervision to discuss these issues is important.
- Many women, including those with a history of mental illness, do not want to take medication while pregnant or breastfeeding. It is important to provide the woman with as much information as she needs to make an informed decision and, unless she or her infant is at great risk (in which case she may be treated under a Mental Health Act), decisions about medication are the woman's choice.

Skills

- The therapeutic relationship is the most important aspect of any treatment success.
- Use the Mental State Examination (MSE) to inform practice (see Chapter 9). This can be a helpful way to formulate care planning and facilitate communication between health professionals using shared language.
- Safety for all. In the postnatal period, as at every time in a woman's life, we need to consider the woman in context, understanding that the baby is both a protective factor and a risk factor, as well as understanding how mental health symptoms may affect a woman's behaviour (including impulsivity). Asking directly, with an empathic tone, is essential. For example: "Are you worried that you are feeling so bad that you might hurt the baby?"
- A family approach is essential to all aspects of care for women in the perinatal period. Including non-birthing parents and extended family/kin in the care planning process is vital to ensure the best outcomes for the woman, her baby and her family/kin.
- Psychoeducation is a valuable tool, particularly concerning issues such as medication use during pregnancy and breastfeeding. This includes not suddenly ceasing medication during pregnancy due to the potential relapse of previous symptoms, or withdrawal symptoms.
- Interprofessional collaboration is crucial. During the perinatal period women often see more health professionals than at any other time in their life. Taking a collaborative approach means that all professionals involved in the woman's care are working together to ensure the best possible outcomes (Psaila & Schmied 2017).
- Accessing ongoing support. Nurses can be pivotal in helping women and their families to access suitable treatment and ongoing support. One of the most helpful things nurses can do is to support mothers to get help from longer term support systems. With modern technology, this can mean accessing mothers' support groups online. Breastfeeding support, sleep and settling support as well as many other resources are often available 24 hours a day, as well as providing information for non-birthing parents.

BOX 28.2 Psychosocial Risk Factors

- Unresolved family-of-origin issues
- History of physical/sexual/emotional abuse, family violence or childhood neglect
- Past pregnancy loss or excess pregnancy concern
- Unplanned or unwanted pregnancy
- Traumatic past pregnancy/delivery
- Mother unable to touch the baby on the day of the birth

- Mother has sole responsibility for the baby's care during the first week of life
- No one else involved in the baby's care
- Availability of emotional/social/practical support
- Amount of time the mother spends away from the baby
- Baby unwell or excessive concern about the baby's wellbeing

EVIDENCE-BASED PRACTICE

Scenario 28.2: Helen

Helen was a 33-year-old woman referred to a perinatal infant mental health service by her general practitioner (GP) for preconception planning. Helen had been diagnosed with bipolar disorder following the birth of her first child (a son) three years previously. He had arrived at 30 weeks' gestation via emergency caesarean delivery and required admission to the neonatal intensive care unit (NICU) for some weeks. Helen felt traumatised by the event and became manic while she was expressing milk constantly to feed him. Her level of exhaustion as well as changing hormone levels contributed to the deterioration of Helen's mental state. When the baby was discharged from the NICU, Helen required a mental health hospital admission. After a trial of several different medications, Helen's mood was stabilised on lithium carbonate (a mood stabiliser) and olanzapine (an antipsychotic). She kept taking the medications after discharge and has remained well. Helen is anxious about having another child, but she and her husband, Joe, always planned to have two children.

As part of her preconception planning, Helen's psychiatrist referred her to "Mother Safe" for consultation, providing a comprehensive history so the consultant was fully informed. It was unclear from Helen's previous history if she had developed bipolar disorder during the pregnancy, which may have contributed to the early and traumatic arrival of her son. Helen did experience psychotic phenomena during the manic episode and had a re-emergence of psychotic symptoms each time olanzapine was ceased. As part of her preconception plan, Helen decided she would continue with lithium and olanzapine during her second pregnancy because she feared a relapse. She chose to be under the care of an obstetrician who specialised in in-utero scan technology. This was important for Helen, who wanted to ensure there were no fetal abnormalities due to taking lithium. And because breastfeeding her first baby had been a traumatic experience for Helen, she decided not to breastfeed with her second baby. Therefore, continuing lithium after delivery did not pose a concern.

Knowledge
Traumatic and Preterm Births
- Traumatic birthing experiences can have lasting effects, not just on the woman but on her partner as well (Thomson et al 2017) and can lead to post-traumatic stress disorder.
- Research by Thomson and colleagues (2017) has highlighted the importance of having support systems in place and good care planning to reduce the risk of further birthing trauma for women.

Helen's first delivery was certainly traumatic – she felt she had no control over the situation and did not feel enough was explained to her about the delivery or risks. She also felt her husband was not included in the decision-making process. This increased her anxiety around the birth of her second baby. In consultation with her obstetrician, a planned caesarean was arranged. Helen felt she was listened to by her health professionals and, because they were working as a team around her (all the clinicians involved in her care worked in different settings but communicated regularly through teleconferencing and written communication), Helen experienced the arrival of her second baby very differently.

- A premature birth is one that occurs before 37 weeks' gestation.
- There are many aspects of infant care in a NICU that can be distressing for parents, such as the potential life threatening situation the family faces, the intrusive tests and procedures that occur, the noise of different machines and witnessing the death of other babies undergoing treatment (Feeley 2017).
- Preterm infants can require hospitalisation for weeks or months, which can lead to mothers experiencing significant separation anxiety from their baby. Helen certainly experienced this with her son; her way of staying connected to him was by producing breastmilk for him. Expressing and

breastfeeding can be difficult for some women, even under the best of circumstances. Helen became obsessed with attempting to produce enough milk and so was awake most of the night trying to express, which contributed to the deterioration in her mental state. When Helen and her son were admitted to a mental health unit, she stopped trying to breast-feed so she could start taking lithium. Helen felt relieved but guilty for not breastfeeding her son.

- In many states in Australia there are no specialist mother–baby units in the public sector, which causes further trauma for mothers requiring a mental health admission postnatally. Helen had private health insurance so was able to be admitted to a specialist mother–baby unit.

> ### ! RED FLAGS
>
> Given Helen's history, nurses who see her during the perinatal period should be aware of her:
> - diagnosis of bipolar disorder during pregnancy, and increased risk of relapse during the perinatal period
> - concerns around medication management during pregnancy and breastfeeding, and worries about potential impact on the fetus
> - previous traumatic delivery of a baby
> - concerns about previous poor communication around her care, in relation to her own understanding, with her partner and between team members. This highlights the need for care planning, including the partner and extended family, as well as interprofessional collaboration to improve outcomes for Helen.

Preconception Planning for Women Diagnosed With Mental Illness
- Preconception planning should begin as soon as a woman of childbearing age is diagnosed with a mental illness (Highet et al 2023). Preconception planning should include discussion of pharmacological treatments to be used during/after the birth, which will involve decision making by the woman about whether she will breastfeed (e.g. if it is planned that lithium be used postnatally) (Highet et al 2023).
- Pregnancy can be a complex process for any woman, with changes in hormonal levels, increased inflammation processes and fluctuations in biorhythms, all of which can cause relapse of a pre-existing mental illness (Kaplan & Erol-Coskun 2019).
- Preconception planning is particularly important for women diagnosed with schizophrenia, bipolar disorder and/or depression, as relapse is common (particularly when medication is ceased) and associated with a range of adverse outcomes (Betcher et al 2019). For example, untreated bipolar disorder has been linked with pregnancy complications such as preterm birth, low birthweight and Apgar scores, induced labour and caesarean section delivery (Sutter-Dallay & Gressier 2019).
- The management of pregnant women with mental illness can be complex for both obstetric and mental health services, suggesting that specific considerations be attended to and monitoring systems followed during the perinatal period. Case conferences may be required depending on the complexity of the presentation and number of services involved (Highet et al 2023).
- There are important aspects to consider in preconception planning, such as the woman's identity and cultural background, health and mental health literacy, partner/family/kinship support, the woman's living/social conditions

Continued

Scenario 28.2: Helen

and the complex issues related to medication use during pregnancy and breastfeeding (Highet et al 2023).

Medication Management During Pregnancy and Breastfeeding

- A clinician should always weigh up the possible risk of the medication against the consequences of untreated maternal psychiatric illness. A discussion regarding those issues, as well as the medical and personal priorities, should be held between the clinician and woman before deciding to start, continue or cease the pharmacotherapy (Kaplan & Erol-Coskun 2019).
- When women are on medication during pregnancy it is essential that there is interprofessional collaboration (Psaila & Schmied 2017).
- Regarding antipsychotic medication during pregnancy, it is recommended that "women who need to take an antipsychotic during pregnancy continue the antipsychotic that has been most effective for symptom remission" (Betcher et al 2019, p. 17). Olanzapine, for example, is a second-generation antipsychotic medication that has not been associated with adverse pregnancy or infant outcomes (Betcher et al 2019). However, given the increased risk of metabolic disorders associated with second-generation antipsychotics (Hirsch et al 2017), this will need to be monitored closely during pregnancy. Monitoring the mother's blood sugar levels is a routine aspect of antenatal care.
- Postpartum psychosis can be the first episode of a mental health condition for many women. Family history of severe mental illness, including bipolar disorder or psychosis, is a risk factor (Highet et al 2023).
- In recent studies, relapse of bipolar disorder was twice as likely for women who have ceased mood stabilisation medication during the perinatal period (Highet et al 2023).
- Women with schizophrenia who stop taking antipsychotic medication experience a 53% increased risk of relapse compared with a 16% relapse rate for women who continue medication (Betcher et al 2019).

Anticonvulsant/Mood Stabilising Medication

- The prescription of valproates is contraindicated during the first trimester of pregnancy. The teratogenic risk is significant, with a global malformation rate around 10% (four times greater than with other antiepileptic drugs), mainly of the central nervous system (Sutter-Dallay & Gressier 2019). In cases of exposure in early pregnancy, some authors consider that the risk of teratogenesis outweighs that of mood decompensation and advocate rapid cessation.
- Highet and colleagues (2023) highlight the importance of monitoring lithium levels during pregnancy because lithium requirements change throughout the pregnancy. The increase in the distribution volume and in renal excretion rates among pregnant women leads to an increase of doses during pregnancy in order to maintain blood levels as low as possible within therapeutic range. It is recommended that serum lithium levels are monitored every 4 weeks up to 36 weeks' gestation and then weekly until birth (Sutter-Dallay & Gressier 2019).
- Thyroid and renal function should be monitored during each trimester, and high-resolution ultrasound and Doppler flow studies for early cardiac assessment should be attended at 16 weeks' gestation due to possible malformation caused by lithium use in pregnancy. Paediatricians should carefully monitor babies during the first 48 hours for fetal goitre, hypotonia, bradycardia, arrhythmias, systolic murmur, hypothermia, cyanosis, tachypnoea and poor sucking reflex (Sutter-Dallay & Gressier 2019).
- A morphology scan at 20 weeks' gestation, with particular attention to a fetal echocardiogram, should be performed (Snellen & Malhi 2014).
- If lithium is prescribed to a pregnant woman, ensure that maternal blood levels are closely monitored and that there is specialist psychiatric consultation.

Lithium levels should be monitored carefully and individual doses adjusted prior to and after delivery (Highet et al 2023).
- It is recommended that lithium not be used while breastfeeding due to the transmission through breastmilk causing infant toxicity. Testing of cord or infant blood could inform decision-making, although exposure across the placenta would already have occurred (Highet et al 2023).

Ethical Considerations and Medication During Pregnancy

There are many ethical considerations when weighing up the risks and benefits of taking medication during pregnancy, including:
- potential risk to the developing fetus exposed to medication in utero
- increased risk of the mother's mental state deterioration without medication, which can also cause risk to the fetus.

Referral to a specialist service such as Mother Safe can provide the opportunity for a woman to weigh up the risks and benefits of continuing medication during pregnancy.

Care Planning for Delivery and Postnatal Care

- Care planning has been highlighted as one of the most important aspects of caring for women with potential mental health problems during the perinatal period (Highet et al 2023).
- All clinicians involved in a woman's care should be involved in the care planning process. This includes her GP, a general practice nurse, an obstetrician, midwives (in the antenatal clinic, delivery suit and in the postnatal ward or visiting service), child and family nurses and other practitioners. In some cases, this may involve the hospital's consultation liaison psychiatry team, including a consultation liaison mental health nurse or an acute mental health team and a perinatal and infant mental health nurse, if one is available.
- Care planning also provides the woman with an opportunity to discuss any worries about the forthcoming delivery or parenting. Given Helen's experiences with a preterm delivery and trauma surrounding the delivery, having a space to process this can be very helpful.
- Including the woman's partner/identified support(s) and extended family/kin in the care planning process is essential for positive outcomes.
- It is important that all information about a woman's health care is communicated in writing to all the health professionals involved. Regular letters to her GP, psychiatrist and obstetrician are necessary to keep everyone informed of her progress and any concerns.

Attitudes

- The role of nurses and midwives is to provide the best possible care to women by ensuring they are as informed as possible about their choices and treatment options in relation to their mental health during the perinatal period.
- All nurses and midwives need to reflect on whether they hold judgemental attitudes and biases about woman who experience mental illness (e.g. bipolar disorder or schizophrenia) choosing to have a baby. Clinical supervision is the appropriate place to consider this.

Nursing Actions and Interventions

- Work with the woman, her partner/chosen support(s) and other members of the multidisciplinary team to avoid a hospital admission, but plan for that outcome should it be required.
- Monitor the woman's mental state by using the MSE and tools such as the EPDS and provide an update to all members of the treating team.
- Providing the team with a written care plan developed in collaboration with the woman and her partner for delivery and immediate aftercare is a high

EVIDENCE-BASED PRACTICE—cont'd

Scenario 28.2: Helen

priority. This would include a brief history of the mother's mental health experiences, medication regimen and preferences.

• Ensure the mother can recommence her medication at the pre-pregnancy dose as soon as possible after the delivery.
• Alert midwives and nursing staff in the maternity unit of the need to monitor the baby for any withdrawal from medication side effects. Including information about the mother's choice not to breastfeed is essential so she is not prompted by staff and feels pressure to do this, particularly when taking medication such as lithium.
• Helping women to develop anxiety management skills and ensuring adequate rest is also very important to reduce the risk of relapse.
• Working with the mother to identify who could take care of the baby overnight for the first few weeks and support her getting enough sleep will reduce the risk of relapse.
• Including a woman's partner/baby's father/identified support(s) is also vital to ensure the woman has adequate post-delivery support. In Helen's case, helping Joe to understand how he could best support Helen after the delivery, as well as highlighting the early warning signs of deterioration in her mental state, would increase his confidence in his ability to help, reduce the chance of relapse and

increase the likelihood of more rapid intervention if relapse or deterioration did occur.

• A psychiatric review in the first few days after delivery can be beneficial. Many hospitals have consultation liaison psychiatry services that provide this and nurses should put in a request if none has been made.
• The mother should be closely monitored for the first few months postnatally, with weekly reviews to ensure she receives timely treatment if her mental state does deteriorate.

Treatment Modalities

Treatment could include a range of therapeutic interventions, such as CBT, interpersonal therapy, dialectical behaviour therapy, parent–infant psychotherapy, couples therapy and parenting training programs as described previously. The most important aspect of care is monitoring the mother's mental state and ensuring her safety with her baby and children – establishing and maintaining a trusting therapeutic relationship is central to this.

In this situation, Helen did not require another mental health hospital admission due to careful preconception planning, care planning and medication management.

CHAPTER SUMMARY

This chapter has considered the importance of early intervention and treatment in the perinatal period. Care planning that includes the woman and her partner/the father/identified supports, the baby, other children and extended family is essential to achieving positive outcomes.

Medication management and good care planning, including interprofessional collaboration, is necessary to improve the outcomes for women and their families.

Slade (2008) suggested that for parents to hold their children in mind, we as health professionals need to hold the parents in mind. This can be for quite a long time.

USEFUL WEBSITES

Beyond Blue: healthyfamilies.beyondblue.org.au/
Centre of Perinatal Excellence (COPE): www.cope.org.au/
Dadvice (website with valuable information for fathers): healthyfamilies.
   beyondblue.org.au/pregnancy-and-new-parents/dadvice-for-new-dads
Embrace – Multicultural Mental Health (Australia): embracementalhealth.org.au/
Gidget Foundation: gidgetfoundation.org.au/
Good Beginnings: www.savethechildren.org.au/
Karitane: karitane.com.au/
Moodgym: www.moodgym.com.au/
Mothersafe: www.seslhd.health.nsw.gov.au/royal-hospital-for-women/services-
   clinics/directory/mothersafe
Parent-Infant Research Institute (PIRI): www.piri.org.au/
Post and Antenatal Depression Association (PANDA): www.panda.org.au/
Tresillian: www.tresillian.org.au/

REFERENCES

Anderson, P., & Tilton, E., 2017. Bringing Them Home 20 years on: An action plan for healing. The Healing Foundation. Online. Available at: healingfoundation.org.au/app/uploads/2017/05/Bringing-Them-Home-20-years-on-FINAL-SCREEN-1.pdf

Austin M-P, Highet N. & the Expert Working Group, 2017. Mental Health Care in the Perinatal Period: Australian Clinical Practice Guideline. Centre of Perinatal Excellence, Melbourne.
Baradon, T., Joyce, A., 2016. The theory of psychoanalytic parent-infant psychotherapy. In: Baradon, T., Biseo, M., Broughton, C., et al. (eds). The Practice of Psychoanalytic Parent-Infant Psychotherapy: Claiming the Baby. Routledge, London.
Betcher, H.K., Montiel, C., Clark, C.T., 2019. Use of antipsychotic drugs during pregnancy. Curr Treat Opin Psychiatry 6(1), 17–31.
Beyond Blue, 2023. New Fathers. Online. Available at: www.beyondblue.org.au/who-does-it-affect/men/what-causes-anxiety-and-depression-in-men/new-fathers
Bowlby, J., 1979. The Making and Breaking of Affectional Bonds. Routledge, London.
Cox, J.L., Holden, J.M., Sagovsky, R., 1987. Detection of postnatal depression. Development of a 10 item Edinburgh Postnatal Depression Scale. Br J Psychiatry, 150, 782–786.
Darwin, Z., & Greenfield, M., 2019. Mothers and others: The invisibility of LGBTQ people in reproductive and infant psychology, J Reprod Infant Psychol, 37(4), 341–343.
Fairbrother, N. Janssen, P., Anthony M.M et al., 2016. Perinatal anxiety disorder prevalence and incidence. J Affect Disord 200, 148–155
Fallon, A.E., Brabender, V.M., 2012. A secure connection, the tethering of attachment and good-enough maternal care. In: Akhtar, S. (ed.), The Mother

and Her Child, Clinical Aspects of Attachment, Separation, and Loss. Rowman & Littlefield, Maryland.

Feeley, N., 2017. Giving birth earlier than expected: Mothers whose new-born requires neonatal intensive care. In: Thomas, G., Schmied, V. (eds), Psychosocial Resilience and Risk in the Perinatal Period: Implications and Guidance for Professionals. Routledge, London.

Fischer, N., 2012. Mother–infant attachment: The demystification of an enigma. In: Akhtar, S. (ed.), The Mother and Her Child, Clinical Aspects of Attachment, Separation, and Loss. The Rowman & Littlefield Publishing Group, Maryland.

Grigoriadis, S. & Peer, M. 2019. Antidepressants in pregnancy. In: F. Uguz, L. Orolini (eds), Perinatal Psychopharmacology. Springer Nature, Switzerland.

Hale, T.W., 2019. Hale's Medications and Mothers' Milk. Springer, New York.

Hartz, D., McGrath, L., 2017. Working with Indigenous families. In: Thomas, G., Schmied, V. (eds), Psychosocial Resilience and Risk in the Perinatal Period: Implications and Guidance for Professionals. Routledge, London.

Highet, N. & the Expert Working Group and Expert Subcommittees, 2023. Mental Health Care in the Perinatal Period: Australian Clinical Practice Guideline 2023 Revision. Centre of Perinatal Excellence, Melbourne.

Hirsch, L., Yang, J., Bresee, L., et al., 2017. Second-generation antipsychotics and metabolic side effects: A systematic review of population-based studies. Drug Saf, 40(9), 771–781.

Hungerford, C., Hodgson, D., Clancy, R., et al., 2021. Mental Health Care: An Introduction for Health Professionals in Australia, 3rd ed. Wiley, Brisbane.

Jomeen, J., Fleming, S.E., Martin, C.R., 2017. Women with a diagnosed mental health problem. In: Thomas, G., Schmied, V. (eds), Psychosocial Resilience and Risk in the Perinatal Period: Implications and Guidance for Professionals. Routledge, London.

Kaplan, Y.C. & Erol-Coskun, 2019. Safety parameters and risk categories used for psychotropic drugs on pregnancy and lactation. In: F. Uguz, L. Orolini (eds), Perinatal Psychopharmacology. Springer Nature, Switzerland.

Kendall-Tackett, K.A., 2017. Depression in New Mothers: Causes, Consequences and Treatment Alternatives. Routledge, London.

Powel, B., Cooper, G., Hoffman, K., et al., 2016. The Circle of Security Intervention: Enhancing Attachment in Early Parent–Child Relationships. The Guilford Press, New York.

Psaila, K., Schmied, V., 2017. Interprofessional collaboration: A crucial component of support for women and families in the perinatal period. In: Thomas, G., Schmied, V. (eds), Psychosocial Resilience and Risk in the Perinatal Period: Implications and Guidance for Professionals. Routledge, London.

PwC Consulting Australia, 2019. The cost of perinatal depression and anxiety in Australia. Gidget Foundation Australia, Sydney.

Sanders, M.R., Mazzucchelli, T.G., 2018. The Power of Positive Parenting: Transforming the Lives of Children, Parents and Communities Using the Triple P System. Oxford University Press, New York.

Scarff, J.R., 2019. Postpartum depression in men. Innov Clin Neurosci, Vol 1; 16(5–6), 11–14.

Scioli, A., Biller, H.B., 2009. Hope in the Age of Anxiety. Oxford University Press, New York.

Slade, A., 2008. Working with parents in child psychotherapy: engaging the reflective function. In: Busch, F.N. (ed.), Mentalization Theoretical Considerations, Research Findings, and Clinical Implications. The Analytic Press, Taylor & Francis Group, New York.

Smith-Nielsen, J., Matthey, S., Lange, T., et al., 2018. Validation of the Edinburgh Postnatal Depression Scale against both DSM-5 and ICD-10 diagnostic criteria for depression. BMC Psychiatry 18, 393.

Snellen, M., Malhi, G.S. 2014. Bipolar Disorder, Psychopharmacology, and Pregnancy. In: Galbally, M., Snellen, M., Lewis, A. (eds), Psychopharmacology and Pregnancy. Springer, Berlin, Heidelberg.

Stephens, S., Ford, E., Paudyal, P., et al., 2016. Effectiveness of psychological interventions for postnatal depression in primary care: A meta-analysis. Ann Fam Med, 14(5), 463–472.

Sutter-Dallay, A. & Gressier, F., 2019. Mood stabilizers in pregnancy. In: F. Uguz & L. Orolini (eds), Perinatal Psychopharmacology, Springer Nature, Switzerland.

Thomson, G., Beck, C., Ayers, S., 2017. The ripple effects of a traumatic birth, risk, impact and implications for practice. In: Thomas, G., Schmied, V. (eds), Psychosocial Resilience and Risk in the Perinatal Period: Implications and Guidance for Professionals. Routledge, London.

29

Forensic Mental Health Nursing

Tessa Maguire and Brian McKenna

KEY POINTS

- The knowledge, skills and attitudes required to work with forensic mental health consumers have been identified.
- Forensic mental health consumers are a heterogeneous group of people with a complex range of needs including offence-related issues.
- Risk assessment, treatment and intervention continue to develop and the associated skills are used by nurses to ensure the safety of all (consumers, staff and the general public).
- Forensic mental health nurses remain focused on recovery-oriented care in partnership with consumers, carers, families and supporters.

KEY TERMS

Coexisting conditions
Criminality and mental illness
Housing and homelessness

Law and prison
Recovery-oriented care
Risk assessment and intervention

Self-awareness
Social justice

LEARNING OUTCOMES

The material in this chapter will assist you to:
- demonstrate awareness of the lived experience and needs of forensic mental health consumers
- identify specific nursing interventions for forensic mental health consumers

- discuss the skills, knowledge and attitudes that are central to forensic mental health nursing
- utilise the structured clinical judgement approach to risk assessment, treatment and intervention.

LIVED EXPERIENCE COMMENT BY JARRAD HICKMOTT
It can be very easy to label someone as "aggressive" without considering context. The authors of this chapter have carefully discussed aggression and violence, acknowledging that the consumer may be experiencing stressful factors that they find distressing, and which result in such behaviour. Stigma, especially the twin contributors of criminality and mental ill health, has flow-on effects and can impact on a person's identity and self-esteem.

INTRODUCTION

For many reasons, people experiencing mental illness are over-represented in the criminal justice system. Forensic mental health services have developed in Australia and Aotearoa New Zealand to provide containment, assessment and treatment for forensic mental health consumers. These services have grown from the recognition that neither the criminal justice system nor the mental health system can adequately provide services for forensic mental health consumers, and that the two systems must work in partnership to meet the needs of consumers and, at times, the need for community safety.

THE CRIMINAL JUSTICE SYSTEM

The criminal justice system includes the police who arrest people alleged to have committed a crime and the courts that are responsible for making determinations of guilt or innocence and for imposing penalties if the person is found guilty. Imprisonment and community-based sentencing options are possible penalties. When the person is thought to be experiencing mental illness, there are options for diversion from police custody, court or prison to mental health services for assessment and treatment. However, most mainstream mental health services do not have the structural security or available treatment and rehabilitation options to contain, assess, treat, care for and manage certain forensic mental health consumers, and therefore forensic mental health services have been developed.

Forensic Mental Health Services

Forensic mental health services are generally independent of the criminal justice system and are managed within the health sector. Components of forensic mental health services include services within police custody centres, prisons and courts (see Perspectives in practice: Nurse's story 29.1 and 29.2 to learn about the experience of forensic mental health nurses working in the court and prison setting). Secure hospitals and community services are also essential components. Forensic mental health services, which have traditionally been custodial and involved in compulsory treatment and care, are being challenged to transform to recovery-oriented services.

Forensic Mental Health Consumers

For forensic mental health consumers, the call is to focus on the lived experience of the individual consumer and their support structure, with the aim that the person leads a satisfying life irrespective of the difficulties imposed by mental health needs and secure services (Chen et al 2022). Integrating an approach which is centred on the person and

their support structure within a custodial environment remains a problematic but essential practice priority for contemporary forensic mental health nurses.

PERSPECTIVES IN PRACTICE

Nurse's Story 29.1: Kevin Seaton, Court Liaison Nurse

I have been employed in the court liaison service for 20 years. Before becoming a court liaison nurse, I had never entered a court and had no dealings with the criminal justice system. On my first day on the job, I helped assess a young man who had been arrested after an unprovoked attack on his neighbours with a knife. He believed they were aliens who had implanted a computer chip in his brain. We had to transfer this man to a secure forensic mental health unit for further assessment and treatment.

I thought to myself, what have I let myself into? I knew nothing about the court process, court protocol, how to address a judge or, more importantly, how to translate a mental health examination (MSE) into a letter to the court that the judge would understand. As a court liaison nurse, I found myself caught between the police who want to convict, the defence lawyers who want the charges withdrawn and the judge who wants advice on the mental health and risk status of the defendant, and guidance as to where they should be placed. I really struggled trying to make sense of the court process, the criminal legislation and trying to do the "right" thing for the consumer/defendant.

I was only two weeks into the role when I found myself in court supporting a mentally ill defendant. The aim, supported by the lawyers and the judge, was to seek bail to the local general mental health facility under mental health legislation. Unfortunately, there were no beds in the region. When this was explained to the judge, with the suggestion of the alternative of a further remand in prison for two days to allow a bed to be secured, the judge's retort was vehement: "Don't expect me to look after your mental cases in prison. You find a bed." I was so embarrassed being spoken to like that in a full courtroom. But I also felt that I should have somehow been able to "find the bed" this person needed, and by not doing so I had failed to provide care for this person.

These are the sorts of challenges you are presented with when working in the courts. Although initially they made me uncomfortable, the challenges

quickly helped me to understand the different agendas in the court context, through which the court liaison nurse is required to stay impartial. The skill is to provide clinical information that is accurate, with a clear rationale as to why certain recommendations are made. Possible responses from the judge need to be anticipated with alternative suggestions being pre-planned. Sound knowledge of legislation and criminal justice processes is imperative.

Court liaison nurses need to be competent and confident not only in their MSE abilities, but also in the recommendations that arise from these assessments. The MSE must also be accompanied by a thorough assessment of risk to self and others.

Court liaison nurses are independent autonomous practitioners, often working in relative professional isolation outside the usual comfort zone of a hospital setting. The court setting is alien territory, working alongside non-health professionals who have a unique professional language and etiquette, which the nurse has to learn to become effective. No senior medical staff are readily on hand for advice and assistance. Peer clinical supervision is imperative. We see and hear horrific details of offending, so support and guidance from colleagues who understand the role and its demands are critical for both competent clinical practice and our own wellbeing.

The work is both challenging and rewarding. Over the years, I have had to hone my clinical skills to enable me to practise at a level of autonomous practice I would not have thought possible 20 years ago. I have had to learn to speak and write in a "legalistic" language rather than just "nurse clinical speak". I get to wear nice professional clothes (no jeans and sandals in court), and work and talk with professionals outside the mental health setting. Judges acknowledge me and listen to and respect my opinion. The stress is high, the hours of work long, but I would work nowhere else.

Source: Adapted from McKenna B, Seaton K 2007. Liaison services to the courts. In: Brookbanks W, Simpson A (eds) Psychiatry and the Law. LexisNexis, Wellington.

PERSPECTIVES IN PRACTICE

Nurse Story 29.2: Katherine Duffy, Clinical Nurse Therapist in a Prison Mental Health Team

My role as a clinical nurse therapist was developed following recognition of the need for specialist psychological interventions for offenders with mental health problems. The remit I was given, as the first clinician to take this role, was to develop and implement group and individual interventions for consumers on the case load. The team covers four separate prison sites, including maximum security, remand and a women's facility, and, as such, the people in these environments have quite diverse issues and circumstances, making the role a challenging and complex one.

It became clear that one of the areas of greatest need was the special needs unit of one of the prisons. This tends to be the area where individuals with severe and chronic mental health issues are housed and often they are unable to attend the programs that they need to meet the requirements of the parole board. This is a consequence of being unable to mix with mainstream prisoners due to their vulnerability. The requirements of the parole board often include education on mental health issues, education about the impact of drugs and alcohol on mental health and offending behaviour, and anger management. If prisoners are unable to attend these programs, they are unable to achieve parole.

It also became clear that there is a group of prisoners with complex mental health needs who are often transferred between prison and forensic mental health in-patient units. While these individuals are in-patients, they are able to attend therapeutic programs, which they often find extremely beneficial. Unfortunately, on their return to prison, they are unable to continue to work on issues that they have begun to address and the initial progress made by this hard work is lost.

It was decided that the first program to be run would be a "recovery" program. This would address the issue of offenders in the special needs unit being unable to attend psycho-education groups; it would also provide some continuity of care between the prison and the in-patient units.

Building on this concept of continuity of care between prison and hospital, a group was devised by the occupational therapist and me on the acute admissions unit. This was a cognitive behavioural therapy (CBT) based group to look at new ways of managing stress. The idea was that we would co-facilitate the program in each environment, providing not only common understanding of concepts and language, but also some continuity in terms of staff working with offenders. The group was a great success and we had unanimous positive feedback from participants, prison staff and the parole board. Not only are these

PERSPECTIVES IN PRACTICE—cont'd

Nurse Story 29.2: Katherine Duffy, Clinical Nurse Therapist in a Prison Mental Health Team

groups now being run on a regular basis on the acute admissions unit and the special needs unit, but they have also been adapted for use at the women's prison.

In addition to the development and implementation of group programs, there have also been a huge number of referrals for individual CBT. The variety of different issues that people can present with was a little overwhelming initially. The consumers have often had very difficult histories with multiple traumas throughout their lives; they also often have coexisting major mental illness and personality disorders. Many of the referrals have been for people experiencing posttraumatic stress disorder related symptoms,

depression, anxiety, obsessive compulsive disorder, hearing voices and self-injury behaviours.

In my time in the role, no two days of that time have ever been the same. One thing that continues to surprise me is the motivation of the offenders that we work with. They attend weekly, having completed tasks that were set for them, and they actively engage in group activities. In fact, they are probably the most motivated group of service users I have ever worked with. Feedback such as "If you don't learn this stuff then your mind is like an untrained monkey in the tree of life" and "I have learned that my mental illness is like a motorcycle and drugs are the fuel that make it go", make the hard work of planning and facilitating these groups worth every minute!

Forensic Mental Health Nurses

Australia and Aotearoa New Zealand do not particularly recognise specialties of nursing, but the term "forensic mental health nurse" is used in this chapter to identify mental health nurses who specialise their practice in criminal justice or forensic mental health settings. Similar to other health fields, there are more nurses than other specialists in these settings. Nurses working in these settings must possess the knowledge, skills and attitudes that are required to provide comprehensive care for complex forensic mental health consumers. The Forensic Mental Health Nursing Standards of Practice 2012 (see Box 29.1) were informed by evidence and practice wisdom and

developed by senior forensic mental health nurses. The standards were developed to identify the knowledge, skills and attitudes required of nurses working in this setting.

Although this chapter focuses on nursing in criminal justice and forensic mental health settings, there is no doubt that nurses in mainstream services will, at some time, work in partnership with consumers to address their physical health, mental health and forensic mental health needs.

Scenarios 29.1 and 29.2 examine the experiences of John, a convicted prisoner facing a long prison sentence, and Stacey, an Australian Aboriginal woman with a history of personal trauma and substance-use issues, two consumers of forensic mental health services.

BOX 29.1 The Forensic Mental Health Nursing Standards of Practice

Standard 1: Structure the treatment environment to integrate security with therapeutic goals.

Standard 2: Apply knowledge of the legal framework to service delivery and individual care.

Standard 3: Conduct forensic mental health nursing practice ethically.

Standard 4: Practise within an interdisciplinary team that may include criminal justice staff.

Standard 5: Establish, maintain and terminate therapeutic relationships with forensic consumers using the nursing process.

Standard 6: Integrate assessment and management of offence issues into nursing care processes.

Standard 7: Assess for the impact of trauma and engage in strategies to minimise the effects of trauma.

Standard 8: Assess and manage risk potential of forensic consumers.

Standard 9: Manage the containment and transition process of forensic consumers.

Standard 10: Promote optimal physical health of forensic consumers.

Standard 11: Minimise potential harm from substance use by forensic consumers.

Standard 12: Practise respectfully with families/carers of forensic consumers.

Standard 13: Advocate for the mental health needs of forensic consumers in a prison or police custodial setting.

Standard 14: Support and encourage optimal functioning of forensic consumers in long-term care.

Standard 15: Demonstrate professional integrity in response to challenging behaviours.

Standard 16: Engage in strategies that minimise the experience of stigma and discrimination for forensic consumers.

Martin et al 2012.

EVIDENCE-BASED PRACTICE

Scenario 29.1: John

John is 25 years old and has been admitted from prison onto an acute forensic mental health unit. He is on remand in prison, accused of stabbing his flatmate. On the day of the stabbing, John had been up all night drinking alcohol and ruminating about his flatmate stealing his belongings. John had become convinced his flatmate had been conspiring with another acquaintance in the thefts. When he confronted his flatmate, John became enraged and attacked him with a kitchen knife. Prior to admission, John had been in a management unit in prison (where prisoners are locked in a cell by themselves) due to repeated threats to kill prison officers. He had refused to speak with the mental health staff, saying he did not have a mental illness.

When John arrived at the hospital he was handcuffed and appeared anxious, hypervigilant, malnourished and would not make eye contact. During the initial

assessment, John said that he knew why he had been transferred but he didn't agree he had a mental illness. He said he came from a large Greek family which he has had no contact with since he was arrested. He attributed the lack of contact with his family to them not knowing how to get in touch with him. On initial assessment, John reported a history of offending, often involving altercations with others. John reported drinking, alcohol use from a young age and "getting around with the wrong crowd". Several years ago, he was in a car accident and received a head injury and has been unable to work since. Although John has had contact with community mental health services in the past, he reported that they hadn't helped because he didn't have a mental illness. This is John's first admission to a mental health service, and he reports that he is worried about the other consumers on the unit.

Continued

Scenario 29.1: John

> **! RED FLAGS**
>
> - Length of stay will determine what care forensic mental health nurses are able to provide. If his stay is short term, the priority will be to stabilise John's mental state and provide him with skills to manage in the prison environment. If John's admission is longer, once his mental state has stabilised, there may be the potential to address offence-related needs in addition to his other needs.
> - The possibility of family contact will need to be explored.
> - Building rapport with John will be necessary to assess his holistic health needs and to work in partnership with him. John may be facing a lengthy prison sentence and therefore it is a possibility that he will be involved with forensic mental health services in a secure hospital or in prison.

Knowledge

Forensic mental health consumers have complex needs that forensic mental health nurses must thoroughly assess in order to provide holistic care, in partnership with consumers and their carers. Apart from the clinical need for treatment, many consumers have recovery needs related to social, cultural and adaptive malfunctioning and patterns of offending that can present as a risk to themselves or others.

On admission, it is important to conduct a comprehensive assessment that includes biopsychosocial factors (e.g. mental state, legal and offence history, substance use history, developmental history, family history, gender/cultural/spiritual/religious needs, physical health, education and employment), but also includes a detailed assessment of risk to self and others. It is also important to consider the impact of incarceration and how this may affect a person's mental, emotional and physical status (e.g. trauma associated with incarceration, inability to exercise, isolation from supports such as family and stress related to pending court issues).

The Legal Status of Forensic Consumers

Forensic mental health consumers are subject to criminal justice legislation and policies that vary greatly between Australian states and territories and between countries.

Defendants appearing in court must be fit to plead. If mental illness prevents a person from meeting certain criteria (including having an understanding of the nature of the charge and the trial, being able to enter a plea and being able to give instructions to the legal practitioner), then that person is likely to be ordered to receive treatment until they are fit to return to court. A small number of consumers are never fit, and other processes are put in place to ensure their treatment and supervision (see Perspectives in practice: Nurse's story 29.1).

Consumers are found not guilty by reason of mental impairment by the court when it has been proved that the person was so unwell at the time of the offence they did not understand the nature and quality of the act (the offence), or did not know that the act was wrong. Consumers who are found not guilty due to mental impairment are required to undertake treatment. The duration and location of the treatment will depend on the severity of the offence and the risk status of the consumer.

A prisoner experiencing symptoms of mental illness may require a transfer to a secure hospital for treatment, if an adequate level of treatment and care cannot be provided at the prison, or if the prisoner is unwilling to accept treatment and meets the criteria for compulsory treatment. The policy in Australia and Aotearoa New Zealand is that prisoners cannot be treated involuntarily in prison because the potential for abuse of mental health treatment is possible in a coercive environment (with the exception of New South Wales).

Some offenders in prison who are experiencing mental illness can adhere to treatment and need an equivalent level of treatment and care to that available in the community, such as outpatient appointments with a nurse (a nurse visiting the person on the prison unit). This service may be provided by prison mental health in-reach teams. Some prisons have mental health units for assessing and treating prisoners. Some high-risk prisoners will be referred to either a forensic mental health hospital or a community team for assessment and treatment following release from prison.

Wherever forensic mental health nurses practise, it is their responsibility to understand the legislation that affects consumers. Forensic mental health consumers and their carers are sometimes confused by the legal processes and requirements. The nurse's knowledge of the law needs to be used proactively to assist forensic mental health consumers and their carers to understand the function and impact of criminal justice legislation and policies, and to optimise care in the context of integrating security, safety and therapeutic intent. The nurse must also provide information to consumers and carers to ensure they are aware of their rights and responsibilities.

Scenario 29.2: Stacey

Stacey is an Australian Aboriginal woman who was exposed to a long history of abuse and victimisation during her childhood and dropped out of school when she was 12. She reported using drugs and alcohol from age 13 to cope with the abuse. Stacey gave birth to her daughter when she was 18 and reported struggling following the birth, feeling as if she had no one to talk to, being estranged from her family and having few friends. In the context of depression with psychotic features, 10 years ago Stacey was found not guilty by reason of mental impairment for the murder of her daughter.

It took 4 years for Stacey's mental illness to stabilise, but following intensive rehabilitation she is currently living in a low-secure forensic mental health unit and has applied for leave to transition to a supported community living arrangement. While Stacey's team feel she is ready to apply for leave, Stacey is anxious about the change. She has also applied for a part-time job, but is anxious about having to disclose her illness and offence to a new employer.

Since her admission, Stacey has gained 30 kg and has recently been diagnosed with type 2 diabetes. Weight gain has also had an impact on her self-esteem.

Stacey hopes that she will be able to address her weight gain by attending a gym near her new housing arrangement.

> **! RED FLAGS**
>
> - Transition periods are stressful and can sometimes result in a relapse of illness.
> - Stigma is an important issue for forensic mental health consumers, who can be disadvantaged by the negative appraisal of others; this can impact on their identity and self-concept.
> - Forensic consumers may be vulnerable to poor physical health for a variety of reasons.

Knowledge

Imprisoned offenders constitute a small proportion of the sentenced population, with the criminal justice system favouring community sentencing options (Forrester & Hopkin 2019). Little is known about the rates of mental illness in this

Scenario 29.2: Stacey

population, although literature from the United Kingdom indicates that approximately 30% of the probation caseload have had formal contact with mental health services (Brooker et al 2020). Consumers who offend and are placed on community-based orders are usually linked to general mental health services. Furthermore, general mental health services engage with consumers with complex needs who may have a forensic history or patterns of behaviour indicative of potential criminal involvement. Specialist community forensic liaison roles involving forensic mental health nurses and psychiatrists have been developed to assist mainstream mental health services to work with this group of consumers.

Specialist community forensic mental health teams have also been established to assist forensic mental health consumers with transitioning to the community from forensic mental health hospitals and prisons. The model of care of these teams often involves intensive case management, with the goal of eventual transfer to general mental health services. Forensic mental health community services provide assessment, consultation and ongoing treatment or shared care with general mental health services.

In Australia, there are numerous sources of referral to community forensic mental health services, including forensic mental health hospitals, justice agencies (courts, prisons, community corrections or the parole boards) and legal aid centres (Forensicare 2023). Forensic mental health consumers are not always well accepted by mainstream community mental health services and tend to be referred to community forensic mental health services if they have a history of violence and other offending, high levels of anger, suspicion or hostility, poor response or non-adherence to treatment and service engagement, or substance misuse.

As case managers in community teams, forensic mental health nurses coordinate necessary services, including health, legal, social, vocational, financial and accommodation services. They assist to manage mental illness, substance abuse, offending and other specific concerns to facilitate clinical recovery and support personal recovery. The community care of forensic consumers also requires working with families and carers. Collaboration is often required for joint management with other agencies to comprehensively address complex needs and avoid duplication in services. Given the over-representation of Aboriginal and Torres Strait Islander people and those from ethnic minorities in such populations, collaboration is also often required with cultural experts (McKenna & Sweetman 2021).

Forensic mental health nurses need to understand, plan for and respond in order to support consumers through difficult transition periods

Mental Health Nursing Actions and Interventions
Pre-Release Planning and Relationship Building

The correct treatment, support and level of supervision are essential to assist forensic mental health consumers to maximise the opportunity for success when transitioning from prison or a forensic mental health hospital to the community. Agencies that will work with the consumer after they leave custody should start building a relationship with them while they are still in prison or hospital. This ensures time for trust to be established, which makes engagement more likely once the consumer is in the community. It also makes recidivism less likely (McKenna et al 2015).

Crucial supports include early, meaningful engagement with mental health services and substance use agencies (Senneseth et al 2022), the involvement of justice agencies if the consumer is on bail or parole, or another order requiring ongoing justice involvement, and assistance to address social care needs (including the need for housing, food, financial assistance, employment and sociocultural supports)

Addressing Stigma and Discrimination

The possible outcome of consumers' engagement with forensic mental health services is double stigma: criminality and mental illness. Community attitudes

towards both are misinformed, ignorant and fearful. The media, through which the public becomes "informed", tends to present offenders with mental health problems in a manner that potentially feeds into this stigma (Vorstenbosch et al 2022). This stigma in turn affects identity, self-concept and self-esteem (West et al 2018).

Forensic mental health nurses need to be aware and provide support, education and advocate where necessary to address stigma and discrimination. It is crucial that forensic mental health nurses work in partnership with forensic mental health consumers in this regard.

Considering Social Disadvantage

When assessing the needs of forensic mental health consumers, forensic mental health nurses must also consider the consumer's sociocultural context. The influences of cultural disadvantage and low socioeconomic status are especially important (Rose et al 2020).

Forensic mental health consumers are more at risk of victimisation compared with the general population. Victimisation includes being subjected to violence, intimidation, sexual exploitation and financial exploitation. Violence may be the reality of high-crime neighbourhoods where people experiencing mental illness often live. There is an indication that people experiencing mental illness move into, or fail to rise out of, low socioeconomic locations because of the impact of the social stigma attached to the illness (Harding & Roman 2017).

Promoting Optimal Physical Health

Forensic mental health nurses must consider risks and the consumer's needs when planning interventions to promote the physical health of consumers. A comprehensive nursing health assessment must include physical health and the forensic mental health nurse must work with the consumer, their family and the multidisciplinary team to develop, implement and evaluate treatment plans that promote and enhance optimal physical health (Maguire, Garvey et al 2022).

Forensic mental health consumers are at a high risk of developing metabolic syndrome and associated physical illnesses, such as diabetes, cardiovascular disease and respiratory problems. Although a key contributing factor is the use of antipsychotic medications, restrictions on activities and lifestyle choices in custodial environments and secure settings also contribute to physical health deficits. Forensic mental health nurses must contribute to an environment that promotes a healthy lifestyle through health education and health-enhancing activities.

Relevant Treatment Modalities and Considerations

Pre-release planning and relationship building bring together a variety of possible supports in partnership with the consumer and should begin many months, even years before a person is released from being detained. Through the pre-release planning process, it is more likely that all involved will clearly understand one another's roles and be able to demonstrate a clear commitment to the consumer following release. Integrated health, justice and social care agency responses are required for this population to attain acceptable levels of social functioning and quality of life (either in prison or in the community) and to avoid reoffending.

In the literature, there are examples of mental health nurses and other disciplines initiating healthy living programs targeted to address physical health care concerns with forensic mental health consumers (Moss et al 2022).

Demographic Characteristics of Consumers

The forensic mental health population tends to be young, male, never married, of low socioeconomic status, unemployed, with poor educational achievement and in itinerant living situations prior to conviction. However,

Continued

Scenario 29.2: Stacey

the number of imprisoned women is increasing and therefore the female forensic consumer population is growing in both Australia and Aotearoa New Zealand (Australian Bureau of Statistics (ABS) 2023; Foulds & Monastario 2018).

There is an over-representation of Indigenous peoples and post-colonisation immigrant populations in forensic mental health services. Colonisation usurped the self-determination of Indigenous peoples and, similarly, immigrant populations are required to adapt to the social reality of the dominant culture. Such social adjustments place considerable pressure on disadvantaged groups. These pressures are reflected in several adverse social indicators, such as poor educational achievement, high unemployment rates, high crime rates and poor health statistics.

In Aotearoa New Zealand, Māori and Pacific Islander ethnicities are over-represented in prisons. Although Māori comprise 16% of the general population and Pacific Islanders 6%, they make up 51% and 12% of the prison population respectively (Foulds & Monastario 2018). In Australia, Aboriginal and Torres Strait Islander peoples are over-represented in prison settings. In 2021 there were 13,039 prisoners who identified as Aboriginal or Torres Strait Islander, and there has been an 8% increase since 30 June 2020 (ABS 2023).

Cognitive and Social Skill Needs

When a person's ability to think clearly and relate constructively to others is compromised by mental illness, the likelihood of antisocial behaviour, including violence and offending, is enhanced (Ghiasi et al 2022). The reasons for compromised cognitive and social ability are complex and may not directly relate to mental illness. They may relate to diminished learning opportunities in the context of the family and environment, harsh or inconsistent parenting, delinquent peer associations or acquired brain injury.

A significant proportion of forensic mental health consumers have a history of traumatic childhood experiences (McKenna et al 2019) and acquired brain injury (Belfry et al 2023). Therefore, the development of cognitive and social skills is a recovery requirement of forensic mental health services. Limitations in cognitive and social skills can militate against a socially positive response to life's challenges (Lambie 2020).

Mental Illness and Risk to Others

Most people who experience mental illness are not violent and are not a risk to others. They are more likely to be the victim of a crime than the perpetrator of it. The relationship between mental illness and criminal behaviour is complex and varies between individuals. Forensic mental health nurses need to identify the unique relationship for each consumer, so they can ascertain the risk and protective factors that need to be addressed in treatment and risk intervention strategies.

Most consumers who progress from assessment to remain on the caseload of forensic mental health nurses experience serious mental illness (a psychotic illness or major depression). A seminal 20-year study undertaken by Wallace and colleagues (2004) found that the overall frequency of violent offences was significantly higher among people experiencing schizophrenia than among the comparison community subjects (8.2% versus 1.8%). The rate of violent offending among people experiencing schizophrenia gradually increased over the years of the study, but there was no difference in the rate of increase when compared with the comparison subjects over the same period. Most people experiencing schizophrenia are not violent and do not commit criminal offences, and the risk might lie in specific symptoms such as paranoia.

International studies have found modest increases in criminal and violent behaviour with serious mental illness, but also note that there is no evidence that mental illness causes criminal behaviour (Ghiasi et al 2022). Rather, exposure to significant adverse childhood events and experiences of being in foster care are strong predictors of offending, and being in forensic mental health services factors include antisocial tendencies of peers and alcohol or drug abuse (Stinson et al 2021).

Substance Use Needs

Substance abuse is common in forensic mental health consumers and the community in general. Researchers consider that the major driver of crime and violence in people (with and without a mental illness) is substance misuse (McFadden et al 2021). There is a high prevalence of prisoners who have a mental illness and who also abuse substances (Baranyi et al 2022). Forensic consumers have high rates of substance abuse and these coexisting conditions have a link to offending and risk of violence (McFadden et al 2021). There is substantial evidence for substance misuse being a significant risk factor for violence and aggression for consumers.

Having a substance use disorder can also present a number of challenges for consumers, including the ability to successfully transition into the community (McFadden et al 2021). While the link between substance abuse and aggression/offending is widely recognised, the mechanisms are poorly understood, resulting from a complex process involving the interaction of the substances' active agents, the substance misuse, the context of the substance misuse and personal factors such as a predisposition to aggression.

See Chapter 13 for more information about substance use and abuse, and their association with coexisting mental disorders.

Attitudes

At some point, most nurses will provide care and treatment for consumers with an offending history or who are at risk of offending. When a consumer has committed an offence and is experiencing mental illness, the forensic mental health nurse is expected to apply the core knowledge, skills and attitudes of nursing generally, mental health nursing specifically and the additional or enhanced

---

BOX 29.2 Groups of Forensic Mental Health Consumers

- Offenders or alleged offenders referred by police, courts, legal practitioners or independent statutory bodies for psychiatric assessment and/or treatment
- Alleged offenders detained, or on conditional release, as being unfit to plead or not guilty by reason of mental impairment
- Offenders or alleged offenders with mental illness ordered by courts or independent statutory bodies to be detained as an in-patient in a secure forensic facility
- Prisoners with mental illness requiring secure in-patient hospital treatment
- Selected high-risk offenders with a mental illness referred by releasing authorities
- Prisoners with mental illness requiring specialist mental health assessment and/or treatment in prison
- People with mental illness in mainstream mental health services who are a significant danger to their carers or the community, and who require the involvement of a specialist forensic mental health service

Australian Health Ministers' Advisory Council 2006, pp. 3–4.

Scenario 29.2: Stacey

skills that are required to work effectively with forensic mental health consumers (see Box 29.2).

For some nurses, the ability to provide care can potentially be compromised by the complex presentation of some forensic mental health consumers. Antisocial personality attributes that are not pleasant to relate to may present as a contributing factor that clouds the nurse's ability to place moral judgement to one side; for example, when the nurse becomes the target of hostile or threatening behaviour. Forensic mental health nursing research has articulated the difficulties that nurses face in confronting moral judgements concerning such behaviour. Poor judgements and bias regarding this behaviour compromise the delivery of nursing care.

A key example of such judgements as framing a consumer as primarily "bad" can result in a total absence of planned care in the form of care plans for this consumer (Maguire et al 2022). It is essential that nurses in general, and forensic mental health in particular, recognise and manage their personal feelings and values related to the offences committed by forensic mental health consumers. Nurses who focus on the offences and allow their feelings and values to dominate their clinical perspective of consumers will be ineffective in providing care.

Often, professional dissonance (an uneasiness that can arise from professional values and job task conflict) is experienced. Equally inappropriate is the belief that the offending behaviour is not a concern of the nurse. In such cases, nurses may choose to ignore an offending behaviour because they find the personal and moral effects distressing. But by ignoring the offending behaviour, a significant forensic mental health consumer need is not addressed.

It is offending and other antisocial behaviours that distinguish consumers within the forensic mental health setting. The professional response is to view offending behaviour as another need to be addressed during therapeutic engagement with the forensic mental health consumer. Consumers need to understand the factors associated with their offending behaviour, in order to increase their personal choice and responsibility.

Cultural Awareness

There is a strong awareness in forensic mental health services of the cultural needs of the communities served and the necessity for an appropriate response to these needs, given that both Indigenous peoples and ethnic minorities are over-represented in such populations. Forensic mental health nurses must pay attention to consumers' cultural and spiritual needs throughout the therapeutic process. Additional cultural and spiritual expertise may be needed to assist this – for example, including local Aboriginal and Torres Strait Islander elders in forensic mental health consultation processes, community outreach and recovery plans.

Forensic mental health nurses must adhere to "cultural safety". Cultural safety focuses on the social determinants of health and the impact of power relationships through social processes, such as colonisation, which are starkly reflected in health inequities. Such power dynamics can filter into the therapeutic relationship and manifest in poor communication, erosion of autonomous decision-making and actions that are perceived as disrespectful, regardless of good intent. Cultural responsivity requires a conscious commitment to the development of long-standing trust initially tainted by injustice and empowerment of those disadvantaged. It requires establishing collaborative relationships with those immersed in the culture to best serve those from that culture (McKenna 2020).

Central to any culture is the family. Family members have the potential to provide a vital link to the community for the consumer and to promote the consumer's wellbeing through supportive relationships. However, mental illness, and the nature of the offence and its consequences, may compromise this potential. For example, family members are more likely to be victims when perpetrators of serious violence have a mental illness (Canning et al 2009). Containment of the consumer can have an impact on family function (emotional, financial or social). The nurse must be part of the multidisciplinary team endeavouring to assist in healing family relationships and maximising the potential of the family to be partners in addressing the needs of forensic mental health consumers.

Forensic Mental Health Nursing Actions and Interventions

Forensic mental health consumers generally have a mental illness, a history of offending and personality attributes and ways of acting and reacting that heighten their potential for risk of harm to self and others. Nurses working in forensic mental health hospitals are likely to be caring for consumers who consistently present with seriously challenging behaviours, including aggression and violence (Maguire et al 2022b). Aggression may be an inevitable outcome of providing treatment to involuntary forensic mental health consumers, some of whom will have limited skills to manage anger that is provoked by the ongoing demands, expectations and conflict of in-patient treatment (Maguire et al 2021).

Forensic mental health nurses working within these facilities undertake assessment, assist with treatment and facilitate recovery. Forensic mental health nurses are obliged to consider the least restrictive alternatives in risk intervention and to reduce the use of restrictive interventions such as seclusion.

Although there are barriers that work against nurses in forensic hospitals being able to safely manage forensic mental health consumers, there are also opportunities; these can include longer admissions, resulting in reduced access to illicit substances and increased access to treatment and therapeutic engagement (Maguire, Ryan et al 2022); a higher staff–consumer ratio, providing the opportunity for nurses to work with consumers to undertake assessment, treatment and other environmental interventions (Barr et al 2022), and access to best-practice risk assessment and intervention approaches.

Risk Assessment

Prevention and management of offending, especially violence, have become the focus of contemporary risk assessment in forensic mental health. Rigorous risk assessment processes are undertaken to identify factors that indicate risk to self or others and the protective factors that mitigate such risk.

Static risk factors cannot be changed by clinical intervention (e.g. gender and age), while **Dynamic risk factors** (e.g. substance use and social support from friends) are factors that are more open to clinical modification and can be altered through risk intervention. **Protective factors** can interact with risk factors and reduce the likelihood of the risk behaviour. Examples of protective factors include having pro-social peers, developed coping skills and employment (de Vries Robbé & Willis 2017). Planning of appropriate interventions is assisted through structured clinical judgement, which includes using validated risk assessment instruments.

In undertaking risk assessments, comprehensive information needs to be collected in a systematic manner. Some of the sources include interviews and, in collaboration with the forensic mental health consumer, to elicit their understanding; interviews with the consumer's family/carers and any person with relevant information to contribute to the process; and a review of the

Continued

EVIDENCE-BASED PRACTICE—cont'd

Scenario 29.2: Stacey

clinical files and other documentation such as legal reports and incident reports.

Nursing Interventions

Assessment alone is unlikely to reduce adverse outcomes of the issue being assessed. For this reason, any type of risk assessment must be followed with strategies to prevent the issue of concern (e.g. aggression or self-harm). In the forensic mental health setting, one of the most common risks encountered is in-patient aggression; however, despite being an issue of concern, there has been limited research investigating nursing intervention following risk assessment (Maguire et al 2021).

In recent years, a program of research has developed a systematic framework to guide nursing practice to reduce aggression and the use of restrictive interventions following assessment using the Dynamic Appraisal of Situational Aggression (DASA) tool. The framework is called the Aggression Prevention Protocol (APP), and together with the DASA (the DASA + APP) can be used to provide structure for nursing interventions, so nurses are guided with recommendations on how to mitigate risk after it has been identified (Maguire et al 2021). See Fig. 29.1.

The APP prioritises the use of the least restrictive interventions (such as one-to-one nursing, distraction and reassurance) and reserves what are considered to be the more restrictive interventions (limit setting, prn medication and close observations) for the high-risk DASA band. Research testing the DASA + APP found that structuring nursing intervention following the assessment of risk using the DASA reduced aggression and the use of restrictive interventions and prn medication (Griffith et al 2021; Maguire et al 2021).

Risk Communication

Risk communication is a very important method of conveying the information that is collected during the risk assessment process, as well as informing interventions and evaluation. Any risk needs must be completed together with the consumer and their support structure, and communicated to all appropriate parties in a timely and accurate way. This also includes contemporaneous documentation in the consumer's files. Failure to do so can have significant negative consequences.

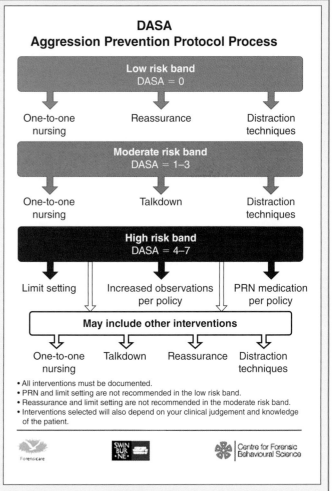

FIG. 29.1 Dynamic Appraisal of Situational Aggression (DASA) and Aggression Prevention Protocol (DPP) outline.

CHAPTER SUMMARY

This chapter has sought to assist nurses to consider the practice reality of forensic mental health nursing. The challenges of this practice reality are characterised by "complexity" relating to the needs of forensic mental health consumers; challenges experienced by nurses when working with significant trauma, offending histories and at times challenging behaviours in a secure setting; the configuration of services to meet these needs, and the law that dictates service provision. All these present as challenges to forensic mental health nursing practice. However, satisfaction with nursing in this area is a direct corollary of this complexity.

The challenges of the complexity can inspire nurses and create a passion for serving some of the most vulnerable and disadvantaged people in our society. The relationships that nurses establish with forensic mental health consumers are pivotal to this work, although there is recognition that forensic mental health consumers often come to the relationship with a history of trauma, distrust and cynicism. Breaking through such barriers and meeting the challenge of recovery-oriented care are possible when nurses maintain therapeutic optimism and an ethical approach to care.

USEFUL WEBSITES

Australia

Australasian Legal Information Institute (Austlii): www.austlii.edu.au/

Each state and territory has different legislation. The following sites may provide a good starting point.

Mental Health Review Tribunal: www.mhrt.qld.gov.au/

Queensland Forensic Mental Health Branch: www.health.qld.gov.au/public-health/topics/mental-health

Victorian Institute of Forensic Mental Health, Forensicare: www.forensicare.vic.gov.au/

New Zealand

Ara Poutama Aotearoa/Department of Corrections: www.corrections.govt.nz/

Mason Clinic (Auckland Regional Forensic Psychiatry Services, including an e-learning package): www.healthpoint.co.nz/public/mental-health-specialty/mason-clinic-regional-forensic-psychiatry/at/mason-clinic/

Ministry of Health New Zealand: www.health.govt.nz
Ministry of Justice: www.justice.govt.nz/

Other Useful Sites

International Association of Forensic Mental Health Services: iafmhs.
  wildapricot.org/
International Association of Forensic Nurses: www.forensicnurses.org/
Statistics New Zealand: www.stats.govt.nz
World Health Organization Mental Health Atlas: www.who.int/mental_health/
  evidence/atlas/profiles/en/

REFERENCES

Australian Bureau of Statistics (ABS), 2023. Prisoners in Australia. Online.
  Available at: www.abs.gov.au/statistics/people/crime-and-justice/prisoners-
  australia/latest-release

Baranyi, G., Fazel, S., Delhey Langerfeldt, S., Mundt, A.P., 2022. The prevalence of comorbid serious mental illnesses and substance use disorders
  in prison populations: A systematic review and meta-analysis. Lancet,
  doi.org/10.1016/S2468-2667(22)00093-7.

Belfry, K.D., Ham, E., Kolla, N.J., & Hilton, N.Z. 2023. Adverse childhood experiences and offending as a function of acquired brain injury among men in a
  high secure forensic psychiatric hospital. Can J Psychiatry, 68(6), 453–460.

Brooker, C., Sirdifield, C., & Marples, R. 2020. Mental health and probation: A
  systematic review of the literature. Forensic Sci Int: Mind Law, doi.org/10.
  1016/j.fsiml.2019.100003.

Chen, S.P., Chang, W.P., Fleet, B., Rai, S., Panteluk, S., et al., 2022. Is a forensic
  cohabitation program recovery-oriented? A logic model analysis. Int J
  Environ Res Public Health, 19(1), 9.

de Vries Robbé, M. & Willis, G.M. 2017. Assessment of protective factors in
  clinical practice. Aggress Violent Behav, 32, 55–63.

Forensicare 2023. Community Forensic Mental Health Service. Online. Available at: www.forensicare.vic.gov.au/our-services/community-forensic-
  mental-health-services/

Forrester, A., & Hopkin, G. 2019. Mental health in the criminal justice system:
  A pathways approach to service and research design. Crim Behav Ment
  Health, 29(4), 207–217.

Foulds, J. A., & Monastario, E. 2018. A public health catastrophe looms: The
  Australian and New Zealand prison crisis. Aust N Z J Psychiatry 52,
  1019–1020.

Ghiasi, N., Azhar, Y., & Singh, J. 2022. Psychiatric illness and criminality.
  [Updated 30 March 2023]. In: StatPearls [Internet]. Treasure Island (FL):
  StatPearls Publishing. Online. Available at: www.ncbi.nlm.nih.gov/books/
  NBK537064/

Harding, C.S., & Roman, C.G. 2017. Identifying discrete subgroups of chronically homeless frequent utilizers of jail and public mental health services.
  Crim Justice Behav, 44(4), 511–530.

Lambie, I. 2020. What were they thinking? A discussion paper on brain and
  behaviour in relation to the justice system in New Zealand. Office of the
  Prime Minister's Chief Science Advisor, Auckland.

Maguire, T., Garvey, L., Ryan, J., Willetts, G., & Olasoji, M. 2022a. Exploration
  of the utility of the nursing process and the clinical reasoning cycle as a
  framework for forensic mental health nurses: A qualitative study. Int J
  Ment Health Nurs, 31(2), 358–368.

Maguire, T., Ryan, J., Fullam, R., & McKenna, B. 2022b. Safewards Secure:
  A Delphi study to develop an addition to the Safewards Model for
  forensic mental health services. J Psychiatric Ment Health Nurs, 29(3),
  418–429.

Maguire, T., McKenna, B., & Daffern, M. 2021. Aggression Prevention
  Protocol User Manual. Centre for Forensic Behavioural Science,
  Swinburne University of Technology and Forensicare, Melbourne.

McFadden, D., Prior, K., Miles, H., Hemraj, S. & Barrett, E.L. 2022. Genesis of
  change: Substance use treatment for forensic patients with mental health
  concerns. DAR, 41(1), 256–259.

McKenna, B. 2020. There is no turning back! J Psychiatric Ment Health Nurs,
  27(5), 495–496.

McKenna, B. & Sweetman, L. 2021. Models of Care in Forensic Mental
  Health Services: A Review of the Literature. Ministry of Health,
  Wellington.

McKenna, B., Skipworth, J., Tapsell, R., et al., 2015. Prison mental health in-
  reach: The impact of innovation on transition planning, community mental health service engagement and re-offending. Crim Behav Ment Health,
  25, 429–439.

McKenna, G., Jackson, N., & Browne, C. 2019. Trauma history in a high secure
  male forensic inpatient population. Int J Law Psychiatry, 66, 101475.

Moss, K., Meurk, C., Steele, M. L., & Heffernan, E. 2022. physical health and
  activity of inpatients under forensic mental health care: A cross-sectional
  survey and audit of patients in a high secure setting in Queensland,
  Australia. Int J Forens Ment Health, 1–12.

Rose, A., Trounson, J.S., Louise, S., Shepherd, S., & Ogloff, J.R. 2020. Mental
  health, psychological distress, and coping in Australian cross-cultural
  prison populations. J Traum Stress, 33(5), 794–803.

Senneseth, M., Pollak, C., Urheim, R., Logan, C., Palmstierna, T. 2022. Personal recovery and its challenges in forensic mental health: Systematic
  review and thematic synthesis of the qualitative literature. BJPsych
  Open 8.1, e17.

Stinson, J.D., Quinn, M.A., Menditto, A.A. & LeMay, C.L. 2021. Adverse
  childhood experiences and the onset of aggression and criminality in
  a forensic inpatient sample. Int J Forens Ment Health, 20(4), 374–385.

Vorstenbosch, E., Masoliver-Gallach, R., & Escuder-Romeva, G. 2022.
  Measuring professional stigma towards patients with a forensic mental
  health status: Protocol for a Delphi consensus study on the design of a
  questionnaire. BMJ open, 12(9), e061160.

Wallace, C., Mullen, P., & Burgess, P. 2004. Criminal offending in schizophrenia over a 25-year period marked by deinstitutionalisation and increasing
  prevalence of comorbid substance use disorders. Am J Psychiatry, 161(4),
  716–727.

West, M.L., Mulay, A.L., DeLuca, J.S., O'Donovan, K., & Yanos, P.T. 2018.
  Forensic psychiatric experiences, stigma, and self-concept: A mixed-
  methods study. J Forens Psychiatry Psychol, 29(4), 574–596.

INDEX

b = box, f = figure, t = table

A

abnormal eating behaviour, 239
Abnormal Involuntary Movements Scale (AIMS),
  331–332, 332b
Aboriginal and Torres Strait Islander people
  mental health, 71–84
  code of conduct for nurses, 76
  consumer's story, 82b
  critical thinking exercise, 74b, 75b, 81b
  cultural considerations, 82b
  culturally appropriate care, 76–78
    cultural differences, 77
    deep listening, 78
    engaging with, 77–78
    fear and lack of trust, 77–78
    use of community and family support, 78
    yarning, 78
  cultural safety, 75–76, 76–77b
  healing, 78–80
    social and emotional wellbeing model,
      79–80, 79f
  historical anecdote, 73b, 74b, 81b
  historical context, 72–74
    colonisation, impacts of, 73
    protectionism and assimilation, 73–74
    terra nullius, 72–73
  nurse's story, 78b
  social and emotional wellbeing
    reflections on, 82
    as strengths-based framework for
      self-determination, 81–82
  social determinants of health and protective
    factors, 80–81
    connection to country, 80
    kinship structures, 80–81
    lore, 80
    traditional healing, 80
    truth-telling, 81
  trauma-informed care, 74–75
Aboriginal health workforce, 81–82
Aboriginal mental health trainee's story, 82b
ABS *see* Australian Bureau of Statistics
absolute neutrophil count (ANC), 333
abstraction, 302
acceptance and commitment therapy (ACT),
  169, 287
ACE-R *see* Addenbrooke's Cognitive
  Examination-Revised
acetylcholinesterase inhibitor, 334
ACT *see* acceptance and commitment therapy
active listening, 44
actuarial risk assessment methods, 49–50
acute agitation, medication for, 338–339, 339f
acute care services, 350
acute dystonic reaction, as side effects of typical
  antipsychotics, 331t
acute intoxication, on alcohol/drugs, 193
acute stress disorder (ASD), 157t, 165, 166
AD *see* adjustment disorder
Addenbrooke's Cognitive Examination-Revised
  (ACE-R), 126t
addiction, pharmacological aspects of, 189,
  189–190b
adjustment disorder (AD), 157t, 165, 166
adolescence
  childhood and
    case study, 271–272b, 272b, 273b, 275b, 276b

adolescence *(Continued)*
  critical thinking exercise, 267b, 273b, 274b,
    276b, 277b, 278b
  depression of, 275
  developmental issues on, 266–267
  eating disorder in, 232
  education and psychosocial intervention in,
    273–274
  engaging with, 270–271
  family work and, 273
  HEEADDSSS assessment for, 277b
  historical anecdote, 266b, 267b
  psychotropic medication use in, 339–340
  risk taking in, 276–277, 277b
  self-harm in, 275–276
  suicide in, 275
  vulnerability in, 269–270
  disorders of, 264–280
    assessment of, 267–268
    behaviour issues of, 274–275
    diagnosis of, 265
    nursing role in, 269–270, 270b
  engaged with, 271
  language and engagement with, 271
  services for, 268–269, 268f
  working with families, 271–273
advance directive, 147b, 152
advanced practice, in expertise development, 109
Adverse Childhood Experiences (ACE) study, 20
adverse events, 31–32
affect, 177
  in mental state assessment, 130–131
ageing
  demography of, 281–282
  older adults care and, 383–386b
ageism, 282, 381b, 383–386b
age, of older adulthood, 381b
aggression, safety in care during, 45–48
agitation, managing of, in emergency care,
  368–370b
agoraphobia, 157t, 163
agranulocytosis, 220–221, 325t, 332, 333
Ahpra *see* Australian Health Practitioner
  Regulation Authority
AIHW *see* Australian Institute of Health and
  Welfare
AIMS *see* Abnormal Involuntary Movements
  Scale
akathisia, 325t, 331t
alcohol, 177, 194t, 199–200t
  consumption, 185–186
  withdrawal, 195, 195f, 196t
"Alcohol & Other Drug" (AOD), 353
Alcohol, Smoking and Substance Involvement
  Screening Test (ASSIST), 201–202
Alcohol Use Disorder Inventory Test (AUDIT),
  126, 126t
Alcohol Use Disorders Identification Test
  (AUDIT), 201–202, 202b
alkalosis, 370–371b
allostatic load, 157, 158f
allostatic state, 158f
alogia, 213
alternative, least restrictive, definition of, 147b
aminoindanes, 191t
amphetamines, 199–200t
  withdrawal, 196–197

AN *see* anorexia nervosa
ANC *see* absolute neutrophil count
anhedonia, 213
anorexia nervosa (AN), 229, 238
  nurse's story, 241b
anosognosia, 325t
antenatal depression, 389–390
antianxiety medications, 325–327
anticholinergic medications, 221
anticholinergic psychosis, 334
anticonvulsants, 326t, 330, 393–395b
  for mood disorder, 180
antidepressant medications, 287, 327–328
antidepressants, 180
antiparkinsonian medications, 333, 334t
antipsychotic medications, 180, 221, 325t,
  330–332, 331t, 332b
  atypical, 332–333, 333b
  in diabetes, 312
antisocial personality disorder, 251–253t
anxiety, 221t, 265
  ASD and, 302
  medications for, 325–327
  nature of, 370–371b
anxiety disorder, 156–172, 282
  aetiology of, 157–158
  agoraphobia, 157t, 163
  assessment of, 160–166
  assessment tools of, 161
  awareness of, 160b
  case study, 164b
  climate change on, 157–158
  comorbidity in, 160
  consumer's story, 162b, 167b
  COVID-19 impacts on, 157–158
  critical thinking exercise, 160b
  definition of, 156
  diagnosis of, 160–166
  epidemiology of, 159–160
  generalised, 157t, 161–162
  in Māori and Pacific peoples, 160
  nurse's story, 161b, 168b
  nursing interventions for, 167–170
  obsessive-compulsive disorder, 157t, 162–163
  in older adults, 285
  panic disorder, 157t, 163
  psychopharmacology of, 170
  social, 157t, 163–164
  specific phobia, 157t, 164–165
  trauma-and stressor-related disorders of
    acute stress disorder, 157t, 166
    adjustment disorder, 157t, 166
    post-traumatic stress disorder, 157t, 165–166
  treatment for, 167–170
    acceptance and commitment therapy, 169
    cognitive behaviour therapy, 168–169, 168t
    cultural support, 169–170
    digital mental health resources, 169
    psychoeducation, 167
    psychological formulations, 167–168
    psychological interventions, 168
    social support, 167
    transdiagnostic approaches, 169
    trauma-informed care, 167–168
Aotearoa New Zealand mental health care, 92–95
  consumer's story, 93–94b
  Te Aka Whai Ora and Te Whatu Ora, 92–94